DISEASES OF THE FETUS AND NEWBORN

DISEASES OF THE FETUS AND NEWBORN

Pathology, imaging, genetics and management

SECOND EDITION

Volume 2

EDITED BY

G.B. Reed,

A.E. Claireaux

and

F. Cockburn

with G.G. Ashmead, S.E. Chambers, S.G. Driscoll, J.P. Neilson and D.K. Stevenson

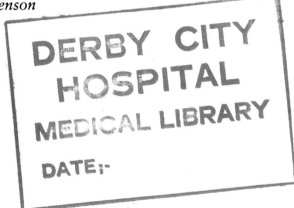
CHAPMAN & HALL MEDICAL

London · Glasgow · Weinheim · New York · Tokyo · Melbourne · Madras

Published by Chapman & Hall, 2–6 Boundary Row, London SE1 8HN,
UK

Chapman & Hall, 2–6 Boundary Row, London SE1 8HN, UK

Blackie Academic & Professional, Wester Cleddens Road, Bishopbriggs,
Glasgow G64 2NZ, UK

Chapman & Hall GmbH, Pappelallee 3, 69469 Weinheim, Germany

Chapman & Hall USA, One Penn Plaza, 41st Floor, New York NY
10119, USA

Chapman & Hall Japan, ITP-Japan, Kyowa Building, 3F, 2-2-1
Hirakawacho, Chiyoda-ku, Tokyo 102, Japan

Chapman & Hall Australia, Thomas Nelson Australia, 102 Dodds Street,
South Melbourne, Victoria 3205, Australia

Chapman & Hall India, R. Seshadri, 32 Second Main Road, CIT East,
Madras 600 035, India

First edition 1989
Second edition 1995

© 1989, 1995 Chapman & Hall

Typeset in 10/12 Sabon by Photoprint, Torquay, Devon
Printed in Hong Kong

ISBN 0 412 39160 0

A catalogue record for this book is available from the British Library

Dr A. Douglas Bain, our co-editor on the first edition, died in January 1987. His sudden death was greatly mourned by colleagues and friends all over the world. We wish to dedicate this book to his memory and his many contributions to pediatric genetic pathology

CONTENTS

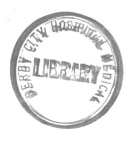

Editorial board   xxix
List of contributors   xxxi
Preface to the second edition   xLi
Preface to the first edition   xLiii
Acknowledgements   xLiv
Introduction – *Aquae Vitae*   xLv

Volume 1

PART ONE   MECHANISMS OF ANTENATAL DISEASE
Edited by G.B. Reed   1

1 An introduction to antenatal and neonatal medicine, the fetal period
   and perinatal ethics   3
   M.D. Bain, D. Gau and G.B. Reed

   1.1 Introduction   3
   1.2 Background   4
   1.3 Risk assessment   5
   1.4 Antenatal screening and prenatal diagnosis   5
   1.5 Antenatal, fetal and neonatal medicine   6
   1.6 The fetal period: the placenta, growth, maturation   11
   1.7 The old and new ethos   17
   1.8 Summary   19
   References   19
   Further reading   20

2 Origins of birth defects   23
   J.M. Opitz

   2.1 Introduction   23
   2.2 Causes   23
   2.3 Pathogenetic effects   26
   2.4 Pathogenetic periods   27
   References   29

3 Molecular biology applied to pathology of the fetus and newborn   31
   G.A. Machin

   3.1 Introduction: application of molecular biology to fetal and
        neonatal pathology   31
   3.2 Diseases caused by abnormal events at the level of the gene   37
   References   52

4 Cytogenetics   55
   M. Vekemans

   4.1 Introduction   55

4.2 Methodology   56
4.3 Chromosomal aberrations   58
4.4 Chromosomal disorders   62
4.5 Impact of chromosome abnormalities on human morbidity and mortality   65
References   66
Further reading   66

5 The prenatal origins of cancer   67
   R.P. Bolande

5.1 Introduction   67
5.2 Heredito-familial cancers   71
5.3 Developmental lesions precursive of cancer   72
5.4 Teratologic conditions predisposing to neoplasia   74
5.5 The prenatal initiation of carcinogenesis   77
5.6 Future considerations   80
References   80

6 Human teratology   83
   T.H. Shepard

6.1 Introduction   83
6.2 Definitions   83
6.3 Identification of human teratogens   83
6.4 Animal tests and human teratogens   85
6.5 Windows of teratogenic susceptibility   86
6.6 Known human teratogens   86
6.7 Possible teratogens   89
6.8 Unlikely teratogens   89
6.9 Sources of teratology information   91
References   91

7 Infections of the fetus and newborn   95
   C.R. Abramowsky and A.J. Nahmias

7.1 Fetal and neonatal host responses to infections   95
7.2 General mechanisms and pathways of infection of the fetus and newborn 101
7.3 Inflammation and healing in the fetus and newborn   114
References   116

8 Human reproduction 0–20 days post coitus   119
   D.M. Boucher and P.M. Iannaccone

8.1 Introduction   119
8.2 Gametogenesis   119
8.3 Fertilization   120
8.4 Preimplantation development   121
8.5 Implantation   123
8.6 Postimplantation development   124
8.7 Reproductive failure   124
8.8 Conclusions   124
References   125

9 Fundamental processes during the period 20–60 days post conception   127
   R.P. Kapur and J.C. Rutledge

9.1 Introduction   127
9.2 Regional differences in molecular composition   127
9.3 Induction and intercellular communication   130

9.4   Cell migration   131
9.5   Cell replication and death   131
9.6   Movements of contiguous cell populations   133
9.7   Mechanics   135
9.8   Circulation and homeostasis   135
9.9   Timing   136
9.10 Examination of the embryo   136
9.11 Final comments   136
References   137

10 Placenta and adnexa in early pregnancy   139
    E. Jauniaux and J. Hustin

    10.1 Introduction   139
    10.2 Uterine anatomical changes associated with placentation 139
    10.3 Anatomy of the early gestational death   141
    10.4 Anatomical–physiological interrelationships   147
    10.5 Concluding remarks   152
    References   157

**PART TWO   PRENATAL PATHOLOGY AND CONDITIONS
PECULIAR TO EARLY LIFE**   159
Edited by S.G. Driscoll

11 Introduction to Part Two   161
    S.G. Driscoll

12 Products of conception and spontaneous abortion   163
    S.G. Driscoll

    12.1 Introduction   163
    12.2 The pathologist's role and responsibility   163
    12.3 Early reproductive wastage   164
    12.4 Ectopic pregnancy   165
    Further reading   166

13 Recurrent abortion: genetic and other non-immune factors 167
    S. Brown and D. Warburton

    13.1 Introduction   167
    13.2 Definition of recurrent abortion   167
    13.3 Epidemiology of recurrent abortion   167
    13.4 Causes of recurrent abortion   168
    13.5 Conclusions   172
    References   172

14 Evaluation of early pregnancy loss   175
    F.R. Bieber and S.G. Driscoll

    14.1 Introduction   175
    14.2 Definitions   175
    14.3 Malformations in human pregnancy   176
    14.4 Morphology and pathology of early fetal loss   176
    14.5 Assessment of fetal death   180
    14.6 Pregnancy exposures (including teratogens)   181
    14.7 New technology   181
    14.8 Genetic counseling in early fetal loss   182
    14.9 Summary and conclusions   183

14.10 Goals of assessment of early fetal loss   183
References   183

15 Trophoblastic disease: pathology of complete and partial moles   187
    A.E. Szulman

    15.1 Introduction   187
    15.2 Complete hydatidiform mole   187
    15.3 Partial hydatidiform mole   192
    15.4 Coda   196
    References   198

16 Twins and their disorders   201
    G.A. Machin

    16.1 Introduction   201
    16.2 Multiple pregnancy   201
    16.3 Placentation in multiple pregnancy   205
    16.4 Pathology of multiple pregnancy   206
    16.5 Prenatal diagnosis, monitoring and intervention in multiple pregnancy 218
    16.6 Examination of the placenta(s) of multiple pregnancies   222
    16.7 Conclusions: the future of twin pathology   222
    References   223

17 Cytogenetic aspects of reproductive loss   227
    G.A. Machin

    17.1 Definition of reproductive loss   227
    17.2 Quantitative and etiologic aspects of reproductive loss   227
    17.3 Cytogenetics of reproductive loss   228
    17.4 Origins of aneuploid chromosomes   253
    17.5 The borderline between cytogenetics and molecular methodology   254
    17.6 Newer techniques in cytogenetics and their applications   255
    References   255

18 Detection of TORCH and TORCH-like infectious syndromes   261
    N.B. Isada and J.H. Grossman

    18.1 Introduction   261
    18.2 Pathophysiology   261
    18.3 Clinical history   262
    18.4 Serologic screening   262
    18.5 Antigen detection   263
    18.6 Ultrasound   263
    18.7 Invasive testing   263
    18.8 Histologic examination   264
    18.9 Specific infections   264
    18.10 Summary   266
    References   266

19 Fetal death: maceration, autolysis and retention   269
    D.R. Genest

    19.1 Introduction: classification, prevalence and causes of fetal death   269
    19.2 Gross evaluation: sequence of fetal maceration   270
    19.3 Histologic evaluation: postmortem autolysis   271
    19.4 Placental evaluation: changes after fetal death   272
    19.5 Ancillary studies in stillborn fetuses: microbiologic, radiologic,
          cytogenetic, biochemical, molecular   272
    References   273

20 Intrauterine growth retardation   275
    S.C. Robson and T.C. Chang

    201   Definitions   275
    20.2 Aetiology   275
    20.3 Diagnosis   276
    20.4 Pathology   277
    20.5 Neonatal assessment   278
    20.6 Outcome   280
    References   282

21 Intrapartum events   285
    J.E. Gillan

    21.1 Introduction   285
    21.2 Normal cardiorespiratory function in the fetus   285
    21.3 Parturition   287
    21.4 Effect of labour on the fetus   290
    21.5 Fetal response to hypoxia   291
    21.6 Causes of intrapartum asphyxia   292
    21.7 Anaesthesia and fetal distress   297
    21.8 Induction and augmentation of labour   297
    21.9 Pathology of birth asphyxia   298
    21.10 Intrapartum trauma   305
    21.11 Infection   312
    References   312

22 Placenta and adnexa in late pregnancy   319
    R.W. Redline

    22.1 Introduction   319
    22.2 Acute perinatal distress   321
    22.3 Placental hemorrhage   323
    22.4 Placental infection   325
    22.5 Chronic placental disease   328
    22.6 Maldevelopment   334
    22.7 Perspective   336
    References   336

23 Maternal–fetal syndromes: immunology and infection   339
    J.R. Voland and E.K. Main

    23.1 Introduction   339
    23.2 Maternal disease states and pregnancy   343
    23.3 Mirror syndromes   344
    23.4 Pre-eclampsia and hypertensive disease of pregnancy   344
    23.5 Maternal infection and fetal loss   345
    References   350

24 The effects of maternal substance abuse on the placenta and fetus 353
    E.J. Larson

    24.1 Introduction   353
    24.2 Alcohol   355
    24.3 Amphetamines   356
    24.4 Cigarettes   356
    24.5 Cocaine   357
    24.6 Heroin   359

24.7 Methadone   361
24.8 Phencyclidine   361
References   361

**PART THREE SYSTEMATIC AND SPECIAL PATHOLOGY
AND NEOPLASMS**   363
Edited by A.E. Claireaux

25 Introduction to antenatal and neonatal pathology   365
    G.B. Reed

    25.1 Introduction   365
    25.2 Antenatal conditions: disturbances, disorders and diseases   365
    25.3 Role of antenatal and neonatal pathology   365
    25.4 Special training in antenatal pathology   366
    25.5 The antenatal landscape: fetal death, birth defects, low birth weight
          and prematurely born infants   366
    25.6 Fetal pathology   367
    25.7 Birth and the neonatal period   368
    25.8 Neonatal adaptations   369
    25.9 Birth injuries   369
    25.10 Fetal origins of adult diseases   370
    25.11 Comments and medicolegal issues   371
    25.12 Summary   372
    References   372
    Further reading   373

26 The genetic implications of autopsy findings in the fetus and newborn
    with structural defects   375
    M.E. Miller

    26.1 Introduction   375
    26.2 Mechanisms of dysmorphogenesis   375
    26.3 Autopsy   376
    26.4 Establishing a diagnosis and communication of this to the parents 376
    References   380

27 Fetal autopsy   381
    H.B. Robinson

    27.1 Introduction   381
    27.2 The history   381
    27.3 The fetal autopsy   382
    27.4 Evaluation of mode and mechanism of fetal death   385
    27.5 Focused laboratory studies   386
    27.6 Conclusions   388
    References   388

28 The uses of human embryonic and fetal tissues in treatment and research 389
    G.B. Reed, K.T. Rajan, P.L. Ballard, T.H. Shepard and L. Wong

    28.1 Introduction   389
    28.2 Worldwide status   389
    28.3 Sources of tissue   389
    28.4 Preservation of cells, tissues and organs   390

28.5   Human embryonic and fetal tissue in research   390
References   395
Further reading   397

29   Congenital anomalies and dysmorphology   399
     E.V.D.K.B. Perrin and E.F. Gilbert-Barness

     29.1   Introduction   399
     29.2   Additional terms and definitions   401
     29.3   Malformations   401
     29.4   Disruptions   402
     29.5   Deformations   405
     29.6   A few non-metabolic dysplasia syndromes   405
     29.7   Metabolic dysplasia syndromes   405
     29.8   Sequences   405
     29.9   Associations   406
     29.10 Autosomal dominant mutations   407
     29.11 Autosomal recessive mutations   407
     29.12 Sporadic defects   408
     29.13 Chromosome anomaly syndromes   408
     References   411

30   The brain   413
     B. Harding

     30.1   Introduction   413
     30.2   Normal development of the brain   413
     30.3   Malformations   416
     30.4   Encephaloclastic developmental lesions   423
     30.5   Haemorrhagic lesions   427
     30.6   White matter lesions   432
     30.7   Hypoxic–ischaemic grey matter lesions   437
     30.8   Infections   440
     30.9   Kernicterus   445
     30.10 Inborn errors of metabolism   445
     30.11 Neuromuscular disorders   450
     30.12 Sudden infant death syndrome   451
     30.13 Congenital tumours   451
     Appendix 30.A Postmortem removal of the brain and cord   453
     References   458

31   The heart   465
     G.M. Hutchins

     31.1   Normal development   465
     31.2   Cardiovascular malformations   480
     31.3   Genetic and other cardiovascular diseases   505
     31.4   Cardiac dysfunction   509
     31.5   The pathology of therapeutic interventions   514
     31.6   Examination of the heart   516
     References   517

32   Respiratory tract and lungs   523
     D.E. deMello and L.M. Reid

     32.1   Introduction   523
     32.2   Normal lung growth   523
     32.3   Disturbed lung growth   527

32.4 Genetic diseases   554
References   556

33 Liver and biliary system   561
R.S. Chandra

33.1 Development and anomalies   561
33.2 Cholestasis in the newborn   563
33.3 Perinatal infection   566
33.4 Subcapsular hemorrhage and hematoma in the newborn   569
33.5 Hereditary and metabolic disorders   569
33.6 Miscellaneous   573
33.7 Cirrhosis   573
33.8 Neoplasms   574
33.9 Gallbladder   577
References   578

34 The pancreas   581
A.E. Claireaux

34.1 Introduction   581
34.2 Congenital malformations   581
34.3 Cystic fibrosis   582
34.4 Infants of diabetic mothers   583
34.5 Tumours   584
References   586

35 The alimentary tract   589
J.P. Barbet and C. Dupont

35.1 Development   589
35.2 Oesophagus and stomach   591
35.3 Small and large intestine   595
35.4 Anorectal malformations   603
35.5 Peritoneal cavity   604
35.6 Abdominal wall defects and hernias   605
References   606

36 Kidneys and lower urinary tract   609
P. Thorner, J. Bernstein and B.H. Landing

36.1 Introduction   609
36.2 Development and embryology   609
36.3 Kidney   610
36.4 Ureter   625
36.5 Bladder and urethra   627
36.6 Prenatal diagnosis   629
36.7 Treatment options   630
Appendix 36.A Renal and urinary tract involvement in heritable disorders and
  malformation syndromes   631
Appendix 36.B Urinary tract malformations reported in chromosomal
  abnormality syndromes   647
Appendix 36.C Apparently etiologically heterogeneous multiple anomaly
  syndromes with renal or urinary tract malformations   648
Appendix 36.D Syndromes associated with renal cystic dysplasia   650
Appendix 36.E Urinary tract calculus syndromes   652
Appendix 36.F Postnatal renal lesions specifically associated with heritable
  syndromes   653
References   658

37 The reproductive systems   663
    The late J.D. Blair

    37.1 Introduction   663
    37.2 Gonadal dysgenesis   666
    37.3 Testicular dysgenesis   675
    37.4 Intersex syndromes: hermaphroditism   680
    37.5 Other malformations and perinatal disorders of the reproductive organs 684
    37.6 Summary and perspective   686
    References   687
    Further reading   691

38 Clinical pathology and the endocrine system   693
    W. Hamilton

    38.1 Endocrine aspects   693
    38.2 Congenital hypothyroidism – athyreosis   696
    38.3 Hyperthyroidism   698
    38.4 Ambiguous genitalia   698
    38.5 Congenital Cushing syndrome   699
    38.6 Anencephaly   700
    38.7 Mammary gland – neonatal mastitis (witch's milk)   701
    38.8 Septo-optic dysplasia   701
    38.9 Neonatal oedema   702
    38.10 Clinical events in the neonate   702
    38.11 Screening for endocrine disease   706
    References   706

39 Blood disorders   709
    V. Mahnovski and Z. Pavlova

    39.1 Introduction   709
    39.2 Anemia in the neonatal period   709
    39.3 Disorders of red cell metabolism   714
    39.4 Disorders of hemoglobin synthesis   715
    39.5 Polycythemia and hyperviscosity   717
    39.6 Blood coagulation   718
    39.7 Disorders of platelets   718
    39.8 Leukocytes   720
    References   727

40 The immune system   729
    C.R. Abramowsky and R.U. Sorensen

    40.1 Organization and development of the immune system   729
    40.2 Evaluation of the immune system in the newborn   740
    40.3 Disorders of the immune system   741
    References   750

41 Antenatal pathology of the skin   755
    V.P. Sybert and K.A. Holbrook

    41.1 Introduction: development of the skin   755
    41.2 Embryogenesis   755
    41.3 The fetal period   755
    41.4 Third trimester   758
    41.5 Fetal skin biopsy for diagnosis   758
    41.6 Amniotic fluid cell culture for diagnosis   764
    41.7 Genodermatoses diagnosed by fetal bood sampling   765

41.8 Summary 765
References 765

42 Neuromuscular disorders in infants 769
K. Bove

42.1 Introduction 769
42.2 Normal muscle development 769
42.3 Muscle biopsy: indications and technique 771
42.4 Disorders of muscle development 771
42.5 Developmental relationships between muscle and other systems 772
42.6 Muscle in intrauterine growth retardation 774
42.7 Muscle diseases due to exogenous agents 774
42.8 Muscular dystrophies 776
42.9 Congenital myopathies 777
42.10 Congenital hypotonia with type 1 fiber size disproportion 779
42.11 Metabolic diseases 780
42.12 Spinomuscular atrophy in infants 782
42.13 Infantile peripheral neuropathy 783
References 784

43 The congenital chondrodysplasias 787
Z. Borochowitz and D.L. Rimoin

43.1 Introduction 787
43.2 Osteochondrodysplasias identifiable at birth 787
43.3 Dysplasias with decreased bone density 800
43.4 Spondylocostal and spondylothoracic dysplasia 800
43.5 Dysplasias with defective mineralization 800
Appendix 43.A Assistance with diagnosis and collection of skeletal tissues 801
References 801

44 Complications of therapy in the prenatal and perinatal period 803
D.J. deSa

44.1 Introduction 803
44.2 Prenatal therapy 803
44.3 Birth trauma 805
44.4 Neonatal therapy 806
44.5 Exchange transfusion 814
44.6 Cardiac complications 814
44.7 Intravenous alimentation 814
44.8 Genitourinary system, adrenals, spleen 815
44.9 Gastrointestinal tract 817
44.10 Skeletal changes 819
44.11 Pituitary lesions 821
44.12 Central nervous system 822
44.13 Eye 823
44.14 Generalized infections 824
44.15 Biopsy complications 825
44.16 Other 826
Appendix 44.A A simplified method for routine study of the major components
of the conduction of the heart in perinatal infants 826
References 828

45 Benign tumours 831
A.E. Claireaux

45.1 Introduction 831

45.2 Teratomas   831
45.3 Hamartomas   834
45.4 Cysts   846
45.5 Polyps   850
References   852

46 Neuroblastoma   855
   J. Chatten

   46.1 Introduction   855
   46.2 General features of neuroblastoma   856
   46.3 Neuroblastoma in the newborn   859
   46.4 Conclusions   861
   References   861

Volume 2

PART FOUR   IMAGING OF THE EMBRYO, FETUS AND NEWBORN   865
Edited by S.E. Chambers

47 Medical ultrasound from A-scan to real-time   867
   J.E.E. Fleming

48 An overview of ultrasound in obstetrics   877
   S.E. Chambers

   48.1 Introduction   877
   48.2 Roles of ultrasound in obstetric practice   877
   48.3 Components of an obstetric ultrasound examination   878
   48.4 Organization of obstetric ultrasound service   878
   48.5 Ultrasound as an adjunct to routine antenatal care 879
   48.6 Safety   881
   References   882

49 Basic physics and instrumentation of ultrasonics   883
   P.R. Hoskins

   49.1 Physics of ultrasound   883
   49.2 B-scan devices   885
   49.3 Doppler ultrasound instrumentation   886
   Further reading   888

50 Biophysical assessment of the at-risk fetus   889
   J.P. Neilson and Z. Alfirevic

   50.1 Introduction   889
   50.2 Ultrasound measurement   890
   50.3 Cardiotocography   891
   50.4 Biophysical profile   892
   50.5 Doppler ultrasound   893
   50.6 Conclusions   894
   References   894

51 Sonoembryology in the structural evaluation of the fetus from 6 to 16 weeks 897
   I.E. Timor-Tritsch, A. Monteagudo and G.M. Brown

   51.1 Introduction   897
   51.2 Dating the gestation   897

51.3 Discriminatory β-human chorionic gonadotrophin zone for vaginal probes 897
51.4 Technical considerations 898
51.5 Structures detected by transvaginal sonography in the first trimester 898
51.6 Structural evaluation at 15 weeks 912
51.7 Summary 915
References 917

52 Ultrasound diagnosis of structural fetal anomalies 919
S.E. Chambers

52.1 Introduction 919
52.2 Central nervous system 919
52.3 Genitourinary system 924
52.4 The abdomen 927
52.5 The fetus with an intrathoracic mass lesion 930
52.6 Abnormalities of liquor volume 932
52.7 The fetus with a short limb dysplasia 933
52.8 Accuracy of antenatal ultrasound diagnosis of fetal anomalies 935
References 936

53 Ultrasound diagnosis of chromosomal disease 939
P. Twining

53.1 Introduction 939
53.2 Trisomy 13 940
53.5 Trisomy 18 941
53.4 Trisomy 21 945
53.5 Turner's syndrome 949
53.6 Triploidy 950
53.7 First trimester diagnosis of chromosomal disease 951
References 951

54 Fetal echocardiography in the diagnosis and management of fetal structural heart disease and arrhythmias 955
A.H. Friedman, J.A. Copel and C.S. Kleinman

54.1 Introduction 955
54.2 Identification of fetal heart disease 956
54.3 Management of the fetus with congenital heart disease 960
54.4 Fetal arrhythmias 963
54.5 Summary 969
References 969

55 The role of ultrasound in the special problems of multiple pregnancy 971
J.P. Neilson

55.1 Introduction 971
55.2 Diagnosis 971
55.3 Selective reduction 972
55.4 Prenatal diagnosis 972
55.5 Placental morphology 973
55.6 Prediction of preterm labour 975
55.7 Intrauterine growth retardation 975
55.8 Labour and delivery 976
References 977

56 In vivo investigations of placental and umbilical cord anatomy 979
E. Jauniaux, G. Moscoso and S. Campbell

56.1 Introduction 979

56.2   Hemodynamics of early placental circulation   979
56.3   Prenatal diagnosis of placental and cord abnormalities   982
56.4   Experimental systems for the study of placental anatomy   989
56.5   Diagnosing iatrogenic lesions of placenta and cord   992
56.6   Concluding remarks   994
       References   994

PART FIVE   GENETIC SCREENING AND PRENATAL DIAGNOSIS   997
Edited by G.G. Ashmead

57   Introduction to genetic screening and prenatal diagnoses   999
     G.B. Reed

     57.1   Introduction   999
     57.2   Comments   1001
     57.3   Summary   1002
            References   1003
            Further reading   1003

58   A biographical sketch of Robert Guthrie   1005
     J.H. Koch

59   Genetic counseling   1007
     K.L. Garver

     59.1   Introduction   1007
     59.2   Definition   1007
     59.3   Who should counsel?   1008
     59.4   Directive or non-directive counseling?   1008
     59.5   Prospective and retrospective counseling   1008
     59.6   Reproductive options   1009
     59.7   Ethics and eugenics   1010
            References   1011

60   Psychosocial aspects of a termination of pregnancy for fetal abnormality   1013
     M.C.A. White-van Mourik and J.M. Connor

     60.1   Introduction   1013
     60.2   Termination of pregnancy for fetal abnormality   1014
     60.3   Psychosocial sequelae of a termination of pregnancy for fetal abnormality   1014
     60.4   Reproductive behaviour after a termination for fetal abnormality   1016
     60.5   Parental needs and perceived management during and after a termination
            of pregnancy for fetal abnormality   1017
     60.6   Further developments and ethical issues   1018
     60.7   Conclusion   1018
            References   1019

61   Screening for genetic disease   1021
     S.F. Cahalane and P.D. Mayne

     61.1   Introduction   1021
     61.2   Range and objectives of genetic screening   1022
     61.3   Prevalence of mendelian disease   1022
     61.4   Approach to prenatal screening   1023
     61.5   Approach to screening for chromosomal disorders   1024
     61.6   Screening for inherited metabolic disorders   1025
     61.7   Phenylketonuria: a model for metabolic screening   1027
     61.8   Screening for cystic fibrosis   1029

61.9   Disorders of fatty acid metabolism   1029
61.10   Cost versus benefit   1029
61.11   Quality assurance of analytical methods   1029
61.12   Computerization and automation   1030
        References   1030

62   Maternal serum screening   1031
        R.E. Falk

62.1   Introduction   1031
62.2   Neural tube defects   1031
62.3   AFP screening for neural tube defects   1032
62.4   Other sources of elevated MSAFP   1034
62.5   Screening for chromosomal abnormalities   1036
62.6   Role of ultrasound in maternal serum screening   1040
62.7   Concluding comments   1041
        References   1041

63   Neonatal screening and carrier detection   1045
        N.R.M. Buist and J.M. Tuerck

63.1   Introduction   1045
63.2   Universal neonatal screening   1046
63.3   Current issues in newborn screening   1051
63.4   The impact of DNA technology   1052
63.5   Heterozygote (carrier) detection   1053
        References   1054

64   Preimplantation genetic diagnosis   1055
        E. Pergament

64.1   Introduction   1055
64.2   Approaches to preimplantation genetic diagnosis   1055
64.3   Patient perspectives   1057
64.4   The future of preimplantation diagnosis   1057
        References   1057

65   Fetal cell isolation from maternal blood   1059
        D.W. Bianchi

65.1   Introduction   1059
65.2   Historical aspects   1059
65.3   Challenges of current research   1059
65.4   Selection of target cell type   1059
65.5   Cell separation methods   1061
65.6   Genetic analysis   1063
65.7   Conclusion   1063
        References   1064

66   Embryoscopy and first trimester prenatal diagnosis   1065
        Y. Dumez, J.-F. Oury, M. Dommergues and L. Mandelbrot

66.1   Introduction   1065
66.2   Technique   1065
66.3   Results   1067
66.4   Indications   1070
66.5   Diagnostic value and obstetric risk   1070
66.6   Future prospects   1070

66.7   Conclusions   1070
References   1070

67   Cordocentesis (percutaneous umbilical blood sampling and
fetal blood sampling)   1071
P. Johnson and D.J. Maxwell

67.1   Introduction   1071
67.2   Methods   1071
67.3   Indications   1072
67.4   Risks of the procedure   1073
67.5   Informed consent   1074
67.6   Conclusions   1074
References   1075

68   Chorionic villus sampling (early and late)   1077
B. Brambati

68.1   Acceptability and benefits of first trimester testing   1077
68.2   Sampling methods   1077
68.3   Multiple pregnancy   1078
68.4   Timing   1078
68.5   Indications   1079
68.6   Transabdominal versus transcervical CVS   1079
68.7   Complications   1080
68.8   Risk evaluation of CVS versus amniocentesis   1081
References   1081

69   Amniocentesis (early and late)   1083
G.G. Ashmead and M.A. Krew

69.1   Introduction   1083
69.2   Mid-trimester amniocentesis   1083
69.3   'Early' amniocentesis   1084
69.4   Amniocentesis after fetal viability   1085
69.5   Therapeutic amniocentesis   1085
69.6   Isoimmunization   1085
69.7   Conclusion   1086
References   1086

70   Histopathological investigation of prenatal tissue samples (excluding skin)   1089
B.D. Lake

70.1   Introduction   1089
70.2   Requirements for prenatal diagnosis   1089
70.3   Microscopic assessment   1089
70.4   Value of investigation   1094
70.5   Turnaround time   1095
70.6   Techniques used   1095
References   1096

71   Chromosomal mosaicism   1099
C.M. Gosden, K. Harrison and D.K. Kalousek

71.1   Introduction   1099
71.2   Mosaicism in the fetus   1101
71.3   Mosaicism in the placenta   1105
71.4   Technical aspects   1111

71.5   Future directions   1111
71.6   Summary   1111
References   1112

72   Fragile X syndrome   1115
      G.R. Sutherland and R.I. Richards

72.1   Introduction   1115
72.2   The syndrome   1115
72.3   Molecular genetics   1116
72.4   Genetics   1117
72.5   Cytogenetics   1117
72.6   Diagnosis   1117
72.7   Prenatal diagnosis   1118
References   1119

73   Molecular cytogenetics   1121
      B.A. Clark and S. Schwartz

73.1   Introduction   1121
73.2   Molecular cytogenetics   1121
73.3   Fluorescence in situ hybridization methodology   1123
73.4   Applications   1123
73.5   Conclusion   1128
References   1128

74   Biochemical and molecular genetics   1131
      D.A. Applegarth, G.T.N. Besley and L.A. Clarke

74.1   Introduction   1131
74.2   Biochemical investigation of small molecule diseases   1132
74.3   Biochemical investigation of large molecule diseases   1141
74.7   Conclusions and general considerations   1147
Appendix 74.A Inherited metabolic disorders   1148
References   1159

75   Hemoglobinopathies   1165
      A. Cao, M.C. Rosatelli, G.B. Leoni and R. Sardu

75.1   Introduction   1165
75.2   α-Thalassemias   1165
75.3   β-Thalassemia and complex β-thalassemia   1167
75.4   Prenatal diagnosis   1175
75.5   Control of β-thalassemia   1182
75.6   Future prospects   1182
References   1183

76   Clinical molecular genetics   1187
      J.M. Connor

76.1   Nucleic acid structure and function   1187
76.2   Nucleic acid pathology   1190
76.3   Nucleic acid analysis   1192
Further reading   1195

77   Compendium of prenatally diagnosable diseases   1197
      J.M. Connor

PART SIX MANAGEMENT OF THE AT RISK FETUS AND NEWBORN 1237
Edited by F. Cockburn, J.P. Neilson and D.K. Stevenson

78 Introduction to management of the high-risk fetus and newborn 1239
    G.B. Reed

    78.1 Introduction 1239
    78.2 Synopsis 1240
    References 1241

79 Oligohydramnios and polyhydramnios 1243
    N.M. Fisk and A.C. Moessinger

    79.1 Introduction 1243
    79.2 Oligohydramnios 1244
    79.3 Polyhydramnios 1248
    79.4 Conclusions 1251
    References 1252

80 Immune and non-immune fetal hydrops 1257
    G. Ryan and M.J. Whittle

    80.1 Definition and history 1257
    80.2 Immune hydrops 1257
    80.3 Non-immune hydrops 1257
    80.4 Conclusions 1264
    References 1264

81 Fetal metabolism 1267
    F. Cockburn

    81.1 Introduction 1267
    81.2 Maternal influences 1267
    81.3 Fetoplacental influences 1275
    References 1277

82 Fetal and neonatal coagulation 1281
    B.E.S. Gibson

    82.1 Development of haemostasis in the newborn 1281
    82.2 Investigation and diagnosis of disorders of haemostasis 1282
    82.3 Inherited haemostatic deficiencies 1283
    82.4 Acquired haemostatic defects 1285
    References 1290

83 Viral infection during pregnancy 1293
    A.B. MacLean

    83.1 History 1293
    83.2 Virology 1293
    83.3 Effects of viral infection on the mother 1293
    83.4 Effects of viral infection on the fetus 1294
    83.5 Individual viruses 1294
    References 1298

84 Rhesus alloimmunization 1301
    K.J. Moise Jr and G.G. Ashmead

    84.1 Introduction 1301
    84.2 Physiologic adaptations in the anemic fetus 1301

84.3   Diagnosis   1302
84.4   Treatment and outcome   1304
84.5   Future therapy   1305
References   1305

85   Direct fetal therapy   1307
     D. Maxwell and P. Johnson

     85.1   Introduction   1307
     85.2   Therapeutic methods   1307
     85.3   Ultrasound-guided therapies   1308
     85.4   Direct vision   1312
     85.5   Therapeutic application   1312
     85.6   Conclusion   1313
     References   1313

86   Shunts in closed fetal surgery   1315
     G.G. Ashmead and W.R. Burrows

     86.1   Overview and history   1315
     86.2   Ethical and medicolegal considerations   1315
     86.3   Obstructive urinary tract lesions   1315
     86.4   Hydrocephalus   1316
     86.5   Pleuritic, ascitic and other fluid collections   1317
     86.6   Conclusions and future directions   1317
     References   1317

87   Congenital diaphragmatic hernia and open fetal surgery   1319
     F. Bargy, E. Sapin, Y. Rouquet, S. Beaudoin, D. Hamza, C. Esteve,
     F. Toubas, F. Lewin and O. Gaudiche

     87.1   Introduction   1319
     87.2   Congenital diaphragmatic hernia   1319
     87.3   Open fetal surgery   1326
     87.4   Conclusions   1329
     References   1330

88   In utero hematopoietic stem cell transplantation   1331
     A.W. Flake

     88.1   Introduction   1331
     88.2   Reconstitution of fetal hematopoietic disease   1331
     88.3   Prenatal tolerance induction   1334
     88.4   Gene therapy   1334
     88.5   Summary   1335
     References   1335

89   Lung maturation in prenatal preparation of the fetus   1337
     R.A. Ballard and P.L. Ballard

     89.1   Pulmonary disease in the preterm infant   1337
     89.2   Agents used to prevent respiratory distress in the preterm infant   1337
     89.3   Glucocorticoid issues affecting efficacy   1338
     89.4   Other effects, risks and benefits of glucocorticoids   1340
     89.5   Recommendations for therapy   1340
     89.6   Long-term outcome after prenatal glucocorticoids   1340
     89.7   Other agents that have been evaluated   1340
     89.8   Summary   1341
     References   1342

90 Intrapartum management of fetal anomalies   1345
    J. Manley and S. Weiner

    90.1 Anomalies affecting the timing of delivery   1345
    90.2 Anomalies affecting the mode of delivery   1345
    90.3 Anomalies affecting the location of delivery   1346
    90.4 Intrapartum monitoring   1347
    References   1348

91 Intrapartum fetal monitoring   1351
    N.C. Smith

    91.1 The high-risk fetus   1351
    91.2 Pathophysiology of intrauterine hypoxia   1351
    91.3 Current methods of intrapartum fetal surveillance   1352
    91.4 Futuristic methods of intrapartum fetal surveillance   1359
    91.5 Conclusions   1359
    References   1360

92 Delivery room care and neonatal resuscitation   1361
    P. Dennery and D.K. Stevenson

    92.1 Etiology of asphyxia in the newborn   1361
    92.2 Pathophysiology of hypoxic–ischemic encephalopathy   1361
    92.3 Pathophysiology of asphyxia   1362
    92.4 Neonatal resuscitation   1363
    92.5 Neurodevelopmental outcome of neonatal asphyxia   1365
    92.6 Methods of evaluation of hypoxic–ischemic encephalopathy and outcome   1367
    References   1369

93 Neonatal intensive care   1373
    I.A. Laing

    93.1 Introduction   1373
    93.2 Organization of neonatal services   1373
    93.3 Recent advances   1374
    93.4 Ethical decisions in the neonatal unit   1376
    93.5 Formulation of a plan   1377
    93.6 Management of neonatal death   1377
    93.7 Autopsy   1378
    93.8 Postbereavement care   1378
    93.9 Summary   1379
    References   1379

94 Ethics of delivery room practice   1381
    A.G.M. Campbell

    94.1 Introduction   1381
    94.2 Communication   1381
    94.3 The place of care   1381
    94.4 The paediatrician in the delivery room   1382
    94.5 Dilemmas of resuscitation and treatment   1382
    References   1385

95 Respiratory problems in the preterm infant   1387
    R.L. Ariagno

    95.1 Introduction   1387
    95.2 Apnea   1387

95.3   Respiratory distress syndrome   1392
References   1396

96   Neonatal cerebrovascular monitoring   1399
      M. Levene

      96.1   Introduction   1399
      96.2   Imaging   1399
      96.3   Assessment of cerebral haemodynamics   1400
      96.4   Measurement of intracranial pressure   1402
      96.5   Neurophysiology   1402
      96.6   Practical monitoring techniques in clinical practice   1404
      References   1404

97   Neonatal metabolism   1407
      F. Cockburn

      97.1   Introduction   1407
      97.2   Anabolism   1407
      97.3   Catabolism   1408
      97.4   Infant feeding   1408
      97.5   Clinical features of inherited metabolic diseases in the newborn   1413
      References   1414

98   Neonatal parenteral nutrition   1417
      J.A. Kerner Jr

      98.1   Introduction   1417
      98.2   Indications   1417
      98.3   Route of administration   1420
      98.4   Requirements   1422
      98.5   Initiating therapy   1431
      98.6   Complications   1431
      98.7   Monitoring   1439
      98.8   Summary   1439
      References   1439

99   Neonatal bacterial and viral sepsis   1445
      C. Sabella and C.G. Prober

      99.1   Introduction   1445
      99.2   Bacterial sepsis   1445
      99.3   Viral sepsis   1448
      References   1450

100   Management of neonatal hemolytic hyperbilirubinemia   1453
      P. Dennery and D.K. Stevenson

      100.1   Bilirubin metabolism and physiology   1453
      100.2   Historical perspective of hemolytic disease and its management   1454
      100.3   Postnatal management of erythroblastosis fetalis   1456
      100.4   Outcome of erythroblastosis fetalis   1458
      References   1458

101   Neonatal obstructive uropathy   1461
      B. Blyth and J.W. Duckett Jr

      101.1   Renal development and sonographic evaluation   1461
      101.2   Incidence of neonatal hydronephrosis   1462
      101.3   Postnatal evaluation of neonatal hydronephrosis   1462

101.4 Indications for prenatal urological intervention   1465
101.5 Indications for postnatal intervention   1465
101.6 Summary   1467
References   1467

102 Extracorporeal membrane oxygenation   1469
     W.D. Rhine

     102.1 History of cardiopulmonary bypass in neonates   1469
     102.2 Indications   1469
     102.3 Techniques of ECMO bypass   1471
     102.4 Physiology of ECMO bypnass   1473
     102.5 Outcome   1474
     102.6 Future modifications and application of extracorporeal membrane
            life support   1476
     References   1476

103 Surgical correction and transplantation in the management of
     congenital heart disease in the neonate   1479
     D. Bernstein

     103.1 Introduction   1479
     103.2 Non-complex congenital heart lesions   1479
     103.3 Complex congenital heart lesions   1480
     References   1483

104 Neonatal necrotizing enterocolitis   1485
     P.A.M. Raine

     104.1 Incidence and aetiology   1485
     104.2 Pathological features and pathogenesis   1485
     104.3 Presentation   1486
     104.4 Diagnosis   1486
     104.5 Management   1488
     104.6 Complications   1489
     104.7 Outcome   1490
     References   1490

105 Omphaloceles and gastroschisis   1493
     E. Sapin and F. Bargy

     105.1 Pathobiology   1493
     105.2 Prenatal pathology   1494
     105.3 Systemic and specialty pathology   1494
     105.4 Obstetric sonography   1495
     105.5 Goals of genetic screening and prenatal diagnosis   1498
     105.6 Management of 'high-risk' fetus and newborn   1498
     References   1501

106 Immunological reconstitution of primary immunodeficiencies in the
     neonatal period   1503
     R.U. Sorensen

     106.1 Introduction   1503
     106.2 Cell and tissue engraftment   1503
     106.3 Cytokine therapy   1508
     106.4 Enzyme replacement therapy   1508
     106.5 Gene therapy   1508

106.6	Treatment of specific immunodeficiency syndromes	1510
	References	1511

107   Basic laboratory support in fetal and neonatal medicine   1513
J. Michaud

107.1	Introduction	1513
107.2	Sampling	1514
107.3	Transportation of samples	1514
107.4	Sample analysis	1515
107.5	Selected specific analyses	1516
107.6	Data reporting	1517
107.7	Final considerations	1518
	References	1522

108   Comments on fetal and neonatal laboratory medicine   1525
G.B. Reed

109   The autopsy and protocols   1529
G.B. Reed

109.1	Introduction	1529
109.2	Organization of the pathology service	1531
109.3	Procedures and documentation	1532
109.4	Tissue sampling	1533
109.5	Brain and spinal cord	1533
109.6	Heart and vascular system	1533
109.7	Conclusions	1533
109.8	Addendum by D.J. deSa	1550
	References	1551
	Further reading	1552

Postscript

110   Two pioneer physician–scientists   1553
S.F. Cahalane

110.1	John William Ballantyne (1861–1923) and antenatal pathology	1553
110.2	Archibald Garrod (1857–1936)	1554
	References	1556

Index   1557

EDITORIAL BOARD

CONTRIBUTORS

CARLOS R. ABRAMOWSKY MD
Department of Pathology
Egleston Hospital
Emory University
1405 Clifton Road
Atlanta, Georgia 30322
USA

ZARKO ALFIREVIC
Department of Obstetrics and Gynaecology
University of Liverpool
PO Box 147
Liverpool L69 3BX
UK

DEREK A. APPLEGARTH PhD
Biochemical Disease Laboratory
Vancouver Children's Hospital
4480 Oak Street
Vancouver, British Columbia V6H 3V4
Canada

RONALD ARIAGNO MD
Neonatology S-222
Stanford University Medical Center
Stanford, CA 94305
USA

GRAHAM G. ASHMEAD MD
OB-Gyn, Room 2123
Fetal Diagnostic Center
MetroHealth Center
2500 MetroHealth Drive
Cleveland, OH 44109
USA

MURRAY D. BAIN MD
Department of Child Health
St George's Hospital Medical School
Cranmer Terrace
London SW17 0RE
UK

PHILIP L. BALLARD MD, PhD
Department of Pediatrics
University of Pennsylvania
Children's Hospital of Philadelphia
34th Civic Center Boulevard
Philadelphia, PA 19104
USA

ROBERTA A. BALLARD MD
Division of Neonatology
Children's Hospital of Philadelphia
34th Civic Center Boulevard
Philadelphia, PA 19104
USA

PROFESSOR JACQUES PATRICK BARBET
Department of Paediatric Pathology
Hospital St Vincent dePaul
74 Avenue Denfert-Rochereau
F-75014 Paris
France

PROFESSOR FREDERIC BARGY MD
Department of Pediatric Surgery
Hospital St Vincent dePaul
74 Avenue Denfert-Rochereau
F-75014 Paris
France

S. BEAUDOIN
Hospital St Vincent dePaul
74 Avenue Denfert-Rochereau
F-75014 Paris
France

DANIEL J. BERNSTEIN MD
Pediatric Cardiology
Stanford University Medical Center
Stanford, CA 94305
USA

JAY BERNSTEIN MD
Research Institute
William Beaumont Hospital
Royal Oak, MI 48073
USA

G.T.N. BESLEY PhD
Willink Biochemical Genetics Unit
Royal Manchester Children's Hospital
Pendlebury, Manchester M27 1HA
UK

DIANA W. BIANCHI MD
Neonatology Division
Department of Pediatrics
New England Medical Center
750 Washington Street, Box 394
Boston, MA 02111
USA

FREDERICK R. BIEBER PhD
Pathology
Brigham and Women's Hospital
75 Francis Street
Boston, MA 02115
USA

JOHN BLAIR MD (deceased)
Department of Pathology
St Louis University Medical Center
St Louis, MO
USA

BRUCE BLYTHE MD
Rocky Mountain Pediatric Urology, P.C.
P/SL Professional Plaza West
160 E. 19th Avenue
Suite 3750
Denver, CO 80218
USA

ROBERT P. BOLANDE MD
Pathology Department
East Carolina Medical School
Greenville, NC 27834
USA

ZVI BOROCHOWITZ MD
The Genetics Institute
B'nai-Zion Medical Center
47 Golomb St
PO Box 4940
Haifa
Israel 31048

DIANE M. BOUCHER
Department of Pathology and Developmental
    Biology T239
Northwestern University Medical School
303 East Chicago Avenue
Chicago, IL 60611
USA

KEVIN BOVE MD
Cincinnati Children's Hospital
Elland and Bethesda
Cincinnati, OH 45229
USA

BRUNO BRAMBATI MD
1 Clinica Obstetrica e Ginecologica
Università di Milano
Via Commenda 12
20122 Milano
Italy

G.M. BROWN MD
Perinatal Unit, Obstetrics/Gynecology
    Department
College of Physicians and Surgeons
Columbia University
630 West 168th Street
New York, NY 10032
USA

STEPHEN BROWN MD
Genetics Laboratory
Babies Hospital, BHS B7
3959 Broadway
New York, NY 10032
USA

NEIL R.M. BUIST MD
Pediatric Metabolic Laboratory L-473
Oregon Health Sciences University
3181 SW Sam Jackson Park Road
Portland, Oregon 97201
USA

WILLIAM R. BURROWS MD
OB-Gyn, Room 2123
Fetal Diagnostic Center
MetroHealth Medical Center
2500 MetroHealth Drive
Cleveland, OH 44109
USA

SEAMUS F. CAHALANE MD, PhD
Department of Pathology
The Children's Hospital
Temple Street
Dublin 1
Ireland

PROFESSOR ALEXANDER G.M.
    CAMPBELL
Department of Child Health
University of Aberdeen
Foresterhill
Aberdeen AB9 2ZD
UK

PROFESSOR STUART CAMPBELL MD
Department of Obstetrics and Gynaecology
King's College Hospital and Medical School
Denmark Hill
London SE5 8RX
UK

PROFESSOR ANTONIO CAO
Istituto di Clinica e Biologia dell'Età
    Evolutiva
Università degli Studi di Cagliari
via Jenner s/n
09121 Cagliari
Italy

SARAH E. CHAMBERS MB
Ultrasound Department
Simpson Memorial Maternity Pavillion
Lauriston Place
Edinburgh EH3 9EF
UK

ROMA S. CHANDRA MD
National Medical Center
Children's Hospital, Pathology
111 Michigan Avenue, NW
Washington DC 20010
USA

THOMAS C. CHANG
Department of Maternal Fetal Medicine
Kandang Kerbau Hospital
1 Hampshire Road
Singapore

JANE CHATTEN MD
Pathology, Children's Hospital
34th and Civic Center Boulevard
Philadelphia, PA 19104
USA

PROFESSOR ALBERT E. CLAIREAUX MD
Histopathology
Hospital for Sick Children
Great Ormond Street
London WC1N 3JH
UK

BRIAN A. CLARK MD, PhD
Departments of Reproductive Biology and
    Genetics
Case Western Reserve University
MetroHealth Medical Center
Cleveland, OH 44109
USA

LORENE A. CLARKE MD
Biochemical Disease Laboratory
Vancouver Children's Hospital
4480 Oak Street
Vancouver, British Columbia V6H 3V4
Canada

PROFESSOR FORRESTER COCKBURN
Department of Child Health
Royal Hospital for Sick Children
Yorkhill
Glasgow G3 8SJ
UK

PROFESSOR J. MICHAEL CONNOR
Duncan Guthrie Institute of Medical Genetics
Royal Hospital for Sick Children
Yorkhill
Glasgow G3 8SJ
UK

JOSHUA A. COPEL MD
Department of Obstetrics and Gynecology
Yale University School of Medicine
PO Box 208063
New Haven, CT 06520-8063
USA

DAPHNE E. DEMELLO MD
Cardinal Glennon Children's Hospital
1465 Grand Boulevard
St Louis, MO 63104
USA

PHYLLIS DENNERY MD
Department of Pediatrics
Division of Neonatology
Stanford University Medical Center
Stanford, CA 94305
USA

DEREK J. DESA MD
Department of Pathology
McMaster University Medical Center
1200 Main Street West
Hamilton, Ontario L8N 3Z5
Canada

M. DOMMERGUES
Gynecologue Accoucher des Hopitaux
Clinique Port Royal University
123 Boulevard Port Royal
F-75014 Paris
France

SHIRLEY G. DRISCOLL MD
10 Bird Hill Avenue
Wellesley, MA 02181
USA

JOHN W. DUCKETT JR MD
Rocky Mountain Pediatric Urology, P.C.
P/SL Professional Plaza West
160 E. 19th Avenue
Suite 3750
Denver, CO 80218
USA

YVES DUMEZ MD
Gynecologue Accoucher des Hopitaux
Clinique Port Royal University
123 Boulevard Port Royal
F-75014 Paris
France

PROFESSOR CHRISTOPHE
    DUPONT MD PhD
Department of Paediatrics
Hospital St Vincent dePaul
74 Avenue Denfert-Rochereau
F-75014 Paris
France

C. ESTEVE
Hospital St Vincent dePaul
74 Avenue Denfert-Rochereau
F-75014 Paris
France

RENA E. FALK MD
Ahmanson Department of Pediatrics
Steven Spielberg Pediatric Research Center
Cedars Sinai MC
8700 Beverley Road
Los Angeles, CA 90048
USA

PROFESSOR NICHOLAS M. FISK
Royal Postgraduate Medical School
Institute of Obstetrics and Gynaecology
Queen Charlotte's and Chelsea Hospital
Goldhawk Road
London W6 0XG
UK

ALLAN W. FLAKE MD
Children's Hospital of Michigan
Department of Surgery
3901 Beaubien Blvd
Detroit, MI 48201-2196
USA

JOHN E.E. FLEMING
Department of Obstetrics and Gynaecology
The Queen Mother's Hospital
University of Glasgow
Glasgow G3 8SH
UK

ALAN H. FRIEDMAN MD
Department of Pediatrics
Yale University School of Medicine
PO Box 333
333 Cedar Street
New Haven, CT 06510
USA

KENNETH L. GARVER MD, PhD
101 Stephens Lane
Verona, PA 15147
USA

DONALD W. GAU MD
11 Stratton Road
Beaconsfield HP9 1HR
UK

O. GAUDICHE
Hospital St Vincent dePaul
74 Avenue Denfert-Rochereau
F-75014 Paris
France

DAVID R. GENEST MD
Pathology
Brigham and Women's Hospital
75 Francis Street
Boston, MA 02115
USA

BRENDA E.S. GIBSON MD
Haematology
Royal Hospital for Sick Children
Yorkhill
Glasgow G3 8SJ
UK

ENID F. GILBERT-BARNESS MD
Department of Pathology
HCHA/Tampa General Hospital
Davis Island
Tampa, FL 33606
USA

JOHN E. GILLAN MB
Department of Pathology
Rotunda Hospital
Dublin 1
Ireland

PROFESSOR CHRISTINE M. GOSDEN
Department of Obstetrics and Gynaecology
University of Liverpool
PO Box 147
Liverpool L69 3BX
UK

JOHN H. GROSSMAN MD, PhD
Fetal Medicine
George Washington University Medical
    School
Washington DC
USA

WILLIAM HAMILTON MD
81 Woodend Drive
Glasgow G13 1QF
UK

D. HAMZA
Hospital St Vincent dePaul
74 Avenue Denfert-Rochereau
F-75014 Paris
France

BRIAN HARDING DPhil, FRCPath
Neuropathology
Hospital for Sick Children
Great Ormond Street
London WC1N 3JH
UK

KAREN HARRISON PhD
Department of Pathology
British Columbia Children's Hospital
4480 Oak Street
Vancouver, British Columbia V6H 3V4
Canada

KAREN A. HOLBROOK PhD
Graduate School
University of Florida
223 Grinter Hall
PO Box 115500
Gainesville, FL 32611-5500
USA

PETER R. HOSKINS
Medical Physics Department
Royal Infirmary
Edinburgh EH3 9YW
UK

PROFESSOR J. HUSTIN PhD
The Morphopathologic Institute of Loverval
  (IMPL)
41 Allée des Templiers
B-6280 Gerpinnes
Belgium

GROVER M. HUTCHINS MD
Department of Pathology, B100
The Johns Hopkins Hospital
600 North Wolfe Street
Baltimore, MD 21287-6901
USA

PHILIP M. IANNACCONE MD, PhD
Department of Pathology and Developmental
  Biology T239
Northwestern University Medical School
303 East Chicago Avenue
Chicago, IL 60611
USA

NELSON B. ISADA MD
Division of Maternal–Fetal Medicine
Hofheimer Hall, Suite 310
825 Fairfax Avenue
Eastern Virginia Medical School
Norfolk, VA 23507-1912
USA

ERIC JAUNIAUX MD, PhD
Department of Obstetrics and Gynaecology
9th Floor New Ward Block
King's College Dental and Medical School
Denmark Hill
London SE5 8RX
UK

PAM JOHNSON MD
c/o D. Maxwell
Fetal Medicine Unit
Guy's Tower, 15th Floor
Guy's Hospital
London SE1 9RT
UK

DAGMAR K. KALOUSEK MD
Department of Pathology
British Columbia Children's Hospital
4480 Oak Street
Vancouver, British Columbia V6H 3V4
Canada

RAJ P. KAPUR MD, PhD
Pathology
Children's Hospital
4800 Sand Point Way NE
Seattle, WA 98105
USA

JOHN A. KERNER Jr MD
Pediatric Gastroenterology and Nutrition
  G310
Stanford University Medical Center
Stanford, CA 94305
USA

CHARLES S. KLEINMAN MD
Department of Pediatrics
Yale University School of Medicine
PO Box 333
333 Cedar Street
New Haven, CT 06510
USA

JEAN H. KOCH
2125 Ames Street
Los Angeles, CA 90027
USA

M.A. KREW MD
c/o G. Ashmead
OB-Gyn, Room 2123
Fetal Diagnostic Center
MetroHealth Medical Center
2500 MetroHealth Drive
Cleveland, OH 44109
USA

IAN A. LAING MD
Neonatal Unit
Simpson Memorial Maternity Pavilion
Lauriston Place
Edinburgh EH3 9EF
UK

PROFESSOR BRIAN D. LAKE PhD, FRCPath
Department of Histopathology
Great Ormond Street Hospital for Children NHS
   Trust
London WC1N 3JH
UK

BENJAMIN H. LANDING MD
Pathology Research
Children's Hospital Los Angeles
4650 Sunset Boulevard
Los Angeles, CA 90027
USA

EUNICE J. LARSON MD
Miller Memorial Children's Hospital
Long Beach Memorial Hospital, POB-1428
2801 Atlantic Avenue
Long Beach, CA 90801
USA

GIOVAN BATTISTA LEONI MD
Ospedale Regionale per le Microcitemie
USL 21
via Jenner s/n
09121 Cagliari
Italy

PROFESSOR MALCOLM LEVENE
Department of Child Health
Clarendon Wing, D Floor
Leeds General Infirmary
Belmont Grove
Leeds LS2 9NS
UK

F. LEWIN
Hospital St Vincent DePaul
74 Avenue Denfert-Rochereau
F-75014 Paris
France

GEOFFREY A. MACHIN MD, PhD
Room 5B4.08
Department of Pathology
W.C. Mackenzie Health Science Center
University of Alberta
Edmonton, Alberta T6G 2B7
Canada

PROFESSOR ALAN B. MacLEAN
Royal Free Hospital
Academic Department of Obstetrics and
   Gynaecology
Pond Street
London NW3 2QG
UK

VLADIMIR MAHNOVSKI MD
Department of Pathology
Children's Hospital of Los Angeles
4650 Sunset Boulevard
Los Angeles, CA 90027
USA

ELLIOT K. MAIN MD
Perinatal Services
California-Pacific Medical Center
c/o California Campus
PO Box 7999
San Francisco, CA 94120
USA

L. MANDELBROT
Gynecologue Accoucher des Hopitaux
Clinique Port Royal University
123 Boulevard Port Royal
F-75014 Paris
France

JAMES MANLEY MD
c/o S. Weiner
Maternal Fetal Medicine
Pennsylvania Hospital
800 Spruce Street
Philadelphia, PA 19107
USA

DARRYL J. MAXWELL
Fetal Medicine Unit
Guy's Tower, 15th Floor
Guy's Hospital
London SE1 9RT
UK

PHILIP D. MAYNE MD
Department of Pathology
The Children's Hospital
Temple Street
Dublin 1
Ireland

PROFESSOR JEAN MICHAUD MD
Pathology, Hospital Ste Justine
3175 Cote Ste-Catherine
Montreal, Quebec H3T 1C5
Canada

MARVIN E. MILLER MD
Children's Medical Center
Medical Genetics Division
1 Children's Plaza
Dayton, OH 45404
USA

ADRIEN C. MOESSINGER MD
Universitats-Frauenklinik
Schanzeneckstr. 1
3012 Bern
Switzerland

KENNETH J. MOISE MD
Department of Obstetrics and Gynecology
Baylor College of Medicine
1 Baylor Plaza
Houston, TX 77030
USA

ANNA MONTEAGUDO MD
Perinatal and Ob/Gyn Ultrasound Unit
Department of Obstetrics and Gynecology
College of Physicians and Surgeons
Columbia University
630 West 168th Street
New York, NY 10032
USA

GONZALO MOSCOSO MD
Early Human Development Research Unit
Pathology
Dulwich Hospital
East Dulwich Grove
London SE22 8PT
UK

ANDRE J. NAHMIAS MD
Division of Infectious Diseases, Epidemiology
  and Immunology
Department of Pediatrics
Emory University School of Medicine
69 Butler Street S.E.
Atlanta, Georgia 30303
USA

PROFESSOR JAMES P. NEILSON
Department of Obstetrics and Gynaecology
University of Liverpool
PO Box 147
Liverpool L69 3BX
UK

JOHN M. OPITZ MD
Foundation of Developmental and Medical
  Genetics
Montana State University
FRB Suite 229
100 Neill Avenue
Helena, MT 59601
USA

J.-F. OURY
Maternité
Hopital Robert Debré
Boulevard Serrurier
75019 Paris
France

ZDENA PAVLOVA MD
Department of Pathology and Pediatrics
LAC-USC Medical Center
1240 North Mission Road
Los Angeles, CA 90033
USA

EUGENE PERGAMENT MD, PhD
Room 1564
Reproductive Genetics
Department of Obstetrics and
  Gynecology
Northwestern Memorial Hospital
333 East Superior
Chicago, IL 60611
USA

EUGENE V.D.K.B. PERRIN MD
Hutzel Hospital
Pathology
Detroit, MI 48201
USA

CHARLES G. PROBER MB, FRCS(Ed), FRCS(Glas)
Pediatrics, A367
Stanford University Medical Center
Stanford, CA 94305
USA

PETER A.M. RAINE MB, FRCS(Ed), FRCS(Glas)
Pediatric Surgery
Royal Hospital for Sick Children
Yorkhill
Glasgow G3 8SJ
UK

K.T. RAJAN MD
Rheumatology
Pontypridd Hospital
Pontypridd CF37 4AL
UK

RAYMOND W. REDLINE MD
Institute of Pathology
Case Western Reserve University
2085 Adelbert Road
Cleveland, OH 44106
USA

GEORGE B. REED MD
133 Via Gayuba
Monterey, CA 93940
USA

LYNNE M. REID MD
Pathology Department
Children's Hospital
Harvard Medical School
300 Longwood Avenue
Boston, MA 02115
USA

WILLIAM D. RHINE MD
Neonatology S-222
Stanford University Medical Center
Stanford, CA 94305
USA

R.I. RICHARDS PhD
Centre for Medical Genetics
Department of Cytogenetics and Molecular
  Genetics
Women's and Children's Hospital
Adelaide, South Australia 5006
Australia

DAVID L. RIMOIN MD, PhD
Department of Pediatrics
Cedars Sinai Medical Center
8700 Beverley Boulevard
Los Angeles, CA 90048
USA

HAYNES B. ROBINSON MD
Pathology
Toledo Hospital
2142 North Cove Boulevard
Toledo, OH 43606
USA

STEPHEN C. ROBSON
Department of Obstetrics and Gynaecology
4th Floor, Leazes Wing
Royal Victorial Infirmary
Newcastle-upon-Tyne NE1 4LP
UK

M. CHRISTINE ROSATELLI MD
Istituto di Clinica e Biologia dell'Età
  Evolutiva
Università degli Studi di Cagliari
via Jenner s/n
09121 Cagliari
Italy

Y. ROUQUET
Hospital St Vincent dePaul
74 Avenue Denfert-Rochereau
F-75014 Paris
France

JOSEPH C. RUTLEDGE MD
Pathology CH-37
4800 Sand Point Way, NE
PO Box C 5371
Seattle, WA 98105
USA

GREG RYAN MB
Perinatal Unit
Mt Sinai Hospital
University of Toronto
600 University Avenue
Toronto, Ontario M5G 1X5
Canada

C. SABELLA MD
Pediatrics, A367
Stanford University Medical Center
Stanford, CA 94305
USA

EMMANUEL SAPIN MD
Department of Pediatric Surgery
Hospital St Vincent dePaul
74 Avenue Denfert-Rochereau
F-75014 Paris
France

R. SARDU MD
Istituto di Clinica e Biologia dell'Età
  Evolutiva
Università degli Studi di Cagliari
via Jenner s/n
09121 Cagliari
Italy

STUART SCHWARTZ PhD
Department of Genetics
Center for Human Genetics
Case Western Reserve University
Cleveland, OH 44106
USA

THOMAS H. SHEPARD MD
Central Laboratory for Human Embryology
Department of Pediatrics, RD-20
University of Washington School of Medicine
Seattle, WA 98195
USA

NORMAN C. SMITH MD
Aberdeen Maternity Hospital
Cornhill Road
Aberdeen AB9 2ZA
UK

RICARDO U. SORENSEN MD
Department of Pediatrics
Louisiana State University Medical Center
1542 Tulane Avenue, Room 827
New Orleans, LA 70112
USA

DAVID K. STEVENSON MD
Neonatology S-222
Stanford University Medical Center
Stanford, CA 94305
USA

GRANT R. SUTHERLAND PhD, DSc
Centre for Medical Genetics
Department of Cytogenetics and Molecular
  Genetics
Women's and Children's Hospital
Adelaide, South Australia 5006
Australia

VIRGINIA P. SYBERT MD
Division of Medical Genetics
Children's Orthopedic Hospital
4800 Sand Point Way, NE
Seattle, WA 98105
USA

PROFESSOR A.E. SZULMAN MB ChB
Pathology
Magee-Women's Hospital
300 Halket St
Pittsburg, PA 15213
USA

PAUL THORNER MD, PhD
Department of Pathology
Hospital for Sick Children
555 University Avenue
Toronto, Ontario M5G 1X8
Canada

I.E. TIMOR-TRISTCH MD
Perinatal and Ob/Gyn Ultrasound Unit
Department of Obstetrics and Gynecology
College of Physicians and Surgeons
Columbia University
630 West 168th Street
New York, NY 10032
USA

F. TOUBAS
Hospital St Vincent dePaul
74 Avenue Denfert-Rochereau
F-75014 Paris
France

M. JUDY TUERCK RN, MS
CDRC Metabolic Clinic
Oregon Health Sciences University
3181 SW Sam Jackson Park Road
Portland, Oregon 97201
USA

PETER TWINING MD
X Ray Department
Queen's Medical Centre
Derby Road
Nottingham NG7 2UH
UK

PROFESSOR MICHEL J.J. VEKEMANS
  MD, PhD
Service of Histology, Embryology and
  Cytogenetics
Hospital Necker-Enfants Malade
149 Rue de Sèvres
F-75743 Paris
France

JOSEPH R. VOLAND MD
UCSD Cancer Center
Warren 303, Q063
University of California at San Diego
La Jolla, CA 92093
USA

DOROTHY WARBURTON PhD
Departments of Genetics and Development,
  and Pediatrics
College of Physicians and Surgeons
Columbia University
701 W-168th Street
New York, NY 10032
USA

STUART WEINER MD
Maternal Fetal Medicine
Pennsylvania Hospital
800 Spruce Street
Philadelphia, PA 19107
USA

M.C.A. WHITE-VAN MOURIK
Duncan Guthrie Institute of Medical Genetics
Royal Hospital for Sick Children
Yorkhill
Glasgow G3 8SJ
UK

PROFESSOR MARTIN J. WHITTLE MD
Department of Fetal Medicine
Birmingham Maternity Hospital
University of Birmingham
Queen Elizabeth Centre
Birmingham B15 2TG
UK

LESLIE WONG MB, CHB
MRC Tissue Bank
Royal Postgraduate Medical School
Hammersmith Hospital
Du Cane Road
London W12 0NN
UK

PREFACE TO THE SECOND EDITION

This book represents a multidisciplinary approach to antenatal and neonatal medicine and pathology. The work is composed of six parts. This second edition of *Diseases of the Fetus and Newborn* includes the various entities that occur during a time span which begins at conception and ends three months postnatally. Genetic and acquired conditions resulting in birth defects, pregnancy loss, fetal and neonatal death are emphasized. As birth defects are often morphologic structural defects, a comprehensive understanding of pathology is essential. In addition, since a great deal of our information is derived from specialized scientific and medical sources, the contributors are encouraged to write in a straightforward fashion. Primary attention is given to the 'at risk' fetus, the family and probable postnatal outcomes.

Currently, a team effort is the most practical approach in practicing fetal and neonatal medicine (also sometimes known as fetal medicine and surgery or perinatal obstetrics). This is a valid idea if one considers the number of disciplines that can be involved in the management of an 'at risk' pregnancy or fetus. In addition, this approach may include preconceptual care, genetic screening, prenatal diagnosis and sonographic surveillance.

Also, currently, in parallel with the 'team approach' is the increased public perception of new medical needs and options. Added to these issues are the rapid advances in molecular and cell biology, genetics, reproductive and developmental biology, and pathology and imaging. These all influence doctors, patients and the practice of medicine.

Considering all these factors in an emerging field, one cannot simply concentrate on the fetus, but must also consider maternal health and, in particular, preconceptual and antenatal health. Furthermore, because of these concerns, options and needs, one must be aware of the ethical, legal and practical issues which are part of daily practice.

Some questions can be posed to the reader:

- What are the 'risks' to the fetus or newborn?
- Which risks produce bad outcomes?
- Can such risks and outcomes be prevented, corrected or modified?
- When is the optimal time to intervene? What are the alternatives?

- What functions are performed by the placental–fetal–maternal unit which can be discovered and used in management?
- Will this 'risk or bad outcome' happen again to this family?

Some of the answers will be found in this book.

Both a mother and conceptus need care. When a bad pregnancy outcome occurs the parents will need support, counsel and after-care. This is true for any family whether the outcome was a pregnancy loss, neonatal death or termination of a pregnancy for teratogenic reasons.

The laboratorian or pathologist fits into this schema by being an important and effective regulator or facilitator. Such a physician can become involved in all stages of the antenatal and neonatal laboratory investigations and can help in management in a variety of ways:

- preconceptual, prenatal screening, diagnosis;
- indirect or invasive methods (maternal markers);
- fetal blood, amniotic fluid or chorionic villus samples;
- infections, teratogens and environmental hazards;
- reproductive and embryopathology, teratology;
- obstetrical and placental pathology;
- fetal pathology, dysmorphology;
- neonatal pathology, hematology, oncology and immunology;
- medical genetics, counselling and after-care;
- molecular, biochemical, cytogenetic and developmental genetics;
- diseases of immaturity and sequelae;
- results of medical, surgical or genetic therapy (*in utero* or *ex utero*), iatrogenic and forensic issues;
- ultrasonography and other imaging techniques, and correlating these observations with anatomical lesions or other data.

Traditional (general) anatomical pathology (morbid anatomy or histopathology) has advanced in many ways; one is by subspecialization and another is by using special techniques or scientific approaches. However, since the 1970s such advances have obscured the need and importance of the practice of antenatal and neonatal pathology in general or tertiary medical centers. In addition few training programs or mentors exist to provide for these ongoing needs. Some alternatives are suggested herein. In an ideal world one would expect well-trained physicians to handle all reproductive, developmental, fetal and neonatology pathology. Sadly such an ideal situation does not very often exist in many centers. The new genetics, obstetrics and neonatology may not be accompanied by many contemporary antenatal pathologists. Such a team approach would be a desirable option for physicians interested in pathology.

Although the multidisciplinary theme may seem a cliché, we hope this book will disprove that notion. This textbook should be useful for a new generation of physicians.

George Reed
Monterey,
July 1994

PREFACE TO THE FIRST EDITION

Our understanding of the pathogenesis of diseases and disorders in the fetus and newborn infant has undergone considerable change during the past decade. Hitherto, most textbooks were concerned with the description of structural changes due to disease processes or developmental abnormalities occurring *in utero*.

In the present volume we attempt to expand our understanding and concepts beyond pure morphology by incorporating studies utilizing new diagnostic and screening techniques in examining the pregnant mother, fetus and newborn child. The opening chapters consider some of the more general aspects of disease, malformation and neoplasia.

This first section is followed by an up-to-date consideration of pathological changes in the more important organs and systems. In this portion of the book the authors do not confine their discussions to pure morphology but include some of the newer types of investigation, including immunology, enzyme histochemistry and molecular biology. The latter has recently made fundamental advances in our knowledge of the haemoglobin molecular defects in sickle cell disease and in thalassaemias.

It is important to remember that a number of abnormalities which are present at birth may not manifest themselves clinically until later infancy or childhood.

The third section is mainly concerned with prenatal screening and diagnostic investigations of the fetus and newborn using a variety of new techniques such as imaging: ultrasonography, MRI and nuclear medicine.

In the final section on medical genetics, the impact of molecular biology and recombinant DNA are emphasized as also are cytogenetics, oncogenes, biochemical genetics and maternal blood markers. The interventional methods of chorionic villous sampling, amniocentesis and fetal tissue sampling are reviewed by experts in their fields.

Some suggestions are given by the authors as to the relative value, usefulness or accuracy of each diagnostic technique. The necessity of correlating findings and of communicating them between the team of experts is stressed.

Several themes recur throughout the book and will become evident to the reader. One is the assumption that biomedical and technical advances have revolutionized obstetrics and medical genetics, and the benefits of these advances enhance the likelihood of improved medical care. Another theme is the basic interdependence of many disciplines, such as enzymology, cytogenetics, ultrasonography, and *in utero* interventional methods and the proper use of pre and postnatal genetic counselling. Finally there is the common thread that ties the DNA molecule in the genome, which may untie or break during gametogenesis. This in turn may lead to such seemingly disparate disorders such as retinoblastoma, Down's syndrome or Huntington's chorea. Therefore despite the genome and its importance we lack information about its relationship to development, maldevelopment or its reaction to the environment. Pathologists can play a pivotal role in such studies and improve the understanding of the pathogenesis of many diseases that remain unsolved. As Douglas Bain wrote:

'. . . Even in those disorders where the metabolic defect is not expressed in the cultured cells, advances in molecular biology . . . [such as fetal DNA] suggest that prenatal diagnosis and carrier detection may prove feasible. These powerful techniques hold great hope for the future but the development of their potential will depend on a supply of appropriate samples.'*

More recently in the Farber lecture† Opitz has drawn attention to the importance of chromosomal abnormalities in total mortality and stresses the need for diagnostic and genetic counselling, appropriate monitoring of the next pregnancy and the possibility of monitoring teratogenic activity or increases in mutation rates.

In a book of this nature, some overlap is inevitable. We have tried to keep this to a minimum and have cross-referenced information where it seemed appropriate.

We hope this book appeals to a wider audience than the pathologist or laboratory scientist. The care of the fetus and future well being of the infant and child can

---

* Editorial (1984) Perinatal pathology. *Lancet*, i, 431–2.
† Opitz, J. (1987) Prenatal and perinatal death. *Pediatr. Pathol.*, 7, 363–74.

only be safeguarded by the concerted effort of a multidisciplinary team, including obstetricians, paediatricians, histopathologists and scientists devoted to that objective.

Increased knowledge increases responsibility. Some of the new techniques may reveal abnormalities in the fetus in early pregnancy. In some instances these abnormalities may be of such a nature that a termination of pregnancy is the only reasonable course to follow. In others the defect may be amenable to treatment either before or after delivery and termina-

tion of pregnancy is not the correct approach. The vigilance by a team of experts devoted to the study of all aspects of each individual case will ensure that in future correct decisions are made.

We would like to thank Mr G.W. Anderson, Mrs S. Chibett and Miss J. Barber and all the staff of the Department of Histopathology, Hospital for Sick Children, Great Ormond Street, London and the Department of Pathology, Royal Hospital for Sick Children, Edinburgh, in particular Sheila Bartholomew, Guy Besley and Patricia Ellis.

ACKNOWLEDGEMENTS

We would like to thank Chapman & Hall for all their efforts in bringing this second edition to publication, especially Dr Peter Altman, Helen Heyes, Sharon Donaghy, Rosaline Crum, Helen MacDonald, Jolyon Philips, Jan Hicks, Jane Sugarman, Alison Jesnick and Hilary Flenley.

A number of people, worldwide, have helped and deserve thanks. These include Janice Klaurens, Dorothy Johnson, Julie Richardson and Allan Baldridge (Monterey); Clare Kellar (Salinas), Mary Clausen (Palo Alto), Nancy Zinn (San Francisco), Caryl Lecznar (Cleveland) and Donna Spitz (Philadelphia). And 'over the water' Fiona Fleming (London) and Sheila Bartholomew (Edinburgh).

In addition, Doctors Vinod Bhutani (Philadelphia), Milan Blaskovics (Los Angeles), Harvey Levy (Boston), and Charles Rodeck and Gillian Gau (London) gave us advice, as did John E. Fleming (Glasgow) and Seamus Cahalane (Dublin). It was a pleasure to deal with Doctors David Hardwick (Vancouver, BC), Kurt Benirschke (San Diego) and the other members of the Editorial Board. Finally, the late John Blair, John Esterley and Douglas Bain continue to be remembered and missed.

INTRODUCTION – *AQUAE VITAE*

'Over the Waters'

This book began 'over the waters', and emerged from various Anglo-American professional associations such as the recent one between the late James B. Arey of Philadelphia and Archibald Douglas Bain of Edinburgh. The earliest contacts began in the colonial period when Benjamin West, Benjamin Rush, John Morgan, William Shippen and others studied in Europe, and since then when many American students attended medical schools and clinics in Leyden, London, Dublin, Edinburgh, Paris or Vienna. Such affiliations have been continuous between 'our' and 'your side of the Water'.

The Fothergill collection of anatomical casts and illustrations at the Pennsylvania Hospital in Philadelphia was an early example of this exchange. Jan Van Rymsdyk was the illustrator of the collection. He prepared drawings or illustrations for a number of prominent physicians or male-midwives. The Rymsdyk 'crayons' produced for Charles Jenty were those purchased by Dr John Fothergill of London. He sent them to Dr Shippen to be used for teaching at the Pennsylvania Hospital.

J. Van Rymsdyk (?1720–?1788) was born in the Netherlands and moved to England, Bristol and to London, where he worked for Wm Smellie on drawings for the *Sett of Anatomical Tables* (1754); for Wm Hunter for drawings in the *Gravid Uterus* (1774); for John Hunter for drawings in the *Natural History of Human Teeth* (1771); for C. Jenty for illustrations in the *Demonstration of the Human Structure* (1757); and for Thomas Denman for illustrations in the *Collection of Engravings* (1787). He and his son, Andrew, wrote, illustrated and published the first 'guide' to the British Museum, *Museum Britanicum* (1778) [1,2] (Figure 1).

The Fothergill collection of anatomical paintings, or 'Van Rymsdyk crayons', was presented to the Pennsylvania Hospital by Dr John Fothergill, a Quaker physician, philanthropist, friend of Benjamin Franklin, a founder of the Hospital and of America in general [2] (Figure 2). Fothergill wrote to the Pennsylvania Hospital board (1762):

'For the want of real Subjects these will have their Use & I have recommended it to Dr. Shippen to give a Course of Anatomical Lectures to such as may attend, he is very well qualified for the Subject & will soon be followed by an able assistant Dr. Morgan both of whom I apprehend will not only be useful to the Province in their Employments but if Suitably countenanced by the Legislature will be able to erect a School for Physic amongst you that may draw many Students from various parts of America & the West Indies & at least furnish them with a better Idea of the Rudiments of their Profession than they have at present the means of acquiring on your side of the Water.'

In the 1750s in London two acquaintances of John Fothergill were the brothers William and John Hunter who established the Anatomical Theatre and Academy on Great Windmill St. The works and students created and trained by the Hunter brothers set English surgery and obstetrics on a scientific path for the next century. William Hunter became famous, rich and philanthropic. He was also jealous, sensitive and unflaggingly industrious. He rediscovered at Windsor Castle (in George the III's collection) Leonardo Da Vinci's anatomical drawings and, in 1774, published his own masterpiece, *The Human Gravid Uterus* [3,4]. John Baskerville, the printer, was introduced to William Hunter by Ben Franklin, also a printer [5].

Not all was sweetness or light in the eighteenth or nineteenth centuries. The harsh realities were depicted by Wm Hogarth and Vincent van Gogh. Jan Van Rymsdyk alluded in his guide to the British Museum to Dr Ibis, who many consider a satirical portrait of William Hunter. Hunter's teacher, William Smellie, was labelled by a midwife competitor, Mrs Nihell of Haymarket, as '. . . a great horse godmother of a he mid-wife' [6].

'Bag of Waters'

'*Amnos*' or '*amnion*' is derived from the Greek 'bowl', 'smooth' or 'lamb'. Empedocles in 500 BC described the membranes around newborn sheep (yean, caul), and J. Pollux in AD 200 used amnion as an anatomical term. However, it was not until the seventeenth century that the amniotic discharge (thought to be a mixture of maternal blood and milk) was described by Francois Mariceau (1637–1709) as 'amniotic fluid' [6,7].

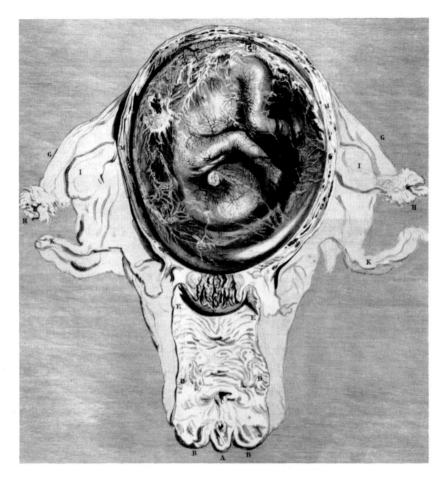

Figure 1 An example of Jan Van Rymsdyk's work: a 5-month-old fetus (Hunter, 1774) [3]. (Reproduced with permission from the Special Collections, University of California at San Francisco, Medical School Library.)

One of the early European 'male-midwives' was Jean Louis Baudelocque who coined the term, 'bag of waters' in 1789. Greenhill and Friedman discussed 'forewaters', and said Baudelocque '. . . defined the bag of waters as that portion of the membranes which pouched into the cervix during uterine contractions. Others apply this term to the portion which is uncovered by the dilating os, while still others call the whole amniotic sac the bag of waters' [8]. The current *William's Obstetrics* gives a description of the amniotic fluid sac as being composed of two compartments: (1) the lower forebag and (2) the upper compartment which is the dome of the sac over the fetus [9].

'Into the Waters'

One of the developers of medical sonography, Ian Donald, who was born in 1910 in Scotland, moved as a child with his family to South Africa. He returned to Fettes School in Edinburgh. After graduation he went on to St Thomas' Hospital Medical School in London, before graduating from the University of London. He worked at the Royal Postgraduate Medical School in Hammersmith and was on the staff at St Thomas' before being appointed Regius Professor of Obstetrics and Gynaecology at the University of Glasgow. His interests outside medicine were music (which he had considered as a career), sailing and biophysical engineering. After service in the British Royal Airforce he became interested in the sonaral applications to medicine, particularly obstetrics. Sonar (*So*und, *Na*vigation, *R*anging) was used in naval encounters during World War I and Radar (*ra*dio *d*etection *a*nd *r*anging) was introduced just before World War II. Donald's first ultrasound paper, entitled 'The investigation of abdominal masses by pulsed ultrasound' appeared in *The Lancet* (**i**, pp. 188–95, 1958). The dream of safe, non-invasive visualization of the embryo and fetus *in utero* became a reality – dreams that J.W. Ballantyne had in 1902, 1904 and 1923 [10]. Ann Oakley wrote that Donald envisioned sonar as seeing 'the fetus as a submarine or seeing with sound' [11] (Chapter 47).

These three Scots permanently changed midwifery, obstetrics and antenatal care. Observations could not be made *in vivo* or *in utero* prior to ultrasound except by X-radiation.

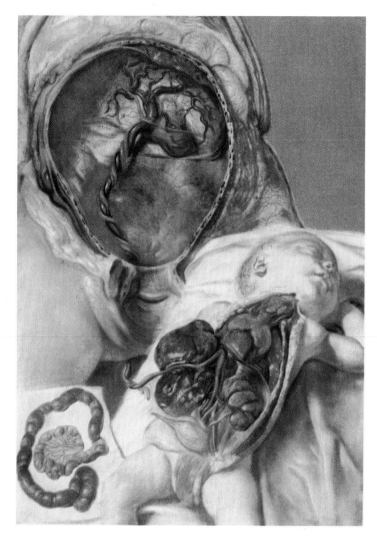

Figure 2 An illustration from the Fothergill Collection: the fetal circulation (1757) [2]. (Reproduced with permission of Pennsylvania Hospital, Philadelphia.)

Each of these medical pioneers, William Hunter, John Ballantyne and Ian Donald, was a tireless, persevering physician, endowed with a measure of genius, gall and luck. They surmounted frustration, prevailing ignorance and attitude and helped prepare the way for what have become everyday matters [12] (Chapter 110).

References

1. Thornton, J.L. (1982) *Jan Van Rymsdyk, Medical Artist of the Eighteenth Century*, Oleander Press, Cambridge, UK.
2. Griem, F. (1952) Anatomical illustrations from the Fothergill Collection of the Pennsylvania Hospital, reprint from 'What's New', April 1952, Abbott Laboratories, N. Chicago, IL.
3. Brock, C. (1990) Dr William Hunter's papers and drawings in the Hunterian Collection, Wellcome Unit for the History of Medicine, Cambridge U. Print-Service, Cambridge, UK.
4. Hunter, William (1718–1783). See Garrison, F. (1966 reprint) *History of Medicine*, W.B. Saunders, Philadelphia, PA.
5. Roberts, K. and Tomlinson, J. (1992) *The Fabric of the Body, European Traditions of Anatomical Illustrations*, Oxford University Press, Oxford, p. 464.
6. Garrison, F. (reprint 1966, 1929) *History of Medicine*, W.B. Saunders, Philadelphia, PA, pp. 338, 350, 399.
7. Wain, H. (1958) *Story Behind the Word*, C. Thomas, Springfield, IL.
8. Greenhill, J. and Friedman, E. (1974) *Obstetrics*, W.B. Saunders, Philadelphia, pp. 190–97.
9. Cunningham, F., Macdonald, P., Gant, N. *et al.* (1993) *William's Obstetrics*, 19th edn, Appleton and Lange, Norwalk, CT, pp. 331–35.
10. Ballantyne, J.W. (1902) *The Manual of Antenatal Pathology and Hygiene*, 2 vols: *The Foetus, The Embryo*, Wm. Green, Edinburgh (*The Embryo* reprint 1991) Stevenson, R. (ed.), Greenwood Genetic Ctr. Jacobs Press, Clinton, SC.
11. Oakley, A. (1986) *The Captured Womb*, Basil Blackwell, Oxford.
12. Dunn, P. (1993) Dr. John Ballantyne (1861–1923). *Arch. Dis. Child*, 68, 66–67.

Further reading

Boyd, J. and Hamilton, W. (1970) *The Human Placenta*, Heffer, Cambridge, pp. 6–14.

Dobson, J. (1969) *John Hunter*, E. Livingstone, Edinburgh, pp. 28, 110, 185, 193–219, 276.

Duden, B. (1993) *Disembodying Women* (translator L. Hoinacki), Harvard University Press, Cambridge, MA, pp. 34–49.

PART FOUR

IMAGING OF THE EMBRYO, FETUS AND NEWBORN

Edited by Sarah E. Chambers

47 MEDICAL ULTRASOUND FROM A-SCAN TO REAL-TIME

J.E.E. Fleming

In 1995 it is impossible to imagine medicine, particularly obstetric and neonatal practice, without ultrasound, yet in 1953 it was barely a dream. A few experimenters were convinced, as inventors and pioneers are, that ultrasound could be useful; how they did not know; with what effort, against what opposition and scepticism they did not know. Ultrasound is now accepted as a basic tool, one which is fundamental to fetal medicine; far beyond any dreams.

When seen as such an important technique it is difficult to realize that there is a history. Indeed all remnants of the past can be quickly overlooked or consigned to the rubbish tip. If this happens a subject loses a sense of perspective and that loss is more than merely sentimental: ideas and understanding disappear and may take a long time to reappear. Fortunately in the last few years there has been a realization that we should record and preserve the history of medical ultrasound. In the UK the British Medical Ultrasound Society has formed an Historical Collection which will soon be taken into the curatorship of Glasgow University's Hunterian Museum. In the USA the American Institute for Ultrasound in Medicine and the National Musuem of Medicine are working together under the guidance of Professor Barry Goldberg. In October 1988 Professor Goldberg organized a Symposium on the History of Medical Ultrasound. This unique and memorable event was attended by 67 pioneers from fifteen countries and acknowledged the work and lives of another 50. This may give the impression that ultrasound only depended on a hundred or so people working in the 1950s, 1960s and 1970s. While these people were responsible for bringing ultrasound into medicine, others had earlier laid the foundations. Well known are the Curies and Paul Langevain. Then there are all those involved in the development of echo sounding and submarine location in the 1910s and 1920s; these are so numerous that acknowledgement is best left to the excellent history of naval sonar by Hackman [1]. If we look deeper we find that advances

in one specialized area like ultrasound rely on a range of discoveries and inventions in other fields and it soon becomes clear that any historical review has to be limited; it is impossible to tell the whole story in one chapter. I will therefore represent the early years by concentrating on the work of Donald, MacVicar and Brown; this will rely heavily on publications by Ian Donald [2] and personal communications from Tom Brown in 1988. This Glasgow group played a significant role and as Donald and MacVicar were obstetricians their work is particularly relevant to this book. Then I will outline the development of real-time imaging which took over as Donald and his contemporaries had reached the point where ultrasound was no longer regarded as an 'eccentricity'.

While the properties of sound have intrigued since the time of Aristotle it was only in the early years of this century that efforts were made to use it for measurement and imaging. The loss of the *Titanic* in 1912 and the threat, and reality, of submarine warfare in two world wars stimulated research on underwater acoustics [1]. Another vital element was the enormous advance in electronics which itself was dependent on development in materials and physics and the stimulus of World War II. By the late 1940s ultrasonic methods, then called supersonics, were being applied to the detection of flaws in metal components and welds. This was happening in the USA where Firestone [3], working in the Sperry Corporation and Michigan University, had patented his Reflectoscope; in Japan Uchida had, in 1949, developed an A-scan instrument and in the UK Sproule at Kelvin and Hughes Ltd had also built A-scan instruments [4]. By 1948 Howry at least had recognized that ultrasound had a potential value in medicine; the seeds were sown and waiting to be nurtured by people like Ian Donald.

Ian Donald was born in 1910, a time of great advance in engineering and technology; the Wright brothers were at the height of their powers, Bleriot had recently flown the English Channel and asdic, or sonar

Diseases of the Fetus and Newborn, 2nd edn, Edited by G.B. Reed, A.E. Claireaux and F. Cockburn. Published in 1995 by Chapman & Hall, London. ISBN 0 412 39160 0

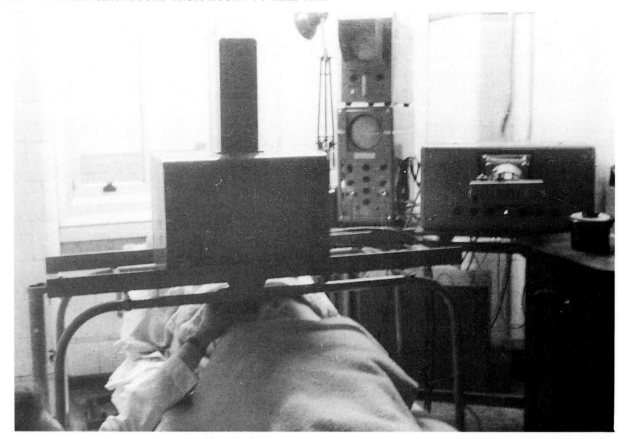

Figure 47.1   The first contact scanner in the Western Infirmary, Glasgow, from 1955 to 1959. Designed by Tom Brown, used by Ian Donald and John MacVicar. From left to right: scanning mechanism mounted on a hospital bed-table over patient, Kelvin & Hughes Mk IV flaw detector, with additional display monitor above, section-scan display unit with 35 mm camera, film developing tank.

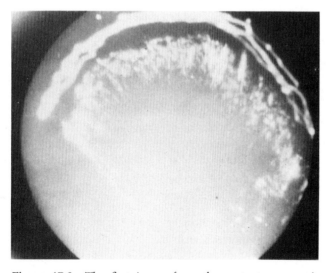

Figure 47.2   The first image from the contact scanner in Figure 47.1. Described by Tom Brown: 'It is a rather unimpressive picture by any standards made by sweeping the transducer three times across the abdomen below the umbilicus without any compounding.'

as it became known, was developing. Later as a young man and a member of the medical branch of the Royal Air Force he was very conscious of the development of radar. Then as Reader in obstetrics at the Hammersmith Hospital, London, he became aware of the medical possibilities of ultrasound from a lecture by J.J. Wild from Minneapolis who had been working in ultrasound from before 1950 [5].

On arriving in Glasgow in 1954 to take up the Regius Chair of Midwifery Donald had, in his own words, 'a rudimentary knowledge of radar and a continuing childish interest in machines, electronic and otherwise – or what my wife would refer to as my "toys"'. In his clinical practice he was commonly faced with the grossly distended female abdomen and the problem of making a differential diagnosis. By chance one of his patients was the wife of a director of Babcock & Wilcox, still a major firm in Glasgow's heavy engineering industry. This contact led to a visit to their works on 21 July 1955 with a quantity of cysts and tumours removed during operations that morning. These were 'tested' using the company's ultrasonic flaw detector. As a camera was not available the A-scan traces were sketched by the company artist; Donald

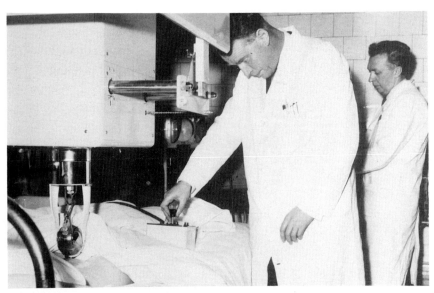

Figure 47.3 The automatic contact scanner in the Western Infirmary, Glasgow, c.1960, being operated by Ian Donald (left) and John MacVicar, shown performing a longitudinal scan. The same electronics were used as in Figure 47.1; A-scan unit just visible by I.D.'s right arm. The British Medical Ultrasound Society's Historical Collection contains a film [9] showing Ian Donald operating this machine and he concludes by saying: 'This apparatus is a prototype but with further refinement it is hoped that sonar will provide an additional aid to diagnosis.'

said 'these (results) were beyond my wildest dreams and clearly showed the difference between a fibroid and an ovarian cyst'. The Babcock equipment had been manufactured by Kelvin & Hughes, also in Glasgow, and through this connection Ian Donald visited Professor Mayneord at the Royal Marsden Hospital. Mayneord had been using a Kelvin & Hughes designed flaw detector in an attempt to examine the brain through the intact skull, but as is now recognized this presents major difficulties [6], so it is no surprise that Donald formed the view 'that they knew a good deal about the subject, enough in fact to be thoroughly discouraged'. Soon after it was agreed that Mayneord's apparatus could be loaned to Donald.

It then happened that an engineer from Kelvin & Hughes was installing an experimental shadowless lamp in Donald's operating theatre in the Western Infirmary, Glasgow, and later mentioned to his colleague Thomas Graham Brown, a young design engineer, that 'the doctor was using a flaw detector on people'. That evening Tom Brown phoned Ian Donald; he later described this 'as the most fateful telephone call I ever made'. It was the start of a fruitful and exciting period. Brown visited Donald at the Western Infirmary and found that the A-scan instrument from Mayneord had, as was common at that time, been designed for use with a transducer having separate transmit and receive elements. Unfortunately it had been inexpertly modified for use with a single transducer. Consequently the system was 'paralysed' for hundreds of microseconds after the transmit pulse. Donald's solution was to use

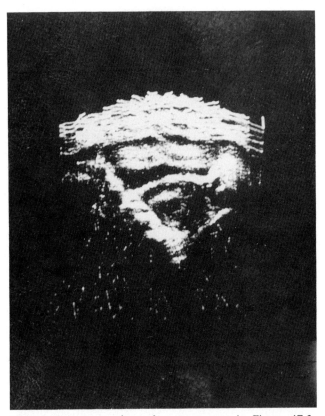

Figure 47.4 Image from the autoscanner in Figure 47.3; note the consistent scanning pattern at the skin surface as the transducer rocked and advanced. Details show: transverse scan, and, in the author's handwriting, 2.5 MHz, transmitter output −5 dB, position 8 cm below umbilicus, 13-week fetus, patient referred from The Queen Mother's Hospital.

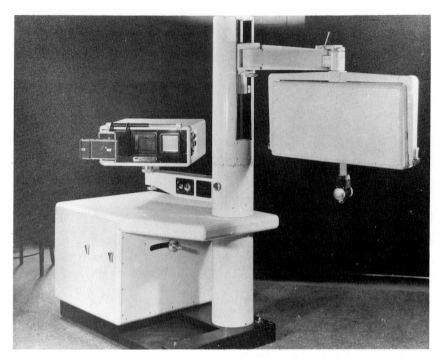

Figure 47.5   The scanner built by Kelvin & Hughes Ltd for Dr Bertil Sunden, Lund, Sweden. Delivered in 1962. A Polaroid camera is used to record the image from short persistence and long persistence cathode ray tubes for viewing during scanning. Industrial design consultant Dugald Cameron was largely responsible for the transformation from experimental systems to this more elegant machine. (Picture by courtesy of Dr B. Sunden.)

clumsy and inconvenient water stand-off devices. Brown however saw past this problem and was struck by the fact that a great deal of echo information was returning from inside the abdomen, it just needed to be interpreted. First something had to be done about the pathetic instrument that Donald was struggling with. Brown unofficially arranged for a brand new Mk IV flaw detector to arrive in Donald's department, and shortly afterwards added a suitable 35 mm camera. The echo patterns from cysts and solid masses and normal bowel could be distinguished but Tom Brown (personal communication, 1988) realized that the A-scope was limited: 'we needed some sort of automatic plotting device' but 'I found it difficult to fire Ian Donald or John MacVicar (Donald's Senior Lecturer) with my "dream"; or even make them understand it.' Then just at this juncture it was suggested to Donald by the physicians at the Western Infirmary that he try his apparatus on a lady 'supposedly dying with massive ascites due to portal obstruction from a radiologically demonstrated carcinoma of the stomach'. The A-scan showed well-separated echoes and MacVicar, who came looking for Donald, said, somewhat embarrassingly, 'Seems like a large cyst'. It turned out that the physicians were uncertain of their diagnosis; after transfer to Donald's care, the lady was operated on and made a rapid recovery. Jokingly Donald [2] said 'For

years afterwards I suffered from this grateful patient's granddaughter who repeatedly subjected me to her experiments in cooking. Mercifully the family finally emigrated to New Zealand'. More seriously this was just what was needed to secure financial support. Initially a sum of £500 was conjured up by Kelvin & Hughes deputy chairman, Bill Slater; it was described later by Tom Brown as 'a rather elastic sum' and allowed him to build his 'dream' – the first contact scanner (Figure 47.1). The transducer could be moved freely in one plane while being kept in contact with the patient thus avoiding the use of a water bath, as thought necessary by all the other experimenters of the time. To explain this departure I quote from Tom Brown: 'I was unaware at the time of Howry's beautiful neck pictures using a water bath, I was aware from my industrial experience, of the reverberation problems. But the most compelling reason was quite unrelated to technical considerations. The patients I was seeing in Donald's gynaecology wards were often elderly, and generally quite unwell, I could not see any technique being well received which involved disturbing these old ladies any more than necessary' (T.G. Brown, personal communication, 1988). I now understand his oft expressed scepticism of 'studying the literature' when seeking a solution to a problem.

The first recorded image from this scanner (Figure

47.2) is of a massive ovarian cystic carcinoma. At the 1988 Symposium Tom Brown said 'I remember it being made and being rather disappointed by it'. Later images from this machine were described in *The Lancet* [7]; the publication was always thought of by Ian Donald as his most important. Brown however could see that the prototype was difficult to use and probably the pictures were influenced by the way in which the operator handled the probe. Howry [8] had similar reservations; he realized that there was a risk of the operator using the controls to produce a picture to meet a preconceived idea. However it was difficult in the still Victorian atmosphere of the 1950s for Tom Brown, an engineer without medical qualification, to take direct control of the scanning. He therefore did so indirectly by designing and building an automatic scanner. This monster of a machine (Figure 47.3) produced thousands of images which are clearly recognizable in publications from Glasgow by the consistent scanning pattern (Figure 47.4). This sort of development cost a great deal of money so that the arrival of a Swedish obstetrician wanting to buy an ultrasound machine must have appeared as a godsend. The machine that Bertil Sunden received (Figure 47.5) in 1962 was based on the original manual contact scanner. This was felt to be satisfactory as experience with the autoscanner had shown that the operator did not unduly affect the images. Sunden provided independent confirmation of

Donald's findings in his MD thesis [10] in 1964. The pictures (Figure 47.6) have a characteristically 'spotty' appearance due to the very low pulse repetition rate of 25/s. This was a result of the desire to maintain a low acoustic output and thus minimize exposure of the patient.

Having sold one machine, the company, by then under the name S. Smith & Sons, saw the prospect of a return on its investment and decided to produce scanners commercially. I was employed as a development engineer and we designed and produced the Diasonograph (Figure 47.7), based in turn on the Sunden machine. Twelve of these 1-ton machines were delivered to hospitals in the UK, USA and Iraq. The scanning frame supported in a substantial gantry gave freedom to scan in virtually any plane with a great degree of stability. The electronic system used thermionic valves; transistors were available then but did not seem to offer any advantage, only problems. In spite of this success and the large potential market (perhaps only evident with hindsight) Smiths decided to close the Glasgow factory. Fortunately in 1967 the medical ultrasound interest was purchased by Nuclear Enterprises, Edinburgh, who went on to produce more to the Smith design. Then they took the bold step of redesigning the system, improved the gantry and took advantage of the revolution in electronics to replace the large unreliable valves with transistors and integrated circuits. Over 200 machines of the new design were built in various versions (NE4102, NE4200, etc.) until they too ran into financial problems. A series of take-overs followed but eventually the activity ceased in the early 1980s. This was partly due to the new technology; 'real-time' was on the ascendant. Looking back we can see that the large slow static scanners had played their part. This was not so obvious at the time, largely because of the shortcomings of real-time — the limited field of view, poor resolution, poor beam shape and gaps in the image [11] — and there was only a gradual realization that real-time could be of value on many parts of the body, not just the heart. Of course it is now clear that real-time had great advantages:

- The image could be adjusted interactively which made the machines easier to use and scanning quicker to learn.
- Images improved because refreshing at 10–20 times per second allowed short persistence display tubes to be used. These gave good grey scale images without the need for photography or complex storage tubes. Soon electronic memory was able to give 'frame freeze' and later scan conversion; this allowed the high quality monitors and recorders developed for television to be used.

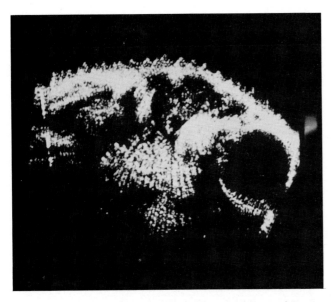

Figure 47.6 Image from Sunden's scanner showing longitudinal section of a fetus taken as a test during the author's visit to Lund to upgrade the machine. The picture has a characteristically 'spotty' appearance due to the very low pulse repetition rate of 25/s. This was a result of the desire to maintain a low acoustic output (here set to −8 dB) and thus minimize exposure of the patient.

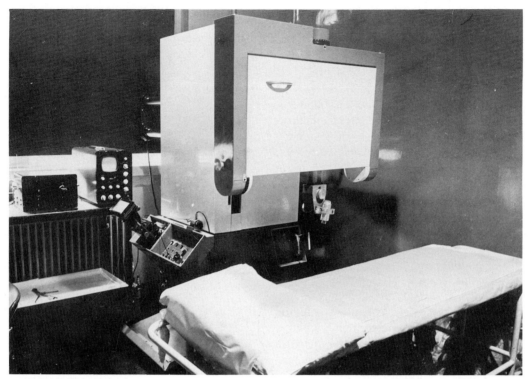

Figure 47.7 The Smith's Diasonograph in The Queen Mother's Hospital, Glasgow. This one small room was the ultrasonic department. Note on the trolley at left an electronic caliper unit and Smith's Mk7 flaw detector (A-scan). This was used by Dr (now Professor) Stuart Campbell in his early work on fetal cephalometry. The switch at bottom of large white panel connected B-scan or A-scan to the transducer.

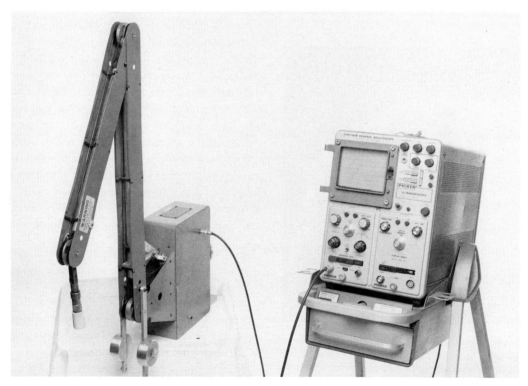

Figure 47.8 The Picker Ultrasonoscope, from the British Medical Ultrasound Society's Historical Collection; the stand to support the scanning mechanism is missing. The electronics unit is basically a Tektronix 564B storage oscilloscope giving bistable images.

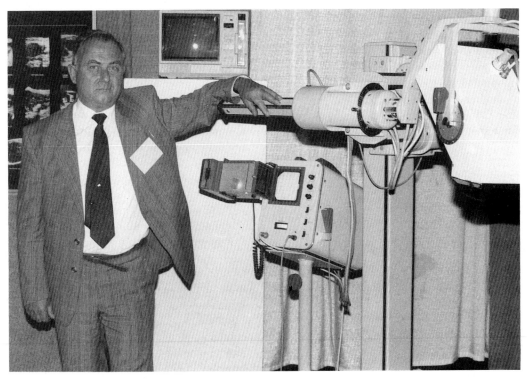

Figure 47.9 The Siemens Vidoson with its designer Richard Soldner at the Symposium on the History of Medical Ultrasound, Washington, DC, 1988.

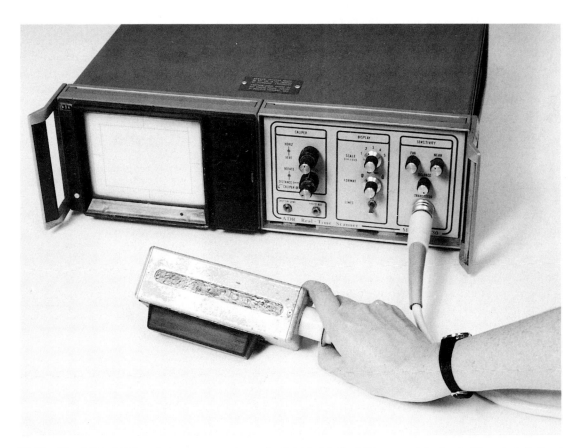

Figure 47.10 The ADR 2130 real-time scanner from the British Medical Ultrasound Society's Historical Collection.

- The massive support used in the Diasonograph or complexity of the articulated arm in the Physionic/Picker scanner (Figure 47.8) was eliminated and replaced by a small hand-held transducer; what had weighed a ton and took a day or more to assemble in a hospital was replaced by a machine which could be moved in by one person. This had a profound commercial advantage as demonstrations were far easier.

These factors made it possible to take advantage of the growing acceptance of ultrasound; the market enlarged, sales increased and the price of machines fell in real terms to about a third between 1976 and 1992 in spite of their greatly increased electronic complexity.

Although real-time appears at first sight to have started in the early 1970s there is evidence of the idea as early as 1950 in the work of Wild [5] and a film exists [12] of the work of Holmes, Howry and Wild showing cross-sections of the neck being scanned with a transducer oscillating at a few sweeps per second as it moves around the patient's neck at the same time. The first array appeared in 1965; this was a ten-element concave array for examining the eye built by Buschmann [13], an East German ophthalmologist, in cooperation with the Kretztechnic company in Austria. It does not seem to have progressed. Then the Siemens Vidoson appeared; this remarkably simple machine (Figure 47.9) was designed by Richard Soldner [14] and had a much greater impact. It used a transducer rotating at the focus of a parabolic mirror in a water-filled enclosure to produce images at 15 frames per second. I first became aware of the Vidoson at an ophthalmic ultrasound conference in Munster during 1966 when Dr Hollander showed a film of obstetric images; I still recall the surprise of seeing movement of a fetus of a few weeks gestation. A large number of Vidosons were sold, particularly in continental Europe. It was somewhat cumbersome and could not be quickly reoriented to locate a particular plane or follow a mobile fetus as can be done with hand-held real-time transducers. This probably accounts for the machine not being seen as a major advance in real-time. However in its own right it was a very important advance and had quite a long life, but it was not developed to any great extent and was overtaken by a return to array transducers.

The return to the array principle arose from an interest in improved cardiac imaging. In 1968 Somer started experimental work on phased arrays, then Bom et al. [15] developed small arrays specifically for cardiac work. The bias mentioned earlier, to use real-time only for the visualization of moving structures, is typified by a paper by King [16] which makes no mention at all of uses other than cardiology. Improvement and progress were fast: by 1974 the Advanced Diagnostic Research Corporation (ADR) put the first commercial linear array scanner on the market. This instrument, the 2130 (Figure 47.10), scanned at 40 frames per second using 64 elements operating in groups of four to give improved resolution. Some idea of the degree of the real-time activity is given in a review by Winsberg [17]. He described 11 forms of real-time transducer 'that have been introduced or are about to be introduced commercially'. Even then, while recognizing the outstanding potential of real-time, he expressed some concern for the loss of the static scanner's large image area – in the Diasonograph approximately 450 × 230 mm. Scans approaching this size are now possible using a curved array but different scanning techniques have provided the answer.

I hope that presenting this limited view of the development of medical ultrasound will give some feel for the early days and some clues to those who wish to look further or in more detail. Similar stories of crude beginnings, fortunate comings together of people and opportunities form the background to Doppler and colour flow imaging. Three-dimensional ultrasound is now advancing rapidly; this too has a long and complex history. I also hope that this chapter will foster sympathy for today's new ideas; they may have a potential just as great as ultrasound had 40 years ago.

One last quotation from Ian Donald [18] who died 19 June 1987: 'In my own old age and looking back over the last thirty years, the innumerable difficulties, set-backs and disappointments have been more than compensated for by those who have turned the subject from a laughable eccentricity (as I have at one time experienced) into a science of increasing exactitude.'

References

1. Hackman, W. (1984) *Seek & Strike – Sonar, Anti-submarine Warfare and the Royal Navy 1914–54*, HMSO, London.
2. Donald, I. (1974) Sonar – the story of an experiment. *Ultrasound Med. Biol.*, 1, 109–117.
3. Firestone, F.A. (1945) The supersonic reflectoscope for interior inspection. *Metal Progress*, 48, 505.
4. Kodak (1988) *Medical Diagnostic Ultrasound: A Retrospective on its 40th Anniversary*, Eastman Kodak, NY.
5. Wild, J.J. (1950) The use of ultrasonic pulses for the measurement of biologic tissues and the detection of tissue density changes. *Surgery*, 27, 183.
6. White, D.N. (1988) Neurosonology pioneers. *Ultrasound Med. Biol.*, 14(7), 541–61.
7. Donald I., MacVicar, J. and Brown, T.G. (1958) Investigation of abdominal masses by pulsed ultrasound. *Lancet*, i, 1188–95.
8. Howry, D.H. (1957) Techniques used in ultrasonic visualisation of soft tissues, in *Ultrasound in Biology and Medicine*, Symposium, June 20–22, 1955, Illinois (ed. E. Kelly). American Institute of Biological Sciences, Washington, pp. 49–65.
9. Donald, I. (1961) *Ultrasonic Echo Sounding*. 16 mm cine film, duration 16 min., University of Glasgow. Copy in British Medical Ultrasound Society Collection, Glasgow.
10. Sunden, B. (1964) On the diagnostic value of ultrasound in obstetrics and gynaecology. *Acta Obstet. Gynecol. Scand.*, 63 (suppl. 6), 1–191.
11. Whittingham, T.A. (1975) A multiple transducer system for heart, abdominal, and obstetric scanning. *Proceedings of the Second European Congress on Ultrasonics in Medicine*, 12–16 May, Munich (eds E. Kazner, M. de Vilieger, H.R. Muller and V.R. McCready). Excerpta Medica, Amsterdam, pp. 59–66.

12. Howry, D.H. and Holmes, J. (1954/5) *A New Diagnostic Tool.* 16 mm cine film, duration 20 min., University of Colorado. Copy in British Medical Ultrasound Society Collection, Glasgow.

13. Buschmann, W. (1964) Ein neues Gerat die Ultraschalldiagnostik. *Proceedings of Symposium Internationale de Diagnostica Ultrasonica in Ophthalmologia,* June 3–5, 1964, Berlin. Augenklinik der Charite, Humboldt-Universitat zu Berlin, pp. 31–35.

14. Krause, W. and Soldner, R. (1967) Ultrasonic imaging technique (B scan) with high image rate for medical diagnosis. *Electromedica* **4**(67), 8–11.

15. Bom, N., Lancee, C.T., Honkoop, J. and Hugenholtz, P.G. (1971) Ultrasonic viewer for cross-sectional analysis of moving cardiac structures. *Biomed. Engineering,* **Nov.,** 500–503.

16. King, D.L. (1973) Real-time cross-sectional ultrasonic imaging of the heart using a linear array multi-element transducer. *JCU,* **1**(3), 196–200.

17. Winsberg F. (1979) Real-time scanners: a review. *Medical Ultrasound,* 3, 99–106.

18. Hansmann, M., Hackeloer, B.J. and Staudach, A. (1986) *Ultrasound Diagnosis in Obstetrics and Gynaecology,* Springer Verlag, Berlin.

48 AN OVERVIEW OF ULTRASOUND IN OBSTETRICS

S.E. Chambers

48.1 Introduction

'The success of obstetric ultrasound, its transformation in 30 years from a rather crazy experimental idea to a routine and welcome part of antenatal care is truly astonishing' [1]. Before the introduction of ultrasound the contents of the pregnant uterus were a virtual mystery until birth. Advances in ultrasound technology have been rapid and now with modern real-time equipment it is possible to visualize and evaluate the fetus in considerable detail and from very early in pregnancy (Chapter 51).

48.2 Roles of ultrasound in obstetric practice

Ultrasound has three major roles in obstetric practice: in the prenatal diagnosis of congenital anomalies; in the identification and assessment of the at-risk fetus; and as an adjunct to routine antenatal care.

48.2.1 PRENATAL DIAGNOSIS

Prenatal diagnosis is one of the most exciting areas of obstetric ultrasound and is covered in Chapters 51–55. Ultrasound is a powerful imaging modality and many structural fetal malformations may be diagnosed. Certain dysmorphic features may point to the presence of a chromosomal defect and prompt fetal sampling (by chorionic villus sampling, amniocentesis or fetal blood sampling) to obtain a karyotype. Direct ultrasound visualization permits accurate needle placement for these techniques and for interventional procedures such as the placement of vesicoamniotic shunts and selective feticide. High resolution transvaginal probes permit diagnosis of some anomalies in the first and early second trimester. Finally, accurate ultrasound dating of pregnancy forms the basis for interpretation of biochemical screening tests, e.g. maternal serum α-fetoprotein screening for neural tube defects and triple biochemical testing for autosomal trisomies (Chapter 62).

48.2.2 IDENTIFICATION AND ASSESSMENT OF THE AT-RISK FETUS

When clinical assessment suggests that a patient is small for dates and intrauterine growth retardation is suspected then fetal size may be estimated by ultrasound measurement of the fetal abdominal circumference, biparietal diameter (BPD) and head circumference. Serial measurements allow assessment of fetal growth. If the clinical suspicion of intrauterine growth retardation is confirmed then the pregnancy may be monitored using the ultrasound based biophysical profiles, which examines fetal breathing movements, gross body movement, fetal tone, fetal heart rate and amniotic fluid volume. These aspects of obstetric ultrasound are covered in Chapter 50. Doppler ultrasound studies of the maternal uteroplacental and fetoplacental circulations and of the fetal cerebral and renal circulations are also of value in high-risk pregnancies as indicators of placental function and the response of the fetus to chronic hypoxaemia. These aspects are covered in Chapters 50 and 54–56. As well as being important in the assessment of the small-for-dates fetus, ultrasound has a role in the assessment of the large-for-dates fetus. Fetal macrosomia is associated with increased perinatal mortality and morbidity and maternal trauma. Antenatal detection of these fetuses is therefore desirable, especially in diabetics, for planning the optimum time and mode of delivery. Measurements which have been used are: individual measurements (usually abdominal circumference), ratios of measurements (head:chest [3], femur length:abdominal circumference [4]) and estimates of fetal weight derived from fetal measurements [5]. Ultrasound detection of the large-for-dates fetus is difficult. The usually acceptable error in ultrasonic fetal weight estimation is 10%, therefore an estimated weight of 4000 g may in

Diseases of the Fetus and Newborn, 2nd edn, Edited by G.B. Reed, A.E. Claireaux and F. Cockburn. Published in 1995 by Chapman & Hall, London. ISBN 0 412 39160 0

reality mean a weight of between 3600 and 4400 g. There is a tendency to underestimate fetal weight with ultrasound. Macrosomic fetuses may show accelerated growth and the rate of growth on serial measurements in the third trimester has been used to identify these fetuses [6]. One of the major complications of macrosomia is shoulder dystocia and computed tomography has been used to measure the distance between the outer margins of the soft tissues overlying each shoulder in the axial plane to try and predict this complication [7].

48.2.3 ULTRASOUND AS AN ADJUNCT TO ROUTINE ANTENATAL CARE

The majority of women will have a normal pregnancy and deliver a normal healthy baby. In ultrasound departments that are not referral centres for high-risk pregnancies or cases with suspected fetal anomaly, examination of normal pregnancies will form the bulk of the workload. Ultrasound is an important adjunct to routine antenatal care and these aspects will be described later in this chapter.

48.3 Components of an obstetric ultrasound examination

In the first trimester the ultrasound examination should confirm viability, identify the number of fetuses, determine gestational age by fetal biometry, assess the fetal form and examine the uterus and adnexae. These are the components of a traditional transabdominal examination. With transvaginal probes high resolution images of the fetus may be obtained (Chapter 51) and it is likely that as the use of these probes becomes more widespread so the first trimester examination will become more detailed. In a normal intrauterine pregnancy using transabdominal ultrasound a gestational sac is visible at 5–6 weeks gestation, and fetal heart activity may be identified at 7 weeks. These structures may be visualized approximately one week earlier with transvaginal ultrasound.

The second and third trimester ultrasound examination should include the following components. The number of fetuses, viability and presentation are determined; the placenta is localized and amniotic fluid volume is assessed; fetal measurements (including BPD, femur length and abdominal circumference) are made to assess gestational age or fetal size and growth. A survey of fetal anatomy is then performed and should include but not necessarily be limited to an assessment of the following: head shape; ventricular size; spine, longitudinal and transverse views; a four-chamber view of the heart; identification of the stomach and cord insertion into the abdominal wall; identification of the

bladder and kidneys. These are the minimum requirements of an ultrasound examination as recommended by various professional bodies [8], the American College of Radiology and the American Institute of Ultrasound in Medicine. Incomplete examinations, that is failure to evaluate fetal anatomy, are considered unacceptable in modern obstetric practice [9]. In cases where the patient is at high risk of fetal anomaly or an initial ultrasound examination has raised the suspicion of a defect then a more detailed examination of fetal anatomy is necessary.

48.4 Organization of obstetric ultrasound services

48.4.1 THE 'TIERED' STRUCTURE OF OBSTETRIC ULTRASOUND

Obstetric ultrasound examinations may be performed in different situations, at different levels of complexity and by operators with differing levels of skill. Although some would wish to eliminate the terms 'level 1', 'level 2' and 'level 3' scanning [10], these terms are nevertheless useful in explaining the tiered structure of obstetric ultrasound services to those not directly involved. A level 1 examination is performed either by non-medical personnel (radiographer, midwife) or a doctor. The basic requirements for this type of examination are given in the previous section. Some doctors will have ultrasound equipment in their surgeries or office for this purpose. A level 2 examination is performed in hospital by a doctor (radiologist or obstetrician); it involves all the components of a level 1 examination together with a detailed survey of fetal anatomy and is performed when there is suspicion or high risk of fetal anomaly. A level 3 examination is performed in a tertiary referral centre; this type of examination is reserved for very high-risk cases and problems which have not been resolved by level 1 or 2 scanning. It includes all the components of level 1 and 2 examinations and in addition the highly experienced medical personnel performing the examination will have special experience in fetal sampling and other diagnostic and therapeutic interventional procedures.

48.4.2 ROUTINE OR SELECTIVE SCANNING?

Ultrasound examinations may be offered to all pregnant women (routine scanning) or may be performed on clinical indication only, a policy of selective scanning. There are several possible advantages of a routine scan [11]. Accurate determination of gestational age permits interpretation of biochemical tests such as maternal serum α-fetoprotein, more reliable diagnosis of intrauterine growth retardation in the third trimester and appropriate interventions for postmaturity. The early diagnosis of multiple pregnancy can be made and some fetal abnormalities may be detected. In addition increased fetal–maternal bonding has been advocated as a benefit of screening. However the cost-effectiveness of routine ultrasound remains to be established. There is debate about the most appropriate timing of routine scans. A scan at the patient's booking visit, which is usually in the first trimester, will confirm viability, establish gestational age and identify multiple pregnancies. If the routine scan is delayed until 18–20 weeks then more information may be obtained; many fetal anomalies may be detected at this gestation and the placenta can be localized, identifying a group at high risk for placenta praevia. Routine examination in the third trimester has the potential benefit of identifying small-for-dates fetuses (Chapter 50).

There is evidence that routine scanning is of benefit in the diagnosis of multiple pregnancies and in the estimation of the expected date of delivery [12–14]. The issues surrounding the use of routine ultrasound at 18–20 weeks for the detection of fetal anomalies are more complex and are discussed in Chapter 52.

There is no consensus view about which is the most appropriate policy, routine or selective scanning, and practices differ. In the UK routine scanning has been advocated by a working party of the Royal College of Obstetricians and Gynaecologists [11] and currently about 70–80% of women will have a routine scan during the course of their pregnancy. In Germany there is legislation which requires mothers to have routine scans. In the USA selective scanning is favoured and the list of indications suggested by the NIH Consensus Panel is widely accepted [15]. It has been suggested that a further indication be added to this list: prenatal informed consent for sonogram [16]. In other words pregnant women should be allowed to decide for themselves whether ultrasonography should be a routine part of their obstetric care. Table 48.1 gives a list of indications for obstetric ultrasound based on these recommendations and those of the Royal College of Obstetricians and Gynaecologists.

48.5 Ultrasound as an adjunct to routine antenatal care

48.5.1 ESTABLISHING THE GESTATIONAL AGE

The gestational age obtained by ultrasound is equivalent to the conceptual age plus 2 weeks, i.e. it is counted from the theoretical first day of the last menstrual period. The weeks are counted as completed weeks, not current weeks. Dating scans should be performed before 20 weeks if possible and ideally not later than 24 weeks. After this gestation biological variability and

Table 48.1 Clinical indications for obstetric ultrasound

- Bleeding or pain in early pregnancy: to exclude ectopic pregnancy and establish viability
- Vomiting in early pregnancy: to diagnose hydatidiform mole and multiple pregnancy
- Patients who have received infertility treatment: to confirm intrauterine pregnancy, viability and number of fetuses
- Estimation of gestational age in patients with unreliable menstrual data, bleeding in early pregnancy or those who have been on the oral contraceptive pill within 2 months of their last menstrual period
- Detailed fetal anatomical examination in patients with a personal or family history of fetal anomaly, raised maternal serum α-fetoprotein, or where there is a condition associated with increased risk of anomaly such as maternal diabetes, twin pregnancies, polyhydramnios or oligohydramnios
- Adjunct to prenatal invasive procedures such as chorionic villus sampling, amniocentesis, fetal blood sampling or prenatal surgical procedures such as placement of vesico-amniotic shunt
- A discrepancy between symphysis–fundal height and gestational age, i.e. small or large for dates
- To monitor fetal growth with serial measurements: when intrauterine growth is suspected; fetal macrosomia is suspected in diabetic pregnancy; in multiple pregnancy
- Antepartum haemorrhage: to diagnose placenta praevia and look for evidence of retroplacental bleeding
- Fetal weight estimation: in circumstances where early delivery is contemplated due to complications such as severe hypertension, intrauterine growth retardation, premature rupture of the membranes
- Determination of fetal presentation when malpresentation is suspected
- Biophysical evaluation for fetal well-being
- Assessment of the cervix in suspected cervical incompetence
- Suspected pelvic mass or uterine abnormality

pathological factors such as intrauterine growth retardation will make dating based on ultrasound measurements inaccurate.

The measurements of choice for the assessment of gestational age are crown–rump length (CRL), BPD and femur length. From the ultrasound measurement gestational age may be predicted using standard curves or tables. Many of these have been produced for each fetal measurement and there may be confusion as to which should be used. The British Medical Ultrasound Society has recently addressed this problem with a report and recommendations on the most appropriate data for ultrasound dating [17]. Even more recently Chitty and Altman have published new charts for fetal measurements [18]. These data merit careful consideration and may become the new standard. Racial or sex differences do not appear to exist for CRL measurements or BPD and femoral length measurements in the first half of pregnancy [19]. Charts are not reproduced here but references are given. Variations in measure-

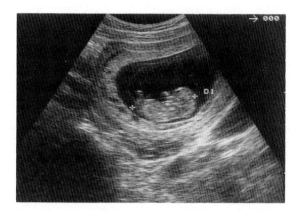

Figure 48.1 CRL measurement in an 11-week fetus.

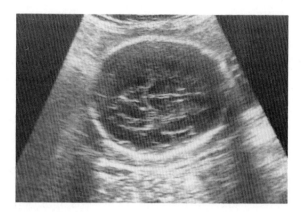

Figure 48.2 Transverse view of the head of a 27-week fetus showing the section for measuring the BPD.

ments due to ultrasound equipment and interobserver and intraobserver variation must be kept to a minimum by regular calibration of ultrasound equipment and meticulous ultrasound technique; the anatomical level at which each measurement should be made is clearly defined. Quality control of measurements should be ongoing in all ultrasound departments.

The CRL (Figure 48.1) is measured from 7 to 14 weeks. Growth at this stage of pregnancy is very rapid, making this an accurate means for estimating gestational age. An image of the longest axis of the fetus is obtained and the measurement is made from the cranial to the caudal end (Figure 48.1). The limbs and yolk sac are not included in the measurement. The traditional charts were produced using static B-scanners [20]; the 95% confidence interval for predicting gestational age between 6 and 14 weeks was found to be ± 5 days. More recently data have been produced using real-time equipment and high resolution transvaginal transducers, and in patients with known dates following *in vitro* fertilization treatment. Although there are some discrepancies these data [21] are remarkably similar to those of Robinson and Fleming [20].

The BPD (Figure 48.2) is appropriate for estimation of gestational age beyond 12 weeks. The measurement is made on a transverse section of the fetal head, at the level of the thalami (Figure 48.2), from the outer edge of the proximal skull vault to the inner margin of the distal vault. Ninety per cent confidence levels in assigning gestational age between 12 and 20 weeks are ± 7 days [18,22,23]. If the head is dolichocephalic in shape the BPD will underestimate gestational age and another parameter should be used.

The femur length is a linear measurement made between the ends of the femoral diaphyses. The femur is identified and the transducer rotated so that the full length of the bone is imaged (Figure 48.3); a foreshortened view will lead to an underestimation of femoral

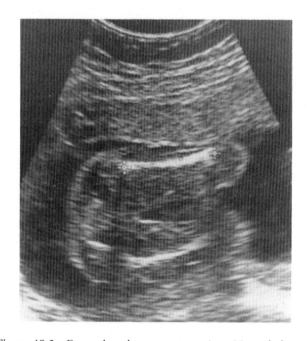

Figure 48.3 Femur length measurement in a 22-week fetus.

length. The femur length is equally as effective as the BPD in the assessment of gestational age and the confidence limits between 12 and 20 weeks are similar [18,24,25].

Gestational age is traditionally calculated from the date of the last menstrual period. If the estimate of gestational age obtained with ultrasound agrees to within 7–14 days of this then it is common practice to accept this as confirmation of the clinical assessment. If the discrepancy between last menstrual period and scanning dates is greater than 14 days then the ultrasound assessment of gestational age is accepted. However menstrual history is unreliable in up to 45%

of women [22]. Even in women who claim to be certain of the date of their last menstrual period, in over half it may be unreliable as a basis for calculating gestation [19]. In addition the timing of ovulation and conception may be inconsistent in relation to the last menstrual period. For these reasons Geirsson argues that the last menstrual period is an insecure basis for estimating gestational age [19]. He advocates the uniform use of mean ultrasound values for estimating gestational age, except in cases where ultrasound before mid-pregnancy is not available.

48.5.2 ASSESSMENT OF AMNIOTIC FLUID VOLUME

Estimation of liquor volume gives an indication of fetal normality since both oligohydramnios and polyhydramnios are associated with fetal anomalies (Chapter 52). In the third trimester it is an indicator for fetal well-being (Chapter 50). There are difficulties in the ultrasound measurement and definition of liquor volumes. Assessment may be subjective, based on the impression of an experienced sonographer, or objective, semiquantitative measurements may be made of pools of liquor. The simplest method is to measure the vertical height of the largest cord and limb-free pool. An alternative method is the four-quadrant technique [26]. The uterine cavity is divided into four quadrants and the vertical height of the largest pool in each quadrant is measured. The sum of these four quadrants is termed the amniotic fluid index. Definitions of oligohydramnios and polyhydramnios are given in Chapters 50 and 52.

48.5.3 PLACENTAL LOCALIZATION

In early pregnancy chorionic villi are present over the entire surface of the gestational sac; at 8 weeks some begin to regress, and by 10–12 weeks a definite placenta may be visualized. Placental localization is important in a number of situations: for procedures such as chorionic villus sampling, amniocentesis and cordocentesis and when antepartum haemorrhage, malpresentation or a high head at term raise the clinical suspicion of placenta praevia. The incidence of placenta praevia at delivery is 0.5%; it is well recognized that ultrasound may overdiagnose this complication in mid-pregnancy [27]. This is due to a number of factors. As pregnancy advances and the lower segment forms then the relationship between the lower placental edge and the internal os will change. A full urinary bladder is necessary for transabdominal examination but an over-full bladder can compress the lower segment and give a false impression of the position of the internal os. In addition focal uterine contractions may mimic placental tissue and lead to the false diagnosis of placenta praevia. Transvaginal ultrasound has a number of advantages over transabdominal examination: a full bladder is not necessary; the transducer is closer to the area of interest and uses a higher frequency, thus images of higher resolution are obtained. With transabdominal examination the acoustic shadowing produced by the fetal head may make it difficult to visualize a posterior placenta; this is not a problem with transvaginal examination. Studies comparing the two methods of examination in clinical practice [28,29] have shown transvaginal examination to be more accurate. In a study of 100 patients with suspected placenta praevia by Leerentveld et al. [29] transvaginal ultrasound resulted in false-positive and false-negative rates of placenta praevia of 1.0% and 2.0%, respectively. This compares with reports on transabdominal examination which gives false-positive and false-negative rates of 7% and 8% respectively. Moreover transvaginal examination has **not** been found to be hazardous in patients with suspected praevia [28,29]; the probe only needs to be inserted a short way into the vagina and does not need to be in contact with the cervix.

48.6 Safety

Careful consideration must be given to the safety of ultrasound as an imaging modality in obstetrics. There is a lack of well-designed, controlled, long-term prospective epidemiological trials and it is therefore necessary to look at the evidence culled from *in vitro* and *in vivo* laboratory studies for possible adverse bioeffects. The following statements are taken from a clinical safety statement by the European Committee for Ultrasound Radiation Safety (European Federation of Societies for Ultrasound in Medicine and Biology) [30].

> Ultrasound imaging for diagnostic purposes in obstetrics has been in extensive clinical use for more than 25 years. Numerous investigations of various degrees of sophistication have been undertaken in an endeavour to detect adverse effects. None of these studies have proved that ultrasound at diagnostic intensities as used today has led to any deleterious effect to the fetus or mother.
>
> Routine clinical scanning of every woman during pregnancy using real-time B mode imaging is not contraindicated by the evidence currently available from biological investigations and its performance should be left to clinical judgement.
>
> However routine examination of every woman during the first trimester of pregnancy using Doppler devices is considered inadvisable at

present. As new instrumentation using higher acoustic outputs and new clinical procedures become widespread, thus giving the potential of higher tissue exposures, it will be necessary to continually re-evaluate the safety of these diagnostic procedures.

There is an increased potential hazard with pulsed Doppler equipment, used for blood flow studies, since the exposure levels with these devices may be considerably higher than those resulting from real-time B-mode equipment. The output parameters with Doppler equipment should therefore be kept to the minimum consistent with good clinical performance. This is the ALARA (as low as reasonably achievable) principle, which is applicable to all ultrasound imaging. In addition every effort should be made to ensure that the time taken for an examination is kept to a minimum.

It has been suggested [31] that the real hazard to patients is not possible adverse bioeffects but the use of ultrasound by poorly trained clinicians with consequent misdiagnoses resulting from improper indications, poor examination technique and errors in interpretation.

References

1. Willox, J. (1993) Ian Donald and the birth of obstetric ultrasound, in *Obstetric Ultrasound*, vol. 1 (eds J.P. Neilson and S.E. Chambers), Oxford University Press, London, pp. 1–18.
2. Tamura, R.K., Sabbagha, R.E., Depp, R. *et al.* (1986) Diabetic macrosomia: accuracy of third trimester ultrasound. *Obstet. Gynecol.*, 67, 828–32.
3. Wladimiroff, J.W., Bloemsma, C.A. and Wallenburg, H.C.S. (1978) Ultrasonic diagnosis of large for dates infant. *Obstet. Gynecol.*, 52, 285–88.
4. Hadlock, F.P., Harrist, R.B., Fearneyhongh, T.C. and Deter, R.L. (1985) Use of femur length/abdominal circumference ratio in detecting the macrosomic fetus. *Radiology*, 154, 503–505.
5. Rosati, P., Exacoustos, C., Cruso, A. and Mancuso, S. (1992) Ultrasound diagnosis of fetal macrosomia. *Ultrasound Obstet. Gynecol.*, 2, 23–29.
6. Landon, M.B., Mintz, M.C. and Gabbe, S.G. (1989) Sonographic evaluation of fetal abdominal growth: predictor of the large-for-gestational age infant in pregnancies complicated by diabetes mellitus. *Am. J. Obstet. Gynecol.*, 160, 115–21.
7. Kitmiller, J., Mall, J.C., Gin, G.D. and Hendriks S.K. (1987) Measurement of fetal shoulder width with computed tomography in diabetic women. *Obstet. Gynecol.*, 70, 941–45.
8. Leopold, G.R. (1986) Antepartum obstetrical ultrasound examination guidelines. *J. Ultrasound Med.*, 5, 241–42.
9. Evans, M.I., Chervenak, F.A. and Eden, R.D. (1991) Report of the Council of Scientific Affairs of the American Medical Association: ultrasound evaluation of the fetus. *Fetal Diagn. Ther.*, 6, 132–47.
10. Platt, L.D. (1991) Leveling out. *Ultrasound Obstet. Gynecol.*, 1, 83–84.
11. Royal College of Obstetricians and Gynaecologists (1984) Report of RCOG Working Party on Routine Ultrasound Examination in Pregnancy. RCOG, London.
12. Grennert, L., Persson, P. and Gennser, G. (1978) Benefits of ultrasound screening of a pregnant population. *Acta Obstet. Gynecol. Scand. Suppl.*, 78, 5–14.
13. Bakketaig, L.S., Eik-Nes, S.H., Jacobsen, G. *et al.* (1984) Randomised controlled trial of ultrasound sonographic screening in pregnancy. *Lancet*, ii, 207–11.
14. Saari-Kemppainen, A., Karjalainen, O., Ylostalo, P. and Heinonen, O.P. (1990) Ultrasound screening and perinatal mortality: controlled trial of systematic one-stage screening in pregnancy. *Lancet*, 336, 387–91.
15. Consensus Conference (1984) The use of diagnostic ultrasound imaging during pregnancy. *JAMA*, 252, 669–72.
16. Chervenak F.A., McCullough, L.B. and Chervenak, J.L. (1989) Prenatal informed consent for sonogram: an indication for obstetric ultrasonography. *Am. J. Obstet. Gynecol.*, 161, 857–60
17. British Medical Ultrasound Society (1990) Fetal Measurements Working Party Report. Clinical Applications of Ultrasonic Fetal Measurements. British Institute of Radiology, London.
18. Chitty, L.S. and Altman, D.G. (1993) Charts of fetal size, in *Ultrasound in Obstetrics and Gynaecology* (eds K. Dewbury, H. Meire and D. Cosgrove), Churchill Livingstone, Edinburgh, pp. 515–95.
19. Geirsson, R.T. (1991) Ultrasound instead of last menstrual period as the basis of gestational age assesment. *Ultrasound Obstet. Gynecol.*, 1, 212–19.
20. Robinson, H.P. and Fleming, J.E.E. (1975) A critical evaluation of sonar 'crown rump length' measurements. *Br. J. Obstet. Gynaecol.*, 82, 702–10.
21. Hadlock, F.P., Shah, Y.P.S., Kanon, D.J. and Lindsey, J.V. (1992) Fetal crown–rump length: reevaluation of relation to menstrual age (5–18 weeks) with high-resolution real-time US. *Radiology*, 182, 501–505.
22. Campbell, S., Warsof, S.L., Little, D. and Cooper, D.J. (1985) Routine ultrasound screening for the prediction of gestational age. *Obstet. Gynecol.*, 65, 613–20.
23. Hadlock, F.P., Deter, R.L., Harrist, R.B. and Park, S.K. (1982) Fetal biparietal diameter: a critical reevaluation of the relationships to menstrual age by means of real time ultrasound. *J. Ultrasound Med.*, 1, 97–104.
24. Hadlock, F.P., Harrist, R.B., Deter, R.L. and Park, S.K. (1982) Fetal femur length as a predictor of menstrual age: sonographically measured. *AJR*, 138, 875–78.
25. Warda, A.H., Deter, R.L. and Rossavik, I.K. (1985) Fetal femur length: a critical reevaluation of the relationship to menstrual age. *Obstet. Gynecol.*, 66, 69–75.
26. Phelan, J.P., Smith, C.V., Broussard, R.N. and Small, M. (1987) Amniotic fluid volume assessment with the four-quadrant technique at 36–42 weeks gestation. *J. Reprod. Med.*, 32, 540–42.
27. Townsend, R.R., Laing, F.C., Nyberg, D.A. and Jeffrey, R.B. (1986) Technical factors responsible for 'placental migration': Sonographic assessment. *Radiology*, 160, 105–108.
28. Farine, D., Fox, H.E., Jakobson, S. and Timor-Tritsh, I.E. (1988) Vaginal ultrasound for diagnosis of placenta previa. *Am. J. Obstet. Gynecol.*, 159, 566–69.
29. Leerentveld, R.A., Gilberts, E.C., Arnold, M.J. and Wladimiroff, J.W. (1990) Accuracy and safety of transvaginal sonographic placental localization. *Obstet. Gynecol.*, 76, 759–62.
30. European Federation of Societies for Ultrasound in Medicine and Biology (1991) Newsletter No. 5.
31. Merritt, C.R.B., Kremau, F.W. and Hobbins, J.C. (1992) Diagnostic ultrasound: bioeffects and safety. *Ultrasound Obstet. Gynecol.*, 2, 366–74.

49 BASIC PHYSICS AND INSTRUMENTATION OF ULTRASONICS

P.R. Hoskins

There are basically two types of information that can be obtained using ultrasound techniques. The first is the depiction of cross-sectional anatomy in real-time and the second is the provision of information related to blood flow. Table 49.1 shows the uses of the different types of ultrasonic device, which are discussed below.

Table 49.1 Clinical uses of different types of ultrasound device

Ultrasonic device	Frequency (MHz)	Use
B-scanner	3.5–5	Routine obstetric examination
	3.5–5	Fetal measurements
	3.5–5	Detailed fetal examination
	3.5–5	Placental examination
	5–7.5	Transvaginal examination
	3.5–5	Biophysical profile
	3.5–5	Fetal echocardiography
M-mode	3.5–5	Fetal echocardiography
Continuous wave Doppler	2–4	Umbilical artery
Duplex/colour Doppler	3–5	Fetal vessels
	3–5	Placental vessels
	3–5	Uterine artery
	3–5	Fetal echocardiography

49.1 Physics of ultrasound

49.1.1 ULTRASOUND

Ultrasound is a term used to describe high-frequency sound waves, and these are usually produced by vibrating crystals within the face of the ultrasound probe. In diagnostic medicine the frequency of ultrasound waves is well above the upper audible limit: typically 2–10 MHz (1 MHz = 1 million vibrations per second). The sound speed of ultrasound in tissue is 1450–1650 m/s. An average value of 1540 m/s is usually taken for ultrasonic scanners. At a frequency of, for example, 3.5 MHz the wavelength is 0.44 mm.

The ultrasonic wave generated by the probe will travel through the tissue. As with any wave there will be reflection, scattering and attenuation (Figure 49.1).

49.1.2 REFLECTION

An important quantity connected with the passage of ultrasound through the tissue is the 'acoustic impedance'. This is the product of the tissue density and the acoustic velocity. The acoustic impedance varies between tissues (Table 49.2) and there are variations within an individual tissue. If adjacent tissues of differing acoustic impedance have dimensions which are large compared with the ultrasonic wavelength then there will be reflections at the boundary between the two tissues. Reflections at boundaries between tissues with differing impedances, such as muscle–bone and artery wall–blood, give rise to the bright lines seen in ultrasonic images. Reflected waves are often of large amplitude, and are highly directional; that is, most of the reflected energy travels in one direction.

If there is an air gap between the transducer and the patient's skin the large difference in acoustic impedance between the transducer material and air prevents the passage of ultrasound into the air. The use of a water-based gel applied between the probe and the patient's skin removes any air gap and enables ultrasound to pass from the transducer to the patient.

49.1.3 SCATTERING

Within an individual tissue there are variations in impedance over distances comparable with or smaller

Diseases of the Fetus and Newborn, 2nd edn, Edited by G.B. Reed, A.E. Claireaux and F. Cockburn. Published in 1995 by Chapman & Hall, London. ISBN 0 412 39160 0

Water   Liver

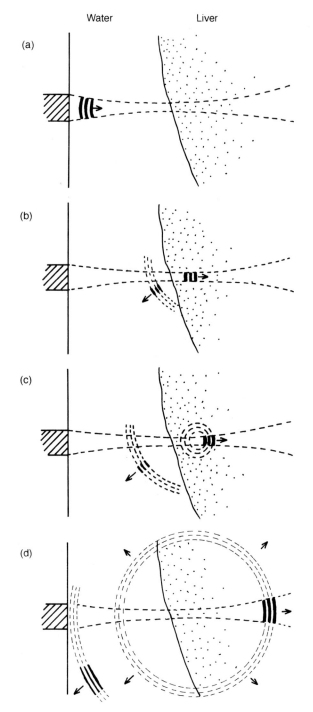

Table 49.2 Acoustic properties of tissue

Tissue	Density (kg/m³)	Sound speed (m/s)	Acoustic impedance (10⁶ kg/m² per s)
Water	1000	1523	1.52
Fat	916	1480	1.36
Muscle	1040	1580	1.64
Liver	1050	1580	1.66
Kidney	1050	1565	1.64
Bone	1900	2000–4000	3.8–7.6

Source: Duck, F.A. (1990) *Physical Properties of Tissue*, Academic Press, London.

than the wavelength of the ultrasound. In this case scattering of ultrasound occurs. The features of this are that the scattering is in all directions, and that the scattered ultrasound is of small amplitude. These scattered waves are seen as the less bright textured pattern within an individual organ or tissue.

49.1.4 ATTENUATION

The amplitude of the ultrasonic wave will decrease as it passes through the tissue. This is due to absorption of the energy of the wave by the tissue, causing heating of the tissue, and also by removal of energy from the wave by scattering and reflection. The ultrasound wave is attenuated on its passage from the transducer, and any reflected or scattered waves which travel back to the transducer are further attenuated. This attenuation means that the amplitude of waves detected by the transducer will be smaller from deeper structures. There comes a depth beyond which the ultrasonic scanner cannot differentiate between the true tissue echoes and noise. The attenuation produced per centimetre of travel is known as the attenuation coefficient (decibels/centimetre). The attenuation coefficient increases linearly with frequency. This means that the depth to which ultrasound can penetrate increases as the frequency decreases. It would seem that the use of a very low frequency would be desirable. Unfortunately the ability of the ultrasonic scanner to distinguish detail decreases as the frequency decreases so that in practice a compromise must be reached between the desired resolution and the desired penetration depth. For the required penetration depth the highest frequency possible is used in order to maximize the resolution for a given study type. Typically studies which require visualization to only a few centimetres, such as transvaginal studies, use relatively high frequencies of 5–7.5 MHz ultrasound, whereas general obstetric scanning, which requires penetration to 20 cm or more, is performed using typically 3.5–5 MHz probes.

Figure 49.1 Propagation of an ultrasonic pulse through a simplified tissue model consisting of water and liver. (a) The pulse of ultrasound travels from the transducer along a well-defined beam. (b) At the boundary between the water and liver there is a strong reflection. If the boundary between the tissues is parallel to the transducer surface the strongest part of the reflected wavefront will travel directly back to the transducer. In the example shown the boundary is not parallel, therefore the strongest part of the wavefront will not strike the transducer. (c) Within the liver there is scattering of ultrasound. Scattering will occur at all points in the liver which are insonated. For the purposes of clarity scattering from only one small region in the liver is shown. (d) The reflected wave is detected by the transducer.

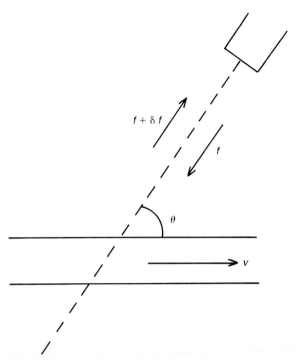

Figure 49.2 Insonation of blood flowing in a vessel. $\delta f =$ Doppler shift; f = transmit frequency; v = velocity of blood; θ = beam–vessel angle.

49.1.5 DOPPLER EFFECT

The change in frequency produced by the scattering of waves by a moving target is a general effect called the Doppler effect. Using ultrasonic equipment the Doppler shift δf is given by the equation (Figure 49.2):

$$\delta f = 2f\,(v/c)\,\cos\,(\theta)$$

where f is the transmit frequency, v is the velocity of blood, c is the speed of sound in tissue and θ is the beam–vessel angle.

Typically the transmitted frequency used in obstetrics is 2–4 MHz. In fetal vessels velocities up to about 1 m/s are common producing Doppler shifts of up to about 5 kHz which is well within the audible range. Doppler ultrasound is used to produce information from moving blood; however any moving object will produce a Doppler shift. High-amplitude low-frequency signals produced by vessel walls during the cardiac cycle are removed using a high-pass filter. For some arteries such as the umbilical artery it is important that the filter level is sufficiently low to enable observation of flow at end-diastole. A filter level of 50–100 Hz is adequate for suppression of vessel wall motion and to enable observation of flow at end-diastole. Occasionally other moving structures such as the fetus itself will produce high amplitude signals which may temporarily obliterate the Doppler signal.

49.2 B-scan devices

49.2.1 B-SCAN INSTRUMENTATION

Virtually all ultrasonic scanning is now performed using real-time devices. A hand-held probe is placed on the skin and pulses of ultrasound are transmitted into the patient along a focused beam. Scattering and reflection of the ultrasound occur in the tissue and a portion of the echo signal is detected by the transducer. The time delay of the received echo is used to derive the depth from which the echo arose, and the amplitude of the echo is used to modulate the brightness of the display. This is called brightness mode or B-mode scanning. The image is built up line by line at a rate sufficient to enable images to be acquired with rapid repositioning of the transducer. This allows large volumes of tissue to be interrogated quickly, and allows visualization of movement such as fetal breathing.

A number of transducer types are used to sweep the beam through the tissue, such as linear or curvilinear arrays, phased arrays and mechanical sector transducers (Figure 49.3). Phased arrays and mechanical sector transducers produce a sector-shaped image. These are most useful in general abdominal scanning and adult cardiac scanning where the small probe size enables images to be obtained through rib spaces and underneath the costal margin. In obstetrics it is desirable to have a wide field of view near to the transducer in order to fully visualize the fetus. Originally linear arrays were used for this purpose. However even with a large linear array the edges of the fetal head are not always visualized. In the last few years the use of curvilinear arrays has enabled visualization of a wide field of view with reduced transducer size.

Improvements in the ultrasonic image quality have occurred over 30 years or more. Many modern scanners have multielement transducers in which the formation and reception of the beam are controlled by computer, giving high resolution images.

49.2.2 B-SCAN MEASUREMENTS

There are two common sets of measurements which are used in routine practice using manually operated cursor facilities on the frozen B-scan image: measurement of linear distances and of circumferences. The calibration of the calliper system can change and it is important to check this regularly using an appropriate test device.

(a) Linear distances

Examples of this include the measurement of biparietal diameter and fetal limb length. Two marker spots are placed manually using joystick or trackerball controls. These are positioned at the edge of the structure of

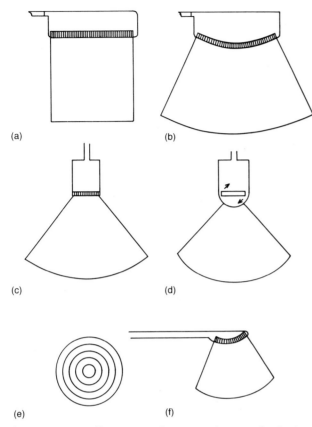

(a)

(b)

(c)

(d)

(e)

(f)

Figure 49.3 Different transducers used in medical ultrasound. The ultrasonic field shape and size is shown directly below the transducer. (a) Linear array. This contains a row of individual elements (typically 128–256). The image is built up line by line by firing groups of elements starting from one side of the array and working to the other side. (b) Curvilinear array. In this transducer the linear array is effectively bent into a curve giving a wide field of view. (c) Phased array. This contains a row of individual elements. In this case all of the elements are fired. Small delays between firing of the elements allows the beam to be fired in a given direction. The beam is swept in this manner from one side of the sector image to the other. (d) Mechanical sector scanner. In this device there is one circular element. Sweeping the beam across the patient is performed by a motor drive. (e) Annular array. This is a mechanical sector probe; however instead of one element there are several elements in the form of rings, perhaps 5–8 rings. Firing of these rings enables superior focusing to be achieved. The illustration shows a typical ring pattern. (f) Transvaginal probe. The most commonly used probe at present is the curvilinear array giving a single scan plane. Transvaginal probes based on a mechanical sector technique have been used, and probes able to provide two scan planes at 90° have also been described.

interest and the distance between the two points is automatically displayed.

(b) Circumference

Examples of this include the circumference of the fetal head and the fetal abdomen. The most common method used is for the operator to manually mark multiple points around the perimeter of the head or abdomen. The machine automatically joins adjacent points with straight lines, and the circumference is calculated from the sum of the individual line lengths. The second method is for the machine to assume that the structure of interest will be an ellipse. One example of the operation of this technique is for two points to be placed opposite each other on the perimeter, usually along the widest diameter. The machine then draws an ellipse through these two points and the minor diameter of the ellipse can be adjusted so that the ellipse coincides closely with the perimeter. The circumference of the ellipse is then calculated and automatically displayed.

Accuracies of a few per cent can be achieved from these measurements. For circumference measurements made using the multiple-point method accuracy improves as the number of points increases.

49.2.3 M-MODE DISPLAY

This display is used to obtain information about moving cardiac structures. A single line of the B-scan image is considered and the change in brightness of the pixels of the line is displayed as a function of time. This mode is used for the study of fetal arrhythmia and for the measurement of cardiac dimensions.

49.3 Doppler ultrasound instrumentation

49.3.1 DISPLAY OF THE DOPPLER SPECTRUM

The most common way of presenting the full Doppler frequency shift information is in the form of a real-time sonogram (Figure 49.4). This is a display of the

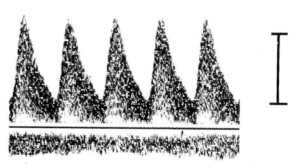

Figure 49.4 Doppler spectrum from the umbilical cord acquired using a 4 MHz continuous wave device. The vertical line at the side of the trace indicates the range for 1 kHz. Blood in the umbilical artery is moving towards the probe and this is displayed as a positive Doppler shift in the upper channel, whereas blood in the umbilical vein is flowing away from the probe and is displayed as a negative Doppler shift in the lower channel.

Doppler frequencies present in the signal against time. The spectrum of Doppler frequency shifts is calculated every 5–10 ms. The intensity at a particular point in the sonogram is related to the amount of blood moving at the corresponding velocity v. Provided that the Doppler beam and the vessel are aligned, and the beam–vessel angle is not near to 90°, it should be possible to acquire Doppler waveforms with a clearly defined outline. If the beam–vessel angle is near 90° or if there is misalignment between beam and vessel then the outline of the waveforms becomes noisy and is difficult to visualize. Waveform indices calculated from inadequate Doppler waveforms acquired under these conditions are likely to be in error.

49.3.2 CONTINUOUS WAVE DOPPLER UNIT

In these devices a simple pencil probe is used. Continuous wave ultrasound is transmitted in a fixed direction by a transmitting element and detected by an adjacent receiving element. Using a stand-alone continuous wave device no information is supplied concerning the depth or location of the vessel. This limits the use of the device to those vessels with well-defined locations or those which show well-defined waveform shapes, such as the umbilical artery.

49.3.3 DUPLEX SYSTEMS

A duplex system is a combination of a B-scan device and a pulsed Doppler device, or occasionally a continuous wave Doppler device. A dotted line on the B-mode image is commonly used to give the direction of the Doppler beam in the field of view. The use of pulsed Doppler enables blood flow information to be acquired from a particular location along the beam, and this location is identified by a cursor which can be moved manually along the line. Visualization of the vessel in relation to the Doppler beam enables the beam–vessel angle to be measured and the sonogram to be calibrated in units of velocity. A number of configurations of duplex system are available commercially. Use of a linear array or phased array allows simultaneous real-time B-scanning and display of Doppler waveforms. Simultaneous display using a mechanical sector scanner is more difficult as the B-scan transducer must move in order to update the B-scan and the vibrations produced are detected by the Doppler device. This usually necessitates switching off the Doppler detector during B-scan update.

49.3.4 COLOUR FLOW SYSTEMS

Using a duplex system blood flow information is obtained from one particular location within the vessel. A colour flow system combines B-scan imaging with a superimposed real-time colour image representing the flow of blood. The basic Doppler information presented at a particular point is the mean Doppler frequency shift. Shades of red and blue are usually used to represent velocities towards and away from the transducer. The Doppler signal processor also produces an index, called variance, related to the variability of the Doppler signal. It is thought that this signal gives an indication of the degree of turbulence present. This index can be displayed separately or combined with the mean velocity information. As with duplex systems there are a number of configurations of colour flow scanner. These all tend to give simultaneous real-time display of the B-scan image and the colour image. For some systems there is also additional simultaneous display of the Doppler spectrum; this is often called triplex scanning. The image quality of colour flow systems has improved greatly since their introduction in 1982. Early colour flow systems were suitable only for high-velocity large amplitude signals which occur in cardiology. The sensitivity and the low-velocity performance have improved to the extent that good colour images can be obtained from fetal vessels.

Colour flow images are used to identify the presence and location of vessels, and are used to guide placement of the sample volume in order to acquire Doppler waveforms.

49.3.5 DOPPLER ULTRASOUND MEASUREMENTS

For a number of vessels such as the umbilical artery and the arcuate/uterine artery, it is the shape of the Doppler waveform which is of interest. The degree of diastolic flow can be quantitated using a number of indices (Figure 49.5). There are often debates about which one of these indices is the 'best' index. In practice these indices describe essentially the same waveform feature, that is the degree of diastolic flow, and as such there is

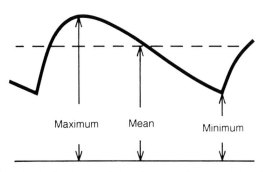

Figure 49.5 Indices used for the quantitation of the degree of diastolic flow of Doppler waveforms: A/B ratio = maximum/minimum; resistance index (RI) = (maximum − minimum)/maximum; pulsatility index (PI) = (maximum − minimum)/mean.

little to choose between them. The only important difference is that for waveforms with absent end-diastolic flow the resistance index (RI) and the A/B ratio reach plateau values of 1.0 and infinity respectively, whereas the pulsatility index (PI) continues to increase as the proportion of the cardiac cycle for which flow is absent increases. It is therefore possible that PI is more useful when monitoring changes over several weeks or months.

Velocity measurements can be made using duplex systems provided that the vessel can be seen sufficiently well to enable the beam–vessel angle to be measured.

Some duplex systems will have the facility to measure volume flow from the cross-sectional area of the vessel and from the mean Doppler frequency shift. Measurement of volume flow in any vessel is fraught with error and it is easy to generate huge errors. This is particularly difficult in very small vessels where the diameter is difficult to assess accurately. Considerable attention to detail must be used if volume flow is to be measured.

Further reading

Introductory texts on the physics and instrumentation of ultrasonics are for example those by Fish (1990) and McDicken (1991). More advanced texts are those by Wells (1977), Hill (1986) and Evans et al. (1989).

Evans, D.H., McDicken, W.N., Skidmore, R. and Woodcock, J.P. (1989) *Doppler Ultrasound*, Wiley, Chichester.

Fish, P.J. (1990) *Physics and Instrumentation of Diagnostic Medical Ultrasound*, Wiley, Chichester.

Hill, C.R. (ed.) (1986) *Physical Principles of Medical Ultrasonics*, Ellis Horwood, Chichester.

McDicken, W.N. (1991) *Diagnostic Ultrasonics*, 3rd edn, Churchill Livingstone, Edinburgh.

Wells, P.N.T. (1977) *Biomedical Ultrasonics*, Academic Press, London.

50 BIOPHYSICAL ASSESSMENT OF THE AT-RISK FETUS

J.P. Neilson and Z. Alfirevic

50.1 Introduction

This short chapter will review the place of commonly used antepartum tests of fetal assessment in a general clinical context. The use of these tests in specific pathological situations may be described in greater detail elsewhere. Biophysical testing has long superseded biochemical assessment and it will, therefore, be highlighted.

Attempts to define the most appropriate use of fetal surveillance tests raise several issues and requirements:

- A focused view of the nature and extent of adverse fetal outcome is important. This is best based on detailed assessment of individual pregnancies, within a defined geographical area, and using forms of classification that give optimal guidance to the clinician. There are various types of adverse outcome that are relevant to tests of fetal well-being. Perinatal death is generally emphasized because of both its importance and also its certainty. Morbidity, while also of obvious relevance (especially if associated with permanent handicap) is more difficult to define precisely. Determination of the causes of perinatal death not only allow appropriate allocation of resources to try to prevent these, but also a realistic view of what is, and what is not achievable using currently available techniques of fetal surveillance.
- Understanding of the technical and pathophysiological bases of fetal assessment tests is required to derive sensible expectations from their performance. Thus, one reason for the disillusionment with biochemical testing, which occurred during the late 1970s and early 1980s, stemmed from its advocacy as a panacea, capable of predicting most complications in most high-risk situations. This view was unrealistic and these tests (notably oestriol and human placental lactogen assays) passed into history.

- Accurate prediction of adverse outcome does not necessarily mean that the outlook for the baby can be improved by any form of intervention – if no effective therapy exists. For example, Figure 50.1 shows a grossly abnormal antepartum cardiotocograph obtained at 32 weeks from a fetus of a woman with pre-eclampsia. The baby was delivered immediately by caesarean section, but was profoundly asphyxiated and died during the first day of life. Similarly, the identification of very early onset intrauterine growth retardation during the second trimester may not allow improved ultimate outcome.
- All tests have the capacity to do harm. The harm may be due to direct trauma by invasive investigations, or exposure of the fetus to toxic agents, or much more commonly because of misleading information produced by the test. Such misinformation could either result in inappropriate intervention, e.g. unnecessary early delivery, or, conversely, dangerous complacency if reassuring results are generated where there is in fact serious fetal compromise.

With the currently low rates of perinatal mortality and morbidity in Western countries it is inconceivable that any future advance in fetal assessment will have such a beneficial impact on outcome that it will need to be rushed into obstetric practice without careful evaluation.

50.1.1 AIMS OF FETAL ASSESSMENT

The aims of fetal assessment are to 'fine tune' antenatal care: to identify the compromised fetus in both high-risk and low-risk pregnancies in sufficient time to permit optimal timing of delivery to maximize the chances of intact survival; to avoid unnecessary intervention in high-risk pregnancies where fetal growth and health are satisfactory; to provide reassurance about

Diseases of the Fetus and Newborn, 2nd edn, Edited by G.B. Reed, A.E. Claireaux and F. Cockburn. Published in 1995 by Chapman & Hall, London. ISBN 0 412 39160 0

fetal health to women who have had an unhappy outcome to previous pregnancies.

50.1.2 RANDOMIZED TRIALS

To demonstrate that a diagnostic test, with apparently useful predictive powers, actually improves outcome and does more good than harm, it is important that the test is evaluated by randomized controlled trial. The use of controls is as vital in clinical trials as it is in any other scientific experiment, and the biases associated with the use of historical or other non-randomized controls should now be well recognized [1]. The process of randomization achieves groups that are matched not only for factors known to influence the outcome of interest, but also for other unknown, but potentially important, variables. In such studies it is important that a clear distinction is made between fetal testing for specific indications in high-risk pregnancies and the use of tests as screening methods for all pregnancies. A technique may be effective in the former situation but not the latter, or vice versa.

There is now an enormous literature on antepartum tests of fetal growth and well-being, and a comprehensive review would not be possible. This chapter will concentrate more on the findings from randomized trials (to assess the effectiveness of testing) than on observational studies (to predict outcome). Systematic reviews of all trials in perinatal medicine are housed in the Oxford Database of Perinatal Trials [2] – now metamorphosed into the Cochrane Collaboration Pregnancy and Childbirth Module; this resource will be cited extensively.

50.2 Ultrasound measurement

Ultrasound is a robust and versatile technique with wide applications during pregnancy. During the first two trimesters of pregnancy ultrasound is mainly used as a screening tool in low-risk women to estimate gestational age and detect fetal anomalies. Later in pregnancy the use of ultrasound is largely restricted to high-risk pregnancies. Serial fetal measurements are performed in order to study intrauterine growth patterns; single measurements may estimate fetal size or weight. Ultrasound can also help in the objective assessment of amniotic fluid volume and placental texture. More recently, its role has expanded to the assessment of fetal behaviour (breathing, tone and movements), investigations of fetomaternal circulation (Doppler) and ultrasonically guided invasive procedures (e.g. umbilical cord blood sampling).

50.2.1 FETAL MEASUREMENT

Nomograms exist for almost all conceivable measurements of the fetus, including head and trunk parameters, abdominal organs, long (and other) bones and even the penis [3]; measurements may be linear, circumferential or of area. The abdominal circumference is the parameter that is most commonly used for the assessment of fetal size in late pregnancy [4]. Repeated measurements of the abdominal circumference (Figure 50.2) are thought to be the most sensitive indicators of both impaired fetal growth because of depleted glycogen deposition in the liver in growth retardation, and of macrosomia, e.g. in diabetic pregnancies. The head:abdominal circumference ratio may be of some value in determining whether the fetus is symmetrically or asymmetrically small, but this is controversial. There are no randomized controlled trials to evaluate the effects of serial fetal measurements on the outcome of pregnancies at high risk of impaired fetal growth. The controlled studies that have been performed have evaluated ultrasound measurements as

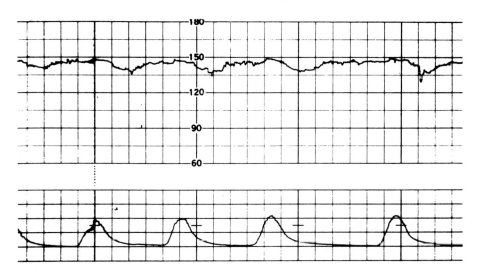

Figure 50.1 Cardiotocograph at 32 weeks. Note the lack of variability of the heart rate and the repetitive late decelerations.

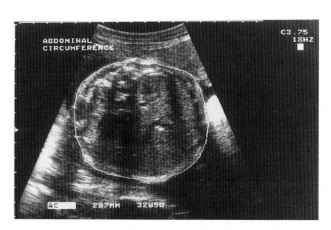

Figure 50.2 Cross-section of the fetal abdomen at the level of the liver. This is a standard plane for the measurement of abdominal circumference.

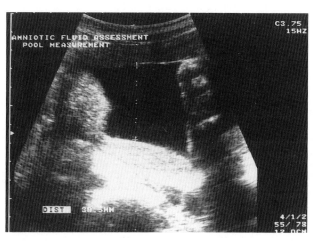

Figure 50.3 Maximum pool depth of amniotic fluid measurement.

a screening technique and provide no evidence to support their routine use during the third trimester in all pregnancies [5].

50.2.2 AMNIOTIC FLUID

Decreased amniotic fluid volume (oligohydramnios) is regarded as a chronic response to hypoxaemic stress. Its use as a marker of chronic fetal compromise has been reinforced by observations of adverse outcome in pregnancies with oligohydramnios [6] and recent Doppler ultrasound studies suggesting decreased fetal renal perfusion in the presence of fetal hypoxaemia [7]. Amniotic fluid volume can be assessed either subjectively or objectively. Objective assessment by ultrasound involves measurement of the maximum depth of the largest pool of amniotic fluid (Figure 50.3); the lower limit of normal is (arbitrarily) 1 or 2 cm [8]. Another technique to assess the volume of amniotic fluid is to measure maximum pool depths in four different uterine quadrants and then add them together to calculate the amniotic fluid index; this has gained popularity since the publication of percentile charts relating the amniotic fluid index to gestational age [9]. However, the actual value of ultrasound assessment of amniotic fluid to guide clinical care remains uncertain because it has not been tested in randomized trials.

50.2.3 PLACENTA

Grannum, Berkowitz and Hobbins [10] classified the characteristic ultrasound patterns which occur in the maturing placenta. This classification, which grades placentas from 0 to 3 according to specific ultrasound findings within the placenta, was initially correlated

with fetal lung maturity. Since then, the classification has been mainly used to identify the 'mature', calcified (grade 3) placenta in which the individual lobules can be seen; this is thought to be associated with complications, especially if found early in the third trimester. One relatively large randomized trial yielded quite strong evidence of improved fetal outcome if clinicians were guided by the ultrasound appearance of the placenta [11]. There were fewer babies with low Apgar score and fewer deaths of normally formed babies during the perinatal period when the ultrasound appearance of the placenta was revealed to clinicians. It would be reassuring if similar findings were to be reported from a different setting so that reliance on the results of a single trial would no longer be necessary. The question of whether routine scanning of all pregnancies during the third trimester for identification of abnormal, early appearances of advanced placental grades is justified needs to be addressed in larger studies.

50.3 Cardiotocography

Cardiotocography is a widely used technique for fetal assessment before, as well as during, labour. The fetal heart rate is recorded simultaneously with contractile activity (if present) of the maternal uterus. Contractions are sometimes deliberately induced to test 'fetal reserve', either by intravenous oxytocin or by tactile stimulation of the mother's nipple. This technique, the 'contraction stress test', has never been popular in some countries, including the UK; its popularity in the USA seems to be decreasing. Cardiotocography in the absence of induced contractions is sometimes called the 'non-stressed test', and the remaining discussion refers exclusively to this.

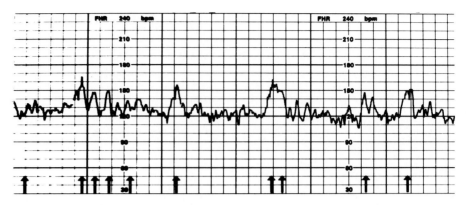

Figure 50.4 Normal cardiotocograph at 42 weeks. Note the accelerations associated with fetal movements (arrows).

The appearances of the cardiotocograph record vary with gestational age and the state of fetal arousal. The normal trace shows a heart rate of between 110 and 150 beats per minute, marked variation in rate/variability, and the occurrence of accelerations of heart rate (Figure 50.4) in association with fetal movement. The heart rate reflects the respective and conflicting influences of the sympathetic and parasympathetic nervous systems in the fetus. The influence of the parasympathetic system becomes stronger as pregnancy advances and the fetal heart rate can, in consequence, be seen to decrease slowly during the third trimester. Heart rate accelerations are also influenced by gestational age and are not seen in some fetuses during the late second trimester. The normal fetus has alternating cycles of 'sleep' and arousal, and these are reflected in the appearances of the cardiotocograph. It is occasionally necessary to wait for 40 minutes or more to see the reactive pattern on the cardiotocograph that is associated with fetal health if the trace has been started during the sleep phase. Fetal vibroacoustic stimulation will decrease the waiting time for the attendants [12].

Despite the widespread use of this technique, the four published randomized controlled trials of antepartum cardiotocography provide no support at all for the use of the technique in high-risk pregnancies; indeed its use appears to be associated with **increased** perinatal mortality [13]. This **might** have resulted from inappropriate inaction because of normal cardiotocography in genuinely compromised pregnancies.

It is interesting to speculate why, in light of these findings, cardiotocography is used so extensively. There was considerable delay in reporting some of the trials, and this may well have diluted their impact. In addition, it can be argued that if antepartum cardiotocography has any validity it is as a method of assessment of immediate fetal health, and not of fetal/placental 'reserve', that provides useful prognostic information. Many of the pregnancies studied in the four trials appeared to have minimal risk features, and it is extremely unlikely that the intermittent performance of cardiotocography, at say weekly intervals, would just happen upon a fetus showing signs of distress. It is likely that more appropriate pregnancies for study would be those in which there is reason to suspect acute fetal hypoxia, e.g. sudden reduction of fetal movements or antepartum haemorrhage.

50.4 Biophysical profile

An alternative method of assessment of fetal well-being is the biophysical profile. The profile includes the assessment of five parameters, and the most commonly used scheme (Table 50.1.) is a (slightly) modified version of the original test [14]. Another, less commonly used, version includes assessment of placental texture by ultrasound examination [15].

There is an association between chronic fetal hypoxaemia and decreased movements (both gross movements and fetal breathing movements). The genuine loss of tone is a late feature and intervention should be effected before this happens. The reduction of amniotic fluid volume is thought to be a consequence of the regional blood flow redistribution associated with fetal hypoxaemia which reduces fetal renal blood flow to produce less urine production and, thus, less amniotic fluid.

Despite the physiological and pathophysiological basis for the biophysical profile, together with the very extensive observational literature that suggests a link between low biophysical scores and poor pregnancy outcome, the available evidence from randomized trials provides no support at all for the use of the biophysical profile as a test of fetal well-being in high-risk pregnancies [16]. We are, therefore, still uncertain about whether the test has any useful role in fetal assessment.

Table 50.1 The biophysical profile [After Ref. 14]

Biophysical variable	Normal (score = 2)	Abnormal (score = 0)
Fetal breathing movements (FBM)	At least one episode of FBM of at least 3 s duration in 30 min observation	Absent FBM or no episode of >30 s in 30 min
Gross body movement	At least three discrete body/limb movements in 30 min (episodes of active continuous movement considered as single movement)	Two or fewer episodes body/limb movements in 30 min
Fetal tone	At least one episode of active extension with return to flexion of fetal limb(s) or trunk. Opening and closing of hand considered normal tone	Either slow extension, with return to partial flexion, or movement of limb in full extension, or total absence of fetal movement
Reactive fetal heart rate (FHR)	At least two episodes of FHR acceleration of > 15 beats/min of at least 15 s duration associated with fetal movement in 20 min	Less than two episodes of acceleration of FHR or acceleration of > 15 beats/min in 20 min
Qualitative amniotic fluid (AF) volume assessment	At least one pocket of AF that measures 2 cm in two vertical axes	Either no AF pocket or largest pocket <2 cm in vertical axis

50.5 Doppler ultrasound

The first Doppler ultrasound studies of the fetoplacental circulation were described in the late 1970s. Initially, they concentrated on volume blood flow measurements, expressed as millilitres per minute, mainly in the umbilical vein. Reduced flow seemed to be strongly associated with pathological pregnancy, especially growth retardation. However, to calculate blood flow volume it is necessary to measure with great accuracy the vessel diameter and the angle between the ultrasound beam and blood vessel. The interobserver and intraobserver variability of these measurements was sufficiently large that this quantitative approach has been largely abandoned.

Currently, clinically relevant Doppler studies in perinatal medicine are restricted to simple and easily reproducible analysis of waveform of pulsatile (arterial) blood flow (Figure 50.5). This particular form of biophysical assessment has been evaluated much more rigorously and extensively than any other test of fetal health or fetoplacental function.

50.5.1 UMBILICAL ARTERY

Most reported Doppler trials have concentrated on the relationship between increased systolic:diastolic blood velocity ratio in the umbilical artery and fetal outcome. The increased systolic:diastolic ratio is a relatively common finding in severely growth-retarded fetuses and has been ascribed to an increased resistance in the umbilical placental bed [17].

The meta-analysis of 11 trials which used pathological flow velocity waveform in the umbilical artery to guide obstetric care showed a significant reduction in perinatal mortality rate and a reduced incidence of

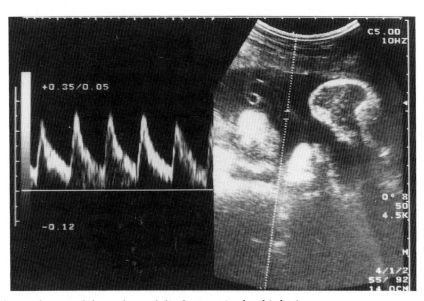

Figure 50.5 Normal Doppler signal from the umbilical artery in the third trimester.

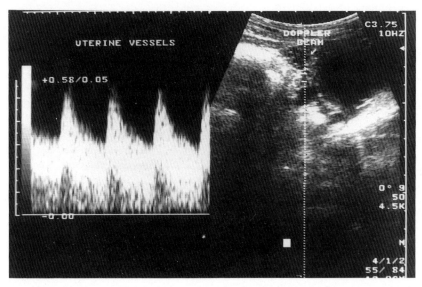

Figure 50.6 Doppler signal from the healthy uterine vessels in the third trimester showing relatively low systolic:diastolic flow ratio.

normally formed stillbirths when Doppler ultrasound results were made available to clinicians during high-risk pregnancies [18]. Despite being the only form of biophysical fetal assessment with beneficial effects confirmed in several randomized trials, most obstetricians still regard Doppler ultrasound as a research method and continue to use traditional but unproven methods like antepartum cardiotocography to assess fetal well-being.

50.5.2 UTEROPLACENTAL CIRCULATION

During pregnancy Doppler waveforms from uterine arteries and their branches show 'low resistance' flow pattern (Figure 50.6). This is a result of 'trophoblast invasion', a two-stage process in which a wave of trophoblast invades the decidual segments of the spiral arteries in the first trimester, and their myometrial segments in the second trimester, thus converting more than 100 uteroplacental arteries into low resistance vessels [19]. High pulsatile waveforms from these vessels imply potential pathology because a lack of trophoblast invasion seems to be a common phenomenon in pregnancies later complicated by intrauterine growth retardation and hypertension.

Doppler studies of uteroplacental vessels have been proposed as an early second trimester screening test to indicate a high-risk pregnancy [20] but the case for this is as yet unconvincing.

50.5.3 FETAL VESSELS

It has been shown in animals that asphyxia *in utero* results in an increased systemic vascular resistance, thus enabling the redistribution of oxygenated blood toward brain and heart. Doppler studies of fetal intracranial circulation, fetal aorta and renal arteries have suggested the presence of the same protective mechanism, so-called 'brain-sparing effect' in humans [21]. The clinical value of this sophisticated form of fetal biophysical assessment remains untested at present but is the focus of considerable research activity

50.6 Conclusions

The main aim of antenatal tests of fetal well-being is to avoid fetal death *in utero*. Evidence from the Cochrane Database of Perinatal Trials suggests that the use of Doppler ultrasound and placental ultrasound grading results in a decreased death rate of normally-formed fetuses. Cardiotocography and biophysical profile scoring, despite their widespread clinical use, have not been shown to be effective techniques by rigorous clinical trials.

References

1. Chalmers, I. (1989) Evaluating the effects of care during pregnancy and childbirth, in *Effective Care in Pregnancy and Childbirth* (eds I. Chalmers, M. Enkin and M.J.N.C. Keirse), Oxford University Press, Oxford, pp. 3–38.
2. Chalmers, I. (1992) *Oxford Database of Perinatal Trials*, disk issue 7, Oxford University Press, Oxford.
3. Johnson, P. and Maxwell, D. (1993) Fetal penile length (abstract). *Br. J. Obstet. Gynaecol.*, **100**, 291.
4. Neilson, J.P. (1992) Abnormalities of fetal growth, in *High-Risk Pregnancy* (eds A.A. Calder and W. Dunlop), Butterworth–Heinemann, Oxford, pp. 362–86.
5. Neilson, J.P. and Grant, A. (1989) Ultrasound in pregnancy, in *Effective Care in Pregnancy and Childbirth* (eds I. Chalmers, M. Enkin and M.J.N.C. Keirse), Oxford University Press, Oxford, pp. 419–39.
6. Chamberlain, P.F., Manning, F.A. and Morrison, I. (1984) Ultrasound evaluation of amniotic fluid volume. I. The relationship of marginal and decreased amniotic fluid volume to perinatal outcome. *Am. J. Obstet. Gynecol.*, **150**, 245–49.

7. Vyas, S., Nicolaides, K.H. and Campbell, S. (1989) Renal artery flow–velocity waveforms in normal and hypoxic fetuses. *Am. J. Obstet. Gynecol.*, **161**, 168–72.

8. Moore, T.R. (1990) Superiority of the four-quadrant sum over the single-deepest-pocket technique in ultrasonographic identification of abnormal amniotic fluid volumes. *Am. J. Obstet. Gynecol.*, **163**, 762–67.

9. Moore, T.R. and Cayle, J.E. (1990) The amniotic fluid index in normal human pregnancy. *Am. J. Obstet. Gynecol.*, **162**, 1168–73.

10. Grannum, P.A.T., Berkowitz, R.L. and Hobbins, J.C. (1979) The ultrasonic changes in the maturing placenta and their relation to fetal pulmonic maturity. *Am. J. Obstet. Gynecol.*, **133**, 915–22.

11. Proud, J. and Grant, A.M. (1987) Third trimester placental grading by ultrasonography as a test of fetal wellbeing. *BMJ*, **294**, 1641–47.

12. Newnham, J.P., Burns, S.E. and Roberman, B.D. (1990) Effect of vibratory acoustic stimulation on the duration of fetal heart rate monitoring tests. *Am. J. Perinatol.*, 7, 232–34.

13. Neilson, J.P. (1992) Cardiotocography for antepartum fetal assessment, in *Oxford Database of Perinatal Trials*, version 1.3, disk issue 7, record 3881 (ed. I. Chalmers), Oxford University Press, Oxford.

14. Manning, F.A., Platt, L.D. and Sipos, L. (1980) Antepartum fetal evaluation: development of a new biophysical profile. *Am. J. Obstet. Gynecol.*, **136**, 787–95.

15. Vintzileos, A.M., Campbell, W.A., Ingardia, C.J. and Nochimson, D.J. (1983) The fetal biophysical profile and its predictive value. *Obstet. Gynecol.*, **62**, 271–78.

16. Neilson, J.P. and Alfirevic, Z. (1993) Biophysical profile for antepartum fetal assessment, in *Pregnancy and Childbirth Module* (eds M.W. Enkin, M.J.N.C. Keirse, M.J. Renfrew and J.P. Neilson), Cochrane Database of Systematic Reviews, review no. 7432, published through Online Journal of Current Clinical Trials.

17. Giles, W.B., Trudiner, B.J. and Baird, P.J. (1985) Fetal umbilical artery flow velocity waveforms and placental resistance: pathological correlation. *Br. J. Obstet. Gynaecol.*, **92**, 31–38.

18. Neilson, J.P. (1992) Doppler ultrasound study of umbilical artery waveforms in high risk pregnancies: overview 7337, in *Oxford Database of Perinatal Trials*, version 1.3, disk issue 7 (ed. I. Chalmers), Oxford University Press, Oxford.

19. Pijnenborg, R., Bland, J.N., Robertson, W.B. and Brosens, I. (1983) Uteroplacental arterial changes related to interstitial trophoblast migration in early human pregnancy. *Placenta*, 4, 387–414.

20. Campbell, S., Pearce, K.M.F., Hackett, G. *et al.* (1986) Qualitative assessment of uteroplacental blood flow: early screening test for high-risk pregnancies. *Obstet. Gynecol.*, **68**, 649–53.

21. Wladimiroff, J.W., Winjgaard, J.A.G.W., Degani, S. *et al.* (1987) Cerebral and umbilical artery flow velocity waveforms in normal and growth retarded pregnancies. *Obstet. Gynecol.*, **69**, 705–709.

51 SONOEMBRYOLOGY IN THE STRUCTURAL EVALUATION OF THE FETUS FROM 6 TO 16 WEEKS

I.E. Timor-Tritsch, A. Monteagudo and G.M. Brown

51.1 Introduction

The high resolution of transvaginal probes, combined with the relative proximity and thin tissue layers between the transducer tip and the targeted fetus, makes transvaginal sonography one of the best imaging modalities to evaluate fetal structures from 6 to 16 weeks. Transvaginal sonography can also be successfully used for dating and early assessment of chorionicity and amnionicity in multifetal pregnancies.

The terms sonoembryology [1–3] and sonoembryography [4] are used to indicate the ability of transvaginal sonography to image with high resolution the small embryonic/fetal structures. Indeed, image interpretation of embryos and fetuses requires knowledge of embryonic/fetal development and the specific terminology used in embryology.

Most chapters on sonoembryology provide the reader with a detailed account of early embryonic and fetal development. The first part of this chapter will focus only on some of the sonographically detected highlights of development up to 14 menstrual weeks. In the second part, and probably the most important section of the chapter, is the description of organs and structures, as well as body parts, seen at the 14th and 15th menstrual weeks. This section will deliberately be more extensive and will focus on the possibilities of very accurate evaluation of the above-mentioned structures and organs, in order to employ them in a formal structural evaluation to ascertain normal fetal anatomy and eventually to be used in the work-up of fetal malformations.

The interested reader is referred to excellent textbooks of embryology [5–10] and detailed texts of transvaginal sonography dealing with scanning of the first and early second trimester fetus [11–14].

51.2 Dating the gestation

When dealing with embryos and fetuses, in terms of their measurements and the sequential appearance of body parts and organs, it becomes important to date the pregnancy accurately. There are three commonly used ways to express the age of the conceptus. (1) **Conceptual age**, used mostly in textbooks of embryology and expressed usually as the number of days from the presumed conception or fertilization. (2) **Gestational age**, usually used when the day of fertilization/conception/insemination is the only date known and computed by adding 14 days to the conceptual age. The gestational age usually compensates for the 2 weeks of a normal menstrual cycle, from the first day of the last menstrual period to the day of ovulation/conception. (3) **Menstrual age**, which expresses the time elapsed from the last menstrual period in weeks. It does not take account of the actual day of ovulation. In clinical obstetrics and gynecology the menstrual age is used to date the pregnancy. Since this is the most applied dating in clinical obstetrics and gynecology, this is the term that we will use in this chapter.

51.3 Discriminatory β-human chorionic gonadotropin (βhCG) zone for vaginal probes

The concept of the discriminatory βhCG zone was developed by Kadar [15] in 1981 and describes the level of the βhCG at which a chorionic sac is consistently

Diseases of the Fetus and Newborn, 2nd edn, Edited by G.B. Reed, A.E. Claireaux and F. Cockburn. Published in 1995 by Chapman & Hall, London. ISBN 0 412 39160 0

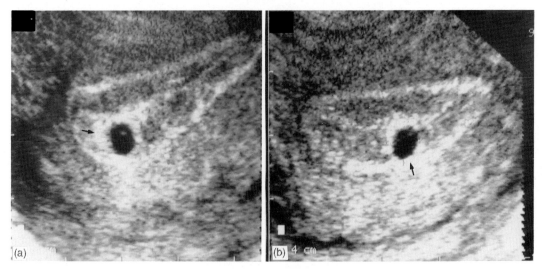

Figure 51.1 At 5 weeks 2 days the hyperechoic chorionic sac (arrow) is embedded in the endometrium lining the posterior wall of the uterine cavity on one side of the cavity line. (a) Sagittal section; (b) transverse section.

seen on ultrasound examination. Above a given discriminatory zone, the chorionic sac of a pregnancy in a normal uterus should be detectable. The introduction of the discriminatory βhCG made a significant impact on the practice of obstetrics and gynecology. The rise of the level of βhCG in a normal intrauterine pregnancy is predictable. The doubling time of the cells is known to be 1.2 days, with a βhCG level doubling about every 2 days [16]. There are several serum βhCG assays expressed in different units of measurement: the First International Reference Preparation (IRP) and the Second International Standard. Values of the Second International Standard are approximately 50% of those of the IRP (2.2 miu/ml Second International Standard = 1 miu/ml First IRP). It is also important to know the differences between the resolution of transabdominal and transvaginal probes. Typically, transabdominal scanning detects a normal intrauterine pregnancy at around 1 cm in diameter. However, transvaginal sonography can depict a clear chorionic sac as small as 2 mm in diameter [17]. The discriminatory zone for transvaginal probes is between 500 and 1000 miu/ml First IRP [17–24]. Typically transvaginal sonography detects the early chorionic sac about 1 week earlier than transabdominal scanning.

It is important to realize that the discriminatory zone for each transvaginal probe is different, and attempts to determine the discriminatory zone for each probe in use should be made as reflected by βhCG values of the laboratory at which the test is carried out.

Discriminatory levels of βhCG can be determined not only for chorionic sacs but also for the appearance of the yolk sac (7200 miu/ml IRP) and the appearance of the embryonic heart beats (10 800 miu/ml IRP) [25].

51.4 Technical considerations

It should be mentioned at the outset that, if accurate determination of fetal anatomy is to be attempted in the first and early second trimester, this should be performed using high frequency transvaginal probes. The higher the frequency of the transducer crystal the higher the resolution of the obtained image. Therefore a 6.5-MHz probe is desirable, though at times clear fetal anatomy can be seen using 5-MHz probes. Since there is no real loss of resolution or detail if higher magnifications are used, one of the requirements of sonoembryology is to be able to magnify the on-screen image. In order to obtain clear pictures on the screen, the embryo/fetus or the targeted organ should be in the focal zone of the transducer. This can be achieved by altering the electronic focusing or by gently pushing or pulling the probe until the structure is clearly seen. The bladder of the patient must be empty if an early pregnancy is scanned. A high quality video-recorder with frame-by-frame advance feature is important. The use of such equipment will not only shorten the examination time but will also enable the entire scanning process to be reviewed off line. The currently introduced 'cineloop' reviews are helpful in retrieving some of the images captured by the machine's memory. However, this is not a replacement for videotaping significant portions of the examination.

51.5 Structures detected by transvaginal sonography in the first trimester

As stated earlier; only the more important and obvious features and structures will be described. The dating will be expressed in menstrual weeks, e.g. the fifth week relates to 4 weeks 0 days to 4 weeks 6 days, and similarly the tenth week expresses the week between 9 weeks 0 days and 9 weeks 6 days.

51.5.1   THE FIFTH WEEK

With most transvaginal probes of at least 5 MHz the chorionic sac is readily detectable embedded in one side or other of the cavity line, within the thick endometrium. The chorionic sac at detection usually measures 2–5 mm. In patients with known dates, all intrauterine gestations in a non-fibroid uterus should be detectable by the end of the fifth week.

51.5.2   THE SIXTH WEEK

During the sixth week, the central sonolucency of the chorionic sac becomes much more evident than during the previous week. The 'double-ring' generated by the rapidly proliferating cytotrophoblast and syncytiotrophoblast as well as the decidua are the hallmarks of this gestational week (Figure 51.1). Towards the end of the 6th week the yolk sac becomes evident and measures 2 mm; however it will quickly achieve its final size, which

is about 4 mm, maintaining this size during the next 6–7 weeks. The fetal heart beats will become visible at around 5 weeks 5–6 days, or 42 days of menstrual age.

Simple rule of thumb: if the yolk sac is seen in a chorionic sac of about 5–6 mm, but no heart activity is seen, the pregnancy is of 5 weeks 2–3 days at most [26].

51.5.3   THE SEVENTH WEEK

The typical transvaginal sonographic picture at the beginning of the seventh week clearly depicts a 4–5-mm yolk sac, with a 4-mm embryonic pole adjacent to the yolk sac and tangentially touching it. The fetal pole contains the beating fetal heart. The embryo will quickly grow during this week, doubling its size towards the end of the seventh menstrual week. The embryo is curled up at this early stage, therefore the measurement performed is not the crown–rump length (CRL) but rather a cross-diameter of the entire embryo [27]. At times, towards the end of the seventh week, the coronal/tangential plane demonstrates the parallel lines of the neural tube.

Simple rule of thumb: if the yolk sac and heart beats are seen but there is no sonolucency yet seen in the cephalic pole of the tiny embryo, the pregnancy is of 6 weeks 3–5 days at most [26].

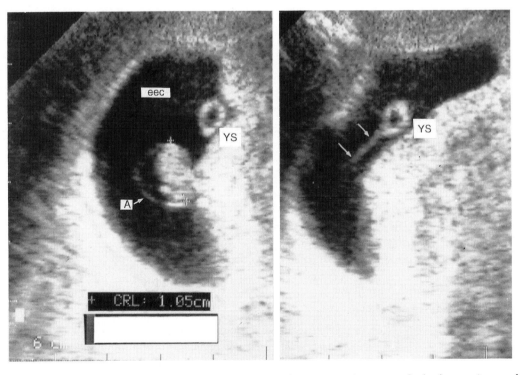

Figure 51.2   The content of the chorionic sac at 7 weeks 2 days. The amnion (A) surrounds the fetus quite snugly (CRL 1.05 cm). The extraembryonic coelom (eec) contains the yolk sac (YS) and the vitelline duct (small arrows).

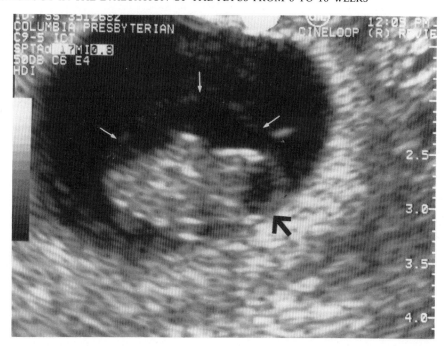

Figure 51.3 An 8-week 1-day pregnancy (CRL 17 mm). The small arrows point to the amnion. The black arrow is directed toward the unilocular sonolucency in the head. This represents the primordial, non-partitioned ventricle.

51.5.4   THE EIGHTH WEEK

At the beginning of the eighth week the amnion can be seen to surround the developing embryo snugly; towards the end of this week it will distance itself from the fetal body and can therefore be distinguished as a separate membrane surrounding the fetus (Figure 51.2). The space between the amnion and the wall of the uterine cavity (lined by the chorion laeve) represents the extraembryonic coelom and is filled with mucinous material. The sonographic echogenicity of this extra-embryonic space is always somewhat greater than the sonolucent amnion. The yolk sac and the vitelline duct are extraembryonic structures and are located in the extraembryonic coelom (Figure 51.2). At the end of this week the rostrally situated unpartitioned telencephalic and mesencephalic vesicles can be depicted for the first time. The limb buds can also be seen for the first time at this age. Towards the end of the 8th week, the incipient features of the convoluted sonolucent ventricles of the central nervous system, with the outstanding pontine and cephalic flexures, can be detected.

   Simple rule of thumb: if the yolk sac and the heartbeats are seen in the embryo and there is a single (unpartitioned) sonolucency in the head which is not larger in size than the yolk sac, the pregnancy is 7–7.5 weeks at most [26].

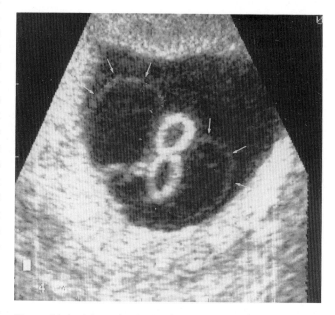

Figure 51.4 Monochorionic, diamniotic twinning at 8 weeks 0 days, showing the two separate amnions (small arrows) and the two yolk sacs which are close to each other.

Figure 51.7 (opposite)   At 10 weeks the posterior and the anterior contours of the body and the head in the sagittal section are crisp enough to lend themselves to evaluation. The arrow points to the physiologic midgut hernia.

Figure 51.5 The structure of the membranes of a triplet gestation is shown. Two of the three fetuses (A and B) were in a monochorionic diamniotic sac. Note the thin amnion between A and B which takes off in a T shape from the chorionic membrane (white arrow). Also note the very different, delta-shaped 'take-off' (black arrow) of the chorion which separates the 'singleton' (C) from the monochorionic diamniotic 'twins' (A and B).

Figure 51.6 Two fetuses of 9 weeks are shown to illustrate imaging the posterior contours. (a) At 9 weeks 3 days the posterior and cephalic contours in the sagittal plane are evident. The sonolucent tortuous brain ventricles and the flexures are also seen. CF = cephalic flexure; PF = pontine flexure; D = diencephalon; Ms = mesencephalon; Mt = metencephalon; My = myelencephalon. (b) To illustrate the feasibility of discerning pathology at 9 weeks, a fetus with a gestational age of 9 weeks 2 days is shown. Note that the posterior contour shows a continuous sonolucent structure of about 2–3 mm beneath the skin of the back. The chromosomal studies revealed normal karyotype.

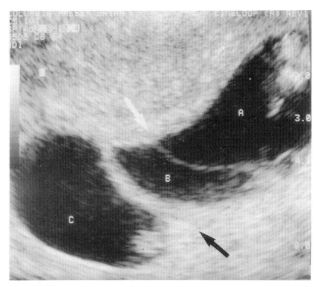

Figure 51.5

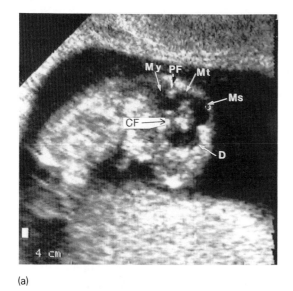

(a)

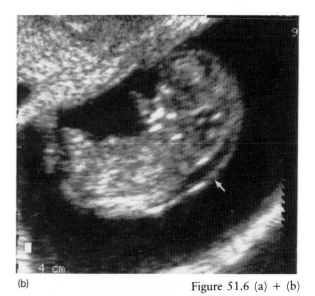

(b)

Figure 51.6 (a) + (b)

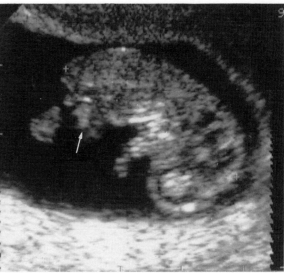

Figure 51.7 (a)   (b)

902

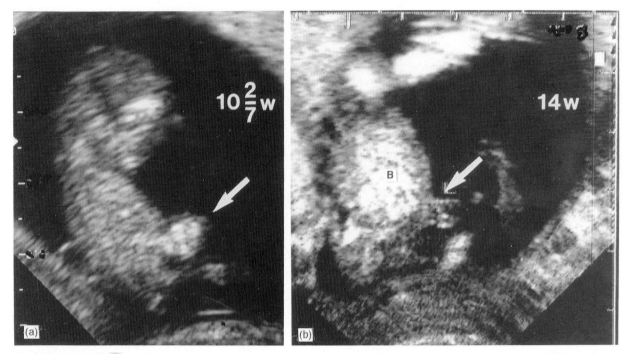

Figure 51.8 The presence and disappearance of the physiologic herniation of the midgut: (a) at 10 weeks 2 days the hyperechoic midgut (arrow) is still present; (b) at 14 weeks the arrow points to the abdominal insertion of the cord. The hyperechoic bowel (B) is now within the abdominal cavity.

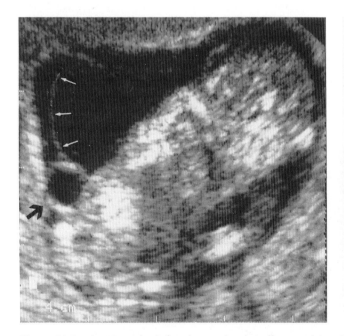

Figure 51.9 At 12 weeks 1 day the amnion (small arrows) is very close to the chorion laeve (lining the inner wall of the uterine cavity), encroaching on the yolk sac (black arrow).

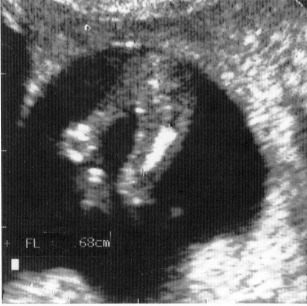

Figure 51.10 At 12 weeks 1 day the femur length is 6.8 mm.

51.5.5   THE NINTH WEEK

At this stage of development the head, trunk and limbs are distinguished using transvaginal sonography. The size of the fetal head surpasses the diameter of the yolk sac towards the end of the ninth week and becomes a distinct anatomical structure. The extra-embryonic coelom is becoming somewhat restricted in size because of the relative expansion of the amnion. The upper and the lower limbs start moving towards the end of this week. The posterior sagittal contour is discernible in most embryos at this time. This is the gestational age at which the physiologic (ventral) midgut hernia is first seen in most embryos [28]. Textbooks of embryology deal extensively with the description of the physiologic midgut hernia [5–7]. The appearance and disappearance of the midgut herniation was previously documented by transabdominal scanning [29,30] and subsequently by transvaginal sonography (Figures 51.7 and 51.8). The hallmark of the ninth week embryonic brain is still the lack of the falx cerebri (Figure 51.3). However, the ventricles are progressively convoluted in the sagittal plane, with only very little lateral protrusion, i.e. telencephalic ventricles. The largest unpartitioned midline sonolucency, typical of the ninth week embryo, is the rhombencephalon.

If multifetal pregnancies are detected or suspected, the ninth to tenth week is probably the ideal gestation when chorionicity and amnionicity can best be determined. The reason for this is that the amnion, the

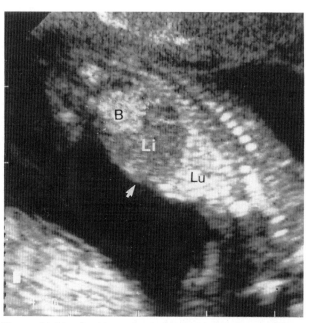

Figure 51.11 At 12 weeks 1 day it is already possible to differentiate between the high echogenicity of the bowel (B) and the lung (Lu) and that of the liver (Li), which not only shows a lower level echogenicity but outlines the diaphragm. Note the normal anterior wall contour (arrow).

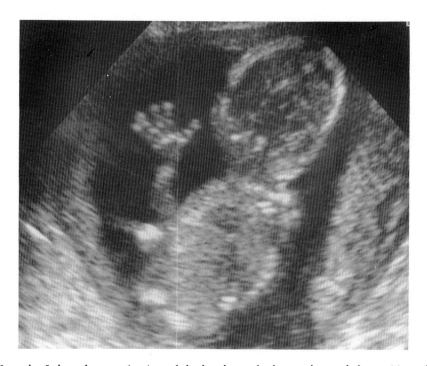

Figure 51.12 At 13 weeks 5 days the examination of the hand reveals the number and the position of the fingers.

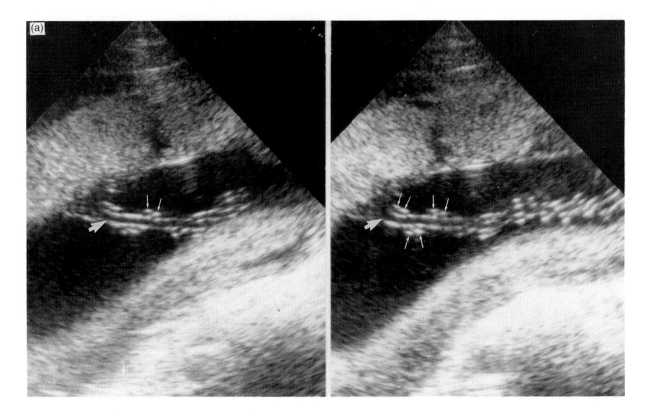

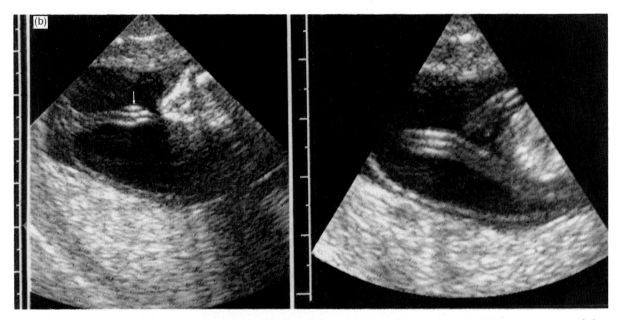

Figure 51.13 The cord. (a) Two serial images of the normal three-vessel cord at 13.5 weeks. The cross-section of the two umbilical arteries (small arrows pointing to the two linear echoes) is shown wrapping multiple times around the wider umbilical vein (larger arrow). (b) For comparison, two pictures of a cord with single umbilical artery at 13 weeks. Note that the walls of the two vessels can be followed for a significant length and if the artery wraps around the vein there is only one linear echo seen, as opposed to the two echoes in a normal cord.

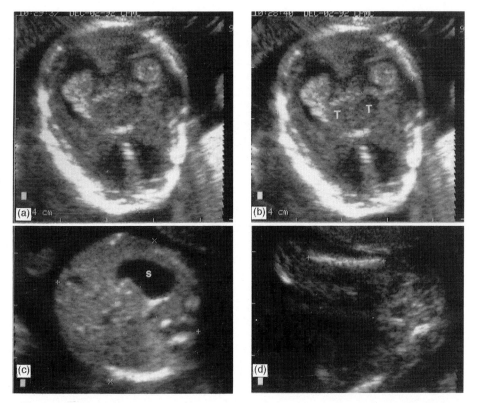

Figure 51.14 Structural evaluation at 15 weeks: biometry. (a) The head circumference is 11.06 cm = 15 weeks 0 days; (b) the BPD is 3.05 cm = 15 weeks 0 days; (c) the abdominal circumference is 9.53 cm = 15 weeks; (d) the femur length is 1.66 cm = 15 weeks 5 days.

chorion and the yolk sacs (Figure 51.4), as well as the insertion of the tiny cords, can be clearly seen due to the relative abundance of sonolucent amniotic fluid surrounding them. There is a basic difference between the appearance of the membranes separating two chorionic sacs (dichorionic/diamniotic) and the membranes separating two amniotic sacs (in a monochorionic/diamniotic sac). This difference is striking at these early gestational ages. The 'take-off' of the dichorionic/diamniotic membrane is wedge-shaped (due to the intervening placental tissue) as opposed to the 'take-off' of the diamniotic membrane which is T-shaped (Figure 51.5).

Simple rule of thumb: if the falx is not yet seen in the unpartitioned, single ventricle within the head, the size of which is still about the size of the yolk sac, but a clear tiny hyperechoic midgut hernia is seen at the ventral insertion of the cord, the pregnancy is about 8.5 weeks but less than 9 weeks [26].

51.5.6 THE TENTH WEEK

Imaging the fetus by transvaginal sonography beginning at and during the tenth week becomes progressively informative and clinically meaningful. The contours of the fetus become extremely clear. The measurements of the crown–rump length are easily obtained. There is a relative abundance of structures that can be depicted by the higher frequency vaginal probes. The posterior and anterior sagittal contours are easy to evaluate because there is constant movement of the fetus which sooner or later will position the optimum scanning planes (Figures 51.6 and 51.7). Even the slightest thickening of the sonolucency along the posterior contours is striking (Figure 51.6b). The abdominal wall still displays the previously described physiologic midgut herniation. The head constitutes almost one-half of the size of the body, and will therefore be the focus of our scanning during this week. Indeed the head contains a large number of structures to be recognized at this gestational age. The transvaginal sonographic hallmark of the tenth week is the appearance of the falx and, on each side, the extremely echogenic choroid plexi [2,13,17,30–32]. The sagittal section through the head depicts in the midsagittal plane the tortuous ventricular system with the prominent cephalic and pontine flexures, around which the various parts of the ventricle are curved (Figure 51.6a).

Imaging the limbs is feasible throughout this week since the arms and the legs stand away from the body

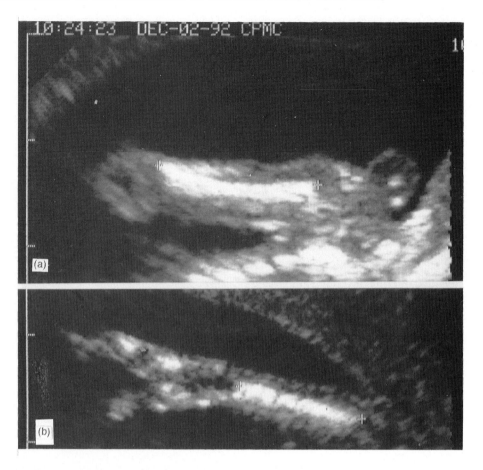

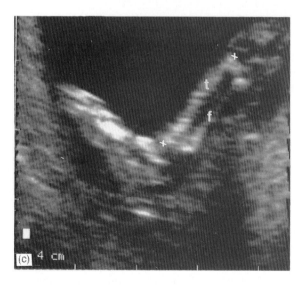

Figure 51.15 Structural evaluation at 15 weeks: measurements of long bones. (a) The humerus measures 1.7 cm; (b) the radius measures 1.33 cm; (c) the tibia (t) measures 1.8 cm. Note the fibula (f) and the silhouette of the foot. By the configuration of the foot and the tibia/fibula, malformations such as club-foot and rockerbottom foot can be ruled out.

and they start to move; even the cross-sections of the fingers are evident. However there is limited clinical importance to be attributed to the structural evaluation of the limbs at this stage of gestation.

Simple rule of thumb: if both the falx and the midgut hernia are seen together, the pregnancy is more than 9–9.5 weeks but less than 12 weeks [26].

51.5.7 THE 11TH WEEK

The growing amniotic cavity 'pushes' the yolk sac to the side against the uterine wall, shrinking the extra-embryonic coelom. The limbs can be scanned with increasing success, and in 25–75% of the fetuses the fingers can be counted. The contours of the fetus during

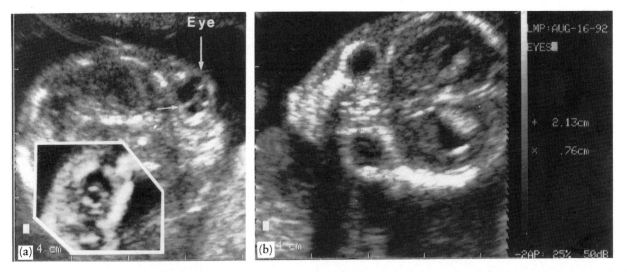

Figure 51.16 Structural evaluation at 15 weeks: the eyes. (a) The left eye: the arrow points at the hyaloid artery which approaches the posterior surface of the lens (axial view). Insert: the orbit and the lens (coronal view); (b) measuring the outer interorbital diameter (2.13 cm) and the inner interorbital diameter (0.76 cm) on a composite coronal–axial plane.

the 11th week are crisp and, if the midsagittal image of the entire fetus is obtained, one can clearly see the outline of the posterior contours, the head and the anterior contours of the body, which will still reveal the physiologic midgut herniation (Figure 51.7). The physiologic midgut hernia is a hyperechoic structure within the cord which, later, by the 12th menstrual week, retracts into the abdominal cavity where the gut retains its relatively high echogenicity (Figure 51.8). Multiple scanning planes of the face and the ventricular system in the brain can now better define these structures. The facial structures can be imaged; however one must remember that even though the hard palate starts the process of fusion at this time it is not completed until the 13th week.

51.5.8 THE 12TH, 13TH AND 14TH WEEKS

A continuous and slow growth is seen throughout the 12–14th weeks and is reflected in a higher percentage of detection of the same structures already described for previous weeks. The yolk sac is pushed more and more to the side of the restricted extraembryonic coelom by the expanding amnion (Figure 51.9).

We undertook a study to evaluate the ability of the high frequency transvaginal scanning method to consistently image fetal structures such as the posterior and anterior body contours, long bones, fingers, face, palate, feet and toes and the four-chamber view. After scanning 97 normal pregnancies between 9 and 14 weeks, the results showed that these structures were consistently detected in all the fetuses scanned at the following weeks: sagittal contours at 9 weeks; long bones at 10 weeks; fingers at 12 weeks; face and palate

at 12 weeks; feet and toes at 13 weeks; and finally the four-chamber view at 14 weeks. This study supported the possibility of searching for specific malformations at or after the menstrual ages mentioned or performing a comprehensive malformation evaluation after the 13th menstrual week [33]. It is evident therefore from the 12th week throughout the 14th week the long bones, the fingers, the face and the palate and finally the feet and the toes can be evaluated since they should be seen in all fetuses at these gestational ages. An example of the picture quality at 12 weeks is shown on Figure 51.10. The four-chamber view could be seen in more than 25% but not all the examined fetuses at these gestational ages. Examining the central nervous system becomes feasible during the 12th, 13th and 14th weeks. Multiple sections can be achieved through each plane. The conventional scanning planes are the axial, coronal, and the sagittal planes; however it should also be noted that most of the time a composite plane is obtained since the 'pure' planes may be hard to obtain. During the 13th week it is expected that the physiologically extruding midgut is already retracted into the abdominal cavity. This is also the time when the different echogenicities of the bowel, liver and lungs as well as the kidneys become evident, enabling the depiction of the exact outlines of structures demarcated by their differential echogenicity (Figure 51.11).

At times when the fetal position permits evaluation of the fingers, a scan at these gestational ages may become extremely important to rule out those anomalies which significantly involve the shape of the fingers. One should also remember that at these gestational ages it is very rare to see all five fingers in the same scanning plane (Figure 51.12). Usually, on one single

908

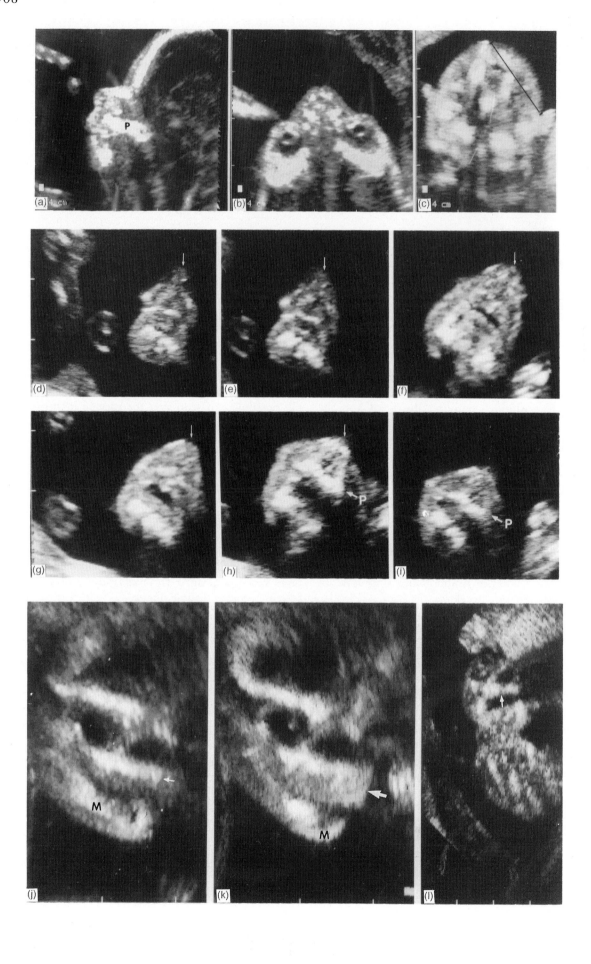

plane, the fingers 2–5 are seen; the thumb appears on a different scanning plane [33].

The umbilical cord is an important marker of chromosomal as well as other structural anomalies. It is therefore important to scrutinize the umbilical cord. Figure 51.13 shows the normal three-vessel cord and the pathological cord with a single umbilical artery, both detected at 13 weeks 3–4 days. It is easier to suspect and verify the number of vessels on a longitudinal scan since the resolution of the equipment employed may not suffice to resolve the two arteries and one vein on a cross-sectional image.

The kidneys are identifiable from 12–14 completed weeks. Tables for use as guides in measuring the kidneys at these gestational ages and their corresponding biparietal diameter (BPD) and CRL measurements are available in the literature [34].

Simple rule of thumb: if a fetus does not have an identifiable physiologic midgut hernia, its gestational age is more than 12 menstrual weeks.

50.5.9 THE 15TH AND 16TH WEEKS

In order to demonstrate the ability of transvaginal sonography to evaluate fetal anatomy at these gestational ages, a fetus with accurate dating at 15 weeks 2 days by certain last menstrual period was selected and scanned. The scanning was recorded by a tape recorder attached to the ultrasound equipment. Pictures were printed on a thermal printer during and subsequently off-line after the completion of the scan from the tape. The first scanning lasted 35 minutes. The patient was rescanned after 5 days in order to complete the imaging and obtain better views of the heart. The second scanning session lasted 45 minutes. The selection of the images obtained throughout the scanning sessions are

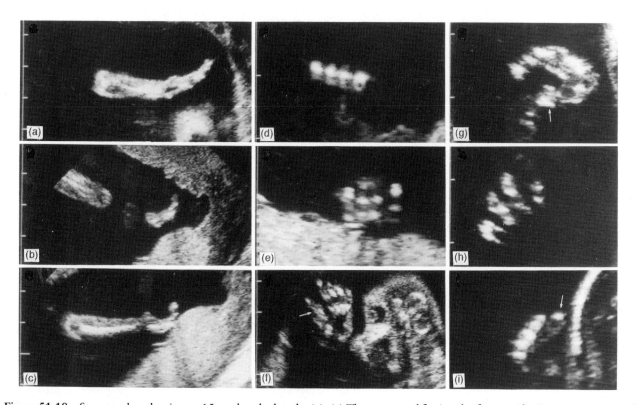

Figure 51.18 Structural evaluation at 15 weeks: the hands. (a)–(c) The process of flexing the fingers; (d)–(i) on transverse and longitudinal sections the fingers are usually seen without the thumb. However, sometimes it can be imaged in a different plane (arrows on (f), (g) and (i)).

Figure 51.17 Structural evaluation at 15 weeks: the palate. (a) The profile in the midsagittal plane (P = palate); (b) axial section of the orbits; (c) coronal section of the head with the bregma-to-ear measurement line; (d)–(i) Successive coronal sections of the lips (mouth), the nose (arrows) and the hard palate (P); (j) this slightly oblique coronal view shows the palate (arrow) and the mandible (M); (k) a more anterior section shows the palate and the alveolar process of the maxilla (arrow) and the tip of the mandible (chin) (M); (l) a symmetrical coronal view shows the normal maxilla (arrow).

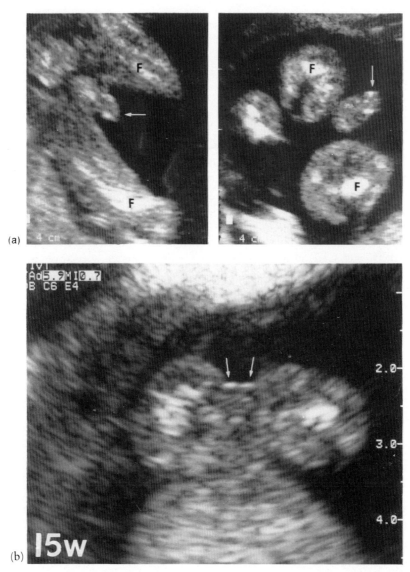

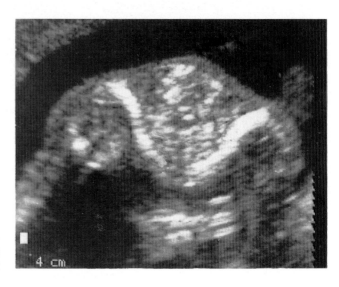

Figure 51.19 Structural evaluation at 15 weeks: the genitalia. (a) It's a boy! The arrow points to the phallus (F = the femur); (b) the arrows point to the labia on this coronal section of a female fetus (this image originates from a different case).

Figure 51.20 Structural evaluation at 15 weeks: the clavicles. This horizontal (transverse) section through the clavicles also shows the normal contours of the back and the lower part of the neck.

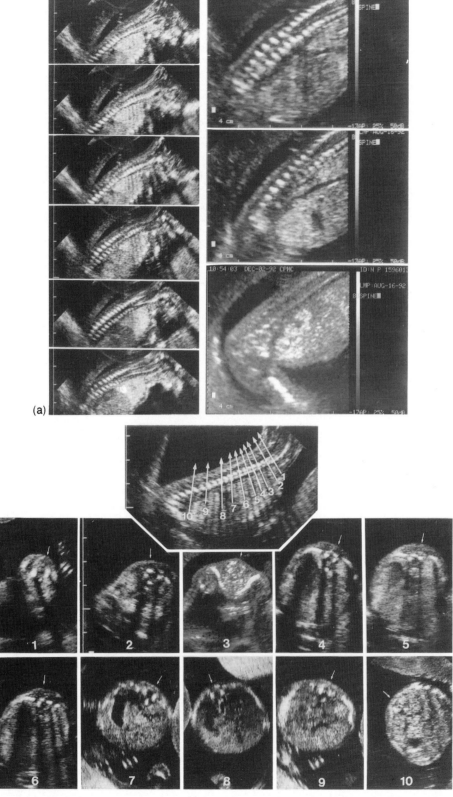

Figure 51.21 Structural evaluation at 15 weeks: the spine. (a) The six sequential images on the left show how the cervical and thoracic spine is evaluated using the slight rocking of the transducer in the sagittal plane. The covering skin, the spinal processes, the spinal canal and the bodies of each vertebra can be studied. The three pictures on the right were selected from many, showing the study of the lumbar and the sacral spine. At times the sections are not aligned with a perfect sagittal plane. (b) Selected coronal sections of the spine: the levels at which each picture was taken are marked by the appropriate number on the top panel.

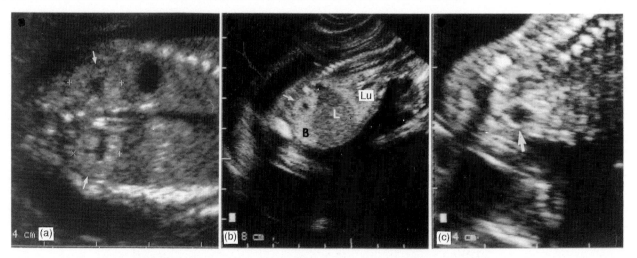

Figure 51.22 Structural evaluation at 15 weeks: the urinary system. (a) Coronal section of both kidneys (arrows). Note the central collecting system in each kidney. (b) On a sagittal section the echogenicity of the kidney (arrow) matches the echogenicity of the lungs (Lu). The low level echogenicity of the liver (L) and the highly echogenic bowel are also seen. (c) A midsagittal section of the lower body reveals the bladder (arrow).

presented in continuation. The reasons for presenting the pictures of this case are to show that a very detailed, in-depth and comprehensive scan of a large number of structures and organ systems can be performed at 15–16 weeks.

51.6 Structural evaluation at 15 weeks

The first task of the sonographer or sonologist is to perform fetal biometry to ascertain that the measurements are consistent with the gestational age of the fetus. Practically every organ can be measured and most of them already have a corresponding table of values for gestational ages of 14 weeks and beyond. The structures measured in most cases are the head circumference, the BPD and the interorbital distance. Measurements of brain structures such as the cerebellum, sometimes measurements to evaluate the position of the ears, the abdominal circumference, and finally the long bones such as the femur, the humerus, the radius and the tibia can all be made (Figures 51.14, 51.15 and 51.16). If fetal structures are evaluated by transvaginal sonography it is essential to use the appropriate tables and graphs that were generated by using transvaginal sonographic measurements. A selection of those graphs can be found in the literature [35].

Evaluation of the face may start with looking at the contours in the sagittal plane (Figure 51.17a) and the orbits in the coronal and axial planes (Figures 51.16 and 51.17b). Even the hyaloid artery can at times be seen (Figure 51.16). The palate and the lips are scanned using the coronal (Figure 51.17d–i) and the midsagittal (Figure 51.17j–l) planes.

One of the most labor-intensive evaluations is that of the hands and the feet. It is rare to image them at will. Usually they 'flash' through the picture and one must be attentive to get the appropriate images. However by reviewing the tape-recorded material it is possible to gather the required pictures for adequate documentation of their anatomy (Figure 51.18).

Evaluation of the genitalia may become extremely important if certain X-linked diseases or structural malformations are evaluated (Figure 51.19). Correct detection of the fetal sex approaches 100% at or after the 15th gestational week, but it is a function of the resolution of the probe and of experience. Early and precise determination of fetal gender is possible and in some of the cases may avoid invasive procedures such as amniocentesis [36].

Evaluation of the spine is almost always the major structural evaluation of a fetus. It is important to realize that the targeted evaluation of the spine cannot always be achieved during a specific and short period of time. At times, the lower spine can be seen and evaluated adequately, and then, due to constant fetal motion, another organ presents itself at the focal range of the probe. Therefore the rest of the spine, e.g. the lumbar, thoracic or cervical region, may have to be evaluated at a later time. The second important fact to note is that, at times, less than perfect and 'clean' planes or sections can be obtained. Thus the three-dimensional reconstruction of the fetal body in the scanner's mind is necessary using the available two-dimensional sequential pictures obtained on the screen. Rocking the transducer, moving the fetus with the abdominal hand, and reconstructing the complete

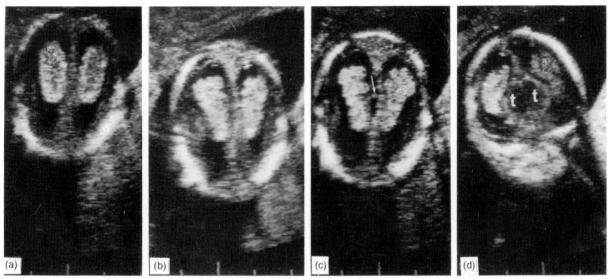

Figure 51.23 Structural evaluation at 15 weeks: the brain. The systematic scanning of the lateral ventricles and choroid plexus can be performed using several axial (a) (b) and (c) and coronal (d) planes. The cavity of the septum pellucidum (arrow in panel (c)) and the thalami (t in panel (d)) are shown.

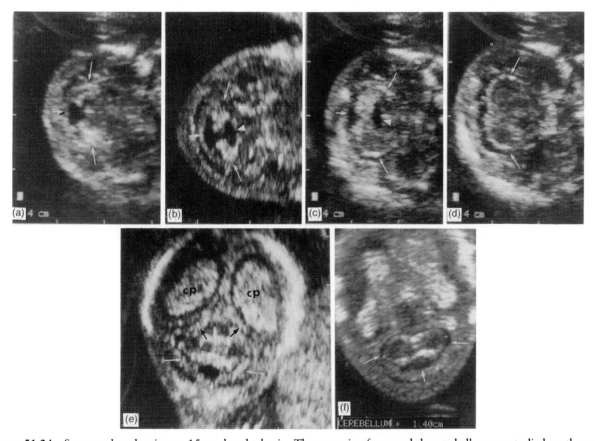

Figure 51.24 Structural evaluation at 15 weeks: the brain. The posterior fossa and the cerebellum are studied on these serial sections. The two slanted arrows on both sides of the cerebellum throughout the six pictures point to the two hemispheres. (a) A low axial section depicting the cisterna magna (small arrow). (b) The higher axial plane reveals the widening cisterna magna (small arrow) and the lower pole of the fourth ventricle (arrowhead). (c) A somewhat 'higher' axial section shows the hemispheres and the fourth ventricle (arrowhead). (d) This is the highest of the axial sections depicting the cerebellum at the level where the bicerebellar measurement usually is taken. Note the hyperechoic cortex surrounded by sonolucent cerebrospinal fluid and the low echogenicity of the medulla. (e) This coronal section shows the cisterna magna (small white arrow in the midline), the inverted funnel-shaped tentorium (two black arrows) and the choroid plexus (cp). (f) A combined slanted axial–coronal section showing the cerebellum measuring 1.4 cm (small arrow in the midline = cisterna magna).

914

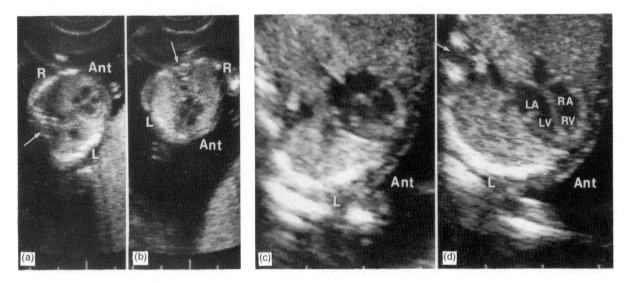

Figure 51.25 Structural evaluation at 15 weeks: the heart. This figure illustrates how the four-chamber view may be obtained. Panels (a) and (b) show the four-chamber view at 15 weeks 0 days. The frequent position changes of the fetus are apparent. The spine (marked by small arrow) is seen at different positions. Panels (c) and (d) show the four-chamber view about 6 days later. At times more than one frame is necessary to depict certain structures, e.g. the atria are better seen on panel (c) but the septum is better imaged on panel (d). See Figure 51.26 for abbreviations.

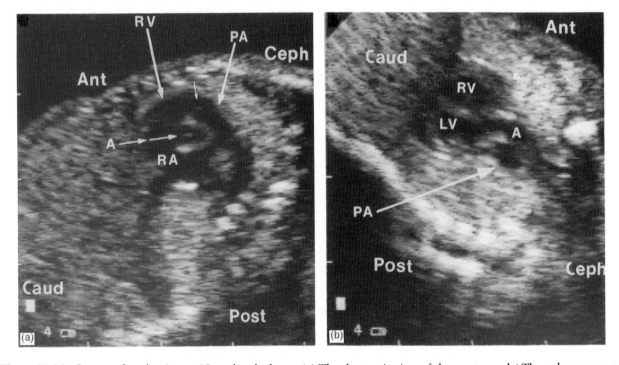

Figure 51.26 Structural evaluation at 15 weeks: the heart. (a) The short axis view of the great vessels. The pulmonary artery (PA) wraps around the cross-section of the aorta (A) after rising from the right ventricle (RV). The right atrium (RA) is also seen. (b) The criss-cross of the great vessels is depicted. The aorta (A) arising from the left ventricle (LV), above which the right ventricle (RV) is seen, which gives rise to the right ventricle outflow tract and the pulmonary artery (PA). The pulmonary outflow tract is not seen since it is not in the plane of this section, only the emerging cross-section of the pulmonary artery is seen. Ant = anterior; Post = posterior; Ceph = cephalad; Caud = caudad.

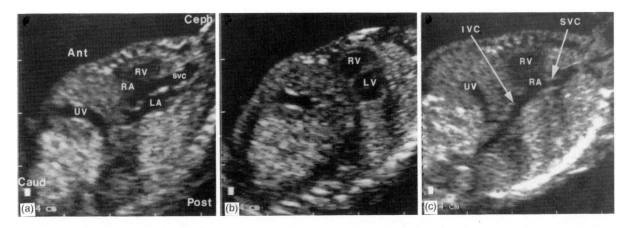

Figure 51.27 Structural evaluation at 15 weeks: the heart. Longitudinal sections are shown. (a) The relationship between the right ventricle (RV), the right atrium (RA) and the left atrium (LA) are shown. The entrance of the umbilical vein (UV) from the anterior abdominal wall through the liver is seen. Ant = anterior; Post = posterior; Ceph = cephalad; Caud = caudad. (b) This is a short axis view of the lower ventricular chambers; the right ventricle (RV) and left ventricle (LV) are shown. (c) This longitudinal picture depicts the inferior vena cava (IVC) and superior vena cava (SVC) and their connection to the right atrium (RA) and right ventricle (RV) is shown. UV = umbilical vein.

scanning of the spine is the ultimate goal and can definitely be achieved throughout the scanning session(s). Figures 51.20 and 51.21 illustrate the way that the spine can be visualized and documented.

To evaluate the urinary system it is necessary to image the two kidneys with the sonolucent pelvis as well as the urinary bladder. At times, slight dilatation of the renal pelvis may be seen. However there are no adequate tables available to use in evaluating the pathology (Figure 51.22).

The evaluation of the fetal brain requires a minimal knowledge of the normal anatomy. However, by using the available descriptions of the developing fetal nervous system, this can be achieved. The fetal head is usually evaluated in the sagittal, coronal and axial planes but as mentioned before, at times only composite planes such as axial–coronal or other slanted non-conventional planes can be obtained. As usual using transvaginal sonography, the three-dimensional picture has to be reconstructed in the mind of the sonographer. Figures 51.23 and 51.24 illustrate only several of the possibilities that depict the feasibility of evaluating the central nervous system in the early second trimester fetus [37].

Evaluation of the fetal heart requires knowledge of more than the conventional standard sections, and often non-conventional sections of the developing fetal heart are needed. The first stage of the examination is to try and obtain the four-chamber view. By doing this, a large number of cardiac malformations can be ruled out (Figure 51.25). However, in order to rule out most cardiac malformations additional sections should be obtained, such as the short axis view of the great vessels (Figure 51.26a), imaging the criss-cross of the large vessels (Figure 51.26b), some longitudinal sections of the heart (Figure 51.27), as well as the left ventricular outflow and the right ventricular inflow of the inferior and superior vena cava. It is possible to evaluate the aortic arch and the larger vessels of the neck and the head emerging from the aortic root (Figure 51.28).

Finally, during the scanning session the number of vessels in the cord should be documented on longitudinal or cross-section (Figure 51.29).

The newly introduced color coded flow imaging enables a somewhat better evaluation of the fetal vascular system, including the fetal heart but the traditional black and white transvaginal scanning is sufficient most of the time to evaluate the fetal vascular system accurately.

51.7 Summary

Transvaginal sonography, employing high frequency probes, enables a closer look at early pregnancy and enables imaging of the different embryonic and fetal structures in great detail. Since this scanning route detects the same anatomic structures up to 3 weeks earlier on the average than the customary transabdominal probe, it is expected that an exhaustive evaluation of the anatomy can be performed at an earlier gestational age.

Before engaging in structural evaluations and early

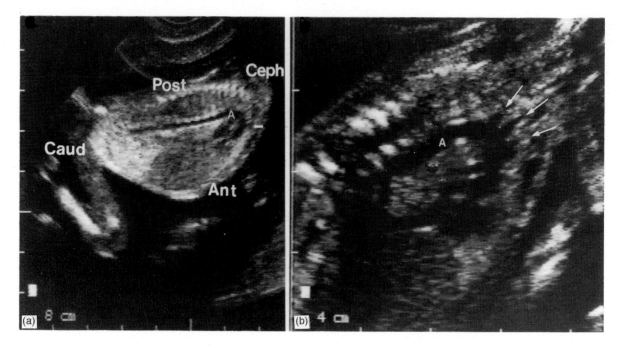

Figure 51.28 Structural evaluation at 15 weeks: the heart. The aortic arch is depicted on the smaller (a) and the larger targeted image (b). The small arrows indicate neck and head vessels emerging from the aortic root (A). Ant = anterior; Post = posterior; Ceph = cephalad; Caud = caudad.

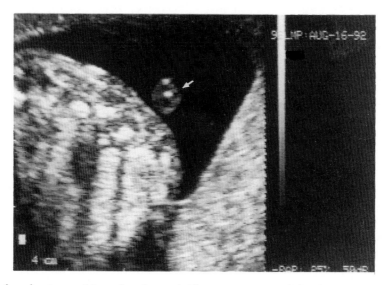

Figure 51.29 Structural evaluation at 15 weeks: the cord. The cross-section of the three-vessel cord (arrow).

diagnosis of fetal anomalies it is important to stress that knowledge of embryonic and fetal structural anatomy is a prerequisite. Using the clear pictures obtained by transvaginal sonography up to the stage of the tenth week of pregnancy, it is possible to follow the normal embryonic and fetal development and detect the slightest pathology leading to pregnancy failure. Past the 10th week there is a possibility of scanning and evaluating fetal anatomy in a clinically meaningful way. As the gestation progresses an increasing number of structures, body parts and organs can be seen with the high frequency transvaginal probe. It seems that the best time to evaluate the largest number of anatomical structures using transvaginal sonography is the 16th week (from 15 weeks 0 days to 16 weeks 0 days). At this period, the fetus will 'fit into' the focal range of the vaginal probe and its frequent movements will enable every organ to be scanned. If needed, an attempt to evaluate the fetus by the vaginal route has to be considered, even at later gestational ages. With progression of gestation the evaluation will be limited to fewer and fewer organs; however the ones that are reached will show an almost unparalleled resolution, which makes transvaginal sonography worth trying. It is also relevant to mention that the primary route for scanning the fetal brain at any gestational age is the transvaginal route, provided the fetal presentation is vertex [37].

The aim of this chapter has been to provide the interested reader with information about the clinical use and the advances of the sonographic evaluation of the fetus. A representative list of references pertaining to the published material regarding the use of transvaginal sonography in describing a large number of malformations detected in the first and the early second trimester is provided [36,38–58].

We believe that the groundwork has been prepared for selective and even routine anatomical work-up of the first and the early second trimester fetus. Sonoembryology or sonofetology has already pushed back the limits of the classical fetal evaluation into the first half of the pregnancy. The value of transvaginal sonography should no longer be doubted, particularly in the evaluation and the early work-up of fetal malformations. We now have to prepare for its routine use. We predict this will happen in the near future, after the necessary personnel and machines become universally available.

References

1. Popp, L.W., Lueken, R.P., Muller-Holne, W. et al. (1983) Gynecologishe Endosonographie. Erste Erfahrungen. Ultraschall Med., 4, 92.
2. Timor-Tritsch, I.E., Peisner, D.B. and Raju, S. (1990) Sonoembryology: an organ-oriented approach using a high frequency vaginal probe. JCU, 18, 286–98.
3. Timor-Tritsch, I.E., Blumenfeld, Z. and Rottem, S. (eds) (1991) Sonoembryology, in Transvaginal Sonography, 2nd edn, Elsevier, NY, pp. 225–98.
4. Neiman, H.L. (1991) Transvaginal ultrasound embryography. Semin. Ultrasound, CT MR, 11, 22–23.
5. England, A.M. (1983) Color Atlas of Life Before Birth; Normal Fetal Development, Year Book Medical, Chicago.
6. Moore, K.L. (1988) The Developing Human, W.B. Saunders, Philadelphia.
7. Crelin, E.S. (1981) Development of the musculo-skeletal system. CIBA Clin. Symp., 33, 2–36.
8. O'Rahilly, R. and Muller, F. (1987) Development Stages in Human Embryos, Carnegie Institution of Washington Publication 637, Washington, DC.
9. Crelin, E.S. (1974) Development of the nervous system. CIBA Clin. Symp., 26, 2–39
10. O'Rahilly, R. and Muller, F. (1992) Human Embryology and Teratology, Wiley–Liss, NY.
11. Goldstein, S.L. (1991) Endovaginal Ultrasound, 2nd edn, Liss, NY.
12. Fleischer, A.C. and Kepple, D.M. (1992) Transvaginal Sonography, Lippincott, NY.
13. Timor-Tritsch, I.E. and Rottem, S. (1991) Transvaginal Sonography, 2nd edn, Elsevier, NY.
14. Nyberg, D.A., Hill, L.M. Bohm-Vélez, M. and Mendelson, E.B. (1992) Transvaginal Ultrasound, Mosby–Year Book, St Louis.
15. Kadar, N., DeVore, G. and Romero, R. (1981) Discriminatory hCG zone; its use in the sonographic evaluation for ectopic pregnancy. Obstet. Gynecol., 58, 156–61.
16. Brauste, G.D., Grodin, J.M., Vaitukastus, J. and Ross, G.T. (1973) Secretory rates of human chorionic gonadotropin by normal trophoblast. Am. J. Obstet. Gynecol., 115, 445–49.
17. Timor-Tritsch, I.E., Farine, D. and Rosen, M.G. (1988) A close look at early embryonic development with the high frequency transvaginal transducer. Am. J. Obstet. Gynecol., 139, 676–81.
18. Goldstein, S. (1988) Very early pregnancy detection with endovaginal ultrasound. Obstet. Gynecol., 72, 200–204.
19. Nyberg, D.A., Filly, R.A., Mahoney, B.S. et al. (1985) Early gestation; correlation of hCG levels and sonographic identification. AJR, 144, 951–54.
20. Timor-Tritsch, I.E., Rottem, S. and Thaler. I. (1988) Review of transvaginal ultrasonography; a description with clinical application. Ultrasound Q., 6, 1–32.
21. Peisner, D.B., Timor-Tritsch, I.E., Margulis, E. et al. (1988) Analysis of beta-hCG and sac size in early pregnancy. J. Ultrasound Med., 7 (suppl.) S106.
22. Fossum, G.T., Dvajan, V. and Kletzky, D.A. (1988) Early detection of pregnancy with transvaginal ultrasound. Fertil. Steril., 49, 788–91.
23. Bernaschek, G., Ruaelstorfer, R. and Csaicsich, P. (1988) Vaginal sonography versus serum human chorionic gonadotropin in early detection of pregnancy. Am. J. Obstet. Gynecol., 158, 608–12.
24. Peisner, D.B. and Timor-Tritsch, I.E. (1990) The discriminatory zone of βhCG for vaginal probes. JCU, 18, 280–285.
25. Bree, R.L. and Marn, C.S. (1990) Transvaginal sonography in the first trimester: embryology anatomy and hCG correlation. Semin Ultrasound, CT MR, 11, 12–21.
26. Warren, W.B., Timor-Tritsch, I.E., Peisner, D.B. et al. (1989) Dating the early pregnancy by sequential appearance of embryonic structures. Am. J. Obstet. Gynecol., 161, 747–53.
27. Goldstein, S.R. (1991) Embryonic ultrasonographic measurements: crown rump length revisited. Am. J. Obstet. Gynecol., 165, 497–501.
28. Timor-Tritsch, I.E., Warren, W.B., Peisner, D.B. and Pirrone, E. (1989) First trimester midgut herniation: a high frequency transvaginal sonographic study. Am. J. Obstet. Gynecol., 161, 831–33.
29. Cyr, D.R., Mack, L.A., Schoenecker, S.A. et al. (1986) Bowel migration in the normal fetus. Radiology, 161, 119–21.
30. Schmidt, W., Yarkoni, S., Crelin, E.S. and Hobbins, J.C. (1987) Sonographic visualization of physiologic anterior abdominal wall hernia in the first trimester. Obstet. Gynecol., 69, 911–15.
31. Timor-Tritsch, I.E., Monteagudo, A. and Warren, W.B. (1991) Transvaginal sonographic definition of the central nervous system in the first and early second trimester. Am. J. Obstet. Gynecol., 164, 497–503.
32. Timor-Tritsch, I.E. and Monteagudo, A. (1991) Transvaginal sonographic evaluation of the fetal central nervous system. Obstet. Gynecol. Clin. North Am., 18, 713–48.
33. Timor-Tritsch, I.E., Monteagudo, A. and Peisner, D.B. (1992) High-frequency transvaginal sonographic examination for the potential malformation assessment of the 9-week to 14-week fetus. JCU, 20, 231–38.
34. Bronshtein, M., Kushnir, O., Ben-Rafael, Z. et al. (1990) Transvaginal sonographic measurement of fetal kidneys in the first trimester of pregnancy. JCU, 18, 299–301.
35. Lasser, D., Vollebergh, J., Peisner, D.B. and Timor-Tritsch, I.E. (1993) First trimester fetal biometry using high-frequency transvaginal ultrasound. Ultrasound Obstet. Gynecol., 3, 104–108.
36. Bronshtein, M., Rottem, S., Yoffe, N. et al. (1990) Early determination of fetal sex using transvaginal sonography: technique and pitfalls. JCU, 18, 302–306.
37. Monteagudo, A., Reuss, M.L. and Timor-Tritsch, I.E. (1991) Imaging the fetal brain in the second and third trimesters using transvaginal sonography. Obstet. Gynecol., 77, 27–32.
38. Reuss, A., Pijpers, L., van Swaaij, E. et al. (1987) First trimester diagnosis of recurrence of cystic hygroma using a vaginal ultrasound transducer. Eur. J. Obstet. Gynecol. Reprod. Biol., 26, 271–73.
39. Bronshtein, M. and Zimmer, E.Z. (1989) Transvaginal ultrasound diagnosis of fetal club feet at 13 weeks menstrual age. JCU, 17, 518–20.
40. Pachi, A., Giancotti, A., Torcia, F. et al. (1989) Meckel–Gruber syndrome: ultrasonographic diagnosis at 13 weeks gestational age in an at risk case. Prenat. Diagn., 9, 187–90.
41. Baxi, L., Warren, W., Collins, M.H. and Timor-Tritsch, I.E. (1990) Early detection of caudal regression syndrome with transvaginal scanning. Obstet. Gynecol., 75, 486–89.
42. Gembruch, V., Knopfe, G., Chatterjee, M. et al. (1990) First trimester diagnosis of fetal congenital heart disease of transvaginal two-dimensional and doppler echocardiography. Obstet. Gynecol., 75, 496–98.
43. Weber, T.M., Hertzberg, B.S. and Bowie, J.D. (1990) Use of endovaginal ultrasound to optimize visualization of the distal fetal spine in breech presentations. J. Ultrasound Med., 9, 519–24.
44. Bronshtein, M., Rottem, S., Yoffe, N. and Blumenfeld, Z. (1990) First-trimester and early second-trimester diagnosis of nuchal cystic hygroma by transvaginal sonography: diverse prognosis of the septated from the nonseptated lesion. Am. J. Obstet. Gynecol., 161, 78–84.

45. Cullen, M.I., Green, J., Whetham, J. *et al.* (1990) Transvaginal ultrasonographic detection of congenital anomalies in the first trimester. *Am. J. Obstet. Gynecol.*, **163**, 466–76.

46. Guzman, E.R. (1990) Early prenatal diagnosis of gastroschisis with transvaginal ultrasonography. *Am. J. Obstet. Gynecol.*, **162**, 1253–54.

47. Rottem, S. and Bronshtein, M. (1990) Transvaginal sonographic diagnosis of congenital anomalies between 9 weeks and 16 weeks, menstrual age. *JCU*, **18**, 307–14.

48. Rottem, S., Bronshtein, M., Thaler, I. and Brandes, J.M. (1990) First trimester transvaginal sonographic diagnosis of fetal anomalies. *Lancet*, i, 444–45.

49. Cullen, M.T., Athanassidiasis, A.P. and Romero, R. (1990) Prenatal diagnosis of anterior parietal encephalocele with transvaginal sonography. *Obstet. Gynecol.*, **75**, 489.

50. Bronshtein, M., Timor-Tritsch, I.E. and Rottem, S. (1991) Early detection of fetal anomalies, in *Transvaginal Sonography*, 2nd edn (eds I.E. Timor-Tritsch and S. Rottem), Elsevier, NY, pp. 327–72.

51. Bronshtein, M., Mashiah, N., Blumenfeld, D.M.D. and Blumenfeld, Z. (1991) Pseudoprognathism: an auxiliary ultrasonographic sign for transvaginal ultrasonographic diagnosis of cleft lip and palate in the early second trimester. *Am. J. Obstet. Gynecol.*, **165**, 1314–22.

52. Bronshtein, M., Zimmer, E.Z., Milo, S. *et al.* (1991) Fetal cardiac abnormalities detected by transvaginal sonography at 12–16 weeks gestation. *Obstet. Gynecol.*, **78**, 374–78.

53. Bronshtein, M., Zimmer, E.Z., Gershoni-Baruch, R. *et al.* (1991) First and second trimester diagnosis of fetal ocular defects and associated anomalies: report of eight cases. *Obstet. Gynecol.*, **77**, 443–49.

54. Szabo, J. and Gellen, J. (1991) Nuchal fluid accumulation in trisomy 21 detected by vaginosonography in first trimester. *Lancet*, **338**, 1133.

55. Maynor, C.H. Herzberg, B.S. and Ellington, K.S. (1992) Antenatal sonographic features of Walker-Warburg syndrome. *J. Ultrasound Med.*, **11**, 301–303.

56. Langrot, H., Sauerbrei, E. and Murray, S. (1991) Transvaginal Doppler sonographic diagnosis of an acardiac twin at 12 weeks gestation. *J. Ultrasound Med.*, **11**, 175–79.

57. Fleming, A.D., Vintzileos, A.M. and Scorza W.E. (1991) Prenatal diagnosis of occipital encephalocele with transvaginal sonography. *J. Ultrasound Med.*, **10**, 285–86.

58. Monteagudo, A. and Timor-Tritsch, I.E. (1992) Cephalocele. *Fetus*, **2**, 4–7.

52 ULTRASOUND DIAGNOSIS OF STRUCTURAL FETAL ANOMALIES

S.E. Chambers

52.1 Introduction

The ultrasound diagnosis of structural fetal malformations is an exciting and challenging area of prenatal diagnosis. Many anomalies will be identified on routine scans so that all those performing obstetric ultrasound examinations are obliged to be well informed about the ultrasound diagnosis of these defects. The dramatic developments of the last two decades in ultrasound technology and expertise have made it possible to diagnose a wide range of congenital anomalies, as illustrated by the comprehensive database by M. Connor in Chapter 77. In this chapter ultrasound diagnosis of the more commonly seen anomalies is described in a problem-orientated approach, the 'problem' being the first indication the sonographer has that the fetus is not normal.

52.2 Central nervous system

52.2.1 THE NORMAL FETAL HEAD AND SPINE

In the fetus the bony structure of the cranial vault may be reliably identified from the 11th week menstrual age [1]. The head is oval in shape. At 10–12 weeks the lateral ventricles, filled with echogenic choroid plexi, occupy most of the cranium. As pregnancy advances the volume of the ventricles relative to the volume of cerebral tissue diminishes until the ventriculohemispheric ratio is similar to that of the neonate. The fetal ventricles are readily measured. The simplest method is to measure the width of the atrium of the lateral ventricle (Figure 52.1a). In the normal fetus this measurement is independent of gestational age from 15 weeks until term and should not exceed 10 mm [2]. Morphological criteria are also helpful in ventricular assessment. In the normal fetus the choroid plexus virtually fills the lumen of the lateral ventricle; when the ventricles are dilated the choroid plexus sinks to the dependent lateral ventricular wall, the 'dangling choroid plexus' sign [3] (Figure 52.2). The posterior

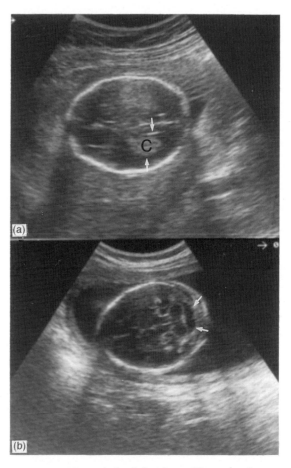

Figure 52.1 Normal fetal head at 18 weeks (transverse sections). (a) Section for measurement of the lateral ventricles; arrows mark the medial and lateral walls of the atrium. c = choroid plexus. (b) Posterior fossa. The cerebellum is seen as a dumb-bell-shaped structure at the back of the fetal head; posterior to it is the cisterna magna (arrows).

fossa may be examined in some detail (Figure 52.1b). The normal cerebellum is seen as a dumb-bell-shaped structure; posterior to it is the cisterna magna whose anteroposterior diameter should measure between 2 and 11 mm [4].

Diseases of the Fetus and Newborn, 2nd edn, Edited by G.B. Reed, A.E. Claireaux and F. Cockburn. Published in 1995 by Chapman & Hall, London. ISBN 0 412 39160 0

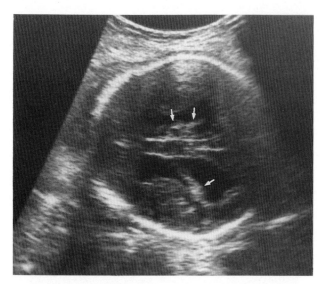

Figure 52.2 Hydrocephalus in a 34-week fetus secondary to intraventricular haemorrhage. There is dilatation of the lateral ventricles and the choroid plexus in the upper ventricle (arrows) is irregular due to the attached haematoma. The dependent ventricle demonstrates the dangling choroid plexus sign (arrow).

Detailed assessment of the fetal spine is possible transabdominally after 16 weeks. At this time three ossification centres can be visualized: one anterior in the vertebral body and two posterior in the neural arch. The spine should be imaged in three planes: a longitudinal sagittal section (Figure 52.3a) shows the curve of the fetal spine and the intact skin over the back; in a coronal longitudinal section (Figure 52.3b) the posterior ossification centres may be seen paralleling each other with flaring of the cervical region, slight widening in the lumbar region and tapering in the sacral region; on the transverse view (Figure 52.3c) the three ossification centres form a ring with the skin intact over the top. Examination of the fetal spine can be difficult and requires meticulous care and attention to scanning technique.

A detailed account of central nervous system anatomy in the first and early second trimester, as visualized by transvaginal ultrasound, is given in Chapter 51. In later pregnancy excellent views of intracranial anatomy may be obtained by transvaginal examination if the vertex is presenting. Similarly transvaginal examination may be helpful in examination of the lower spine when the fetus is presenting by the breech.

52.2.2 THE PREGNANCY WITH AN ELEVATED MATERNAL SERUM α-FETOPROTEIN (MSAFP)

The MSAFP screening programme is fully described in Chapter 62; only the role of ultrasound is described here. Accurate knowledge of gestational age is vital for

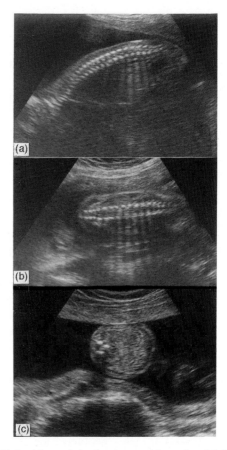

Figure 52.3 Normal fetal spine at 18 weeks. (a) Longitudinal sagittal view; (b) longitudinal coronal view; (c) transverse view, the spine is marked with arrows.

correct interpretation of the MSAFP. In as many as 15–20% of patients found to have a raised level the cause is underestimated gestation [5]. Multiple pregnancy, threatened abortion and intrauterine death may account for up to 25% of abnormal results [5]. Table 52.1 lists the fetal abnormalities found in 2289 patients with an elevated MSAFP; the figures are derived from four studies [6–9]. Defects were identified in 232 of the fetuses, illustrating that in the majority of pregnancies with an elevated MSAFP the fetus is structurally normal. Neural tube defects were the most common defect found but there were also a significant number of anterior abdominal wall defects.

An elevated MSAFP identifies a pregnancy as high risk and a careful examination of the fetus and placenta, with special attention to the central nervous system, is mandatory.

(a) Anencephaly

The ultrasonic appearances of anencephaly are typical (Figure 52.4): the facial structures are visible but the cranial vault is absent. There may be complete absence

Table 52.1 Fetal abnormalities diagnosed in 2289 patients with an elevated MSAFP [After Refs 6–9]

Abnormality	Number
Neural tube defects	
Open spina bifida	75
Anencephaly	43
Encephalocele	7
Anterior abdominal wall defects	51
Urinary tract anomalies	13
Chromosomal defects	7
Cystic hygroma/hydrops	6
Multiple anomalies and syndromes	5
Isolated hydrocephalus	3
Fetal masses	2
Cardiac defects	2
Gastrointestinal anomalies	2
Congenital adenomatoid malformation	2
Congenital infection	1
Agenesis of the corpus callosum	1
Unspecified anomalies	12
Total	232

It is likely that some of these anomalies were incidental and not related to the elevated MSAFP.

of cerebral tissue, or some disorganized tissue, the area cerebrovasculosa, may be present. Exencephaly is defined as absence of the cranium in the presence of cerebral hemispheres. This entity probably progresses to classical anencephaly as the exposed neural tissue degenerates. Its significance and the reason for distinguishing it from anencephaly lies in the potential for ultrasound misdiagnosis in the late first trimester since the cephalic pole of a fetus with exencephaly may appear remarkably normal. Thus while the diagnosis of anencephaly may be made as early as 11–12 menstrual weeks, the defect may be difficult to diagnose before 14 weeks [10]. In centres where a first trimester booking scan is performed, most cases of anencephaly will be detected before MSAFP testing.

(b) Spina bifida

The recognition that the vast majority of fetuses with open spina bifida have abnormalities of the head, which act as a pointer to the spinal lesion, has been a major advance in the ultrasound diagnosis of spina bifida [11]. In a fetus with a meningomyelocele the head may have an abnormal lemon configuration (Figure 52.5) and the ventricles may be dilated. The associated Arnold–Chiari malformation results in abnormalities of the posterior fossa: obliteration of the cisterna magna, an abnormal banana configuration of the cerebellum (Figure 52.5) or failure to visualize the cerebellum. In a recent study [12] of 1561 patients at high risk for neural tube defects, in which there were 130 affected fetuses, the lemon sign was present in 98% of those under 24 weeks, 94% had evidence of ventricular dilatation and 96% had abnormalities of the posterior fossa. Of those fetuses that were normal nine had the lemon sign, a false-positive rate of 1%. There were no false-positive posterior fossa signs.

The ultrasonic appearance of a meningomyelocele depends on the size of the lesion, the presence of a sac and the amount of bony anatomical disruption. The most reliable sign is widening of the distance between the posterior ossification centres, which produces a

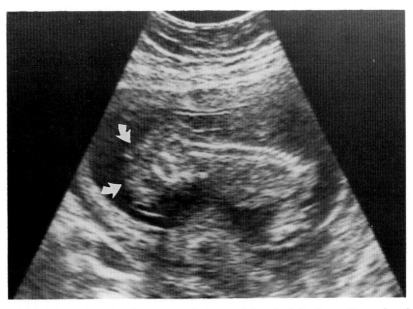

Figure 52.4 Anencephalic fetus at 12 weeks. Arrows mark the cranial end of the fetus. (Reproduced with permission from Chambers S.E. (1990) Prenatal ultrasound diagnosis I: neural tube defects. *Radiology Now*, 7(2), 20–23.)

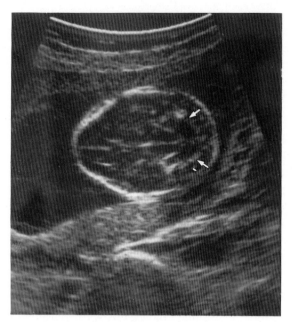

Figure 52.5 Lemon head shape ·and banana cerebellum (arrows) in an 18-week fetus with a lumbosacral myelomeningocele. (Reproduced with permission from Chambers S.E. (1990) Prenatal ultrasound diagnosis I: neural tube defects. *Radiology Now*, 7(2), 20–23.)

saucer-shaped configuration on the transverse view and may also be seen on the coronal view (Figure 52.6). The sac of a meningomyelocele may be seen as a fluid-filled structure. Some lesions are easy to identify; others, in particular low sacral lesions with little bony disorganization, can be extremely difficult to identify. In these cases it is the abnormalities of the fetal head that alert the sonographer to the presence of the spinal lesion.

(c) Encephaloceles

Most encephaloceles are skin covered and the MSAFP is not elevated. In the Western world they occur most commonly in the occipital region. A cystic swelling is identified at the back of the neck; herniated brain will appear as solid tissue within the sac (Figure 52.7). The skull defect may be identified and there are frequently associated intracranial malformations [13]. They are also associated with malformations outside the central nervous system, most notably cystic kidneys in the Meckel–Gruber syndrome.

(d) Can detailed ultrasound replace amniocentesis in patients with an elevated MSAFP? How accurate is the ultrasound diagnosis of neural tube defects in high-risk patients?

The positive predictive value of an elevated MSAFP for the diagnosis of neural tube defects is 2–4%, depending on the cut-off level used and whether there is a policy of second sample testing [14]. Therefore the MSAFP screening programme generates a large number of false positives. Assays of amniotic α-fetoprotein (AAFP) and acetylcholinesterase (AChE) have a sensitivity and specificity approaching 100% [14] in the diagnosis of neural tube defects but amniocentesis carries a significant risk of miscarriage. Women with a raised MSAFP have an increased risk of miscarriage and amniocentesis exposes these women to an additional procedure-related risk. Tabor *et al.* [15] found a 1% increase in miscarriage rate following amniocentesis, a raised MSAFP before amniocentesis being associated with an increased risk of spontaneous abortion. Details of recent studies [7,8,12,16,17] reporting the accuracy of ultrasound in the diagnosis of neural tube defects in high-risk patients are given in Table 52.2. All centres show a high level of diagnostic accuracy, but in most centres cases of open spina bifida were missed. Those confident in their ultrasound [8,12] do not advocate routine amniocentesis in patients with raised MSAFP. Platt *et al.* [17] on the other hand advise against relying on ultrasound alone. The decision as to whether to perform amniocentesis in patients with an elevated MSAFP must be taken at a local level and be based on the population prevalence of neural tube defects, the level of ·MSAFP, the detection rate of diagnostic ultrasound in individual departments and the wishes of the patient. Such calculations have been formally expressed as tables for estimation of individual risk by Thornton, Lilford and Newcombe [18]. In centres where the detection rate approaches 100% it seems reasonable to rely on ultrasound with biochemical amniotic fluid assessment as a complementary technique in cases of doubt.

(e) Can ultrasound screening replace MSAFP testing? How accurate is ultrasound in the diagnosis of neural tube defects in a low-risk population?

In general the sensitivity of MSAFP screening is 95–100% for anencephaly and 70–80% for open spina bifida [14]; thus MSAFP misses some cases of neural tube defect which might potentially be diagnosed by ultrasound. The head signs of spina bifida have been shown to be sensitive and specific in a high-risk population and are suitable for application to a low-risk population. Recent published studies [19–23] show a detection rate for ultrasound (open spina bifida) in a low-risk population of between 76 and 100%. However the study numbers are small and in some MSAFP screening was also available, making it impossible to assess the diagnostic performance of ultrasound independently.

Diagnostic ultrasound in a patient with an elevated MSAFP will be performed by an experienced sono-

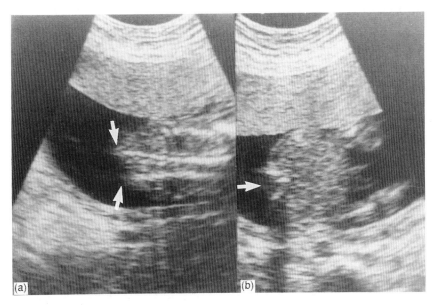

Figure 52.6 Lumbosacral myelomeningocele (arrows) in an 18-week fetus. (a) Longitudinal coronal view; (b) transverse view. (Reproduced with permission from Chambers S.E. (1990) Prenatal ultrasound diagnosis I: neural tube defects. *Radiology Now.* 7(2), 20–23.)

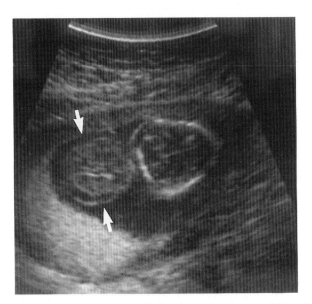

Figure 52.7 Occipital encephalocele (arrows) in an 18-week fetus.

grapher with good equipment, the index of suspicion will be high because the patient has already been identified as high risk and the prevalence of disease is high. On the other hand routine ultrasound in a low-risk patient will be performed by a less experienced sonographer, perhaps with poorer equipment and the prevalence of disease is low. A screening examination cannot therefore be expected to be as accurate as a diagnostic examination. The most success is likely to be obtained when biochemical testing is used in conjunction with ultrasound.

52.2.3 THE FETUS WITH VENTRICULOMEGALY AND AN INTACT SPINE

Causes of fetal ventriculomegaly are given in Table 52.3. Approximately 30% of cases occur in association with spina bifida. The incidence of congenital hydrocephalus with an intact spine has been estimated to be in the order of 4.9/10 000 deliveries (including live births, fetal deaths and induced abortions) [24]. If the fetal spine is intact then every attempt should be made to identify the specific cause of the hydrocephalus. Fetal hydrocephalus is often associated with other malformations and a careful search for associated structural abnormalities is essential. Some disorders, especially holoprosencephaly, are associated with chromosomal disorders and fetal karyotyping is indicated. Maternal screening for TORCH infection should also be considered. Cases of fetal ventriculomegaly form a heterogeneous group: the prognosis depends on the anatomical lesion and the presence or absence of other intracranial and extracranial malformations.

In the presence of fetal hydrocephalus it is rare for the biparietal diameter to be increased before 28 weeks. If the pregnancy continues then serial ultrasound should be performed to monitor head growth. Cerebral Doppler ultrasound studies of the middle cerebral artery may be of value in identifying those fetuses where hydrocephalus has led to raised intracranial pressure [25].

Table 52.2   Accuracy of ultrasound diagnosis of neural tube defects (NTD) in high-risk patients

| Study | No. of patients | Detection rate (%) | | False-positive rate (%) |
		All NTD	Spina bifida	
Lindfors *et al.* [7]	681	91(29/32)	73(8/11)	0.3 (2[a]/649)
Morrow *et al.* [8]	905	98(48/49)	97(38/39)	0
Van den Hof *et al.* [12]	1561	100(176/176)	100(130/130)	0
Hogge *et al.* [16]	225	100(21/21)	100(10/10)	0
Platt *et al.* [17]	–	–	92(148/161)	–

[a] Equivocal ultrasound results.
The detection rate is the proportion of affected pregnancies with an ultrasound diagnosis of NTD.
The false-positive rate is the proportion of unaffected pregnancies with an ultrasound diagnosis of NTD.

Table 52.3   Causes of fetal ventriculomegaly

Neural tube defects
Congenital hydrocephalus with an intact spine
  Aqueduct stenosis
  Communicating hydrocephalus
  Dandy–Walker malformation
Holoprosencephaly
Hydranencephaly
Agenesis corpus callosum
Porencephaly
Arachnoid cysts
Vein of Galen aneurysm
Neoplasms
Infection
Intraventricular haemorrhage (Figure 52.2)

(a)   Aqueduct stenosis

There is symmetrical dilatation of both lateral ventricles and of the third ventricle in the presence of a normal posterior fossa.

(b)   Dandy–Walker malformation (Figure 52.8)

The classical sonographic features of this disorder are absence of the cerebellar vermis with a posterior fossa cyst. There may be complete absence of the cerebellar vermis or the defect may be more subtle, involving only the inferior portion. The size of the posterior fossa cyst is also variable [26]. Hydrocephalus is not always present; in a recent review of 15 cases diagnosed antenatally it was present in 53% of fetuses [27]; in a further study of 34 cases [26] 88% showed evidence of ventricular dilatation.

(c)   Holoprosencephaly

Holoprosencephaly is characterized by failure of division of the forebrain in early embryonic development and is often associated with facial abnormalities. The ultrasound appearances depend on the severity of the lesion. In the lobar and semilobar forms there is a single ventricle, with no visible midline structures, arching over the fused thalami [28]. In the lobar form the cavum septum pellucidum is absent and the fused frontal horns of the lateral ventricles communicate centrally with the slightly dilated third ventricle. The superior aspects of the frontal horns have a characteristic squared appearance [29]. Careful examination of the fetal face, including measurement of the interorbital diameter, is essential [30].

(d)   Agenesis of the corpus callosum

In this disorder the cavum septum pellucidum is absent and there is lateral displacement of the bodies of the lateral ventricles. The pattern of ventricular dilatation is characteristic, being most marked in the posterior and occipital horns, and there may be upward displacement and enlargement of the third ventricle [31].

52.3   Genitourinary system

The fetal kidneys may be reliably visualized transabdominally from 18 weeks. They appear as relatively hypoechoic structures lying on either side of the fetal spine; the renal pelvis may be visualized as a central transonic area. The fetal bladder is seen as a fluid-filled structure in the fetal pelvis which fills and empties in an approximately 60–90-min cycle.

The reported incidence of fetal uropathies varies. In a recent study of 46 775 pregnancies [32] 78 important urinary tract anomalies were identified, giving an incidence of 1 in 600 pregnancies.

In a study of 62 antenatally diagnosed uropathies Greig *et al.* [33] reported an accurate diagnosis in 74% of cases. One of the main roles of ultrasound is to identify a group of fetuses with a probable uropathy who require investigation in postnatal life; many of these lesions would otherwise only have come to light later in life as a result of infection or renal impairment. This is illustrated by a recent review of 145 liveborn babies with a prenatally diagnosed uropathy [34]: 121 (83%) had no physical signs of urological disease at birth.

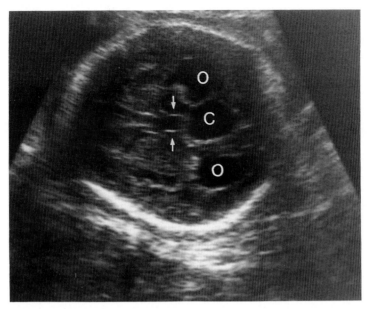

Figure 52.8 Dandy–Walker malformation in a 34-week fetus. There is a posterior fossa cyst (c) and dilatation of the occipital horns (o) and third ventricle (arrows).

Table 52.4 Causes of a dilated fetal urinary tract

Obstructive uropathies (unilateral or bilateral)
   Pelviureteric obstruction
   Vesicoureteric obstruction
   Ureteroceles
   Bladder outlet obstruction
      Urethral atresia
      Posterior urethral valves
Vesicoureteric reflux
Prune-belly syndrome
Megacystis–microcolon–intestinal hyperperistalsis syndrome

52.3.1 THE FETUS WITH A DILATED URINARY TRACT

Causes of a dilated fetal urinary tract are given in Table 52.4; dilatation frequently but not always indicates obstruction (Figure 52.9). Urinary tract dilatation may present at different gestations. In severe cases with urethral atresia it may be apparent early in pregnancy on the booking scan (Figure 52.10). Routine mid-trimester scans will reveal cases but it is well documented that at this gestation the urinary tract may appear normal even in the presence of an obstructive lesion [35]. Cases presenting later in pregnancy are often fortuitous findings on scans performed for obstetric indications. Measurement of the anteroposterior diameter of the renal pelvis is the simplest and most sensitive technique for diagnosis of fetal hydronephrosis [36]. A diameter of greater than 10 mm is the measurement most widely used [37,38] for the diagnosis of hydronephrosis; however Corteville, Gray and

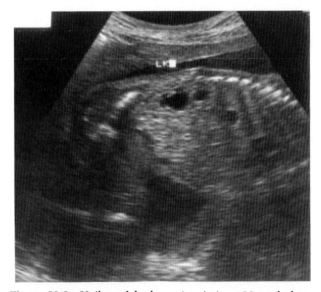

Figure 52.9 Unilateral hydronephrosis in a 20-week fetus. Postnatal investigations revealed a duplex kidney with grade IV vesicoureteric reflux.

Crane [36] recommend smaller diameters – 4 mm or greater before 33 weeks and 7 mm or greater after 33 weeks.

Once dilatation is identified serial examinations are necessary: the hydronephrosis may remain stable, improve and in some cases resolve completely, or it may progress. The kidneys are assessed to see if the hydronephrosis is unilateral or bilateral and an attempt is made to identify the level of obstruction. Pelviureteric

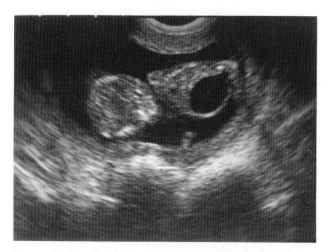

Figure 52.10 Urethral atresia in a 13-week fetus (transvaginal scan). There is marked dilatation of the fetal bladder.

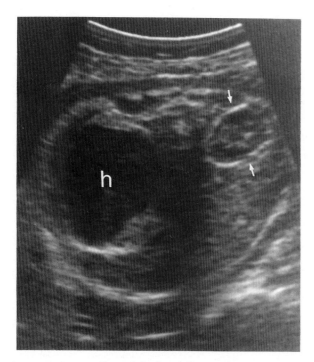

Figure 52.11 Unilateral hydronephrosis (h) in a 34-week fetus (transverse view of the abdomen) due to pelviureteric junction obstruction; normal contralateral kidney (arrows).

obstruction is identified as dilatation of the renal pelvis (Figure 52.11); in vesicoureteric junction obstruction the ureters are dilated in addition to the hydronephrosis. Ureteroceles are seen as thin-walled fluid collections in the bladder. The classical picture of bladder outlet obstruction is of a dilated bladder with bilateral hydroureter and hydronephrosis; the bladder outlet

may have a 'funnelled' appearance due to the dilated posterior urethra. Certain features may help to assess the severity of the condition: oligohydramnios carries a very poor prognosis; the width of the renal cortex can be measured; if the renal parenchyma is echogenic this indicates renal dysplasia in association with the obstruction.

A careful search for other structural abnormalities should be made and fetal karyotyping is appropriate in some cases. The role of fetal urine sampling for biochemistry and vesicoamniotic shunting is discussed in Chapter 86.

When renal dilatation is marked ultrasound assessment is relatively straightforward; more minor degrees of dilatation are more problematic and lead to dilemmas in counselling. Some of these fetuses will be normal and unnecessary anxiety is caused, but if these cases are not followed significant pathology may be missed. In many published series a proportion of fetuses with antenatally diagnosed hydronephrosis have no abnormality on postnatal investigation: Mandell *et al.* [39] 23%, Corteville, Gray and Crane [36] 29%. These 'false positives' may reflect transient fetal hydronephrosis; some may have a prominent extrarenal pelvis [40]. Transient urinary tract dilatation is often seen in mid-pregnancy and it is not known yet if this is a manifestation of undiagnosed vesicoureteric reflux. An additional consideration is the reported association between mild hydronephrosis and Down's syndrome [41].

52.3.2 THE FETUS WITH CYSTIC KIDNEYS

The differential diagnosis of fetal renal cystic disorders is given in Table 52.5.

Macroscopic cysts of the kidney may be identified on ultrasound as fluid-filled collections. Microscopic cysts are too small to resolve with ultrasound but the walls of the cysts act as multiple reflectors, resulting in diffuse increased echogenicity of the kidney. Both types of cystic lesion are included in this discussion.

As a first step cystic lesions of the kidney must be differentiated from dilatation of the renal collecting

Table 52.5 Major causes of fetal cystic kidneys

1. Renal dysplasia
    Multicystic dysplasia
    Dysplasia with congenital lower urinary tract
      obstruction
2. Polycystic kidney disease
    Autosomal recessive polycystic kidney disease
      (ARPKD)
    Autosomal dominant polycystic kidney disease
      (ADPKD)
3. Cystic disease associated with malformation syndromes

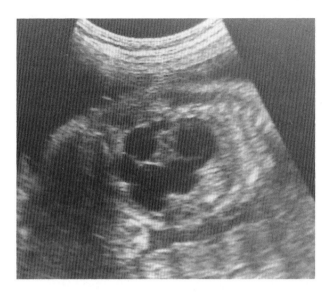

Figure 52.12 Unilateral multicystic dysplastic kidney in a 20-week fetus (longitudinal view).

systems. This is possible by careful examination and consideration of the anatomy of the pelvicalyceal system.

Multicystic dysplastic kidney (Figure 52.12) may be unilateral or bilateral. The kidneys are enlarged, with disruption of the normal renal architecture, and non-communicating cysts of varying sizes are present throughout the kidney. The renal parenchyma may show increased echogenicity. The earliest recognizable feature may be a single cyst, with an increase in the number and size of cysts as pregnancy advances. Later in pregnancy the cysts may regress and rarely complete involution *in utero* has been described [42]. Lethal disease (bilateral multicystic dysplastic kidneys or unilateral multicystic dysplastic kidney with unilateral renal agenesis) will be associated with absent bladder filling and oligohydramnios. Unilateral disease may be associated with abnormalities of the contralateral kidney, particularly pelviureteric junction obstruction. Associated extrarenal anomalies are common with bilateral disease but rare with unilateral disease.

Cystic dysplasia of the kidneys may result from severe *in utero* obstruction: the gestation at which the obstruction develops is critical to the development of the dysplasia. Typically the renal parenchyma is echogenic, there may be small cortical cysts and there is evidence of renal tract dilatation.

The classical appearances of autosomal recessive polycystic kidney disease (ARPKD) are bilateral enlarged and diffusely echogenic kidneys (Figure 52.13). Oligohydramnios is characteristic but is not an invariable finding [43]. There are however a number of potential pitfalls in making this diagnosis. The disorder has a wide spectrum of severity and only the most

severe forms of the perinatal type are likely to be diagnosed *in utero*. Ultrasound examination of the kidneys at 20 weeks may be normal, with the characteristic changes only developing after fetal viability in the late second or third trimester. There is also the potential for false-positive diagnosis [44] and caution should be exercised when there is no family history of the disorder.

Many individuals with autosomal dominant polycystic kidney disease (ADPKD) will be born with ultrasonically normal kidneys. There are, however, now several reports in the literature of the prenatal ultrasound diagnosis of this disorder [45–48] which presumably represent a more severe form in the spectrum of disease. Most reports describe enlarged echogenic kidneys, in some cases with macroscopic cysts. McHugo *et al.* [46] describe two cases in which the kidneys were enlarged with accentuation of the corticomedullary junction but no cystic changes. The appearances may be indistinguishable from ARPKD. As with ARPKD the kidneys may be normal at 20 weeks, with changes only developing later in pregnancy. A positive family history is crucial in making the diagnosis and the chance finding of abnormal fetal kidneys is an indication for renal ultrasound of the parents.

Many syndromes are associated with cystic kidneys, e.g. Meckel's syndrome and chromosomal disorders. The finding of cystic kidneys should therefore always prompt a careful examination of the fetus, looking for other malformations which might indicate the diagnosis of a syndrome (Chapter 36).

52.4 The abdomen

52.4.1 THE FETUS WITH AN ANTERIOR ABDOMINAL WALL DEFECT

The incidence of exomphalos and gastroschisis is in the order of 2.7 in 10 000 and 0.9 in 10 000 deliveries (fetal deaths, induced abortions and live births) [24] respectively. Complex body wall defects are less common, with an incidence of approximately 1 in 25 000 deliveries. Defects of the anterior abdominal wall commonly present with an elevated MSAFP. Exomphalos is less likely to present in this way since the defect is covered, preventing the leakage of protein.

The ultrasonic appearances are characteristic and gastroschisis may be reliably distinguished from exomphalos. In the former the defect is paramedian (usually to the right), the umbilical cord inserts normally into the abdominal wall and loops of bowel may be seen floating free in the amniotic cavity (Figure 52.14). In exomphalos the abdominal contents herniate into the base of the umbilical cord and are therefore covered by a sac. The umbilical cord inserts into the apex of this sac and there may be ascites. The diagnosis of exom-

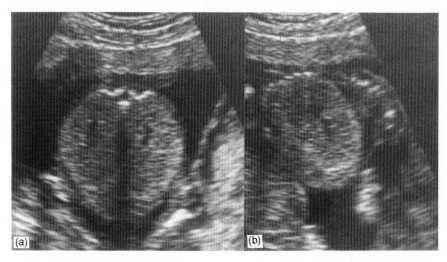

Figure 52.13 Autopsy proven ARPKD in a 20-week fetus. The kidneys are enlarged with increased echogenicity. The fetal abdomen is distended. (a) Transverse view; (b) longitudinal view.

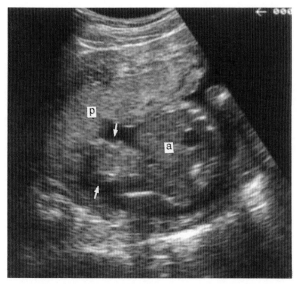

Figure 52.14 Gastroschisis (arrows) in an 18-week fetus. A = Fetal abdomen; p = placenta.

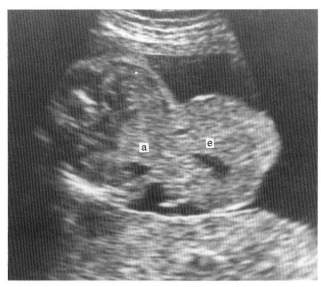

Figure 52.15 Large exomphalos (e) in a 20-week fetus. a = Fetal abdomen.

phalos should not be made before 12 menstrual weeks because of the normal physiological gut herniation prior to this gestation. The appearances of exomphalos are variable depending on the contents of the sac. Those containing only bowel are smaller and harder to detect than those containing bowel and liver (Figure 52.15). It has been suggested that small lesions are more commonly associated with chromosomal defects [49]. Polyhydramnios may be seen in about one-third of patients with exomphalos and is associated with a poor fetal prognosis [49]. Complex body wall defects may be associated with spinal, cranial and limb defects

and failure to identify the fetal bladder should suggest cloacal exstrophy.

It must be remembered that associated structural anomalies are common with exomphalos. They are present in up to 70% of cases [50–52], the most frequent being cardiac defects, seen in up to 55% of cases [50,51]. Detailed echocardiography and fetal karyotyping are therefore essential in the assessment of these fetuses. The most common defects seen in association with gastroschisis affect the bowel. Ischaemic lesions or areas of atresia are present in up to 30% of cases [50,52,53]. In fetuses with gastroschisis the bowel should be monitored by ultrasound in the third trimester. The finding of bowel dilatation and thickening of the bowel wall correlates well with bowel complications postnatally [54]. Other structural anomalies are uncommon in association with gastroschisis: cardiac defects are the most common with a reported incidence of up to 12% of cases [50,52,53]. Chromosomal anomalies are rarely seen in association with gastroschisis.

The prognosis of anterior abdominal wall defects depends on the presence of associated abnormalities. In isolated defects the postnatal surgical results are excellent for both gastroschisis and exomphalos, with survival rates of 90%. Current opinion favours vaginal delivery in these patients.

52.4.2 THE FETUS WITH AN INTRA-ABDOMINAL CYSTIC MASS

Table 52.6 lists the major differential diagnoses for an intra-abdominal cystic structure. A careful examination of the abdominal anatomy is necessary to differentiate these from the normal fluid-filled stomach and bladder and to attempt to identify the source of the abnormality.

Duodenal obstruction occurs in approximately 1 in 10 000 pregnancies and may be due to either complete or partial obliteration of the lumen. The classical sonographic appearance is of dilatation of the stomach and duodenum giving the double-bubble appearance (Figure 52.16). Polyhydramnios is present in about half of cases [55,56]. Patients may also present after spontaneous rupture of the membranes, in which case liquor volume is reduced and the diagnosis is apparent because of the dilated stomach and duodenum. In the

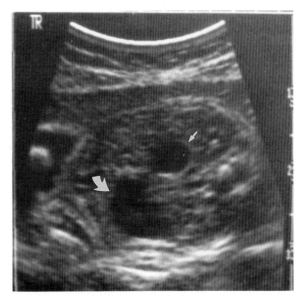

Figure 52.16 Duodenal atresia. Transverse view of the fetal abdomen showing the dilated stomach (large arrow) and duodenum (small arrow).

majority of cases the diagnosis is not made until after 24 weeks but earlier diagnosis has been reported [56,57]. In a recent series [56] an antenatal diagnosis of duodenal obstruction was made in 15 of the 34 cases. In the same series concurrent anomalies were present in 65% of cases. It is associated with the VACTERL syndrome and about 30% of cases have Down's syndrome. Outcome is influenced by prematurity (54%), low birth weight and associated congenital anomalies. Antenatal diagnosis leads to earlier postnatal surgery but Hancock and Wiseman [56] found that it did not otherwise change the outcome of affected infants.

The estimated incidence of jejunoileal atresias is between 1 in 3000 and 1 in 5000 [57]. Ultrasonic appearances of jejunoileal atresias are dilated small bowel loops (these may show strong peristalsis) proximal to the obstruction and there is often associated polyhydramnios. The overall sensitivity of ultrasound in the diagnosis of small bowel atresias is unknown but is probably low [57]. Associated extraintestinal anomalies are uncommon; there are however frequently associated bowel anomalies, including malrotation, volvulus, anterior abdominal wall defects, meconium ileus and peritonitis, enteric duplications and other bowel atresias.

Anal atresia occurs in approximately 1 in 5000 births. Bowel dilatation is the primary ultrasound finding. However this is variable (Harris et al. [58] found it in only 5/12 (42%) of cases) and the lesion

Table 52.6 Causes of a fetal intra-abdominal cystic mass

Gastrointestinal system
Dilated bowel loops (duodenal, jejunoileal atresias, anal atresia)
Meconium peritonitis

Genitourinary system
Dilated renal tract
Renal cysts

Other
Ovarian cysts
Mesenteric cysts
Choledochal cysts
Hepatic cysts
Presacral teratoma

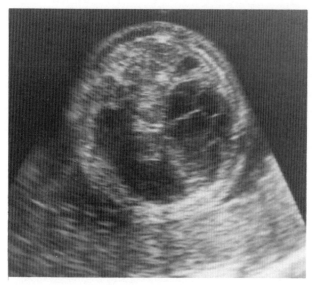

Figure 52.17 Cystic meconium peritonitis in a 28-week fetus. Transverse view of the abdomen showing multiloculate cystic spaces.

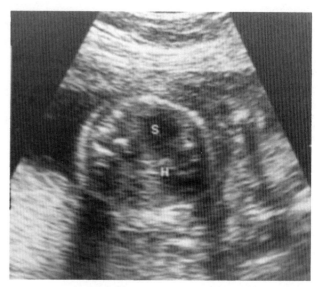

Figure 52.18 Diaphragmatic hernia. Transverse view of the thorax showing the stomach (S) and heart (H) in the same plane.

may not present any ultrasound features which are detectable antenatally. Associated anomalies are common, in particular those related to the VACTERL syndrome or the caudal regression syndrome.

Meconium peritonitis may be diagnosed antenatally [59]. In the cystic form (Figure 52.17) single or multiple cystic or hypoechoic masses may be seen in the abdomen, often with a calcified rim and associated ascites. In the diffuse form hyperechoic calcific foci may be seen together with ascites and polyhydramnios.

Fetal ovarian cysts appear as well-defined fluid collections, usually to one side of the midline, in a female fetus. The antenatal diagnosis must however be presumptive since rare lesions such as mesenteric cysts will have a similar appearance. Ovarian cysts may remain static or regress *in utero*. Torsion of the cysts may result in particulate material forming within the cyst and layering in the bottom. In a series of 15 cases [60] this appearance was seen in six fetuses and the diagnosis of torsion was confirmed in all at postnatal surgery (Chapter 35).

52.5   The fetus with an intrathoracic mass lesion

Table 52.7 gives the main differential diagnoses of an intrathoracic mass. A lesion may be identified by its mass effect (mediastinal displacement) and echogenicity, if this differs significantly from the surrounding tissues. Cystic lesions, e.g. stomach in a left-sided congenital diaphragmatic hernia and bronchogenic cysts, are relatively easy to identify but solid lesions,

Table 52.7   Major causes of an intrathoracic fetal mass

Hydrothorax
Congenital diaphragmatic hernia
Cystic adenomatoid malformation
Bronchopulmonary sequestration
Bronchogenic cysts
Bronchial atresia
Teratomas
Neuroblastoma
Hamartoma
Foregut duplication cyst
Mediastinal cystic hygroma

e.g. herniated liver in a right-sided congenital diaphragmatic hernia, are more difficult to identify. The potential life-threatening complications of chest masses are pulmonary hypoplasia secondary to compression and hydrops secondary to obstruction of venous return. Spontaneous regression of lung lesions *in utero* has been reported in a few cases [61–63].

Congenital diaphragmatic hernia (Figure 52.18) occurs in between 1 in 2000 and 1 in 5000 deliveries. The defect is usually posterolateral at the foramen of Bochdalek; the majority occur on the left side. In a recent series [64] of 65 cases, 92% were Bochdalek hernias (78% left, 14% right), 1.5% were Morgagni hernias and 1.5% involved complete absence of the diaphragm. There was insufficient information to classify the remainder. In this series 28% of the fetuses had major associated defects (structural and chromosomal).

In another large series [65] (94 cases), 16% of fetuses had associated lethal defects. A careful search should therefore be made for other structural defects and fetal karyotyping is indicated. Adzick *et al.* [66] found a 16% incidence of chromosomal anomalies in a series of 38 cases. Nicolaides, Gosden and Snijders [67] report a similar incidence: 20% in a series of 79 cases. The ultrasound features of congenital diaphragmatic hernia are the presence of herniated abdominal viscera in the thorax, resulting in distortion of the upper abdominal anatomy and mediastinal shift. Movement of herniated viscera in and out of the chest has been noted in several fetuses [65], suggesting that congenital diaphragmatic hernia is a dynamic process. Attempts have been made to assess the prognosis on the basis of the ultrasonic features. Early herniation of a large volume of viscera through a large defect results in severe pulmonary hypoplasia [65]. In a later study by this group [66], 14 fetuses diagnosed prior to 24 weeks all died. Poly-hydramnios, present in approximately 70% of cases [65,66] has been associated with poor prognosis. Fetuses with congenital diaphragmatic hernia may show disproportion in the size of the cardiac ventricles with apparent reduction in the size of the left ventricle due either to compression by the herniated organs or altered haemodynamics. Crawford *et al.* [68] found this to be associated with a poor prognosis. In a series of 19 cases the presence of ventricular disproportion in the second trimester was associated with 100% mortality; the absence of ventricular disproportion in the third trimester suggested a good prognosis. Finally the prognosis will of course be influenced by the presence of associated malformations. For discussion of the outcome and surgical implications of congenital dia-phragmatic hernia the reader is referred to Chapter 87.

Fetal pleural effusions (Figure 52.19) have been estimated to occur in approximately 1 in 15 000 pregnancies [69]. They are seen on ultrasound as transonic collections lying between the chest wall and lung edge. They may be unilateral or bilateral and vary in size from just a thin rim of fluid to much larger collections causing mediastinal shift and lung compres-sion. There is commonly associated polyhydramnios. They are seen in association with generalized fetal hydrops (with ascites and skin oedema) or as an isolated finding. Fetal hydrops may occur as a con-sequence of a large pleural effusion. The most common cause of isolated effusions is chylothorax; they may also be seen in association with chromosomal anomal-ies and pulmonary lymphangiectasia and may develop secondary to intrathoracic mass lesions. The overall perinatal mortality associated with pleural effusions is 46% [70], the prognosis being worse in fetuses with hydrops than in those where effusions are isolated. *In utero* drainage of effusions is possible. The diagnosis of chylothorax may be made by lipoprotein electrophor-

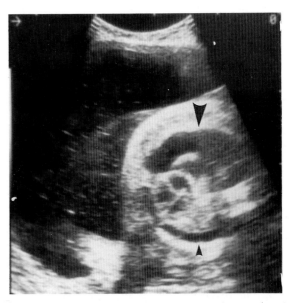

Figure 52.19 Transverse view of the fetal thorax showing bilateral pleural effusions (arrows). In addition there is subcutaneous oedema and polyhydramnios.

esis of the pleural fluid [71]. Pleural fluid tends to reaccumulate rapidly after thoracocentesis; indwelling pleuroamniotic shunts provide better long-term drainage [69]. The aims of drainage are to prevent pulmonary compression and the development of pul-monary hypoplasia. There is no consensus view about the most appropriate management of isolated effusions. Many fetuses survive with conservative management; spontaneous resolution has been documented in a number of cases [69,72] and drainage procedures are not without risk [72]. A recent meta-analysis of 124 cases [70] found that fetuses who had drainage pro-cedures had a better outcome.

The ultrasonic appearances of cystic adenomatoid malformation depends on the size of the cysts. Diag-nosis of all types has been reported at 20 weeks [73–75]. Type 1 lesions [76] (cyst size greater than 2 cm) appear as single or multiple cysts within the chest. This type of lesion has the best prognosis, and is the most commonly reported lesion antenatally. Type 2 lesions (cyst size less than 1 cm) create a mass with numerous small cysts; at 20 weeks these lesions show a prepon-derance of echogenic tissue [74]. This type is often associated with other anomalies (Stocker, Madewell and Drake [76]: 9 out of 16 cases) and is the most infrequently reported antenatally. Type 3 lesions (cyst size less than 0.5 cm) appear as echogenic solid lesions. There may be complete bilateral involvement, in which case the main differential diagnosis is from laryngeal atresia. The prognosis of this type of lesion is poor. As with all intrathoracic masses cystic adenomatoid mal-formation may be associated with hydrops and poly-hydramnios. *In utero* regression of apparent cystic adenomatoid malformation has been described in a few cases [60,61]. *In utero* surgical intervention is reported – both resection of the lesion [77] and drainage of large cysts to avoid compressive complications [78].

Bronchopulmonary sequestration appears sonographically as a well-defined echogenic mass. Intralobar sequestrations occur with equal frequency on the left and right; approximately 80% of extralobar sequestrations occur in the left hemithorax. Approximately 5% of sequestrations occur below the diaphragm [73]. Associated malformations are common with extralobar sequestration (60%) but less so with the intralobar type (14%). Both types may be complicated by hydrops and pleural effusion. Diagnosis at 19 weeks by demonstration of feeding vessels originating from the aorta has been reported [79] (Chapters 32 and 87).

52.6 Abnormalities of liquor volume

52.6.1 THE FETUS WITH POLYHYDRAMNIOS

Amniotic fluid volume is assessed in every ultrasound examination and the experienced observer can subjectively diagnose polyhydramnios or oligohydramnios. Objective assessment is based on measurement of the vertical height of pools of liquor. Mild polyhydramnios is defined as a maximum vertical height of 8–12 cm, moderate as 12–16 cm and severe as greater than 16 cm [80,81]. An alternate method is to sum the vertical heights of liquor pools in the four quadrants. The total is referred to as the amniotic fluid index; a value of 24 cm or greater is considered to indicate polyhydramnios [82]. Caution should be exercised in diagnosing polyhydramnios before the third trimester because an apparent increase in liquor volume in the second trimester may be normal.

The prevalence of polyhydramnios is between 0.4 and 1.0%; mild forms occur more often than severe forms. In a series of 102 cases, Hill *et al.* [80] found 79% of cases to be mild, 19% moderate and 4% severe. The causes of polyhydramnios are given in Table 52.8. The incidence of malformations is greater in cases with severe hydramnios.

Table 52.8 Causes of polyhydramnios

Cause	Incidence (%)
Idiopathic	34–66.7
Maternal causes	
Diabetes	15–24.6
Pre-eclampsia	up to 17
Fetal causes	
Malformations	13–43
Multiple pregnancy	5–8.5

These figures are derived from several studies [80,83,84,85] and therefore do not sum. Some may reflect selection bias.

Table 52.9 Malformations resulting in polyhydramnios

Type	Incidence (%)
Central nervous system	23–52
Gastrointestinal system	10–47
Cardiovascular system	9–30
Skeletal system	4.5–11.5
Renal	14–16
Hydrops	18–21
Chromosome	4–22

These figures are derived from several studies [80,82,83,84] and therefore do not sum.

Once it has been established that there is polyhydramnios a careful search for anomalies should be made, keeping in mind the possible sites of defects (Table 52.9). Mild polyhydramnios makes ultrasound examination easier. Severe forms can hamper the examination since, due to the large volume of amniotic fluid, the fetus may lie posteriorly, outwith the focal range of the transducer.

The gastrointestinal defects which commonly give rise to polyhydramnios are the foregut atresias. The classical features of oesophageal atresia are increased liquor volume and absent stomach bubble. However in 90% of cases there is an associated fistula and the ultrasound findings will depend on the size and ability of the fistula to cope with the transit of liquor. If the fistula is wide the stomach will fill and liquor volume will be normal. In a series of 22 cases Pretorius *et al.* [86] found the combination of absent stomach bubble and polyhydramnios in only 32% of cases.

The ultrasound features of duodenal atresia are described in section 52.4.2.

Renal abnormalities have been associated with polyhydramnios; these are usually unilateral (multicystic dysplastic kidney and pelviureteric junction obstruction) but bilateral disorders have also been reported [81].

Chromosome disorders should not be forgotten and fetal karyotyping should be considered in pregnancies complicated by severe polyhydramnios [82,87].

52.6.2 THE FETUS WITH OLIGOHYDRAMNIOS (Table 52.10)

Between 0.5 and 5.5% of pregnancies are complicated by oligohydramnios, depending on the criteria used for

Table 52.10 Causes of oligohydramnios

Fetal anomaly
Intrauterine growth retardation
Premature rupture of the membranes
Post-term pregnancy
Presumed placental insufficiency and elevated MSAFP
Drugs

diagnosis [88]. Oligohydramnios may be diagnosed by subjective criteria or by objective assessment of liquor pools. There are several criteria in the literature for the semiquantitative assessment of oligohydramnios. The most widely used measurement has been the vertical height of the largest cord and limb-free pool. Manning, Hill and Platt [89] defined oligohydramnios as being present when this measurement was less than 1 cm; other workers have used 2 cm or 3 cm [90–92]. Fisk et al. [93] defined severe oligohydramnios as the deepest liquor pool of less than 1 cm, moderate 1.1–2 cm and mild 2.1–3.0 cm. Using the amniotic fluid index, Phelan et al. [94] defined oligohydramnios as a measurement of less than 5.

Ultrasound examination of the fetus is severely hampered by oligohydramnios. The normal acoustic window and fetal–fluid interfaces which aid imaging are lost and the fetus lies in a flexed position with crowding of the small parts, making examination difficult. The improved resolution and proximity to the fetus which transvaginal ultrasound provides may be helpful in this situation [95]. Another approach is to inject warmed isotonic fluid into the amniotic cavity, a procedure known as amnioinfusion [93,96]. In a series of 61 patients with oligohydramnios, Fisk et al. [93] were able to revise the diagnosis of the underlying aetiology in 13% of patients, either as a result of improved visualization or determination of membranous integrity. The procedure may be followed by vaginal leakage and there is some debate as to whether this is the result of the amnioinfusion or is due to unmasking of pre-existing ruptured membranes [93].

In the presence of oligohydramnios the ultrasonographer must attempt to answer three questions. Is there evidence of a fetal malformation to account for the reduced liquor? Is fetal size appropriate for dates; could the reduced liquor be due to intrauterine growth retardation? Has the oligohydramnios resulted in pulmonary hypoplasia? The emphasis placed on these questions depends on the gestation at which the patient presents.

Renal abnormalities are most frequently associated with oligohydramnios. Severe obstructive uropathy, bilateral renal agenesis, ARPKD, and lethal forms of multicystic dysplastic kidney may all be seen in association with severe oligohydramnios. The ultrasonic diagnosis of renal agenesis is particularly difficult since it is harder to diagnose the absence of a structure than the presence of an abnormal structure. Hypertrophied adrenal glands filling the renal fossae may give the false impression of kidneys.

Severe oligohydramnios may be seen in the second trimester with or without fetal malformations. In some cases this is associated with an elevated MSAFP. Severe oligohydramnios at this gestation carries a very poor prognosis regardless of the aetiology. In a review of 94

cases published in the literature [97] there were only eight survivors. Between 5 and 10% of fetuses with second trimester oligohydramnios will have a chromosomal anomaly [98] and karyotyping should be considered. Doppler studies of the uteroplacental and fetal circulations may also help to define the aetiology of the oligohydramnios [98].

Fetal pulmonary hypoplasia is a severe consequence of prolonged oligohydramnios and reliable antenatal detection is desirable for obstetric management and counselling of the parents. Blott et al. [99] suggested fetal breathing movements as a predictor of favourable outcome in pregnancies complicated by premature rupture of the membranes and oligohydramnios. Moessinger et al. [100] did not confirm these findings: they observed fetal breathing movements in eight fetuses who died in the neonatal period with a necropsy diagnosis of pulmonary hypoplasia. Measurements of fetal chest size, which reflect lung mass, ratios reflecting cardiothoracic disproportion and ratios demonstrating disproportion with other parts of the body have also been used to diagnose pulmonary hypoplasia in the fetus. Vintzileos et al. [101] studied six parameters: chest circumference, chest area, chest area minus heart area, chest circumference to abdominal circumference ratio, chest area to heart area ratio and chest area minus heart area divided by chest area ratio. They found the last parameter to be the most sensitive and specific in the diagnosis of lethal pulmonary hypoplasia. It also has the advantage of being gestation independent (Chapter 79).

52.7 The fetus with a short limb dysplasia

The birth prevalence of skeletal dysplasias has been estimated as 2.4 per 10 000 births [102]. Table 52.11 lists short limb dysplasias which have been diagnosed antenatally by ultrasound. This list is not exhaustive; for information about other dysplasias the reader is referred to the database in Chapter 77. Thanatophoric dysplasia and achondrogenesis together account for approximately 62% of all lethal skeletal dysplasias; heterozygous achondroplasia is the most common non-lethal dysplasia [103] (Chapter 43).

A full discussion of the ultrasound antenatal diagnosis of skeletal dysplasias is beyond the scope of this chapter; more detailed accounts are available in longer works [103,104,106,107].

Fetuses with a short limb dysplasia are usually identified at examinations performed because of a previous affected sibling or by a shortened femur length found on routine ultrasound examination in a patient with no prior history (Figure 52.20). Accurate knowledge of gestational age is necessary for the interpretation of limb lengths. In patients with uncertain gestational age comparison may be made between limb

Table 52.11 Major short limb dysplasias which have been diagnosed *in utero* [After Refs 103–105]

Dysplasia	Pattern of limb shortening	Small thorax	Large head	Bone density	Bone shape	Other features
Thanatophoric dysplasia	Severe micromelia	+	May be cloverleaf skull + hydrocephalus	−	Bowed, telephone receiver-shaped femora	May be polyhydramnios and hydrops
Heterozygous achondroplasia	Rhizomelia	−	+ May be hydrocephalus	Normal	−	Limb growth may be normal until late second trimester
Homozygous achondroplasia	Severe micromelia	+	+ May be hydrocephalus	−	−	−
Osteogenesis imperfecta						
Type I	Mild shortening or normal	−	−	Decreased	Bowed femora	10% have intrauterine fractures
Type II	Severe micromelia	+	−	Markedly decreased	Severe bowing; multiple fractures	−
Type III	Mild micromelia	+	−	Decreased	Severe bowing; fractures	−
Achondrogenesis	Severe micromelia	+	+	Markedly decreased	−	May be hydropic
Asphyxiating thoracic dysplasia	Mild micromelia	+	−	Normal	−	Renal dysplasia common; polydactyly
Camptomelic dysplasia	Mild micromelia	+	+ May be hydrocephalus	Decreased	Bowed femora and tibia	Scapula may be small; micrognathia
Hypophosphatasia	Severe micromelia	+	−	Markedly decreased	Fractures	
Short rib polydactyl syndromes	Severe micromelia	+	−	−	Bowed long bones	Kidneys may be dysplastic; polydactyly
Robert's syndrome	Hypoplastic or absent long bones	−	−	Normal	−	May be microcephaly, cleft lip, polydactyly
Diastrophic dysplasia	Mild micromelia	+	−	−	Bowing of all long bones	Hitchhiker thumb; kyphosis
Chondroectodermal dysplasia	Mild micromelia	+	−	Normal	−	50% congenital heart disease; polydactyly
Mesomelic dysplasias	Mesomelia[a]	−	−	−	−	−

[a] Langer, Nievergelt, Reinhardt, Robinow and Werner syndromes (see database in Chapter 77 and Chapter 43).

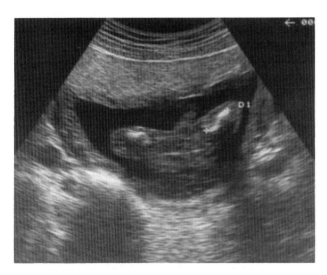

Figure 52.20 Shortened bowed femur in a 20-week fetus with a severe lethal short limb dysplasia.

lengths and head measurements [103]; this will of course be invalidated if the head is involved in the dysplasia and abnormal in size. In heterozygous achondroplasia limb growth may be normal until the late second or third trimester and serial examinations should therefore be performed.

Once it has been established that there is evidence of a skeletal dysplasia then the fetus should be examined in a systematic way to try and establish the precise nature of the disorder. All limb bones should be identified and measured and the measurements related to nomograms of limb length [103,106]. Comparison should be made between the length of the segments of the limbs to determine if the dysplasia is rhizomelic (shortened humerus, femur), mesomelic (shortened tibia/fibula, radius/ulna) or micromelic (all segments shortened). The bones should then be evaluated for fractures, bowing and mineralization. Assessment of mineralization is difficult; useful signs include unusual clarity of intracranial anatomy and compressibility of the fetal head, decreased bone echogenicity with weak acoustic shadowing and absent or decreased visualization of the spine. The head should be examined and may show enlargement with normal intracranial anatomy, hydrocephalus or rarely a clover-leaf skull deformity with symmetrical protrusion in the temporal regions. The chest size should be evaluated since lethal pulmonary hypoplasia is associated with many short limb dysplasias. The hands and feet should be examined, looking for polydactyly and syndactyly. Polyhydramnios may be present; Pretorius et al. [107] found this in 12 of a series of 13 fetuses with short limb dysplasias, and in the same series five (38%) of the fetuses were hydropic. Fetal radiology may further help to define the skeletal abnormalities.

It may not be possible to reach a specific diagnosis but ultrasound examination will provide sufficient information for appropriate management of the pregnancy and counselling of the parents. A definitive diagnosis, with its implications for future pregnancies, can then be made after delivery on clinical, pathological and radiological examination.

52.8 Accuracy of antenatal ultrasound diagnosis of fetal anomalies

The accuracy of ultrasound antenatal diagnosis must be considered in two ways. Firstly, if a well-defined community-based pregnant population is offered ultrasound examination then what proportion of the anomalies occurring in that population will be detected by ultrasound? Secondly, how precise is ultrasound diagnosis and how does the prenatal diagnosis correlate with the postnatal diagnosis?

Before discussing these two options consideration must be given to factors which impose limitations on ultrasound diagnosis. Ultrasound is an operator dependent modality and results are related to the experience of the operator. Results are also dependent on the equipment used. Modern real-time equipment is capable of producing high resolution images of fetal anatomy but not all departments will have 'state of the art' machines. A distinction must be made between diagnostic examinations and screening examinations. The former will be performed by a highly experienced ultrasonographer using good equipment, the patient has already been identified as 'high risk', the prevalence of disease is high and the index of suspicion will be high. In comparison, a screening examination is performed in a low-risk population, the prevalence of disease is low, the index of suspicion will be low, the ultrasonographer will probably have less experience of anomalies and may be using poorer equipment. For these reasons a screening examination cannot be expected to achieve the same results as a diagnostic examination. A detailed examination of the fetus is time consuming and meticulous care as well as skill is required; if fetal position is unfavourable for visualization of a particular area and the fetus cannot be manoeuvred into a more favourable position, then the ultrasonographer must be prepared to reschedule the examination. The examination may also be limited by maternal obesity. The problems involved in imaging the fetus with oligohydramnios have already been discussed. Lesions which result in a major disorganization of fetal anatomy or marked changes in echo pattern (e.g. large exomphalos, cystic lesions) are relatively easy to identify. Lesions however which result in only a minor disruption of the anatomy (e.g. small atrial or ventricular septal defects) will be very difficult or impossible to detect. Timing of the examination is also important as some lesions may not manifest until the late second or third trimester (e.g. microcephaly, some obstructive uropathies, duodenal atresia) and affected fetuses may be 'ultrasonically normal' at 18–20 weeks when most detailed scans are performed.

52.8.1 ULTRASOUND DETECTION OF FETAL ANOMALIES IN A COMMUNITY-BASED POPULATION

An ultrasound service for the detection of fetal anomalies may be used alone or in conjunction with MSAFP screening. There are two main models for the provision of ultrasound in this context. In the first, an examination is offered to all pregnant women irrespective of their risk factors (routine fetal anomaly scanning). This examination is best performed between 18 and 20 weeks, a gestation which offers the best compromise between early detection and a fetal size and stage of development which permits ultrasound diagnosis. Since the majority of fetal anomalies will occur in women with no identifiable risk factors such a policy should have the best chance of high fetal anomaly detection rates. There is however no consensus view and there is still debate about the validity of such scans as screening tests [108–111]. Several concerns have been expressed. Not all anomalies are currently amenable to diagnosis at 18–20 weeks; the cost-effectiveness is uncertain; there is incomplete understanding of the natural history of some anomalies; dilemmas in counselling and unnecessary patient anxiety may result from the finding of minor abnormalities such as choroid plexus cysts and mild hydronephrosis; and there are difficulties involved in ensuring a universally high standard of ultrasound examination. There are now a number of studies reporting the accuracy of routine scanning for congenital malformations: Levi et al. [21] reported a detection rate of 21% of anomalies when scanning was conducted before 22 weeks, with a specificity of 99.9%; Brocks and Bang [20] detected 36% of anomalies in the second trimester with a specificity of 99.9%. Other studies [22,23] report detection rates of 70–74%, with specificities again of 99.9%.

An alternative way in which ultrasound is used for the detection of malformations is to perform examinations only on those patients considered to be at high risk of fetal anomaly, a policy of selective scanning. The concerns with this type of ultrasound provision are that anomalies will be missed in those patients with no identifiable risk factors and when an anomaly is diagnosed after 24 weeks the parents will be denied the full range of management options, principally termination [112]. We recently reviewed our own experience [113] (of 19 497 deliveries) in which selective scanning was combined with MSAFP screening. Thirty-five per cent of anomalies were diagnosed by ultrasound prior to 24 weeks and 20% after 24 weeks. Forty per cent of anomalies were not diagnosed antenatally. These cases, together with those where an antenatal diagnosis was only made after 24 weeks, were reviewed. In 69% of these cases it was considered that the anomaly was not one which was likely to have been detected on an 18–20 week screening examination. Of the remaining 31% of cases (in whom the lesion might have been detected on a routine anomaly scan) half had defects which were lethal, half of the babies survived, many with no major handicap, and in many of these cases earlier diagnosis would not have altered management. The primary aim of prenatal diagnosis is the early detection of chronically handicapping disorders. Early detection of lethal anomalies may be desirable but its value is debatable, the final outcome is not altered and earlier diagnosis must be justified in terms of improved obstetric decision making and reduction in parental suffering. It is doubtful whether a policy of routine scanning applied to our population would achieve the primary aim of a significant reduction in the incidence of chronic handicapping disorders in childhood.

52.8.2 THE PRECISION OF ULTRASOUND DIAGNOSIS

Several studies from secondary and tertiary referral centres have addressed this topic. A common theme emerges: prenatal ultrasound diagnoses are accurate overall but may be insensitive to associated anomalies. False-positive rates are low. In a study reported by Manchester et al. [114], 99% of antenatal diagnoses were confirmed; however 37% of those infants born with anomalies had additional problems not diagnosed by ultrasound. The false-positive rate was 1.5%. In two studies comparing prenatal ultrasound diagnoses with autopsy findings [115,116], additional findings relevant to parental counselling were found in 46% and 42% of cases. Similarly Clayton-Smith et al. [117] in their series found that 40% of antenatal diagnoses were revised after termination in a way which affected genetic counselling. In a further recent series [118], 89% of diagnoses were confirmed after delivery or termination but in 36% of these cases there were additional anomalies not diagnosed antenatally; in 1.7% of cases a false-positive diagnosis was made. In the remaining 9.3% of cases a full postnatal examination had not been made; in many cases this was because there had been a suction termination of the pregnancy.

References

1. Rottem, S. and Bronshtein, M. (1990) Transvaginal sonographic diagnosis of congenital anomalies between 9 and 16 weeks menstrual age. *JCU*, 18, 307–14.
2. Cardoza, J.D., Goldstein, R.B. and Filly, R.A. (1988) Exclusion of fetal ventriculomegaly with a single measurement: the width of the lateral ventricular atrium. *Radiology*, 169, 711–14.

3. Cardoza, J.D., Filly, R.A. and Podrasky, A.E. (1988) The dangling choroid plexus: a sonographic observation of value in excluding ventriculomegaly. *AJR*, **151**, 767–70.

4. Filly, R.A., Cardoza, J.D., Goldstein, R.B. and Barkovich, A.J. (1989) Detection of fetal central nervous system anomalies: a practical level of effort for the routine sonogram. *Radiology*, **172**, 403–408.

5. Ferguson-Smith, M.A. (1983) The reduction of anencephalic and spina bifida births by maternal serum alphafetoprotein screening. *Br. Med. Bull.*, **39**(4), 365–72.

6. Romero, R., Mathieson, J.M., Ghidini, A. *et al.* (1989) Accuracy of ultrasound in the prenatal diagnosis of spinal anomalies. *Am. J. Perinatol.*, **6**, 320–23.

7. Lindfors, K.K., Gorcyza, D.P., Hanson, F.W. *et al.* (1991) The roles of ultrasonography and amniocentesis in evaluation of elevated maternal serum alphafetoprotein. *Am. J. Obstet. Gynecol.*, **164**, 1571–76.

8. Morrow, R.J., McNay, M.B. and Whittle, M.J. (1991) Ultrasound detection of neural tube defects in patients with elevated maternal serum alphafetoprotein. *Obstet. Gynecol.*, **78**, 1055–57.

9. Milunsky, A., Jick, S., Bruell, C.L. *et al.* (1989) Predictive values, relative risks, and overall benefits of high and low maternal serum alphafetoprotein screening in singleton pregnancies: new epidemiologic data. *Am. J. Obstet. Gynecol.*, **161**, 291–97.

10. Goldstein, R.B., Filly, R.A. and Callen, P.W. (1989) Sonography of anencephaly; pitfalls in early diagnosis. *JCU*, **17**, 397–402.

11. Nicolaides, K.H., Campbell S., Gabbe, S.G. and Guidetti, R. (1986) Ultrasound screening for spina bifida: cranial and cerebellar signs. *Lancet*, **ii**, 72–74.

12. Van den Hof, M.C., Nicolaides, K.H., Campbell, J. and Campbells, S. (1990) Evaluation of the lemon and banana signs in one hundred and thirty fetuses with open spina bifida. *Am. J. Obstet. Gynecol.*, **162**, 322–27.

13. Goldstein, R.B., Laidus, A.S. and Filly, R.A. (1991) Fetal cephaloceles: diagnosis with ultrasound. *Radiology*, **180**, 803–808.

14. Connor, J.M. (1989) Screening for genetic abnormality. *Fetal Med. Rev.*, **1**, 13–25.

15. Tabor, A., Philip, J., Madsen, M. *et al.* (1986) Randomised controlled trial of genetic amniocentesis in 4606 low risk women. *Lancet*, **i**, 1287–92.

16. Hogge, W.A., Thiagarajah, S., Ferguson, J.E. *et al.* (1989) The role of ultrasonography and amniocentesis in the evaluation of pregnancies at risk for neural tube defects. *Am. J. Obstet. Gynecol.*, **161**, 520–24.

17. Platt, L.D., Feutchtbaum, L., Filly, R.A. *et al.* (1992) The California maternal serum alphafetoprotein screening programme: the role of ultrasonography in the detection of spina bifida. *Am. J. Obstet. Gynecol.*, **166**, 1328–29.

18. Thornton, J.G., Lilford, R.J. and Newcombe, R. (1991) Tables for estimation of individual risks of fetal neural tube and ventral wall defects, incorporating prior probability, maternal serum alphafetoprotein levels, and ultrasonographic examination results. *Am. J. Obstet. Gynecol.*, **164**, 154–60.

19. Neven, P., Ricketts, R.T., Geirsson, R.T. *et al.* (1991) Screening for neural tube defects with maternal serum alphafetoprotein and ultrasound without the use of amniocentesis. *J. Obstet. Gynaecol.*, **11**, 5–8.

20. Brocks, B. and Bang, J. (1991) Routine examination by ultrasound for the detection of fetal malformation in a low risk population. *Fetal Diagn. Ther.*, **6**, 37–45.

21. Levi, S., Hyjazi, Y., Schaaps, J.P. *et al.* (1991) Sensitivity and specificity of routine antenatal screening for congenital anomalies by ultrasound: the Belgian multicentric study. *Ultrasound Obstet. Gynecol.*, **1**, 102–110.

22. Chitty, L.S., Hunt, G.H., Moore, J. and Lobb, M.O. (1991) Effectiveness of routine ultrasonography in detecting fetal structural abnormalities in a low risk population. *BMJ*, **303**, 1165–69.

23. Luck, C.A. (1992) Value of routine ultrasound scanning at 19 weeks: a four year study of 8849 deliveries. *BMJ*, **304**, 1471–78.

24 Eurocat Report 4 (1991) *Surveillance of Congenital Anomalies 1980–88*. Eurocat Central Registry, Department of Epidemiology, Catholic University of Louvain, Brussels.

25. Voight, H.J. and Brauns, S. (1992) Cerebral doppler velocimetry and fetal hydrocephalus. *Ultrasound Obstet. Gynaecol.*, **2** (suppl. 1), 255.

26. Pilu, G., Goldstein, I., Reece, E.A. *et al.* (1992) Sonography of fetal Dandy–Walker malformation: a reappraisal. *Ultrasound Obstet. Gynecol.*, **2**, 151–57.

27. Russ, P.D., Pretorius, D.H. and Johnson, M.J. (1989) Dandy–Walker syndrome: a review of fifteen cases evaluated by prenatal sonography. *Am. J. Obstet. Gynecol.*, **161**, 401–406.

28. Greene, M.F., Benacerraf, B.R. and Frigoletto, F.D. (1987) Reliable criteria for the prenatal sonographic diagnosis of alobar holoprosencephaly. *Am. J. Obstet. Gynecol.*, **156**, 687–89.

29. Pilu, G., Sandri, F., Perolo, A. and Giangaspero, F. (1992) Prenatal diagnosis of lobar holoprosencephaly. *Ultrasound Obstet. Gynecol.*, **2**, 88–94.

30. McGahan, J.P., Nyberg, D.A. and Mack, L.A. (1990) Sonography of facial features of alobar and semilobar holoprosencephaly. *AJR*, **154**, 143–48.

31. Pilu, G. and Bovicelli, L. (1989) Sonography of the fetal cranium. *Clin. Diagn. Ultrasound*, **25**, 221–58.

32. Arthur, R.J., Irving, H.C., Thomas, D.F.M. and Watters, J.K. (1989) Bilateral fetal uropathy: what is the outlook? *BMJ*, **298**, 1419–20.

33. Greig, J.D., Raine, P.A.M., Young, D.G. *et al.* (1989) Value of antenatal diagnosis of abnormalities of the urinary tract. *BMJ*, **298**, 1417–19.

34. Thomas, D.F.M. and Gordon, A.C. (1989) Management of prenatally diagnosed uropathies. *Arch. Dis. Child.*, **64**, 58–63.

35. Wheeler, T. and Jeanty, P. (1993) The dilated fetal renal tract: imaging and prenatal management, in *Obstetric Ultrasound*, vol. 1 (eds J.P. Neilson and S.E. Chambers), Oxford University Press, London, pp. 102–116.

36. Corteville, J.E., Gray, D.L. and Crane, J.P. (1991) Congenital hydronephrosis: correlation of fetal ultrasonographic findings with infant outcome. *Am. J. Obstet. Gynecol.*, **165**, 384–88.

37. Arger, P.H., Coleman, B.G. and Mintz, M.L. (1985) Routine fetal genitourinary tract screening. *Radiology*, **156**, 485–89.

38. Grignon, A., Filion, R. and Filiatrault, D. (1986) Urinary tract dilatation in utero: classification and clinical applications. *Radiology*, **160**, 645–47.

39. Mandell, J., Blyth, B.R., Peters, C.A. *et al.* (1991) Structural genitourinary defects detected in utero. *Radiology*, **178**, 193–96.

40. Livera, L.N., Brookfield, D.S.K., Egginton, J.A. and Hawnaur, J.M. (1989) Antenatal ultrasonography to detect fetal renal abnormalities: a prospective screening programme. *BMJ*, **298**, 1421–33.

41. Benacceraff, B.R., Mandell, J., Estroff, J.A. *et al.* (1990) Fetal pyelectasis: a possible association with Down syndrome. *Obstet. Gynecol.*, **76**, 58–60.

42. Dungan, J.S., Fernandez, M.T., Abbitt, P.L. and Thiagarajah, S. (1990) Multicystic dysplastic kidney: natural history of prenatally diagnosed cases. *Prenat. Diagn.*, **10**, 175–82.

43. Zerres, K., Hansmann, M., Mallmann, R. and Gembruch, U. (1988) Autosomal recessive polycystic kidney disease. Problems of prenatal diagnosis. *Prenat. Diagn.*, **8**, 215–19.

44. Lilford, R.J., Irving, H.C. and Allibone, E.B. (1992) A tale of two prior probabilities: avoiding the false positive diagnosis of autosomal recessive polycystic kidney disease. *Br. J. Obstet. Gynaecol.*, **99**, 216–19.

45. Pretorius, D.H., Lee, M.E., Manco-Johnson, M.L. *et al.* (1987) Diagnosis of autosomal dominant polycystic kidney disease in utero and in the young infant. *J. Ultrasound Med.*, **6**, 249–55.

46. McHugo, J.M., Shafi, M.I., Rowlands, D. and Weaver, J.B. (1988) Prenatal diagnosis of adult polycystic kidney disease. *Br. J. Radiol.*, **61**, 1072–74.

47. Ceccherini, I., Lituania, M., Cordone, M.S. *et al.* (1989) Autosomal dominant polycystic kidney disease: prenatal diagnosis by DNA analysis and sonography at 14 weeks. *Prenat. Diagn.*, **9**, 751–58.

48. Journel, H., Guyot, C., Barc, R.M. *et al.* (1989) Unexpected ultrasonographic prenatal diagnosis of autosomal dominant polycystic kidney disease. *Prenat. Diagn.*, **9**, 663–71.

49. Hughes, M.D., Nyberg, D.A., Mack, L.A. and Pretorius, D.H. (1989) Fetal omphalocele: prenatal detection of concurrent anomalies and other predictors of outcome. *Radiology*, **173**, 371–76.

50. Nyberg, D.A. and Mack, L.A. (1990) Abdominal wall defects, in *Diagnostic Ultrasound of Fetal Anomalies* (eds D.A Nyberg, B.S. Mahony and D.H. Pretorius), Year Book Medical, Chicago, pp. 395–432.

51. Gilbert, W.M. and Nicolaides, K.H. (1987) Fetal omphalocele: associated malformations and chromosomal defects. *Obstet. Gynecol.*, **70**, 633–35.

52. Sipes, S.L., Weinĕr, C.P., Sipes, D.R. *et al.* (1990) Gastroschisis and omphalocele: does either antenatal diagnosis or route of delivery make a difference in perinatal outcome. *Obstet. Gynecol.*, **76**, 195–99.

53. Stringer, M.D., Brereton, R.J. and Wright, V.M. (1990) Controversies in the management of gastroschisis: a study of 40 patients. *Arch. Dis. Child.*, **66**, 34–6.

54. Bond, S.J., Harrison, M.R., Filly, R.A. and Callen, P.W. (1988) Severity of intestinal damage in gastroschisis: correlation with prenatal sonographic findings. *J. Pediatr. Surg.*, **23**, 520–25.

55. Miro, J. and Bard, H. (1988) Congenital atresia and stenosis of the duodenum: the impact of a prenatal diagnosis. *Am. J. Obstet. Gynecol.*, **158**, 555–59.

56. Hancock, B.J. and Wiseman, N.E. (1989) Congenital duodenal obstruction: the impact of an antenatal diagnosis. *J. Pediatr. Surg.*, **24**, 1027–31.

57. Nyberg, D.A. (1990) Intrabdominal abnormalities, in *Diagnostic Ultrasound of Fetal Anomalies* (eds D.A. Nyberg, B.S. Mahony and D.H. Pretorius), Year Book Medical, Chicago, pp. 342–94.

58. Harris, R.D., Nyberg, D.A., Mack, L.A. and Weinberger, E. (1987) Anorectal atresia: prenatal sonographic diagnosis. *AJR*, **149**, 395–400.

59. Pennell, R.G. and Kurtz, A.B. (1989) Fetal intrathoracic and gastrointestinal anomalies. *Clin. Diagn. Ultrasound*, **25**, 111–38.

60. Meizner, I., Levy, A., Katz, M. *et al.* (1991) Fetal ovarian cysts: prenatal ultrasonographic detection and postnatal evaluation and treatment. *Am. J. Obstet. Gynecol.*, **164**, 874–78.

61. Saltzman, D.H., Adzick, N.S. and Benacerraf, B.R. (1988) Fetal cystic adenomatoid malformation of the lung: apparent improvement in utero. *Obstet. Gynecol.*, **71**, 1000–1002.

62. Fine, C., Adzick, N.S. and Doubilet, P.M. (1988) Decreasing size of congenital adenomatoid malformation *in utero*. *J. Ultrasound Med.*, 7, 405–408.

63. Sonek, J.D., Foley, M.R. and Iams, J.D. (1991) Spontaneous regression of a large intrathoracic fetal lesion before birth. *Am. J. Perinatol.*, 8, 41–43.

64. Wenstrom, K.D., Weiner, C.P. and Hanson, J.W. (1991) A five year statewide experience with congenital diaphragmatic hernia. *Am. J. Obstet. Gynecol.*, 165, 838–42.

65. Adzick, N.S., Harrison, M.R., Glick, P.L. *et al.* (1985) Diaphragmatic hernia in the fetus: prenatal diagnosis and outcome in 94 cases. *J. Pediatr. Surg.*, 20, 357–61.

66. Adzick, N.S., Vancanti, J.P., Lillehei, C.W. *et al.* (1989) Fetal diaphragmatic hernia: ultrasound diagnosis and clinical outcome in 38 cases. *J. Pediatr. Surg.*, 24, 654–58.

67. Nicolaides, K.H., Gosden, C.M. and Snijders, R.J.M. (1993) Ultrasonographically detectable markers of fetal chromosomal defects, in *Obstetric Ultrasound*, vol. 1 (eds J.P. Neilson and S.E. Chambers), Oxford University Press, London, pp. 41–82.

68. Crawford, D.C., Wright, V.M., Drake, D.P. and Allan, L.D. (1989) Fetal diaphragmatic hernia: the value of fetal echocardiography in the prediction of postnatal outcome. *Br. J. Obstet. Gynaecol.*, 96, 705–710.

69. Longaker, M.T., Laberge, J.M., Danserau, J. *et al.* (1989) Primary fetal hydrothorax: natural history and management. *J. Pediatr. Surg.*, 24, 573–76.

70. Weber, A.M. and Philipson, E.H. (1992) Fetal pleural effusion: a review and meta-analysis for prognostic indicators. *Obstet. Gynecol.*, 79, 281–86.

71. Benacerraf, B.R., Frigoletto, F.D. and Wilson, M. (1986) Successful midtrimester thoracocentesis with analysis of the lymphocyte population in the pleural effusion. *Am. J. Obstet. Gynecol.*, 155, 398–99.

72. Pijpers, L., Reuss, A., Stewart, P. and Wladimiroff, J.W. (1989) Noninvasive management of isolated bilateral fetal hydrothorax. *Am. J. Obstet. Gynecol.*, 161, 330–32.

73. Nyberg, D.A. (1993) The fetal lung, in *Obstetric Ultrasound*, vol. 1 (eds J.P. Neilson and S.E. Chambers), Oxford University Press, London, pp. 83–101.

74. Catanzarite V., Mendoza, A., Chapman, T. *et al.* (1992) Early prenatal diagnosis of type II cystic adenomatoid malformation of the lung: sonographic and histological findings. *Ultrasound Obstet. Gynecol.*, 2, 129–32.

75. Chou, M.M., Ho, E.S.C., Lee, H.S. *et al.* (1992) Early prenatal diagnosis of type III bilateral congenital cystic adenomatoid malformation of the lung. *Ultrasound Obstet. Gynecol.*, 2, 126–28.

76. Stocker, J.T., Madewell, J.E. and Drake, R.M. (1977) Congenital cystic adenomatoid malformation of the lung. *Hum. Pathol.*, 8, 155–71.

77. Harrison, M.R., Adzick, N.S., Jennings, R.W. *et al.* (1990) Antenatal intervention for congenital cystic adenomatoid malformation. *Lancet*, 336, 965–67.

78. Dumez, Y. (1992) *Prenatal Management of Congenital Cystic Adenomatoid Malformation of the Lung: Experience of 24 Cases.* Proceedings of the Second World Congress of Ultrasound in Obstetrics and Gynaecology, 1992, Bonn.

79. Hernanz Schulman, M., Stein, S.M., Neblett, W.W. and Atkinson, J.B. (1991) Pulmonary sequestration: diagnosis with colour doppler sonography and a new theory of associated hydrothorax. *Radiology*, 180, 817–21.

80. Hill, L.M., Breckle, R., Thomas, M.L. and Fries, J.K. (1987) Polyhydramnios: ultrasonically detected prevalence and neonatal outcome. *Obstet. Gynecol.*, 69, 21–25.

81. Hill, L.M. (1990) Abnormalities of amniotic fluid, in *Diagnostic Ultrasound of Fetal Anomalies* (eds D.A. Nyberg, B.S. Mahony and D.H. Pretorius), Year Book Medical, Chicago, pp. 38–66.

82. Carlson, D.E., Platt, L., Medearis, A.L. and Horenstein, J. (1990) Quantifiable polyhydramnios: diagnosis and management. *Obstet. Gynecol.*, 75, 989–93.

83. Barkin, S.Z., Pretorius, D.H., Beckett, M.K. *et al.* (1987) Severe polyhydramnios: incidence of anomalies. *AJR*, 148, 155–59.

84. Desmedt, E.J., Henry, O.A. and Beischer, N.A. (1990) Polyhydramnios and associated maternal and fetal complications in singleton pregnancies. *Br. J. Obstet. Gynaecol.*, 97, 1115–22.

85. Queenan, J.T. and Gadow, E.C. (1970) Polyhydramnios: chronic versus acute. *Am. J. Obstet. Gynecol.*, 108, 349–55.

86. Pretorius, D.H., Drose, J.A., Dennis, M.A. *et al.* (1987) Tracheoesophageal fistula *in utero*: twenty two cases. *J. Ultrasound Med.*, 6, 509–13.

87. Stoll, C.G., Alembik, Y. and Dott, B. (1991) Study of 156 cases of polyhydramnios and congenital malformations in a series of 118 265 consecutive births. *Am. J. Obstet. Gynecol.*, 165, 586–90.

88. Peipert, J.F. and Donnenfeld, A.E. (1991) Oligohydramnios: a review. *Obstet. Gynecol. Surv.*, 46, 325–39.

89. Manning, F.A., Hill, L.M. and Platt, L.D. (1981) Qualitative amniotic fluid determination by ultrasound: antepartum detection of intrauterine growth retardation. *Am. J. Obstet. Gynecol.*, 139, 254–58.

90. Goldstein, R.B. and Filly, R.A. (1988) Sonographic estimation of amniotic fluid volume: subjective assesment versus pocket measurements. *J. Ultrasound Med.*, 7, 363–69.

91. Chamberlain, P.F., Manning, F.A. and Morrison, I. (1984) Ultrasound evaluation of amniotic fluid volume: the relationship of marginal and decreased amniotic fluid volumes to perinatal outcome. *Am. J. Obstet. Gynecol.*, 150, 245–49.

92. Halpern, M.E., Fong, K.W., Zalev, A.H. *et al.* (1985) Reliability of amniotic fluid volume estimation from ultrasonograms: intraobserver and interobserver variation before and after the establishment of criteria. *Am. J. Obstet. Gynecol.*, 153, 264–67.

93. Fisk, N.M., Ronderas-Dumit, D., Soliani, A. and Nicolini, U. (1991) Diagnostic and therapeutic transabdominal amnioinfusion in oligohydramnios. *Obstet. Gynecol.*, 78, 270–77.

94. Phelan, J.P., Vernon-Smith, C., Bronssard, P. and Small. M. (1987) Amniotic fluid volume assessment with the four quadrant technique at 36–42 weeks gestation. *J. Reprod. Med.*, 32, 540–42.

95. Benaceraff, B. (1990) Examination of the second-trimester fetus with severe oligohydramnios using transvaginal scanning. *Obstet. Gynecol.*, 75, 491–93.

96. Gembruch, U. and Hansmann, M. (1988) Artificial installation of amniotic fluid as a new technique for the diagnositic evaluation of cases of oligohydramnios. *Prenat. Diagn.*, 8, 33–45.

97. Gillet, J.H., Boog, G., Dumez, Y. *et al.* (1990) Anomalies du volume du liquide amniotique, in *Echographie des Malformations Foetales*, Vigot, Paris, pp. 370–76.

98. Hackett, G.A., Nicolaides, K.H. and Campbell, S. (1987) Doppler ultrasound assessment of fetal and uteroplacental circulations in severe second trimester oligohydramnios. *Br. J. Obstet. Gynaecol.*, 94, 1074–77.

99. Blott, M., Nicolaides, K.H., Gibb, D. *et al.* (1987) Fetal breathing movements as a predictor of favourable pregnancy outcome after oligohydramnios due to membrane rupture in the second trimester. *Lancet*, i, 129–31.

100. Moessinger, A.C., Higgins, A., Fox, H.E. *et al.* (1987) Fetal breathing movements are not a reliable predictor of continued lung development in pregnancies complicated by oligohydramnios. *Lancet*, ii, 1297–99.

101. Vintzileos, A.M., Campbell, W.A., Rodis, J.F. *et al.* (1989) Comparison of six different ultrasonographic methods for predicting lethal fetal pulmonary hypoplasia. *Am. J. Obstet. Gynecol.*, 161, 606–12.

102. Camera, G. and Mastroiacovo, P. (1982) Birth prevalence of skeletal dysplasias in the Italian multicentric monitoring system for birth defects, in *Skeletal Dysplasias* (eds C.J. Papadatos and C.E. Bartsocas), Liss, NY, p. 441.

103. Romero, R. and Sirtori, M. (1989) The prenatal diagnosis of skeletal dysplasias. *Clin. Diagn. Ultrasound*, 25, 163–202.

104. Spirt, B.A., Oliphant, M., Gottlieb, R.H. and Gordon, L.P. (1990) Prenatal sonographic evaluation of short limb dwarfism: an algorithmic approach. *Radiographics*, 10, 217–36.

105. Donnenfeld, A.E. and Mennuti, M.T. (1987) Second trimester diagnosis of fetal skeletal dysplasias. *Obstet. Gynaecol. Surv.*, 42, 199–217.

106. Brons, J.T.J. and van den Harten, H.J. (1988) *Skeletal Dysplasias. Pre- and Postnatal Identification.* Free University Hospital, Amsterdam.

107. Pretorius, D.H., Rumack, C.M., Manco-Johnson, M.L. *et al.* (1986) Specific skeletal dysplasias *in utero*: sonographic diagnosis. *Radiology*, 159, 237–42.

108. Whittle, M.J. (1990) Routine fetal anomaly screening, in *Antenatal Diagnosis of Fetal Abnormalities* (eds J.O. Drife and D. Donnai), Springer, Berlin, pp. 35–44.

109. McNay, M. (1991) Clinical considerations in screening for fetal abnormalities. *Br. Med. Ultrasound Bull.*, 63, 23.

110. Pitkin, R.M. (1991) Screening and detection of congenital malformation. *Am. J. Obstet. Gynecol.*, 164, 1045–48.

111. Whittle, M.J. (1992) Value of routine ultrasound (letter). *BMJ*, 305, 583–84.

112. Hegge, F.N., Franklin, R.W., Watson, P.T. and Calhoun, B.C. (1989) An evaluation of the time of discovery of fetal malformations by an indication-based system for ordering obstetric ultrasound. *Obstet. Gynecol.*, 74, 21–24.

113. Chambers, S.E., Geirsson, R.T., Stewart, R.J. *et al.* (1994) Audit of a screening service for fetal abnormalities using early ultrasound scanning and maternal serum alphafetoprotein estimation combined with selective detailed scanning. *Ultrasound Obstet. Gynecol.* (in press).

114. Manchester, D.K., Pretorius, D., Avery, C. *et al.* (1988) Accuracy of ultrasound diagnosis in pregnancies complicated by suspected fetal anomalies. *Prenat. Diagn.*, 8, 109–17.

115. Schen Schwartz, S., Neisch, C. and Hill, L.M. (1989) Antenatal ultrasound for fetal anomalies: importance of perinatal autopsy. *Pediatr. Pathol.*, 9, 1–9.

116. Keeling, J.W., Manning, N. and Chamberlain, P. (1990) Accuracy of fetal anomaly scanning. *Pediatr. Pathol.*, 10, 653.

117. Clayton-Smith J., Farndon, P.A., McKeown, C. and Donnai, D. (1990) Examination of fetuses after induced abortion for fetal abnormality. *BMJ*, 300, 295–97.

118. Grant, H.W., MacKinlay, G.A., Chambers, S.E. *et al.* (1993) Prenatal ultrasound diagnosis: a review of fetal outcome. *Pediatr. Surg. Int.*, 8, 469–71.

53 ULTRASOUND DIAGNOSIS OF CHROMOSOMAL DISEASE

P. Twining

53.1 Introduction

For thousands of years the fetus has been an inaccessible patient protected by the uterus and cushioned by warm amniotic fluid. The advent of ultrasound has meant that fetal disease can now be diagnosed. Although chromosomal disease as such cannot be treated, if a diagnosis is made before viability then a termination of pregnancy can be offered to the mother. When the diagnosis is made late in pregnancy it can be useful in deciding the mode of delivery. In particular a caesarian section for fetal distress may be avoided as this is a frequent complication in certain chromosomal abnormalities [1]. In addition the antenatal diagnosis gives the patient time to come to terms with the diagnosis and prepare for the possibility of surgery to the baby in the neonatal period.

The antenatal diagnosis of chromosomal disease is based on the detection of certain fetal abnormalities and these are outlined in Table 53.1. Nicolaides *et al.*

Table 53.1 Ultrasound findings indicating detailed scanning and/or karyotyping and likely chromosomal anomaly [After Ref. 2 with permission]

Finding	Chromosomal anomaly
Head/body	
Holoprosencephaly, hydrocephalus, Dandy–Walker syndrome	Trisomy 13, triploidy, trisomy 18
Choroid plexus cysts – when other anomaly present	Trisomy 18, 21
Strawberry head	Trisomy 18
Cystic hygroma, nuchal oedema	Turner's syndrome, trisomy 21
Cardiac anomalies – ventricular septal defect, atrioventricular canal defect	Trisomy 18, 21
Diaphragmatic hernia	Trisomy 18, 13
Omphalocele	Trisomy 18, 13
Duodenal atresia	Trisomy 21
Hands/feet	
Overlapping fingers, flexion deformities	Trisomy 18
Polydactyly	Trisomy 13
Radial aplasia	Trisomy 18
Clinodactyly – fifth finger	Trisomy 21
Rockerbottom feet	Trisomy 18
Increased gap between first and second toes	Trisomy 21
Face	
Facial clefting	Trisomy 13, 18
Micrognathia	Trisomy 18
General	
Intrauterine growth retardation of whatever type, if other anomalies present	Trisomy 13, 18, triploidy
Hydrops	Turner's, trisomy 18, 13, 21
Multiple abnormalities	Trisomy 13, 18, 21, triploidy
Polyhydramnios – when other anomaly present	Trisomy 13, 18, 21

Diseases of the Fetus and Newborn, 2nd edn, Edited by G.B. Reed, A.E. Claireaux and F. Cockburn. Published in 1995 by Chapman & Hall, London. ISBN 0 412 39160 0

[3] have shown a high correlation between multiple abnormalities and chromosomal disease. For example if two or more abnormalities are seen then the risk of chromosomal disease is 29%, whereas when five abnormalities are seen in a fetus this risk rises to 70% [3]. There are however a number of patterns of abnormalities that are well established in indicating a specific chromosomal syndrome [4]. In effect then, not only are we looking for multiple abnormalities but also a series of specific abnormalities, a constellation of findings which fit together like pieces in a jigsaw puzzle to form the final picture [2].

Another important point is that for a given malformation the risk of a chromosomal abnormality may be inversely related to the severity of the defect [3]. For example fetuses with a small omphalocele (containing bowel only) have a much higher risk of a chromosomal defect than those with large omphaloceles which may contain bowel and liver [5]. Similarly fetuses with mild ventriculomegaly or mild dilatation of the renal pelvises have a higher risk of chromosomal disease than fetuses with established hydrocephalus or hydronephrosis [6,7].

In addition to specific abnormalities there are a number of non-specific findings that can suggest the presence of chromosomal disease. Intrauterine growth retardation is a common finding in chromosomal disease, occurring in up to 51% of fetuses with trisomy 18 [8], and can occur early in the second trimester in triploidy [2]. The type of growth retardation is not specific for chromosomal disease, i.e. symmetrical or asymmetrical, far more important is the presence of fetal abnormalities.

One other non-specific finding is the presence of polyhydramnios which, in isolation, has a low incidence of chromosomal disease. However, if growth retardation and/or fetal abnormalities are present then this finding not only carries a high suspicion of a chromosomal defect but should always prompt the search for fetal abnormalities associated with chromosomal disease [9].

In the UK most women are offered a routine ultrasound scan at 18–20 weeks' gestation [10] and this has proven to be effective in detecting fetal abnormalities [11,12]. It involves a full anatomical scan of the fetus including assessment of the head, thorax and abdomen. Detailed ultrasound scans are reserved for high-risk pregnancies and are usually carried out at tertiary referral centres. These involve closer scrutiny of the fetus with special attention placed on visualizing the fetal face, hands, feet and heart. It is often the face, heart and extremities that may give the clue to the presence of a chromosomal defect.

When a chromosomal defect is suspected it must always be confirmed by cytogenetic analysis. Although amniocentesis has long been the mainstay for karyotyping fetuses the main disadvantage is a 2–3-week delay in obtaining the result. This situation has been revolutionized with the development of chorion villus sampling or placental biopsy whereby under ultrasound guidance a small amount of placental tissue is removed for cytogenetic evaluation. The advantage of this technique is that a result can be obtained in under 2 days [13], which is extremely important when an ultrasound diagnosis is made at 18–20 weeks' gestation.

Cordocentesis is another technique that can be used to obtain a fetal karyotype [14], with a result available within 2–4 days. In this procedure a sample of fetal blood is obtained by puncturing the umbilical vein under ultrasound control. The overall loss rate is approximately 1–2% [15]; however this can rise to as much as 14–25% in the presence of severe growth retardation and hydrops [16].

There are however new cytogenetic techniques, such as fluorescence *in situ* hybridization [17], which can deliver a rapid karyotype, i.e. within 2 days from an amniocentesis sample [18]. Furthermore the application of this technique to fetal cells harvested from the maternal circulation [19] holds the promise of a non-invasive means of obtaining a fetal karyotype in the future (Chapter 73).

53.2 Trisomy 13 (Table 53.2)

This condition was first described by Patau *et al.* in 1960 [20]. The incidence is 1 in 5000 and the prognosis for a baby with this condition is extremely poor. Fifty per cent of babies with trisomy 13 will die within the first month, 75% die within 6 months and less than 5% survive to 3 years of age [21]. As stated earlier the important ultrasound findings are seen in the head, face, hands and heart.

Intracranial abnormalities are common in fetuses with trisomy 13, in particular holoprosencephaly (Figure 53.1). In one series of antenatally diagnosed holoprosencephaly, trisomy 13 occurred in 40% of cases [22]. The other common intracranial abnormalities are agenesis of the corpus callosum, the Dandy–Walker syndrome and hydrocephalus [2]. Occasionally neural tube defects may be seen in trisomy 13.

Facial clefting is a frequent observation in trisomy 13 and this is often associated with holoprosencephaly [23]. The facial appearances in this condition range from cyclopia with proboscis to hypotelorism with midline facial clefting, and it is often stated that 'the face predicts the brain' as the changes are so characteristic. Facial clefting may also occur in trisomy 13 without the presence of holoprosencephaly [24]. Postaxial polydactyly is another common finding in trisomy 13 and this may affect both hands and feet (Figure

Table 53.2 Frequency of abnormalities in fetuses with trisomy 13

Abnormality	Incidence (%)
Head	
Holoprosencephaly	75
Agenesis of corpus callosum	22
Dandy–Walker syndrome	20
Hydrocephalus	13
Face	
Cleft lip/palate	75
Low-set ears	
Hands/feet	
Polydactyly	65
Heart	
Ventricular septal defect	
Atrioventricular septal defect	80
Hypoplastic left heart	
Kidney	
Renal cyst dysplasia	30
Hydronephrosis	
Abdomen	
Omphalocele	30
General	
Growth retardation	>90

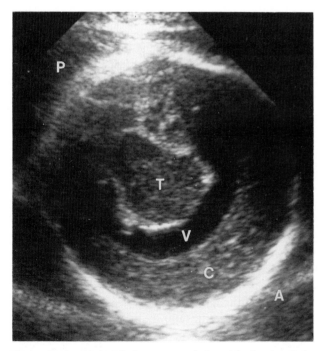

Figure 53.1 Alobar holoprosencephaly with the fused thalami (T) protruding into the single ventricular cavity (V). The rim of cortex (C) is well demonstrated. A = anterior; P = posterior.

53.2). Less frequently one may see flexion of the fingers with or without overlapping.

These fetuses often demonstrate cardiac abnormalities, the most important of which are ventricular septal defect, atrioventricular septal defect and hypoplastic left heart syndrome [25,26].

In the abdomen an omphalocele is the most common abnormality and is likely to contain bowel only [5]. Renal cystic disease and hydronephrosis are also seen in approximately 30% of fetuses. In this context it is important to differentiate from Meckel's syndrome which may present with renal cystic disease, polydactyly and occipital encephalocele with posterior fossa abnormalities [27]. The outlook for both conditions is equally poor; however Meckel's syndrome, which has a normal karyotype, is an autosomal recessive inheritance and so an accurate diagnosis is essential in terms of counselling for future pregnancies. This point highlights the importance of obtaining a karyotype in fetuses with multiple abnormalities and its bearing on future pregnancies and genetic counselling.

As mentioned earlier the vast majority of fetuses with trisomy 13 will also show growth retardation.

53.3 Trisomy 18 (Table 53.3)

Trisomy 18 was first described by Edwards in 1960 [28] and has an incidence of 1 in 3000. The prognosis is extremely poor and most babies die from severe cardiac abnormalities within the first few days of life [29].

One of the most striking abnormalities and a hallmark of the syndrome is fixed flexion of the fingers with overlapping (Figures 53.3 and 53.4). The classical configuration is the index finger over the third finger and the fifth finger over the fourth. Radial aplasia may also be seen in the hands [30] (Figure 53.5). The feet often show talipes or rockerbottom deformity. Less common findings in the hands include hypoplasia or absence of the thumb (Figure 53.3) and syndactyly. Polydactyly, although much more common in trisomy 13, is occasionally seen in trisomy 18 [4].

The most common abnormality in the face is micrognathia (Figure 53.6) [31] and this may be seen in up to 70% of cases [2]. Facial clefting is also seen but is not so frequent as in trisomy 13. Low-set 'pixie-type' ears are also a feature but may be more obvious in the neonatal period.

As in all chromosomal abnormalities cardiac disease is a frequent finding and a ventricular septal defect is the most common defect (Figure 53.7) seen in trisomy 18 [32]. Unfortunately this abnormality is the most likely to be missed. Routine four-chamber scanning will detect only 38–40% of major cardiac anomalies [12,33]. The additional visualization of the outflow tracts increases this figure to 78% [34].

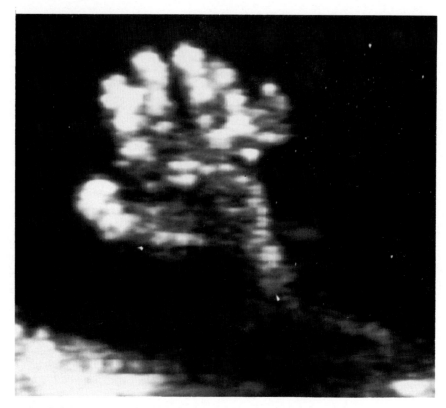

Figure 53.2   Postaxial polydactyly. Scans through the hand of a 28-week fetus showing postaxial polydactyly. (Reproduced with permission from Twining and Zuccollo [2].)

Even in expert hands ventricular septal defects are seen in only 65% of cases [35]. This underlines the point that, although the fetal heart is a common setting for abnormality in chromosomal disease, it is often one of the most difficult organs to assess in the fetus and so extra special care is needed in assessing the fetal heart when a chromosomal defect is suspected. In this respect colour flow imaging may prove useful in assessing the patency of the fetal ventricular septum in the future.

The other main cardiac abnormalities seen in trisomy 18 are atrioventricular septal defects [36] and double outlet right ventricle [25].

Scanning the fetal head often reveals a number of anomalies suggestive of trisomy 18. The shape of the head is important because a characteristic appearance known as the 'strawberry skull' (Figure 53.8) may be seen in up to 45% of trisomy 18 fetuses [37]. This appearance is produced by a flattened occiput and narrow frontal bones and is common in neonates with trisomy 18 [4,28].

Choroid plexus cysts are another common finding in trisomy 18 [38–43] (Figure 53.9). First described in 1984 [44], they occur in 25–30% of fetuses with trisomy 18 [9,45] but also occur in 1% of normal fetuses. The cysts vary in size between 3 and 16 mm, appear at about 14–16 weeks gestation and resolve by 22 weeks [30,45]. The vast majority of fetuses with choroid plexus cysts and trisomy 18 have other fetal abnormalities present. However 17–20% of fetuses with trisomy 18 will have no abnormalities detectable on ultrasonography [9,46]. It is possible, therefore, and a few cases have been documented where choroid plexus cysts were the only abnormality present in a fetus with trisomy 18 [41,47,48]. Because of this certain groups have advocated karyotyping all fetuses with choroid plexus cysts whether abnormalities are present or not [49–51]. At present one would certainly offer a karyotype if choroid plexus cysts are seen in the presence of other abnormalities [30,41,43] as this carries a high risk of chromosomal disease. The risk of a fetus with isolated choroid plexus cysts having trisomy 18, although small, is not insignificant and has been calculated to be approximately 1 in 200 [48]. Unfortunately this is identical to the risk of miscarriage following a karyotype procedure and so counselling patients in this situation is very difficult.

Enlargement of the cisterna vena magna is also associated with trisomy 18 [52], as is the Dandy–

Table 53.3 Frequency of abnormalities in fetuses with trisomy 18

Abnormality	Frequency (%)
Head	
Strawberry skull	45
Choroid plexus cysts	30
Enlarged cisterna vena magna	19
Neural tube defects	
Agenesis of corpus callosum	
Hydrocephalus	
Face/neck	
Micrognathia	70
Low set 'pixie' ears	40
Cleft lip/palate	15
Hands/feet	
Flexed/overlapping fingers	80
Rockerbottom/club foot	20
Radial aplasia	10
Heart	
Ventricular septal defect	
Atrioventricular septal defect	80
Double outlet right ventricle	
Kidney	
Cystic dysplasia	
Horseshoe kidney	15
Hydronephrosis	
Abdomen	
Omphalocele	20
Thorax	
Diaphragmatic hernia	20
General	
Single umbilical artery	13
Growth retardation	59
Polyhydramnios	21

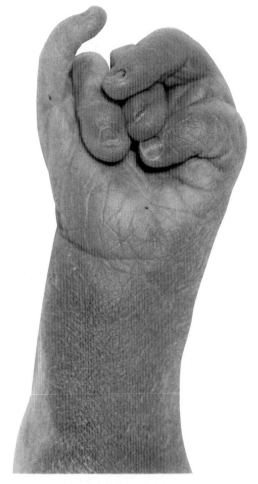

Figure 53.3 Trisomy 18. Appearances in the hand of a term fetus showing overlapping of the fingers. The most characteristic configuration is the second finger overlapping the third and the fifth finger overlapping the fourth. (Reproduced with permission from Twining and Zuccollo [2].)

Walker syndrome [53,54]. The degree of associated ventricular dilatation is also important as minimal or no ventricular dilatation carries a much higher risk of chromosomal disease, 77% compared with 9%, when ventriculomegaly is present [52].

Less common cranial abnormalities seen in trisomy 18 are agenesis of the corpus callosum and hydrocephalus [6,55]. Neural tube defects are also seen but occur in less than 10% of fetuses with trisomy 18 [31].

In the chest and abdomen, diaphragmatic hernia [56] and omphalocele [57,58] are often seen and it is the smaller omphaloceles, i.e. containing bowel only, that are more likely to be associated with chromosomal disease [59]. A diaphragmatic hernia produces displacement of the heart and this can make assessment of the heart difficult: extra vigilance is required in this situation.

Also seen in the abdomen are renal abnormalities, which can occur in up to 15% of cases and range from cystic dysplasia to hydronephrosis and horseshoe kidney [9,60].

As mentioned earlier, growth retardation is seen in over 50% of fetuses with trisomy 18 [61] and although it can be seen in the second trimester it is more obvious in the third trimester. The presence of associated polyhydramnios is an ominous sign and can be seen in up to 21% of fetuses with trisomy 18 [9,62].

In a small number of fetuses a cystic hygroma may be identified, and occasionally generalized hydrops is seen [63].

944

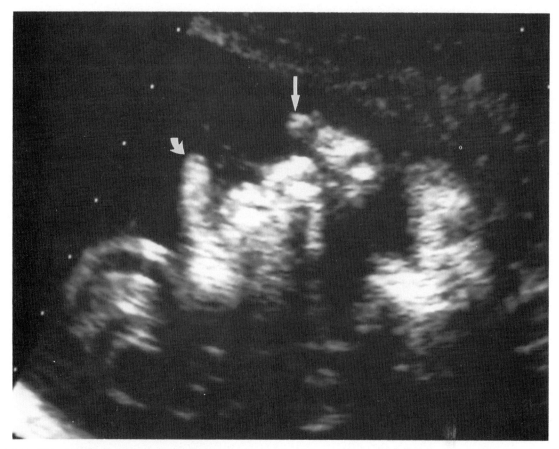

Figure 53.4 Trisomy 18. Coronal scans through the hand of a 28-week fetus. The fifth finger overlaps the fourth (curved arrow) and the second finger overlaps the third (straight arrow).

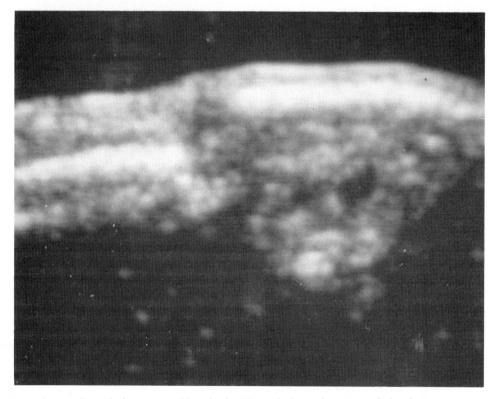

Figure 53.5 Sagittal scan through forearm and hand of a 20-week fetus showing radial aplasia.

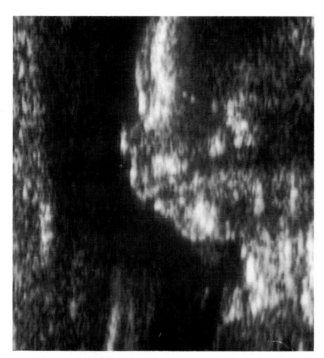

Figure 53.6 Profile view of an 18-week fetus with trisomy 18 showing micrognathia. (Reproduced with permission from Turner and Twining [23].)

53.4 Trisomy 21 (Table 53.4)

Trisomy 21 or Down's syndrome is the most common chromosomal abnormality, with an incidence of 1.3 in 1000, but it is also the most difficult to detect using antenatal ultrasound. In the best hands fetal abnormalities will be seen in only 33% of affected fetuses [2,69]. Many of these abnormalities will be subtle changes in hands and feet, requiring detailed ultrasound evaluation. At present amniocentesis is routinely offered to all women over 35 years of age; however, using this basis for screening only 15% of affected pregnancies are likely to be detected [64]. The introduction of the triple test, comprising analysis of serum levels of α-fetoprotein, unconjugated oestriol and human chorionic gonadotrophin, has meant that up to 48% of fetuses with Down's syndrome may be detected [65]. In addition assessment of serum concentrations of pregnancy-associated plasma protein hold promise of a screening test in the first trimester [66].

Although the ultrasound diagnosis of Down's syndrome has limitations [67,68], there are a number of reliable ultrasound findings and recent studies have revealed new markers for the syndrome [69–72].

The most reliable ultrasound findings in trisomy 21 are duodenal atresia (Figure 53.10) and atrioventricular septal defects. Although duodenal atresia only occurs in

5% of fetuses with Down's syndrome [69], its detection in a fetus carries a 30% risk of the syndrome [73]. Unfortunately duodenal atresia can rarely be detected with confidence before 24 weeks gestation [69] so its use as an early sign of Down's syndrome is limited.

Congenital heart disease occurs in about 40% of neonates with Down's syndrome [31]; the most common abnormalities detected antenatally are atrioventricular septal defects and ventricular septal defects [25,26].

Due to the difficulty in making an ultrasound diagnosis of trisomy 21 considerable attention has been placed on finding other ultrasound signs of the syndrome. Thickening of the nuchal tissues at the back of the fetal neck (Figure 53.11) is a useful sign in Down's syndrome [74–77] and occurs in approximately 16% of fetuses [70]. This increased nuchal thickening may be caused by a previous cystic hygroma which has resolved [78].

It is well documented that persons with Down's syndrome have shortened long bones and there has been considerable debate in the literature as to the usefulness of the detection of a shortened femur in the second trimester diagnosis of Down's syndrome. Early papers demonstrated a clear link between the syndrome and a shortened femur [79,80]; however later papers [68,81,82] have not confirmed these findings as there is considerable overlap with the normal population. At present one would not routinely offer a karyotype on the basis of a shortened femur alone.

Benacerraf, Neuberg and Frigoletto [70] have also proposed that a shortened humerus may be useful in the antenatal diagnosis of Down's syndrome. However this sign requires larger studies to confirm this finding.

Certain subtle findings may be seen in the hands and feet: clinodactyly of the fifth finger caused by absence or hypoplasia of the middle phalanx has been described in a number of fetuses antenatally in Down's syndrome [83] (Figure 53.12), as has a widened gap between the first and second toes [3].

In the head mild dilatation of the lateral ventricles may be seen [6] and in one study [69] occurred in 3% of Down's syndrome fetuses. This is likely to be caused by a degree of cerebral atrophy or decreased brain mass. Similarly, another recent study demonstrated reduced frontal lobe dimensions in fetuses with Down's syndrome, again indicating reduced brain mass [84].

In the abdomen mild dilatation of the renal pelves carries a risk of Down's syndrome and has been estimated to be in the region of 0.3% in a fetus demonstrating this appearance [85]. Omphaloceles are also occasionally seen and these are usually small, containing only bowel. Echogenic bowel is another recent finding that has been reported and may occur in up to 5% of fetuses [69]. Some workers however have found no link between echogenic bowel and

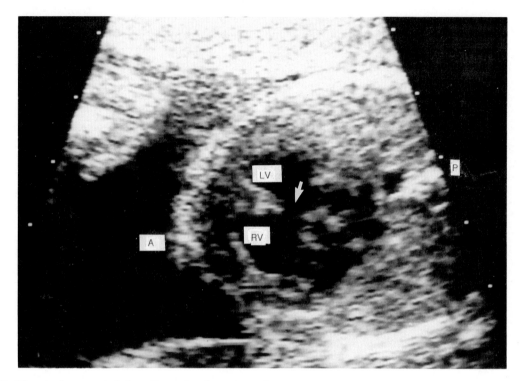

Figure 53.7 Ventricular septal defect. Four-chamber view of a 28-week fetus showing a large ventricular septal defect (arrow). LV = left ventricle; RV = right ventricle; A = anterior; P = posterior. (Reproduced with permission from Twining and Zuccollo [2].)

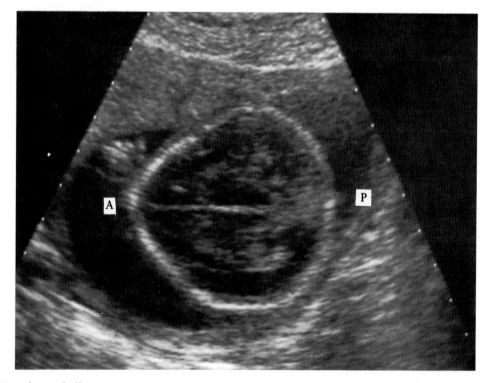

Figure 53.8 Strawberry skull. Transverse section through head of an 18-week fetus with trisomy 18. Note occipital flattening and frontal pointing typical of this appearance. A = anterior; P = posterior.

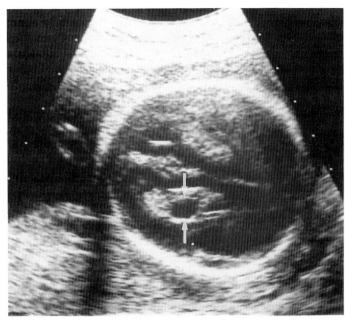

Figure 53.9 Choroid plexus cysts. Transverse section through head of an 18-week fetus showing a unilocular choroid plexus cyst (arrows).

Table 53.4 Frequency of abnormalities in trisomy 21

Abnormality	Incidence (%)
Head	
Mild ventriculomegaly }	3
Small frontal lobes }	
Face/neck	
Macroglossia	
Snub nose, prominent lips	
Cystic hygroma	4
Nuchal oedema	16
Hands/feet	
Clinodactyly – fifth finger	
Wide gap between first and second toes	
Heart	
Atroventricular septal defect }	40
Ventricular septal defect }	
Kidney	
Mild dilatation of renal pelves	
Abdomen	
Duodenal atresia	5
Omphalocele	2
Echogenic bowel	5
Thorax	
Pleural effusion	1
General	
Growth retardation	6
Polyhydramnios	3
Hydrops	2

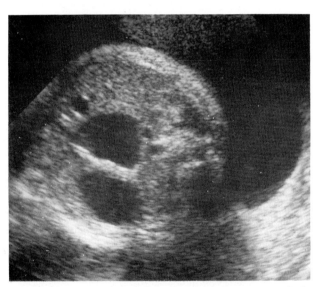

Figure 53.10 Duodenal atresia. Transverse scan through the abdomen of a 28-week fetus showing typical double-bubble appearance.

chromosomal disease [86,87] so its significance remains controversial.

The face may also reveal clues to the presence of Down's syndrome as macroglossia may be present [3], and in the third trimester a characteristic profile with a snub nose and prominent lips may be seen [23].

A small proportion of Down's syndrome fetuses will

948

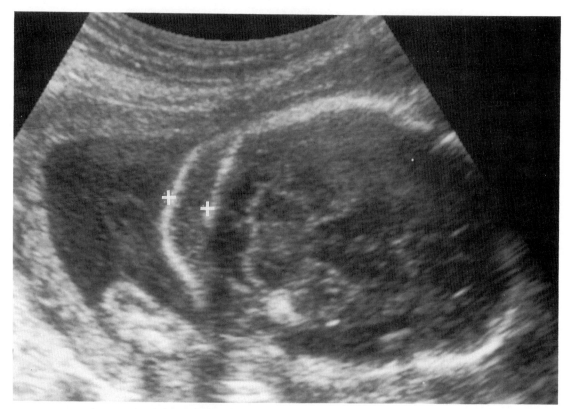

Figure 53.11 Increased nuchal thickening. Transverse scans through the head of a 20-week fetus showing increased nuchal thickening as measured by the electronic callipers.

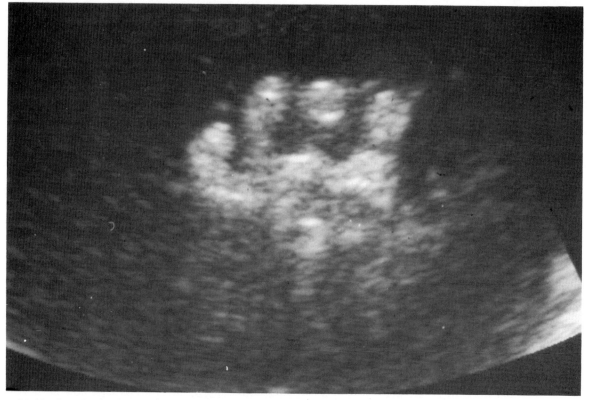

Figure 53.12 Longitudinal scan through the hand of a 28-week fetus showing clinodactyly of the fifth finger.

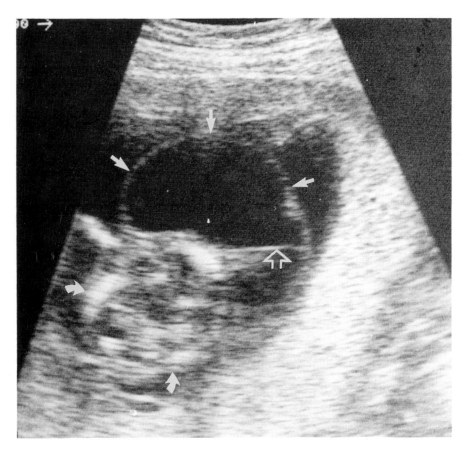

Figure 53.13 Cystic hygroma. Transverse scans through the neck of an 18-week fetus. Curved arrows indicate the anterior fetal neck; straight arrows outline the cystic hygroma; open arrow shows septum within the cystic hygroma.

demonstrate a degree of growth retardation which may occur in the late second and early third trimester.

As alluded to earlier, cystic hygromas occurring in the first trimester can resolve and this can be a useful early marker for Down's syndrome; however, a cystic hygroma is far more common in Turner's syndrome.

Finally a fetus with Down's syndrome may present with generalized hydrops and/or pleural effusions. These occur in approximately 1–2% of fetuses with trisomy 21 [69]. Although the diagnosis of Down's syndrome is difficult, many new ultrasound markers are being developed and, together with the use of biochemical markers, the rate of detection should improve.

53.5 Turner's syndrome

First described by Turner in 1938, the incidence of this syndrome is approximately 1 in 5000 live births but it accounts for up to 10% of first trimester miscarriages.

Neonates with Turner's syndrome are often indistinguishable from normal babies and the diagnosis is often not made until short stature or delayed puberty becomes apparent [31].

The hallmark of the antenatal diagnosis of Turner's syndrome is the presence of a cystic hygroma [2] (Figure 53.13). This abnormality is caused by an obstruction in the cervical lymphatic vessels so that lymphatic fluid collects at the back of the fetal neck; the classical appearance is of a multiseptate fluid collection in the posterior nuchal space [88] (Figure 53.13). These cystic hygromas can be very large and may be associated with generalized hydrops.

In this setting the outlook is extremely poor [21]. It is important to differentiate cystic hygroma from an occipital encephalocele; however the head shape, appearances of the intracranial contents and the presence of an occipital bony defect are all important signs of an encephalocele [89].

The presence of a cystic hygroma is not however totally specific for Turner's syndrome: approximately 70% of fetuses with a cystic hygroma will have this syndrome [90]. As mentioned previously, 5% will have trisomy 18, 5% trisomy 21 and approximately 20% will have a normal karyotype [90]. Cystic hygromas which present at other sites on the body, for example the anterior abdominal wall, have a low incidence of

Table 53.5 Frequency of abnormalities in fetuses with triploidy

Abnormality	Incidence (%)
Head	
Hydrocephalus	
Holoprosencephaly	50
Agenesis of corpus callosum	
Face	
Micrognathia	30
Low-set ears	50
Cleft lip/palate	25
Hands/feet	
Syndactyly of third and fourth fingers	60
Club-foot	
Heart	
Ventricular septal defect	60
Tetralogy of Fallot	
Kidney	
Renal cystic dysplasia	15
Hydronephrosis	
Abdomen	
Omphalocele	20
General	
Early growth retardation	100
Oligohydramnios	95
Hydropic placenta	40

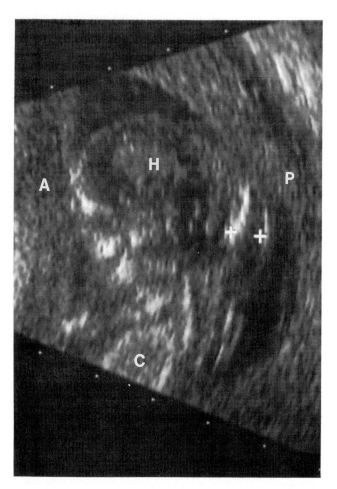

Figure 53.14 Fetal nuchal translucency. Sagittal scan through the head and neck of a 14-week fetus showing increased nuchal translucency (as measured by electronic callipers). H = head; C = chest; A = anterior; P = posterior.

chromosomal disease and do not usually require karyotyping.

The other malformations which can occur in Turner's syndrome are usually cardiac malformations, which can occur in 15% of fetuses, and the most common anomaly is coarctation [31].

The only other abnormality of note is renal and occasionally one sees hydronephrosis, renal agenesis and renal hypoplasia.

It has been estimated that up to 35% of liveborn individuals may have a mosaic chromosomal defect and this may account for the relatively mild clinical signs seen in liveborn infants [31]. In view of this, and in view of the fact that not all fetuses with a cystic hygroma have Turner's syndrome, it is mandatory that a chromosomal analysis be carried out if a cystic hygroma is identified on antenatal ultrasound.

53.6 Triploidy (Table 53.5)

This condition occurs when there are three sets of chromosomes present instead of the normal two sets.

The extra set can be paternal in origin (69,XXY), which is the most common, accounting for 60% of cases, or maternal (69,XXX), seen in 37%. A third karyotype (69,XYY) is seen in about 3% [91].

The vast majority of triploid fetuses will however abort in the first trimester and such fetuses account for approximately 10% of all first trimester abortuses. Of those that survive, the most common finding is early growth retardation associated with oligohydramnios [92,93]. The patients often present as 'small for dates' in the second trimester and abnormalities in the placenta may also be demonstrated. Hydatidiform change, although not always present in triploidy, should always prompt a karyotype if seen with growth retardation and oligohydramnios [2]. Occasionally the placenta may be enlarged and the hydropic changes may vary from solitary large cysts to multiple small cysts [21,94,95].

The presence of growth retardation and oligohydramnios makes scanning the fetus difficult and the absence of any specific patterns of abnormalities compounds the problem. Having said that cranial abnormalities are common, in particular holoprosencephaly, hydrocephalus and agenesis of the corpus callosum. Facial clefting can occur but is often difficult to demonstrate due to the oligohydramnios, as are the abnormalities of the hands and feet. In the hands syndactyly of the third and fourth fingers can be seen in up to 50% of fetuses and club-foot may also be present. Cardiac abnormalities are less common, as are abdominal anomalies such as an omphalocele and renal cystic dysplasia.

The outcome is extremely poor, with most fetuses aborting during early pregnancy. Only rarely has prolonged survival been reported [96].

53.7 First trimester diagnosis of chromosomal disease

The presence of a cystic hygroma, presenting in the first trimester and then resolving, in fetuses with chromosomal disease is well documented [78] and the cystic hygroma has a clear-cut association with Turner's syndrome. It may also be associated with other chromosomal abnormalities such as trisomy 13, 18 or 21 [63]. This knowledge, together with the development of the use of transvaginal sonography, has prompted further evaulation of markers of chromosomal disease in the late first and early second trimesters of pregnancy.

Nicolaides et al. [97] using transabdominal ultrasound found a high correlation between a fetal nuchal translucency (fluid behind the fetal head) (Figure 53.14) of greater than 3 mm and chromosomal abnormalities, most commonly trisomy 21. Bronshtein et al. [98] however further refined the definition of cystic hygromata, using transvaginal ultrasound, into septated and non-septated types. The septated cystic hygroma was found to have a much higher incidence of chromosomal disease and hydrops and was less likely to resolve spontaneously. Together with biochemical markers [66], an early scan in the late first trimester may hold important clues to the presence of chromosomal disease which may have resolved by the second trimester. There may therefore be a return to early scanning, not only for accurate dating of the pregnancy but also to look for markers of chromosomal disease.

References

1. Schneider, A.S., Mennut, M.T. and Zackai, E.M. (1981) High caesarian section rate in trisomy 18 births: a potential indication for late prenatal diagnosis. American Journal of Obstetrics and Gynecology, 140, 367–70.
2. Twining, P. and Zuccollo, J. (1993) The ultrasound markers of chromosomal disease: a retrospective study. British Journal of Radiology, 66, 408–14.
3. Nicolaides, K.H., Snijders, R.J.M., Gosdon, C.M. et al. (1992) Ultrasonographically detectable markers of fetal chromosomal abnormalities. Lancet, 340, 704–707.
4. Jones, K.L. (1988) Smiths Recognizable Patterns of Human Malformation, 4th edn, W.B. Saunders, Eastbourne.
5. Getachew, M.M., Goldstein, R.B., Edge, V. et al. (1991) Correlation between omphalocoele contents and karyotypic abnormalities: sonographic study in 37 cases. AJR, 158, 133–36.
6. Nicolaides, K.H., Berry, S., Snijders, R.J.M. et al. (1990) Fetal lateral cerebral ventriculomegaly: associated malformations and chromosomal defects. Fetal Diagnosis and Therapy, 5, 5–14.
7. Benacerraf, B.R., Mandell, J., Estroff, J.A. et al. (1990) Fetal pyelectasis: a possible association with Down's syndrome. Obstetrics and Gynecology, 76, 58–60.
8. Benacerraf, B.R. (1991) Prenatal sonography of autosomal trisomies. Ultrasound in Obstetrics and Gynecology, 1, 66–75.
9. Nyberg, D.A., Kramer, D., Resta, R.G. and Kapur, R. (1993) Prenatal sonographic findings of trisomy 18. Journal of Ultrasound in Medicine, 2, 103–13.
10. Royal College of Obstetricians and Gynaecologists (1984) Working Party Report on Routine Ultrasound Examination in Pregnancy, RCOG, London, p. 10.
11. Chitty, L.S., Hunt, G.H., Moore, J. and Lobb, M.O. (1991) Effectiveness of routine ultrasonography in detecting fetal structural abnormalities in a low risk population. BMJ, 303, 1165–69.
12. Luck, C.A. (1992) Value of routine ultrasound scanning at 19 weeks: a four year study of 8849 deliveries. BMJ, 304, 1474–78.
13. Ledbetter, D.H., Martin, A.O., Verlinsky, Y. et al. (1990) Cytogenetic results of chorionic villus sampling. High success rate and the diagnostic accuracy in the United States collaborative study. American Journal of Obstetrics and Gynecology, 162, 495–501.
14. Nicolaides, K.H., Rodeck, C.H. and Gosden, C.M. (1986) Rapid karyotyping in non-lethal fetal abnormalities. Lancet, i, 283–86.
15. Daffos, F., Capella Pav Bovsky, M. and Forester, F. (1985) Fetal blood sampling during pregnancy with use of a needle guided by ultrasound: a study of 606 consecutive cases. American Journal of Obstetrics and Gynecology, 153, 655–60.
16. Maxwell, D.J., Johnson, P., Hurley, P. et al. (1991) Fetal blood sampling and pregnancy loss in relation to indication. British Journal of Obstetrics and Gynaecology, 98, 892–97.
17. Evans, M.J., Klinger, K.W., Nelson, B. et al. (1992) Rapid prenatal diagnosis by fluorescent in situ hybridization of chorionic villi. An adjunct to long term culture and karyotype. American Journal of Obstetrics and Gynecology, 167, 1522–25.
18. Ried, T., Landes, G., Dackowski, W. et al. (1992) Multicolour fluorescence in situ hybridization for the simultaneous detection of probe sets for chromosome 12, 18, 21, X and Y in uncultured amniotic fluid cells. Human Molecular Genetics, 1, 307–13.
19. Roberts, L. (1991) FISHing cuts the angst in amniocentesis. Science, 254, 378–79.
20. Patau, K., Smith, D.W., Therman, E. et al. (1960) Multiple congenital anomaly caused by an extra chromosome. Lancet, i, 790–93.
21. Nyberg, D.A. and Crane, J.P. (1990) Chromosome abnormalities, in Diagnostic Ultrasound of Fetal Anomalies, Text and Atlas (eds D.A. Nyberg, B.S. Mahoney and D.M. Pretorius), Mosby Year Book, St Louis, pp. 676–724.
22. Greene, M.F., Benacerraf, B.R. and Frigoletto, F.D. (1987) Reliable criteria for the prenatal sonographic diagnosis of alobar holoprosencephaly. American Journal of Obstetrics and Gynecology, 156, 687–89.
23. Turner, G. and Twining, P. (1993) The facial profile in the diagnosis of fetal abnormalities. Clinical Radiology, 47, 389–95.
24. Benacerraf, B.R., Frigoletto, F.D. and Greene, M.F. (1986) Abnormal facial features and extremities in human trisomy syndromes: prenatal ultrasound appearances. Radiology, 159, 243–46.
25. Brown, D.L., Emerson, D.S., Shulman, L.P. et al. (1993) Predicting aneuploidy in fetuses with cardiac anomalies. Journal of Ultrasound in Medicine, 3, 153–61.
26. Paladini, D., Calabro, R., Palmieri, S. and D'Andrea, T. (1993) Prenatal diagnosis of congenital heart disease and fetal karyotyping. Obstetrics and Gynecology, 81, 679–82.
27. Meckel, S. and Passarge, E. (1971) Encephalocoele, polycystic kidneys and polydactyly as an autosomal recessive trait simulating certain other disorders: the Meckel syndrome. Annals of Genetics, 14, 97–103.
28. Edwards, J.H. (1960) A new trisomic syndrome. Lancet, i, 787.
29. Carter, P.E., Pearn, J.H., Bell, J. et al. (1985) Survival in trisomy 18: life tables for use in genetic counselling and clinical paediatrics. Clinical Genetics, 27, 59–61.
30. Twining, P., Zuccollo, J., Clewes, J. and Swallow, J. (1991) Fetal choroid plexus cysts: a prospective study and review of the literature. British Journal of Radiology, 64, 98–102.
31. Donnenfield, A.E. and Mennut, M.T. (1988) Sonographic findings in

fetuses with common chromosome abnormalities. *Clinical Obstetrics and Gynecology*, **31**, 80–96.

32. Allan, L.D., Sharland, G.K. and Chita, S.K. (1991) Chromosomal abnormalities in fetal congenital heart disease. *Ultrasound in Obstetrics and Gynecology*, **1**, 8–11.
33. Shirley, I.M. Bottomley, F. and Robinson, V.P. (1992) Routine radiographer screening for fetal abnormalities by ultrasound in an unselected low risk population. *British Journal of Radiology*, **65**, 564–69.
34. Achiron, R., Glaser, J. and Gelernter, I. (1992) Extended fetal echocardiographic examination for detecting cardiac malformations in low risk pregnancies. *BMJ*, **304**, 671–74.
35. Crawford, D.C., Chita, S.K. and Allan, L.D. (1988) Prenatal detection of congenital heart disease factors affecting obstetric management and survival. *American Journal of Obstetrics and Gynecology*, **159**, 352–56.
36. Copel, J., Cullen, M., Green, J.S. *et al.* (1988) The frequency of aneuploidy in prenatally diagnosed congenital heart disease: an indication for fetal karyotype. *American Journal of Obstetrics and Gynecology*, **158**, 409–13.
37. Nicolaides, K.H., Salveston, D.R., Snidjers, R.J.M. and Gosden, C.M. (1992) Strawberry shaped skull in fetal trisomy 18. *Fetal Diagnosis and Therapy*, **7**, 132–37.
38. Bundy, A.L., Saltzman, D.M., Prober, B. *et al.* (1986) Antenatal sonographic findings in trisomy 18. *Journal of Ultrasound in Medicine*, **5**, 361–64.
39. Furness, M.E. (1987) Choroid plexus cysts and trisomy 18. *Lancet*, **ii**, 693.
40. Chitkara, U., Cogswell, C., Norton, K. and Wilkins, I.A. (1988) Choroid plexus cysts in the fetus: a benign anatomic variant or pathological entity? *Obstetrics and Gynecology*, **72**, 185–89.
41. Ostlere, S.J., Irving, H.C. and Lilford, R.J. (1990) Fetal choroid plexus cysts: a report of 100 cases. *Radiology*, **175**, 753–55.
42. Thorpe-Beeston, J.G., Gosden, C.M. and Nicolaides, K.H. (1990) Choroid plexus cysts and chromosomal defect. *British Journal of Radiology*, **63**, 783–86.
43. Nadel, A.S., Bromely, B.S., Frigeletto, F.D. *et al.* (1992) Isolated choroid plexus cysts in the second trimester fetus: is amniocentesis really indicated? *Radiology*, **185**, 545–48.
44. Chudleigh, P., Pearce, J.M. and Campbell, S. (1984) The prenatal diagnosis of transient cysts of the fetal choroid plexus. *Prenatal Diagnosis*, **4**, 135–37.
45. Benacerraf, B.R., Harlow, B. and Frigoletto, F.D. (1990) Are choroid plexus cysts an indication for second trimester amniocentesis? *American Journal of Obstetrics and Gynecology*, **162**, 1001–1006.
46. Benacerraf, B.R., Miller, W.A. and Frigoletto, F.D. (1988) Sonographic detection of fetuses with trisomies 13 and 18: accuracy and limitation. *American Journal of Obstetrics and Gynecology*, **158**, 404–409.
47. Perpignano, M.C., Cohen, H.L., Klein, V.R. *et al.* (1992) Fetal choroid plexus cysts: beware the smaller cyst. *Radiology*, **182**, 715–17.
48. Chudleigh, T., Chitty, L., Campbell, S. and Pembrey, M. (1992) Choroid plexus cysts, incidence and clinical significance in low risk pregnancies. *British Journal of Radiology*, **65**, 636.
49. Platt, L.D., Carlson, D.E. and Medeans, A.L. (1991) Fetal choroid plexus cysts in the second trimester, a cause for concern. *American Journal of Obstetrics and Gynecology*, **164**, 1652–56.
50. Gabrielli, S., Reece, E.A. and Pilu, G. (1989) The clinical significance of prenatally diagnosed choroid plexus cysts. *American Journal of Obstetrics and Gynecology*, **160**, 1207–10.
51. Achiron, R., Barkal, G., Katznelson, B. and Maschiach, S. (1991) Fetal lateral ventricle choroid plexus cysts: the dilemma of amniocentesis. *Obstetrics and Gynecology*, **78**, 815–18.
52. Nyberg, D.A., Mahoney, B.S., Hegge, F.N. *et al.* (1991) Enlarged cisterna vena magna and the Dandy–Walker malformation: factors associated with chromosome abnormalities. *Obstetrics and Gynecology*, **77**, 436–42.
53. Cornford, E. and Twining, P. (1992) The Dandy–Walker syndrome: the value of antenatal diagnosis. *Clinical Radiology*, **45**, 172–74.
54. Pilu, G., Romero, R. and DePalma, L. (1986) Antenatal diagnosis and obstetric management of Dandy–Walker syndrome. *Journal of Reproductive Medicine*, **31**, 1017–22.
55. Twining, P., Zuccollo, J. and Jaspan, T. (1994) The outcome of fetal ventriculomegaly. *British Journal of Radiology*, **67**, 26–31.
56. Thorpe-Beeston, G., Gosden, C.M. and Nicolaides, K.H. (1989) Congenital diaphragmatic hernia, associated malformations and chromosomal defects. *Fetal Therapy*, **4**, 21–28.
57. Nyberg, D.A., Fitsimmons, J. and Mack, L.A. (1989) Chromosomal abnormalities in fetuses with omphalocele: significance of omphalocele contents. *Journal of Ultrasound in Medicine*, **8**, 299–308.
58. Nicolaides, K.H., Snijders, R.J.M., Cheng, H. *et al.* (1992) Fetal abdominal wall and gastrointestinal tract defects: associated malformations and chromosomal defects. *Fetal Diagnosis and Therapy*, **7**, 102–15.
59. Benacerraf, B.R., Saltzman, D.H., Estroff, J.A. and Frigeletto, F.D. (1990) Abnormal karyotype of fetuses with omphalocoele: prediction based on omphalocoele contents. *Obstetrics and Gynecology*, **75**, 317–19.
60. Nicolaides, K.H., Cheng, H., Snijders, R.J.M. and Gosden, C.M. (1992) Fetal renal defects, associated malformations and chromosomal defects. *Fetal Diagnosis and Therapy*, **7**, 1–11.
61. Dicke, J.M. and Crane, J.P. (1991) Sonographic recognition of major

malformations and aberrant fetal growth in trisomic fetuses. *Journal of Ultrasound in Medicine*, **10**, 433–38.
62. Landy, M.J., Isada, N.B. and Larsen, J.W. (1987) Genetic implications of idiopathic hydramnios. *American Journal of Obstetrics and Gynecology*, **157**, 114–17.
63. Pearce, J.M., Griffin, D. and Campbell, S. (1984) Cystic hygromata in trisomy 18 and 21. *Prenatal Diagnosis*, **4**, 371–75.
64. Wald, N.J., Cuckle, H.S., Densem, J.W. *et al.* (1988) Maternal serum screening for Down's syndrome in early pregnancy. *BMJ*, **297**, 883–87.
65. Wald, N.J., Kennard, A., Densem, J.W. *et al.* (1992) Antenatal maternal serum screening for Down's syndrome: results of a demonstration project. *BMJ*, **305**, 391–94.
66. Wald, N.J., Stone, R., Cuckle, H.S. *et al.* (1992) First trimester concentrations of pregnancy associated plasma protein A and placental protein 14 in Down's syndrome. *BMJ*, **305**, 28.
67. Tongue, M. and Rodeck, C. (1989) Commentary. Is ultrasound of any value in screening for Down's syndrome? *British Journal of Obstetrics and Gynaecology*, **96**, 1369–72.
68. Lynch, L., Berkowitz, G.S., Chitkara, U. *et al.* (1989) Ultrasound detection of Down's syndrome: is it really possible? *Obstetrics and Gynecology*, **73**, 267–70.
69. Nyberg, D.A., Resta, R.G., Luthy, D.A. *et al.* (1990) Prenatal sonographic findings of Down's syndrome: review of 94 cases. *Obstetrics and Gynecology*, **76**, 370–77.
70. Benacerraf, B.R., Neuberg, D. and Frigoletto, F.D. (1991) Humeral shortening in second trimester fetuses with Down's syndrome. *Obstetrics and Gynecology*, **77**, 223–27.
71. Perella, R., Duerinckx, A.J., Grant, E.G. *et al.* (1988) Second trimester sonographic diagnosis of Down's syndrome: role of femur length shortening and nuchal fold thickening. *American Journal of Radiology*, **151**, 981–85.
72. Ginsberg, N., Cadkin, A., Pergament, E. and Verlinsky, Y. (1990) Ultrasonographic detection of the second trimester fetus with trisomy 18 and 21. *American Journal of Obstetrics and Gynecology*, **163**, 1186–90.
73. Nelson, L.H., Clark, C.E., Fishburne, J.I. *et al.* (1982) Value of serial sonography in the *in utero* detection of duodenal atresia. *Obstetrics and Gynecology*, **59**, 657–60.
74. Crane, J.P. and Gray, D.L. (1991) Sonographically measured nuchal skinfold thickness as a screening tool for Down's syndrome: results of a prospective clinical trial. *Obstetrics and Gynecology*, **77**, 533–36.
75. Benacerraf, B.R. and Frigoletto, F.D. (1987) Soft tissue nuchal fold in the second trimester fetus: standards for normal measurements compared to those in Down's syndrome. *American Journal of Obstetrics and Gynecology*, **157**, 1146–49.
76. Nicolaides, K.H., Azar, G., Snijders, R.J.M. and Gosden, C.M. (1992) Fetal nuchal oedema, associated malformations and chromosomal defects. *Fetal Diagnosis and Therapy*, **7**, 123–31.
77. Benacerraf, B.R., Laboda, L.A. and Frigoletto, F.D. (1992) Thickened nuchal fold in fetuses, not at risk for aneuploidy. *Radiology*, **184**, 239–42.
78. Rodis, J.F., Vintzileos, A.M., Campbell, W.A. *et al.* (1988) Spontaneous resolution of fetal cystic hygroma in Down's syndrome. *Obstetrics and Gynecology*, **71**, 976–77.
79. Benacerraf, B.R., Galman, R. and Frigoletto, F.D. (1987) Sonographic identification of second trimester fetuses with Down's syndrome. *New England Journal of Medicine*, **317**, 1371–76.
80. Lockwood, C., Benacerraf, B.R. and Hansky, A. (1987) A sonographic screening for Down's syndrome. *American Journal of Obstetrics and Gynecology*, **157**, 803–808.
81. Nyberg, D.A., Resta, R.G. and Hickok, D. (1990) Femur length shortening in the detection of Down's syndrome: is prenatal screening feasible? *American Journal of Obstetrics and Gynecology*, **162**, 1247–52.
82. Twining, P., Whalley, D.R., Lewin, E. and Foulkes, K. (1991) Is a short femur length a useful marker for Down's syndrome? *British Journal of Radiology*, **64**, 990–92.
83. Benacerraf, B.R., Osathanondh, R. and Frigoletto, F.D. (1988) Sonographic demonstration of hypoplasia of the middle phalanx of the 5th digit: a finding associated with Down's syndrome. *American Journal of Obstetrics and Gynecology*, **159**, 181–83.
84. Bahado-Singh, R.O., Wyse, L., Dorr, M.A. *et al.* (1992) Fetuses with Down's syndrome have disproportionately shortened frontal lobe dimensions on ultrasonographic re-examination. *American Journal of Obstetrics and Gynecology*, **167**, 1009–14.
85. Chitty, L., Chudleigh, T., Campbell, S. and Pembrey, M. (1992) Incidence, natural history and clinical significance of mild fetal pyelectasis. *British Journal of Radiology*, **65**, 636.
86. Fakhry, J., Reiser, M., Shapiro, L.R. *et al.* (1986) Increased echogenicity in the lower fetal abdomen: a common normal variant in the second trimester. *Journal of Ultrasound in Medicine*, **5**, 489–92.
87. Dicke, J.M. and Crane, J.P. (1992) Sonographically detected hyperechoic fetal bowel: significance and implications for pregnancy management. *Obstetrics and Gynecology*, **80**, 778–82.
88. Obrien, W.F., Cefalo, R.C. and Bair, D.G. (1980) Ultrasonographic diagnosis of fetal cystic hygroma. *American Journal of Obstetrics and Gynecology*, **138**, 464–66.

89. Goldstein, R., Lapidus, A.S. and Filly, R.A. (1991) Fetal cephalocoeles: diagnosis with ultrasound. *Radiology*, **180**, 803–808.

90. Chervenak, F.A., Isaacson, G. and Blakemore, K.J. (1983) Fetal cystic hygroma: cause and natural history. *New England Journal of Medicine*, **309**, 822–25.

91. Uchida, I.A. and Freeman, V.C.P. (1985) Triploidy and chromosomes. *American Journal of Obstetrics and Gynecology*, **151**, 65–69.

92. Edwards, M.T., Smith, W.L., Hanson, J. and Abu Yousef, M. (1986) Sonographic diagnosis of triploidy. *Journal of Ultrasound in Medicine*, **5**, 279–81.

93. Lockwood, C., Sciosa, A. and Stiller, R. (1987) Sonographic features of the triploid fetus. *American Journal of Obstetrics and Gynecology*, **157**, 285–87.

94. Szulman, A.E., Philipp, E., Bone, J.G. and Bone, A. (1982) Human triploidy: association with partial hydatidiform moles and non-molar conceptuses. *Human Pathology*, **12**, 1016.

95. Rubenstein, J.B., Swayne, L.C., Dise, C.A. *et al.* (1986) Placental changes in fetal triploidy syndrome. *Journal of Ultrasound in Medicine*, **5**, 545–50.

96. Sherard, J., Bean, C. and Bove, B. (1986) Long survival in an 69XXY triploid male. *American Journal of Human Genetics*, **46**, 223–24.

97. Nicolaides, K.H., Azar, G., Byrne, D. *et al.* (1992) Fetal nuchal translucency: ultrasound screening for chromosomal defects in first trimester of pregnancy. *BMJ*, **304**, 867–69.

98. Bronshtein, M., Bar Hava, I., Blumenfield, I. and Bijar, J. (1993) The difference between septated and non-septated nuchal cystic hygroma in the early second trimester. *Obstetrics and Gynecology*, **81**, 683–87.

54 FETAL ECHOCARDIOGRAPHY IN THE DIAGNOSIS AND MANAGEMENT OF FETAL STRUCTURAL HEART DISEASE AND ARRHYTHMIAS

A.H. Friedman, J.A. Copel and C.S. Kleinman

54.1 Introduction

54.1.1 GENERAL BACKGROUND

Non-invasive ultrasound imaging has become the principal diagnostic tool in the prenatal detection of fetal malformations. With the development of 'real-time' imaging, *in utero* evaluation of fetal heart structure, function and rhythm has become possible as well. Congenital heart disease, with a live birth incidence of 0.8%, constitutes one of the most common fetal malformations [1,2].

In this chapter we will outline the evolution of fetal echocardiography as a tool used for the diagnosis of abnormal fetal cardiovascular structure and physiology, focus on the current capabilities and applications of these techniques to diagnose structural fetal heart disease and fetal arrhythmias, and report on the current management of the fetus with cardiovascular disease.

Ultrasonographic imaging of the fetal heart has evolved from the early scanning techniques of M-mode to the current technical capabilities which include two-dimensional imaging, M-mode, pulsed Doppler, steerable continuous wave Doppler and, most recently, Doppler color flow mapping. These advances in sonographic instrumentation and analysis permit detailed anatomic and physiologic study of the normal and abnormal fetal heart.

The early and accurate detection of cardiac structural and rhythm abnormalities *in utero* has become an important aspect of fetal diagnosis and care for several reasons. First, precise prenatal diagnosis of critical congenital heart disease permits planning for early postnatal medical interventions intended to maintain fetal shunt pathways, which may be necessary for systemic perfusion, pulmonary perfusion or intracardiac mixing. For example, congenital heart diseases which are dependent on patency of the ductus arteriosus for systemic or pulmonary blood flow can be managed with early postnatal therapy with prostaglandin E_1 (PGE_1). If intracardiac mixing of blood is required, early balloon atrial septostomy can be performed. These timely interventions can potentially avoid the development of subsequent profound organ ischemia or hypoxia with associated acidemia. Second, prenatal diagnosis of congenital heart disease permits appropriate planning of obstetrical care. This may include prenatal maternal transfer so that delivery can occur in a tertiary center where neonatal management can be optimized. Third, early detection of cardiac abnormalities should prompt evaluation of the fetal karyotype and examination for other fetal structural abnormalities which may alter the prognosis. Finally, the continued progress being made in fetal therapy has allowed *in utero* management options to increase dramatically. For these reasons, we believe that the routine obstetric ultrasonographic examination of the fetus should include imaging of the fetal heart.

54.1.2 TEAM APPROACH

The health care team providing prenatal and early postnatal care to the patient with congenital heart disease can be quite large in number. Members of this team include the sonographer, nurse, obstetrician, geneticist and genetic counselor, neonatologist, pediatrician, pediatric cardiologist and cardiac surgeon. The

Diseases of the Fetus and Newborn, 2nd edn, Edited by G.B. Reed, A.E. Claireaux and F. Cockburn. Published in 1995 by Chapman & Hall, London. ISBN 0 412 39160 0

importance of a well-organized team approach cannot be overemphasized. Some institutions have established a Fetal Management Board to function as a multi-disciplinary group which reviews each case of fetal malformation, refining the diagnosis, establishing management plans and facilitating issues relating to the delivery of the patient [3]. The concept of the team approach capitalizes on the knowledge and expertise of the participants in their respective fields, and also broadens the team's competence in parental counseling, as well as coordinating the planning of the prenatal and postnatal care of the patient.

54.2 Identification of fetal heart disease

54.2.1 EPIDEMIOLOGY

As noted above, the incidence of cardiac structural abnormalities in newborns is approximately 8 per 1000 live births [1,2]. However, the mid-trimester incidence of congenital heart disease is higher than the live birth incidence. This is the result of several factors. First, the incidence of congenital heart disease is higher among stillbirths (27.5/1000) when compared to live births (7.7/1000) [2]. Second, some severely complex cardiac anomalies may be associated with an increased incidence of fetal wastage [4]. Third, the demise of the fetus with congenital heart disease may result from the increased frequency of associated karyotype abnormalities [5]. Finally, some congenital heart diseases and fetal arrhythmias can lead to the development of non-immune hydrops fetalis, which may represent *in utero* congestive heart failure and is a condition associated with fetal loss [6,7].

Some physicians believe that all pregnancies should have fetal imaging studies, including a specific evaluation of the fetal heart. Some countries have adopted mandatory prenatal ultrasound screening, including imaging of the heart, as a routine part of prenatal care. However, when no such protocol exists, a decision regarding performance of a fetal echocardiogram must be made for each individual pregnancy. Which pregnancies should undergo fetal echocardiography? Our efforts have been focused on studying pregnancies with identifiable risk factors, as well as those with suspected abnormalities found during routine prenatal sonography (Chapter 31).

54.2.2 INDICATIONS FOR STUDY

Most patients referred for fetal echocardiography have one or more risk factors. These risk factors can be categorized into three groups, and are presented in detail in Table 54.1 [8]. Fetal risk factors include the presence of extracardiac anomalies which can be either chromosomal or anatomic. Our experience at the Yale

Table 54.1 Indications for fetal echocardiography

Fetal risk factors
  Extracardiac anomalies
    Chromosomal
    Anatomic
    Fetal cardiac arrhythmia
      Irregular rhythm
      Tachycardia (>200 beats/min)
      Bradycardia (non-periodic)
    Non-immune hydrops fetalis
    Suspected cardiac anomaly on level 1 scan

Maternal risk factors
  Congenital heart disease
  Cardiac teratogen exposure
    Lithium carbonate
    Amphetamines
    Alcohol
    Anticonvulsants
      Phenytoin
      Trimethadione
      Carbamazepine
      Valproate
      Isotretinoin
  Maternal metabolic disorders
    Diabetes mellitus
    Phenylketonuria
  Polyhydramnios

Familial risk factors
  Congenital heart disease
    Previous sibling
    Paternal
  Syndromes (examples)
    Noonan
    Tuberous sclerosis

Reprinted with permission from Ref. 8.

Fetal Cardiovascular Center has demonstrated that the presence of extracardiac anomalies places the fetus at increased risk for having concurrent cardiac anomalies [9]. While some extracardiac malformations have a higher incidence of associated cardiac disease than others, we have found an overall incidence of 11% of congenital heart disease in fetuses who underwent fetal echocardiography because of the presence of extra-cardiac malformations over the past 9 years. The greatest statistical fetal risk factor, however, is the suspicion of a cardiac anomaly raised during a basic scan [10–13]. In our laboratory, the yield of congenital heart disease from fetuses suspected of having abnormal cardiac structure by the referring sonographer during the past 9 years is approaching 50%, and was 74% for patients referred during 1992 [14]. Table 54.2 outlines the relative frequencies and incidence of structural heart disease in the major indication categories seen at Yale over a 9-year period, based upon the primary indication for fetal cardiac evaluation [14].

Table 54.2 Fetal echocardiographic frequency and relative yield of structural congenital heart disease found by indication category over a 9-year period at the Yale Fetal Cardiovascular Center

Indication	No. (%)	No. positive	Relative yield (%)
Family history	1063 (30)	15	1.4
Arrhythmia	520 (15)	5	1
Extracardiac anomaly	524 (15)	60	11
Maternal diabetes	366 (10)	9	2.5
Teratogen exposure	288 (8)	3	1
Suspicious level 1 scan	187 (5)	84	45
Aneuploidy	155 (4)	19	12
Hydrops	64 (2)	15	23
Other	339 (10)	4	1.2

Reprinted with permission from Ref. 14.

Among the maternal risk factors which should prompt a fetal echocardiographic study are a maternal history of congenital heart disease, a history of a specific cardiac teratogen exposure and maternal metabolic disorders such as diabetes mellitus and phenylketonuria. Potential cardiac teratogens include medications such as lithium, anticonvulsants such as phenytoin, valproic acid and carbamazepine and substances such as alcohol.

Familial risk factors carry a low statistical risk but usually affect the largest number of patients. This group includes families in whom there has been a previous child with congenital heart disease or in whom there is a history of paternal congenital heart disease. Although the statistical risk to the fetus with familial risk factors is low, significant anxiety is frequently experienced by these families, who have previously dealt with congenital heart disease. The reassurance which can be provided to a family by a normal fetal echocardiogram should not be underestimated. Additionally, the presence of familial syndromes which are associated with congenital heart disease and inherited in mendelian patterns such as Noonan's syndrome, Williams' syndrome or tuberous sclerosis should prompt a fetal echocardiographic study.

54.2.3 EXAMINATION TECHNIQUES

The fetal echocardiographic examination usually begins with two-dimensional imaging of the cardiac anatomy. Although it may not always be possible, it is suggested that the sonographer follow a generally established approach or routine to obtain the standard views of the fetal heart in a sequential fashion. Frequently, however, the operator must be flexible, as fetal position and movement may alter the order in which the standard views are obtained [15]. In addition to an unfavorable fetal lie, other factors which may affect the study and limit visualization include maternal obesity and oligohydramnios [16,17]. The complete fetal echocardiographic examination should incorporate the following standard views: the four-chamber view; the left ventricular long axis view with visualization of the aortic outflow tract; the short axis view with visualization of the pulmonary outflow tract and ductus arteriosus; and the longitudinal view of the aortic arch [16–21].

As the study commences, the operator should determine the position of the fetus in the uterus and ascertain abdominal situs by identifying the right and left sides of the trunk. In the normal situation, the stomach should be visualized in the left side of the abdomen. Once the orientation of the fetus has been established, the transducer can be tilted from the fetal abdominal view toward the fetal head. As a result of this maneuver, images of the fetal heart in the four-chamber view are usually obtained. It is important to ensure that the fetal heart is situated in the middle of the chest with the cardiac apex on the same side of the body as the stomach. Further, the fetal heart should not have a pronounced deviation to either the right or left thorax as this could be an indication of a situs abnormality or other intrathoracic congenital malformations.

The four-chamber view is useful to assess the relative sizes of the cardiac chambers as well as to identify individual chamber anatomy. In the heart with normal structure, the chamber closest to the ventral wall is the right ventricle, while the most posterior chamber (closest to the spine) is the left atrium (Figure 54.1). In addition, the right ventricle has coarse muscular trabeculations, including the moderator band, which may be visible toward its apex and which appears to foreshorten the right ventricular cavity. The tricuspid valve annulus is noted to be located slightly more apically than that of the left-sided mitral valve. The left atrium can be identified by the presence of the undulating septum primum or flap valve of the foramen ovale. Whenever possible, it is important to see the four-chamber view from more than one orientation, including one that is perpendicular to the interventricular septum, since the upper portion of the septum may be quite thin in normal fetuses, giving rise to a false-positive suspicion of a ventricular septal defect [8].

Next, the operator should define the origins of the great arteries by means of the long axis view of the left ventricle. When the fetus is in the vertex position with the left side down, this view can be obtained by a slight clockwise rotation of the transducer. In general, this rotation will change the plane of imaging from the four-chamber view to a view of the long axis of the left ventricle with its outflow. In the normal situation, the

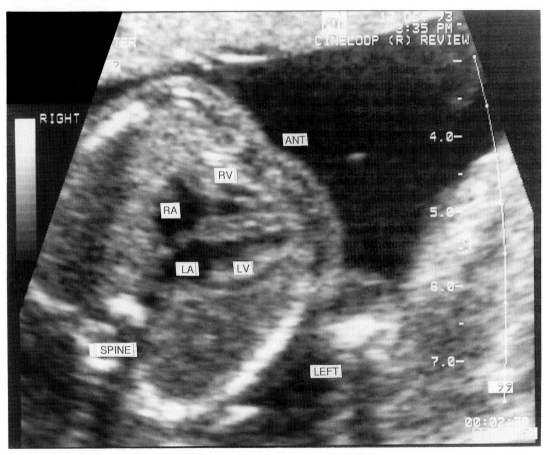

Figure 54.1 The normal fetal four-chamber view demonstrates the integrity of the atrioventricular septum. The two fetal ventricles have approximately equal sizes. The interatrial septum is seen between the fetal right and left atria (RA, LA) and has a defect in its midportion, representing the normal fetal foramen ovale. The left atrium receives the pulmonary veins and is the most posterior cardiac chamber, most closely approximated to the fetal spine. The cardiac apex should be localized to the same side of the fetal body as the stomach bubble. LV = left ventricle; ANT = anterior.

anterior wall of the aorta will be noted to be continuous with the ventricular septum while the posterior wall of the aorta will be in continuity with the anterior leaflet of the mitral valve (Figure 54.2a). From this view, if the transducer is angled slightly toward the fetal head, the pulmonary artery should be seen exiting the anterior right ventricle and crossing over the aorta (Figure 54.2b). The bifurcation of this great vessel (into ductus arteriosus and right pulmonary artery) defines it as the pulmonary artery. To obtain a short axis view of the fetal heart, the transducer is rotated counterclockwise. This view demonstrates the aorta in cross-section, the right ventricular outflow tract, the pulmonary artery and ductus arteriosus. In the short axis view, the right heart structures appear to partially encircle the aorta at the cardiac base (Figure 54.3). This view, along with a longitudinal view of the aortic arch and ductus arteriosus, should confirm the normal crossing relationship of the great arteries and effectively exclude the possibility of transposition of the great arteries. In this

latter lesion, the great arteries arise in a parallel fashion and have a discordant relationship with their ventricle of origin (Figure 54.4).

54.2.4 UTILITY OF FETAL ECHOCARDIOGRAPHY

The usefulness of echocardiography in helping to evaluate the structure, function and hemodynamics of the fetal heart has been noted by many investigators [16,22–25]. The findings from these studies have been validated by confirmatory autopsy results from fetuses examined previously by echocardiography [26]. In general, adequate imaging of cardiovascular structure can be obtained from the middle of the second trimester forward, though with the use of high-frequency trans-vaginal probes, accurate cardiac scanning may be feasible as early as the 11th week of pregnancy [27]. While there is clear agreement on the virtues of fetal echocardiography as a screening tool, there continues to be some question as to the degree of its sensitivity.

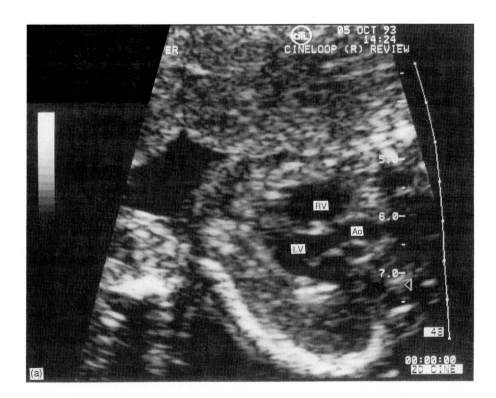

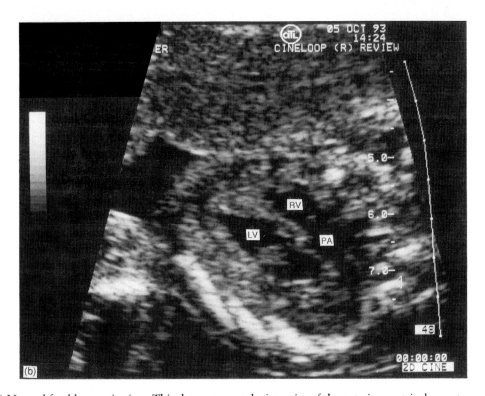

Figure 54.2 (a) Normal fetal long axis view. This demonstrates the integrity of the anterior ventricular septum, separating the right and left ventricles (RV, LV). There is fibrous continuity between the interventricular septum and the anterior wall of the aorta (Ao). The anterior mitral valve leaflet is in fibrous continuity with the posterior aspect of the aorta (with the non-coronary aortic valve leaflet). (b) Long axis view of the right ventricular outflow tract to the pulmonary artery (PA) in the same fetus. Note that the sweep of the outflow tract to the pulmonary artery results in a crossing of the pulmonary artery across the plane of the aorta. This 'cross-over' of the great arteries is present when the great arteries arise in a concordant fashion from the appropriate ventricles, and is not seen when the great arteries are malposed or transposed (arising in a discordant ventriculoarterial connection).

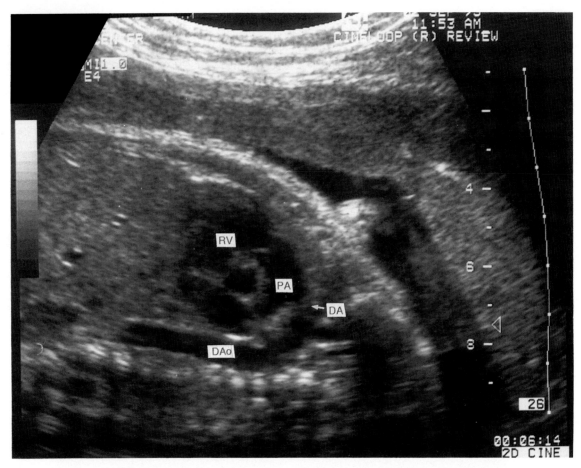

Figure 54.3   Normal cross-sectional view of the fetal great arterial origins. The circular cross-section of the aorta at the level of the aortic valve is seen in the center of the heart. The crescent-shaped sweep of the right ventricular outflow tract (RV) to the anterior and leftward pulmonic valve is seen. The main pulmonary trunk is confluent with the descending thoracic aorta (DAo) via the ductus arteriosus (DA). PA = pulmonary artery.

Previous work from our center has suggested the potential utility and importance of the four-chamber view when screening for congenital heart disease [28]. However, this report was retrospective in nature and more recent reports have suggested that the true sensitivity of the four-chamber screening technique may be somewhat lower than we initially reported [29]. Recently, Vergani and co-workers [30] in Italy reported an 81% sensitivity and 99.9% specificity for fetal congenital heart disease in a large ultrasonographic screening study utilizing the four-chamber view.

While the four-chamber view may elucidate many cardiac structural defects, it is most effective in detecting lesions that alter the central anatomy of the heart (Figure 54.5). This is evidenced by the variety of cardiac malformations diagnosed in our laboratory compared with the postnatal incidence reported from our geographic region, and is presented in Table 54.3 [13]. Clearly, our experience is affected by referral patterns for abnormal four-chamber screening examinations,

and this is reflected in the types of different defects which we most frequently encounter in our laboratory.

Although the most common cardiac malformation encountered postnatally is the ventricular septal defect, small ventricular septal defects may be missed in the fetus [24]. As a result, patients with small or moderate ventricular septal defects, who comprise a large segment of the pediatric population with congenital heart disease, may not be detected by prenatal studies, as their defects may be too small to be noted prenatally or be without sufficient interventricular flow to be observed by Doppler color flow mapping.

54.3   Management of the fetus with congenital heart disease

When the fetal echocardiogram reveals a cardiac anomaly, salient issues such as the presence of extracardiac anomalies, fetal karyotype and the presence of associated cardiac failure must be addressed. These

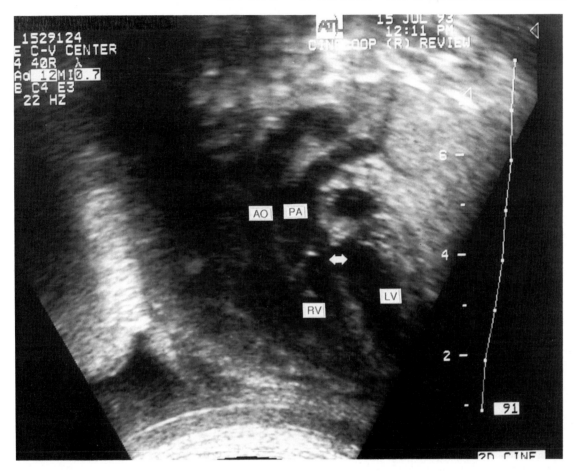

Figure 54.4 Outflow view of the great arteries in a fetal patient with transposition of the great arteries with ventricular septal defect (arrow). In transposition, the great arteries arise in abnormal fashion and are parallel to one another rather than demonstrating the normal 'criss-crossed' relationship to one another. AO = aorta; PA = pulmonary artery; RV = right ventricle; LV = left ventricle.

factors have important implications for the prenatal and postnatal management of the fetus with cardiac disease [13,31,32].

54.3.1 STRUCTURAL MALFORMATIONS

The fetus found to have an abnormality of cardiac structure should undergo a thorough evaluation for the presence of associated extracardiac defects. Allan and colleagues [26] reported that more than half of all fetuses found to have cardiac disease also had an extracardiac malformation. There are numerous reports in the literature that list the extracardiac malformations which have been associated with structural congenital heart disease [9,33–35]. The etiology of the association between the occurrence of congenital heart disease with extracardiac malformations is not always evident, but may be the result of: (1) an exposure to a teratogen; (2) an underlying chromosomal abnormality; (3) a combined morphological expression as components of a recognized syndrome; or perhaps (4) a purely coincidental occurrence. Regardless of the reason for the association, it is clear that all fetuses found to have congenital heart disease should undergo a complete, comprehensive and careful general fetal ultrasound evaluation. Likewise, all fetuses noted to have extracardiac malformations should also receive a thorough fetal echocardiographic study to exclude cardiac anomalies.

54.3.2 CHROMOSOMAL ABNORMALITIES

Whenever fetal cardiac disease is found, fetal chromosomal abnormalities must be considered. The occurrence of chromosomal abnormalities among **pediatric** patients with congenital heart disease is significantly less than that of the **fetal** population with congenital heart disease [5,36]. Berg and colleagues [37] have suggested that this may result from a high rate of fetal wastage during the second and third trimesters when

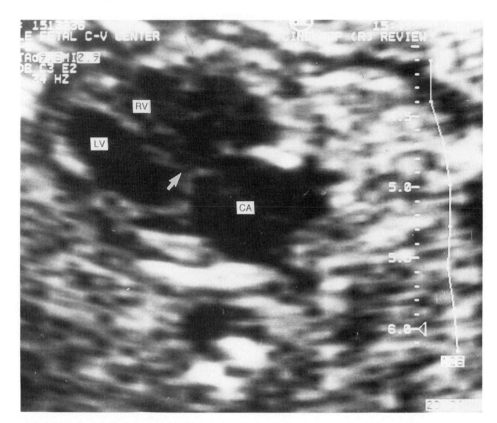

Figure 54.5 Abnormal four-chamber view of the heart of a fetal patient with complete atrioventricular septal defect. There is a common atrium (CA) with a common atrioventricular orifice and a large defect of the inflow portion of the interventricular septum (arrow). This is the most common single defect that is diagnosed on our fetal echocardiographic service. RV = right ventricle; LV = left ventricle.

aneuploidy exists. While the incidence of abnormal chromosomes is high in both groups, our experience has demonstrated a higher rate of aneuploidy when congenital heart disease is found in association with extracardiac malformations (28%) compared with those fetuses with isolated structural heart disease (15%) [13].

We recommend fetal karyotyping to any patient who is found to have an abnormal fetal echocardiogram, regardless of the patient's gestational age or attitude regarding pregnancy termination. Knowledge of the fetal chromosomal structure allows for a well-defined postnatal surgical intervention strategy which may be altered by the finding of a devastating aneuploidy. In addition, prenatal knowledge of the fetal karyotype may help avoid procedures which carry an increased risk for the pregnant woman, such as an emergency cesarean section for fetal distress, when the fetus is rendered non-viable by virtue of its chromosomal structure (e.g. trisomy 13, trisomy 18 or triploidy).

For the family planning to continue a pregnancy with an identified chromosomal abnormality (e.g. trisomy 21 found from screening for advanced maternal age) a complete fetal echocardiogram should be obtained to exclude coexisting congenital heart disease [9,36]. For example, when trisomy 21 is found, 40–50% of fetuses will have concurrent congenital heart disease, with the most common defects being those of the atrioventricular septum and ventricular septum [38,39]. Similarly, the finding of 45X (Turner's syndrome) should prompt fetal echocardiography because up to 35% of such fetuses will have coarctation of the aorta and/or other left heart malformations [38,39]. Both of these examples illustrate how early knowledge of the fetal karyotype allows both the family and the health care team to make appropriate decisions regarding the logistics of delivery and postnatal management.

54.3.3 NON-IMMUNE HYDROPS FETALIS

In many cases, non-immune hydrops fetalis is a manifestation of end-stage congestive heart failure, and is generally due to the presence of either pressure or volume load on the right side of the heart [7]. Non-immune hydrops can result from fetal arrhythmia, structural heart disease, such as atrioventricular valve

Table 54.3 Incidence of structural heart disease found by fetal echocardiography compared to incidence noted postnatally in the same geographic region

	Prenatal		Postnatal	
	N	%	N	%
Atrioventricular septal defect	37	21.7	119	5.3
Hypoplastic left heart syndrome	22	12.9	177	7.9
Double outlet right ventricle	15	8.8	35	1.6
Ventricular septal defect	14	8.2	374	16.7
Tetralogy of Fallot	11	6.5	212	9.5
Critical aortic stenosis	11	6.5	45	2.0
Ebstein anomaly	7	4.1	0	0
Univentricular connection	7	4.1	58	2.6
Transposition of great arteries	6	3.5	252	11.2
Atrial isomerism	6	3.5	95	4.3
Pulmonary atresia	5	2.9	75	3.4
Coarctation	5	2.9	179	8.4
Pulmonary stenosis	4	2.4	79	3.5
Tricuspid atresia	4	2.4	61	2.7
Truncus arteriosus	3	1.8	33	1.6
Other	13	7.3	1867	50.9
Total	170		3661	

Prenatal data are from Yale Fetal Cardiovascular Center. Postnatal data are from New England Regional Infant Cardiac Program. Frequencies are significantly different ($P < .001$) by chi-squared test. Reprinted with permission from Ref. 8.

regurgitation, or from a combination of the two. Occasionally, this may be transient as there may be myocardial adaptation with augmentation of the low cardiac output and resolution of the hydrops. This myocardial adaptation is thought to occur by the Frank–Starling mechanism. In general, however, the presence of a chronic or progressive non-immune hydrops fetalis suggests a poor prognosis, and when it is found in the patient with structural heart disease, it is almost always fatal. When non-immune hydrops results from a fetal arrhythmia, therapy, as outlined below, can often result in a more favorable outcome.

54.3.4 MATERNAL DIABETES MELLITUS

The fetus of the diabetic mother is at risk for congenital anomalies including neural tube defects, the caudal regression syndrome, renal malformations and congenital heart disease. Maternal diabetes increases the risk of fetal cardiac malformations fivefold compared with the non-diabetic [40,41], with the most common abnormalities being ventricular septal defects and trans-

position of the great arteries [42]. Over weeks, the degree of maternal hyperglycemia is reflected by the glycosylated hemoglobin level (HbA_{1c}). Miller and colleagues [43] have shown that an elevated HbA_{1c} level in the first trimester is associated with an increased risk for diabetic embryopathy. Fetal echocardiography is an important tool for evaluation of the pregnant woman with diabetes since abnormalities of cardiac structure resulting from such a diabetic embryopathy can be found with a mid-trimester scan.

Fetal hypertrophic cardiomyopathy can also occur as the result of maternal diabetes. This entity, however, is most often encountered during the third trimester, and thus is not an embryopathy but a fetopathy. The echocardiographic features of the fetus with diabetic hypertrophic cardiomyopathy include restricted ventricular filling, dynamic left ventricular outflow tract obstruction and global myocardial hypertrophy [44,45] (Figure 54.6). This process may result from the growth stimulation caused by high circulating levels of fetal insulin, which occur in response to maternal hyperglycemia [46]. Because it appears that the amount of cardiac hypertrophy is related to the degree of maternal hyperglycemia, strict metabolic control has been suggested for the pregnant woman with diabetes [44]. It has also been shown that, even with strict control of maternal glucose levels, fetuses of diabetic mothers have measurable cardiac hypertrophy, although not necessarily to a clinically significant degree [47].

We have developed a protocol for patients with maternal diabetes which includes a fetal echocardiogram at 20–24 weeks to define the structural integrity of the heart, and a follow-up study at 32–34 weeks both to re-evaluate cardiac structure and to evaluate for ventricular hypertrophy. To obtain consistent and reproducible wall thickness measurements, the M-mode cursor must be placed just below the atrioventricular valves, perpendicular to the ventricular septum in a four-chamber view. Failing to do this may lead to an exaggerated value for septal thickness. The ventricular septum should measure less than 6 mm during the third trimester [47].

54.4 Fetal arrhythmias

There are several reports in the literature describing the natural history of fetal cardiac rhythm disturbances [48–50]. Fetal echocardiography, using a variety of techniques, has been established as the principal means by which fetal arrhythmias can be assessed and defined [22,24,51–54]. The prenatal assessment of fetal cardiovascular status and fetal well-being has progressed with the growth of available technology in recent years, as has the attention given to the evaluation of the fetal cardiac rhythm. Approximately 15% of referrals to our laboratory are for abnormalities of cardiac rhythm

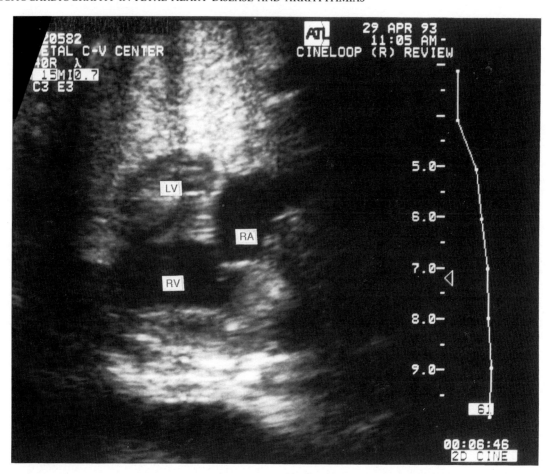

Figure 54.6 Abnormal fetal heart with large right ventricle (RV) and right atrium (RA) and markedly abnormal left ventricle (LV). The left ventricle has a very hypoplastic cavity with a markedly hypertrophic ventricular wall.

[13]. Fetal arrhythmias can be defined as any rhythm irregularity or any sustained regular rhythm outside the range of 100–160 beats/min [8]. Certain non-cardiac conditions, such as chorioamnionitis, can also be associated with sinus tachycardia to rates of 180–190 beats/min.

Echocardiographic analysis of the fetal rhythm can be accomplished with M-mode imaging and/or pulsed wave Doppler evaluation. When a two-dimensional image of the four-chamber view is obtained, the M-mode cursor can be positioned so that it simultaneously traverses the walls of the atrium and ventricle (Figure 54.7). This dual chamber M-mode permits simultaneous recording of atrial and ventricular wall motion, and the relative timing of their respective wall movements can be compared. Because these recordings reflect the mechanical responses to preceding electrical stimulation, they can be used to analyze the underlying arrhythmia [8]. If color flow mapping is available, it can be applied to the M-mode image so that temporally-resolved measurements of both mechanical function and blood flow can be made. In addition, placing the pulsed Doppler sample volume in the left

ventricle just distal to the atrioventricular valve, at a point that captures both diastolic filling and systolic emptying of the chamber, permits assessment of blood flow against time. The combination of these two techniques provides evaluation of both cardiac motion and hemodynamic data necessary for complete rhythm analysis.

54.4.1 SPECIFIC FETAL ARRHYTHMIAS

Fetal cardiac arrhythmias currently account for a significant number of patients who are referred to our laboratory. Fetal echocardiography has been essential to the diagnostic process, and with the growing availability of therapeutic options, fetal echocardiography can provide the basis by which any intervention is monitored. Table 54.4 lists the various arrhythmias which have been diagnosed at the Yale Fetal Cardiovascular Center through 1991.

(a) Isolated extrasystoles

The most common fetal arrhythmias are isolated extrasystoles. These extrasystoles are usually detected

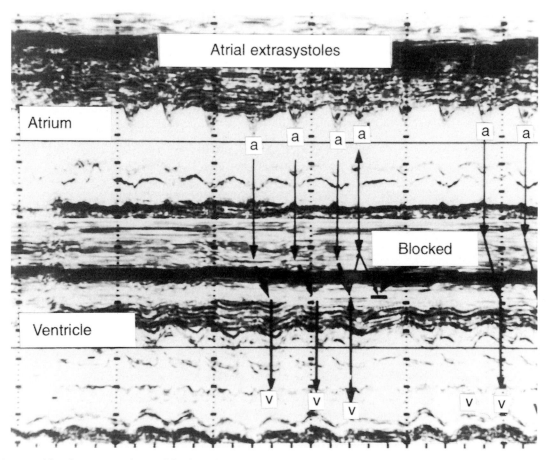

Figure 54.7 Ladder diagram analysis of fetal cardiac rhythm using dual M-mode echocardiographic recording of atrial and ventricular activity. Upper tracing represents atrial wall motion. Lower tracing represents ventricular wall motion. Each normal atrial wall motion (a) is followed by a ventricular contraction (v). The delay between the two represents the electrical delay imparted at the level of the atrioventricular node. Occasional early atrial extrasystoles (a′) are blocked at the atrioventricular node and are not followed by a ventricular contraction. (Reproduced with permission from Creasy, R.K. and Resnik, R. (1989) *Maternal–Fetal Medicine: Principles and Practice*, 2nd edn, W.B. Saunders, Philadelphia, p. 345.)

Table 54.4 Fetal cardiac arrhythmias diagnosed at Yale [After Ref. 8]

Isolated extrasystoles	878
Supraventricular tachycardia	47
Atrial flutter	12
Atrial fibrillation	2
Sinus tachycardia	6
Junctional tachycardia	1
Ventricular tachycardia	4
Second-degree atrioventricular block	7
Complete heart block	26
Sinus bradycardia	1
Total	984

as post-extrasystolic pauses during auscultation of the fetal heart in a routine obstetrical examination. It has been our experience that these arrhythmias are almost exclusively supraventricular in origin. Occasionally, however, the origin of these extrasystoles can be junctional or ventricular [55]. This isolated ectopy is a self-limited process and, just as in the neonate, it almost always carries a benign prognosis [49,50,56,57]. Interestingly, these arrhythmias usually resolve before labor or shortly after delivery [54].

We have found that 1% of fetuses with premature atrial contractions have concomitant structural heart disease [58]. As a result, we recommend that all patients demonstrating such ectopy have a complete fetal echocardiographic evaluation. Furthermore, 0.5% of such patients will develop a re-entrant tachycardia later in pregnancy [49,58,59], which is the basis for our recommendation that any fetus with premature extrasystoles be auscultated weekly until the extrasystoles resolve, to rule out the possible development of a sustained tachycardia.

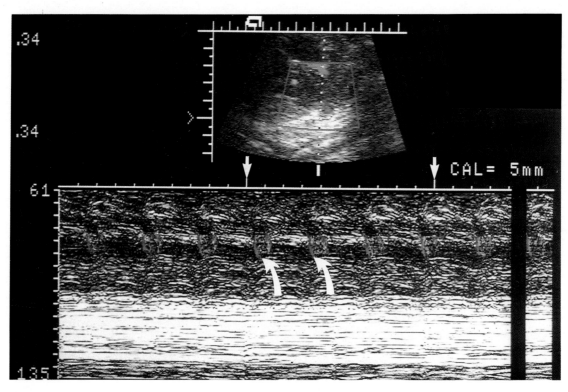

Figure 54.8 Color-encoded M-mode echocardiogram demonstrating transatrioventricular valve flow (curved arrow). Vertical arrows denote 1-s time calibrations. Heart rate is monotonous at 240 beats/min. The rhythm is sustained supraventricular tachycardia.

(b) Supraventricular tachycardia

As shown in Table 54.4, fetal supraventricular tachycardia accounts for 5% of fetal arrhythmias referred to our unit. Fetal re-entrant supraventricular tachycardia most frequently presents with a ventricular rate of 240 beats/min and can be recognized using M-mode echocardiography (Figure 54.8). Among the mechanisms which have been implicated as possible etiologies of fetal supraventricular tachycardias are:([1] a re-entrant or reciprocating mechanism, related to a 'circus' or circular movement of electrical energy, arising at the atrioventricular junction with a monotonous 1:1 ratio of atrial to ventricular rate; (2) 'an automatic focus' above the bundle of His which is separate from, and faster than, the sinus nodal pacemaker; and (3) atrial flutter or fibrillation with typically high atrial rates of 300–500 beats/min and a variable degree of atrioventricular nodal block, yielding lower ventricular rates [8,60].

(c) Ventricular tachycardia

Unlike fetal supraventricular tachycardia, fetal ventricular tachycardia may have a highly variable rate. With this arrhythmia, the rate can be as fast as 400 beats/min or as slow as 170 beats/min. The diagnosis of ventricular tachycardia can be made using M-mode echocardiography with the beam of interrogation transecting the atrium and the ventricle. This technique may reveal atrioventricular dissociation with the ventricular chamber contracting at a faster pace than the atrial chamber. It is our belief that not all of these fetuses will require antiarrhythmic therapy. In addition, ventricular tachycardia that is misdiagnosed as supraventricular tachycardia leading to maternal administration of digoxin for the fetus may cause life-threatening fetal ventricular fibrillation [60]. Therefore, of primary importance for the fetus with an abnormal tachycardia is a thorough analysis of the cardiac rhythm to define accurately whether it is supraventricular or ventricular in origin.

(d) Bradyarrhythmias

Fetal complete heart block is the most common etiology of fetal bradyarrhythmias with ventricular rates less than 90 beats/min [61,62] (Figure 54.9).

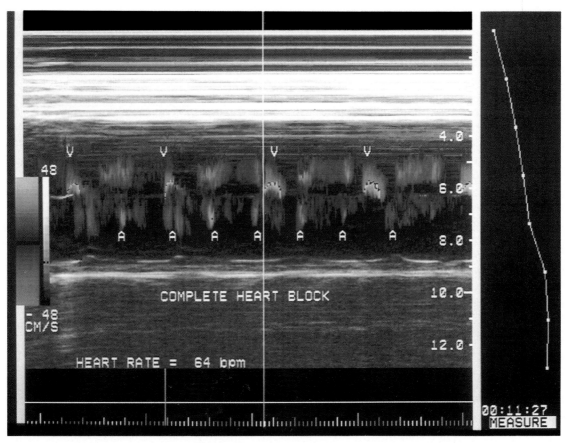

Figure 54.9 Color-encoded M-mode echocardiogram in a fetus with a fixed bradycardia at 64 beats/min. Multicolored signals (V) represent aliased higher velocity flow signals in the ascending aorta. Red signals (A) within atrial cavity represent flow related to atrial contractions reflecting an atrial rate of 140 beats/min. The atrial (A) and ventricular (V) contractions do not relate to one another. The rhythm is complete atrioventricular block.

Complete heart block is a rare prenatal condition with an incidence of about 1 in 20 000 live births [63]. Of the 55 cases of fetal atrioventricular block which were compiled in a recent multicenter study [64], approximately half were found to have associated complex cardiac structural malformations, the most common being either atrioventricular discordance or one of the heterotaxy syndromes (i.e. polysplenia, asplenia). When fetal atrioventricular block was found in conjunction with normal cardiac structure, there was a high incidence of maternal autoimmune antibodies such as anti-ro (SS-A) or anti-la (SS-B) [64].

The experience at the Yale Fetal Cardiovascular Center has demonstrated that all mothers of fetuses with normal cardiac structure and complete atrioventricular block can be found to have circulating autoantibodies with the use of sensitive assays [65]. A ventricular rate of 55 beats/min or greater has been correlated with a favorable outcome. Approximately 85% of the fetuses with complete atrioventricular block and a structurally normal heart will survive the neonatal period [64]. Once a fetus has been shown to have complete atrioventricular block, close echocardiographic follow-up is necessary to evaluate the patient for the development of hydrops fetalis, a condition which, as discussed above, can have ominous prognostic implications.

54.4.2 THERAPY OF FETAL ARRHYTHMIAS

Many pharmacological agents have been used to treat the fetus with arrhythmias. Among these are digoxin, adenosine, flecainide, procainamide and amiodarone [66–69]. Even when indications for use are clear, it must be remembered that each of these therapies carries with it inherent risks both for the fetus and for the mother. Whenever treatment of fetal arrhythmias is undertaken, a detailed discussion of the risks and benefits should be held with the parents. If fetal arrhythmias are to be treated effectively via maternal administration, it is essential that the drug have adequate maternal absorption and reliable transplacental transfer and achieve therapeutic levels in the fetus without causing toxicity or severe side-effects to either the mother or fetus. Some of these clinical problems can be avoided with direct administration of the medication into the fetus via cordocentesis. The small but finite risk of this procedure must be balanced against the potential need for multiple drug doses.

We advocate a team approach to the management of the fetus with an arrhythmia, with the principal emphasis placed upon the accurate diagnosis of the abnormality and a clear understanding of the electrophysiologic basis of the particular arrhythmia. When this information is known, an attempt to select the most appropriate therapeutic intervention for both the mother and fetus can be made [60]. We prefer this approach rather than a rigid algorithm for guiding the decision-making process for the therapy of fetal arrhythmias.

(a)   Supraventricular tachycardia

When a reciprocating supraventricular tachycardia is found in a fetus at term, we suggest delivery and postnatal management of the tachycardia. If the fetus is preterm, and without evidence of hydrops, we use observation with a fetal monitor for an extended period of time (6–12 hours) to demonstrate the proportion of time that the fetus experiences the tachycardia. When the amount of time spent in supraventricular tachycardia is relatively short compared with the time spent in sinus rhythm, the team may determine that intervention is unnecessary, whereas a more aggressive approach would be undertaken if the tachycardia is incessant. In the latter case, a reasonable first-line therapy is intravenous maternal digoxin loading, with subsequent oral digoxin sufficient to achieve a high therapeutic level in the mother. If there is no response observed after therapeutic maternal trough levels are documented, other strategies may be warranted. It is beyond the scope of the current chapter to discuss the potential risks and benefits of the various therapeutic regimens which have been proposed, and which have recently been extensively reviewed [60].

If fetal hydrops is present, fetal blood sampling for drug levels as well as for direct introduction of medications may be performed [8]. Adenosine, which has an extremely short half-life and few side-effects, blocks conduction through the atrioventricular node and can be an effective, albeit transient, therapy if directly administered to the fetus with supraventricular tachycardia. It is not useful, however, when maternally administered, because its half-life and rapid protein binding render it ineffective to the fetus. In addition, adenosine is not effective against recurrent tachycardia.

If cordocentesis is performed, the fetus can also be directly loaded through the umbilical blood sampling catheter with digoxin at a dose of 10 µg/kg (estimated fetal 'dry' body weight). This direct loading can then be followed by maintenance therapy through maternal dosing. It is important to remember that the physiologic changes of pregnancy act to increase the maternal metabolism of digoxin so that relatively high doses may be needed to achieve a therapeutic level. Although digoxin is usually transferred across the placenta efficiently, transplacental passage of digoxin has also been reported to be impaired when placental edema resulting from fetal hydrops is present [70,71].

Other therapeutic strategies may be considered if the above regimen is unsuccessful in controlling fetal supraventricular tachycardia, including direct fetal administration of procainamide followed by oral maternal therapy or maternal oral administration of flecainide. However, the potential benefits of these antiarrhythmics must be balanced against the potential risks to both the mother and the fetus.

Digoxin is our first-line therapy in the management of fetal atrial flutter. We administer the medication either by intravenous maternal loading or by direct fetal injection through the umbilical vessels. If cardioversion does not occur with this single therapy, we next administer oral quinidine to the mother. One must bear in mind that quinidine alters the metabolism of digoxin, leading to increased serum digoxin levels. Because of this interaction, the digoxin dose should be decreased by approximately half when it is given in conjunction with quinidine and both the mother and fetus should be closely monitored for any detrimental effects. When atrial flutter is resistant to therapy with digoxin and quinidine, one may consider maternal amiodarone administration. An intravenous form of amiodarone can be infused directly to the fetus [69], although this form is not currently available in the USA. Amiodarone has a half-life of several weeks, making it an attractive therapy for fetal arrhythmias since it needs to be given much less often than other drugs. However, the complications of this drug, including profound fetal hypothyroidism, should not be disregarded.

(b)   Ventricular tachycardia

Although the experience with fetal ventricular tachycardia is limited, it appears that the primary indication for therapeutic intervention is the presence of hydrops fetalis and a ventricular rate in excess of 200 beats/min. When therapy is necessary, lidocaine may be given directly to the fetus by umbilical vessel injection. If this therapy is successful, maternal administration of the type 1B agent, mexiletine, or a type 1A agent such as quinidine or procainamide, can be used [8]. It is imperative that the diagnosis of ventricular tachycardia be accurate and not be confused with supraventricular tachycardia, as standard therapy for the latter is digoxin, which can be potentially dangerous if administered to the fetus with ventricular tachycardia.

(c) Bradyarrhythmias

A variety of management strategies have been employed to treat fetal complete atrioventricular block. Included among these are the administration of steroids, maternal terbutaline therapy, plasmapheresis and fetal pacemaker placement [72–75]. The most promising of these therapies stems from several reports which have demonstrated that maternal antibodies and fetal inflammatory cells are deposited in the fibrosed atrioventricular nodal tissue of the fetus with complete atrioventricular block and an otherwise structurally normal heart [76–78]. This evidence strongly implicates an antibody-mediated inflammatory process as the principal etiology of disease in these fetuses. We have given steroids known to have transplacental passage, such as dexamethasone, to the mother, with the intention of interfering with the ongoing inflammatory process in the cardiac conduction tissue of these fetuses. We have used this therapy alone or in combination with terbutaline which stimulates the adrenergic receptors in the heart, thereby increasing heart rate. To date, our preliminary results have been encouraging; however further study is necessary to confirm the efficacy of this therapy.

When complete atrioventricular block is found in the fetus near term, delivery may be indicated for neonatal therapy. Both fetal heart rate monitoring and fetal echocardiography can be used to assess atrial rate reactivity, and may allow for a vaginal delivery of some of these patients [65]. Gembruch and colleagues [40] have suggested frequent fetal scalp blood pH measurements and/or the continuous measurement of transcutaneous carbon dioxide partial pressure to assess fetal well-being during the vaginal delivery of the patient with complete atrioventricular block. Postnatally, evaluation of ventricular rate, morphology and duration of the QRS complex as well as evaluation for the signs and symptoms of congestive heart failure should be made serially. As the neonatal clinical picture develops, individual management strategies can be determined.

54.5 Summary

During the past 15 years, the ultrasound examination of the fetal heart has become increasingly sophisticated. The fetal echocardiographic examination now permits the early and accurate assessment of cardiovascular structure and function, as well as the diagnosis and management of fetal rhythm disturbances. The challenge to the fetal echocardiographer has been rivaled by the burgeoning technology. Today, a complete fetal echocardiographic study includes use of two-dimensional and M-mode imaging, as well as Doppler analysis by pulsed wave, continuous and color flow mapping. The horizon promises capabilities for earlier cardiovascular imaging during pregnancy and advances such as three-dimensional reconstruction of structures.

The information obtained from the fetal echocardiogram can have a profound impact on both the expectant family and the health care team. With a normal examination, the reassurance to the family can be immeasurable; when an abnormality is found, appropriate planning, counseling and management strategies can be implemented.

References

1. Hoffman, J.I.E. and Christianson, R. (1978) Congenital heart disease in a cohort of 19 502 births with long-term follow-up. Am. J. Cardiol., 42, 641–47.
2. Mitchell, S.C., Korones, S.B. and Behrends, H.W. (1971) Congenital heart disease in 56 109 births: incidence and natural history. Circulation, 43, 323–32.
3. Porter, K.B., Wagner, P.C. and Cabainiss, M.L. (1988) Fetal board: a multidisciplinary approach to management of the abnormal fetus. Obstet. Gynecol., 72, 275–78.
4. Allan, L.D., Crawford, D.C., Anderson, R.H. et al. (1985) Spectrum of congenital heart disease detected echocardiographically in prenatal life. Br. Heart J., 54, 523–26.
5. Copel, J.A., Cullen, M., Green, J. et al. (1988) The frequency of aneuploidy in prenatally diagnosed congenital heart disease: an indication for fetal karyotyping. Am. J. Obstet. Gynecol., 158, 409–13.
6. Silverman, N.H., Kleinman, C.S., Rudolph, A.M. et al. (1985) Fetal atrioventricular valve insufficiency associated with nonimmune hydrops: a two-dimensional echocardiographic and pulsed Doppler ultrasound study. Circulation, 72, 825–32.
7. Kleinman, C.S., Donnerstein, R.L., DeVore, G.R. et al. (1983) Fetal echocardiography for evaluation of in utero congestive heart failure: a technique for the study of non-immune hydrops fetalis. N. Engl. J. Med., 306, 568–75.
8. Baumann, P., Copel, J.A. and Kleinman, C.S. (1992) Management of the fetus with cardiac disease. Ultrasound Q., 10(2), 57–78.
9. Copel, J.A., Pilu, G. and Kleinman, C.S. (1986) Congenital heart disease and extracardiac anomalies: associations and indications for fetal echocardiography. Am. J. Obstet. Gynecol., 154, 1121–32.
10. Allan, L.D., Crawford, D.C., Chita, S.K. et al. (1986) Prenatal screening for congenital heart disease. BMJ, 292, 1717–19.
11. Copel, J.A. and Kleinman, C.S. (1986) The impact of fetal echocardiography on perinatal outcome. Ultrasound Med. Biol., 12, 327–35.
12. Fermont, L., de Geeter, B., Aubry, J. et al. (1986) A close collaboration between obstetricians and pediatric cardiologists allows antenatal detection of severe cardiac malformations by 2D echocardiography, in Pediatric Cardiology. Proceedings of the Second World Congress (eds E.F. Doyle, M.E. Engle, W.M. Gersony et al.), Springer, NY, p. 34
13. Smythe, J.F., Copel, J.A. and Kleinman, C.S. (1992) Outcome of prenatally detected cardiac malformations. Am. J. Cardiol., 69, 1471–74.
14. Friedman, A.H., Copel, J.A. and Kleinman, C.S. (1992) Fetal echocardiography and fetal cardiology: indications, diagnosis and management. Semin. Perinatol., 17(2), 76–88.
15. Reed, K.L., Anderson, C.F. and Shenker, L. (1988) Methods of examination: two-dimensional, in Fetal Echocardiography. An Atlas. Alan R. Liss, NY, pp. 11–45.
16. Benacerraf, F.R., Pober, B.R. and Sanders, S.P. (1987) Accuracy of fetal echocardiography. Radiology, 165, 847–49.
17. Shime, J., Bertrand, M., Hagen-Ansert, S. et al. (1984) Two-dimensional and M-mode echocardiography in the human fetus. Am. J. Obstet. Gynecol., 148, 679–85.
18. Axel, L. (1983) Real-time sonography of fetal cardiac anatomy. AJR, 41, 283–88.
19. DeVore, G.R., Donnerstein, R.L., Kleinman, C.S. et al. (1982) Normal anatomy as determined by real-time-directed M-mode ultrasound. Am. J. Obstet. Gynecol., 144, 249–60.

20. Huhta, J.C., Hagler, D.J. and Hill, L.M. (1984) Two-dimensional echocardiographic assessment of normal fetal cardiac anatomy. *J. Reprod. Med.*, **29**, 162–67.

21. Nimrod, C., Nicholson, S., Machin, G. *et al.* (1984) *In utero* evaluation of fetal cardiac structure: a preliminary report. *Am. J. Obstet. Gynecol.*, **148**, 516–18.

22. Kleinman, C.S., Hobbins, J.C., Jaffe, C.C. *et al.* (1980) Echocardiographic studies of the human fetus: prenatal diagnosis of congenital heart disease and cardiac dysrhythmias. *Pediatrics*, **65**, 1059–67.

23. Kleinman, C.S. and Santulli, T.V. (1983) Ultrasonic evaluation of the fetal human heart. *Semin. Perinatol.*, **7**, 90–101.

24. Kleinman, C.S., Weinstein, E.M., Talner, N.S. *et al.* (1984) Fetal echocardiography: applications and limitations. *Ultrasound Med. Biol.*, **10**, 747–55.

25. Silverman, N.H. and Golbus, M.S. (1985) Echocardiographic techniques for assessing normal and abnormal fetal cardiac anatomy. *J. Am. Coll. Cardiol.*, **5**, 20S–29S.

26. Allan, L.D., Crawford, D.C., Anderson, R.H. and Tynan, M.J. (1984) Echocardiographic and anatomical correlations in fetal congenital heart disease. *Br. Heart J.*, **52**, 542–48.

27. D'Amelio, R., Giorlandino, C., Masala, L. *et al.* (1991) Fetal echocardiography using transvaginal and transabdominal probes during the first period of pregnancy: a comparative study. *Prenat. Diagn.*, **11**, 69–75.

28. Copel, J.A., Pilu, G., Green, J. *et al.* (1987) Fetal echocardiographic screening for congenital heart disease: the importance of the four-chamber view. *Am. J. Obstet. Gynecol.*, **157**, 648–55.

29. Eik-Nes, S.H. (1991) Four chamber view of the fetal heart: part of the routine scan? Presentation at the International Perinatal Doppler Society, Malmo, Sweden.

30. Vergani, P., Silvana, M., Ghidini, A. *et al.* (1992) Screening for congenital heart disease with the four-chamber view of the heart. *Am. J. Obstet. Gynecol.*, **167**, 1000–1003.

31. Crawford, D.C., Chita, S.K. and Allan, L.D. (1988) Prenatal detection of congenital heart disease: factors affecting obstetric management and survival. *Am. J. Obstet. Gynecol.*, **159**, 352–56.

32. Kleinman, C.S. and Donnerstein, R.L. (1985) Ultrasonic assessment of cardiac funtion in the intact human fetus. *J. Am. Coll. Cardiol.*, **5**, 84S–94S.

33. Gallo, P., Nardi, F. and Marinozzi, V. (1976) Congenital extracardiac malformations accompanying congenital heart disease. *G. Ital. Cardiol.*, **6**, 450–59.

34. Greenwood, R.D., Rosenthal, A., Parisi, L. *et al.* (1975) Extracardiac abnormalities in infants with congenital heart disease. *Pediatrics*, **55**, 485–92.

35. Wallgren, E.I., Landtman, B. and Rapola, J. (1978) Extracardiac malformations associated with congenital heart disease. *Eur. J. Cardiol.*, **7**, 15–24.

36. Wladimiroff, J.W., Stewart, P.A., Sachs, E.S. and Niermeijer, M.F. (1985) Prenatal diagnosis and management of congenital heart defects: significance of associated fetal anomalies and prenatal chromosome studies. *Am. J. Med. Genet.*, **21**, 285–90.

37. Berg, K.A., Clark, E.B., Astemborski, J.A. and Baugham, J.A. (1988) Prenatal detection of cardiovascular malformations by echocardiography: an indication for cytogenetic evaluation. *Obstet. Gynecol.*, **159**, 477–81.

38. Nora, J.J., Fraser, F.C., Bear, J. *et al.* (1994) Clinical consequences of autosomal chromosome abnormalities, in *Medical Genetics, Principles and Practice*, 4th edn, Lea & Febiger, Philadelphia, pp. 35–54.

39. Bulbul, Z.R., Rosenthal, D. and Brueckner, M. (1993) Genetic aspects of heart disease of the newborn. *Semin. Perinatol.*, **17**, 61–75.

40. Gembruch, U., Hansmann, M., Redel, D.A. *et al.* (1989) Fetal complete heart block: antenatal diagnosis, significance and management. *Eur. J. Obstet. Gynecol. Reprod. Biol.*, **31**, 9–22.

41. Gabbe, S.G. and Cohen, A.W. (1982) Diabetes mellitus in pregnancy, in *Perinatal Medicine* (eds R.J. Bolognese, R.H. Schwarz and J. Schneider), Williams and Wilkins, Baltimore, MD.

42. Rowland, T.W., Hubbell, J.P. and Nadas, A.S. (1973) Congenital heart disease in infants of diabetic mothers. *J. Pediatr.*, **83**, 815–20.

43. Miller, E., Hare, J.W., Cloherty, J.P. *et al.* (1981) Elevated maternal hemoglobin A1c in early pregnancy and major congenital anomalies in infants of diabetic mother. *N. Engl. J. Med.*, **304**, 1331–34.

44. Mace, S., Hirschfeld, S.S., Riggs, T. *et al.* (1979) Echocardiographic abnormalities in infants of diabetic mothers. *J. Pediatr.*, **95**, 1013–19.

45. Gutgessell, H.P., Speer, M.E. and Rosenberg, H.S. (1980) Characterization of the cardiomyopathy in infants of diabetic mothers. *Circulation*, **61**, 441–50.

46. Breitweser, J.A., Meyer, R.A., Sperling, M.A. *et al.* (1980) Cardiac septal hypertrophy in hyperinsulinemic infants. *J. Pediatr.*, **96**, 535–39.

47. Weber, H.S., Copel, J.A., Reece, E.A. *et al.* (1991) Cardiac growth in fetuses of diabetic mothers with good metabolic control. *J. Pediatr.*, **118**, 103–107.

48. Bergmans, M.G.M., Jonker, G.J. and Kock, H.C.L.V. (1985) Fetal supraventricular tachycardia. Review of the literature. *Obstet. Gynecol. Surv.*, **40**, 61–68.

49. Kallfelz, H.C. (1979) Cardiac arrhythmias in the fetus – diagnosis, significance and prognosis, in *Heart Disease in the Newborn* (eds M.J. Godman and R.M. Marquis,), Churchill Livingstone, Edinburgh.

50. Southall, D.P., Richards, J., Hardwick, R.A. *et al.* (1980) Prospective study of fetal heart rate and rhythm pattern. *Arch. Dis. Child.*, **55**, 506–11.

51. Allan, L.D., Anderson, R.H., Sullivan, I.D. *et al.* (1983) Evaluation of fetal arrhythmias by echocardiography. *Br. Heart J.*, **50**, 240–45.

52. Crowley, D.C., Dick, M., Rayburn, W.F. *et al.* (1985) Two-dimensional and M-mode echocardiographic evaluation of fetal arrhythmia. *Clin. Cardiol.*, **8**, 1–10.

53. DeVore, G.R., Siassi, B. and Platt, L.D. (1983) Fetal echocardiography, III. The diagnosis of cardiac arrhythmias using real-time directed M-mode ultrasound. *Am. J. Obstet. Gynecol.*, **146**, 792–99.

54. Kleinman, C.S., Donnerstein, R.L., Jaffe, C.C. *et al.* (1983) Fetal echocardiography: a tool for evaluation of *in-utero* cardiac arrhythmias and monitoring of *in-utero* therapy: analysis of 71 patients. *Am. J. Cardiol.*, **51**, 237–43.

55. Kleinman, C.S. (1986) Prenatal diagnosis and mangement of intrauterine arrhythmias. *Fetal Ther.*, **1**, 92–95.

56. Bernstine, R.L., Winler, J.E. and Callagan, D.A. (1968) Fetal bigeminy and tachycardia. *Am. J. Obstet. Gynecol.*, **101**, 856–57.

57. Kendall, B. (1967) Abnormal fetal heart rates and rhythms prior to labor. *Am. J. Obstet. Gynecol.*, **99**, 71–78.

58. Kleinman, C.S., Copel, J.A., Weinstein, E.M. *et al.* (1985) *In utero* diagnosis and treatment of fetal supraventricular tachycardia. *Semin. Perinatol.*, **9**, 113–29.

59. Gillette, P.C. (1976) The mechanism of supraventricular tachycardia in children. *Circulation*, **54**, 133–39.

60. Kleinman, C.S. and Copel, J.A. (1991) Electrophysiological principles and fetal antiarrhythmic therapy. *Ultrasound Obstet. Gynecol.*, **1**, 286–97.

61. Crawford, D., Chapman, M. and Allan, L. (1985) The assessment of persistent bradycardia in prenatal life. *Br. J. Obstet. Gynaecol.*, **92**, 941–44.

62. Shenker, L., Reed, K.L., Anderson, C.F. *et al.* (1987) Congenital heart block and cardiac anomalies in the absence of maternal connective tissue disease. *Am. J. Obstet. Gynecol.*, **157**, 248–53.

63. Michaelsson, M. and Engle, M.A. (1972) Congenital complete heart block: an international study of the natural history. *Cardiovasc. Clin.*, **4**, 85–101.

64. Schmidt, K.G., Ulmer, H.E., Silverman, N.H. *et al.* (1991) Perinatal outcome of fetal complete atrioventricular block: a multicenter experience. *J. Am. Coll. Cardiol.*, **17**, 1360–66.

65. Kleinman, C.S., Copel, J.A. and Hobbins, J.C. (1987) Combined echocardiographic and Doppler assessment of fetal congenital atrioventricular block. *Br. J. Obstet. Gynaecol.*, **94**, 967–74.

66. Allan, L.D., Chita, S., Maxwell, D. and Priestley, K. (1990) Use of flecainide in fetal atrial tachycardia. *Br. Heart. J.*, **64**, 90–91.

67. Arnoux, P., Seyral, P., Llurens, M. *et al.* (1987) Amiodarone and digoxin for refractory fetal tachycardia. *Am. J. Cardiol.*, **59**, 166–67.

68. Dumesic, D.A., Silverman, N.S., Tobias, S. and Golbus, M.S. (1982) Transplacental cardioversion of fetal supraventricular tachycardia with procainamide. *N. Engl. J. Med.*, **307**, 1128–31.

69. Hansmann, M., Gembruch, U., Bald, R. *et al.* (1991) Fetal tachyarrhythmias: transplacental and direct treatment of the fetus – a report of 60 cases. *Ultrasound Obstet. Gynecol.*, **1**, 162–70.

70. Ward, R.M. (1992) Maternal drug therapy for fetal disorders. *Semin. Perinatol.*, **16**, 12–20.

71. Younis, J.S. and Granat, M. (1987) Insufficient transplacental digoxin transfer in severe hydrops fetalis. *Am. J. Obstet. Gynecol.*, **157**, 1268–69.

72. Barcaly, C.S., French, M.A., Ross, L.D. and Sokol, R.J. (1987) Successful pregnancy following steroid therapy and plasma exchange in a woman with antiro (SS-A) antibodies. *Br. J. Obstet. Gynaecol.*, **94**, 369–71.

73. Bierman, F.Z., Baxi, L., Jaffe, I. and Driscoll, J. (1988) Fetal hydrops and congenital complete heart block: response to maternal steroid therapy. *J. Pediatr.*, **112**, 646–48.

74. Buyon, J.P., Swersky, S.J., Fox, H.E. *et al.* (1987) Intrauterine therapy for presumptive fetal myocarditis with acquired heart block due to systemic lupus erythematosus. *Arthritis Rheumatol.*, **30**, 44–49.

75. Carpenter, R.J., Strasburger, J.F., Garson, R. *et al.* (1986) Fetal ventricular pacing for hydrops secondary to complete atrioventricular block. *J. Am. Coll. Cardiol.*, **8**, 1434–36.

76. Lee, L.A., Coulter, S., Erner, S. and Chu, H. (1987) Cardiac immunoglobulin deposition in congenital heart block associated with maternal anti-Ro autoantibodies. *Am. J. Med.*, **83**, 793–96.

77. Litsey, S.E., Noonan, J.A., O'Connor, W.N. *et al.* (1985) Maternal connective tissue disease and congenital heart block: demonstration of immunoglobulin in cardiac tissue. *N. Engl. J. Med.*, **312**, 98–100.

78. Taylor, P.V., Scott, J.S., Gerlis, L.M. *et al.* (1986) Maternal antibodies against fetal cardiac antigens in congenital complete heart block. *N. Engl. J. Med.*, **315**, 667–72.

55 THE ROLE OF ULTRASOUND IN THE SPECIAL PROBLEMS OF MULTIPLE PREGNANCY

J.P. Neilson

55.1 Introduction

Although the rate of perinatal loss from multiple pregnancies is now substantially higher than that among fetuses of diabetic women, the challenge of multiple pregnancy has not been met with similar commitment or organization of specialized perinatal services. The most important causes of perinatal death are preterm delivery, intrauterine growth retardation, and twin–twin transfusion syndrome. Preterm delivery, in particular, is not only a major cause of mortality and morbidity, but is also a major drain on human and financial resources. Thus, the provision of neonatal intensive care has been, at times, severely restricted by the preterm delivery of babies from multiple (and especially higher multiple) pregnancies [1]. This is of increasing concern because multiple pregnancy has become more common with greater use of assisted reproduction techniques.

The specific pathologies of multiple pregnancy are discussed in Chapter 16; this chapter, by concentrating on the contributions that ultrasound can make to the care of women with multiple pregnancies, is complementary. Ultrasound is of especial importance as a diagnostic technique because it permits the separate assessment of each fetus in a multiple pregnancy, in contrast to biochemical assessment, for example, in which the combined outputs of both fetoplacental units are assessed together. Aspects of the management of multiple pregnancies have been reviewed elsewhere recently, including general clinical care [2,3], prenatal diagnosis [4], preterm labour [5] and assessment of fetal growth and well-being [6].

55.2 Diagnosis

Formerly, when the diagnosis of multiple pregnancy depended on a high degree of clinical suspicion followed by careful abdominal palpation, usually then confirmed by radiology, in about one-fifth of cases the presence of two or more fetuses remained undetected until delivery, and sometimes the diagnosis was not made or suspected until after the first baby had been delivered [3]. Nowadays proficient ultrasound scanning provides a sure method of diagnosing multiple pregnancies as early as possible. Clearly, the detection rate is best when an ultrasound examination is a routine procedure, either at first antenatal clinic visit or, as is often the policy, at 18 weeks' gestation. The early diagnosis of multiple pregnancy by routine ultrasound has been claimed to reduce the risk of preterm delivery and of perinatal mortality [7] but it seems unlikely that diagnosis alone will improve outcome. Earlier detection of multiple pregnancies is one of the proven benefits of routine (i.e. screening) ultrasound in early pregnancy [8], although this has not been translated into a lower perinatal mortality rate in randomized controlled trials [9]; the need for improvements in subsequent management is emphasized. Nevertheless, early diagnosis identifies what is undeniably a high-risk group, and allows the setting of appropriate priorities in the antepartum management of multiple pregnancies, i.e.:

1. accurate prenatal diagnosis;
2. detection and management of the abnormal consequences of monochorionic placentation;
3. early detection of maternal hypertension;
4. prediction and prevention of preterm labour;
5. detection of fetal growth retardation.

Potential pitfalls in ultrasound diagnosis occur with discordant anencephaly (if excessive attention is paid to counting heads), high multiple pregnancies, arrested development of one of the embryos (the 'vanishing twin'), and late gestation at presentation. It used to be said that there was a 'window' at 12–14 weeks gestation during which ultrasound diagnosis was more difficult; this was never true.

Diseases of the Fetus and Newborn, 2nd edn, Edited by G.B. Reed, A.E. Claireaux and F. Cockburn. Published in 1995 by Chapman & Hall, London. ISBN 0 412 39160 0

55.3 Selective reduction

The risk of preterm labour and delivery, and of perinatal mortality, rises with the number of fetuses in multiple pregnancies. Perinatal mortality rates of 63, 164, 200, 214 and 416 per 1000 births have been recently reported for, respectively, twins, triplets, quadruplets, quintuplets and sextuplets [10]. While nothing can be done to prevent naturally conceived multifetal pregnancies, measures can be taken to prevent this undesirable side-effect of assisted reproduction. It is now recommended that no more than three pre-embryos are transferred in any treatment cycle unless there are exceptional clinical circumstances [11]. The use of embryo cryopreservation has been an important advance in *in vitro* fertilization programmes by allowing the transfer of a single pre-embryo during a treatment cycle without jeopardizing other pre-embryos.

While it is obvious that high multiple pregnancies should be avoided wherever possible by the careful monitoring of ovulation induction, and by rigorous (and statutory) control of assisted reproduction, high multiple pregnancies will continue to occur from time to time. The very high rate of associated loss may make the procedure of 'selective reduction' the best of a poor choice of options. The procedure usually involves the injection of potassium chloride into the thorax to cause death of the embryo or embryos. This may not, of course, be morally acceptable to some couples, nor indeed to some clinicians. Selective reduction of quadruplet pregnancy to twin pregnancy may improve the eventual outcome [12] despite the immediate risks of the procedure, although this is controversial. The desirability of 'reducing' triplets is certainly very unclear.

55.4 Prenatal diagnosis

There is controversy about whether or not multiple pregnancy is associated with an increased risk of fetal malformation. The generally accepted view is that there is no increased risk in dizygotic pregnancies, but that the unusual circumstances surrounding cleavage of the conceptus to produce monozygotic twins does carry an increased chance of abnormality. A recent large epidemiological study [13] in fact reported no overall increased incidence of anomaly among 76 000 newborn twins (no information was available about zygosity). Certain conditions were found more commonly in twins than in singletons: anencephaly, patent ductus arteriosus, exomphalos, hydrocephalus and atresias and stenoses of the gastrointestinal tract; some of these are commonly associated with polyhydramnios.

55.4.1 ULTRASOUND

In obstetric units in which ultrasound anomaly scanning is not performed routinely at 18 weeks, selective examination is often done in the case of multiple pregnancies [14].

55.4.2 INVASIVE PROCEDURES

Invasive procedures may be more difficult to perform in multiple pregnancies; all should be guided by simultaneous ultrasound imaging.

(a) Amniocentesis

Amniocentesis can be done by either double-needle insertion or a single insertion [15], traversing the membrane that divides the two amniotic cavities. The quality of imaging by modern ultrasound equipment is such that where there is a dichorionic placenta it seems to me unnecessary to resort to the simultaneous insertion of two needles into the same imaging field (as has been advocated recently [16]), or to the installation of a dye to exclude the possibility of sampling the same amniotic sac twice. The use of methylene blue for this purpose has been linked to subsequent jejunal atresia in the fetus [17–19]. Where the placenta appears to be monochorionic (and the twins are therefore presumed to be monozygotic) and there are no dysmorphic features seen on detailed ultrasonography in either fetus, a single puncture will suffice.

There remains controversy about the additional risk of amniocentesis in multiple pregnancies. A recently reported large series [20] quoted a loss rate up to 28 weeks of 3.6% in multiple pregnancies after amniocentesis, compared with 0.6% in singleton pregnancy amniocentesis controls. The lack of extensive epidemiological data about the mid-trimester loss of multiple pregnancies makes it difficult to estimate what is merely 'background loss' and what is the excess price to be paid for amniocentesis in multiple pregnancies.

(b) Chorion villus sampling

Chorion villus sampling can be successfully accomplished in almost 100% of multiple pregnancies using transcervical, transabdominal or combined approaches [21,22]. As with amniocentesis, where the placenta appears monochorionic on ultrasound examination a single sample is done. Where the placenta appears dichorionic, double sampling is required. If placentation is dichorionic but the placentas are contiguous and the fetuses are of like sex, a specific search should be made in the laboratory for cytogenetic or DNA polymorphisms. If reassurance cannot be obtained by these methods that each placenta has been sampled separately, back-up amniocentesis is required [21]. Identical results indicate either monozygotic twins with dichorionic placentation, or that both samples were obtained from the same placenta.

Another potential source of diagnostic confusion after chorion villus sampling is the false result attributed to unrecognized twinning in what appears a singleton pregnancy [23]. Here, it is hypothesized that one twin undergoes very early arrest of embryonic development to produce an apparently single pregnancy at the time of sampling. Residual viable trophoblastic tissue from the arrested embryo continues to exist for some time, however, and may be sampled and analysed to give a different karyotype (perhaps of different gender) from that of the survivor.

(c) Cordocentesis

Disruption of the dividing membrane has been described after transmembrane cordocentesis in a twin pregnancy [24]. It has been recognized recently that this can also occur without iatrogenic interference producing, in effect, a single monochorionic monoamniotic cavity with the accompanying risk of entanglement of the umbilical cords [25].

(d) Clinical practice

The decision about whether it is desirable to perform any invasive procedure in an individual multiple pregnancy requires careful thought and raises several issues.

- As the incidence of dizygotic twinning and the incidence of major chromosomal abnormalities both increase with age, a significant number of women requesting prenatal diagnosis for advanced age will have a multiple pregnancy.
- Because there are two fetuses in a twin pregnancy, there is probably a greater risk of one baby having Down's syndrome than in a singleton pregnancy to a mother of similar age [26].
- However, there are probably greater risks in multiple pregnancies from invasive procedures, as has been discussed.
- The potential problems of interpretation of the laboratory results (especially after chorion villus sampling) need to be discussed in advance (especially the possible need for back-up amniocentesis).
- Difficult human dilemmas are produced by the demonstration of non-lethal but handicapping abnormality in only one of twin fetuses. Available options are to continue the pregnancy, to terminate the entire pregnancy, or to perform 'selective feticide' to destroy the anomalous fetus (usually by the ultrasound-guided intracardiac injection of potassium chloride). Because of the inherent risks of invasive procedures in multiple pregnancies, these

are best avoided unless the parents would wish active intervention if one or both results were to prove abnormal.

55.5 Placental morphology

Aside from the increased risk of malformation, the excess incidence of fetal death and damage in monozygotic compared with dizygotic pregnancies can be attributed to the adverse consequences of monochorionic placentantion – the factors of most importance being:

- the occasional presence of a single amnion;
- the almost universal presence of vascular anastomoses connecting the circulations of the two twins [27].

55.5.1 MONOCHORIONIC MONOAMNIOTIC PLACENTATION

This is the least common type of twin pregnancy placentation, accounting for only 1% of cases, but associated with the highest perinatal mortality rate, 30–70% [25], mainly due to cord entanglement. Several publications in recent years have confirmed that the type of placentation (monochorionic or dichorionic) can be predicted with substantial accuracy by the ultrasound inspection of the dividing membrane in early or mid-pregnancy. Failure to find a dividing membrane at all does not, however, necessarily indicate a monoamniotic placenta, as the dividing membrane may be thin and difficult to see in some monochorionic diamniotic pregnancies [28]. Positive diagnosis of monoamnionicity have been made by the intra-amniotic injection of indigo carmine dye, and by amniography with or without computed tomographic scanning but whether antepartum diagnosis has improved fetal outcome is unclear [4].

Monoamnionicity indicates late cleavage of the conceptus. At this time, cleavage can be incomplete, producing conjoined twins (which always have a monoamniotic placenta). Ultrasound features of conjoined twinning include inseparable bodies and skin contours, and constant relative positions (although this may be absent occasionally in omphalopagus twins joined by a narrow and pliant bridge of tissue) [29]. Transvaginal ultrasound can facilitate early diagnosis.

55.5.2 ABNORMAL CONSEQUENCES OF MONOCHORIONIC PLACENTATION

(a) Twin reversed arterial perfusion (TRAP)

The TRAP sequence is rare and is unique to multiple pregnancies with monochorionic placentas with both artery–artery and vein–vein anastomoses. Acardiac twins display a spectrum of abnormality extending

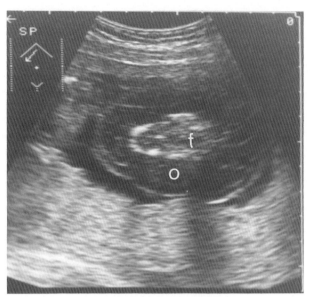

Figure 55.1 Acardiac fetus. There is extensive subcutaneous oedema (o) surrounding the fetal body (f).

from some development of the head and thorax, with well-formed limbs, to amorphous masses that reveal little semblance to human fetuses; some acardiac twins differ chromosomally from their co-twins (heterokaryotypic monozygotic twinning). The continuing existence of the acardiac fetus depends on a blood supply from its co-twin. Arterial (and therefore poorly oxygenated) blood from the normal twin passes in a pulsatile and retrograde fashion through the umbilical artery to the acardiac twin – thus the reversed perfusion. This phenomenon has now been observed by colour flow Doppler ultrasound [30]. The blood returns (even more poorly oxygenated) via the umbilical vein to the normal twin.

The ultrasound appearances of the acardiac fetus depend on the degree of structural organization; gross and progressive subcutaneous oedema is often seen on repeated examination (Figure 55.1). There is a poor prognosis for the normal (pump) twin, with a mortality rate of around 50%. Death usually occurs either because of cardiac overload and failure (signs of hydrops fetalis may appear on ultrasound), or through very preterm delivery associated with polyhydramnios. Treatment has been attempted with some apparent success by inserting a thrombogenic coil into the umbilical artery of the acardiac twin [30], by administering indomethacin to the mother [31], and even by performing hysterotomy to remove the acardiac fetus [32].

(b) Twin–twin transfusion syndrome

In contrast to the TRAP syndrome, the vascular connection in the twin–twin transfusion syndrome is arteriovenous, producing anaemia and growth retardation in the donor twin and polycythaemia in the recipient. Typical ultrasound features include extreme oligohydramnios in the sac of the donor twin producing the so-called 'stuck twin' (the fetus is enmeshed in the dividing membrane which is no longer visible ultrasonically), while in the sac of the recipient there is gross polyhydramnios. The recipient twin is typically larger, has an unusually obvious bladder and a thick umbilical cord. Although imaging ultrasound appearances are characteristic, reports about the value of Doppler ultrasound have been confusing and conflicting. It is difficult to understand from first principles if, or why, there should be a consistent pattern of flow velocities in the umbilical arteries. Previous disagreements are perpetuated in the most recent publications which report both discordant [33] and concordant [34] umbilical artery waveform patterns in the presence of twin–twin transfusion syndrome.

Imprecise definition of twin–twin transfusion syndrome has occurred in a number of publications and has made the subject more opaque than it need be. In the neonate, the syndrome is usually diagnosed by finding an intertwin difference in haemoglobin of greater than 5 g/dl, and a birth weight difference of greater than 20%. However, the majority of twin pregnancies which demonstrate these differences have dizygotic placentas, and the differences reflect not the twin–twin transfusion syndrome but rather the chronic hypoxaemia-induced polycythaemia of a discordantly growth retarded twin fetus [35]. To confirm the diagnosis of twin–twin transfusion syndrome it is therefore vital that investigators both inspect the placenta and ensure that the smaller twin has the lower haemoglobin. The report of Giles and colleagues [34], which does include rigorous diagnostic criteria, describes similar umbilical artery waveforms in both fetuses.

Of the various attempts made to try to improve the outcome of twin–twin transfusion syndrome, the most popular has been repeated therapeutic amniocentesis, aiming at a reduction of amniotic fluid volume to normal levels. This may necessitate the removal of around 2 litres of fluid three times a week. Varying reports of success have appeared [36,37]. Some have also used indomethacin to attempt prolongation of these pregnancies and to try to decrease the polyhydramnios. It is far from clear whether or not these treatments are beneficial.

(c) Intrauterine death

Where there is both a shared monochorionic placenta and also intrauterine death of one of twin fetuses, cerebral and renal damage may occur in the survivor, probably by the passage of thromboplastins through vascular connections [38]. This has been thought of as predominantly a third trimester problem, but recent evidence points to these mechanisms operating during the second trimester as well [39]. Repeated ultrasound examination is therefore desirable after the death of one fetus when the placenta is thought to be monochorionic (cerebral damage may be identified by the appearance of porencephalic cysts), and it may in any case be appropriate to consider delivery from 34 weeks of gestation.

There has been a report of the characteristic infarctive lesions of brain and kidney in a fetus in whom there was no evidence of coagulation defect [40]; the ischaemia was instead attributed to acute twin–twin transfusion. Thus, there may be several mechanisms producing similar damage.

55.6   Prediction of preterm labour

While some multiple pregnancies are obviously at especially high risk of preterm delivery (e.g. higher multiples, TRAP sequence, twin–twin transfusion syndrome), the majority of pregnancies that end early (and make the largest contribution to perinatal mortality and morbidity) are unremarkable (except that they are multiple). Effective prediction of preterm labour therefore requires a screening technique.

55.6.1   CERVICAL ASSESSMENT

In parts of continental Europe, clinical digital examination of the cervix is routinely performed on all women at each antenatal clinic visit. Observation of early cervical ripening by such cervical assessment does help identify a group of women with twin pregnancies at especially high risk of preterm labour [41,42].

Some clinicians have been anxious that digital examination of the cervix might itself provoke preterm labour or rupture of the membranes. A recent trial [43] of routine repeated cervical assessments at term found no greater risk of spontaneous rupture of membranes after this examination, but this did not exclude an effect on high-risk pregnancies preterm. Ultrasound has been favoured by a number of workers as an alternative method of examining the cervix. Unfortunately technical difficulties exist with transabdominal scanning (especially the effects of the full bladder) and there is little firm evidence that it is genuinely helpful [44]. Transvaginal ultrasound provides better images of the cervix than transabdominal scanning, and possibly less interference with the cervix than by digital examination. Reports of this technique are awaited with interest.

55.6.2   UTERINE VOLUME MEASUREMENTS

It is frequently assumed that the increased incidence of preterm labour in multiple pregnancies results simply from uterine overdistension, like polyhydramnios. It is thought that uterine contractions commence at a critical degree of myometrial stretch and then increase in frequency and strength to cause, ultimately, progressive dilatation of the cervix in labour [45]. If this simple explanation is correct, one would expect to find the uterine size to be greater in those pregnancies which deliver preterm. Tape measurement of symphysis–fundal height has shown the reverse of what was expected – that the fundal height was on average greater in those pregnancies going on to term than in those ending preterm [46]. Although tape measurement is a crude way of assessing uterine size, these findings are consistent with a small study of measurement of uterine size by ultrasound [47] and suggest that the commonly accepted theory that preterm labour in twin pregnancies results simply from uterine overdistension may not be correct.

55.7   Intrauterine growth retardation

The following issues have to be addressed in any discussion of fetal growth in multiple pregnancies.

- Should normal singleton, or separate twin, standards be used to define normal and abnormal growth, size and birth weight?
- What is more important – the absolute size of the fetus or the difference in size between two twin fetuses (discordance)?

I believe that singleton standards should be used for practical clinical purposes [48]. We accept that if a singleton fetus is unable to achieve its intrinsic growth potential because of uteroplacental insufficiency, it is at increased perinatal risk. There is no reason at all to think that dizygotic twins have inherited different growth potentials than have singleton fetuses; for them, at least, it therefore seems sensible to apply singleton standards. It is theoretically possible that the unusual circumstances surrounding the cleavage of a conceptus to form monozygotic twins could produce a diminished growth potential in the embryos. Our ultrasound studies, however, found no difference in abdominal circumference measurement between monozygotic and dizygotic twin fetuses from 16 weeks onwards [49]. I conclude that it is appropriate to use normal singleton standards for both dizygotic and monozygotic twins. This view, although disputed by some, is endorsed by others [e.g. 50].

The converse argument (i.e. to recommend separate twin growth standards) seems akin to recommending separate standards for the fetuses of women with severe proteinuric pre-eclampsia. It is especially important, in view of the high perinatal mortality rate, that we do not use less stringent criteria in twin pregnancies than we do in singleton pregnancies. It is distressing to hear from time to time of the intrauterine death of a growth retarded twin fetus despite ultrasound evidence of impaired growth which would, in a singleton pregnancy, have provoked intensive monitoring of fetal well-being and, ultimately, earlier delivery. This was not done because of the prevalent, but erroneous, view that twins 'should' be smaller.

Discordancy of size (and weight) should also be noted but not to the exclusion of actual weight (as occurred in many early ultrasound reports). There is a mean difference of birth weight between twins of 12%, and 10% of twin pairs have a discordancy of more than 25% [50]. Intertwin birth weight differences (expressed as a percentage) are relatively constant across the birth weight range but large differences (>15%) are not associated with adverse outcome at term unless the smaller twin weighs less than 2.5 kg (i.e. is small for gestational age). Low birth weight for gestational age is a better prediction of poor outcome than is discordancy [50].

55.7.1 FETAL MEASUREMENT

Detection of small for gestational age twin fetuses by abdominal palpation is inevitably made more difficult by the presence of the other baby. Tape measurement of symphysis–fundal height can detect about 60% of pregnancies in which both babies are small for gestational age [46] and is therefore worthwhile, but it is very poor, for obvious reasons, at identifying pregnancies in which only one of the twins is small for gestational age. Again, there is a need for a method of assessment that assesses each twin individually – thus the important role of ultrasound.

As in singleton pregnancies, the best single fetal measurement for assessing fetal size and growth during the second half of pregnancy is the abdominal circumference [48]. Unfortunately, fetal measurement is more difficult and probably less accurate in twin than in singleton fetuses. We have systematically studied, during a 4-year period, all twin fetuses from 16 to 18 weeks gestation by abdominal circumference measurement. Prediction of small for gestational age fetuses proved better than by tape measurement of symphysis–fundal height but the sensitivity fell short of results we have previously obtained in singleton pregnancies by abdominal circumference measurement. A plausible explanation is that mechanical flexion of the trunk increases the measured abdominal circumference, and mechanical flexion is common in twin fetuses during late pregnancy. This is especially a problem in the second twin.

Where size discrepancy is detected by ultrasound measurement there is sometimes a tendency to assume that this is because of twin–twin transfusion, especially

when found during the second trimester. This is not necessarily so: it may be due to uteroplacental insufficiency, fetal abnormality or constitutional factors [6].

55.7.2 DOPPLER ULTRASOUND

Another method of predicting babies that are small for gestational age is by Doppler ultrasound examination of flow velocity waveforms in the umbilical artery, and this is the focus of intense interest and debate at present. The fetoplacental circulation should be of low vascular resistance with forward flow of blood throughout the cardiac cycle. In some compromised pregnancies the resistance increases, producing reduced velocities during diastole. Continuous wave Doppler ultrasound, although simple and relatively inexpensive, does not (in contrast to pulsed Doppler ultrasound) permit range gating and precise identification of the vessel generating the recorded waveforms. Considerable care is therefore required by prior imaging to ensure separate waveform sampling in multiple pregnancies. Simultaneous imaging has been recommended to allow simultaneous fetal heart rate measurement but this can produce unacceptable interference with the Doppler signal. Pulsed Doppler ultrasound, with or without colour flow imaging, has obvious advantages in multiple pregnancies.

We have studied the value of Doppler ultrasound in twin pregnancies to predict small for gestational age fetuses, taking care to study each umbilical cord separately [51]. Between 32 and 35 weeks the sensitivities and specificities were 39% and 79%; between 36 and 39 weeks the corresponding figures were 50% and 86%. Thus, in our experience of 89 consecutive twin pregnancies, this is not an effective method of predicting small for gestational age fetuses. Only persistently absent end-diastolic velocities proved useful in predicting adverse fetal outcome. It may be that the placental pathophysiology in these twin pregnancies is different from that typically seen in singleton intrauterine growth retardation. Other workers have, however, been more optimistic about the place of Doppler ultrasound in the assessment of twin pregnancies [52], and further studies are awaited with interest.

55.8 Labour and delivery

There has been an increasing trend towards delivery of twins by caesarean section. In one Canadian study, the caesarean section rate rose from 3% between 1963 and 1972 to 51% between 1978 and 1984 [56]. Evidence that this has had a markedly beneficial impact on fetal outcome is lacking [53]. Delivery of twins, and especially the second twin, is one of the remaining manipulative challenges of modern obstetrics. The ready availability of ultrasound equipment in the delivery suite can be helpful if there is uncertainty about fetal lie or presentation. It can also assist optimal intrapartum monitoring by identifying the position of the fetal hearts. As many twin fetuses are preterm or small for gestational age, or both, at the time of delivery, they are at especially high risk of intrapartum asphyxia. Continuous or intermittent recording of the heart rate of both twins, the first by scalp electrode and the second by external recording, is therefore required. It is essential that attendants ensure that both traces are not obtained from the one fetus. From time to time the progressive asphyxia of a twin (usually the second) goes unrecognized for this reason.

References

1. Levene, M.I., Wild, J. and Steer, P. (1992) Higher multiple births and the modern management of infertility in Britain. *Br. J. Obstet. Gynaecol.*, 99, 607–13.
2. Crowther, C.A. (1994 Multiple pregnancy: including delivery, in *High Risk Pregnancy Management Options* (eds D.K. James, P.J. Steer, C.P. Weiner and B. Gouik), W.B. Saunders, London (in press).
3. Neilson, J.P. (1994) Multiple pregnancy, in *Dewhurst's Textbook of Obstetrics and Gynaecology for Postgraduates* (ed. C.R. Whitfield), Blackwell, Oxford, (in press).
4. Neilson, J.P. (1992) Prenatal diagnosis in multiple pregnancies. *Curr. Opin. Obstet. Gynecol.*, 4, 280–85.
5. Neilson, J.P. and Crowther, C.A. (1994) Preterm labour in multiple pregnancies. *Fetal Med. Rev.* (in press)
6. Neilson, J.P. (1994) Fetal assessment in multiple pregnancies, in *Contributions to Obstetrics and Gynaecology 3* (eds S.S. Ratnam, S.-C. Ng, S. Arulkumaran and D.K. Sen), Churchill Livingstone, Edinburgh, (in press).
7. Persson, P. and Grennert, L. (1979) Towards a normalisation of the outcome of twin pregnancy. *Acta Genet. Med. Gemellol.*, 28, 341–46.
8. Neilson, J.P. (1992) Routine ultrasonography in early pregnancy, in *Oxford Database of Perinatal Trials*, version 1.3, disk issue 7, record 3872 (ed. I. Chalmers), Oxford University Press, Oxford.
9. Waldenstrom, U., Axelsson, O., Nilsson, S. *et al.* (1988) Effects of routine one-stage ultrasound screening in pregnancy: a randomised controlled trial. *Lancet*, ii, 585–88.
10. Botting, B.H., McDonald-Davies, I. and McFarlane, A.J. (1987) Recent trends in the incidence of multiple births and associated mortality. *Arch. Dis. Child.*, 62, 941–50.
11. Interim Licensing Authority (ILA) (1990) The Fifth Report of the Interim Licensing Authority for Human *in vitro* Fertilisation and Embryology. Medical Research Council/Royal College of Obstetricians and Gynaecologists, London.
12. Melgar, C.A., Rosenfeld, D.L., Rawlinson, K. and Greenberg, M. (1991) Perinatal outcome after multifetal reduction to twins compared with nonreduced multiple gestations. *Obstet. Gynecol.*, 78, 763–67.
13. Doyle, P.E., Beral, V., Botting, B. and Wale, C.J. (1991) Congenital malformations in twins in England and Wales. *J. Epidemiol. Community Health*, 45, 43–48.
14. Allen, S.R., Gray, L.J., Frentzen, B.H. and Cruz, A.C. (1991) Ultrasonographic diagnosis of congenital anomalies in twins. *Am. J. Obstet. Gynecol.*, 165, 1056–60.
15. Jeanty, P., Shah, D. and Roussis, P. (1990) Single-needle insertion in twin amniocentesis. *J. Ultrasound Med.*, 9, 511–17.
16. Bahado-Singh, R., Schmitt, R. and Hobbins, J.C. (1992) New technique for amniocentesis in twins. *Obstet. Gynecol.*, 79, 304–307.
17. Nicolini, U. and Monni, G. (1990) Intestinal obstruction in babies exposed *in utero* to methylene blue. *Lancet*, 336, 1258–59.
18. McFadyen, I. (1992) The dangers of intra-amniotic methylene blue. *Br. J. Obstet. Gynaecol.*, 99, 89–90.
19. Van der Pol, J.G., Wolf, H., Boer, K. *et al.* (1992) Jejunal atresia related to the use of methylene blue in genetic amniocentesis in twins. *Br. J. Obstet. Gynaecol.*, 99, 141–43.
20. Anderson, R.L., Goldberg, J.D. and Golbus, M.S. (1991) Prenatal diagnosis in multiple gestation: 20 year's experience with amniocentesis. *Prenat. Diagn.*, 11, 263–70.
21. Brambati, B., Tului, L., Lanzani, A. *et al.* (1991) First-trimester genetic diagnosis in multiple pregnancy: principles and potential pitfalls. *Prenat. Diagn.*, 11, 767–74.
22. Pergament, E., Schulman, J.D., Copeland, K. *et al.* (1992) The risk and efficacy of chorionic villus sampling in multiple gestations. *Prenat. Diagn.*, 12, 337–84.
23. Reddy, K.S., Petersen, M.B., Antonarakis, S.E. and Blakemore, K.J. (1991) The vanishing twin: an explanation for discordance between chorion villus karyotype and fetal phenotype. *Prenat. Diagn.*, 11, 679–84.
24. Megory, E., Weiner, E., Shalev, E. and Ohel, G. (1989) Pseudomono-amniotic twins with cord entanglement following genetic funipuncture. *Obstet. Gynecol.*, 78, 915–17.
25. Gilbert, W.M., Stanley, S.E., Kaplan, C. *et al.* (1991) Morbidity associated with prenatal disruption of the dividing membrane in twin gestations. *Obstet. Gynecol.*, 78, 623–30.
26. Rodis, J.F., Egan, J.F.X., Craffey, A. *et al.* (1990) Calculated risk of chromosomal abnormalities in twin gestations. *Obstet. Gynecol.*, 76, 1037–41.
27. Robertson, E.G. and Neer, K.J. (1983) Placental injection studies in twin gestation. *Am. J. Obstet. Gynecol.*, 147, 170–73.
28. Neilson, J.P., Danskin, F. and Hastie, S.J. (1989) Monozygotic twin pregnancy: diagnostic and Doppler ultrasound studies. *Br. J. Obstet. Gynaecol.*, 96, 1413–18.
29. Barth, R.A., Filly, R.A., Goldberg, J.D. *et al.* (1990) Conjoined twins: prenatal diagnosis and assessment of associated malformations. *Radiology*, 177, 201–207.
30. Porreco, R.P., Barton, S.M. and Haverkamp, A.D. (1991) Occlusion of umbilical artery in acardiac, acephalic twin. *Lancet*, 337, 326–27.
31. Ash, K., Harman, C.R. and Gritter, H. (1990) TRAP sequence: successful outcome with indomethacin treatment. *Obstet. Gynecol.*, 76, 960–62
32. Ginsberg, N.A., Applebaum, M., Rabin, S.A. *et al.* (1992) Term birth after midtrimster hysterotomy and selective delivery of an acardiac twin. *Am. J. Obstet. Gynecol.*, 167, 33–37
33. Yamada, A., Kasugai, M., Ohno, Y. *et al.* (1991) Antenatal diagnosis of twin–twin transfusion syndrome by Doppler ultrasound. *Obstet. Gynecol.*, 78, 1058–61
34. Giles, W.B., Trudinger, B.J., Cook, C.M. and Connelly, A.J. (1990) Doppler umbilical artery studies in the twin–twin transfusion syndrome. *Obstet. Gynecol.*, 76, 1097–99.
35. Danskin, F.H. and Neilson, J.P. (1989) Twin-to-twin transfusion syndrome: what are appropriate diagnostic criteria? *Am. J. Obstet. Gynecol.*, 161, 365–69.
36. Mahony, B.S., Petty, C.N., Nyberg, D.A. *et al.* (1990) The 'stuck twin' phenomenon: ultrasonographic findings, pregnancy outcome and management with serial amniocenteses. *Am. J. Obstet. Gynecol.*, 163, 1513–22.
37. Saunders, N.J., Snijders, R.J.M. and Nicolaides, K.H. (1992) Therapeutic amniocentesis in twin–twin transfusion syndrome appearing in the second trimester of pregnancy. *Am. J. Obstet. Gynecol.*, 166, 820–24.
38. Hanna, J.H. and Hill, J.M. (1984) Single intrauterine fetal demise in multiple gestation. *Obstet. Gynecol.*, 63, 126–30.
39. Anderson, R.L., Golbus, M.S., Curry, C.J.R. *et al.* (1990) Central nervous system damage and other anomalies in surviving fetus following second trimester antenatal death of co-twin. *Prenat. Diagn.*, 10, 513–18.
40. Fusi, L., McParland, P., Fisk, N. *et al.* (1991) Acute twin–twin transfusion: a possible mechanism for brain-damaged survivors after intrauterine death of a monochorionic twin. *Obstet. Gynecol.*, 78, 517–20.
41. Neilson, J.P., Verkuyl, D.A.A., Crowther, C.A. and Bannerman, C. (1988) Preterm labor in twin pregnancies: prediction by cervical assessment. *Obstet. Gynecol.*, 72, 719–23.
42. Newman, R.B., Godsey, R.K., Ellings, J.M. *et al.* (1991) Quantification of cervical change: relationship to preterm delivery in the multifetal gestation. *Am. J. Obstet. Gynecol.*, 165, 264–71.
43. McDuffie, R.S., Nelson, G.E., Osborn, L. *et al.* (1992) Effect of routine cervical examinations at term on premature rupture of the membranes: a randomized controlled trial. *Obstet. Gynecol.*, 79, 219–22.
44. Michaels, W.H., Schrieber, F.R., Padgett, R.J. *et al.* (1991) Ultrasound surveillance of the cervix in twin gestations: management of cervical incompetency. *Obstet. Gynecol.*, 78, 739–44.
45. Quilligan, E.J. (1981) Pathologic causes of preterm labor, in *Preterm Labor* (eds M.G. and C.H. Hendricks), Butterworth, London, pp. 61–74.
46. Neilson, J.P., Verkuyl, D.A.A. and Bannerman C. (1988) Tape measurement of symphysis–fundal height in twin pregnancies. *Br. J. Obstet. Gynaecol.*, 95, 1054–59.
47. Redford, D.H.A. (1982) Uterine growth in twin pregnancy by measurement of total intrauterine volume. *Acta Genet. Med. Gemollol.*, 31, 145–48.
48. Neilson, J.P. (1981) Detection of the small-for-dates twin fetus by ultrasound. *Br. J. Obstet. Gynaecol.*, 88, 27–32.
49. Neilson, J.P. and Hastie, S.J. (1988) Ultrasound studies of monozygotic and dizygotic twin pregnancies, in *Fetal and Neonatal Development* (ed. C.T. Jones) Perinatology Press, Ithaca, NY, pp. 541–43.
50. Bronsteen, R., Goyert, G. and Bottoms, S. (1989) Classification of twins and neonatal morbidity. *Obstet. Gynecol.*, 74, 98–101.
51. Hastie, S.J., Danskin, F., Neilson, J.P. and Whittle, M.J. (1989) Prediction of the small-for-gestational age fetus by Doppler umbilical artery waveform analysis. *Obstet. Gynecol.*, 74, 730–33.
52. Giles, W.B., Trudinger, B.J., Cook, C.M. and Connelly, A.J. (1988) Umbilical artery flow velocity waveforms and twin pregnancy outcome. *Obstet. Gynecol.*, 72, 894–97.
53. Bell, D., Johansson, D., McLean, F.H. and Usher, R.H. (1986) Birth asphyxia, trauma and mortality in twins; has cesarean section improved outcome? *Am. J. Obstet. Gynecol.*, 154, 235–39.

56 IN VIVO INVESTIGATIONS OF PLACENTAL AND UMBILICAL CORD ANATOMY

E. Jauniaux, G. Moscoso and S. Campbell

56.1 Introduction

Research on placental function and morphology has probably been undertaken since Ancient Egyptian times; however the first detailed descriptions of placental anatomy were only published by Leonardo da Vinci and by Vesalius at the beginning of the sixteenth century [1]. Arantius, a distinguished pupil of Vesalius, was the first to publish a formal statement of the hypothesis that maternal and fetal circulations are separate within the human placenta [2]. The second half of the eighteenth century was crucial in the development of the understanding of the human placental circulations [2]. By injection of melted wax into the uterine arteries of a woman dying at the end of pregnancy, John and William Hunter conclusively demonstrated that maternal and fetal circulations were not anastomosed end-to-end in the placenta. The nineteenth and early twentieth centuries saw very rapid growth in knowledge of placental anatomy. Histological and ultrastructural studies elucidated the nature of the different placental components and, in particular, the structure of the chorionic villi [2].

Determining placental position *in utero* was the first aim of placental routine examination *in vivo*. Visualization and localization of the placenta by ultrasound became rapidly superior to all other imaging techniques such as radiographic placentography or scintigraphy [3,4] and is now an essential part of routine prenatal examinations. The information which can now be obtained by high resolution ultrasound or Doppler techniques places additional demands on the clinician, who requires more extensive knowledge of the anatomy and physiology of the vascular circulatory changes that occur during pregnancy. The prenatal diagnosis of placental and cord abnormalities is reviewed and their pathophysiology and potential clinical implications are discussed in this chapter.

56.2 Hemodynamics of early placental circulation

Until recently Doppler ultrasound studies of the uteroplacental circulation have been limited to the late second and third trimesters of pregnancy. The introduction of transvaginal transducers has enabled studies of uteroplacental and fetal circulation physiology in the first trimester.

56.2.1 UTEROPLACENTAL CIRCULATION

Implantation and subsequent placental development in the human requires complex adaptive changes of the uterine wall constituents, i.e. endometrium, myometrium and branches of the uterine arteries. In the early weeks of human pregnancy the spiral arteries undergo major morphologic changes. They become the uteroplacental arteries, which are distended, low-resistance channels capable of increasing the blood supply to the fetoplacental unit at term to ten times that of the non-pregnant uterus [2]. These pregnancy vascular changes have been closely related to the trophoblastic infiltration of the placental bed (Chapter 10). However, in some animal species such as horses, pigs and all ruminants, no erosion of the spiral arteries occurs and the developing pregnancy is adequately supplied by maternal blood [5]. The vascular transformation secondary to placentation is probably also influenced by variations in circulating steroid and protein hormones. Correlation of Doppler measurements and standard hormonal parameters suggest that maternal serum 17β-estradiol levels have a significant influence on uterine resistance to blood flow [6].

The various branches of the uterine circulation can be reliably distinguished by means of color imaging (Figures 56.1 and 56.2) and the overall Doppler features correlate well with the classical anatomic

Diseases of the Fetus and Newborn, 2nd edn, Edited by G.B. Reed, A.E. Claireaux and F. Cockburn. Published in 1995 by Chapman & Hall, London. ISBN 0 412 39160 0

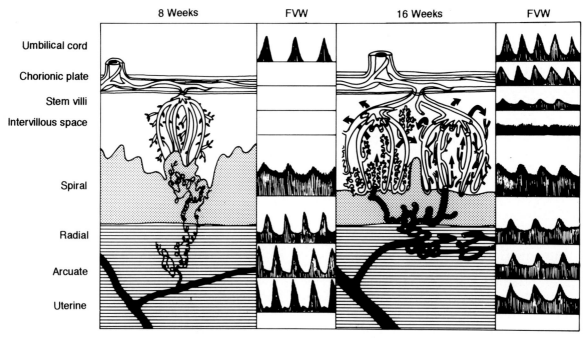

Figure 56.1 The various flow velocity waveforms (FVW) obtained from both placental circulations at 8 and 16 weeks of gestation, respectively. (Reproduced from Jauniaux, Jurkovic and Campbell [7].)

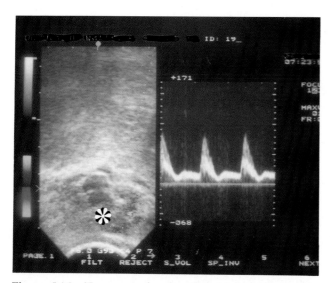

Figure 56.2 Transvaginal color Doppler mapping at the level of uterine cervix (*) and spectral analysis of blood velocity waveforms obtained from the main uterine artery at 8 weeks of gestation. Note the well defined protodiastolic notch.

towards the placental implantation site, low impedance findings [7–9]. Blood flow velocity waveforms from the main uterine arteries in normal pregnancies are characterized by a well-defined protodiastolic 'notch' (Figure 56.2) which disappears around 18–20 weeks of gestation [10]. When the Doppler gate is moved turbulent flow, which characterizes the transformed spiral arteries, is detected [7]. Continuous non-pulsatile flow on color imaging, with a venous pattern on spectral analysis, can only be detected between 12 and 14 weeks of gestation when the Doppler gate is placed over intraplacental sonolucent spaces [11]. This flow pattern is assumed to derive from maternal intervillous blood flow which enters the intervillous space when the trophoblastic plugs no longer obliterate the utero-placental arteries (Chapter 10).

Studies using either continuous wave or pulsed Doppler have demonstrated a progressive decrease in downstream resistance to blood flow (Figure 56.3) in the uterine arterial circulation during the first trimester of pregnancy [12–15]. This decrease continues during the second and the third trimesters and can be observed in all segments of the uterine arteries [7,16]. Doppler studies at an angle of insonation of less than 10° eliminate angle-dependent errors in maximum and mean velocity calculations [7,8,14]. These studies demonstrate an exponential increase in the mean peak systolic velocity of the main uterine artery (Figure 56.4). This increase is maximal between 13 and 14 weeks and has been related to the establishment of the intervillous circulation [7,11].

56.2.2 UMBILICAL CIRCULATION

Umbilical flow velocity waveforms before 14 weeks of gestation are mainly characterized by the absence of

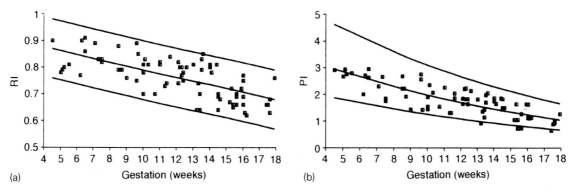

Figure 56.3 Individual values and reference ranges (mean and 95% confidence interval) of (a) the resistance index (RI) ($r = -0.69$, $P < 0.001$, $n = 76$) and (b) the pulsatility index (PI) ($r = -0.77$, $P < 0.001$, $n = 76$) in the main uterine artery with gestational age. (Reproduced from Jauniaux, Jurkovic and Campbell [7].)

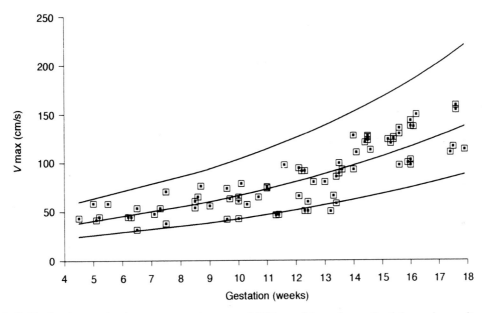

Figure 56.4 Individual values and reference ranges (mean and 95% confidence interval) of the peak systolic velocity (cm/s) in the main uterine artery with gestational age ($r = 0.83$, $P < 0.001$, $n = 76$). (Reproduced from Jauniaux, Jurkovic and Campbell [7].)

end-diastolic velocities [7,17,18]. Pulsatility index values from the umbilical artery remain almost constant, which suggests minor changes in umbilical placental vascular resistance during the first trimester [17]. Between 12 and 14 weeks, end-diastolic velocities develop rapidly (Figure 56.5). Diastolic flow is incomplete and/or inconsistently present until 14 weeks of gestation [7]. After this, pandiastolic frequencies are consistently present. End-diastolic velocities are present at the level of the intracerebral artery 2 weeks earlier than in the umbilical artery [19,20]. The lack of correlation between fetal heart rate and Doppler measurements in the different fetal vessels suggests heart rate

independency of the fetal waveforms at the end of the first trimester [19].

Cardiac and extracardiac arterial and venous flow studies have demonstrated the presence of a high fetal placental vascular resistance in normal late first trimester pregnancy, followed by a marked reduction in resistance in early second trimester pregnancy [20]. The anatomic changes in the villous vasculature, which are characterized by the progressive increase in the number and surface area occupied by the fetal vessels (Chapter 10), must have a key role in the gradual fall in blood flow impedance in the umbilical circulation. However, the appearance of end-diastolic frequencies in the

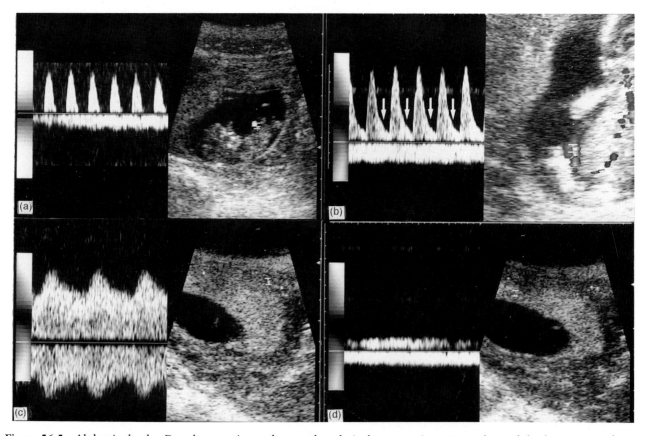

Figure 56.5   Abdominal color Doppler mapping and spectral analysis demonstrating: (a) regular umbilical artery waveforms with no end-diastolic flow at 8 weeks of gestation; (b) continuous end-diastolic flow (arrows) in the umbilical artery at 14 weeks (same case as in (a)); (c) continuous blood flow with a venous pattern (i.e. intervillous flow) at 13 weeks of gestation; (d) uteroplacental artery waveforms near the basal placental plate at 13 weeks of gestation showing a typical flow with an irregular and spiky outline.

umbilical circulation also coincides with an abrupt and significant increase in uterine artery peak systolic velocity, together with the presence of a continuous intervillous flow within the whole placental mass (Figure 56.5). The establishment of the intervillous circulation may be associated with changes in the pressure gradient due to the expansion of the inter-villous space and/or with modification in blood gases and metabolite concentrations which could cause the rapid appearance of end-diastolic frequencies in the umbilical circulation [11].

56.3   Prenatal diagnosis of placental and cord abnormalities

The interval between the development of a lesion *in utero* and delivery can result in marked differences between the sonographic and the pathologic findings. The ultrasound features of most placental or cord vascular lesions may undergo major changes within a few days. When a placental abnormality which could

be associated with perinatal complications is suspected, serial sonographic examinations should be performed. Many inaccurate and misleading expressions have been used by ultrasonographers to describe placental lesions. This is probably due to the fact that little attempt has been made to compare ultrasound and pathologic findings. One should always refer to the classical pathologic terminology to categorize these lesions and evaluate their clinical significance.

56.3.1   ULTRASONOGRAPHIC ASSESSMENT AND CLASSIFICATION

(a)   Placental maturation and grading

Sonographic changes in placental texture have been reported during the second half of pregnancy [21–24]. A sonographic classification system for grading placentas *in utero* according to maturational changes was developed by Grannum and associates [22]. The placentas were graded from 0 to III on the basis of compound B-scan changes in placental structures and the results were correlated with fetal pulmonary maturity evaluated by amniotic fluid lecithin:sphingomyelin (L:S) ratios. However, their results were not confirmed by other authors and subsequent reports showed that a grade III placenta was associated with an immature L:S ratio in 8–42% of the cases and was, therefore, not accurate enough to replace amniocentesis in predicting fetal pulmonary maturity [25]. A very well-conducted randomized controlled trial has demonstrated that pregnant women presenting with mature placental sonographic features (grade III) between 34 and 36 weeks gestation have an increased risk of problems during labor and their babies have an increased risk of low birth weight, intrapartum distress and perinatal death [26].

(b)   Current placental abnormalities

A sonographic classification of placental lesions based on their location, size, echogenicity and number has recently been proposed (Table 56.1).

Circumvallate placentas are characterized by a transition of membranous to villous chorion within the placental disc and are associated with a relatively high rate of premature rupture of the membranes, antepartum bleeding and preterm onset of labor [25]. These complications are probably due to a non-adaptation of the rigid placental edge with tearing of the membranes as the uterine wall stretches in the second half of gestation. Multiple subamniotic sonolucent areas of

various size and shape, located in the periphery of the placenta (Figure 56.6a,b) are the main ultrasound features of this form of placentation [27].

Cytotrophoblastic cysts are isolated from the placental circulation and appear sonographically as single sonolucent areas (Figure 56.6c,d) showing no blood flow on color imaging and have little or no clinical significance [28]. In contrast, subamniotic hematomas which are due to the rupture of a fetal vessel are sometimes complicated by fetal growth retardation and abnormal Doppler measurements [27]. Sonographically, they appear as a single mass protruding from the fetal plate and surrounded by a thin membrane. The newly formed clot is echogenic (Figure 56.6e) but the lesion becomes less so as the clot resolves (Figure 56.6f,g).

Chorioangiomas are associated with an increased incidence of polyhydramnios and fetal growth retardation [28]. Large tumors are sometimes complicated by fetal cardiac failure with hydrops due to the shunting of blood through the tumor [27]. The fetal risk depends probably more on the proportion of angiomatous versus mixoid tissue inside the tumor than on its exact size. On ultrasound, chorioangiomas appear as well-circumscribed lesions with a different echogenicity from the rest of the placental tissue. They protrude into the amniotic cavity (Figure 56.7) or are located inside the placental mass (Figure 56.8). The echogenicity varies according to the degree of degenerative change present in the tumor. The vascular nature of the tumor can easily be evaluated in utero with color Doppler imaging [16].

Table 56.1   Differential diagnosis of the principal placental sonographic features

Location	Sonographic features	Pathologic classification
Fetal plate	Multiple sonolucent areas to the placental periphery (Figure 56.6a)	Circumvallate placenta Circummarginate placenta
	Single sonolucent or hypoechoic area surrounded by a thin membrane (Figure 56.6c,f)	Subamniotic cyst Old subamniotic hematoma
	Single hyperechoic area surrounded by a thin membrane (Figure 56.6e)	Recent subamniotic hematoma
	Heterogeneous mass protruding into the amniotic cavity (Figure 56.7a)	Chorioangioma Teratoma
Placental tissue	Small sonolucent area in the center of the cotyledon	Centrocotyledonary cavity
	Hypoechoic round mass well circumscribed (Figure 56.8)	Chorioangioma Old infarct
	Large sonolucent area (Figure 56.9a)	Cavern Septal cyst Recent thrombosis
	Large hyperechoic area (Figure 56.9c,e)	Old thrombosis Recent infarct
	Multiple sonolucent areas of various sizes and shapes (Figure 56.10)	Hydatidiform-like transformations
Maternal plate	Large hyperechoic area	Recent retroplacental hematoma
	Large hypoechoic area (Figure 56.11)	Old retroplacental hematoma

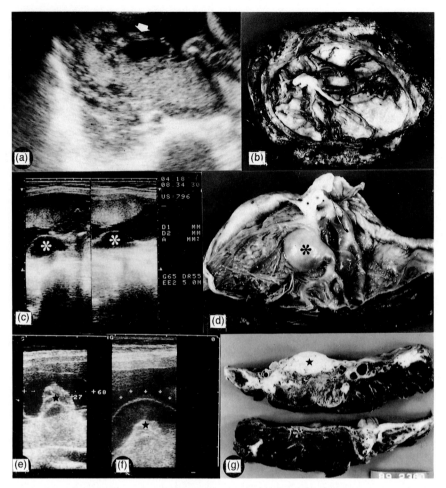

Figure 56.6 (a) Transverse scan at 20 weeks of gestation of the marginal zone of the placenta, showing sonolucent areas over the fetal plate (arrow). These abnormalities were found only near the placental edge. (b) Pathologic examination demonstrated a circumvallate placenta. (c) Transverse and longitudinal scans of a single sonolucent subamniotic area (*) at 32 weeks corresponding to (d) a subamniotic cyst (*). (e) and (f) Longitudinal sonograms at 24 and 32 weeks, respectively, showing a hyperechogenic placental lesion on the top of the fetal plate (stars), surrounded by a thin membrane (arrows). The lesion becomes less echogenic as the clot resolves. (g) Pathologic examination revealed an old subamniotic hematoma (star). (Reproduced from Jauniaux and Campbell [25].)

Placental thromboses are the result of focal coagulation of blood in the intervillous spaces and occur more frequently in pregnancies complicated by rhesus isoimmunization [28]. Large hypoechoic areas, with low flow laterally and relatively high flow in the central part on real-time imaging, can be observed in the early stages of the development of an intervillous thrombosis (Figure 56.9a). Abnormal hemodynamic flow in the intervillous space may result from the failure of the cotyledon to expand in response to the increasing flow of the corresponding uteroplacental artery and compression of the surrounding villi with gradual atrophy as fibrin is laid down in the periphery [29,30]. This process causes a progressive increase in the echogenicity of the lesion (Figure 56.9c,d). Finally, the maternal blood coagulates in the placental tissue, obliterating,

focally, the intervillous circulation. Placental infarcts are the result of obstruction of a uteroplacental artery leading to focal degeneration of the overlying villous tissue [28]. Extensive infarcts are found in pregnancies complicated by pre-eclampsia or essential hypertension and are associated with an increase in perinatal mortality and intrauterine growth retardation [28]. Sonographically, placental infarcts appear as large intraplacental areas, irregular and hyperechoic in the acute stage [31] and isoechoic in a more advanced stage (Figure 56.9e,f).

Hydatidiform transformation (Figure 56.10) of the villous tissue is a common finding in placental trophoblastic tumors. Complete or classic hydatidiform moles are characterized by generalized swelling of the villous tissue and no embryonic or fetal tissue [25]. Sono-

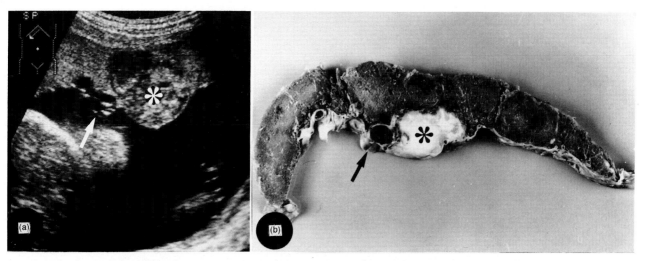

Figure 56.7   (a) Heterogeneous placental mass at 32 weeks (*) protruding from the fetal plate near the cord insertion (arrow). The pregnancy was complicated by polyhydramnios. (b) Pathologic examination demonstrated a chorioangioma (*) showing generalized degenerative changes. (Reproduced from Jauniaux and Campbell [25].)

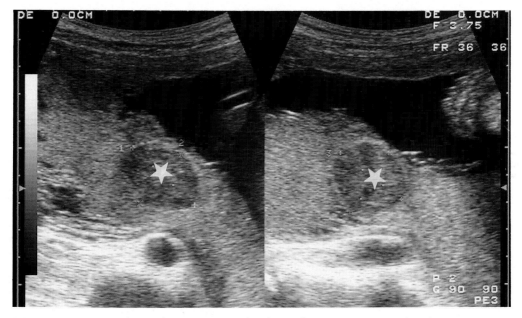

Figure 56.8   Heterogeneous intraplacental mass (star) under the cord insertion at 25 weeks of gestation, corresponding to a cellular chorioangioma after delivery.

graphically, the uterus is filled with sonolucent spaces (snowstorm appearance) of various sizes and shapes. Partial hydatidiform moles are characterized by focal swelling of the villous tissue and embryonic or fetal tissue [25]. Molar changes of the placenta are not always pathognomonic of trophoblastic disorders and can be found in other placental pathologies such as benign diffuse mesenchymal hyperplasia (Figure 56.10)

or in prolonged placental retention *in utero* after fetal death [32].

Retroplacental hematomas cause a wide spectrum of sonographic features depending on the location of the lesion and on the degree of organization of the blood clot. Sonographic investigations are mainly used in non-acute cases to confirm the clinical diagnosis and to exclude the presence of a placenta previa [25]. Acute

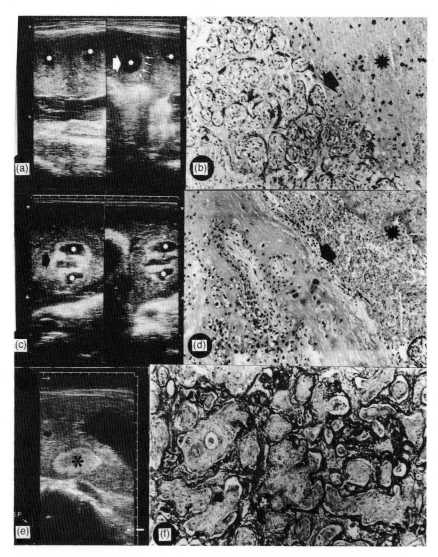

Figure 56.9 (a) Sonograms at 35 weeks showing small and large placental sonolucent spaces (*) containing turbulent blood flow. Note the increased echogenicity of the surrounding villi (small arrows); (b) histological section (H and E, 50×) at the level of the large arrow showing a recent intervillous thrombosis (*) and normal villi (arrow). The villi surrounding the lesion at the level of the small arrows were compressed and infarcted. (c) Sonograms at 39 weeks showing a large placental lesion (*) corresponding (d) to an organized intervillous thrombosis (*) with extensive fibrin deposition (large arrows) in periphery (H and E, 50×). (e) Large placental hyperechoic area (*) located near the basal plate at 32 weeks of gestation corresponding (f) to a chronic infarct (H and E, 50×). (Reproduced from Jauniaux and Campbell [25].)

hemorrhage is hyperechoic to isoechoic compared with placental tissue, while resolving hematomas are hypoechoic (Figure 56.11).

(c) Major cord abnormalities

The umbilical cord anatomy can often be visualized around 20 weeks gestation by gray scale imaging but a precise diagnosis of a particular cord abnormality may be difficult and time consuming [33]. At the end of the second trimester or during the third trimester of pregnancy the umbilical cord anatomy can be examined in detail without difficulty (Figure 56.12). However, various factors such as oligohydramnios or multiple loops in the cord can make accurate visualization of the cord vessels impossible, even near term. High resolution color Doppler imaging has an important role in early and accurate diagnosis of cord abnormalities [34,35] and is also of clinical value in difficult invasive procedures.

The absence of one umbilical artery is among the most common congenital fetal malformations, with an

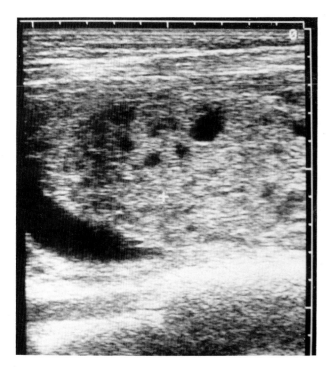

Figure 56.10 Longitudinal sonogram at 22 weeks of gestation showing an enlarged placenta containing multiple sonolucent spaces. The fetus was anatomically normal and pathologic examination demonstrated diffuse mesenchymal hyperplasia with myxoid degeneration of the stem villi and dilatation of the main fetal vessels.

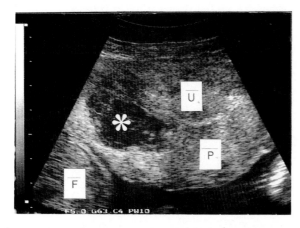

Figure 56.11 Sonogram at 32 weeks of gestation, 2 weeks after cordocentesis, showing a large hypoechoic area (*) separating the placenta (P) from the uterine wall (U) and corresponding to a retroplacental hematoma. F = fetal body.

incidence of approximately 1% of all deliveries [36]. Fetal major anatomic defects are largely responsible for the high fetal and neonatal loss from this pathology [36,37]. Fetal malformations are present in about

50% of the cases of single umbilical artery and can affect any organ system. The incidence of intrauterine growth retardation is significantly elevated among fetuses with only one umbilical artery and may be present without other congenital anomalies in 15–20% of cases [36].

Color Doppler imaging can easily demonstrate the cord location early in pregnancy. Looping of the cord may occur around the fetal neck, body or shoulder but is an uncommon cause of fetal death. However in monoamniotic twins a significant portion of the high mortality can be attributed to umbilical cord problems [38]. Velamentous insertion of the cord or placenta velamentosa is a well-defined pathologic entity with a frequency of around 1% of pregnancies [28]. From a clinical point of view, attachment of the cord to the extraplacental membranes is important because of the risk of severe fetal hemorrhage during labor [33]. Antenatal diagnosis of attachment of the cord to the membranes rather than the placental mass can be easily performed before labor by means of color Doppler imaging [39,40].

Umbilical cord tumors are infrequent perinatal findings [33]. From a pathologic point of view, primary cord tumors can be divided into angiomyxomas or hemangiomas derived from embryonic vessels, teratomas derived from germ cells and vestigial cysts derived from remnants of the allantois or of the omphalomesenteric duct [28]. A cord angiomyxoma appears sonographically as a heterogeneous mass made of a strong echogenic area, embedding the umbilical vessels (Figure 56.13) and surrounded by large echopoor areas [41]. The prenatal diagnosis of a cord teratoma has never been reported but this type of tumor should be mainly composed of dense tissue [28]. Conversely, vestigial cysts appear sonographically as a single fluid-filled mass. Vestigial cysts and pseudocysts can sometimes be associated with small abdominal wall defects and a precise early prenatal diagnosis can be more difficult to establish [42,43]. Several conditions causing simple or complex multicystic cord masses can mimic a tumor on gray scale imaging. These conditions include cord hematomas, ectasia of the umbilical vein, pseudocysts and true knots [33].

56.3.2 BIOCHEMICAL MARKERS

The two principal biochemical indicators in the maternal serum (MS) of a placental pathology are the human chorionic gonadotropin (hCG) and the α-fetoprotein (AFP) levels. Elevated MShCG levels are suggestive of trophoblastic disorders, while elevated MSAFP levels are less specific of a typical placental lesion but indicate a breakdown of the maternal barrier such as may occur with infarcts or thrombosis [25,44]. Most

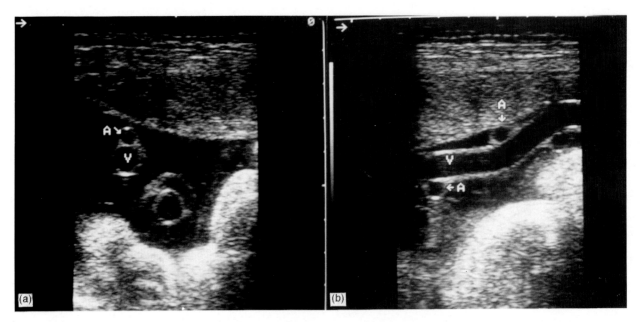

Figure 56.12   Transverse (a) and longitudinal (b) sonograms at 32 weeks demonstrating only one artery (A) and one vein (V). The fetus was growth retarded with no associated malformation.

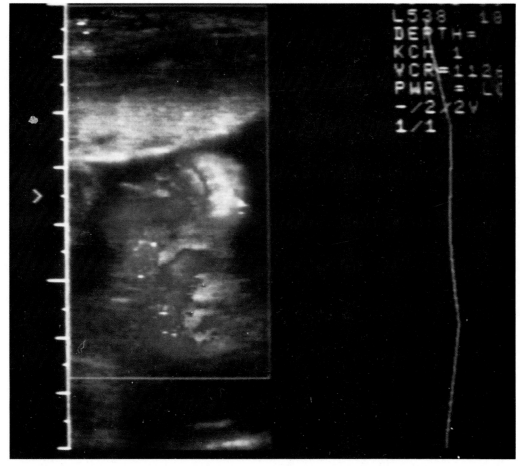

Figure 56.13   Color flow image of the cord angiomyxoma showing an abnormal vascular pattern at the placental insertion. (Reproduced from Jauniaux, Campbell and Vyas [35].)

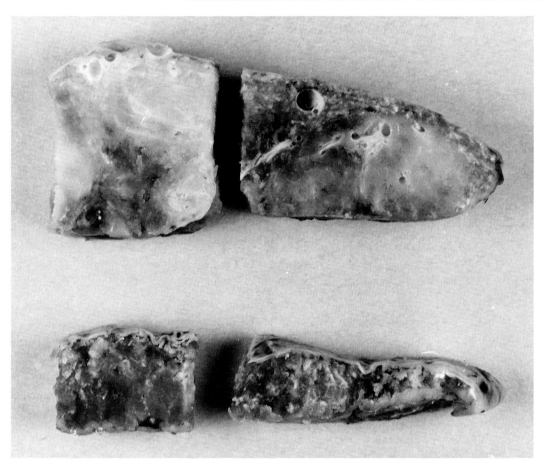

Figure 56.14 Macroscopic appearance of perfused-fixed (upper slices) and immersed-fixed (lower slices) parts of the same placenta. Perfusion fixation restores the initial thickness and general anatomy that may be observed *in vivo* by ultrasound. (Reproduced from Jauniaux *et al.* [49].)

other placental products such as human placental lactogen or estriol, which were very popular in the 1970s and 1980s for the screening of placental insufficiency and fetal growth retardation, have now been supplanted by ultrasound techniques.

It is accepted that complete hydatidiform moles are almost always associated with very high MShCG levels. The most common karyotype found in cases of partial mole is triploidy, and published biologic findings indicate that most of the triploidy cases also present with elevated MShCG levels [25]. There is a strong correlation between the origin of the extra set of chromosomes, the survival rate of the pregnancies and the degree of the placental molar change, and therefore probably also with the biological changes.

A large range of placental and cord abnormalities are associated with elevated MSAFP and are potentially diagnosable by routine sonographic examination at the time of AFP screening [45,46]. Chorioangiomas are lesions classically associated with elevated MSAFP levels in the literature [47]. However, cellular chorio-

angiomas, which consist of loose mesenchymal tissue and few vessels, and therefore little or no shunting of fetal blood through the tumor and fetal protein leakage in the maternal circulation, may be associated with normal MSAFP levels [48].

56.4 Experimental systems for the study of placental anatomy

The correlation of *in vivo* and *in vitro* features is a fundamental step for better comprehension of the pathophysiology of various maternal–fetal diseases, in particular those involving the placental circulations.

56.4.1 PERFUSION FIXATION OF HUMAN PLACENTA

Due to unavoidable placental collapse during delivery, important details of the placental morphology are obscured. Perfusion fixation is of particular interest for pathophysiologic studies of placental function related

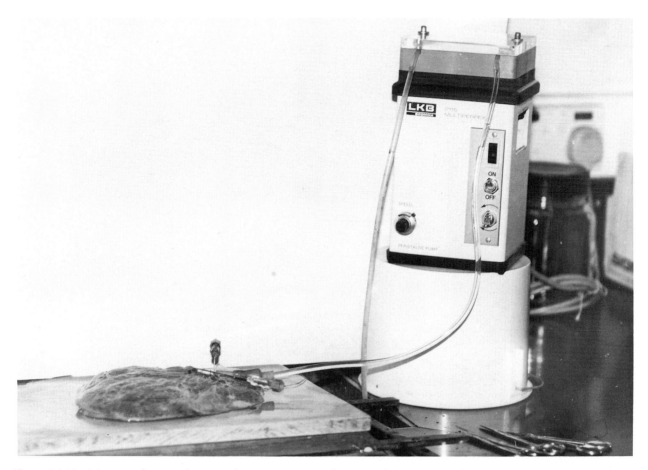

Figure 56.15   Montage showing the peristaltic pump connected to an umbilical artery. The placenta is subsequently placed in a bath containing physiologic solution and perfused with fixative.

to anatomy (Figure 56.14). Several authors have attempted to reproduce *in vitro* the sonographic morphologic features observed *in vivo* [21,23]. In these studies, however, the placentas were not always fixed immediately after delivery, some changes observed *in vivo* were not found *in vitro* and new features could have been created during placental collapse. More satisfactory results were obtained using gravity [24] or mechanical perfusion systems (Figures 56.15 and 56.16). Sonolucent areas or echo-free spaces, frequently observed in the center of the cotyledon or under the fetal plate of the placenta during the second half of pregnancy, have been correlated with avillous zones and the peripheral echoes with septal calcification and fibrin deposition [24,29].

Unfixed placental tissue deteriorates rapidly after delivery [50]. Within a few minutes of total ischemia, ultrastructural alterations can be found in the syncytiotrophoblastic layer; these are similar to those observed in placentas from pregnancies complicated by intrauterine growth retardation associated with partial occlusion of the uteroplacental arteries [50]. Perfusion fixation of

the placenta allows faster histologic examination of the specimens than simple fixation by immersion. If the perfusion pressure is carefully controlled, no histologic artifacts are created during the procedure [49,50]. Placental collapse considerably influences the histomorphometric data. Compared to perfused-fixed placental tissue, immersed-fixed placental villi show an important degree of fetal capillary collapse and present with a significant increase of the mean trophoblastic and barrier thickness [49,50]. Significant histomorphometric differences are also found between placentas from cesarean section and placentas from vaginal delivery [49]. These findings should be taken into account when correlation between Doppler ultrasound measurements and placental histologic changes are attempted.

56.4.2   DOPPLER INVESTIGATIONS

During the second half of gestation, the vascular network with the lowest resistance in the entire fetal circulatory system is at the level of the placental

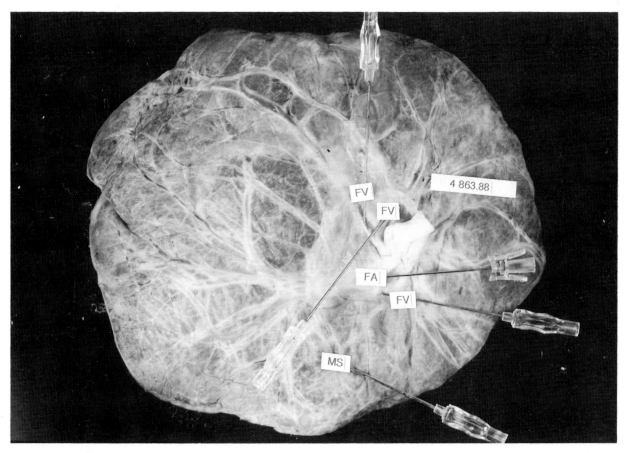

Figure 56.16   Needle placement for placental perfusion fixation. The fixative enters the placental circulation via a main fetal artery (FA) and leaves it via fetal veins (FV). The maternal villous space (MS) can also be perfused by inserting needles through the chorionic plate.

vascular bed [51]. Electrical circuit and mathematical equivalent models depict the vascularization of the placenta by a two-level resistance system. The first level is represented by the resistance of the main umbilical arteries and the second level is composed of a large number of small resistances (branching arteries) in parallel [52]. It is important to underline that Doppler investigations of the placental villous tree in normal pregnancies are limited to the vessels of the main stem villi [16]. Because of their small size, the terminal villi are not accessible by this method.

Several authors have reported placental lesions in pregnancies complicated by abnormal umbilical artery Doppler indices [53–58]. A significant relationship has been found between an increased pulsatility index and a decrease in the number of small arterioles of tertiary stem villi, suggesting an obliterative process [53–55,58]. An increased incidence of various macroscopic anomalies, including major placental vascular lesions and hypermaturity or shape anomalies, has also been described in these cases [55,57]. As most of these placental lesions are detectable by ultrasonography,

detailed antenatal placental morphologic investigation should be performed in all pregnancies complicated by abnormal Doppler indices.

56.4.3   PLACENTAL BIOPSIES

Sampling of placental villi *in utero* was first performed by Acosta-Sison [59] and Alvarez [60] for the clinical diagnosis of hydatidiform mole. The procedure consisted of a blind transabdominal biopsy and was subsequently carried out from 6 weeks of gestation to term in order to investigate *in vivo* normal placental anatomy and development [60]. Ultrasound guidance has indubitably improved the safety of chorionic villous sampling. The procedure is now routinely performed from 6 weeks of gestation until delivery for prenatal genetic diagnosis [61,62]. Microscopic examination of fresh villous tissue sampled *in utero* has not been used for the routine management of complicated pregnancies. Its usefulness, in particular, in cases of fetal intrauterine growth retardation (Figure 56.17) needs to

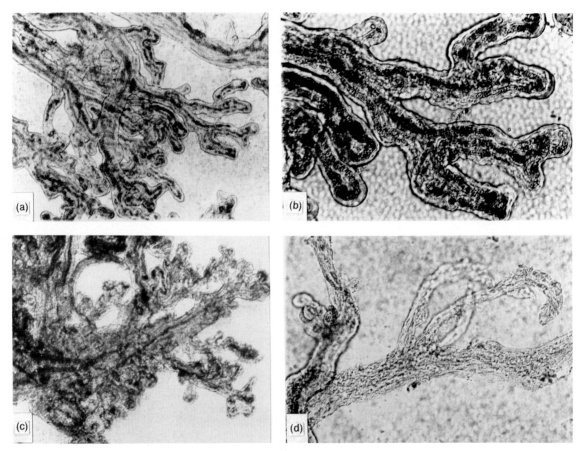

Figure 56.17   Phase contrast micrographs of fresh villous tissue sampled *in utero* during percutaneous umbilical blood sampling procedure for karyotyping at 35 weeks of gestation: (a) (25×) and (b) (100×) from a normally growing fetus with normal Doppler measurements showing a well-developed villous vascular network; (c) (25×) and (d) (100×) from a poorly growing fetus with abnormal Doppler features (absent end-diastolic flow in the umbilical artery circulation) showing poorly vascularized and degenerated villous trees.

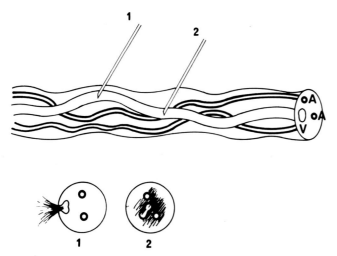

Figure 56.18   Possible cord damage due to umbilical cord puncture *in utero*: (1) laceration of a superficial vessel with hemorrhage in the amniotic cavity; (2) hematoma due to direct injection of blood in the Wharton's jelly during transfusion or secondary to the leakage of fetal blood by the opening created by the needle. A = artery; V = vein.

be evaluated by means of modern histomorphometric techniques.

56.5   Diagnosing iatrogenic lesions of placenta and cord

Increasing use of invasive prenatal procedures has resulted in an increase in adverse cord and placental damage with potential consequences for the fetus. Amniocentesis has been the most frequently used, but is now being progressively replaced by chorionic villus sampling and percutaneous umbilical blood sampling or cordocentesis.

Cord and placental trauma associated with severe fetal distress or fetal death were described during the early days of amniocentesis when no ultrasound guidance was used [29]. Uncontrolled movements of the needle in percutaneous umbilical blood sampling are reduced by precise insertion of the needle in the cord under ultrasound guidance and by the larger

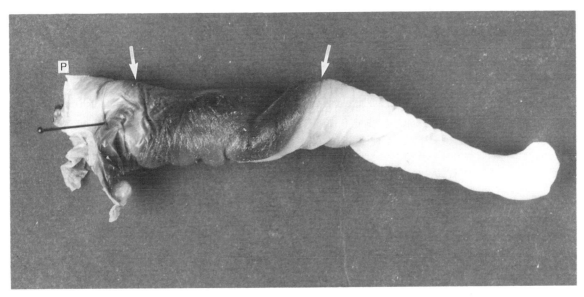

Figure 56.19 Macroscopic appearances of the cord near its placental (P) insertion showing a large hematoma (in between arrows) developed after fetal transfusion *in utero*.

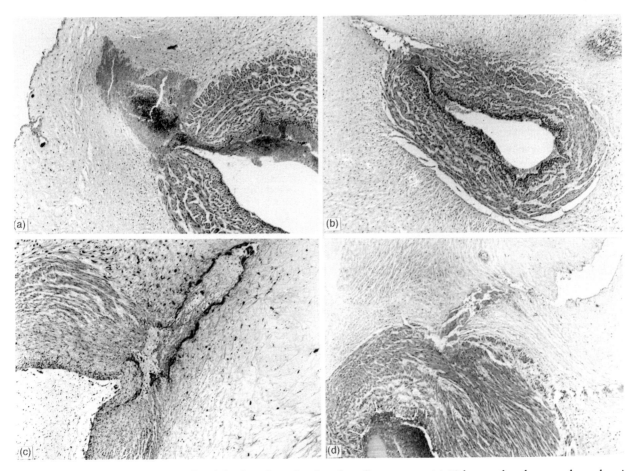

Figure 56.20 Microscopic aspects of umbilical cords at the site of needle puncture: (a) 12 hours after the procedure, showing extravasation of erythrocytes (H and E, 100×); (b) 1 week after the needle puncture (H and E, 100×); (c) 1 month after the puncture, showing partial regeneration of the vessel wall (H and E, 125×); (d) 17 weeks after percutaneous umbilical blood sampling showing only fibrin deposition into the Wharton jelly (H and E, 125×). (Reproduced from Jauniaux *et al.* [65].)

experience of the perinatal teams in these invasive procedures [29]. Lacerations of superficial umbilical vessels may lead to substantial hemorrhage into the amniotic sac with severe hemodynamic consequences. A small hematoma will probably not affect fetal umbilical circulation because the blood can drain into the amniotic cavity via the needle entry (Figure 56.18). The extension of the hematoma is probably also limited by the tension created by the Wharton's jelly and the amniotic cavity [29]. The end-result of a cord hematoma may range from complete occlusion of the cord vessels, with inevitable fetal death, to varying degrees of fetal distress, either acute or chronic [63]. Macroscopic examination of the cord after delivery may help to elucidate how often procedure-related bradycardia is associated with specific cord damages (Figure 56.19). Microscopic examination of the cord of fetuses born after percutaneous umbilical blood sampling [64] demonstrates a rapid regeneration of the vessel wall within a week after the procedure (Figure 56.20). As for amniocentesis, amnionitis, puncture of subchorionic vessels or retroplacental hematoma (Figure 56.11) are also possible complications of percutaneous umbilical blood sampling.

56.6 Concluding remarks

The recent emphasis placed on fetal medicine and on prenatal investigation of fetoplacental abnormalities has resulted in an increased demand for rapid postnatal placental examinations. An important goal in contemporary perinatal research is to define more accurately the pathophysiologic basis of the different gestational complications involving the placental circulation and/or function. With improvement of ultrasound equipment, obstetricians are able to examine the placenta and the cord in detail before delivery and to investigate the placental circulations *in vivo*. The differential diagnosis of placental anomalies is now possible *in utero* but still requires detailed pathologic correlation after delivery. Pathologic examination of the placenta and umbilical cord is also recommended in all complicated invasive procedures so that the consequences of these techniques may be more fully documented.

References

1. Boyd, J.D. and Hamilton, W.J. (1970) *The Human Placenta*, Heffer, Cambridge.
2. Ramsey, E.M. and Donner, N.W. (1980) *Placental Vasculature and Circulation*, Georg Thieme, Stuttgart.
3. Gottesfeld, K.R., Thomspon, H.E., Holmes, J.H. and Taylor, E.S. (1966) Ultrasonic placentography: a new method for placental localization. *Am. J. Obstet. Gynecol.*, 96, 539–47.
4. Campbell, S. and Kohorn, E.I. (1968) Placental localization by ultrasonic compound scanning. *J. Obstet. Gynaecol. Br. Commonw.*, 75, 1007–13.
5. Burton, G.J. (1992) Human and animal models: limitations and comparisons, in *The First Twelve Weeks of Gestation: A New Frontier for Investigation and Intervention* (eds E. Barnea, J. Hustin and E. Jauniaux), Springer, Heidelberg, pp. 469–85.

6. Jauniaux, E., Jurkovic, D., Delogne-Desnoek, J. and Meuris, S. (1993) Influence of human chorionic gonadotropin, oestradiol and progesterone on uteroplacental and corpus luteum blood flow in normal early pregnancy. *Hum. Reprod.*, 7, 1467–73.
7. Jauniaux, E., Jurkovic, D. and Campbell, S. (1991) *In vivo* investigations of the anatomy and the physiology of early human placental circulations. *Ultrasound Obstet. Gynecol.*, 1, 435–45.
8. Jurkovic, D., Jauniaux, E. and Campbell, S. (1992) Doppler ultrasound investigations of pelvic circulation during the menstrual cycle and early pregnancy, in *The First Twelve Weeks of Gestation: A New Frontier for Investigation and Intervention* (eds E. Barnea, J. Hustin and E. Jauniaux), Springer, Heidelberg, pp. 78–96.
9. Jauniaux, E., Jurkovic, D., Kurjak, A. and Hustin, J. (1991) Assessment of placental development and function, in *Transvaginal Color Doppler* (ed. A. Kurjak), Parthenon, Carnforth, pp. 53–65.
10. Cohen-Overbeek, T.E., Pearse, J.M. and Campbell, S. (1985) The antenatal assessment of uteroplacental blood flow using Doppler ultrasound. *Ultrasound Med. Biol.*, 11, 329–39.
11. Jauniaux, E., Jurkovic, D., Campbell, S. and Hustin, J. (1992) Doppler ultrasonographic features of the developing placental circulations: correlation with anatomic findings. *Am. J. Obstet. Gynecol.*, 166, 585–87.
12. Schulman, H., Fleisher, A., Farmakides, G. *et al.* (1986) Development of uterine artery compliance as detected by Doppler ultrasound. *Am. J. Obstet. Gynecol.*, 155, 1031–36.
13. Deutinger, J., Rudelstorfer, R. and Bernaschek, G. (1988) Vaginosonographic velocimetry of both main uterine arteries by visual recognition and pulsed Doppler method during pregnancy. *Am. J. Obstet. Gynecol.*, 159, 1072–76.
14. Jurkovic, D., Jauniaux, E., Kurjak, A. *et al.* (1991) Transvaginal color Doppler assessment of uteroplacental circulation in early pregnancy. *Obstet. Gynecol.*, 77, 365–69.
15. Jaffe, R. and Warsof, S.L. (1991) Transvaginal color Doppler imaging in the assessment of uteroplacental blood flow in the normal first-trimester pregnancy. *Am. J. Obstet. Gynecol.*, 164, 781–85.
16. Jauniaux, E., Jurkovic, D., Campbell, S. *et al.* (1991) Investigation of placental circulations by color Doppler ultrasound. *Am. J. Obstet. Gynecol.*, 164, 486–88.
17. Loquet, Ph., Broughton-Pipkin, F., Symonds, E.M. *et al.* (1988) Blood velocity waveforms and placental vascular formation. *Lancet*, ii, 1252–53.
18. Guzman, E.R., Schulman, H., Karmel, B. and Higgins, P. (1990) Umbilical artery Doppler velocimetry in pregnancy of less than 21 weeks' duration. *J. Ultrasound Med.*, 9, 655–59.
19. Wladimiroff, J.W., Huisman, T.W.A. and Stewart, P.A. (1991) Fetal and umbilical flow velocity waveforms between 10–16 weeks' gestation: a preliminary study. *Obstet. Gynecol.*, 78, 812–14.
20. Huisman, T.W.A., Stewart, P.A. and Waladimiroff, J.W. (1992) Doppler assessment of normal early fetal circulation. *Ultrasound Obstet. Gynecol.*, 2, 300–305.
21. Winberg, F. (1973) Echogenic changes with placental aging. *J. Clin. Ultrasound*, 1, 52–55.
22. Grannum, P.A.T., Berkowitz, R.L. and Hobbins, J.C. (1979) The ultrasonic changes in the maturing placenta and their relation to fetal pulmonic maturity. *Am. J. Obstet. Gynecol.*, 133, 915–22.
23. Fisher, C.C., Garrett, W. and Kossoff, G. (1976) Placenta aging monitored by gray scale echography. *Am. J. Obstet. Gynecol.*, 124, 483–88.
24. Vermeulen, R.C.W., Lambalk, N.B., Exalto, N. and Arts, N.F.T. (1985) An anatomic basis for ultrasound images of the human placenta. *Am. J. Obstet. Gynecol.*, 153, 806–10.
25. Jauniaux, E. and Campbell, S. (1990) Sonographic assessment of placental abnormalities. *Am. J. Obstet. Gynecol.*, 163, 1650–58.
26. Proud, J. and Grant, A.M. (1987) Third trimester placental grading by ultrasonography as a test of fetal wellbeing. *BMJ*, 294, 1641–44.
27. Jauniaux, E., Avni, F.E., Donner, C. *et al.* (1989) Ultrasonographic diagnosis and morphological study of placentas circumvallate. *J. Clin. Ultrasound*, 16, 126–31.
28. Fox, H. (1978) *Pathology of Placenta*, W.B. Saunders, Philadelphia.
29. Jauniaux, E. and Campbell, S. (1993) Perinatal assessment of placental and cord abnormalities, in *Textbook of Obstetrics and Gynecologic Ultrasound* (eds F.A. Chervenak, G. Isaacson and S. Campbell), Little, Brown, Boston, pp. 327–44.
30. Jauniaux, E., Avni, F.E., Elkazen, N. *et al.* (1989) Etude morphologique des anomalies placentaires echographiques de la deuxieme moitié de la gestation. *J. Gynécol. Obstet. Biol. Reprod.*, 18, 601–13.
31. Jauniaux, E. and Campbell, S. (1991) Antenatal diagnosis of placental infarcts by ultrasound. *J. Clin. Ultrasound*, 19, 58–61.
32. Moscoso, G., Jauniaux, E. and Hustin, J. (1991) Placental vascular anomaly with diffuse mesenchymal stem villous hyperplasia of the placenta: a new clinico-pathological entity? *Pathol. Res. Pract.*, 187, 324–28.
33. Jauniaux, E. and Campbell, S. (1993) Ultrasonographic diagnosis of placental and cord abnormalities, in *Clinical Ultrasound. A Comprehensive Text*, vol. III (eds H. Meire, D. Cosgrove and K. Dewbury) Churchill Livingstone, London, pp. 435–62.
34. Jeanty, P. (1989) Fetal and funicular vascular anomalies: identification with prenatal US. *Radiology*, 173, 367–70

35. Jauniaux, E., Campbell, S. and Vyas, S. (1989) The use of color Doppler imaging for prenatal diagnosis of umbilical cord anomalies: report of three cases. *Am. J. Obstet. Gynecol.*, **161**, 1195–97.

36. Jauniaux, E., De Munter, C., Pardou, A. *et al.* (1989) Evaluation échographique du syndrôme de l'artère ombilicale unique: une série de 80 cas. *J. Gynécol. Obstet. Biol. Reprod.*, **18**, 341–48.

37. Nyberg, D.A., Mahony, B.S., Luthy, D. and Kapur, R. (1991) Single umbilical artery: prenatal detection of concurrent anomalies. *J. Ultrasound Med.*, **10**, 247–53.

38. Jauniaux, E., Mawissa, C., Peellaerts, C. and Rodesch, F. (1992) Nuchal cord in normal third trimester pregnancy: a color Doppler imaging study. *Ultrasound Obstet. Gynecol.*, **2**, 417–19.

39. Nelson, L.H., Melone, P.J. and King, M. (1990) Diagnosis of vasa previa with transvaginal and color flow Doppler ultrasound. *Obstet. Gynecol.*, **76**, 506–509.

40. Harding, J.A., Lewis, D.F., Major, C.A. *et al.* (1990) Color flow Doppler: a useful instrument in the diagnosis of vasa previa. *Am. J. Obstet. Gynecol.*, **163**, 1566–68.

41. Jauniaux, E., Moscoso, G., Chitty, L. *et al.* (1990) An angiomyxoma involving the whole length of the umbilical cord: prenatal diagnosis by ultrasonography. *J. Ultrasound Med.*, **9**, 419–22.

42. Jauniaux, E., Donner, C., Thomas, C. *et al.* (1988) Umbilical cord pseudocyst in trisomy 18. *Prenat. Diagn.*, **8**, 557–63.

43. Jauniaux, E., Jurkovic, D. and Campbell, S. (1991) Sonographic features of an umbilical cord abnormality combining a cord pseudocyst and a small omphalocele. *Eur. J. Obstet. Gynecol. Reprod. Biol.*, **38**, 245–48.

44. Jauniaux, E., Moscoso, G., Campbell, S. *et al.* (1990) Correlation of ultrasound and pathologic findings of placental anomalies in pregnancies with elevated maternal serum alpha-fetoprotein. *Eur. J. Obstet. Gynecol. Reprod. Biol.*, **37**, 219–30.

45. Kelly, R.B., Nyberg, D.A., Mack, L.A. *et al.* (1989) Sonography of placental abnormalities and oligohydramnios in woman with elevated alpha-fetoprotein levels: comparison with control subjects. *Radiology*, **153**, 815–19.

46. Jauniaux, E., Gibb, D., Moscoso, G. and Campbell, S. (1990) Sonographic diagnosis of a large intervillous thrombosis associated with elevated maternal serum alpha-fetoprotein. *Am. J. Obstet. Gynecol.*, **163**, 1558–60.

47. Thomas, R.L. and Blakemore, K.J. (1990) Chorioangioma: a new inclusion in the prospective and retrospective evaluation of elevated maternal serum alpha-fetoprotein. *Prenat. Diagn.*, **10**, 691–96.

48. Jauniaux, E., Kadri, R., Donner, C. and Rodesch, F. (1992) Not all chorioangiomas are associated with elevated maternal serum alpha-fetoprotein. *Prenat. Diagn.*, **12**, 73–74.

49. Jauniaux, E., Moscoso, G., Vanesse, M. *et al.* (1991) Perfusion fixation for placental morphologic investigation. *Hum. Pathol.*, **22**, 442–49.

50. Burton, G.J., Ingram, S.C. and Palmer, M.E. (1987) The influence of mode of fixation on morphometrical data derived from terminal villi in the human placenta at term: a comparison of immersion and perfusion fixation. *Placenta*, **8**, 37–51.

51. Fouron, J.C., Teyssier, G., Maroto, E. *et al.* (1991) Diastolic circulatory dynamics in the presence of elevated placental resistance and retrograde diastolic flow in the umbilical artery: a Doppler echographic study in lambs. *Am. J. Obstet. Gynecol.*, **164**, 195–203.

52. Thompson, R.S. and Trudinger, B.J. (1990) Doppler waveforms pulsatility index and resistance, pressure and flow in the umbilical placental circulation: an investigation using a mathematical model. *Ultrasound Med. Biol.*, **16**, 449–58.

53. Gilles, W.B., Trudinger, B.J. and Baird, P.J. (1985) Fetal umbilical artery flow velocity waveforms and placental resistance: pathological correlation. *Br. J. Obstet. Gynaecol.*, **92**, 31–38.

54. McCowan, L.M., Mullen, B.M. and Ritchie, K. (1987) Umbilical artery flow velocity waveforms and the placental vascular bed. *Am. J. Obstet. Gynecol.*, **157**, 900–902.

55. Nessmann, C., Huten, Y. and Uzan, M. (1988) Placental correlations of abnormal umbilical Doppler index. *Trophoblast Res.*, **3**, 309–24.

56. Jimenez, E., Vogel, M., Arabin, B. *et al.* (1988) Correlation of ultrasonographic measurements of the utero-placental and fetal blood with the morphological diagnosis of placental function. *Trophoblast Res.*, **3**, 325–34.

57. Jauniaux, E. and Campbell, S. (1990) Fetal growth retardation with abnormal blood flows and placental sonographic lesions. *J. Clin. Ultrasound*, **18**, 210–14.

58. Fok, R.Y., Pavlova, Z., Benirschke, K. *et al.* (1990) The correlation of arterial lesions with umbilical artery Doppler velocimetry in the placentas of small-for-dates pregnancies. *Obstet. Gynecol.*, **75**, 578–83.

59. Acosta-Sison, H. (1958) Diagnosis of hydatidiform mole. *Obstet. Gynecol.*, **12**, 205–208.

60. Alvarez, H. (1965) Diagnosis of hydatidiform mole by transabdominal placental biopsy. *Fetus Newborn*, **95**, 538–41.

61. Alvarez, H. (1968) Phase contrast microscopic observations of the human placenta from six weeks to term. *Am. J. Obstet. Gynecol.*, **32**, 28–39.

62. Brambati, B. (1992) Prenatal diagnosis and invasive techniques in the first trimester of pregnancy, in *The First Twelve Weeks of Gestation: A New Frontier for Investigation and Intervention* (eds E. Barnea, J. Hustin and E. Jauniaux), Springer, Heidelberg, pp. 393–418.

63. Nicolaides, K.H., Rodeck, C.H., Soothill, P.W. *et al.* (1986) Why confine chroionic villus (placental) biopsy to the first trimester? *Lancet*, i, 543–44.

64. Jauniaux, E., Nicolaides, K.H., Campbell, S. and Hustin, J. (1990) Hematoma of the umbilical cord secondary to cordocentesis for intrauterine fetal transfusion. *Prenat. Diagn.*, **10**, 477–78.

65. Jauniaux, E., Donner, C., Simon, P. *et al.* (1989) Pathologic aspects of the umbilical cord after percutaneous umbilical blood sampling. *Obstet. Gynecol.*, **73**, 215–18.

PART FIVE

GENETIC SCREENING AND PRENATAL DIAGNOSIS

Edited by G. Ashmead MD

57 INTRODUCTION TO GENETIC SCREENING AND PRENATAL DIAGNOSES

G.B. Reed

D'où venous-nous? Que sommes-nous? Où allons-nous? (Paul Gaugin) [1]

57.1 Introduction

The morbid anatomy of the human genome is being defined and is presently being mapped. Victor McKusick [2] has described three developmental periods of contemporary medical genetics: (1) chromosomology (1960s); (2) somatic cell genetics (1970s); and (3) molecular genetics (1980s). McKusick posed several questions similar to those posed by Paul Gauguin, asking: 'What is wrong?' (diagnosis), 'What is going to happen?' (prognosis), 'What can be done?' (treatment) and 'Why did it happen?' (prevention, progress).

The present medical genetic armamentarium, as compared with that of 1950, has increased and continues to do so. The concerns, here, are the 'high-risk' fetus and newborn, and particularly those who are at risk genetically or due to an insult *in utero* or a major birth defect. The chapters in this part deal with advances in genetic screening and prenatal diagnosis in the last decade. These advances have provided 'access to the other patient' [3].

However, little progress could or did occur until the late 1960s when Ian Donald's sonographic window opened to scrutiny the gravid uterine environment and its gestational passenger(s) and baggage. In the early 1900s fetal X-rays were performed, but such access was infrequent and limited. Subsequently, biopsy of the placenta, fetoscopy and sampling of the amniotic fluid were occasionally carried out. However, when D.C.A. Bevis (1951) studied fetal hydrops due to rhesus (iso-immunization) disease by amniocentesis, it became feasible to do prenatal diagnoses, surveillance and therapy *in utero*. Since 1980, reproductive and obstetrical genetics have emerged lumbering toward Bethesda, Baltimore, Boston and Elsewhere.

57.1.1 OUTLINE OF PART FIVE

This part concentrates on three main topics: (1) genetic counselling and aftercare; (2) genetic screening and prenatal diagnosis and the procedures and methodologies involved; and (3) some important conditions seen in the perinatal period.

The cellular and molecular conversations which occur between mother and embryo are critical to normal development. [4]

57.1.2 BACKGROUND

Whatever the formulation, the powerful technologies and sciences that make up the new medicine must be given life by a constant flow of memory and meaning. [5]

The origins and beginnings of human life have always been intriguing. The story of the high-risk fetus and newborn involves life, death and diseases during gestation. The present concepts are embroidered into the fabric of human reproductive, cell and developmental biology – that is, human embryology, teratology, obstetrics, perinatology and neonatology.

Since John and William Hunter in the 1780s, and since the late 1800s when scientific works became public knowledge (such as those of R. Koch, L. Pasteur, E. Metchnikoff, P. Ehrlich, G. Mendel, T. Boveri, C. Darwin and S. Freud), and subsequently in the 20th century after major discoveries by A. Garrod, T. H. Morgan, A. Einstein and others became well known, our concepts and views of the universe, earth, psyche and soma, life, death and disease have changed dramatically from those held in the past [6]. Now, 'progress' seems to be incremental, sporadic and cyclical. Often there may be long periods between discovery, appli-

Diseases of the Fetus and Newborn, 2nd edn, Edited by G.B. Reed, A.E. Claireaux and F. Cockburn. Published in 1995 by Chapman & Hall, London. ISBN 0 412 39160 0

cation and practical results. After Louis Pasteur and Robert Koch had defined bacterial diseases, Alexander Fleming helped produce penicillin at a much later date. A similar lag phase may occur for gene therapy. These subtle aspects of history are often imperceptible and it is especially true when one considers preventive medical measures, and specifically human reproductive biology and genetics. One can ask: Who did the first obstetrical screen? Aubinais in 1864 [7]? Who made the first prenatal diagnosis? MacFarland in 1929 [8]?

The concepts of life, disease and wellness have cultural and ideological overtones, and, today, many couples wish to have a perfect baby. In the past, newborn survival was an achievement compared with the present circumstances in the Western World [9].

57.1.3 'GENETIC SCREENING' AND 'DIAGNOSIS'

Screening is an ancient and honorable medical procedure; one still screens urine specimens as Chaucer's Doctor of Physic did when scanning urine flasks. However, uroscopists have been replaced by dipsticks. Soon molecular biologists may be replaced by DNA dipsticks (Tables 57.1 and 57.2).

Screening can be an observational and morphological study as with sonography (Part Four). Videotape records help, in live replay or at later review. To

Table 57.1 Basic elements of genetic counselling

Diagnosis:	ascertainment, confirm results
Risk estimation:	pedigree, pattern
Communication:	time, timing
Back-up to counselling:	availability, education, prevention

Based on patient's or couple's autonomy, rights to information and confidentiality

Source: Ref. 13 and Harper (1983).

Table 57.2 Basic indications for genetic screening and prenatal diagnosis

Maternal:	Age – <20, >35 years
	MSAFP elevated or depressed levels
	exposure – to teratogen or mutagen
	TORCHS, diabetes, epileptic drugs
	consanguinity, life style – drug abuse
	serendipity, paternal age
	past history – personal, familial
	carrier – premarital (couple)
	recurrent abortion, preconceptual 'positive' sonogram

MSAFP = maternal serum α-fetoprotein (based on multiples of the mean) (Chapter 62); TORCHS = toxoplasmosis, other (human immunodeficiency virus, hepatitis B virus), rubella, cytomegalovirus, herpes and syphilis (Chapter 7).

'screen' means to separate an individual from a population. Results of a screen can be positive, negative or 'falsely' positive or negative.

A diagnostic 'test' is a procedure performed with a reagent (probe) in order to identify a specific quality or quantity of a substance or object and its character or function. The diagnostic test may confirm a screening result. Diagnostic test results can be diagnostic or lead to a differential diagnosis. Screening test results always need to be confirmed by a diagnostic or confirmatory 'test', including whatever standards or controls are necessary to verify the 'positive' screen. As an example, a 'positive' urine ferric chloride reaction nowadays requires a more definitive analysis (see discussion on phenylketonuria (PKU) and its variants in Chapter 61).

Genetic screening is performed as a public health measure and for individual well-being. In general, screening should be voluntary, based on informed consent, and the results should be kept confidential.

57.1.4 ADVERSITIES AND ADVANCES

Recent controversies related to *in vitro* fertilization and pre-embryo (preimplantation) diagnoses have been published, as well as reports of pre-embryos being implanted into older women who are over 50 years of age. Similarly the 'rise and fall' of chorionic villus sampling has been alleged to be associated with lesions due to the procedure, i.e. the limb reduction syndromes. Another concern is the laboratory contamination of the polymerase chain reaction procedure by technicians' DNA. It should be emphasized that no procedure is totally foolproof, nor should one offer such procedures or tests as 100% free of complication(s).

Several advances in genetic diagnosis may be anticipated: (1) three-dimensional imaging and Doppler; (2) a 'practical' medical gene map; (3) the beginnings of gene therapy; and (4) specific probes to detect severe monogenic or multifactorial disorders prior to conception.

Sherlock Holmes: 'Never trust to general impressions, my boy, but concentrate yourself on details.' [10]

57.1.5 SIMPLE GOALS

The simple goals are to detect birth defects by genetic screening and prenatal diagnosis, whether anatomical or molecular. The process of detection should be stepwise, precise and linked to the patient (embryo/fetus/infant) or mother's risks. By using deduction, induction and intuition, one may use the four following steps, i.e. choose:

1. appropriate, sensitive and economic screening protocols; informed consent;

2. precise confirmatory tests by indirect or invasive methods; patient's rights to information and education are presumed;

3. appropriate, timely and confidential counselling; peer review and consultations when indicated;

4. options and management based on the mother's or couple's decision(s); aftercare and follow-up sessions.

These steps are inseparably linked to genetic counselling, genetic screening and prenatal diagnostic methods and procedures. Appropriate fetal samples need to be obtained in order to establish a definitive, accurate and timely diagnosis. Consultation prior to special sampling procedures or diagnostic tests is usually necessary.

Perhaps everything terrible is in its deepest being something helpless that wants help from us. [11]

57.2 Comments

57.2.1 REPRODUCTIVE MEDICINE

Ideally, preconceptual or premarital genetic screening and testing of individuals or couples might avoid many birth defects as well as adverse pregnancy outcomes. Avoidance and primary or secondary preventive measures are practices still not fully appreciated or utilized. Community genetic centers may be able to provide more help in this area in the future.

The 'screens', non-invasive or invasive 'procedures' and diagnostic 'tests' described in this part of the book, lead on to Part Six which discusses clinical management. A century from now, the 'new' genetics may be looked upon as passé, as we look upon Chaucer's uroscopist and the impressive genomic maps of 1994 [12] may be crude scientific mandalas in 2094. When genomic maps are refined and markers are available it may be possible to screen, preconceptually or very early during gestation, for many more monogenic disorders and multifactorial conditions than can be detected at present [13–15].

However the real and present concern is based on the notion that one should not allow one's dreams to be turned into nightmares. Professor Emeritus Neil Macintyre, a pioneer in genetic counselling and prenatal diagnosis (Case Western Reserve University Medical School, Anatomy and Cytogenetics, Cleveland, Ohio), gave an annual lecture at our hospital. The talk was given to young men and women during their training in laboratory technology. The lecture began with a story about the hopes and dreams of a young couple and their elation over the impending birth of their first baby. A little later during the talk the newborn baby's photograph was projected; on the screen was the face of a baby with trisomy 13. The happy mood of the audience turned to tears. To resolve the students'

responses took up much of the remaining hour. One moral of this story was and is to remind people to take care and time when doing such laboratory work. These tests are not just routine. The accuracy or inaccuracy of the results can be devastating for both the infant and parents. The long-term sequelae in situations for such couples and their psychic, emotional and reproductive morale can be unpredictable and prolonged (Chapters 59 and 60).

In the context of the following chapters in which genetic screening or prenatal diagnostic tests are described, whether *in vitro*, *in utero* or *in vivo*, it should be emphasized that there are two underlying basic assumptions: 'informed consent' and 'ethical principles and conduct'. Informed consent varies worldwide but honesty, solid data (truth) and the ability to communicate and consult with experts exist. The couple or mother should be informed about the options during gestation. George Annas describes the 'doctrine of informed consent' as 'the recognition that people are not all the same and that physicians must let patients decide about . . . options' [16].

Medical ethics in genetics or 'genethics' vary (for example, Chapters 1, 59 and 60. The issues of confidentiality, autonomy and the social implications that may affect a person's job, insurance and status are being debated. Neil Holtzman stresses that one should 'proceed with caution' [17].

57.2.2 MOLECULES, MAPS AND MEN

The principles of informed consent and ethics can be considered in historical terms. The following ideas are obtained from Isaiah Berlin's writings [18,19]. Any society (in public or in private) must weigh means against ends. There is a universal wish to live in a 'decent society'. In the nineteenth and twentieth centuries, Berlin noted two dominant features. First, science and technology. Second, storms of the intellect. The latter arose from the human mind, for example Tolstoy, Hegel, Hitler, Marx, Lenin. Many of these storms continue, such as racism, bigotry, nationalism. The human fabric is dyed, and color is a well-known characteristic of ethnicity, family, culture and secular trends. The human fabric is made of molecules and is being mapped sequence by sequence. Patterns in the fabric may be helpful, but it is clear the path from genotype (G) to phenotype (P) is variable and the genotype and phenotype can be heterogeneous. Thus, for the near future, clinical studies will continue to be necessary, in spite of the ability to discover 'new genes'. Table 57.3 indicates some of the factors which are involved in early human life and development. The denominators of the G to P path are shown. One may conclude that individuals' genetic essence and expression are complex. The gene sits in a cell but it does not do so in isolation.

Table 57.3   Links in early human life

♂, ♀	G→ → →P	♂, ♀
Gamete	Time →	Fetus
Zygote	Environment, development	Newborn
Embryo	Maternal–placental–fetal unit	Child

57.2.3 HEDGEHOGS AND FOXES

When the hedgehogs and foxes and lumpers and splitters join forces to advance medicine, then there may be progress [20].

> The fox knows many things, but the hedgehog knows one big thing. [19,21]

In our time Isaiah Berlin [19] has discussed these two human proclivities or 'mind sets' and the two great historical forces (science and technology and 'isms'). Berlin concluded that all 'great goods' may not be compatible between various cultures during recorded history (*circa* 10 000 years).

Berlin [19] wrote: choices and action are reality. 'We cannot legislate for the unknown consequences of consequences of consequences' (p. 14). Ethical and legal discussions sometimes end in trivial results. 'In short . . . one cannot have everything . . .' Or know and be able to do everything. 'Priorities, never final or absolute must be established' (p. 17). With economic constraints and equity. 'The first public obligation is to avoid extremes of suffering' (p. 17). Both mental and physical. 'The best that can be done . . . is to maintain a precarious equilibrium . . . that is the first requirement for a decent society . . .' (p. 18) and a society which is open and stable. 'To force people into the neat uniforms demanded by dogmatically believed-in schemes is almost always the road to inhumanity' (p. 18). The reader should refer to Daniel Kevles on eugenics [2] and one may also wish to consider C.P. Snow's *The Two Cultures and the Scientific Revolution* (1959).

'Hedgehogs' are names for drosophila genes, which are also found in chicks, zebra fish and mice. There are families of hedgehog genes. One recently described [15] is a 'sonic' hedgehog ('sonic' taken from a video game). These terms are colorful, but at times acronyms and alpha–beta soup become hard to understand.

57.3 Summary

This introduction has focused on the reproductive and societal implications associated with genetic screening and prenatal diagnosis. These issues will affect medical practice. Common sense includes the recognition that advice can be easily given and may be complied with, but ultimately the choices and burdens rest with the mother or parents. Rights, obligations, needs and responsibilities should be balanced. Society should provide decent support.

Charles Dickens spoke at a dinner in support of the Hospital for Sick Children at Great Ormond Street in London in 1858. His words still carry a message over a

Table 57.4   Genetic screening and prenatal diagnosis

Diseases, disorders types of conditions	*Optimal technology, samples, conditions and timing*
Mendelian inheritance (AR, AD, XL)	Non-invasive, economical
Predisposition (susceptible, vulnerable)	Risks, accuracy, alternatives
Carrier (mosaic, chimera, other)	Verification, repeat sample
Presymptomatic	Heterogeneity, variants
Late onset	Meiotic, interphase samples
	Molecular and biochemical methods: probes, PCR RFLP, Southern blots
Non-traditional inheritance	*In vitro* – cell cultures
Mitochondrial (maternal)	Probes, kits, libraries
Uniparental disomy	Predictability, statistics
Trinucleotide repeats	Archival material: databases, computer databases,
Unaffected parent (germinal mosaicism)	Reference laboratories and consultations – clinical or
Imprinting (developmental)	laboratory
Somatic cell mutation	
Retrotransposition (RNA, hemophilia A)	
Cis and *trans* mechanisms	
Nuclear and mitochondrial DNA	

Cis (acting locus) = A genetic region affecting genes on same DNA molecule (same chromosome) serve as attachment sites for DNA binding proteins (e.g. enhancers, operators and promoters); *trans* (acting locus) = a genetic element, encodes diffusible product(s) affecting other genes, can be on a different DNA molecule (different chromosome) to those genes controlled (e.g. regulator gene); PCR = polymerase chain reaction; RFLP = restriction fragment length polymorphism; DNA, RNA = nucleotides.
See also Chapters 61, 74, 75 and 76.
Source: Kazazian (1994).

century later. Today, knowledge and technology may have outstripped custom, but as Charles Dickens said 'his dumb speech to me . . . Why, in the name of a gracious God, such things should be?' [23] We are now 'seeing with sound' the dream child: 'dumb but visible, perfectly formed or misshapen, in natural sleep or already addicted'. Today, medicine is being heavily influenced by technology, corporate interests and molecular biology. There is no doubt that the pioneers of antenatal medicine would welcome our current abundances and opportunities. However the real concern is not to allow our dreams to be turned into nightmares. The chapters which follow are written by optimists; their contributions have been produced to help the reader.

The current 'working model' of clinical genetics is a 'team approach'. A similar concept is used in management (Part Six). The genetic team consists of a medical geneticist, nurse, genetic counsellor and various medical specialists, who may include psychologists and social workers. As individuals with inheritable disorders are evaluated, tested, etc., ethical dilemmas are resolved and informed consent obtained.

With medical knowledge increasing, access to the unborn expanding and the ability to intervene *in utero*, there are still unknown frontiers to be solved and mapped. Although the scope of medical genetics continues to grow (Table 57.4), in each patient's 'case' the physician, team and field of genetics should 'proceed with caution'.

References

1. Coles, R. (1990) *The Spiritual Life of Children*, Houghton Mifflin, NY, p. 37.
2. McKusick, V. (1993) Medical genetics: a 40-year perspective. *JAMA*, 270, 2351–56.
3. Daffos, F. (1989) Access to the other patient. *Semin. Perinatol.*, 13, 252–59.
4. Johnson, M. (1977) Development in mammals. *Dev. Mamm.* 1, 1.
5. Jonsen, A. (1990) *The New Medicine and the Old Ethos*. Harvard University Press, Cambridge, MA, p. 158.
6. Tauber, A. (1994) Darwinian aftershocks: repercussions in late twentieth century medicine. *J. R. Soc. Med.*, 87, 27–31.
7. Bradley, R. *et al.* (1989) cited in *Diseases of the Fetus and Newborn*, 1st edn (eds G. Reed, A. Claireaux and A. Bain), Chapman & Hall, London, p. 661.
8. Weaver, D. (1989) *Catalog of Prenatally Diagnosed Conditions*, 1st edn, Johns Hopkins University Press, Baltimore, p. XIII.
9. Wertz, R. and Wertz, D. (1989) *Lying-In*, Yale University Press, New Haven, CT.
10. Conan Doyle, A. (1930, (1901–4)) Case of identity, in *Illustrated Sherlock Holmes* (Strand Magazine), Avenel Books, NY, p. 37.
11. Rilke, R.M. (1956) *Letters to a Young Poet* (translated by M. Norton), W. Norton, NY, p. 69.
12. Elmer-Dewitt, P. (1994) The genetic revolution. *Time*, 143, 46–53.
13. Modell, B. and Modell, R. (1992) *Towards a Healthy Baby*. Oxford University Press, Oxford.
14. Redline, R., Neish, A., Holmes, L. and Collins, T. (1992) Homeobox genes and congenital malformations, *Lab. Invest.*, 66, 659–70.
15. Echelard, Y., Epstein, D., and St-Jacques, B. *et al.* (1993) Sonic Hedgehog mediates the polarizing activity of the ZPA. *Cell*, 75, 1417–30.
16. Annas, G. (1994) Informed consent, cancer, and the truth in prognosis. *N. Engl. J. Med.*, 330, 223–25.
17. Holtzman, N. (1989) *Proceed with Caution: Predicting Genetic Risks in the Recombinant DNA Era*. Johns Hopkins University Press, Baltimore, MD.
18. Berlin, I. (1993) *The Hedgehog and the Fox. An Essay on Tolstoy's View of History*, I. Dee, Chicago, pp. 3–4.
19. Berlin, I. (1991) *The Crooked Timber of Humanity*, A. Knopf., NY, pp. 1–19.
20. McKusick, V. (1969) On lumpers and splitters, or the nosology of genetic disease. *Perspect. Biol. Med.*, 12, 298–312.
21. Archilochus, in *Encylopaedia Britannica*, 15th edn, 1980, vol. 1, University of Chicago Press, Chicago, p. 489.
22. Kevles, D. (1985) *In the Name of Eugenics*, A. Knopf., NY.
23. Johnson, E. (1952) *Charles Dickens*, vol. 2, Simon & Schuster, NY, pp. 912–13.

Further reading

Wald, N. (1990) The meaning of 'screening' (letter). *Lancet*, 336, 1587.
Harper, P. (1983) Genetic counselling and prenatal diagnosis. *Br. Med. Bull.*, 39, 302–309.
Kazazian, H. (1994) Human gene mutation (book review). *Science*, 263, 255–56.
McGinnis, W. and Kuziova, M. (1994) The molecular architects of body design, *Sci. Am.*, 270, 58–66.
Wulfsberg, E., Hoffman, D. and Cohen, M. (1994) Alpha 1 antitrypsin deficiency – impact of genetic discovery on medicine and society, *JAMA*, 271, 217–22.
Brock, D. (1993) *Molecular Genetics for the Clinician*, Cambridge University Press, Cambridge.
Brock, D., Rodeck, C. and Ferguson-Smith, M. (eds) (1992) *Prenatal Diagnosis and Screening*, Churchill Livingstone, Edinburgh.
Jonsen, A., Siegler, M. and Winslade, W. (1992) *Clinical Ethics*, 3rd edn, McGraw, NY.
Institute of Medicine (1993) *Assessing Genetic Risks*, National Academic Press, Washington, DC.
Nuffield Foundation (1993) *Genetic Screening, Ethical Issues*, Council on Bioethics, London.
King, R. and Stansfield, W. (1990) *A Dictionary of Genetics*, 4th edn, Oxford University Press, Oxford.
Anonymous (1994) Less equal than other (editorial). *Lancet*, 343, 805–806.
Khaur K-T. (1994) Genetics and environment: Geoffrey Rose revisited. *Lancet*, 343, 838–39.

58 A BIOGRAPHICAL SKETCH OF ROBERT GUTHRIE

J.H. Koch

Robert Guthrie is best known in the field of biochemistry for his development of the newborn screening test for phenylketonuria (bacterial inhibition assay) [1]. Anyone who knows Bob Guthrie, however, knows this is only one of his prodigious accomplishments. Bob has been called 'an evangelist for the prevention of mental retardation', a most fitting title. Eventually he and his laboratory personnel developed tests for more than 30 different treatable conditions that cause mental handicap or death, all of which could be done on the single newborn blood specimen collected for phenylketonuria screening. Bob attributes his interest in preventing mental handicap to the fact that Johnnie, one of his six children, is mentally handicapped. Although the cause of Johnnie's disability has never been diagnosed, Bob has not let this deter him from doing everything in his power to prevent mental handicap in others.

Bob Guthrie (Figure 58.1) was born in 1916 in Marionville, Missouri, a small town in the Ozark mountains, the younger son of Reginald and Ina Ledbetter Guthrie. His father traveled throughout Minnesota and Wisconsin wholesaling White sewing machines to furniture stores. Bob, as everyone has always called him, grew up and attended school in Minneapolis where the family moved when he was six years old. He recalls accompanying his father on one or two of his sales trips during the summer and perhaps that is where he learned the art of selling, a talent he later used tirelessly in his never-ending campaign to prevent mental handicap.

In school, Bob did not distinguish himself academically, but had an active social life. It was not until he had graduated from high school that he realized the value of a higher education. He worked his way through college, for although his father was a successful salesman, these were depression years and his family was not wealthy. At one point, he decided to become a chemical engineer and he sported a sweat shirt and leather jacket and carried a slide rule, as all engineers

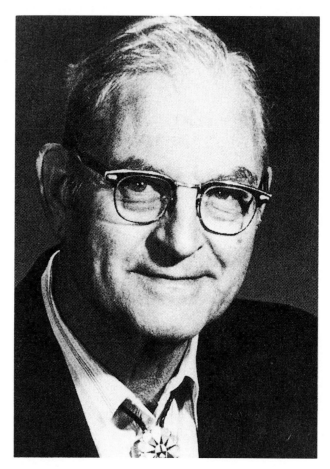

Figure 58.1 Robert Guthrie.

did. Finally, because of a challenge from a girl friend, he applied to medical school and, to his surprise, was accepted. He never gave up his ambition of getting a PhD, however, and he completed the courses for a degree in bacteriology and took his oral exams while he was in medical school. By 1946, he had earned an MD and a PhD degree from the University of Minnesota.

Bob began his professional career doing cancer research at the Sloan Kettering Institute in New York,

Diseases of the Fetus and Newborn, 2nd edn, Edited by G.B. Reed, A.E. Claireaux and F. Cockburn. Published in 1995 by Chapman & Hall, London. ISBN 0 412 39160 0

but after the birth of Johnnie he became increasingly interested in preventing mental handicap. He has waged a battle from Kuwait to California against lead poisoning. For years, he sported a lapel button, 'Get the Lead Out', long before the general public or even the medical community became concerned about lead exposure. Bob was instrumental in starting a newborn screening program in New Zealand and the Pacific Islands in 1969, traveling to many remote areas to spread his gospel. He was willing to talk with three people or twelve or several hundred, whoever he could mesmerize by his spellbinding zeal. He has been active in numerous organizations, such as the International League of Societies for the Mentally Handicapped, where for a number of years he served as chairman of the Prevention Committee, traveling the world over, often to developing countries.

Bob's concern and enthusiasm has also included local issues, such as the passage of school bonds when additional classrooms were needed in his community, serving on committees in the Association for Mentally Retarded Citizens, developing a National Science Foundation summer program for high-achieving high school students and visiting the local elementary school with microscopes to talk about what it is like to be a scientist. He has worked to combat racism and pro-

mote integration. He has campaigned to end nuclear testing. Bob has done all this, and much more.

Bob Guthrie, the son of a traveling salesman, who is himself something of a traveling salesman at heart, is well deserving of the honors he has received. Among many others, he has twice been nominated for a Nobel peace prize. But the award of which he is most proud is the bronze plaque permanently installed at the Mill Middle School in Williamsville, New York. It says, 'This school is dedicated to Robert Guthrie whose high expectations and constant endeavor to attain excellence in education provided an unyielding challenge for its accomplishment in the Williamsville school district.'

Bob Guthrie's dedication and enthusiasm have inspired many others to become involved. Probably no one will ever know how many changes have been made, how many lives have been influenced and how many children are well and healthy instead of mentally handicapped because of Bob Guthrie. He has accomplished much [2].

References

1. Guthrie, R. (1961) Blood screening for phenylketonuria. *JAMA*, 178, 863.
2. Guthrie, R. (1992) The origin of newborn screening. *Screening*, 1, 5–15.

Photograph courtesy Harvey Levy.

59 GENETIC COUNSELING

K.L. Garver

59.1 Introduction

The role of genetics in providing care to our patients increases on a daily basis. During the past 40 years there has been an explosion of new knowledge in human genetics which has been applied in various ways [1–3]. In the 1950s, population and quantitative genetics primarily involved public health physicians. After Tjio and Levan's publication in 1956 [4], there was much new information delineated concerning the etiology of birth defects and mental retardation by the advances in cytogenetics. In the 1970s, cytogenetics became more and more sophisticated because of the introduction of banding techniques. Somatic cell and biochemical genetics were also developed at this time. In the 1990s and continuing into the 21st century, we shall see the greatest breakthrough of all, namely the utilization of molecular genetic techniques to aid in diagnosing and treating our patients [3].

Although the science of medical genetics is new, the art of genetic counseling is ancient. Genetic diseases such as congenital adrenal hyperplasia have been described in the Bible [5]. A very precise description of an X-linked disease, namely hemophilia, was described in the Talmud [6]. Jewish rabbis, more than 1000 years ago, described a situation in which a woman had her first child circumcised and he died (as a result of bleeding from the operation) and a second son also died (similarly); she must not circumcise her third child. Although nothing was known at that time about the science of hemophilia, it is still the same advice we give women in this situation today.

One of our newer techniques, which is described in many chapters in this book, is prenatal diagnosis. However, the first written account of prenatal diagnosis was given over 3500 years ago by the Egyptians in the ancient Berol papyrus [7]. This was a technique for diagnosing the sex of the fetus when the mother was 8–10 weeks pregnant, and required a bag of wheat and a bag of barley. Each day several drops of urine from the woman were placed in each bag. If the wheat sprouted first, it indicated a boy; if the barley sprouted first, it indicated a girl. In 1933 an American obstetrician repeated this test in a controlled manner, and found it to be 80% predictive [7].

59.2 Definition

Genetic counseling is now an important part of medical care. It involves an accurate diagnosis, delineation of risk for genetic disease, and, very importantly, the chance of not developing a particular genetic disease. If a patient is identified as being at an increased risk for a genetic disease, counseling entails advice to the patient, particularly from the standpoint of removing environmental factors that might increase the patient's risk. Also, with the availability of more knowledge in molecular genetics in the future, it will be possible to supply missing enzymes, other proteins and to transplant genes to successfully treat or cure serious genetic diseases. If an infant, child or adult does have a genetic disease, the obstetrician should identify community and professional resources, such as early stimulation programs, parent-to-parent groups, specialized educational facilities, rehabilitation facilities and newer technologies, that might enable the patient to lead a more normal life.

The Committee on Genetic Counseling of the American Society of Human Genetics has defined genetic counseling as follows [8].

> Genetic counseling is a communication process which deals with the human problems associated with the occurrence, or the risk of occurrence, of a genetic disorder in a family. This process involves an attempt by one or more appropriately trained persons to help the individual or family to (1) comprehend the medical facts, including the diagnosis, probable course of the disorder, and the available management; (2) appreciate the way heredity contributes to the disorder, and the risk of recurrence in specified relatives; (3) understand the alternatives for dealing with the risk of recurrence; (4) choose the course of action which seems to them appropriate in view of their risk,

Diseases of the Fetus and Newborn, 2nd edn, Edited by G.B. Reed, A.E. Claireaux and F. Cockburn. Published in 1995 by Chapman & Hall, London. ISBN 0 412 39160 0

their family goals, and their ethical and religious standards, and to act in accordance with that decision; and (5) make the best possible adjustment to the disorder in an affected family member and/or to the risk of recurrence of that disorder.

59.3 Who should counsel?

All physicians, particularly and including primary care physicians such as obstetricians, pediatricians, internists and family practitioners, should take an active role in providing genetic counseling for their patients [9–12]. Other health professionals such as genetic counselors, nurses, social workers and medical educators should also take an active role. The level of counseling depends on the individual's knowledge of and interest in human genetics. With the daily increase in knowledge of human genetics, particularly in molecular genetics, it is not possible for those trained in medical genetics (i.e. clinical geneticists, medical geneticists or genetic counselors) to identify and counsel all those in need of information. Therefore, the primary care physician must identify and recognize patients requiring further genetic evaluation. Hopefully, more physicians will take the responsibility of counseling the patient themselves. In lieu of this, the physician should be able to seek help from MD, PhD or MS genetic professionals.

One of the problems with current medical care is its fragmentation into various subspecialities, so that sometimes the patient receives opinions from many health professionals, with no one seemingly in charge. In the case of reproductive genetics, it is important that the obstetrician act as the coordinator and dispenser of genetic information. In difficult situations the obstetrician can have the patient seen by a clinical geneticist or a genetic counselor for a consultation, but the continued care of the patient should return to the obstetrician. In order to make this work, the obstetrician has to have an interest in and knowledge of medical genetics. The most important factors in giving adequate genetic counseling are an accurate and specific diagnosis. Two of our most important tools are a complete medical, obstetric and family history, plus a thorough physical examination. This still is and must be the responsibility of the obstetrician [10,11].

59.4 Directive or non-directive counseling?

In reproductive genetics the concern is for three individuals, namely the mother, father and fetus. It is important when counseling, if at all possible, to have both parents present. Even in a situation where there is not an increased risk of a birth defect or genetic disease to the fetus, it is an anxious and psychologically traumatic time for the parents. They are concerned about the outcome of the initial history and physical and, particularly if testing is involved, the outcome of the tests and what this will mean for the third person, namely the fetus.

In non-directive counseling, the consultands are instructed in all aspects of the particular genetic situation, whether it be advanced maternal or paternal age, a previously affected child, history of genetic disease in the family, or an environmental influence on the pregnancy. The consultands are then given the risk of having an affected child, the chance of having a normal child, then an ensuing discussion of all possible prenatal testing to make their risk more definitive. When all reproductive options are discussed with the patients, it should be clearly indicated that the choice is theirs because many of these decisions require moral and ethical values that are different with each patient. The counselor assists in making a decision; however, the final decision must be that of the consultand [11–17].

Each of our patients has a different moral, ethical and ethnic background, as does each obstetrician. Each patient has a different need to have his or her own children, and it requires a strong commitment to care for a child with a birth defect. Counselors should not interject their own biases into the decision making of their patients. Genetic information given to patients is only part of the information they need for decision making. In many cases the decision is a very difficult one, and the consultands should be given time to talk privately with each other and, in many cases, to seek outside help. This may involve speaking to respected family members, friends, clergy, or possibly obtaining another medical opinion.

With directive counseling the obstetrician takes a more assertive attitude and indicates to the patient that she should or should not have additional children, should have an amniocentesis, or should or should not have an abortion. In other aspects of medicine, physicians have been trained to take an authoritarian approach, when, for example, recommending an antibiotic, surgery, or even in some situations invasive testing. However, because of the moral and ethical implications, reproductive genetic counseling is entirely different; the counselor must act as a conduit of information and support and let the patients make their own decisions.

59.5 Prospective and retrospective counseling

Another way of categorizing genetic counseling is by it being either prospective or retrospective. Prospective genetic counseling is anticipatory in that an individual or a couple are identified as being at an increased risk for developing a genetic disease or birth defect, or of having a child with a similar problem before its occurrence in the couple being counseled. Examples of prospective genetic counseling would be of a couple where either the father or mother is older, or where one of the couple is at risk for having a particular disease that is more prevalent in their ethnic or racial group (e.g. Caucasians, cystic fibrosis; blacks, sickle-cell disease; Ashkenazim, Tay–Sachs disease; Mediterraneans, β-thalassemia; Orientals, α-thalassemia).

Other examples of prospective genetic counseling would include: a woman who is planning a pregnancy and is taking a medication which is potentially teratogenic; a woman who has successfully treated phenylketonuria and has reverted to a normal diet so that she has high blood phenylalanine levels; a woman who has insulin-dependent diabetes mellitus; or a woman who has no history of rubella and has a non-immune rubella titer.

Retrospective counseling is given after an individual develops a genetic disease or a couple has a child with a particular birth defect or genetic disease. Until recently, most obstetrical genetic counseling was retrospective. At present, more at-risk situations can be identified before conception, and the individual or couple can be given prospective counseling.

Genetic counseling can be given at many different times and situations. An excellent time to do prospective counseling is during the premarital examination. A few questions can delineate whether an individual is at an increased risk because of age, medication, ethnic group or family history. Experience in taking a history can enable the family physician or obstetrician to do this, and eliminate some of these major groups as causes of concern. Every physician should have a series of five or six genetically oriented questions that can also be included in routine office visits, annual physical examinations, or when a couple comes in for contraceptive advice. Unfortunately, much counseling is still done in a retrospective manner. Either a child is born with a birth defect or an individual develops a genetic disease before it is realized that they have been at an increased risk.

A very difficult time to give genetic counseling is immediately after the birth of a child with birth defects. When parents are seen at this time it is important to understand that they are going through a period described by psychiatrists as the 'mourning process.' The first goal of the obstetrician should be to help the couple through this very trying emotional period. Parents may react with anger, guilt, depression or denial, and in some instances with rejection of the baby. If parents ask about the genetic cause and risk of recurrence during the postpartum period answers should be given, but a follow-up appointment should be made for 4–6 weeks thereafter. At this time most

parents have, to some extent, dealt with their emotional problems and are then ready to ask the questions: 'Why did this occur? What chance of recurrence is there for us and what chance do our normal children and other collateral relatives have of having a similarly affected child?'

59.6 Reproductive options

It is important that the obstetrician gives a thorough explanation of reproductive options that are available to an at-risk couple. Each couple will react differently to the risk that they are given. One couple, considered by the obstetrician to be in a high-risk category, may interpret their risk as low. Conversely, a couple in a low-risk category may consider this risk to be extremely high. Therefore, all reproductive options should be discussed with a couple without the obstetrician indicating personal bias [11].

The obstetrician should also be non-directive and impartial to the couple and their decision should not be made solely on the basis of the genetic information but should also depend on their moral and ethical beliefs. There are many reproductive options available to at-risk couples, however not all may be acceptable because of the couple's needs. It is necessary for the obstetrician to support the couple in the decision they make. The following reproductive options should be discussed.

59.6.1 NO CHANGE IN REPRODUCTIVE PATTERNS

After the obstetrician has discussed the genetic information, implications of the disease and a review of all options, the couple may decide to make no modifications in their future reproductive plans. This is seen more commonly in couples with a low risk of recurrence, particularly if the burden of the disease is low. Occasionally, even a couple with a high risk of recurrence and a high burden of the disease will make no change in their reproductive plans because of their moral or ethical beliefs.

59.6.2 CONTRACEPTION

After the birth of a child with a birth defect, physicians, other health care workers and well-intentioned friends may advise a couple to have another baby as soon as possible to replace the child with the birth defect with another child. In most instances, this advice is unsound because the couple needs to adjust to the child with the birth defect or to the death of their affected child. The obstetrician should counsel the patient accordingly.

59.6.3 STERILIZATION

The birth of a child with a birth defect is devastating to most couples. Occasionally, their first reaction is to request sterilization because they do not want any other children. This is particularly true if the birth defect is a heavy burden; that is, the defect is severe and the child may live for a long time.

The decision to be sterilized should be discussed thoroughly with the couple. If the child dies, this couple may decide to have other children, or, as sometimes happens, the couple may divorce and wish to start a family with another spouse. Since sterilization is not readily reversible, the couple may not be able to have further children. Sterilization should be postponed until all options are considered. The decision for sterilization should be mutual between the couple.

59.6.4 ADOPTION

Adoption is an acceptable and fulfilling way of having a family; however, there are associated problems. The greatest problem is that there are few babies available for adoption. Even though a couple have a high genetic risk, they usually have trouble obtaining a baby through an adoption agency. Occasionally a couple can obtain a baby through an obstetrician or family practitioner. If adoption proceedings are started early in pregnancy the natural mother can be prepared psychologically, by appropriate counseling, to relinquish her baby. A lawyer knowledgeable in the adoption laws of a particular locality should discuss all the legal details with the natural mother. In the ideal situation, the adoption is arranged before the baby is born. If the baby is normal, the adoption can then be completed shortly after birth [18–20].

59.6.5 ARTIFICIAL INSEMINATION

Couples can increase their chances of having a normal child through donor insemination. This is suitable when a father or one of his parents is affected with an autosomal dominant condition, or when the father is the carrier of a balanced translocation or another balanced chromosomal rearrangement. By selecting a suitable donor, the risk of transmitting the disease is eliminated. It is important to completely evaluate any donor for artificial insemination. An adequate family and medical history, along with a thorough physical examination, is imperative. If the donor is of a particular ethnic or racial group, that is Ashkenazim (Tay–Sachs disease), blacks (sickle-cell anemia), Mediterraneans (β-thalassemia), Caucasians (cystic fibrosis) or Orientals (α-thalassemia), appropriate heterozygote testing could be performed.

59.6.6 IN VITRO FERTILIZATION

In vitro fertilization, although still expensive, is now available in most major cities. Depending upon the situation in the particular couple, the mother's egg and the donor sperm, donor egg and father's sperm, or, in some situations, a donor egg and donor sperm, may be used.

59.6.7 PRENATAL DIAGNOSIS

During the past 25 years prenatal diagnosis has grown from a technique that required 30 ml of amniotic fluid to diagnose a chromosomal condition using an unbanded chromosome technique, to one that can diagnose a specific metabolic disease by obtaining only one cell from a preimplantation embryo. This has been associated with tremendous advances in the techniques of cell culture, cytogenetics, molecular genetics and more sophisticated sonar and echocardiography. Preimplantation diagnosis is now available at a few centers and will probably expand its role. All of these techniques are discussed in more detail in other chapters in this book [21–29].

59.7 Ethics and eugenics

It is sometimes difficult to reflect objectively concerning our current actions and practices; particularly, how new advances in science and technology and their applications to genetic counseling and clinical care in medical genetics can possibly be deleterious to our patients [30–38]. In the past, however, rather innocuous medical practices or public policies have been distorted to be applied as negative eugenics, aggravating the rights and privacy of millions of individuals. Examples are the distortion of the German Racial Hygiene program of the late 1800s, the Johnson Restriction Immigration Act of 1924, and the Involuntary Sterilization Laws in the USA. It is painful to realize that some of our accepted practices today (for example, prenatal diagnosis and maternal serum α-fetoprotein/β-chorionic gonadotropin screening) can be considered as negative eugenics [30,39,40]. When these technologies were introduced into medical practice, it was on the basis of patient/physician relationships. Now it is being suggested that changes in public policy be made so that the individual patients can lose, in many instances, their right to make a decision. This may not be their choice but will be dictated by the subtle influences of economic pressures and the increasing reliance of utilitarian cost-effective criteria for making genetic decisions.

A disturbing development has been suggestions for the financial audit of genetic services. Everyone would agree that services provided for our patients' health, whether through a University or private practitioner, should have some means of audit for quality, correct information and effectiveness. Traditionally, the goal was to have the patients understand the genetic disease, and their risk of having an affected child – or their chance of having a normal child. Now it has been suggested in Great Britain that for a genetic clinic to continue to be funded it should show that the birth prevalence of a particular disease or malformation is declining, and that the termination of pregnancies because of a particular disease is increasing in the population [41]. In other words, the notion has now shifted to a cost-effective or utilitarian method regarding genetic counseling. This cost-effective attitude of genetic counseling is against the present purpose of most clinics in the USA, namely that the patient be informed and educated and then make a decision based on his or her needs and ethical background, not because of economic measures. Utilitarian reasoning was the basis of the Nazi eugenic policies [42–50].

Genetic technology will increase in scope and effectiveness with each subsequent year. It is important that obstetricians realize the necessity of protecting their patients' rights to make decisions, and of protecting the confidentiality of their genetic records in the work place, in relation to third-party carriers, the government and other individuals. A recent review article reported 41 incidents of possible discrimination because of a genetic predisposition, not because of a genetic disease [38]. Human life must be protected, and those with birth defects and genetic disease can be protected by providing support with care and educational opportunities. A monumental step in this direction was the signing into law by President Bush on 26 July 1990 of the Americans with Disabilities Act. This new law will help an estimated 43 million Americans with disabilities, and has the force of a national law.

The years ahead will be exciting and challenging for all health care professionals. As new technologies are developed, they will produce many benefits, including more information about the so-called complex diseases such as insulin-dependent diabetes mellitus, arteriosclerosis, hypertension and many of the psychiatric illnesses. Hopefully, with each passing year, new genetic information can be used in a way familiar to all physicians, namely to ease suffering and prevent and cure disease in our patients. Information from these new technologies should never be used to discriminate genetically against any individual, ethnic group or race.

References

1. Garver, K.L. and LeChien, K.A. (1992) End of an era (editorial). *Am. J. Hum. Genet.*, **51**, 209–10.
2. Garver, K.L. and LeChien, K.A. (1992) Geneticists' responsibility to other health care professionals and the lay public. *Am. J. Hum. Genet.*, **52**, 922–23.
3. McKusick, V.A. (1992) Presidential address, Eighth International Congress of Human Genetics: The last 35 years, the present, and the future. *Am. J. Hum. Genet.* **50**, 663–70.
4. Tjio, J.H. and Levan, A. (1956) The chromosome number in man. *Hereditas*, **42**, 1–6.
5. Greenblat, R.B. (1963) *Search the Scriptures: A Physician Examines Medicine in the Bible*, Lippincott, Philadelphia.
6. Rosner, F. (1969) Hemophilia in the Talmud and Rabbinic writings. *Ann. Intern. Med.*, **70**, 833–38.
7. Cederquist, L. (1970) Antenatal sex determination – a historical view. *Clin. Obstet. Gynecol.*, **13**, 159–177.
8. Ad Hoc Committee on Genetic Counseling (1975) Genetic counseling. *Am. J. Hum. Genet.* **27**, 240.
9. Garver, K.L. (1977) Genetic counseling in the delivery of health care. *Pa. Med.*, **80**, 40–43.
10. Garver, K.L. (1979) Genetic counseling in primary obstetric care. *Obstet. Gynecol. Ann.*, **8**, 87–121.
11. Garver, K.L. and Marchese, S.G. (1986) *Genetic Counseling for Clinicians*, Year Book Medical, Chicago.
12. Clarke, A. (1991) Is non-directive genetic counseling possible? *Lancet*, **338**, 998–1001.
13. Super, M. (1991) Non-directive genetic counseling (letter). *Lancet*, **338**, 1266.
14. Pembrey, M. (1991) Non-directive genetic counseling (letters). *Lancet* **338**, 1266–67.
15. Morrison, P.J. and Nevin, N.C. (1991) Non-directive genetic counseling (letters). *Lancet*, **338**, 1267.
16. Harris, R. and Hopkins, A. (1991) Non-directive genetic counselling (letters). *Lancet*, **338**, 1267–68.
17. Simms, M. (1991) Non-directive genetic counseling (letter). *Lancet*, **338**, 1268.
18. Morris, M., Harper, P.S. and Tyler, A. (1988) Adoption and genetic prediction for Huntington's disease. *Lancet*, **ii**, 1069–70.
19. Omenn, G.S., Hall, J.G. and Kansen, K.D. (1980) Genetic counseling for adoptees at risk for specific inherited disorders. *Am. J. Med. Genet.*, **5**, 157–64.
20. Plomin, R. and DeFries, J.C. (1983) The Colorado adoption project. *Child Dev.*, **54**, 276–89.
21. Frets, P.G. and Niermeijer, M.F. (1990) Reproductive planning after genetic counselling: a perspective from the last decade. *Clin. Genet.*, **38**, 295–306.
22. Goldberg, J.D. (1990) Basic principles of recombinant DNA use for prenatal diagnosis. *Semin. Perinatol.*, **14**, 439–45.
23. Seashore, M.R. (1990) Prenatal diagnosis of hematologic disorders. *Semin. Perinatol.*, **14**, 343–45.
24. Lubin, M.B., Lin, H.J., Vadheim, C.M. and Rotter, J.I. (1990) Genetic counseling of common diseases of adulthood. Implications for prenatal counseling and diagnosis. *Clin. Perinatol.*, **17**, 889–910.
25. Iafolla, A.K. and McConkie-Rosel, A. (1990) Prenatal diagnosis of metabolic disease. *Clin. Perinatol.*, **17**, 761–77.
26. Bieber F.R. and Hoffman, E.P. (1990) Duchenne and Becker muscular dystrophies: genetics, prenatal diagnosis, and future prospects. *Clin. Perinatol.*, **17**, 845–65.
27. Christian, C.L. (1990) Prenatal diagnosis of cystic fibrosis. *Clin. Perinatol.*, **17**, 779–91.
28. Simpson, J.L. (1992) Preimplantation genetics and recovery of fetal cells from maternal blood. *Curr. Opin. Obstet. Gynecol.*, **4**, 295–301.
29. Verlinsky, Y., Rechitsky, S., Evsikov, S. *et al.* (1992) Preconception and preimplantation diagnosis for cystic fibrosis. *Prenat. Diagn.*, **12**, 103–10.
30. Garver, K.L. and Garver, B. (1991) Eugenics: past, present, and the future. *Am. J. Hum. Genet.*, **49**, 1109–18.
31. Murray, T.H. (1991) Ethical issues in human genome research. *FASEB J.*, **5**, 55–60.
32. Wilford, B.S. and Frost, N. (1990) The cystic fibrosis gene: medical and social implications for heterozygote detection. *JAMA*, **263**, 2777–83.
33. Juengst, E.T. (1991) The human genome project and bioethics. *Kennedy Inst. Ethics J.*, **13**, 71–74.
34. Gostin, L. (1991) Genetic discrimination: the use of genetically based diagnostic and prognostic tests by employers and insurers. *Am. J. Law Med.*, **17**, 109–44.
35. Holtzman, N.A. and Rothstein, M.A. (1992) Eugenics and genetic discrimination (invited editorial). *Am. J. Hum. Genet.*, **50**, 457–59.
36. Harper, P.S. (1992) Huntington disease and the abuse of genetics. *Am. J. Hum. Genet.*, **50**, 460–64.
37. Natowicz, M.R., Alper, J.K. and Alper, J.S. (1992) Genetic discrimination and the law. *Am. J. Hum. Genet.*, **50**, 465–75.
38. Billings, P.R., Kohn, M.A., de Cuevas, M. *et al.* (1992) Discrimination as a consequence of genetic testing. *Am. J. Hum. Genet.*, **50**, 476–82.
39. Garver, K.L. and Garver, B. (1992) Eugenics, euthanasia and genocide. *Linacre Q.*, **59**, 24–51.
40. Garver, K.L. (1991) Update on maternal serum alpha fetoprotein screening (letter). *Am. J. Hum. Genet.*, **48**, 1203–204.
41. Clark, A. (1990) Genetics, ethics and audit. *Lancet*, **335**, 1145–47.
42. LaChat, M.R. (1975) Utilitarian reasoning in Nazi medical policy: some preliminary investigations. *Linacre Q.*, **Feb.**, 14–37.
43. Alexander, L. (1949) Medical science under dictatorship. *N. Engl. J. Med.*, **241**, 39–47.
44. Mitscherlich, A. (ed.) (1949) *Doctors of Infamy: The Story of the Nazi Medical Crimes*, Henry Schuman, NY.
45. Motulsky, A.G. (1986) Presidential address. Human and medical genetics:

past, present and future, in *Human Genetics*, Proceedings of the Seventh International Congress, Berlin (eds F. Vogel and K. Sperling) Springer, NY, pp. 3–13.

46. Muller-Hill, B. (1988) *Murderous Science*, Oxford University Press, Oxford.

48. Proctor, R.N. (1988) *Racial Hygiene*, Harvard University Press, Cambridge, MA.

49. Weiss, S.F. (1987) *Race, Hygiene and National Efficiency*, University of California Press, Berkeley.

50. Lifton, R.J. (1986) *The Nazi Doctors*, Basic Books, NY.

60 PSYCHOSOCIAL ASPECTS OF A TERMINATION OF PREGNANCY FOR FETAL ABNORMALITY

M.C.A. White-van Mourik and J.M. Connor

60.1 Introduction

The Abortion Act (1967) in the UK legalized the selective termination of pregnancy, and subsequent developments in obstetrics, biochemistry and cytology made the possibility of offering prenatal screening and diagnosis a reality. The element of choice regarding child rearing, seen by many as a positive development, may have brought with it emotional and social costs.

This chapter investigates the practical, ethical, emotional and social issues involved in the sequelae of a second trimester termination for fetal abnormality, and will look into measures designed to alleviate some of the consequent stress and confusion.

60.1.1 PSYCHODYNAMICS OF PREGNANCY AND EMOTIONAL ADJUSTMENT

To understand the reaction to pregnancy loss it may be prudent to explore how a couple adapts to pregnancy. Pregnancy has frequently been viewed as a psychobiological crisis akin to puberty or the menopause [1]. Emotional disturbance in pregnancy is a normal, not a pathological, response and in most cases women regain a state of equilibrium spontaneously [2]. Adjustment to pregnancy may follow various stages. What is first experienced as 'putting on weight' and an enlarging abdomen changes into empathy with the developing child and an awareness of the fetus as an independent human being. The conclusion of pregnancy, regardless of its outcome, challenges emotional stability and requires psychological adjustment. Even after an uneventful, fullterm delivery, maternal postpartum depression is commonly observed [2,3].

60.1.2 PARENTAL–FETAL BONDING

Although the 'infant–mother' relationship develops gradually in pregnancy, current techniques make fetal life audible (fetal heart monitor) and visible (ultrasonography) from weeks 8 to 10 or even earlier, and present the parents-to-be with undeniable evidence of fetal life well before quickening occurs (maternal awareness of the fetal movements) [4,5], thus enabling the parents to start the psychological preparation for their offspring at an early stage [1,6]. In spite of this, Western cultures still have not decided officially on the moral status of the human embryo [7,8]. Other cultures have traditionally had a personification of the fetus before birth [9]. The relationship with the fetus starts after the awareness of conception and continues after delivery in a modified way. The Siriono of Eastern Bolivia, for instance, perform the same bereavement ritual for a miscarried fetus as for a deceased adult and thereby formalize its status. Cranley [10], reporting on her research into the relationship of parents with their unborn in Western society, observed a wealth of interaction between the mother and her fetus and noted that both father and mother developed 'bonding behaviour', in which the fetus is experienced as a future child and not simply as a composite of developing cells.

60.1.3 GRIEF AFTER PREGNANCY LOSS

With increased parental awareness of the fetus as an independent identity it is not surprising that the loss of a wanted and planned pregnancy is experienced as the loss of a child. Many women who abort spontaneously experience anguish, loneliness and depression following the realization of pregnancy loss [11,12]. The fetal loss is viewed as an experience of bereavement [13,14] and thus grieving is not a pathological symptom but a normal and even necessary reaction [15]. Bereavement follows a pattern of indistinct phases and the bereaved may pass between them or become locked into one or another. Shock, numbness and disbelief may give way

Diseases of the Fetus and Newborn, 2nd edn, Edited by G.B. Reed, A.E. Claireaux and F. Cockburn. Published in 1995 by Chapman & Hall, London. ISBN 0 412 39160 0

to anger, protest, despair and pining. The duration of grieving varies greatly and depends on the parents' perception of their loss, and on the success with which the individuals do the 'grief work', which chiefly entails the acceptance of the feelings of intense distress. Avoiding this and denying what has happened may lead to 'morbid grief' which is either a delayed reaction precipitated by specific circumstances or events, sometimes years later, or a distorted reaction which may be difficult to recognize as the original grief. This unresolved grief may in turn have an adverse affect on health [16].

It is often assumed that the longer the period of gestation, the closer the bonding to the fetus and therefore the greater the feelings of bereavement after pregnancy loss. However, just as not all births of live, healthy babies result in immediate, ideal attachment, so women with first or second trimester pregnancy loss must not be assumed to have a less severe reaction to bereavement. A more important criterion is the significance of the pregnancy to the parents, their previous experience of loss and adaptation to it, their personalities and their perception of social support.

60.2 Termination of pregnancy for fetal abnormality

With burgeoning technology lengthening the list of adverse conditions that can be recognized in the fetus comes a greater awareness that there now is some choice in the avoidance of genetic disease and congenital malformations. Prenatal diagnosis is available for many couples with a family history of genetic disease, thereby enabling them to dare to consider further pregnancies and the option of a termination of pregnancy for an affected fetus. Ultrasonography and antenatal maternal serum screening programmes identify fetuses at risk. The emotional implications of screening and prenatal diagnosis are many and complex, but in this chapter we will concentrate on the couples who were subjected to the acute trauma produced by the discovery of a fetal defect and who chose the option of termination of pregnancy.

Realization of an unfavourable result triggers an immediate grief response that may be characterized by disbelief, shock and anger [1,17–19]. Hopes and expectations are dashed by the revelation of the fetal abnormality. The medicolegal necessity of a quick decision to maintain or to terminate the pregnancy adds to the burden of the already distressed couple. Abstract attitudes towards abortion provide little guidance for couples trapped in this moral dilemma. The parents' understanding of the specific defect affecting the fetus is a significant determinant of their course of decision and action [6].

60.3 Psychosocial sequelae of a termination of pregnancy for fetal abnormality

In contrast to the mostly positive reactions of women after abortion for psychosocial indications [20,21] many authors [1,6,13,17,22–25] observed the opposite after a termination for fetal abnormality. Research into this subject started in the mid-seventies [17] and, although studies were small and with some design flaws [26], the researchers observed acute grief reactions, depression and social disruption. When the couples were compared with other parents who had experienced spontaneous fetal loss, their reactions were found to be more akin to the grief which followed stillbirth or neonatal death than that which followed miscarriages [13]. Only Jones et al. [27] reported fewer negative sequelae in this, post-termination, group but they stressed the low response rate of 39% and the probability that coping problems were the main reasons for non-participation. When the findings in the literature are collated, the reasons for this increased distress emerge. In the majority of women who agreed to antenatal screening or prenatal diagnosis, the termination of pregnancy had the psychological meaning tantamount to the loss of a wanted child. Loss implies mourning, yet coping and grieving were complicated by by other problems which needed attention.

There was a **loss of biological self-esteem**, because producing a handicapped child (or fetus) is still, if only subconsciously, perceived as a reproductive failure. Matters were further complicated by the fact that there may be an increased incidence of fetal abnormality in subsequent pregnancies.

A further complication to the grief was a **loss of moral self-esteem**. This was produced by the awareness of the parents' own contribution to the pregnancy loss. This loss was not passive but one of their own choosing. Even the knowledge that the fetus would not be viable was not found to take away the overwhelming feeling of parental responsibility [28]. This ethical conflict and the moral pain of having to choose either against life, or for suffering, produced in many couples a strong spiritual disturbance [25].

Loss of social self-esteem was often a result of the marked ambivalence which further complicated matters. Couples reported both rationally recognizing the prevention of the birth of a handicapped child and emotionally mourning the wanted baby. They felt supported but at the same time isolated, grateful but angry, and so on. These conflicting feelings were instrumental in the couples' reluctance to instigate discussion. Coping is hindered by paradox, conflict and ambivalence, and mourning may not succeed if couples fail to unravel the complexity of the situation. Consequently they may continue to experience anxiety and depression.

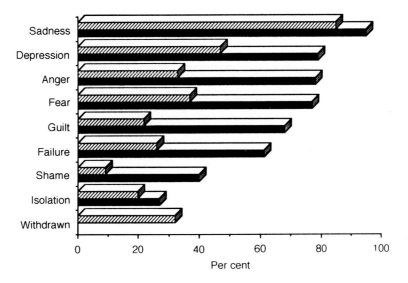

Figure 60.1 Emotional feelings after a termination for fetal abnormality: differences between men (▨) and women (■).

The general public, and even many professionals, prefer to shun issues of handicap and abortion. This meant that couples who already felt reticent about discussing their confusing feelings after the intervention were actively discouraged from doing so by their surroundings. When voicing their feelings of grief they were often reminded how lucky they were to have had the choice, or pointedly told that it had been their own decision. This exacerbated feelings of guilt and failure [25]. Outsiders may deduce that a strong grief reaction was linked to regretting the decision to terminate the pregnancy. The trauma of the diagnosis triggered an immediate grief response, characterized by disbelief, shock and anger, and it was in this frame of mind that couples had to make decisions about their fetus. It was therefore not unusual for some newly bereaved parents to experience doubts shortly after the termination of pregnancy. A recent study [25] showed that 48% of the women admitted to being unsure about their decision in the first weeks or months after the termination of pregnancy. They were worried that the medical professionals might have made a mistake, or that they were being disapproved of for agreeing to an abortion. Mothers whose fetal abnormality had been detected by 'routine' antenatal screening had frequently only a vague comprehension of the fetal condition for which they had been offered the intervention. Doubts were particularly common in very young women (16–20 years) and those belonging to a lower socioeconomic group. Doubts were significantly lessened if, at a post-termination consultation, time was taken to explain the condition of the fetus, the nature of the malformation or illness and the possible prognosis, especially were this was backed up by the evidence of a post-mortem report or a picture of the fetus. Two years after the

intervention, even where there had been initial doubts, the vast majority of couples felt at peace with their decision [23,25]. Society frequently fails to comprehend that it is possible to grieve sorely over a loss and at the same time be grateful that a tragedy was avoided [28].

60.3.1 PARENTS' SUBJECTIVE ASSESSMENT OF EMOTIONAL AND SOMATIC REACTIONS IN THE FIRST 6 MONTHS AFTER THE TERMINATION OF PREGNANCY

It is common for a feeling of deep sadness to be shared by both partners after the termination of pregnancy. Depression, anger, fear, guilt and failure were the most frequently mentioned strong emotions. The anger was often a reaction to the feeling of helplessness for not having been able to protect their child from harm. The feeling of responsibility for this new life was mentioned by some men, but was expressed principally by women. The differences in the feelings expressed by men and women are illustrated in Figure 60.1. When describing their feelings of fear, couples stressed the possibility of recurrence of the abnormality and the idea of having to repeat the whole decision-making process again. Some women complained of prolonged numbness, panic spells and palpitations, but only men admitted to feeling withdrawn and excluded [23]. In our society reproduction and reproductive failure are still frequently perceived as the woman's province. As well as coping with strong feelings many couples reported somatic symptoms. Of these, listlessness, loss of concentration, irritability and crying are mentioned most frequently, as shown in Figure 60.2. Male partners found that a lack of concentration in the first few

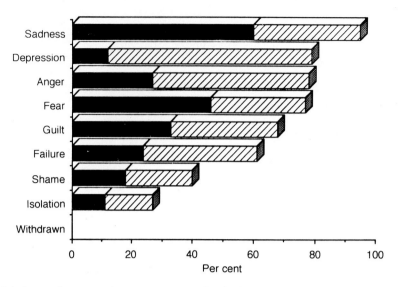

Figure 60.2 Emotional feelings of women after a termination for fetal abnormality: ▨ = reported in the first 3–12 months; ■ = remaining after 2 years.

months led to mistakes at work and to unexpected failures in exams.

Nightmares commonly have one or more of three elements: (1) replay, in which the termination procedure is repeated night after night, and sometimes continues intermittently for up to a year after the termination of pregnancy; (2) persecution, in which the parent runs away to prevent pursuers from taking the baby; and (3) blame, in which the baby, or family members, would appear and accuse the parent of murder.

Despite these dissonant feelings and complaints many couples feel reluctant to bring them up in discussion with health professionals, family or friends for fear of being judged mentally unstable and thus exposed to unwanted psychiatric treatment [25].

60.3.2 ASPECTS OF SEQUELAE AFTER 2 YEARS

Two years after the intervention most couples reported that they had regained equilibrium despite continued feelings of deep sadness about the loss of the baby and the fear of recurrence of the condition in a subsequent pregnancy. A feeling of continuing relief was especially mentioned by those families familiar with a distressing handicap or genetic disease. However, some studies [23,25] showed that about 20% of women continued to feel anger, guilt, failure, irritability and tearfulness (Figure 60.2). They felt that these strong emotions had a disruptive impact on their lives and relationships. Men appeared to come to terms with their loss more quickly than their spouses (Figure 60.3). The same analysis was made by Martinson, Modow and Henry [29], who observed that after the loss of a child fathers

were twice as likely as mothers to report that the most intensive part of grieving was over in a few weeks. However, their response may have reflected the social expectations of the father 'to take it like a man'. Men appear to have greater need to keep their grief private [30], and this may even give their partners the impression that they are not affected by the loss. Although the termination often produces an initial closeness in the marital relationship, disparate grieving patterns or sexual needs often evoked friction 3–6 months after the intervention, for which few sought help or counselling.

60.4 Reproductive behaviour after a termination for fetal abnormality

As one of the factors which affected couples after a termination for fetal abnormality was a loss of biological self-esteem, a new pregnancy may be presumed to be of great importance. Most couples have a planned family size but the procreative wish may be amended depending on circumstances. In the past, couples at risk of genetic disease were often deterred from planning further pregnancies [31–34]. Authors reported changed reproductive behaviour after the introduction of prenatal diagnosis [35–40], in that couples dared to try to achieve their planned family size. However, the decision-making process in couples deciding to have children with the option of prenatal diagnosis was perceived as more burdensome than in those for whom prenatal diagnosis was not available [41]. The literature about the sequelae of a termination for fetal abnormality provides anecdotal information about couples refraining from further pregnancy. Two studies [23,42] examined the reproductive behaviour of couples after a

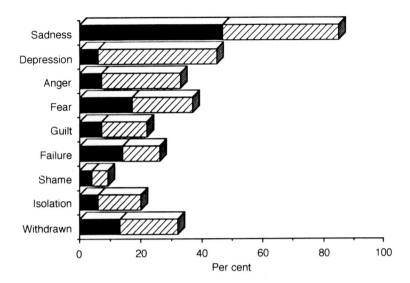

Figure 60.3 Emotional feelings of men after a termination for fetal abnormality: ▨ = reported in the first 3–12 months; ■ = remaining after 2 years.

termination for fetal abnormality and observed a reproductive conflict in 14% of younger women and 40% of the older women. A reproductive conflict is where the desired family size is not realized, yet, despite this, the couple do not dare to try for further children.

The actual recurrence risk alone did not necessarily deter couples from further reproduction [43], nor did single factors such as religious conviction, negative feeling about the termination procedure or lack of postintervention support. The deciding factors in the reproductive conflict after the intervention appeared to be maternal age, an unexpected diagnosis, the presence of healthy children in the family, and a subtle combination of multiple elements. Frets *et al.* [41] made similar observations in genetic counsellees. Help could be offered to couples with such a conflict by providing focused counselling in which the counsellor concentrates on the feelings concerning the reproductive decision, accepts apparently irrational considerations (because these feelings indicate the influence of unconscious motives) and understands the role which guilt plays in the decision.

All women who subsequently became pregnant in two studies [23,42] chose prenatal diagnosis.

60.5 Parental needs and perceived management during and after termination of pregnancy for fetal abnormality

In two studies [25,44] hospital staff were reported to be kind and caring but few hospitals appeared to have a protocol concerning the discharge and follow-up procedures after the termination of pregnancy. This meant that it was not uncommon for the woman to turn up in the surgery of her family doctor, only to be asked how the pregnancy was progressing.

Even though there was kindness, ambivalence towards abortion was shown in subtle ways. After the delivery the fetus was handled by some staff with lack of respect, which on reflection was perceived as very painful by the mother. Further ambivalence towards abortion was also evident in some hospitals where parents were refused access to a memorial book. This book is frequently kept to acknowledge babies lost after late miscarriage, stillbirth or neonatal death. Posttermination parents were rarely accompanied to the door on leaving hospital, which was in marked contrast to those who left with a baby. Couples were very sensitive to the mood of the professionals who cared for them, and translated slightly brusque behaviour as disapproval, even if this behaviour was due to pressure of work [45].

Parents found it helpful if they were prepared for decisions they had to face. These included considering the psychosocial implications of a termination of pregnancy before the procedure, whether or not to hold and look at the fetus, the possibility of a religious blessing, and the choice between a funeral or a cremation. Studies of patients following perinatal death emphasized the importance of ceremonially recognizing the end of the preparation for parenthood.

Not all men and women want to see their fetus and many feel at peace with this decision. Women who regretted not seeing the fetus after delivery were those who were too frightened by the suspected abnormality or those who were too exhausted after the delivery. Those who had been frightened often imagined the fetal abnormality to be much worse then the reality. Many women requested a photograph of the fetus months or even 8 years after the event. This included women who had not wanted to see the fetus or had refused a picture of the fetus after the termination of pregnancy. A picture of the fetus, especially showing a severe abnormality, was perceived as particularly helpful in coming to terms with the termination of pregnancy by those who wondered if they had made the right decision. Support after the termination of pregnancy was particularly appreciated if the painful psychosocial sequelae were recognized and help given in finding appropriate coping strategies for individual parents.

Parental dissatisfaction, when reported, appeared to be centred on short-term and long-term after care. This may be partly due to the reluctance of both men and women to report emotional disturbances or somatic complaints to the family doctor for fear of being put on addictive tranquillizers or antidepressants, or even for fear of psychiatric hospital admission. The most frequently mentioned complaints were **lack of information, lack of preparation, lack of understanding and lack of communication between caring agencies.**

60.6 Further developments and ethical issues

Chorionic villus sampling, which facilitates termination of pregnancy at an earlier gestation, may alter the sequelae of a termination of pregnancy because it reduces the time of parental–fetal bonding, the waiting time for results and frequently the more traumatic second trimester termination procedure. The sadness and disappointment about the pregnancy loss would remain. There are, unfortunately, still difficulties attached to this procedure [46]. Test results may be ambiguous, thus necessitating amniocentesis, and the procedure is not suitable for many fetal abnormalities (neural tube defects, congenital heart defects). Even so, there is some indication that early intervention could reduce the duration of painful sequelae [24]. The greater availability of antenatal maternal serum screening with biochemical markers for chromosomal disorders and possible antenatal or preconceptional screening for cystic fibrosis will expose more couples to the dilemmas discussed in this chapter.

Do our facilities for optimum care match our eagerness and willingness to implement new developments in genetics and obstetrics? The issue which couples brought up most frequently after the termination for fetal abnormality was a feeling of confusion. Medical and social responsibility frequently seemed to have come to an end after the damaged fetus was terminated. A choice had been given and the couples themselves had made the decisions. At this time, for many couples and especially for those unfamiliar with the diagnosed fetal abnormality, the long process of realization, grieving, learning to live with the grief and striving for resolution is just starting. Unfortunately, few hospitals have a protocol for aftercare and long-term follow-up. Few couples are given the information about the psychosocial sequelae of the intervention or are helped to explore coping strategies for coming to terms with the decision. Barbara Katz Rothman [28] observed that 'these women are victims of a social system that fails to take collective responsibility for the needs of its members, and leaves individual women to make impossible choices. We individualize the problem and make it the woman's own. Whatever the cost, she has chosen, it is her problem not ours.'

Surely it must be part of any antenatal screening programme and prenatal diagnostic service not only to provide choice but also to prevent subsequent morbidity and help couples to learn to live with their choice?

60.7 Conclusion

Within the context of continuing medical care, professionals have a responsibility to understand this new kind of grief and to recognize the signs that may indicate a need for further counselling or professional mental health intervention. In view of the ambivalence to abortion and handicap in our society, the couples' reticence and lowered self-esteem must be recognized. A standard protocol designed to counteract this reticence would facilitate better short-term and, where required, long-term care and would ensure consistency of care. The protocol should be based on couples' perception of good management [44]. When couples' recommendations were collated they fell into three themes: recognition, information and hope.

Recognition was described in several ways: as a perception and comprehension of the grief: as an insight of the fact that choice is often perceived as no choice at all but the only action feasible under the circumstances; as an understanding of the fear of social disapproval and the subsequent reticence in asking for help when required; as a perception of the turmoil of ambiguous feelings and the time it may take to come to terms with the event. Recognition prevents trivialization and the use of platitudes.

Information and communication were found to be of enormous value in coming to terms with the termination of pregnancy for fetal abnormality. Explanations using appropriate language about the fetal abnormality and the termination of pregnancy procedure and preparation for the physical, psychosocial, short-term and long-term sequelae were considered essential. Better and continuing communication minimized the feeling of being out of control and reduced misunderstanding.

Hope for another pregnancy was felt to be of great importance to those wishing to achieve their planned family. A successful subsequent pregnancy counterbalanced the loss of biological self-esteem and to some extent restored a sense of social competence. Couples attached great importance to discussions about the implications of the fetal abnormality for further pregnancies, the prenatal diagnosis available and preconception health care.

Research and development of new prenatal procedures and screening programmes must surely include studies into the psychosocial consequences so that provisions for information, care and counselling can be made simultaneously with implementation of these procedures. Finally, regional audit of patient care will ensure that the standards are being upheld.

References

1. Donnai, P., Charles, N. and Harris, R. (1981) Attitudes of patients after genetic termination of pregnancy. *BMJ*, **282**, 621–22.
2. Bibring, B.L. and Valenstein, A.F. (1967) The psychological aspects of pregnancy. *Clin. Obst. Gynecol.*, **19**, 357–71.
3. Nott, P.N., Franklin, M., Armitage, C. and Gelder, M.G. (1976) Hormonal changes and mood in puerperium. *Br. J. Psychiatry*, **128**, 379.
4. Lumley, J. (1980) The image of the fetus in the first trimester. *Birth. Fam.*, **7**, 5–14.
5. Fletcher, J.C. and Evans, M.I. (1983) Maternal bonding in early fetal ultrasound examinations. *N. Engl. J. Med.*, **308**, 392–93.
6. Blumberg, B.D. (1984) The emotional implications of prenatal diagnosis, in *Psychological Aspects of Genetic Counselling* (eds A.E.H. Emery and I.M. Pullen), Academic Press, London, pp. 202–17.
7. Dunstan, G.R. (1984) The moral status of the human embryo; a tradition recalled. *J. Med. Ethics*, **1**, 38–44.
8. Dunstan, G.R. (1988) Screening for fetal and genetic abnormality: social and ethical issues. *J. Med. Genet.*, **25**, 290–93.
9. Cranley, M.S. (1981) Roots of attachment: the relationship of parents with their unborn, in *Perinatal Parental Behaviour: Nursing Research and Implications for the Newborn Health* (eds R.P. Lederman, B.S. Baff and P. Carrol), Alan R. Liss, NY, pp. 59–83.
10. Cranley, M.S. (1981) Development of a tool for measurement of maternal attachment during pregnancy. *Nurse Res.*, **30**, 281–84.
11. Borg, S. and Lasker, J. (1982) *When Pregnancy Fails: Coping with Miscarriage, Stillbirth and Infant Death*, Routledge & Kegan Paul, London.
12. Le Roy, M. (1988) *Miscarriage*, Macdonald Optima, London.
13. Lloyd, J. and Laurence, K.M. (1985) Sequelae and support after termination of pregnancy for fetal malformation. *BMJ*, **290**, 907–909.
14. Morris, D. (1976) Parental reactions to perinatal death. *Proc. R. Soc. Med.*, **69**, 837–38.
15. Pedder, J.R. (1982) Failure to mourn, and melancholia. *Br. J. Psychiatry*, **141**, 329–37.
16. Stroebe, W. and Stroebe, M. (1987) *Bereavement and Health: the Psychological and Physical Consequences*, Cambridge University Press, Cambridge, pp. 168–223.
17. Blumberg, B.D., Golbus, M.C. and Hanson, K. (1975) The psychological sequelae of abortion performed for a genetic indication. *Am. J. Obstet. Gynecol.*, **122**, 799–808.
18. Blumberg, B.D. (1974) Psychic sequelae of selective abortion. Yale University, MD thesis.
19. Adler, B. and Kusnick, T. (1982): Genetic counselling in prenatally diagnosed trisomy 18 and 21. *Paediatrics*, **69**, 94–99.
20. Doane, B.K. and Quigley, B.G. (1981) Psychiatric aspects of therapeutic abortion (review). *Can. Med. Assoc. J.*, **125**, 427–32.
21. Adler, N.E., Henry, P.D., Major, B.N. *et al.* (1990) Psychological responses after abortion. *Science*, **248**, 41–44.
22. Becker, J., Glinski, L. and Laxova, R. (1984) Long-term emtional impact of 2nd trimester pregnancy termination after detection of fetal abnormality. *Am. J. Hum. Genet.*, **36**, 122s.
23. Thomassen-Brepols, L.J. (1985) Psychosociale aspecten van prenatale diagnostiek (Psycho-social aspects of prenatal diagnosis). Erasmus University, Rotterdam, PhD thesis.
24. Black, R.B. (1989) A 1 and 6 month follow-up of prenatal diagnosis patients who lost pregnancies. *Prenat. Diagn.*, **9**, 795–804.
25. White-van Mourik, M.C.A., Connor, J.M. and Ferguson-Smith, M.A. (1992) The psychosocial sequelae of a second-trimester termination of pregnancy for fetal abnormality. *Prenat. Diagn.*, **19**, 189–204.
26. Hollerbach, P.E. (1979) Reproductive attitudes and the genetic counsellee, In *Counselling in Genetics* (eds Y.E. Hsia, K. Hirschorn, R.L. Silverberg and L. Godmillow), Alan R. Liss. NY, pp. 155–222.
27. Jones, O.W., Penn, N.E., Schuchter, S. *et al.* (1984) Parental response to mid-trimester therapeutic abortion following amniocentesis, *Prenat. Diagn.*, **4**, 249–56.
28. Rothman, B.K. (1986) *The Tentative Pregnancy*, Viking Penguin, NY.
29. Martinson, I., Modow, D. and Henry, W. (1980) *Home Care for the Child with Cancer*, Final report (Grant no. Ca 19490) National Cancer Institute, US Department of Health and Human Services, Washington DC.
30. De Frain, J., Taylor, J. and Ernst, L. (1982) *Coping with Sudden Infant Death*, Lexington Books, D.C. Heath, Lexington Ma.
31. Emery, A.E.H., Watt, M.S. and Clark, E.R. (1972) The effects of genetic counselling in Duchenne muscular dystrophy. *Clin. Genet.*, **3**, 147–50.
32. Emery, A.E.H., Watt, M.S. and Clark, E.R. (1973) Social effects of genetic counselling. *BMJ*, **i** 724–26.
33. Reynolds, B.D., Puck, M.H. and Robinson, A. (1974) Genetic counselling: an appraisal. *Clin. Genet.*, **5**, 177–78.
34. Klein, D. and Wyss, D. (1977) Retrospective and follow up study of approximately 1000 genetic consultations. *J. Hum. Genet.*, **25**, 47–57.
35. Modell, B., Petrou M., Ward, R.H. *et al.* (1984) Effect of fetal diagnostic testing on birthrate of thalassaemia major in Britain. *Lancet*, **ii**, 1383–86.
36. Kaback, M., Zippin, D., Boyd, P. *et al.* (1984) Attitudes towards prenatal diagnosis of cystic fibrosis amongst parents of affected children, in *Cystic Fibrosis; Horizons* (ed. D. Lawson), Wiley, NY, pp. 6–28.
37. Wyss-Hutin, D. (1979) Consequences du conseil génétique. *J. Genet. Hum.*, **27** (suppl. 1), 53–96.
38. Scriver, C.R., Bardanis, M., Cartier, L. *et al.* (1984) Beta-thalassemia disease prevention; genetic medicine applied. *Am. J. Hum. Genet.*, **36**, 1024–38.
39. Modell, B. and Bulyzhenkov, V. (1988) Distribution and control of some genetic disorders. *World Health Stat. Q.*, **41**, 209–18.
40. Evers-Kiebooms, G., Denayer, L., Cassiman, J.J. and van den Berghe, H. (1988) Family planning decisions after the birth of a cystic fibrosis child: impact of prenatal diagnosis. *Scan. J. Gastroenterol. Suppl.*, **143**, 38–46.
41. Frets, P.G., Duivenvoorden, H. J., Verhage, F. *et al.* (1991) Analysis of problems in making the reproductive decision after genetic counselling. *J. Med. Genet.*, **28**, 194–200.
42. White-van Mourik, M.C.A. (1989) The psycho-social sequelae of a termination of pregnancy for fetal abnormality. University of Glasgow, MSc thesis.
43. Lippman-Hands, A. and Fraser, F.C. 1979) Genetic counselling: the provision and perception of information. *Am. J. Med. Genet.*, **3**, 113–27.
44. White-van Mourik, M.C.A., Connor, J.M. and Ferguson-Smith, M.A. (1990) Patient care before and after termination of pregnancy for neural tube defect. *Prenat. Diagn.*, **10**, 497–505.
45. Leschot, N.J., Verjaal, M. and Treffers, P.E. (1982) Therapeutic abortion on genetic indication: a detailed follow-up study of 20 patients. *J. Psychosom. Obstet. Gynecol.*, **1**, 47–56.
46. Canadian Collaborative CVS–Amniocentesis Clinical Trial Group (1989) Multicentre randomised clinical trial of chorion villus sampling and amniocentesis. *Lancet*, **i**, 1–6.

61 SCREENING FOR GENETIC DISEASE

S.F. Cahalane and P.D. Mayne

61.1 Introduction

The several thematic strands which have been brought together in this book have remote and disparate origins which began to interweave in the early years of this century. Around that time, in London, Garrod was channelling his profound insights into his *Inborn Errors of Metabolism* [1], while in Edinburgh, Ballantyne was bringing his meticulous observations to a focus in *The Antenatal Pathology of the Foetus and Embryo* [2]. Theodor Schwann, the German physiologist, had previously cobbled the word 'metabolism' from the Greek roots 'to change' and 'to cast into'; before that the abbé Mendel had pondered the formulary of inheritance, in a Silesian monastery garden. Meanwhile, the cousins Darwin and Galton were propounding their theories of evolution and natural selection.

This chapter will deal with the application of mass or population screening and individual screening for inherited diseases, some of which have been described earlier. Since the patients may be either unborn or but lately delivered the parents are integral and, as the disorders are familial, so the immediate relatives and even remoter kin may be drawn into the investigative process. Many scientific and medical disciplines are involved in the investigation, diagnosis and treatment which follows. Modern medicine, in its preventive preoccupation, extols preclinical diagnosis, while genetic screening activities have drawn central and local government into the panoply.

Since screening for chromosomal disorders has not achieved the widespread application of its metabolic sister, the emphasis in this chapter will be on the latter. Prenatal and neonatal screening is the investigation of the products of flawed generations; both the living and the dead are involved (Figure 61.1).

For a long time the pace of progress was measured and gradual, but the recent conceptual and technological cascade in molecular genetics has overtaken events, so that now the retrospective view is an uneven one. It is more than 60 years since Folling [3] detected phenylketoacids in the urines of mentally handicapped children, leading to the discovery of the enzymatic metabolism of phenylalanine and ultimately to insights into and treatment of conditions as disparate as endogenous depression and parkinsonism. There are now some 6000 confirmed or suspected monogenic disorders [4]. Over 40 years ago the genetic material of most organisms had been identified as DNA, but during the last decade recombinant techniques have elicited the precise intragenic loci for many inherited metabolic disorders including phenylketonuria, cystic fibrosis and Duchenne muscular dystrophy. For some disorders there is a correlation between the clinical phenotype and the genotype but for others there is no complete pathogenetic chain to link the defective enzyme activity with abnormal brain function. To paraphrase Clayton [5], the study of cases accumulated from genetic screening has highlighted the deficiencies in our knowledge of the natural history of many of the inherited metabolic disorders, and what had previously seemed straightforward has become complex and heterogeneous.

Apart from the severe clinical impact, there is, as yet, inevitable loss of life from genetic disorders, whether occurring as early or late fetal death, as neonatal or infant death or from death in later childhood, adolescence or, rarely, adult life. Deaths from chromosomal disorders predominate prenatally, while those from monogenic disorders occur in infants, and those from polygenic conditions are more common in adults. The screening and diagnostic techniques used in the living, whether before or after birth, are applicable to the autopsy and must be so used in order to enable accurate genetic counselling, to avert subsequent sibling deaths, establish the prevalance of the disorder within a population (enumeration) and to promote research.

There is now an unprecedented opportunity to harness such diverse disciplines as those of genetics, biochemistry and cell biology to the older one of anatomic pathology [6].

Diseases of the Fetus and Newborn, 2nd edn, Edited by G.B. Reed, A.E. Claireaux and F. Cockburn. Published in 1995 by Chapman & Hall, London. ISBN 0 412 39160 0

61.2 Range and objectives of genetic screening

Genetic screening is an important public health and clinical activity, almost a discipline in its own right, with aspirations and attributes using simple and complex technologies and governed by ethical, economic and legal constraints.

The traditional goals of genetic screening are to provide the following:

- management: medical intervention at the stage of incipient disease;
- reproductive options: appropriate genetic counselling for parents or potential parents;
- enumeration and research.

These three aims promote the search for abnormal phenotypes, in both the heterozygotic and homozygotic state, among the unborn (prenatal), the newborn (neonatal) and the adult (heterozygote). The laboratory techniques of screening and confirmation exploit sequential steps of mutant genetic expression, which are as follows.

1. Identification of gene defect: heterozygote determination; confirmatory and possibly eventual screening procedures.
2. Disordered protein (enzyme and other) function: for confirmatory procedures and prenatal primary screening programmes.

Figure 61.1 is a graphic synthesis of the multifaceted

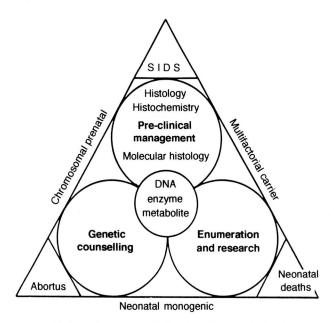

Figure 61.1 A 'tryptogram' showing the association between goals of screening methods and causes of death. SIDS = sudden infant death syndrome.

but constantly interlinking characteristics of screening which will be discussed in later paragraphs. Screening programmes can be either voluntary or mandatory but both require informed consent and counselling.

The definition of screening, distinguishing between the three terms, screening, surveillance and testing, has been discussed. Screening benefits the individual, whereas community surveillance and testing are population based and are done to protect the community.

Previous chapters in Part Four reviewed screening for malformations, chromosomal syndromes and twins by sonography; the next two chapters in this part are devoted to prenatal and maternal screening (Chapter 62) and neonatal and earlier screening (Chapter 63).

61.3 Prevalence of mendelian disease

Before discussing screening for inherited disease, a summary of the size of the problem, its geography and geology is indicated.

The McKusick catalogue of *Mendelian Inheritance in Man* [4] has shown, in successive editions, the expansion of this terrain, and relevant 1992 figures are reproduced (Table 61.1).

Thus, there are more than 5750 unifactorial disorders, the majority of which are autosomal dominant. Against this, some 400 chromosomal disorders have been described; the divergence is understandable when one considers that each individual hands on an endowment of a mere 23 chromosomes, but some 100 000 genes. Nevertheless, each of the monogenic disorders is rare, but as a group they constitute an important cause of morbidity and mortality, accounting for some 10% of all paediatric hospital admissions. The overall population frequency of monogenic disorders is about 10 per 1000 livebirths, comprising rates of 7 for dominant, 2.5 for recessive and about 0.5 for X-linked disorders. Of the inherited metabolic diseases whose biochemical basis has been defined, approximately 80% have proven enzyme abnormalities [4].

61.3.1 RESPONSE TO TREATMENT

A comprehensive analysis, from Montreal [7,8], of the effects of inherited disease, as measured by longevity,

Table 61.1 Number of unifactorial inherited disorders identified by 1992 [After Ref. 4]

Type	Confirmed	Suspected	Total
Autosomal dominant	2500	1200	3700
Autosomal recessive	650	1000	1650
X-linked	200	200	400
Total	3350	2400	5750

reproducibility and intellectual and physical growth, showed that in only 12% was there complete response to treatment and that in 48% response was totally lacking. Most deaths in dominant conditions occurred in the reproductive phase of life while those in lethal recessive disorders occurred earlier; deaths from X-linked disorders were almost evenly distributed over the prereproductive and intrareproductive eras.

61.3.2 IMPACT OF SCREENING

There are no such objective measures of the impact of screening, but rather more subjective parameters are proposed, as shown in Table 61.2.

Galactosaemia is one of the conditions considered in the above-mentioned reviews; Table 61.3 is compiled from the information given therein on the effect of early treatment on its outcome [8]. Table 61.3 shows that there was a marked reduction in the cumulative predictive score in those patients receiving early treatment compared with those who did not. Since galactosaemia is one of the more serious of the conditions that can be screened for in neonatal programmes it is reasonable to infer that the benefits of early treatment also represent those of screening. Presenting in the neonate with abnormal liver function, death may occur from sepsis or hypoprothrombinaemic haemorrhage.

Table 61.2 Impact of genetic screening

Quality of life improved
Health costs reduced
Natural history unfolded
Gene frequencies altered
Technology improved
New disorders discovered

Table 61.3 Effect of treatment on disadaptive phenotypes in classical galactosaemia

	Without treatment	With early treatment
Lifespan	3	0
Reproducibility	3	1
Somatic growth	3	0
Mental handicap	3	1
Learning capacity	3	1
Normal work capability	3	1
Cosmetic effect	1	0
Complete score	19	4

A score ranging from 0 for normal phenotype to 3 for death or severe disability was applied. Compiled from the information given in the second of the Montreal papers [8].

Survivors may be blind, as a result of cataracts, mentally retarded, or infertile if female. Yet the simple expediency of avoiding galactose-containing foods may avert some of these catastrophies.

This is an example of the importance and likely impact of newborn screening in those conditions for which it is currently practised.

61.4   Approach to prenatal screening

The approach to prenatal screening or intrauterine detection of genetic disease emphasizes the confusion that exists between a diagnostic and a screening procedure. In effect, screening is a less common approach than the purely diagnostic one, in which a specific disease is sought on the basis of either an established abnormality in a previously seriously affected or dead sibling or the parents having been unequivocally diagnosed as carriers. Most amniotic, fetal or chorionic villous samplings for metabolic disease are for a single disorder. If prenatal diagnosis of such a disorder is routinely offered to particular populations, e.g. Tay–Sachs disease in Ashkenazi Jews, then it is legitimate screening. Testing of amniotic fluid samples by α-fetoproteins (AFPs) for neural tube defects in the fetus is a screening exercise. Simple biochemical screening procedures on maternal blood, such as AFP and free β-human choriogonadotrophin (βhCG) for Down syndrome, may determine high-risk individuals or groups requiring confirmation by amniocentesis.

Karyotyping, because it seeks abnormality in any of 23 pairs of chromosomes, is a screening procedure unless it is undertaken for a given disorder on specific indications. Prenatal chromosomal examination, on fetal or placental tissues, is most probably a diagnostic but may be a screening procedure. The search for unbalanced chromosomes in the fetuses of older expectant mothers is an example of the latter. The techniques of invasive prenatal procedures and the ensuing laboratory assays are described elsewhere. A brief introduction to the current practice of prenatal screening is all that is proposed at this point.

The clinical geneticist, obstetrician, paediatrician, cytogeneticist, biochemist and molecular biologist should all be involved in such screening programmes and the family doctor must be kept fully informed. Ethical principles and safety considerations must be gone into and the latter fully explained to the parents. The expectation of parents to have normal children may conflict with medical inclinations to carry out prenatal diagnosis only for disorders of relatively sinister import. Some of the prenatally detectable conditions are benign and management for many metabolic disorders are still experimental.

Galactosaemia poses a special problem in that prenatal fetal damage may occur [9]; long-term follow-up studies of congenital hypothyroid patients diagnosed shortly after birth suggest a similar possibility [10]. Prenatal diagnosis for these two conditions in high-risk groups may need to be considered so that therapy can be instituted *in utero*.

Prenatal diagnosis may also be carried out to plan immediate therapy after elective delivery in deleterious disorders, such as the organic acidurias. Thus abortion is not the only indication for prenatal diagnosis. However, prevention of conception seems a less demanding approach than abortion, which is only an interim measure. There is a real need in screening terms for procedures on maternal blood, such as AFP assay, that can determine the mothers who should proceed to prenatal diagnosis. It is not good enough that young parents should have to suffer at least one infant death before a genetic condition is anticipated and a precise diagnosis made.

A short list of guidelines for preliminary studies to prenatal diagnosis is given.

1. Full investigation of a previously affected infant, abortus or neonatal/infant death.
2. Parents or other siblings may be investigated by skin fibroblast culture, blood cell enzyme assays and/or DNA analyses.
3. Some group screening can be carried out for erythrocyte or leucocyte enzymes on fetal blood samples but a reasonable shortlist of suspected disorders should be made available to the laboratory. Some obvious limitations to this approach may arise either because enzyme activity in cultured fibroblasts and other amniotic cells is not uniform or may not be expressed or because enzyme activity is non-specific between 10 and 26 weeks [1].
   (a) There are large differences between the activity of some enzymes in cultured fibroblasts and in cultured amniotic cells.
   (b) It has been shown that a number of enzymes have similar activity at any time between 10 and 36 weeks gestation [11].
   (c) Weeks 14–16 are generally most suitable for sampling as prior to this the number of cells present is small.
   (d) The time of amniocentesis is more critical for metabolic disorders than for chromosomal anomalies as longer periods of cell study are required, 3–4 weeks between amniocentesis and final result being average. This can be reduced by ultramicroenzyme assays on smaller cell populations [12].
   (e) A control sample which undergoes identical processing and has been acquired under the same conditions is desirable in order to assess the reliability of the assay.
   (f) There are variations in enzyme activities from culture to culture and subcultures generally give more predictable levels than do primary cultures.
   (g) Molecular biological techniques can often be used to identify homozygous, heterozygous and X-linked state, particularly if the carrier status and genotype of the parents is known (Chapters 74, 75 and 77).

61.5 Approach to screening for chromosomal disorders

Routine neonatal screening for chromosomal disorders has not been implemented despite the fact that the overall incidence of such anomalies in neonates is quite considerable (0.62%) [13]. The rate of unbalanced karyotypes in the offspring of parents, one of whom has a balanced structural arrangement, varies according to the method of ascertainment. In one study involving 1349 pregnancies it was found that among 496 pregnancies monitored because of a segregating robertsonian translocation there were no abnormal fetuses when the father was the carrier, but there were 4.8% unbalanced fetuses if the carrier was the mother [14].

61.5.1 SELECTIVE CHROMOSOMAL SCREENING

Selective genetic chromosomal screening is indicated in a number of situations.

- In children with multiple congenital anomalies, with mental defects of unknown cause, with peculiar dysmorphic facies, or with failure to grow for unknown reasons.
- In all children with suspected Down syndrome and in their parents, if a balanced translocation is shown to exist.
- In women who abort repeatedly.
- In families producing many congenitally abnormal children.
- In individuals with ambiguous genitalia.

The birth risk of trisomy 21 (Down syndrome) increases with maternal age from 0.7 per 1000 live-births for mothers in their early twenties to 18.6 per 1000 livebirths for mothers of 40 years of age or over [15]. Chromosomal analysis for this disorder has largely been replaced by screening the mother during the second trimester with a combination of assays, such as AFP and free βhCG and relating these to the relative risk, depending on maternal age [16].

61.5.2 RECOMMENDATIONS FOR FUTURE CHROMOSOMAL SCREENING

There are indications that besides the already known high-risk groups, such as Down syndrome and fragile

X syndrome, other still unidentified groups exist with a higher risk of producing chromosomally abnormal offspring. Medical Research Councils from EU member states have made proposals which, among other aims, addressed the problem of identifying additional high-risk groups [17]. Two projects were designed and recommended:

- a population screening of all conceptions in a certain area over a given time frame; this to include stillbirths and abortions;
- a study of all perinatal and infant deaths.

A careful study of probands including autopsy chromosomal studies, with an evaluation of family data against background population data, was recommended as being potentially valuable in pinpointing at-risk factors.

61.6 Screening for inherited metabolic disorders

The onset of inherited metabolic disorders is overt: (1) at birth or during the neonatal period in 37% of instances; (2) during infancy in 46%; (3) in childhood in 12% and (4) in later life in 5% [7]. Prenatal diagnosis is available for 46% of these conditions, and treatment for some 66%. The response to treatment has been discussed already and the treatment modalities used consisted of prevention of substrate accumulation, replacement of product and enzyme or coenzyme infusion. Gene insertion is under evaluation for a number of disorders. Non-specific and surgical procedures have also been used.

Screening is part of a diagnostic process, and as such it is inseparable from the confirmatory procedures, treatment, monitoring and long-term follow-up of the patient and the informed support of the family.

The psychological aspects of screening for both parents and child is often overlooked. Particularly important is the stress of awaiting confirmatory assays on provisionally positive screening tests, a problem which is compounded in the case of false-positive tests. Naturally, a false-negative test is of more lasting effect if there is ensuing serious disease. Also important is the effect on parents if they know that their child's disorder might have been prevented had screening been made available at an appropriate time.

The screening technologies vary depending on whether the test is for prenatal, neonatal or heterozygote detection, and whether they involve selective or non-selective programmes. However, there is considerable overlap with a logical process from simple spot tests to complex high technological investigations.

Prenatal detection of inherited metabolic disorders is based mainly on enzyme assay of cultured amniotic, fetal or chorionic villus cells, but may also include molecular biological techniques when the carrier status of the parents is known.

Furthermore, genetic variants can be identified as well as genetic compounds. Linkage analysis of restriction fragment length polymorphism (RFLP) markers has enabled gene mutations to be located. Polymerase chain reaction amplified DNA extracted from dried blood spots followed by allele specific hybridization has enabled many gene defects to be detected; the ultimate implication for individual genotyping has exceeded the most optimistic predictions. Such techniques may be used to confirm a diagnosis in an individual, but it is unlikely that they will be applicable for mass population screening in the near future due to the diversity of genotype variation for the majority of inherited disorders. Such procedures only become feasible as a screening test if a 95% level of carrier detection can be achieved; this would involve screening for a minimum of six mutations for cystic fibrosis despite the fact that the most common mutation (ΔF508) has a frequency of about 70% in western Europe.

The point should be made that, whatever the technology, the present situation is that a screening result is merely provisional, should only lead to provisional treatment and must be subject to definitive procedures on repeat specimens of serum, blood cells or other biological fluids or tissue. Non-selective neonatal screening has depended for a quarter of a century on the ever widening repertoire of the dried blood spot assays using either the semiquantitative microbiological Guthrie-type inhibition assays or thin layer amino acid chromatographic techniques. However, these are gradually being replaced by automated enzyme linked assays.

61.6.1 APPROACH TO NEONATAL SCREENING FOR METABOLIC DISORDERS

The approach is twofold.

1. The condition is expected on the basis of previous sibling history; it may be clearly defined or identified only in general or group terms.
2. The condition is unexpected and has been detected by non-selective mass screening.

The diagnosis of an inherited metabolic disorder depends on both the clinical and laboratory findings in (1), but only on the results of laboratory investigations in (2).

(a) Approach to screening in the sick infant

Clinical approach to sick infant screening

An acutely ill neonate is most likely to be suffering from sepsis, hypoxia, or haemorrhagic or other forms

Table 61.4 Identification of sick neonates and infants at risk of inherited metabolic disorders

History of neonatal illness or death in sibling
Initial symptom-free period
Change of diet precedes illness
Unresponsive to treatment of symptoms
More common causes ruled out

Initial symptoms
    Respiratory distress
    Diminished reflexes
    Hypotonia
    Vomiting
    Aversion to food
    Altering consciousness
    Seizures

Continuing symptoms
    Downward spiral
    Poor suction
    Coma
    Hypertonia
    Tonic and clonic movements

Table 61.5 Histological and histochemical screen for metabolic disorder

Tissue tested	Metabolic disease screened for:
Blood film	Gangliosidoses, lipidoses, Pompe's disease, Batten's disease, I-cell disease, mucopolysaccharidoses, Wolman's disease, abetalipoproteinaemia
Bone marrow	Lipidoses, gangliosidoses, mucopolysaccharidoses, cystinosis
Urine	Metachromatic leukodystrophy, Fabry's disease, mucopolysaccharidoses
Rectal biopsy	Gangliosidoses, Batten's disease, lipidoses

Also liver, brain, adrenal, hair, muscle, peripheral nerve, conjunctiva and skin

of shock, but the possibility of an inherited metabolic disorder should be borne in mind. Table 61.4 presents a list of clinical symptoms which should arouse suspicion and prompt appropriate investigation.

Laboratory approach to sick infant screening

The metabolic laboratory investigation of the sick neonate begins with broad, generally routine, eliminating procedures on blood and urine, and proceeds by stages to more sophisticated technology for definitive diagnosis. These latter investigations are generally only available in special centres.

Some infants with inherited metabolic disorders are not protected *in utero* so the disorder presents clinically shortly after birth, e.g. non-ketotic hyperglycinaemia and pyridoxine-dependent convulsions.

The approaches to the critically ill infant or unexpectedly dead infant, with suspected inherited metabolic disease, are similar. It is not possible to screen for all inherited metabolic conditions so the clinical ability to subdivide and select is essential. Even at autopsy it is difficult to anticipate so that it is best to ensure against all eventualities by correct sample collection techniques. Thus, the first step in the elucidation of an inherited disorder may well be careful autopsy examination of unexpected and unexplained deaths. Urine, plasma and cerebrospinal fluid should be collected. Snap-frozen liver and muscle samples should be collected as soon as possible for histology and histochemistry; if necessary needle aspiration will suffice. The rule is to fix some, freeze some and retain some for electron microscopy.

Skin is taken and fibroblasts cultured and stored for possible enzyme assay later.

It should not be forgotten that histological and histochemical procedures have a place in screening for inherited metabolic disorders, and are particularly useful techniques in the elucidation of some lysomal storage disorders (Table 61.5).

Molecular biological techniques are also available, such as fluorescent *in situ* hybridization, and these procedures can be done on stored tissue or paraffin sections.

(b) Approach to mass neonatal screening

A wide variety of disorders fulfil the criteria for screening using dried blood spot sampling, but for practical reasons they are reduced to only a few. The approach is dictated by the following factors:

- education and support groups;
- professional awareness;
- rapid communication of positive tests;
- unequivocal confirmatory testing on a second specimen;
- minimal hospitalization for confirmation and management, e.g. dietary;
- counselling parents regarding implications of positive tests and management;
- latency of positive diagnosis and phenotypic expression, e.g. α_1-antitrypsin deficiency and familial hypercholesterolaemia;
- if no therapy is available, e.g. Duchenne muscular dystrophy, neonatal screening is not deemed appropriate at the present time;
- parents and siblings should be tested;
- a protocol for baseline and follow-up studies should be available.

61.6.2 CHOICE OF CONDITIONS AND TESTS FOR NEONATAL SCREENING

The disorders sought in newborn screening programmes have been governed by a set of criteria which states that they should: (1) be treatable; (2) not be clinically apparent in the newborn; (3) require immediate therapy; and (4) have a reasonable frequency within the population to be tested (Chapter 63).

Before embarking on a screening programme a pilot study should have been carried out and the screening test evaluated by standard criteria, whereby it should reach the entire population at risk, be sufficiently sensitive to detect a high proportion of affected individuals, be sufficiently specific to detect few unaffected individuals, be safe and acceptable to patients, parents and medical attendants, be rapidly and safely transportable, and be relatively inexpensive.

The back-up services should be immediately available in order to provide discriminative confirmatory tests on a second specimen, appropriate treatment and long-term monitoring facilities.

61.6.3 SCREENING 'RECOMMENDATIONS'

On the basis of current information, conditions for neonatal screening should probably be limited to hyperphenylalaninaemia, congenital hypothyroidism, galactosaemia and cystic fibrosis.

Other conditions for which screening should be optional, depending on local frequencies, include maple syrup urine disease, medium chain acyl-CoA dehydrogenase deficiency, sickle-cell disease and glucose-6-phosphate dehydrogenase deficiency.

A group of conditions for which mass screening by dried blood spot is possible, but currently questionable, includes: congenital adrenal hyperplasia, Duchenne muscular dystrophy, α_1-antitrypsin deficiency and some of the urea cycle defects.

An example of a screening programme is given in Table 61.6. This programme for phenylketonuria began in the Republic of Ireland in 1966 [18] and was the first nationwide metabolic screening service. Subsequently screening for a number of other conditions was added. The screening laboratory is located within the service pathology department of a children's hospital which also provides confirmatory and follow-up procedures as well as high-risk neonatal screening.

61.6.4 FACTORS INFLUENCING NEONATAL SCREENING

- Medicolegal considerations: newborn screening is not governed by legislation in any of the European countries but is mandatory for certain conditions in some states of the USA.
- Confidentiality becomes an issue as the traditional patient and doctor relationship is altered.
- Missed cases: if there is 100% compliance with computerized surveillance, no baby should fail to have a screening sample taken and the screening laboratories should be in a position to check specimens submitted against birth registers. Sampling may be neglected or forgotten in home deliveries or when the baby becomes ill and is transferred from one unit or hospital to another.
- False-negative results may occur because of change of diet. Some proprietary diets are known to contain little or no methionine so that tests based on the presence of this metabolite in blood, e.g. for homocystinuria, may give a false-negative reaction. The practice of early hospital discharge may lead to false negative screening results because of lack of protein challenge to the infant's homoeostasis.

61.7 Phenylketonuria: a model for metabolic screening

Phenylketonuria is an autosomal recessive disorder caused by a deficiency of phenylalanine hydroxylase (PAH) activity. PKU was discovered 60 years ago by Folling [3] and mass newborn screening was instituted with the Guthrie test 30 years ago [19]. Considerable advances in the understanding of the disorder were made in between the two events, but the impact of cases detected by newborn screening on research into the biochemical pathogenesis of hyperphenylalaninaemia has been potent.

PKU is unique in screening in that it was the first inherited disorder for which mass newborn screening was undertaken and it gave rise to two secondary

Table 61.6 Results of national newborn screening in the Republic of Ireland until 1993

Condition	Commenced	No. screened	No. detected	Incidence
Phenylketonuria	1966	1 721 600	386	1: 4 460
Homocystinuria	1971	1 422 812	24	1: 59 284
Galactosaemia	1972	1 335 792	70	1: 19 083
Maple syrup urine disease	1972	1 351 915	12	1: 112 660
Congenital hypothyroidism	1979	878 528	251	1: 3 550

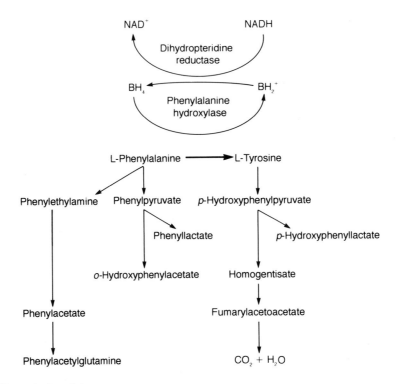

Figure 61.2 Metabolism of phenylalanine. BH_4 = tetrahydrobiopterin; BH_2 = dihydrobiopterin.

screening programmes, one for maternal PKU and the other for tetrahydrobiopterin deficiency. This latter is carried out as a screen within a screen on the original dried blood spot for all cases with hyperphenylalaninaemia [20]. Classical PKU results from severe deficiency of PAH activity to levels less than 1% of normal. The classical disorder has virtually disappeared as a clinical entity, following preclinical detection and treatment. However, problem areas have continued to arise and cause concern.

- Early termination of dietary treatment has been followed by clinical regression in some individuals.
- Between 0.5 and 3% of cases with hyperphenylalaninaemias detected by primary screening did not respond to dietary treatment. These individuals either underwent severe deterioration and death, or responded to treatment with neurotransmitter amine precursors (pterins) [21].
- Other variant forms did not require so rigorous a regimen of phenylalanine restriction, suggesting a wide spectrum of atypical variants, probably allelomorphic.
- Female patients gave birth to offspring who had intrauterine growth retardation and microcephaly, were mentally handicapped and had various severe congenital malformations. This occurred despite careful dietary control before and after conception; the severity of the congenital malformations

appeared to be directly related to the maternal plasma phenylalanine levels [22]. The milder variant forms of maternal PKU can have less severe teratogenic effects than those of the classical forms.

Figure 61.2 is a simplified schema of the metabolic pathway by which phenylalanine is normally converted to tyrosine but undergoes alternative catabolism to ketoacids when there is deficient PAH function. However, PAH is a complex enzyme which requires tetrahydrobiopterin as a co-factor. This co-factor is common to two other pathways with a crossover effect on tyrosine hydroxylase and tryptophan hydroxylase; consequently there are inter-related consequences of derangement of each of the three pathways.

61.7.1 MOLECULAR BASIS OF PKU

The PAH gene has been sequenced and mapped to the long arm of chromosome 12, many mutations being associated with RFLP haplotypes [23]. Eight different mutations account for approximately 60% of the PKU cases, the majority of the patients being compound heterozygotes, inheriting different mutations from their parents [24]. Recent evidence suggests a correlation between the genotype and the phenotype, some mutations being associated with lower PAH activities and thus a more severe form of the disorder [24]. RFLP haplotype analysis has facilitated population studies and the postulation of 'founder effects' and the spread of the PKU mutations [25].

61.8 Screening for cystic fibrosis

Cystic fibrosis is the most common inherited disorder in people of north-western European descent, having a carrier status of 1 in 25 individuals. Screening programmes have been established measuring immunoreactive trypsin concentrations on dried blood spots [26]. However, this method has resulted in a high false-positive rate, with a consequent high recall rate, resulting in increased parent anxiety. A second-line mutation analysis technique identifying the presence of the most common mutation, ΔF508, which is present in up to 70% in some populations, has significantly reduced the number of false-positive results, but has resulted in the identification of the carrier status as the allele is present in about 95% of the cases. A sweat test is then required to confirm the diagnosis. The screen for cystic fibrosis remains controversial [27], but the outcome of trials involving methods of gene insertion may change this outlook.

61.9 Disorders of fatty acid metabolism

Disorders of β-oxidation of fat metabolism, particularly medium chain acyl-CoA dehydrogenase deficiency, are now well recognized and may present acutely with non-ketotic hypoglycaemia and encephalopathy; other features include hepatomegaly similar to Reye's syndrome, sudden infant death and 'near miss' sudden infant death [28]. Because of the high incidence of the disorder in some countries, the possible poor outcome and the good response to treatment involving high carbohydrate intake and the avoidance of fasting, newborn screening for medium chain acyl-CoA dehydrogenase deficiency has been suggested [29]. The gene for this enzyme has been characterized and up to 85% of patients with the deficiency are homozygous for a single mutation. DNA analysis of dry blood spots has been proposed, although not all affected individuals will be identified. Other possible tests include the measurement of octanoyl carnitine or cis-4-decenoic acid, but both methods require sophisticated technology such as gas chromatography mass spectroscopy [30].

However, the application of automated tandem mass spectroscopy is under development for the detection of disorders of amino acids and acylcarnitines from dry blood spots [31]; the latter may occasionally be associated with a dilated cardiomyopathy [32]. This technique has the potential for mass screening of such diverse inherited conditions as PKU, maple syrup urine disease, urea cycle disorders, methylmalonic and propionic acidurias, as well as the fat oxidation defects.

61.10 Cost versus benefit

Delineation of what constitutes benefit has always proved difficult as many costs are lost in general laboratory and hospital budgets [31].

Prenatal detection is cost-effective in that the birth of a seriously disadapted individual is avoided and maintenance and treatment costs are thus precluded. There are many intangibles involved which make objective assessments of the effects of prenatal genetic screening difficult. For newborn congenital hypothyroidism and PKU screening programmes, with average frequencies of 1 in 4000 and 1 in 10 000 worldwide, the salvage of individuals from institutionalization over a predicted 30 years has been seen as cost-beneficial. However, long-term effects, such as impaired intellectual and social achievements, were not then being considered, nor was the cost of maternal PKU anticipated. Recent work has also shown that there is curtailed life span in many untreated inborn errors of metabolism [7]. Less certainty attends the benefits of salvaging patients with rare disorders such as maple syrup urine disease or tyrosinosis. Since the tests for these are easily incorporated in established dried blood spot programmes, there should be little additional detection cost. However, so many cases of transient tyrosinaemia have been detected and the treatment of maple syrup urine disease is so expensive that such unanticipated effects now need to be taken into account. In the ultimate analysis the attainment parameters must include social adaptation and productivity, normal reproducibility, as well as the more conventional quotients of physical and mental attainment.

61.11 Quality assurance of analytical methods

Quality control measures for the screening and confirmatory procedures are an essential component for ensuring accuracy and continued efficiency.

It is important that all laboratories which undertake the more sophisticated assays associated with antenatal screening or the confirmatory procedures in neonatal screening and those for primary diagnosis in cytogenetics should be subject to intensive quality control measures. Enzyme assay procedures for extremely rare conditions pose a special problem in quality control. One solution is to nominate a few supraregional centres for particular (rare) disorders, perhaps one or two each for western Europe and Asia and three or four for North America, thus increasing the number of analyses performed and the information gained for enumeration and research.

International and regional advisory groups with broad medical, laboratory, administrative and legislative representation have already been established for the purpose of formulating screening policy.

It is clear that the demand for early screening of a great number of new disorders will increase and this potential already exists. Pressure will come from lay groups as well as from medical sources. It is therefore imperative that there should be objective evaluation of each disorder in terms of the need for and advisability of screening.

61.12 Computerization and automation

The earliest development in the automation of screening came with the introduction of automatic punching machines for the distribution of dried blood discs on agar trays. Automated scanning with computerized reporting were added later.

The Guthrie-type tests, which have served so well for so long, and amino acid chromatographic techniques will gradually be replaced by quantitative fully automated enzymatic assays. Some of these techniques may themselves be replaced by fully automated tandem gas chromatography mass spectroscopy.

However, caution must be exercised as technological advances may outstrip the clinicians' ability to treat some conditions appropriately. Consideration must also be given to the consequences of increasing the mutant gene pool.

References

1. Garrod, A. (1908) Inborn errors of metabolism. The Croonian lectures. *Lancet*, ii, 1, 73, 142, 214.
2. Ballantyne, J. (1902, 1904) *Antenatal Pathology and Hygiene*, vol. 1 Foetus and vol. 2 Embryo, W. Green, Edinburgh.
3. Folling, A. (1934) Uber Ausscheidung von Phenylbrenztraubensaure in den Harn als Stoffwechselanomalie in Verbindung mit Imbezillitat. *Z. Physiol. Chem.* 227, 169–76.
4. McKusick, V. (1992) *Mendelian Inheritance in Man*, 8th edn, Johns Hopkins University Press, Baltimore.
5. Clayton, B.E. (1980) Repercussions of screening, in *Inborn Errors of Metabolism in Humans* (eds F. Cockburn and R. Gitzelmann), MTP Press, Lancaster, pp. 255–65.
6. Kornberg, A. (1977) Pathology, pathologists and the new biology (editorial). *Arch. Pathol. Lab. Med.*, 101, 397–99.
7. Costa, T., Scriver, C. and Childs, B. (1985) The effect of mendelian disease in human health: a measurement. *Am. J. Med. Genet.*, 21, 231–42.
8. Hayes, A., Costa, T., Scriver, C. and Childs, B. (1985) The effect of mendelian disease on human health. II: Response to treatment. *Am. J. Med. Genet.*, 21, 243–55.
9. Allen, J.T., Gillett, M.G., Holton, J.B. *et al.* (1980) Evidence of galactosaemia *in utero. Lancet*, i, 603.
10. Barnes, N. (1985) Screening for congenital hypothyroidism: the first decade. *Arch. Dis. Child.*, 60, 587–92.
11. Nadler, H. (1968) Patterns of enzyme development utilizing cultivated human fetal cells derived by amniotic fluid. *Biochem. Genet.*, 2, 119–26.
12. Galjaard, H., Mekes, M., De Josselin, J.E. *et al.* (1973) A method for rapid prenatal diagnosis of glycogenosis II (Pompe's disease). *Clin. Chim. Acta*, 49, 361–75.
13. Weatherall, D.J. (1985) *The New Genetics and Clinical Practice*, 2nd edn, Oxford University Press, Oxford.
14. Boue, A. and Gallano, P. (1984) A collaborative study of the segregation of inherited chromosome structural rearrangements in 1356 prenatal diagnoses. *Prenat. Diagn.*, 4, 45–67 (special issue).
15. Mikkelsen, M. (1982) Down's syndrome: current state of cytogenetic epidemiology, in *Human Genetics*, Part B Medical Aspects, Alan R. Liss, NY, pp. 297–309.
16. Macri, J. N., Kasturi, B.E., Krantz, B.S. *et al.* (1990) Maternal serum Down syndrome screening: free beta protein is a more effective marker than human chorionic gonadotropin. *Am. J. Obstet. Gynecol.*, 163, 1248–53.
17. Ermans, A. and Lafontaines, A. (1976) *Prospectives for a Common Action in Pre and Neonatal Screenings of Inborn Metabolic Disease and of Chromosome Abnormalities*. Proceedings of a Symposium of the Council of Medical Research and Council of European Communities, October 4–5, Brussels.
18. Cahalane, S.F. (1969) Phenylketonuria: mass screening of newborns in Ireland. *Arch. Dis. Child.*, 43, 141–44.
19. Guthrie, R. and Susi, A. (1963) A simple phenylalanine method for detecting phenylketonuria in large populations of newborn infants. *Pediatrics*, 32, 338–43.
20. Leeming, R., Barford, P., Blaire, J. and Smith, I. (1984) Blood spots on Guthrie cards can be used for inherited tetrahydrobiopterin deficiency screening in hyperphenylalaninaemic infants. *Arch. Dis. Child.*, 59, 58–61.
21. Smith, I., Clayton, B. and Wolff, O. (1975) A new variant of phenylketonuria with a progressive neurological illness unresponsive to phenylalanine restriction. *Lancet*, i, 1108–1111.
22. Levy, H.L. and Waisbren, S.E. (1983) Effects of untreated maternal phenylketonuria and hyperphenylalaninaemia on the fetus. *N. Engl. J. Med.*, 309, 1269–75.
23. Woo, S.L.C., Lidsky, A.S., Guttler, F. *et al.* (1983) Cloned human phenylalanine hydroxylase gene allows prenatal diagnosis and carrier detection of classical phenylketonuria. *Nature*, 306, 151–55.
24. Okano, Y., Eisensmith, R.C., Guttler, F. *et al.* (1991) Molecular basis of phenotype heterogeneity in phenylketonuria. *N. Engl. J. Med.*, 324, 1232–38.
25. Woo, S.L.C., Okano, Y., Dasovich, M. *et al.* (1991) Molecular population dynamics of phenylketonuria among Caucasians: multiple founding populations in Europe. *Am. J. Hum. Genet.*, 51, 1355–65.
26. Bowling, F.G., Rylatt, D.B., Bunch, R.J. *et al.* (1987) Monoclonal antibody-based enzyme immunoassay for trypsinogen in neonatal screening for cystic fibrosis. *Lancet*, i, 826–27.
27. Wilcken, B. (1993) Newborn screening for cystic fibrosis: its evolution and a review of the current situation (review). *Screening*, 2, 43–62.
28. Anonymous (1986) Sudden infant death and inherited disorders of fat oxidation. *Lancet*, i, 1073–75.
29. Gregersen, N., Andresen, B.S., Bross, P. *et al.* (1991) Molecular characterization of MCAD deficiency. *Hum. Genet.*, 86, 545–51.
30. Millington, D., Terada N. and Chace, D.N. (1992) *Diagnosis of Metabolic Diseases by Tandem Mass Spectrometry*. Proceedings of an International Conference on Biology and Mass Spectrometry (ed. T. Matsuo), San-ei, Kyoto, pp. 94–595.
31. Komrower, G. (1990) Structure of the system required to handle problems in the European Community related to inborn errors of metabolism, in *Neonatal Screening for Inborn Errors of Metabolism* (eds H. Bickel, R. Guthrie and G. Hammsen), Springer, Berlin, pp. 281–83.
32. Stanley, C.A. (1987) New genetic defects in mitochondrial fatty acid oxidation and carnitine deficiency. *Adv. Pediatr.*, 34, 59–88.

62 MATERNAL SERUM SCREENING

R.E. Falk

62.1 Introduction

The development of a battery of screening procedures which would identify women at higher risk of bearing a malformed or otherwise abnormal child has long been a goal of pediatric and obstetrical care providers. Identification of at-risk couples or individuals on the basis of ethnicity is well-established for conditions such as Tay–Sachs disease and sickle-cell anemia. However, such an approach does not provide a useful basis for the detection of most common disorders. Provision of specific prenatal diagnostic testing to couples who have already had one affected child is an effective means of decreasing recurrence risk within families but has little effect on the incidence of the condition in the general population. Similarly, when prenatal diagnosis is offered to pregnant women solely on the basis of advanced maternal age, which is known to correlate with increased risk for Down syndrome and other chromosome disorders, the procedures can detect only about 20% of Down syndrome fetuses even with 100% utilization by eligible women [1]. Since many women do not elect to undergo such testing, age-based programs detect only a small proportion of fetuses with Down syndrome and other chromosomal disorders.

In keeping with its public health role, the World Health Organization (WHO) defined screening as the identification within a low-risk population of individuals at higher risk for the occurrence of a given condition [2]. The WHO guidelines for screening programs outlined in the section on neonatal screening (Chapter 63) are equally applicable to maternal screening. Briefly, in order to justify screening one must define a problem of sufficient importance in which identification of an affected fetus may prevent or ameliorate symptoms. Screening tests should be voluntary, readily available, rapid, inexpensive, reproducible, and should have adequate sensitivity and specificity to provide an acceptable cost–benefit ratio. Accuracy and reliability of laboratory results must be guaranteed, preferably by means of centralized regional laboratories and regular participation in quality assurance programs. Specific diagnostic procedures which can readily distinguish affected from normal fetuses must be available to all individuals with positive screening tests. Finally, effective education, patient counseling and medical management services must be in place prior to the implementation of large scale screening programs.

The use of maternal serum markers in the detection of fetal abnormality has largely been confined to two major categories. The association of elevated maternal blood levels of a fetal blood α-globulin, α-fetoprotein (AFP), with open (not skin-covered) neural tube defects (NTDs) has provided a basis for successful general population NTD screening programs in many Western countries. The more recent observation that low maternal serum AFP (MSAFP) levels predict fetal chromosome anomalies has produced numerous studies in which MSAFP levels and maternal age have been correlated to provide a rationale for the detection of Down syndrome. Other maternal markers have recently been identified. Used alone or in concert with MSAFP, these markers greatly increase the efficacy of maternal screening for Down syndrome. This chapter will focus on the development and application of maternal screening for NTDs and Down syndrome, and will also present data related to the coincidental identification of pregnancies at high risk for other adverse outcomes.

62.2 Neural tube defects

62.2.1 DEFINITION AND SCOPE OF THE PROBLEM

Neural tube defects comprise the second most common group of malformations after congenital heart defects. NTDs result from defective primary neurulation in which the neural groove fails to fuse dorsally to form a neural tube by the end of the fourth week of gestation. Defective anterior neural tube closure results in anencephaly because of resultant degeneration of the unfused forebrain and incomplete development of the calvarium. Meningomyelocele (spina bifida cystica)

Diseases of the Fetus and Newborn, 2nd edn, Edited by G.B. Reed, A.E. Claireaux and F. Cockburn. Published in 1995 by Chapman & Hall, London. ISBN 0 412 39160 0

results from faulty closure of the more caudal portion of the neural tube [3]. Of note, a recent study in a mouse model found initial closure of the neural tube with subsequent rupture through a necrotic roof plate generating a spina bifida and meningomyelocele [4]. Open NTDs comprise the group with neural elements or meninges exposed to the amniotic fluid or covered by a thin membrane, which may rupture at delivery. Closed defects are skin covered and account for only 5–10% of meningomyeloceles. Many meningoceles, all encephaloceles, and most minor distal lesions are skin covered as well.

Problems associated with NTDs include paralysis and sensory loss below the level of the lesion, hydrocephaly, seizures, mental retardation, bowel and bladder dysfunction, chronic urinary tract infections, sexual dysfunction, and scoliosis with consequent cardiac and respiratory compromise [5,6]. Surviving children often require multiple surgical procedures, physical and occupational therapy and special education. Thus, this group of malformations accounts for a significant proportion of fetal and pediatric mortality, morbidity and health costs. One estimate of the financial burden of medical/surgical care for American spina bifida patients exceeded $200 million in 1985 dollars [7].

62.2.2 ETIOLOGY OF NTDS

The etiology of NTDs is unclear. Numerous environmental factors have been implicated including low parity, low socioeconomic status, poor nutrition, potato blight, maternal vitamin or zinc deficiency, maternal diabetes, maternal hyperthermia, and prenatal exposure to ethanol, valproic acid or carbamazepine [8]. Seasonal variation in NTD incidence has caused speculation regarding infectious etiology. Ethnic and geographic differences are well known. Although the NTD incidence is 1–2:1000 in the USA and Canada, there is a significant excess of cases on the east coast and in southern Appalachia. The incidence is significantly higher in the UK and Ireland, particularly in some north-west regions where NTD incidence approaches 1%. NTDs are relatively uncommon in Blacks, Scandinavians and some other groups [9]. Consanguinity may play a role, but genetic influence is not clear-cut. Recurrence risk is 3–5% in the offspring of an affected parent or the siblings of an affected child, but rises to 10–15% when there are two first-degree relatives (Table 62.1). These factors, as well as data from twin studies, suggest a multifactorial mode of inheritance [9]. Observations in the curly tail mouse confirm the interaction of environmental factors with an autosomal recessive locus for spinal dysraphism in that species [10].

Table 62.1 Recurrence risk of NTDS

Affected	Risk to fetus (%)	
Sibling	2–3	(US data)
	5	(UK data)
Parent	4–5	
Two siblings	10	
Parent and sibling	10–15	

Combined data from various published sources

62.2.3 PREVENTION OF NTDS

Efforts toward primary prevention of NTDs have centered on dietary supplementation with vitamins and trace metals. Despite some controversy, the aggregate data now implicate folic acid deficiency [11] or unusual folic acid metabolism in the pathogenesis of NTDs and favors periconceptional supplementation. Although the minimum effective dosage remains unclear, periconceptional folic acid supplementation with up to 4 mg/day may result in a 50–80% reduction in the recurrence of NTD [12–17]. A recent prospective study in Hungary demonstrated a substantial overall reduction in birth defects and a highly significant decrease in NTDs in offspring of women supplemented with 0.8 mg/day of folic acid [18]. A subsequent controlled trial suggested a 60% reduction in occurrence of NTD in association with a daily periconceptional folic acid dosage of 0.4 mg/day [19]. The Centers for Disease Control and other agencies now recommend that all fertile American women of child-bearing age consume 0.4 mg of folic acid daily as a supplement or in fortified foods [20,21].

62.3 AFP screening for neural tube defects

62.3.1 α-FETOPROTEIN

α-Fetoprotein is a phase-specific antigen which is abundant in fetal blood, liver, intestine and neural tissues. Belonging to the class of α-globulins, AFP is synthesized initially in the yolk sac. Subsequently, most AFP is produced in the fetal liver, but there is a small intestinal contribution as well [22,23]. AFP has a molecular weight of about 70 000 Da and considerable sequence homology with albumin [24]. Despite evidence of hormone binding, low antigenicity in maternal serum and immunosuppressive properties, its major biologic function in humans remains unclear [22]. AFP is detectable in fetal tissue as early as 4 weeks, peaks in the mid-trimester, decreases near term, and rapidly disappears after delivery. Amniotic fluid AFP (AFAFP) steadily increases during early pregnancy, reaching maximum levels at 13–14 weeks. AFAFP levels decline subsequently, maintaining a near linear relationship with gestational age from 14–22 weeks. In contrast, MSAFP levels, which are measured in nanograms, increase steadily during the same period, becoming widely scattered thereafter [22,23]. As AFAFP occurs in microgram amounts, there is a gradient between amniotic fluid and maternal serum. The MSAFP is approximately 250 times lower than AFAFP during the mid-trimester. Refinements in AFP determination led to the development of an inexpensive, rapid, reproducible radioimmunoassay system which is commercially available as a test kit. Nevertheless, variations in standardized normative data and single sample analysis among different laboratories prevents useful comparison of values expressed in standard units and standard deviation. Therefore, for ease and accuracy of comparison, MSAFP values are generally expressed in multiples of the median (MoM).

62.3.2 ELEVATION OF AFAFP IN NTD PREGNANCIES

In 1972 Brock and Sutcliffe first reported the association of elevated AFAFP with anencephaly and spina bifida [25]. This finding was rapidly confirmed in large prospective studies in the UK and the USA [26], leading to the implementation of AFAFP determination as a standard analysis for all women undergoing amniocentesis, regardless of the indication for the procedure. The Second Report of the UK Collaborative Study presented data representing 385 pregnancies complicated by fetal NTD, including 222 with anencephaly, 152 with open spina bifida and 11 with encephalocele, as well as 13 105 singleton pregnancies without fetal NTD. Using cut-offs at progressively higher MoM for more advanced gestational age ranges, the overall detection efficiency was 98.2% for anencephaly and 97.6% for open spina bifida. The corrected false-positive rate (excluding pregnancies complicated by other major malformations or ending in miscarriage) was 0.48% [26]. However, the finding of elevated AFAFP in the absence of ultrasound-detectable malformation, and the occurrence of blood-contaminated amniotic fluid specimens posed serious problems of interpretation.

62.3.3 CONFIRMATORY TESTING FOR NTDS

Chubb and colleagues' [29] observation of neural origin of a specific acetylcholinesterase (AChE) isozyme led to the development of a qualitative gel electrophoresis technique for evaluation of amniotic fluid AChE [30]. Numerous studies established the efficacy of this assay as a confirmatory test for NTDs in cases of elevated AFAFP [28,31,32]. Moreover, the density and sharpness of the AChE band differed in amniotic fluid from

pregnancies complicated by NTD, ventral wall defects, twins and fetal demise [28,33,34]. Finally, the AChE assay usually discriminated between elevated AFP due to NTD and/or other defects and elevations secondary to fetal blood contamination of the amniotic fluid [32,35,36]. Implementation of quantitative monoclonal immunoassay systems for AChE may provide a higher open NTD detection rate than AFAFP [37], and may offer a more efficient primary test, particularly in situations where detailed fetal ultrasound evaluation is not available [38]. Currently, the use of AFAFP testing, implementation of AChE determination on samples with elevated AFAFP using a relatively conservative cut-off (2.0 MoM), and the availability of detailed ultrasound assessment of the fetus allows accurate diagnosis of open NTD in >99% of pregnancies in which amniocentesis is performed, and 100% detection of anencephaly in those pregnancies.

62.3.4 POPULATION SCREENING FOR NTDs

The availability of accurate prenatal diagnostic testing for NTDs suggested the possibility of screening relatively low-risk populations by means of MSAFP determination. The UK Collaborative Study Group evaluated the efficacy of MSAFP screening in 18 684 normal singleton and 163 normal twin pregnancies as well as 301 singleton pregnancies affected with a fetal NTD. They concluded that the ideal timing of MSAFP screening was from 16 to 18 weeks of gestation, and found no benefit of first trimester screening [39]. This multicenter trial determined that the distribution curves of MSAFP values from normal, spina bifida and anencephalic pregnancies overlapped such that the three groups could not be distinguished absolutely at any specific cut-off level. The curve for anencephaly was significantly higher than the spina bifida curve, and values for twin gestations were higher than those from singleton pregnancies, such that a separate distribution curve or different cut-off level was required for interpretation of MSAFP values in twins [39].

62.3.5 EFFICACY OF NTD SCREENING

With a cut-off level (action line) of 95% of the normal range, MSAFP screening detected nearly 90% of affected cases in the UK Collaborative Study population. Raising the cut-off level resulted in a lower detection rate for NTDs, especially spina bifida, but also lowered the false-positive rate. Thus, an action line could be selected arbitrarily in order to obtain acceptable sensitivity and specificity of the procedure (Figure 62.1). Cut-offs of 2, 2.5 and 3 MoM resulted in detection rates of open spina bifida of 91%, 79% and 70%, respectively, while overall NTD detection rate was 83%, 69% and 60% for those three cut-offs. Similarly, the false-

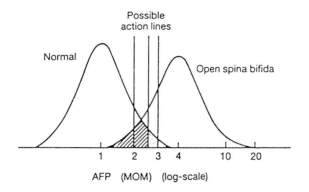

Figure 62.1 Overlap of maternal serum AFP distributions for normal and open spina bifida pregnancies, indicating the likely effects of the selection of action lines at 2, 2.5 and 3 MoM. (Reproduced with the permission of the author from Brock [40].)

Table 62.2 NTD detection rate (%) at varying action lines [After Ref. 40]

	2.0 MoM	2.5 MoM	3.0 MoM
Anencephaly	90.0	88.0	84.0
Open spina bifida	91.0	79.0	70.0
All spina bifida	83.0	69.0	60.0
False-positive rate	7.7	3.6	1.6

positive rates for those cut-offs were 7.7, 3.6 and 1.6% (Table 62.2) [39].

Numerous later studies confirmed the efficacy of MSAFP screening and resulted in adjustment of cut-off values or calculation of risk for a variety of maternal factors, including body weight [41,42], race [42,43] and presence of diabetes mellitus [44,45], which is associated with a tenfold increase in NTDs and a significantly lower (about 40%) MSAFP distribution curve in the mid-trimester of pregnancy [45]. In an early report of a relatively high-risk population in South Wales, in which 70% of eligible women elected MSAFP testing, detection rates for open NTD were 79.6% and 77.5% for cut-off levels at the 90th and 95th centiles, respectively. However, while all detected anencephalic fetuses were terminated, only 11 of 17 open spina bifida fetuses were terminated. The report suggested that maximal efficacy for general screening programs was unlikely to exceed 65% [46]. Screening a lower-risk American population with a cut-off at 2.5 MoM, Burton, Sowers and Nelson reported a detection rate of 83%. Of their screen-positive patients, 1.2% were offered amniocentesis and 10% of these women had a fetus with an NTD. Milunsky *et al.* reported results of screening 21 000 non-diabetic and 442 diabetic women. Detection rates were 85.7% for

anencephaly and 62.5% for spina bifida (open and closed defects). The report emphasized the importance of an interdisciplinary team in the evaluation and management of screened women, as well as the benefits of genetic counseling. A multicenter study of 28 062 women in Denmark resulted in amniocentesis in 0.9% of women screened. The authors stressed the importance of ultrasound in the detection of NTDs in this group, and also emphasized the presence of other significant abnormalities in pregnancies associated with elevated MSAFP [48].

62.3.6 COST–BENEFIT ASSESSMENT

In virtually all of the voluntary studies of low-risk populations, screening was accepted by 50–60% of eligible women. Loss of normal fetuses through misclassification was rare, and spontaneous miscarriage after amniocentesis was not increased compared with high AFP controls [49]. Similarly, identification of relatively benign meningoceles was generally avoided as these lesions tend to be skin covered and associated with normal MSAFP values. A combined study of over 50 000 women in Germany underscored the feasibility and acceptance of AFP screening in low-risk populations and also stressed the positive cost–benefit ratio in terms of both economic and human factors [50]. Data from British Columbia, where NTD incidence was 0.94 per 1000 livebirths, yielded a cost–benefit ratio of 1:1.6 [51]. Milunsky and Alpert estimated the benefit to be in excess of 10:1 in purely economic terms [52]. Nevertheless, many authors have questioned the economic benefit of screening low-risk populations for NTD since anencephaly is lethal, overall NTD incidence appears to be diminishing, and more aggressive obstetrical management combined with newer surgical techniques may improve the prognosis for patients with open spina bifida [53,54]. Some have also raised concerns about the anxiety associated with screening in general, and with elevated MSAFP results. Of note, Burton, Sowers and Nelson [47] reported decreased anxiety and improvement in attitude toward pregnancy in a population of women screened with MSAFP compared with a group of unscreened women. Even in a very low-risk Chinese population, in which anencephaly is the predominant NTD, the potential value of providing reassurance to the majority of participant women and alternatives to the group with detected malformations seemed to justify the cost of mass screening [55].

62.4 Other sources of elevated MSAFP

62.4.1 FETAL ABNORMALITIES

In addition to multiple gestation and NTD, elevated MSAFP may reflect a variety of adverse fetal or maternal conditions, as well as other fetal malformations. The association of ventral wall defects [56,57] and congenital nephrosis [58,59] with elevated AFAFP suggested the possibility that these conditions would also result in elevated MSAFP levels. The latter observation led to implementation of an effective MSAFP screening program in Finland where the birth prevalence of congenital nephrosis is as high as 1:2600 in some districts [60]. In that population, MSAFP screening for nephrosis is more efficacious than screening for NTDs, which occur at relatively low frequency. While virtually every large MSAFP screening program has reported cases of gastroschisis and omphalocele among the fetuses identified because of an elevated MSAFP level, the relative frequency of detection of NTDs versus ventral wall defects varies from about 5:1 to greater than 10:1, depending on the population incidence of NTDs versus ventral wall defects, which are significantly less prevalent. However, the distribution curves for MSAFP in pregnancies complicated by fetal ventral wall defects tend to be higher than those for NTD pregnancies. Therefore, the detection rate is quite high for this group of malformations, particularly when combined with careful ultrasound assessment of the fetus.

Other malformations associated with elevated AFP include Meckel–Gruber syndrome, which presents with ventral wall defects and posterior encephalocele [61,62], urethral agenesis [63], renal agenesis [64], cystic adenomatoid malformation of the lung [65], and a variety of other defects including hydrocephaly, sacrococcygeal teratoma, exstrophy of the bladder or cloaca, and some congenital lesions of the skin (Table 62.3) [66]. The observation of elevated AFAFP in association with nuchal bleb or frank cystic hygroma in the Turner syndrome fetus [67] was quickly confirmed in multiple reports of AFAFP and MSAFP screening. Other chromosomal disorders which may present with elevated MSAFP include triploidy [68] and trisomies 13 and 18, usually associated with ventral wall defects, NTDs, or both. Virtually every large series reports occasional instances of XXX and XXY fetuses in pregnancies with increased MSAFP. The mechanism for this association is unclear, raising the possibility of coincidental concordance of two common events. Abnormalities of the umbilical cord, membranes, or placenta may lead to increased MSAFP [69,70] Finally, outcome of pregnancy is particularly poor in pregnancies with both elevated MSAFP and oligohydramnios [71,72].

62.4.2 EXTRAFETAL CAUSES

Even small fetomaternal bleeds can result in significant, transient elevation of MSAFP [73]. This poses a major interpretation problem which only rarely remains un-

Table 62.3 Selected abnormalities associated with elevated MSAFP

Fetoplacental factors

Neural tube defects
Central nervous system malformation; hydrocephaly
Omphalocele; gastroschisis
Exstrophy of bladder or cloaca
Congenital nephrosis
Renal agenesis, dysgenesis; polycystic kidneys
Urethral agenesis; obstructive uropathy
Sacrococcygeal teratoma
Cystic hygroma; nuchal bleb
Cystic adenomatoid malformation of lung
Congenital skin defects (variable)

Fetomaternal hemorrhage
Placental, membrane or cord defects
Infection (? parvovirus)

Maternal factors

Hepatoma; germ cell or gastrointestinal tumors
Hepatitis; other liver disease
Immunodeficiency disorders
Hypertension
Hereditary persistence of AFP

resolved following AFAFP and AChE assessment, as well as detailed fetal ultrasound. Maternal hepatoma, germ cell tumors, primary gastrointestinal tract tumors, liver metastases and a number of non-malignant hepatic diseases have been associated with elevated MSAFP [74]. An autosomal dominant condition, hereditary persistence of AFP, may result in false-positive elevated MSAFP levels in otherwise uncomplicated pregnancies [75]. The observation of elevated MSAFP prior to onset of hydrops fetalis suggested that MSAFP may also be a marker for fetal aplastic crisis in pregnancies complicated by parvovirus infection [76]. Maternal immunodeficiency disorders such as ataxia telangiectasia and adenosine deaminase deficiency have been associated with elevated blood AFP levels [77]. Finally, an association between elevated MSAFP and maternal hypertension has been noted by several groups [78,79], while low MSAFP has been associated with complications in hypertensive pregnancy in one study [80]. A report of third trimester MSAFP values in hypertensive women suggested that elevated MSAFP may be a sensitive indicator of fetal distress and impending fetal demise in pre-eclampsia. [81]

62.4.3 SIGNIFICANCE OF ELEVATED MSAFP

As NTD screening programs have become standard in numerous Western countries, it has become evident that there are many unexpected benefits, including identification of twin pregnancies as well as those at risk for adverse outcome unrelated to NTDs. However, the major concern of the pregnant woman with an elevated mid-trimester MSAFP value is the immediate likelihood of finding a fetal NTD by ultrasound or amniocentesis. Assuming a birth prevalence of 1:1000 for open spina bifida, Wald and Cuckle [82] note that a cut-off of ≥2.5 MoM will result in detection of 75% of open spina bifida and a somewhat lower (65%) detection rate when closed defects are included. The false-positive rate is 3.8%, and the approximate risk of open spina bifida in a woman who tests positive (i.e. MSAFP value ≥2.5 MoM) is 1:44. However, the true risk varies with the population incidence and MSAFP level (i.e. greater risk at successively higher MoM) and risk calculations should be adjusted accordingly.

62.4.4   INCREASED FETAL WASTAGE

As early as 1975, Seppala [83] noted an association between elevated MSAFP and *in utero* fetal demise. In a series of 51 women with second or third trimester fetal demise, 30 (59%) had significantly elevated MSAFP values. Subsequently, Wald and co-workers reported a greater than sixfold increase in miscarriage risk in women with second trimester MSAFP values at or above 2.8 MoM compared with women with lower values [84]. Although this study suggests that elevated MSAFP predicted recent or impending fetal demise, an assessment of data from the California MSAFP Screening Program confirmed a dramatic increase in late fetal loss when elevated second trimester MSAFP remained unexplained after ultrasound and amniocentesis. In this case-control study, the relative risk for fetal death was 10.4 for women with MSAFP ≥3 MoM and 2.4 when MSAFP was in the range of 2.0–2.9 MoM (95% confidence) [85]. A similar association of increasing adverse outcome rates with increasingly elevated MSAFP levels was described by Robinson, Grau and Crandall [86] who reported later loss rates of 5% and 11% in women with normal amniocentesis and ultrasound whose MSAFP levels were 3.0–3.9 MoM and ≥4.0 MoM, respectively. Overall, adverse outcome rate was 38% in women with unexplained MSAFP elevation ≥2.5 MoM, while adverse outcome affected 45% of pregnancies with MSAFP ≥4.0 MoM and 86% of pregnancies with values ≥6.0 MoM.

62.4.5   LOW BIRTH WEIGHT

The earliest reports of low birth weight associated with elevated MSAFP described an average reduction of birth weight of 357 g in 94 singleton non-NTD fetuses whose mothers had mid-trimester MSAFP of ≥3.0 MoM [87]. Other investigators described low birth weight associated with prematurity and intrauterine growth retardation [88], and with placental abruption [89]. Possible

explanations for the association of low birth weight and elevated MSAFP include various types of placental pathology, particularly chronic villitis, vascular lesions such as infarction or intervillous hemorrhage, and consequent development of vascular lakes [90,91]. Salafia *et al.* [91] suggested that chronic villitis may represent an inflammatory response to viral infection or an immunologic process which could recur in subsequent pregnancies.

62.5   Screening for chromosomal abnormalities

62.5.1   LOW MSAFP

The chance observation of an undetectable AFP level in the serum of a woman who delivered a trisomy 18 infant led to a retrospective study in which Merkatz and associates [92] analyzed mid-trimester levels in 43 mothers of infants with autosomal trisomies. Excluding two cases with concurrent NTDs, they found a dramatic and highly significant decrease in the MSAFP distribution compared with the distribution curve of controls. A larger retrospective study verified that the median mid-trimester MSAFP level in 61 Down syndrome pregnancies was 0.72 MoM for 36 652 normal singleton pregnancies. The authors suggested implementation of screening using maternal age combined with MSAFP levels and a system of age-dependent action lines. Using a cut-off of ≤0.5 for women ≤31 years, and increasing cut-offs (higher MoM) until age 38 years, the authors estimated that they could detect 40% of Down syndrome pregnancies, while selecting 8% of non-affected pregnancies (Table 62.4) [93]. A similar review of German MSAFP screening data for 36 428 pregnancies with known outcome confirmed the lower MoM value in Down syndrome pregnancies [94]. The authors noted that a cut-off value of ≤0.5 MoM would have resulted in an amniocentesis rate of 3.7%

Table 62.4 Down syndrome detection rates using maternal age-adjusted MSAFP cut-offs [After Ref. 93 with permission]

MA at delivery (years)	AFP level (MoM)	Down syndrome (%)	Unaffected fetus (%)	Relative risk
>38	N/A	20.0	2.1	9.2
37	<1.0	2.9	0.4	6.8
36	0.9	2.6	0.5	5.4
35	0.8	2.2	0.4	5.1
34	0.7	1.8	0.4	4.2
32–33	0.6	3.0	0.7	4.4
25–31	0.5	7.5	2.2	3.4
Overall		40.0	6.8	5.8

MA = maternal age; N/A = not available.

and a Down syndrome detection rate of 21%. The ratio of amniocenteses to Down syndrome cases was about 150:1 which represents a higher detection rate than the ratio expected when maternal age ≤35 years is the sole indicator for amniocentesis [94].

The finding of low MSAFP in Down syndrome fetuses was mirrored by the documentation of low values in cord blood [95] and amniotic fluid [96,97]. Although the pathophysiologic mechanism is unclear, reduced hepatic AFP synthesis by the Down syndrome fetus has been demonstrated and may occur on the basis of delayed liver maturation [98]. In a retrospective study of 180 women with an MSAFP level ≤0.25 MoM, Davenport and Macri [99] noted a 38% fetal loss rate and suggested that much of the fetal wastage could be attributed to chromosome abnormalities. Low MSAFP levels have now been reported in pregnancies complicated by trisomy 18, trisomy 13, several rare structural chromosomal abnormalities, sex chromosome disorders, triploidy, molar pregnancy, blighted ovum, fetal death and other conditions [66,100]. The lower MSAFP curves for normal pregnancies in insulin-dependent diabetic women may also be related to decreased fetal growth and relative hepatic immaturity [100]. As more data have become available, it has become apparent that screening programs should provide risk data for all chromosome abnormalities, rather than risk for Down syndrome alone, as the overall risk may be twice that reported for Down syndrome at any specific age-adjusted low MSAFP cut-off [101].

62.5.2 LOW MSAFP SCREENING EXPERIENCE

A number of prospective screening programs have now reported data on the use of MSAFP and maternal age for the detection of chromosomal disorders. These studies generate slightly different Down syndrome risk figures for MSAFP cut-offs adjusted for maternal age [102–104]. Most studies suggest use of an age-dependent cut-off which results in selection of women with Down syndrome risk between 1:350 and 1:400 at birth. This generally corresponds to a risk of 1:270 in the mid-trimester. Cuckle, Wald and Thompson [104] developed six screening protocols and demonstrated that use of maternal age and MSAFP levels is more efficient than use of either parameter alone. Using age-adjusted cut-offs which generated Down syndrome predictive risks of 1:400 at term, Tabor et al. [105] noted that a policy of offering amniocentesis to all women selected (i.e. risk ≥1:400) regardless of age would detect 53% of affected fetuses compared with a 28% detection rate for age ≥35 years.

Three major prospective series have reported screening experience in large populations. DiMaio et al. [106] analyzed data on 34 354 women who were screened positive (e.g. selected for possible amniocentesis) if the Down syndrome risk was ≥1:270. Of 1451 women with risk ≥1:270 and ultrasound confirmation of gestational age, nine had a fetus with Down syndrome and four fetuses had trisomy 13 or 18. The detection rate per total number of amniocenteses was 1:161 for Down syndrome and 1:112 for all autosomal trisomies. A total of 23 autosomal trisomies (18 Down syndrome) would have been missed at that action line. Using the same cut-off, the New England Regional Genetics Group [107] offered amniocentesis to 2.7% of 77 273 <35-year-old women screened, yielding a detection rate of 1:89 for Down syndrome and 1:69 for all autosomal trisomy. Of note, nearly one-quarter of the indicated women declined further intervention so that only 2.1% of the screened population underwent amniocentesis. In the first 12 months of the California AFP Screening Program [108] 174 784 women were screened and 3939 (2.25%) were subsequently evaluated at an AFP follow-up center (prenatal diagnosis center) because of a risk of Down syndrome estimated at ≥1:350 at term. Of these, 13% were reinterpreted as normal following ultrasound dating, 20% were noted to have had blood drawn before 15 weeks of gestation (too early), 2% were non-pregnant or had fetal demise and <1% had gestations too far advanced for further testing (Table 62.5). Amniocentesis was offered to 2552 women (65%) and performed on 1940. Detection rate for Down syndrome was 1:121 while detection of all 'significant chromosome abnormalities' was 1:78, including XXY and 45,X. It is notable that the refusal rate of 24% was consistent with that reported for New England [108].

62.5.3 MATERNAL SERUM CHORIONIC GONADOTROPIN

The desire to increase the efficacy of Down syndrome screening has resulted in a search for other maternal markers which are predictive of fetal trisomy. Bogart, Pandian and Jones [109] described elevation of maternal serum chorionic gonadotropin, which has subsequently proven to be the single most discriminatory mid-trimester Down syndrome marker in current usage. Human chorionic gonadotropin (hCG) is a 39 500 molecular weight glycoprotein hormone comprising two different subunits, each of which also occurs free (unbound) in serum. Of interest, the α-subunit is common to other hormones including luteinizing hormone, follicle stimulating hormone, and thyrotropin stimulating hormone [82], while the β-subunit is unique to hCG. Synthesized by the syncytiotrophoblast, hCG is stimulated or inhibited by a variety of other hormones [100]. A marker of viable pregnancy, hCG can be detected in maternal blood soon after implantation, rises rapidly until 8–10 weeks of gestation, then declines steadily until 16–18 weeks [82,100]. Both hCG

Table 62.5 Outcome of low MSAFP screening in California [Data abstracted from Ref. 108]

Category	Number	(%)
Women screened	174 784	
Women seen for PDC follow-up	3 939	(2.25)
US redated – AFP reinterpreted negative	518	(13.15)
US redated – blood drawn too early	772	(19.60)
US redated – too late for testing	26	(0.66)
Fetal demise or not pregnant	71	(1.80)
Screen remained positive after US	2 552	(64.79)
Amniocentesis performed	1 940	(76.02)
Down syndrome fetus detected	17[a]	
Trisomic fetus, not Down syndrome	5	
Triploid fetus	1	
Fetal sex chromosome abnormality	8	

PDC = prenatal diagnosis center; US = ultrasound.
[a] 16 cases detected at a PDC = 1/121 amniocentesis procedures; 17/1940 = 1 Down syndrome fetus per 114 amniocenteses overall. Detection rate for non-mosaic abnormalities was 1/78.

subunits and total hCG can be measured using sensitive monoclonal antibody assay systems. A recent observation of increasing β-subunit fractions in stored serum samples underscores the importance of timely analysis [10]. Although it is present at levels equivalent to only 0.5% of bound hCG, the free β-subunit may be particularly elevated in mid-trimester Down syndrome pregnancies [11]. Nevertheless, the benefit of screening with the β-subunit remains controversial.

The initial report of hCG screening described elevated total hCG values in 56% of sera from Down syndrome pregnancies [109]. Using stored maternal samples from 77 Down syndrome pregnancies and 385 controls, Wald et al. [112] noted a twofold increase in median level of total maternal serum hCG in Down syndrome pregnancies compared with sera from unaffected pregnancies. This relative increase in MoM was confirmed in summary data from 17 additional studies [82]. The authors demonstrated better Down syndrome detection rates for maternal serum hCG plus maternal age than for MSAFP and maternal age, and highest detection rate when AFP, hCG and maternal age were considered. In another retrospective study of 614 women under age 35, Suchy and Yeager [113] observed a 62.5% detection rate for Down syndrome with a 4.7% false-positive rate (amniocentesis with normal results) when both serum markers and maternal age were assessed. In these and other studies, detection rate increased with increasing maternal age, and the false-positive rate increased with detection rate when successively lower-risk cut-offs were selected. Prospective data from 27 167 pregnancies in <35-year-old women confirmed a Down syndrome detection rate of 65% and false-positive rate of 4.5% when pregnancies were selected using a risk cut-off of 1:270. The

detection rate for other significant abnormalities was 57% [100].

62.5.4 MATERNAL SERUM UNCONJUGATED ESTRIOL (MSuE3) [100]

An early observation of low maternal urinary estriol excretion in third trimester pregnancies complicated by fetal Down syndrome [114] provided the basis for evaluation of MSuE3 for the mid-trimester detection of Down syndrome. Unconjugated estriol is produced by syncytiotrophoblasts from precursors derived from the fetal adrenal gland and further modified by fetal liver [82]. Immaturity of either fetal organ may lead to lowered production of estriol and consequent reduction in MSuE3 [115]. Canick et al. [115] documented MSuE3 levels of 0.79 MoM in 22 Down syndrome pregnancies compared with the median for 110 controls, suggesting possible benefit of Down syndrome screening with MSuE3. They also found that the uE3 level was independent of maternal age, though later studies disputed this point [116]. Wald et al. [117] reported a lower false-positive rate (12%) using MSAFP, MSuE3 are maternal age compared with MSAFP and maternal age alone (20%) when cut-offs were selected to achieve a Down syndrome detection rate of 60% [112]. This study confirmed that the three markers were largely independent of each other. A later study of 41 Down syndrome pregnancies and 441 controls suggested that MSuE3 screening was not helpful in the detection of Down syndrome [118]. A recent prospective study of 10 000 women under age 35 years evaluated effectiveness of Down syndrome screening using hCG, uE3 and maternal age. With a Down syndrome risk cut-off of 1:125, amniocentesis

Table 62.6 Triple marker screening for trisomy

	MSAFP	MShCG	MSuE3
Trisomy 21	Low	High	Low
Trisomy 18	Low[a]	Low	Low

MShCG = maternal serum hCG.
[a] MSAFP may be elevated in association with neural tube or ventral wall defects.

was offered to 446 women, and completed in 412. Six Down syndrome cases were identified in this group, while four cases were later confirmed among the offspring of women who screened negative. Screening with hCG and age would have resulted in detection of only four of the six cases. Among women ≥38 years who were screened but offered amniocentesis, there were 13 cases of Down syndrome, all of which would have been detected at a risk cut-off of 1:125. The authors concluded that the hCG:uE$_3$ ratio was a more effective screening tool than either marker alone [119].

62.5.5 TRIPLE MARKER SCREENING

The major mid-trimester maternal serum markers for Down syndrome are clearly hCG, AFP, and uE3, which can be combined with maternal age to provide a basis for triple marker screening (Table 62.6). In a combined retrospective and prospective study, Milunsky noted an 81.3% detection rate for Down syndrome and a 62.9% detection rate for all chromosomal defects in women <35 years undergoing triple marker screening. This compared with detection rates of 56.3% and 48.1%, respectively, when AFP and hCG were used [100]. The largest prospective study published to date evaluated triple screening in 25 207 women and compared efficiency of a 1:190 Down syndrome risk cut-off to that of a 1:270 cut-off in a subset of the women. Of 1661 (6.6%) women who initially screened positive, 962 (3.8%) remained positive and were offered amniocentesis after ultrasound assessment. A total of 20 cases of Down syndrome and seven other chromosomal conditions were found in the 760 pregnancies of women who elected amniocentesis. One more Down syndrome case was born to a woman who declined the procedure. The authors cited a detection rate of 58% and described odds of 1:38 for identification of a Down syndrome fetus in women undergoing amniocentesis [120].

62.5.6 OTHER MATERNAL SERUM MARKERS

A number of other fetal or placental proteins have been evaluated for possible use as maternal screening markers. Elevated maternal serum levels of a pregnancy specific β$_1$-glycoprotein (SP-1), which is also produced

in the syncytiotrophoblast, have been reported in six studies [82,121]. Graham et al. [121] noted that Down syndrome screening using age, AFP and SP-1 was less effective than screening with age, AFP and hCG. The addition of SP-1 did not increase the Down syndrome detection rate for the latter protocol. Elevation of the placental protein inhibin may also prove useful in Down syndrome screening [122]. Elevations of maternal serum antithyroid antibodies [123] and progesterone [124] appear to be less effective screening tools. Finally, the epithelial ovarian cancer marker, CA 125, has been proposed to have both elevated and low curves in second-trimester Down syndrome gestations, while sera from 9–11-week pregnancies have not differed significantly from controls [125].

The most efficient marker for fetal Down syndrome may be urea-resistant neutrophil alkaline phosphatase (UR-NAP), which had a median value of 1.65 MoM in 72 Down syndrome pregnancies when compared with maternal sera from 156 controls. Detection rate for Down syndrome was 79% at a cut-off of 1.4 MoM, which corresponds to a false-positive rate of about 5% [126]. However, as the UR-NAP assay is labor intensive and subjective [82] it may not be valuable for mass screening.

62.5.7 SCREENING FOR TRISOMY 18

In contrast to the elevated values reported for Down syndrome, MShCG levels are extremely low in pregnancies associated with fetal trisomy 18 [109,127,128]. Also, while MSAFP is generally low in this condition, it may be normal or elevated in the 25% of trisomy 18 fetuses who have an associated NTD or ventral wall defect. Therefore, screening for this condition, which represents the second most common autosomal trisomy, depends on a different interpretation of multiple marker results. Palomaki, Knight and Haddow [129] recently described a prospective study of 19 491 women screened with AFP, uE3 and hCG, and evaluated using a separate screening protocol, which labeled a screen positive if the values fell at or below 0.75 MoM, 0.60 MoM, and 0.55 MoM, respectively. Of 98 women identified using the trisomy 18 algorithm, 92 were offered amniocentesis. Six cases of trisomy 18 and one 45,X fetus were identified, yielding an odds ratio of one trisomy 18 fetus identified for every 14 unaffected pregnancies selected for amniocentesis, and an estimated detection rate of 85%. This multivariate approach was much more effective than a protocol based on hCG alone [130].

62.5.8 OTHER CONSIDERATIONS IN MULTIPLE MARKER SCREENING

As in MSAFP screening, hCG and uE3 levels are affected by a variety of fetal, maternal and placental factors. Sufficient data now exist to warrant correction of MShGG levels for maternal weight [112], insulin-dependent diabetes [131], and African–American or Asian heritage [132,133]. MSuE3 levels are minimally affected by weight [115] and unaffected by race [133]. Both hCG [115,134] and uE3 [115] levels are lowered by cigarette smoking, but AFP levels are elevated [135]. While the effect of smoking has not been sufficient to warrant correction of MSAFP values for NTD screening, a correction factor appears to be indicated for uE3 and hCG. Specific formulas for weight and smoking adjustments have recently been proposed by Bartels *et al.* [136]. However, the value of multiple complex adjustments remains controversial. [87]

Maternal serum hCG and uE3 levels are elevated in twin gestations as are MSAFP values. Adjustment must be made for the interpretation of all three analytes in multiple gestation [137]. Similarly, MSAFP values are higher in pregnancies with a male fetus [138]. Low MSAFP selects a slightly greater number of Down syndrome females, as demonstrated by DiMaio *et al.* [106], who noted 57% females in their report of AFP screening. The sex ratio may be affected more significantly when selecting with hCG. In a report of 477 singleton fetuses from pregnancies selected by elevated MShCG, Leporrier, Herrou and Leymarie [139] noted ascertainment of 46% males overall, 36% in pregnancies studied at 18–20 gestation weeks and 50% in pregnancies evaluated at 16–17 weeks. Because the effect of fetal sex on hCG levels was noted only after 17 weeks of gestation, and reliable determination of fetal sex is limited, the authors suggested that MShCG screening be performed prior to week 18 [139].

62.5.9 ADVERSE OUTCOME AND MULTIPLE MARKER SCREENING

Davenport and Macri's [99] report of 38% fetal wastage in pregnancies with very low MSAFP reflects the data obtained from later studies. Gravett *et al.* [140] evaluated pregnancy outcome in 3000 women screened with hCG and found adverse outcome in 4 of 7 with MShCG $\geq$ 5 MoM. Outcomes included severe pre-eclampsia, placental abruption and preterm labor. Although the number of women in this category was small, representing 0.23% of the total, and the cut-off value was relatively high, the 57% adverse outcome rate underscores the sensitivity of hCG as a determinant of placental insufficiency. Very low MShCG and MSuE3 have also been described in 14 cases of triploidy, which may be associated with normal or elevated MSAFP [141]. Mason *et al.* [142] also reported fetal loss in 11 of 163 women with elevated or low hCG and uE3. They suggested the importance of ultrasound evaluation in women who fall in either category and suggested increased ultrasound monitor-

ing of such pregnancies. Finally, Canick *et al.* [143] noted no significant differences in hCG or uE3 levels in association with open spina bifida but described very low MSuE3 and somewhat reduced MShCG in pregnancies associated with anencephaly, presumably on the basis of pituitary–adrenal dysfunction.

62.5.10 FIRST TRIMESTER SCREENING

As described earlier, the UK Collaborative Study data found little benefit for MSAFP screening for NTDs in the first trimester [40]. A recent report by Fuhrman *et al.* [144] confirmed prior observations of low MSAFP values, but suggested that MSAFP values are not sufficiently low to effectively predict Down syndrome or trisomy 18 in early gestation. Although a number of reports document low uE3 and hCG levels in Down syndrome pregnancies, neither is an adequate indicator to warrant first trimester screening currently [82]. During the first trimester, the free β-subunit of hCG is very low while the free α-subunit is elevated, producing a very low free β to free α ratio in trisomy 18 pregnancies [100]. The most promising maternal serum marker for early Down syndrome screening appears to be pregnancy-associated plasma protein A, which may detect $\geq$ 60% of Down syndrome fetuses [145]. Finally, transvaginal ultrasonography may play a role in early detection of chromosomal abnormalities [146].

62.6 Role of ultrasound in maternal serum screening

The role of ultrasound in antenatal detection of NTD and chromosome anomalies relates to two independent functions. Even routine screening sonography will generally detect multiple pregnancy, blighted ovum, fetal demise and anencephaly. Moreover, some cases of open spina bifida, ventral wall defect or other malformation will be detected, as will moderate–severe oligohydramnios. More detailed sonographic studies performed by experienced sonographers now lead to the detection of fetal abnormalities even in the absence of abnormal maternal serum screening. Multiple ultrasonographic signs have been described which facilitate detection of early hydrocephaly and Arnold–Chiari malformation associated with open spina bifida [147–150], or the identification of the trisomic fetus [150,151]. Therefore, the role of ultrasound in the detection of complications of pregnancy or fetal abnormality is now well established. The major role of sonography in screening programs, however, is in the assignment of gestational age [152,153]. As the major maternal serum markers vary significantly with gestational age, accurate dating of the pregnancy is critical in the correct interpretation of analyte levels [82]. Wald *et al.* [152] emphasized the smaller biparietal diameter in the fetus with open spina bifida at the mid-trimester. The smaller biparietal diameter results in the ascertainment of a larger proportion of open spina bifida pregnancies when ultrasonography is used to establish gestational age (i.e. the fetus will be assigned an earlier gestational age and MSAFP will be interpreted as relatively higher). Wald notes that the detection rate for open spina bifida increased from 75 to 90% and the false-positive rate decreased from 3.3 to 2.8% when biparietal diameter dating and an MSAFP cut-off of ≥2.5 MoM were used [82]. Cuckle and Wald [154] described a similar benefit from the use of biparietal diameter to establish gestational age and avoid earlier redating of the Down syndrome pregnancy. Finally, the accuracy of gestational age assignment may be especially critical for triple marker screening, for which a misassignment of only 2 weeks may result in as much as a ten-fold change in the calculated risk [100].

62.7 Concluding comments

Prenatal screening protocols have been suggested by various authors and have received widespread acceptance [82,100]. Most rely on complex computer-based algorithms which correct for weight, race, diabetes and cigarette smoking, assess each analyte for gestational age, and generate a maternal age-specific risk for open spina bifida, Down syndrome and, sometimes, trisomy 18. Nevertheless, there are a number of issues which remain controversial or await further data for clarification. In addition, there are numerous ethical, social, economic and even medicolegal ramifications of antenatal screening. As there are few prospective studies of multiple marker screening in women ≥35 years [155, 156], there is some disagreement regarding extension of screening services to this high-risk group. Some authors strongly favor triple screening for all age groups [82], while others hesitate to abandon primary testing (amniocentesis) in this group, noting that the economic savings may not outweigh the social burden associated with missing an affected fetus in a particularly high-risk population (B.F. Crandall, personal communication). Similarly, the screening protocols do not all agree on the use of weighted markers (e.g. the risk assessment for Down syndrome is more heavily determined by age and hCG than by AFP and uE3).

Researchers in antenatal diagnosis recognized the importance of participant and practitioner education, reliable laboratory procedures and an organized screening program including ultrasound assessment, genetic counseling and access to experienced practitioners for follow-up diagnostic services (targeted ultrasound and amniocentesis). Such recommendations were emphasized by an Antenatal Diagnosis Working Group which particularly stressed the necessity and difficulty of education and genetic counseling of screening participants [157]. Cost–benefit issues remain, particularly with regard to multiple marker screening, though preliminary data suggests that benefit will outweigh risks/costs in monetary, medical and social terms [158]. A recent cost–benefit analysis of a prospective hCG screening program calculated that the cost of screening 100 000 women would reach $8.3 million, while the savings from pregnancy termination would exceed $32 million for Down syndrome alone. The authors suggested that financial considerations clearly favor widespread screening and would even support lower (more liberal) cut-off values, such that a higher number of amniocentesis procedures would be performed [159].

Triple screening may prove to be the best early indicator of later fetal or placental compromise, thus providing early detection of an otherwise apparently low-risk pregnancy, and subsequent fetal monitoring. Similarly, early detection of infants with malformation may allow improved management with resultant decreased fetal morbidity for pregnancies continuing to term. The efficacy of first trimester screening and utilization of new or additional markers awaits further research. Nevertheless, it is clear that current techniques allow for the detection of at least 60% of Down syndrome fetuses, a higher fraction of other autosomal trisomies and 75–80% of fetuses with open spina bifida at risk cut-offs which select 5–6% of pregnancies for amniocentesis.

References

1. Adams, M.M., Erickson, J.D. Layde, P.M. and Oakley, G.P. (1981) Down's syndrome: recent trends in the United States. *JAMA*, **246**, 758–60.
2. World Health Organization (1972) Genetic disorders: preventions, treatment and rehabilitation. *WHO Tech. Rep. Ser. 681*.
3. Volpe, J.J. (1987) *Neurology of the Newborn*, W.B. Saunders, Philadelphia.
4. Park, C.H., Pruitt, J.H. and Bennett, D. (1989) A mouse model for neural tube defects: the curtailed (T^c) mutation produces spina bifida occulta in T^c/ + animals and spina bifida with meningomyelocele in T^c/t. *Teratology*, **39**, 303–312.
5. Lemire, R.J. (1988) Neural tube defects. *JAMA*, **259**, 558–62.
6. Hunt, G.M. (1990) Open spina bifida: outcome for a complete cohort treated unselectively and followed into adulthood. *Devel. Med. Child Neurol.*, **32**, 108–118.
7. CDC (1989) Economic burden of spina bifida – United States, 1980–1990. *MMWR*, **38**, 264–67.
8. Holmes, L.B., Driscoll, S.B. and Atkins L. (1976) Etiologic heterogeneity of neural-tube defects. *N. Engl. J. Med.*, **294**, 365–69.
9. Carter, C.O. (1974) Clues to the aetiology of neural tube malformations. *Dev. Med. Child Neurol.*, **16** (6 suppl. 32), 3–15.
10. Seller, M.J. and Adinolfi, M. (1981) The curly-tail mouse: an experimental model for human neural tube defects. *Life Sci.*, **29**, 1607–15.
11. Economides D.L., Ferguson, J., Mackenzie, I.Z. *et al.* (1992) Folate and B$_{12}$ concentrations in maternal and fetal blood, and amniotic fluid in second trimester pregnancies complicated by neural tube defects. *Br. J. Obstet. Gynaecol.*, **99**, 23–25.
12. MRC Vitamin Study Research Group (1991) Prevention of neural tube defects: results of the Medical Research Council Vitamin Study. *Lancet*, **338**, 131–37.
13. Smithells, R.W., Sheppard, S., Schorah, C.J. *et al.* (1981) Apparent prevention of neural tube defects by periconceptional vitamin supplementation. *Arch. Dis. Child.*, **56**, 911–18.
14. Bower, C. and Stanley, F.J. (1989) Dietary folate as a risk factor for

neural tube defects: evidence from a case-control study in Western Australia. *Med. J. Aust.*, **150**, 613–19.

15. Milunsky, A., Jick, H., Jick, S.S. *et al.* (1989) Multivitamin folic acid supplementation in early pregnancy reduces the prevalence of neural tube defects. *JAMA*, **262**, 2847–52.

16. Mulinare, J., Cordero, J.F., Erickson, J.D. and Berry, R.J. (1988) Periconceptional use of multivitamins and the occurrence of neural tube defects. *JAMA*, **260**, 3141–45.

17. CDC (1991) Use of folic acid for prevention of spina bifida and other neural tube defects, 1983–1991. *MMWR*, **40**, 513–16.

18. Czeizel, A.E. and Dúdas, I. (1992) Prevention of the first occurrence of neural-tube defects by periconceptional vitamin supplementation. *N. Engl. J. Med.*, **327**, 1832–35.

19. Werler, M.M., Shapiro, S. and Mitchell, A.A. (1993) Periconceptional folic acid exposure and risk of occurrent neural tube defects. *JAMA*, **259**, 1257–61.

20. Rosenberg, I.H. (1992) Folic acid and neural-tube defects – time for action? *N. Engl. J. Med.*, **327**, 1875–77.

21. CDC (1993) Recommendations for use of folic acid to reduce number of spina bifida cases and other neural tube defects. *JAMA*, **269**, 1233–38.

22. Adinolfi, A., Adinolfi, M. and Lessof, M.H. (1975) Alpha-feto-protein during development and disease. *J. Med. Genet.*, **12**, 138–51.

23. Seller, M.J. (1974) Alpha-fetoprotein and the prenatal diagnosis of neural tube defects. *Develop. Med. Child Neurol.*, **16**, 369–71.

24. Abelev, G.I. (1971) Alpha-fetoprotein in ontogenesis and its association with malignant tumors. *Adv. Cancer Res.*, **14**, 295–358.

25. Brock, D.J.H. and Sutcliffe, R.G. (1972) α-Feto-protein in the antenatal diagnosis of anencephaly and spina bifida. *Lancet*, **ii**, 197–99.

26. Second Report of the UK Collaborative Study on Alpha-fetoprotein in Relation to Neural Tube Defects (1979) Amniotic fluid alpha-fetoprotein measurement in the antenatal diagnosis of anencephaly and open spina bifida in early pregnancy. *Lancet*, **ii**, 651–62.

27. Milunsky, A. (1980) Prenatal detection of neural tube defects. VI. Experience with 20 000 pregnancies. *JAMA*, **244**, 2731–35.

28. Crandall, B.F. and Matsumoto, M. (1984) Routine amniotic fluid α-fetoprotein measurement in 34 000 pregnancies. *Am. J. Obstet. Gynecol.*, **149**, 744–47.

29. Chubb, I.W., Pilowsky, P.M., Springell, H.J. and Pollard, A.C. (1979) Acetylcholinesterase in human amniotic fluid: an index of fetal neural development? *Lancet*, **i**, 688–90.

30. Smith, A.D., Wald, N.J., Cuckle, H.S. *et al.* (1979) Amniotic-fluid acetylcholinesterase as a possible diagnostic test for open neural-tube defects in early pregnancy. *Lancet*, **i**, 685–88.

31. Wald, N.J. and Cuckle, H.S. (1981) Report of the Collaborative Acetylcholinesterase Study. Amniotic fluid acetylcholinesterase electrophoresis as a secondary test in the diagnosis of anencephaly and open spina bifida in early pregnancy. *Lancet*, **ii**, 321–24.

32. Seller, M.J. and Cole, K.J. (1980) Polyacrylamide gel electrophoresis of amniotic fluid cholinesterases: a good prenatal test for neural tube defects. *Br. J. Obstet. Gynaecol.*, **87**, 1103–108.

33. Goldfine, C., Miller, W.A. and Haddow, J.E. (1983) Amniotic fluid gel cholinesterase density ratios in fetal open defects of the neural tube and ventral wall. *Br. J. Obstet. Gynaecol.*, **90**, 238–40.

34. Aitken, D.A., Morrison, N.M. and Ferguson-Smith, M.A. (1984) Predictive value of amniotic acetylcholinesterase analysis in the diagnosis of fetal abnormality in 3700 pregnancies. *Prenat. Diagn.*, **4**, 329–40.

35. Zeisel, S.H., Milunsky, A. and Blusztajn, J.K. (1980) Prenatal diagnosis of neural tube defects. V. The value of amniotic fluid cholinesterase studies. *Am. J. Obstet. Gynecol.*, **137**, 481–85.

36. Barlow, R.D., Cuckle, H.S., Wald, N.J. and Rodeck, C.H. (1982) False positive gel-acetylcholinesterase results in blood-stained amniotic fluids. *Br. J. Obstet. Gynaecol.*, **89**, 821–26.

37. Brock, D.J.H. and Barron, L. (1988) Prospective prenatal screening for fetal abnormalities using a quantitative immunoassay for acetylcholinesterase. *J. Med. Genet*, **25**, 605–608.

38. Loft, A.G.R., Hogdall, E., Larsen, S.O. and Norgaard-Pederson, B. (1993) A comparison of amniotic fluid and alpha-fetoprotein in the prenatal diagnosis of open neural tube defects and anterior abdominal wall defects. *Prenat. Diagn.*, **13**, 93–109.

39. UK Collaborative Study on Alpha-fetoprotein in Relation to Neural Tube Defects (1977) Maternal serum AFP measurement in antenatal screening for anencephaly and spina bifida in early pregnancy. *Lancet*, **i**, 1323–32.

40. Brock, D.J.H. (1989) Maternal blood markers (alphafetoprotein), in *Diseases of the Fetus and Newborn* (eds G.B. Reed, A.E. Claireaux and A.D. Bain), C.V. Mosby, St Louis.

41. Wald, N.J., Cuckle, H.S., Boreham, J. *et al.* (1980) The effect of maternal weight on maternal serum alpha-fetoprotein levels. *Br. J. Obstet. Gynaecol.*, **88**, 1094–96.

42. Crandall, B.F., Lebherz, T.B., Schroth, P.C. and Matsumoto, M. (1983) Alphafetoprotein concentrations in maternal serum: relation to race and body weight. *Clin. Chem.*, **29**, 531–33.

43. Macri, J.N., Kasturi, R.V., Hu, M.G. *et al.* (1987) Maternal serum α-fetoprotein screening. III. Pitfalls in evaluating Black gravid women. *Am. J. Obstet. Gynecol.*, **157**, 820–22.

44. Wald, N.J., Cuckle, H.S., Boreham, J. *et al.* (1979) Maternal serum alpha-fetoprotein and diabetes mellitus. *Br. J. Obstet. Gynaecol.*, **86**, 101–105

45. Milunsky, A., Alpert, E., Kitzmiller, J.L. *et al.* (1982) Prenatal diagnosis of neural tube defects. VIII. The importance of serum alpha-fetoprotein screening in diabetic pregnant women. *Am J. Obstet. Gynecol.*, **142**, 1030–32.

46. Roberts, C.J., Elder, G.H., Lawrence, K.M. *et al.* (1983) The efficacy of a serum screening service for neural tube defects: the South Wales experience. *Lancet*, **i**, 1315–16.

47. Burton, B.K., Sowers, S.G. and Nelson, L.H. (1983) Maternal serum α-fetoprotein screening in North Carolina: experience with more than twelve thousand pregnancies. *Am. J. Obstet. Gynecol.*, **146**, 439–44.

48. Norgaard-Pederson, B., Bagger, P., Bang, J. *et al.* (1985) Maternal-serum-alphafetoprotein screening for fetal malformations in 28 062 pregnancies. *Acta Obstet. Gynecol. Scand.*, **64**, 511–14.

49. Lester, C.A. and Farrow, S.C. (1987) Serum α-fetoprotein and amniocentesis. *J. Obstet. Gynecol.*, **7**, 245–58.

50. Fuhrman, W. and Weitzel, H.K. (1985) Maternal serum alpha-fetoprotein screening for neural tube defects. *Hum. Genet.*, **69**, 47–61.

51. Sadovnick, A.D. and Baird, P.A. (1983) A cost–benefit analysis of a population screening program for neural tube defects. *Prenat. Diag.*, **3**, 117–26.

52. Milunsky, A. and Alpert, E. (1978) Maternal serum AFP screening. *N. Engl. J. Med.*, **298**, 738–39.

53. Seller, M.J. (1983) Is routine maternal serum α-fetoprotein testing a waste of time in an area of low incidence of neural tube defects? *J. Obstet. Gynecol.*, **3**, 139–43.

54. Tosi, L.L., Detsky, A.S., Roye, D.P. and Morden, M.L. (1987) When does mass screening for open neural tube defects in low-risk pregnancies result in cost savings? *Can. Med. Assoc. J.*, **136**, 255–65.

55. Ghosh, A., Tang, M.H.Y., Tai, D. *et al.* (1986) Justification of maternal serum alphafetoprotein screening in a population with low incidence of neural tube defects. *Prenat. Diagn.*, **6**, 83–87.

56. Kunz, J. and Schmid, J. (1976) Amniotic alpha-fetoprotein and omphalocele. *Lancet*, **i**, 47.

57. Ainbender, E. and Hirschhorn, K. (1976) Routine alpha-fetoprotein studies in amniotic fluid. *Lancet*, **i**, 597–98.

58. Kjessler, B., Johansson, S.G.O., Sherman, M. *et al.* (1975) Alpha-fetoprotein in antenatal diagnosis of congenital nephrosis. *Lancet*, **i**, 432–33.

59. Seppala, M., Aula, P., Rapola, J. *et al.* (1976) Congenital nephrotic syndrome: prenatal diagnosis and genetic counselling by estimation of amniotic-fluid and maternal serum alpha-fetoprotein, *Lancet*, **ii**, 123–25.

60. Ryynanen, M., Seppala, M., Kuusela, P. *et al.* (1983) Antenatal screening for congenital nephrosis in Finland by maternal serum α-fetoprotein. *Br. J. Obstet. Gynaecol.*, **90**, 437–42.

61. Seller, M.J. (1975) Prenatal diagnosis of a neural tube defect: Meckel syndrome. *J. Med. Genet.*, **12**, 109–10.

62. Aula, P., Karjalainen, O., Rapola, J. *et al.* (1977) Prenatal diagnosis of the Meckel syndrome. *Am. J. Obstet. Gynecol.*, **129**, 700–702.

63. Nevin, N.C., Ritchie, A., McKeown, F. and Roberts, G. (1978) Case report: raised alpha-fetoprotein levels in amniotic fluid and maternal serum associated with distension of the fetal bladder caused by absence of urethra. *J. Med. Genet.*, **15**, 61–63.

64. Seller, M.J. and Berry, A.C. (1987) Amniotic-fluid alpha-fetoprotein and fetal renal agenesis. *Lancet*, **i**, 660.

65. Petit, P., Bossens, M., Thomas, D. *et al.* (1987) Type III congenital cystic adenomatoid malformation of the lung: another cause of elevated alpha-fetoprotein? *Clin. Genet.*, **32**, 172–74.

66. Main, D. and Mennuti, M.T. (1986) Neural tube defects: issues in prenatal diagnosis and counseling. *Obstet. Gynecol.*, **67**, 1–16.

67. Hunter, A., Hammerton, J.L., Baskett, T. and Lyons, E. (1976) Raised amniotic-fluid alpha-fetoprotein in Turner syndrome. *Lancet*, **i**, 598.

68. O'Brien, W.F., Knuppel, R.A., Kousseff, B. *et al.* (1988) Elevated maternal serum alpha-fetoprotein in triploidy. *Obstet. Gynecol.*, **71**, 994–95.

69. Schnittger, A., Liedgren, S., Radberg, C. *et al.* (1980) Raised maternal serum and amniotic fluid alpha-fetoprotein levels associated with a placental haemangioma. *Br. J. Obstet. Gynaecol.*, **87**, 824–26.

70. Read, A.P., Donnai, D. and Brandreth, C. (1982) Abnormalities of the umbilical cord or membranes leading to raised amniotic AFP. *J. Med. Genet.*, **19**, 64.

71. Dyer, S.N., Burton, B.K. and Nelson, L.H. (1987) Elevated maternal serum α-fetoprotein levels and oligohydramnios: poor prognosis for pregnancy outcome. *Am. J. Obstet. Gynecol.*, **157**, 336–39.

72. Los, F.J., Hagenaars, A.M., Marrink, J. *et al.* (1992) Maternal serum alpha-fetoprotein levels and fetal outcome in early second-trimester oligohydramnios. *Prenat. Diagn.*, **12**, 285–92.

73. Los, F.J., de Wolf, B.T.H.M. and Huisjes, H.J. (1979) Raised maternal serum-alpha-fetoprotein levels and spontaneous fetomaternal transfusion. *Lancet*, **ii**, 1210–12.

74. Haddow, J.E., Thompson, D.K. and Kloza, E.M. (1980) Maternal hepatoma detected during serum AFP screening. *Lancet*, **ii**, 806–807.

75. Ferguson-Smith, M.A. (1983) The reduction of anencephalic and spina bifida births by maternal serum alpha-fetoprotein screening. *Br. Med. Bull.*, **39**, 365–72.

76. Carrington, D., Whittle, M.J., Gibson, A.A.M. *et al.* (1987) Maternal serum α-fetoprotein – a marker of fetal aplastic crisis during intrauterine human parvovirus infection. *Lancet*, **i**, 433–35.

77. Ammann, A.J., Cowan, M., Wara, D. *et al.* (1986) Alpha-fetoprotein levels in immunodeficiency. *N. Engl. J. Med.*, **314**, 717–18.

78. Khalil, F.K., Bonnet, M., Guiloaud, S. *et al.* (1979) Alpha-fetoprotein levels in placenta, maternal, and cord blood in normal and pathologic pregnancy. *Obstet. Gynecol*, **54**, 117–19.

79. Wald, N.J. and Cuckle, H.S. (1980) Alphafetoprotein in the antenatal diagnosis of open neural tube defects. *Br. J. Hosp. Med.*, **23**, 473–89.

80. Rodeck, C.H., Campbell, S. and Biswas, S. (1976) Maternal plasma alpha-fetoprotein in normal and complicated pregnancies. *Br. J. Obstet. Gynaecol.*, **83**, 23–32.

81. Clayton-Hopkins, J.A., Olsen, P.N. and Blake, A.P. (1982) Maternal serum alpha-fetoprotein levels in the pregnancy complicated by hypertension. *Prenat. Diagn.*, **2**, 47–54.

82. Wald, N.J. and Cuckle, H.S. (1992) Biochemical screening, in *Prenatal Diagnosis and Screening* (eds D.J.H. Brock, C.H. Rodeck and M.A. Ferguson-Smith), Churchill Livingstone, London, pp. 563–77.

83. Seppala, M. (1975) Fetal pathophysiology of human alphafetoprotein. *Ann. N. Y. Acad. Sci.*, **259**, 59–73.

84. Wald, N.J., Barker, S., Cuckle, H. *et al.* (1977) Maternal serum alphafetoprotein and spontaneous abortion. *Br. J. Obstet. Gynaecol.*, **84**, 285–89.

85. Waller, K., Lustig, L.S., Cunningham, G.C. *et al.* (1991) Second-trimester maternal serum alpha-fetoprotein levels and the risk of fetal death. *N. Engl. J. Med.*, **325**, 6–10.

86. Robinson, L., Grau, P. and Crandall, B.F. (1989) Pregnancy outcomes after increasing maternal serum alpha-fetoprotein levels. *Obstet. Gynecol.*, **74**, 17–20.

87. Wald, N., Cuckle, H., Stirrat, G.M. *et al.* (1977) Maternal serum alphafetoprotein and low-birth-weight. *Lancet*, **ii**, 268–70.

88. Brock, D.J.H., Barron, L. and Raab, G.M. (1980) The potential of midtrimester maternal plasma alpha-fetoprotein measurement in predicting infants of low birth weight. *Br. J. Obstet. Gynaecol.*, **87**, 582–85.

89. Purdie, D.W., Young, J.L., Guthrie, K.A. *et al.* (1983) Fetal growth achievements and elevated maternal serum alpha-fetoprotein. *Br. J. Obstet. Gynaecol.*, **90**, 433–36.

90. Perkes, E.A., Baim, R.S., Goodman, K.J. and Macri, J.N. (1982) Second-trimester placental changes associated with elevated maternal serum α-fetoprotein. *Am. J. Obstet. Gynecol.*, **144**, 935–38.

91. Salafia, C.M., Silberman, L., Herrera, N.E. and Mahoney, M.J. (1988) Placental pathology at term associated with elevated mid-trimester maternal serum α-fetoprotein concentration. *Am. J. Obstet. Gynecol.*, **158**, 1064–68.

92. Merkatz, I.R., Nitowsky, H.M., Macri, J.N. and Johnson, W.E. (1984) An association between low maternal serum α-fetoprotein and fetal chromosomal abnormalities. *Am. J. Obstet. Gynecol.*, **148**, 886–94.

93. Cuckle, H.S., Wald, N.J. and Lindenbaum, R.H. (1984) Maternal serum alpha-fetoprotein measurement: a screening test for Down syndrome. *Lancet*, **i**, 926–29.

94. Fuhrman, W., Wendt, P. and Weitzel, H.K. (1984) Maternal serum-AFP as screening test for Down sydrome. *Lancet*, **ii**, 413.

95. Cuckle, H.S., Wald, N.J. and Lindenbaum, R.H. (1986) Cord serum alpha-fetoprotein and Down syndrome. *Br. J. Obstet. Gynaecol.*, **93**, 408–10.

96. Davis, R.O., Cosper, P., Huddleston, J.F. *et al.* (1985) Decreased levels of AF alpha-fetoprotein associated with Down syndrome. *Am J. Obstet. Gynecol.*, **153**, 541–44.

97. Crandall, B.F., Matsumoto, M. and Perdue, S. (1988) AF-AFP in Down syndrome and other chromosomal abnormalities. *Prenatal Diagn.*, **8**, 255–62.

98. Kronquist, K.E., Dreazen, E., Keener, S.L. *et al.* (1990) Reduced fetal hepatic alpha-fetoprotein levels in Down syndrome. *Prenat. Diagn.*, **10**, 739–51.

99. Davenport, D.M. and Macri, J.N. (1983) The clinical significance of low maternal serum α-fetoprotein. *Am J. Obstet. Gynecol.*, **146**, 657–61.

100. Milunsky, A. (1992) The use of biochemical markers in maternal serum screening for chromosome defects, in *Genetic Disorders and the Fetus*, 3rd edn (ed. A. Milunsky), Johns Hopkins University Press, Baltimore, pp. 565–92.

101. Drugan, A., Dvorin, E., Koppitch, F.C. *et al.* (1989) Counseling for low maternal serum alpha-fetoprotein should emphasize all chromosome anomalies, not just Down syndrome. *Obstet. Gynecol.*, **73**, 271–74.

102. Martin, A.O. and Liu, K. (1986) Implications of 'low' maternal serum alpha-fetoprotein levels: are maternal age risk criteria obsolete? *Prenat. Diagn.*, **6**, 243–7.

103. Hershey, D.W., Crandall, B.F.C. and Perdue, S. (1986) Combining maternal age and serum α-fetoprotein to predict the risk of Down syndrome. *Obstet. Gynecol.*, **68**, 177–80.

104. Cuckle, H.S., Wald, N.J. and Thompson, S.G. (1987) Estimating a woman's risk of having a pregnancy associated with Down syndrome using her age and serum alpha-fetoprotein level. *Br. J. Obstet. Gynaecol.*, **94**, 387–402.

105. Tabor, A., Larsen, S.O., Nielsen, J. *et al.* (1987) Screening for Down's syndrome using an isorisk curve based on maternal age and serum alpha-fetoprotein level. *Br. J. Obstet. Gynaecol.*, **94**, 636–42.

106. DiMaio, M.S., Baumgarten, A., Greenstein, R.M. *et al.* (1987) Screening for fetal Down syndrome in pregnancy by measuring maternal serum alpha-fetoprotein levels. *N. Engl. J. Med.*, **317**, 342–46.

107. New England Regional Genetics Group Prenatal Collaborative Study of Down Syndrome Screening (1989) Combining maternal serum α-fetoprotein measurements and age to screen for Down syndrome in pregnant women under 35. *Am. J. Obstet. Gynecol.*, **3**, 575–81.

108. Lustig, L., Clarke, S., Cunningham, G. *et al.* (1988) California's experience with low MS-AFP results. *Am J. Med. Genet.*, **31**, 211–22.

109. Bogart, M.H., Pandian, M.R. and Jones, O.W. (1987) Abnormal maternal serum chorionic gonadotropin levels in pregnancies with fetal chromosome abnormalities. *Prenat. Diagn.*, **7**, 623–30.

110. Knight, G. and Cole, L.A. (1991) Measurement of choriogonadotrophic free β subunit: an alternative to choriogonadotrophin in screening for fetal Down syndrome? *Clin. Chem.*, **37**, 779–82.

111. Macri, J.N., Kasturi, R., Krantz, D. *et al.* (1990) Maternal serum Down syndrome screening: free β-protein is a more effective marker than human chorionic gonadotropin. *Am. J. Obstet. Gynecol.*, **163**, 1248–53.

112. Wald, N.J., Cuckle, H.S., Densem, J.W. *et al.* (1988) Maternal serum screening for Down syndrome in early pregnancy. *BMJ*, **297**, 883–87.

113. Suchy, S.F. and Yeager, M.T. (1990) Down syndrome screening in women under 35 with maternal serum hCG. *Obstet. Gynecol.*, **76**, 20–24.

114. Jorgensen, P.I. and Trolle, D. (1972) Low urinary oestriol excretion during pregnancy in women giving birth to infants with Down's syndrome. *Lancet*, **ii**, 782–84.

115. Canick, J.A., Knight, G.J., Palomaki, G.E. *et al.* (1988) Low second trimester maternal serum unconjugated oestriol in pregnancies with Down's syndrome. *Br. J. Obstet. Gynaecol.*, **95**, 330–3.

116. McDonald, M.L., Wagner, R.M. and Slotnick, R.N. (1991) Sensitivity and specificity of screening for Down syndrome with alpha-fetoprotein, hCG, unconjugated estriol and maternal age. *Obstet. Gynecol.*, **77**, 63–68.

117. Wald, N.J., Cuckle, H.S., Densem, J.W. *et al.* (1988) Maternal serum unconjugated oestriol as an antenatal screening test for Down syndrome. *Br. J. Obstet. Gynaecol.*, **95**, 334–41.

118. Macri, J.N., Kasturi, R.V., Krantz, D.A. *et al.* (1990) Maternal serum Down syndrome screening: unconjugated estriol is not useful. *Am. J. Obstet. Gynecol.*, **162**, 672–3.

119. Herrou, M., Leporrier, N. and Leymarie, P. (1992) Screening for fetal Down syndrome with maternal serum hCG and oestriol: a prospective study. *Prenat. Diagn.*, **12**, 887–92.

120. Haddow, J.E., Palomaki, G.E., Knight, G.J. *et al.* (1992) Prenatal screening for Down's syndrome with use of maternal serum markers. *N. Engl. J. Med.*, **327**, 588–93.

121. Graham, G.W., Crossley, J.A., Aitken, D.A. and Connor, J.M. (1992) Variation in the levels of pregnancy-specific β-1-glycoprotein in maternal serum from chromosomally abnormal pregnancies. *Prenat. Diagn.*, **12**, 505–12.

122. Van Lith, J.M.M., Pratt, J.J., Beekhuis, J.R. and Mantingh, A. (1992) Second-trimester maternal serum immunoreactive inhibin as a marker for fetal Down's syndrome. *Prenat. Diagn.*, **12**, 801–806.

123. Cuckle, H.S., Wald, N.J., Stone, R. *et al.* (1988) Maternal serum thyroid antibodies in early pregnancy and fetal Down's syndrome. *Prenat. Diagn.*, **8**, 439–45.

124. Cuckle, H.S., Wald, N.J., Densem, J. *et al.* (1990) The effect of smoking in pregnancy on maternal serum alpha-fetoprotein, unconjugated oestriol, human chorionic gonadotrophin, progesterone and dehydroepiandrosterone sulphate levels. *Br. J. Obstet. Gynaecol.*, **98**, 272–6.

125. Norton, M.E. and Golbus, M.S. (1992) Maternal serum CA 125 for aneuploidy detection in early pregnancy. *Prenat. Diagn.*, **12**, 779–81.

126. Cuckle, H.S., Wald, N.J., Goodburn, S.F. *et al.* (1990) Measurement of activity bf urea resistant neutrophil alkaline phosphatase as an antenatal screening test for Down's syndrome. *BMJ*, **301**, 1024–26.

127. Ozturk, M., Milunsky, A., Brambati, B. *et al.* (1990) Abnormal serum levels of human chorionic gonadotropin free subunits in trisomy 18. *Am. J. Med. Genet.*, **36**, 480–83.

128. Bartels, I., Thiele, M. and Bogart, M.H. (1990) Maternal serum hCG and SP1 in pregnancies with fetal aneuploidy. *Am. J. Med. Genet.*, **37**, 261–64.

129. Palomaki, G.E., Knight, G.J. and Haddow, J.E. (1992) Prospective intervention trial of a screening protocol to identify fetal trisomy 18 using maternal serum alpha fetoprotein, unconjugated oestriol, and human chorionic gonadotropin. *Prenat. Diagn.*, **12**, 925–30.

130. Blitzer, M., Carmi, R., Blakemore, K. *et al.* (1991) Low maternal serum human chorionic gonadotropin (MS-hCG) in second trimester trisomy 18 pregnancies (abstract). *Am. J. Hum. Genet.*, **49**, 211.

131. Wald, N.J., Cuckle, H.S., Densem, J.W. et al. (1992) Maternal serum unconjugated oestriol and human chorionic gonadotrophin in pregnancies with insulin-dependent diabetes: implications for Down's syndrome screening. Br. J. Obstet. Gynaecol., 99, 51–53.

132. Bogart, M.H., Jones, O.W., Felder, R.A. et al. (1991) Prospective evaluation of maternal serum human chorionic gonadotropin levels in 3428 pregnancies. Am. J. Obstet. Gynecol., 165, 663–67.

133. Kulch, P., Keener, S., Matsumoto, M. and Crandall, B.F. (1993) Racial differences in maternal serum human chorionic gonadotropin and unconjugated oestriol levels. Prenat. Diagn., 13, 191–5.

134. Bernstein, L., Pike, M.C., Lobo, R.A. et al. (1989) Cigarette smoking in pregnancy results in marked decrease in maternal hCG and oestradiol levels. Br. J. Obstet. Gynaecol., 96, 92–96.

135. Thomsen, S.G., Isager-Sally, L., Lange, A.P. et al. (1983) Smoking habits and maternal serum α-fetoprotein levels during the second trimester of pregnancy. Br. J. Obstet. Gynaecol., 90, 716–17.

136. Bartels, I., Hoppe-Sievert, B., Bockel, B. et al. (1993) Adjustment formulae for maternal serum alphafetoprotein, human chorionic gonadotropin, and unconjugated oestriol to maternal weight and smoking, Prenat. Diagn., 13, 123–130.

137. Wald, N.J., Cuckle, H.S., Wu, T. and George, L. (1991) Maternal serum unconjugated oestriol and human chorionic gonadotrophin levels in twin pregnancies: implications for screening for Down's syndrome. Br. J. Obstet. Gynaecol., 98, 905–908.

138. Wald, N.J., Cuckle, H.S. and Boreham, J. (1984) Alpha-fetoprotein screening for open spina bifida: effect of routine biparietal diameter measurement to estimate gestational age. Rev. Epidemiol. Santé Publique, 32, 62–69.

139. Leporrier, N., Herrou, M. and Leymarie, P. (1992) Shift of the fetal sex ratio in hCG selected pregnancies at risk for Down syndrome. Prenat. Diagn., 12, 703–704.

140. Gravett, C.P., Buckmaster, J.G., Watson, P.T. and Gravett, M.G. (1992) Elevated second trimester maternal serum β-hCG concentrations and subsequent adverse pregnancy outcome. Am. J. Med. Genet., 44, 485–86.

141. Mason G., Lindow, G., Cuckle, H. and Holding, S. (1992) Low maternal serum chorionic gonadotrophin and unconjugated oestriol in a triploid pregnancy. Prenat. Diagn., 12, 545–47.

142. Mason, G., Lindow, S., Ramsden, C. et al. (1993) Low maternal serum oestriol and chorionic gonadotropin in prediction of adverse pregnancy outcome. Prenat. Diagn., 13, 223–25.

143. Canick, J.A., Knight, G.J., Palomaki, G.E. and Haddow, J.E. (1990) Second-trimester levels of maternal serum unconjugated oestriol and human chorionic gonadotropin in pregnancies affected by fetal anencephaly and open spina bifida. Prenat. Diagn., 10, 733–37.

144. Fuhrman, W., Altland, K., Jovanovic, V. et al. (1993) First-trimester alpha-fetoprotein screening for Down syndrome. Prenat. Diagn., 13, 215–18.

145. Brambati, B., MacIntosh, M.C.M., Teisner, B. et al. (1993) Low maternal serum levels of pregnancy-associated plasma protein A (PAPP-A) in the first trimester in association with abnormal fetal karyotype. Br. J. Obstet. Gynaecol., 100, 324–26.

146. Bronshtein, M. and Blumenfeld, Z. (1992) Transvaginal sonography-detection of findings suggestive of fetal chromosomal anomalies in the first and early second trimesters. Prenat. Diagn., 12, 587–93.

147. Campbell, S., Johnstone, F.D. and Holt, E.M. (1972) Anencephaly: early ultrasound diagnosis and active management. Lancet, ii, 1226–27.

148. Rose, J.S. (1977) The ultrasonic diagnosis of fetal neural tube abnormalities. Ann. Radiol., 20, 19–24.

149. Allen, L.C., Doran, T.A., Miskin, M. et al. (1982) Ultrasound and amniotic fluid alpha-fetoprotein in the prenatal diagnosis of spina bifida. Obstet. Gynecol., 60, 169–73.

150. Campbell, J., Gilbert, W.M., Nicolaides, K.N. and Campbell, S. (1987) Ultrasound screening for spina bifida: cranial and cerebellar signs in a high risk population. Obstet. Gynecol., 70, 247–50.

151. Benacerraf, B., Miller, W.A. and Frigoletto, F.D. (1988) Sonographic detection of fetuses with trisomies 13 and 18: accuracy and limitations. Am. J. Obstet. Gynecol., 158, 404–409.

152. Wald, N.J., Cuckle, H.S., Boreham, J. and Stirrat, G. (1980) Small biparietal diameter of fetuses with spina bifida: implications for antenatal screening. Br. J. Obstet. Gynaecol., 87, 219–21.

153. Persson, P.H., Kullander, S., Gennser, G. et al. (1983) Screening for fetal malformations using ultrasound and measurements of α-fetoprotein in maternal serum. BMJ, 286, 747–49.

154. Cuckle, H.S. and Wald, N.J. (1987) The effect of estimating gestational age by ultrasound cephalometry on the sensitivity of alpha-fetoprotein screening for Down's syndrome. Br. J. Obstet. Gynaecol., 94, 274–76.

155. Zeitune, M., Ben-Tovim, T., Fejgin, M. et al. (1991) Screening for Down's syndrome in older women based on maternal serum alpha-fetoprotein levels and age: preliminary results. Prenat. Diagn., 11, 393–98.

156. Haddow, J.E., Palomaki, G.E., Knight, G.J. et al. (1994) Reducing the need for amniocentesis in women 35 years of age or older with serum markers for screening. N. Engl. J. Med., 330, 1114–18.

157. Results of a Consensus Meeting (1985) Maternal serum alpha-fetoprotein screening for neural tube defects. Prenat. Diagn., 5, 77–83.

158. MacRae, A.R. (1990) Screening for high-risk pregnancies with maternal serum alpha-fetoprotein (MSAFP). The Canadian Society of Clinical Chemists' Task Force on MSAFP Screening. Clin. Biochem., 23, 469–76.

159. Seror, V., Muller, F., Moatti, J.P. et al. (1993) Economic assessment of maternal serum screening for Down's syndrome using human chorionic gonadotropin. Prenat. Diagn., 13, 281–92.

63 NEONATAL SCREENING AND CARRIER DETECTION

N.R.M. Buist and J.M. Tuerck

63.1 Introduction

The panoply of modern medical technology has made it progressively easier to detect diseases much earlier than before. Indeed, it is now standard medical practice to screen for a large variety of conditions before they begin to cause symptoms or irreparable damage. Screening of adults for hypertension, glaucoma, malignant disease and numerous biochemical abnormalities is expected by patients, but in each case is done on an individual basis, with consent or at least with tacit approval, in an attempt to improve an individual's health.

In contrast to this approach, the last 30 years has seen the development of over 50 tests which have been devised for routine newborn screening. About ten of these are in routine use in different combinations in different programs. The primary tests are for phenylketonuria (PKU) and hypothyroidism. Guthrie's blood test to detect PKU in infants, first routinely deployed in April 1961 in Oregon and Massachusetts, led the way to 'one of the successes of modern medicine' [1]. His revolutionary idea that blood constituents might be stable in samples dried on absorbent paper presaged the discovery that not only amino acids and other small metabolites, but also hormones, polypeptides and a large variety of cellular and plasma proteins including enzymes and antibodies, were stable and could be reliably detected and quantitated in dried samples equivalent to 2–6 μl of whole blood. Many of the tests often reflect the interests and expertise of their designers rather than their true value as screening tests for general use. Many have indeed been tried for mass screening, some being dropped, others incorporated permanently into a screening battery, sometimes without critical evaluation. For example, after 27 years of screening for galactosemia, there is still deep disagreement about its value [2]. Clearly, all new tests need to evolve through a rigorous review to ensure that they meet the requirements of the society which is involved.

Concern over the growing menu of tests, and the possibility of their uncritical inclusion into formal screening programs, led the World Health Organization (WHO) to formulate some general guidelines regarding these issues (Table 63.1) [3].

In the last 10 years, the new technology of genetic diagnosis by detection of defects in enzymes, proteins and even DNA and RNA now provides the means to detect an even larger array of inherited conditions. This technology, while still clearly in the realm of research and development, will ultimately provide the ability to detect DNA mutations in both homozygous and heterozygous individuals routinely – a development which has

Table 63.1 Recommendations of WHO regarding screening [After Ref. 3]

1. Appropriate techniques and methods for general screening and certain high risk populations should be developed
2. Automatic procedures for sample analysis and handling should be developed
3. The long-term storage of biological specimens should be standard
4. Large scale pilot studies should be made to evaluate and compare screening methods
5. Selected populations should be studied to obtain data on frequency of these diseases and traits
6. Multidisciplinary groups are needed to study the short and long-term social and biological consequences of screening programs
7. A careful estimate should be made of the cost of the program and of personal facilities and equipment needed
8. Central laboratories specializing in screening procedures should be created on a regional basis and existing laboratories should be assisted
9. There should be special regional centers for the study and management of patients
10. Collaborative studies on the management of patients should be done
11. International cooperation is needed for exchange and training of personnel and exchange of information, materials and comparison of results and outcome

Diseases of the Fetus and Newborn, 2nd edn, Edited by G.B. Reed, A.E. Claireaux and F. Cockburn. Published in 1995 by Chapman & Hall, London. ISBN 0 412 39160 0

profound implications for communal and personal decisions in the coming century.

In this chapter we will confine ourselves to a review of the major screening tests which are performed on newborn infants through the use of filter paper samples. In addition we will review the new directions for genetic screening which can be envisaged through the use of filter paper or other blood samples.

63.2 Universal neonatal screening

It is hard for thee to kick against the pricks.

Acts 8:5

All the current tests for newborn screening identify abnormal metabolites, hormones or hemoglobin patterns in an otherwise asymptomatic infant; therefore, if all affected infants are to be found, all infants must be screened. In the USA recognition of this basic premise has led most states to enact legislation mandating screening of every newborn [4]. Even in states or countries where it is voluntary, participation in newborn screening is high, reflecting the widespread acceptability and benefits of screening [5].

When screening is mandated, it is not necessary for practitioners to obtain informed consent from parents, and specimens are routinely collected prior to discharge from the newborn nursery. Once in the laboratory, all specimens are tested for all the disorders covered in a given state or region. Although it has been proposed, there is usually no choice in the selection of tests; this leads to major cost savings and liability protection for both practitioners and the laboratory, in that decisions regarding 'at-risk' infants are not made by practitioners, and laboratory personnel do not have to sort samples, which is a time consuming and error prone activity.

Since its inception, neonatal screening has been viewed as a preventive public health program and as such has been guided by criteria designed to maximize the benefits (i.e. prevention of mental handicap) while minimizing the costs and complexities for participants. Many of these criteria are now being challenged in light of burgeoning technology and community expectations.

63.2.1 ORGANIZATION OF NEONATAL SCREENING PROGRAMS

Newborn screening programs are complex systems in which private care providers, laboratory personnel, administrative follow-up personnel and tertiary care providers all play different and critical roles and have different responsibilities for the success of the overall program (Figure 63.1).

Practitioners are responsible for ensuring correct collection and handling of screening specimens, parent

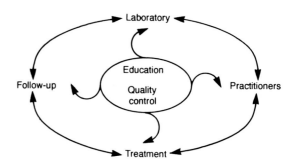

Figure 63.1 Model for a newborn screening system.

education, prompt follow-up in the event of an abnormal result and that every baby is tested.

Central screening laboratory personnel are responsible for testing, record keeping, quality control of laboratory methods, notification of results and tracking of abnormal and unresolved results.

Follow-up personnel are responsible for ensuring confirmation tests are obtained on infants with abnormal results, practitioner and lay education and for program quality assurance and evaluation.

Tertiary care providers are responsible for treatment and long-term management of confirmed cases.

It cannot be emphasized strongly enough that newborn screening should not be a laboratory-driven program but an integrated system. Without the enthusiastic and educated compliance of each participant the system readily breaks down, in which case the legal liabilities for missed cases are often assigned to everyone connected with the program.

Most screening programs are administered through state or national health systems which may supply some or all of the costs, although many programs in the USA are now completely supported by fees.

63.2.2 CRITERIA FOR SELECTION OF SCREENING TESTS

There have been several attempts to codify recommendations for adoption of newborn screening tests, but criteria which can be applied in diverse societies have been difficult to develop. While the tenets developed by WHO (Table 63.1) [3] certainly remain valid, societal, political, financial and moral issues have emerged and other attempts have been made to formulate guidelines for evaluating the benefits of a screening test. One such set, which seems more in tune with the 1990s, is summarized in Table 63.2 [6]. However, it must be emphasized that all such proposals are strongly colored by national or regional realities and that what applies in one country may have little relevance elsewhere. The

Table 63.2 Amended guidelines for newborn screening [After Ref. 4]

1. Newborn screening is a public health act of preventive medicine
2. Tests should be of immediate health benefit to the infant, i.e. intervention should prevent or ameliorate symptoms
3. Tests should be universally available for the target population
4. Tests should not be done if facilities for evaluation, treatment and counseling are not available
5. Tests should be done with appropriate methods for the population being tested and the methods should have appropriate sensitivity and specificity
6. Pilot studies should be done to demonstrate efficacy and benefits in the population to be tested
7. Screening programs should inform parents and the public of the goals, scope and objectives of the tests being performed
8. Screening tests results should be confirmed by specific assays
9. No tests should be introduced until matters of quality control in the laboratory, a follow-up treatment program and screening practices have been identified and addressed
10. Use of anonymous samples for disease surveillance is acceptable provided that (a) voluntary access to such testing is also available, (b) the test results are also unlinked, and (c) that sample or program requirements for the anonymous testing do not impinge upon the primary reasons for obtaining the screening samples in the first place
11. Newborn screening programs could use DNA typing as a test procedure when genetic heterogeneity in populations becomes technically interpretable

diversity of newborn screening programs even within the USA demonstrates how personal and local issues determine their design and execution. It is for this reason that no recommendations for global deployment of any screening test exist.

Few tests meet all of these criteria, and none really qualifies **before** being deployed in mass screening since the full clinical spectrum and the effect of treatment may not be known for years after a test is introduced. For example, the variants of PKU and hypothyroidism were not known at the outset, and there was serious debate whether early treatment would change the outcome. Galactosemia screening seemed to be remarkably effective by preventing early death from hepatocellular damage and Gram-negative sepsis. However, a recent survey of 350 cases indicates that most patients, even when well diagnosed and treated from birth, have lower IQs, speech and motor dysfunction, and growth and ovarian failure [2]; screening, therefore, prevents death but not the long-term sequelae. Likewise, treatment of sickle-cell disease with prophylactic penicillin prevents death from sepsis but does little to ameliorate the sickling crises or their debilitating effects.

63.2.3 THE TOP TEN TESTS

Well over 50 newborn screening tests have been described; the most common are named in Table 63.3, together with some of the initial screening practice considerations. In fact each of the methods entails a large number of such considerations which must be well understood before any routine or pilot program is started.

63.2.4 COST/BENEFITS

In the last few years most newborn screening programs in the USA have begun to charge fees for performing the tests. The actual cost for collection and prelaboratory processing is calculated to be between $3 and $7 per specimen. Laboratory costs vary depending upon which tests are used but range from about $3 to $10 per sample. A few programs in the USA charge more than the laboratory costs in order to cover the costs of other aspects of the program, such as medical consultation, follow-up, education, treatment, or, in some cases, support for other genetic services. Such a model could result in a major improvement in the quality of screening and other genetic services across the USA.

Screening programs, whether of newborn infants or of other populations, must be viewed in the context of national health priorities and available budgets. A well-executed immunization program can affect the health of the whole population, whereas screening for PKU or congenital hypothyroidism (both entirely justifiable in many societies) may only benefit the health of 35–40 infants per 100 000 births (Table 63.4). Filter paper screening for toxins such as lead or drug exposures, infectious diseases or immune status, or for nutritional hypothyroidism or other nutritional deficiencies, might be more valuable than screening for a congenital or hereditary condition. The ability to monitor tuberculosis, parasitic or other communicable diseases through a centralized screening program might have profoundly beneficial effects in certain societies and many are certainly technically feasible at this time.

63.2.5 CONSIDERATIONS FOR SPECIMEN COLLECTION AND HANDLING

A bird in the hand is worth two in the bush.

Anonymous

(a) Timing of the test

Postnatal care practices vary enormously in different parts of the world. In many parts of the USA over 50% of infants are discharged home within 24 hours of birth. In other countries, infants may not leave the hospital for 3–7 days. In Britain, all infants are

Table 63.3 Neonatal screening tests performed in North America

Condition/major symptoms	Type of test	Special screening practice considerations
Aminoacidopathies (phenylalanine, tyrosine, methionine, leucine)		Abnormal blood levels develop after birth and depend on the severity of the defect and the protein intake Transient elevations are not uncommon, especially in sick or premature infants Hyperalimentation can raise blood levels (usually of several amino acids) Antibiotics can affect the assays Need to retest all 'early' tested infants
PKU, hyperphenylalaninemia Incidence: 1:12 000 Symptoms: mental handicap	B,C,F	Variants not uncommon
Maple syrup urine disease Incidence: 1:250 000 Symptoms: acidosis, CNS damage, death	B	Rapid onset of symptoms Screen before 3 days for rapid detection
Homocystinuria Incidence: 1:250 000 Symptoms: Late onset mental handicap, dislocated lenses, liver damage, osteoporosis, thromboses	B,C	Methionine may not be elevated in all forms of this disorder Methionine slow to rise after birth No neonatal symptoms

Tyrosinemia
Incidence: 1:150 000
  Type 1: liver/kidney damage, failure to thrive, death
  Type 2: eye and skin lesions
	B,C	Tyrosine may be slow to rise after birth
		Methionine rises later still and only in type 1
		Type 1 has acute infantile and later onset chronic forms
		Transient tyrosinemia of newborn is common

Hypothyroidism Incidence: 1:4000 Symptoms: mental handicap, cretinism, growth delay	I	Different physiologic values in premature and sick infants Late onset of disorder in 10% of cases Thyroid binding globulin deficiency (1:5000) gives low T_4, normal TSH, raised T_3 resin binding Hypopituitary hypothyroidism (3–5% of cases) have normal TSH Effect of maternal medications or antibodies or iodine on infant's thyroid
Galactosemia Incidence: 1:60 000 Symptoms: liver, kidney, CNS damage, sepsis, death, late onset speech and ovarian dysfunction	β (galactose or galactose 1-phosphate) F Enzyme (Beutler) test	Galactose only rises after lactose ingestion Galactose can be increased in liver diseases Antibiotics affect the metabolite assays Assays may become 'normal' after transfusions In classic galactosemia, galactose 1-phosphate is elevated without galactose ingestions and even in cord blood. Enzyme test is also abnormal In 'benign' variants of galactosemia both the enzyme test and galactose 1-phosphate may be abnormal Enzyme test affected by heat, storage and transfusions In galactokinase deficiency only the galactose test is valid
Biotinidase deficiency Incidence: 1:250 000 Symptoms: acidosis, skin rashes, growth failure, death	F (biotinidase)	Enzyme affected by heat, storage and transfusions
Sickle-cell diseases Incidence: 1:400 (African–American) Symptoms: sepsis, anemia, vascular occlusion, bone, kidney damage, death	C,E (Hb)	Specimen must be obtained before transfusion Heterozygote detection can create problem of follow-up and counseling
Congenital adrenal hyperplasia Incidence: 1:12 000 Symptoms: virilization, electrolyte imbalances, shock, death	I (17-OH-progesterone)	Rapid onset of shock in severe cases Affected female patients more likely to be detected clinically by virilization
Cystic fibrosis Incidence: 1:2500 (Caucasian) Symptoms: meconium ileus, pancreatic and respiratory dysfunction, malnutrition, death	I (trypsin) D (only specific mutations)	High incidence of false-positive results Appreciate incidence of false-negative results Continuing debate over long-term benefits Trypsin test is only applicable in early infancy

B = bacterial; C = chromatography; D = DNA analysis; E = electrophoresis; F = fluorescent/colorimetric assay; I = immunoasay. Other tests that have been developed and that might be under trial in some programs include Duchenne dystrophy (creatine phosphokinase assay), α_1-antitrypsin deficiency, c-esterase deficiency, hyperlipidemia, congenital infection (IgM), toxoplasmosis, syphilis, peroxisomal diseases (very long chain fatty acids), protoporphyrins (lead poisoning), red cell enzyme defects such as glucose-6-phosphate dehydrogenase deficiency, and adenosine deaminase deficiency.

Table 63.4 Costs (1985 US$) per 100 000 infants
[After Ref. 7]

	Screen and treat	Immunize	
	PKU/CH	MMR	HIB
Cases	35–40	100 000	
Costs ($ million)	1.7	2.6	0.3
Savings ($ million)	3.2	3.8	9.0

CH = congenital hypothyroidism; MMR = measles, mumps, rubella; HIB = *Haemophilus influenzae* B.

routinely visited at home shortly after discharge. If only one specimen is to be collected, such differences profoundly affect the decision of when it should be collected. The decision is further complicated by the fact that in disorders such as PKU the test does not become totally reliable for 48–72 hours, although most cases can be detected by 24 hours. On the other hand, disorders such as maple syrup urine disease, galacto-semia or congenital adrenal hyperplasia cause life-threatening symptoms within a few days; effective screening for these disorders needs to be done within 24–72 hours of birth.

In the UK and other countries in Europe the normal practice is to postpone testing until 5–9 days after birth **because** the community follow-up systems are so efficient. In the USA the situation is very different and universal predischarge testing is recommended since many infants do not return for routine postnatal care. While routine discharge screening assures that every infant is tested, it does not ensure that all infants with PKU will be detected, in view of the high rate of early discharge before 24 hours of protein and lactose ingestion. In order to address these problems, the American Academy of Pediatrics has made the follow-ing recommendations.

- All infants should be screened before discharge.
- All infants screened before 24 hours of age should be rescreened before 14 days of age.
- All infants should be tested before the 7th day of life.

Some programs are more conservative and require or advise rescreening of all infants initially tested before 48 hours of age. It is the authors' firm conviction that discharge screening constitutes a fundamental standard of care for all infants. The question of whether all children in the USA should be rescreened is addressed later in this chapter.

(b) Type of blood sample

Cord blood is not acceptable for a routine specimen because most metabolites do not accumulate until after

birth. It is collected in some states, partly for research and partly because it can be used to detect abnormal proteins such as antibodies, red cell enzyme defects and some hormone deficiencies. Thus, the red cell enzyme (Beutler) test for galactosemia and the tests for biotini-dase deficiency, hemoglobinopathies and various anti-bodies can be performed on cord blood samples because they do not depend on the age or intake of the infant. At least 90% of cases of congenital hypothyroidism also can be detected in cord blood by a low thyroxine (T_4) and elevated thyroid stimulating hormone (TSH) because T_4 does not cross the placenta from the mother.

(c) Filter paper application

Thou shalt bruise his heel

Genesis 3:15

Blood should be applied from only one side of the paper; it is best obtained from a heel stick and ideally should collect in one large drop on the infant's heel, sufficient to fill the entire circle. Venous blood is also acceptable because it may be more accessible in sick newborns; care should be taken to ensure that intra-venous lines are clear of heparin or hyperalimentation and that blood from a syringe is applied to the filter paper without the needle to prevent hemolysis. Blood may be collected in capillary tubes but the glass should not touch the filter paper because it may cause microscopic tears. Most assays are calibrated to a 1/8-inch filter paper disk, which contains only 3 μl of blood, so uniform saturation of the paper is critical [8].

(d) Specimen handling

Contamination of the filter paper with fingers, body oils, urine, stool, alcohol, milk or other substances can interfere with saturation, cause dilution of the blood, or interfere with assays. For example, contamination with milk causes galactose elevations. Specimens should be individually air dried at room temperature in a horizon-tal position; hanging or vertical drying results in uneven concentration of blood within the spots, and specimens stacked on top of each other can cause cross-contamination. Enzymes are easily destroyed by expo-sure to heat; common sources include sunlight, heaters, microwaves, and mailboxes in summer. Samples collected on weekends or holidays are best stored at room temperature and sent express mail, rather than spending the weekend in a hot mailbox.

(e) Demographic data

The information requested on the screening requisition form varies from program to program. All the data items are needed, however, not only to identify the infant and the submitter, but to determine the follow-up in the event of an abnormal result. Omission of information can result in delayed or missed diagnosis. In some areas, 25% of samples are missing critical data such as name, birthdate, sample date or feeding history [9]. The automatic imprinting devices commonly used for laboratory requisitions are one of the most common causes of unreadable data items.

(f) Transit to the screening laboratory

Transit delays are a frequent screening practice problem; all specimens should be mailed within 24 hours of collection. Enzyme activity can decrease within a few days, which results in false-positive results for the Beutler and biotinidase tests. Some laboratories refuse to test specimens more than a few days old.

Most specimens in North America are sent through the regular mail, which is usually adequate, but even when daily courier services are used, preventable transit delays still can occur. Batching specimens in the wards, offices or laboratories for several days is common. Moreover, specimens batched in large envelopes may go by third class mail unless otherwise marked. The savings on postage must be balanced against potential liability. Egress from the hospital can be delayed by cumbersome in-laboratory tracking systems; although these are clearly important, all personnel must recognize the priority nature of newborn screening specimens.

(g) Premature or sick infants

These infants should have their first test taken before 7 days of age, regardless of health or feeding status. Normal premature infants may have low T_4 results that gradually normalize over the first 5 weeks, but serial tests may be required. Transient hypothyroidism can occur in infants exposed to topical iodinated antiseptic agents [10].

(h) Hyperalimentation and antibiotic therapy

Hyperalimentation and antibiotic therapy are not contraindications to testing, but samples should not be taken from the lines used for alimentation or drugs. High levels of plasma amino acids can occur during hyperalimentation, and antibiotics can inhibit growth of the bacteria used in some assays. These therapies must be specified on the request slip.

(i) Transfusions

A screening specimen should be taken before any transfusion, regardless of the age, health or feeding status of the infant. Donor blood provides plasma and cells that can negate the assays for several conditions, particularly the hemoglobinopathies, galactosemia and biotinidase deficiency. Transfusions only transiently affect the levels of abnormal metabolites such as the amino acids or galactose.

(j) Transfer of infants between hospitals

Some programs specify either the sending or the receiving hospital to be responsible for obtaining the specimen; however, practitioners must remain alert that these infants have a high risk of not being screened during all the activity that usually surrounds such transfers.

63.2.6 FOLLOW-UP OF SCREENING RESULTS

Failure to provide appropriate follow-up is a common reason for affected infants to be missed [11].

Before discharge, hospital and birth unit personnel, or even administrators, may be designated by law and listed on the request slip as the physician of record. In the event of an abnormality the screening laboratory must refer to the physician of record although the infant is no longer under his or her care and may not even be known to him or her. Responsibility for follow-up remains with the physician of record until it is actively accepted by another practitioner. This requires extra vigilance for the highly mobile segments of our society, including the armed forces.

In cases in which an infant cannot be located, local and state public health departments or laboratory assistance can be enlisted. Efforts to find an infant should be carefully documented before a case can be closed as 'lost to follow-up'.

(a) Normal results

The laboratory should mail all results to the submitter on a regular basis, although this is not standard practice in many places. Sometimes two copies are sent, one for the hospital and the other for the physician of record. It is critical for each submitter, whether hospital, birth center or private care provider, to ensure that a report has been received for *every* infant. Failure to receive a report implies that the specimen may have been lost and places the onus on the submitter and the practitioner to determine that an infant's test results were normal.

(b) Unsatisfactory specimens

There is wide variation among screening laboratories as to what constitutes an unsatisfactory specimen. In some programs, any of the problems discussed in section

63.2.5 may cause the sample to be rejected without testing and automatically triggers a request for a repeat specimen. In others, as many tests as possible are run while a repeat sample is being obtained. In all such cases the practitioner of record must ensure that repeat specimens are redrawn as quickly as possible.

(c)   Abnormal results

Presumptive positive results or significant abnormalities are generally reported by telephone to the practitioner of record; in most programs, lesser abnormalities are usually reported by mail. Instructions regarding the appropriate follow-up and confirmation testing vary, depending on the kind and degree of abnormality and the condition of the infant. Practitioners must ensure that the appropriate confirmation tests are obtained on every infant when requested and that the results are reported to the screening program.

63.3   Current issues in newborn screening

(a)   Quality control issues

It has been found to be inefficient, costly and even dangerous to run newborn screening tests in small-volume laboratories. It is extremely hard to maintain high quality control for tests that only have a genuinely abnormal result in between 1:5000 and 1:50 000 samples. Most lawsuits for missed cases have originated under such circumstances. Optimally, a single laboratory should handle at least 50 000–200 000 newborn screening samples per year. Quality control of laboratory functions is now standard, with national regulations provided for most laboratory activities. It is only recently, however, that any quality assurance measures have been applied to the other, interconnected parts of newborn screening systems (Figure 63.1).

(b)   Targeted screening

This term indicates that a test is used only for a specific group of people and not for everyone. For example, some states have targeted screening of blacks for hemoglobinopathies and universal screening for PKU, although the latter occurs predominantly in whites. In the USA there has been a huge amount of racial admixture so that 'ethnic' diseases such as PKU, cystic fibrosis or sickle-cell disease, while much commoner in certain populations, can occur in anyone. In targeted screening, practitioners must decide which infants belong to the high-risk group and indicate on the request slip that hemoglobin testing should be done. This clearly puts an impossible demand upon practitioners and exposes the program to considerable medicolegal risk. In the USA the National Institutes of Health have recognized this liability and have recommended universal screening for hemoglobinopathies.

(c)   Is every infant screened?

Even though most patients are screened, cases are still missed, with resulting disease, disability and major legal battles. The greatest responsibility of a screening program, therefore, is to assure that every infant is properly tested, that the results are known and filed in the infant's record, that follow-up samples or information requested by the screening program are supplied promptly and that treatment is properly initiated. In 1990 there were about 4.4 million births in North America; for each 1% not tested, three patients with PKU and ten with hypothyroidism may be missed. In some areas, up to 50% of infants are discharged before 24 hours of age. Moreover, up to 5% of births in the USA now occur out of hospital, half of them being attended by unlicensed midwives. Such situations create potential pitfalls for unwary practitioners.

(d)   Routine rescreening

The increasing trend towards early discharge in the USA has precipitated tremendous debate regarding routine rescreening of all infants. In some areas it may be feasible for practitioners to track and retest all the infants who were screened early. In other areas, however, 50–80% of infants are discharged and tested early and require retesting, in which case routine rescreening becomes more practical and economical.

In a program where routine rescreening is practiced, 10% of infants with hypothyroidism were detected only on the second test [12]. All these infants had initial T_4 levels that were normal; only 20% had an abnormal TSH by retrospective analysis. All would therefore have been missed if a single T_4 was the primary screening test, and 80% would have been missed if TSH was the primary test. In places where only a single test is recommended, practitioners must be aware of the necessity for rescreening infants tested early and must always remain alert to the possibility of hypothyroidism in older children.

(e)   Human immunodeficiency virus testing

Antibody to human immunodeficiency virus (HIV) crosses the placenta and can be detected in the infant's blood. Detection of the antibody implies that the mother has been infected but does not indicate whether she or her infant is actively infectious or whether either will necessarily develop acquired immunodeficiency syndrome. In the last 5 years, routine testing of newborn screening specimens for maternal antibodies to HIV has been introduced in many states in order to provide ongoing surveillance on the HIV status of fertile heterosexual females [13]. This program was introduced only after assurances that it would not compromise existing newborn screening priorities, and is therefore done anonymously. Currently samples are batched in such a way that the HIV status of the community can be tracked, but no individual patient can be identified. It has proved to be a very powerful public health tool and has provided the best available means for tracking the HIV in the heterosexual population. In some hospitals in the USA more than 2% of samples are abnormal and there is increasing pressure to de-anonymize the procedure so that individual cases can be identified. In the current climate, and with lack of curative therapy, this could seriously compromise the public's acceptance of newborn metabolic screening.

(f) Is consent necessary?

Where screening for PKU is required by law, no prior consent would seem to be necessary. In the USA a few states require screening for other metabolic diseases. When such conditions are added to the screening battery it is often without the knowledge or consent of either the families or the practitioners involved. Some explanation of all the screening tests should be provided before they are performed; in some instances, a form of parental assent might seem appropriate. Screening for Duchenne muscular dystrophy is a poignant example. Proponents argue on the benefits of early recognition, treatment and genetic counseling. Opponents point out that no treatment or cure is possible and grave distortions of emotional bonding and behavior may result from such early, unsolicited and unwelcome information. In this kind of situation there is no single right solution.

63.3.1 OTHER USES FOR FILTER PAPER TECHNOLOGY

In several places, including Japan, routine screening of infants' urine for neuroblastoma is offered. Urine is collected on filter paper at several months of age and screened for catecholamine metabolites. There is no question that many presymptomatic cases are detected, and the program has many firm proponents [14]. Pilot trials have been reported from North America but the consensus is that this program should not be introduced on a wide scale until issues are resolved regarding the costs, detection ratio and clinical significance of some of the tumors that are detected.

There is no reason why filter paper technology should not be used for other conditions and other age groups. For example, hypothyroidism is far more common in the elderly than in infants, and the cost of

the testing is small compared with tests on liquid blood samples in regular laboratories. Similarly, an argument could be made for wide-scale screening for drugs or infectious diseases such as infectious hepatitis, syphilis, toxoplasmosis, HIV or other infections of public health concern, including many tropical diseases. Indeed, multiplex methods could be developed so that several such disorders could be detected simultaneously. Routine filter paper specimens could be obtained at school entry or leaving. Currently available methods for lead poisoning, hyperlipidemia, α_1-antitrypsin deficiency, or other new tests – for example, islet cell antibodies to detect presymptomatic juvenile onset diabetes – could be justified, particularly if presymptomatic therapy was effective.

63.4 The impact of DNA technology

Although small pricks
To their subsequent volumes, there is seen
The baby figure of the giant mass
of things to come
                    Troilus and Cressida, I. iii. 343

It is now possible to use the polymerase chain reaction to amplify specific portions of DNA with great speed and accuracy. This has profound implications for the future in regard to detection of both homozygous and heterozygous conditions and is discussed further below.

Since most of the conditions discussed above are autosomal recessive traits, the following discussion relates to them as well. Indeed genetic testing by DNA analysis is already well established on an individual basis for PKU, cystic fibrosis, muscular dystrophy and sickle-cell disease, among others. For two of these, cystic fibrosis and sickle-cell hemoglobinopathy, routine carrier identification is already a public health issue.

For the most part, diagnosis of genetic disease and of genetic risks is initiated with an enquiry from an individual or a family regarding a specific condition. Evaluation starts with obtaining an accurate pedigree that is as complete as possible. From this, statistical genetic risks can usually be assigned to individuals, depending upon their relationship to an affected proband. The pedigree information is usually refined by physical examination or by special laboratory tests. While this sounds simple, the spectrum and variability of genetic disorders is so wide that most such counseling is done in genetic clinics which specialize in this area.

It is now possible to use the polymerase chain reaction to amplify the DNA from a Guthrie blood spot or a single hair, or even from a single cell, to quantities which can be analyzed by standard laboratory techniques provided the specific DNA information which is required is known. This has already been done in pilot projects for several disorders and is being proposed as a possible alternative approach to the current methods for hemoglobin screening [15]. However, this has the disadvantage that other forms of hemoglobinopathy would not be detected.

We now know that some conditions, such as sickle cell disease, are only caused by one specific single base pair mutation, whereas most others can be caused by a huge variety of mutational changes with deletions, duplications, additions, inversions, insertions of huge chunks of DNA or by apparently minor changes which may affect only one base pair. Moreover many conditions which appear to be homogeneous clinically may be caused by defects of a number of completely different genes (Chapter 75).

Certain conditions such as sickle-cell disease, Tay–Sachs and Gaucher's disease occur predominantly in specific racial groups, while many others have strong geographic or national associations. In such instances it is more likely that specific mutations may be found in these populations, but even among Ashkenazi Jews there are several common Tay–Sachs mutations, so that one single DNA probe cannot detect every case. In medium chain acyl-CoA dehydrogenase deficiency, one mutation accounts for about 90% of all the homozygotes, so that using only one probe could identify most homozygotes and heterozygotes. In cystic fibrosis and PKU there are hundreds of mutations, but about a dozen account for the majority of the cases. It would be possible to achieve reasonably complete homozygote detection by deploying a battery of different gene probes.

Readers should realize that this technology will render other kinds of genetic diagnoses feasible. DNA diagnosis of dominantly inherited diseases, such as neurofibromatosis, tuberous sclerosis, Huntington's disease and a host of other diseases, should become possible, and later it may be possible to detect genes for familial cancer, environmentally related disorders, or even diseases of aging by similar approaches. Samples also could be used for forensic purposes, for example to compare the DNA found in the stored sample from a baby with that of a grown individual suspected of a crime.

63.5 Heterozygote (carrier) detection

The same DNA technology that detects homozygotes can also detect heterozygotes. It is a primary tenet of genetics that information on one's genetic risks is a private matter and that this must be voluntarily sought. Heterozygote detection by DNA analysis can be done for many conditions in specific families when the mutation has already been identified. In most disorders the mutations occur in all segments of the gene so that it is unlikely that simple, universal screening for carriers of any disease will be contemplated in the near future.

For an autosomal recessive trait, such as PKU, with an incidence of 1:10 000, it can be calculated by the Hardy–Weinberg equation that 1:50 people is a heterozygote; for disorders which occur within an incidence of 1:1 000 000, the carrier rate is 1:500. Since there are thousands of genetic conditions it can be seen that every single person must carry several dozen deleterious or even lethal mutations. Society has not begun to grapple with the idea of universal screening for carriers of such disorders but it must be expected that, with the new DNA technology, this will become an increasingly urgent area of public health concern.

Voluntary, consented screening performed on individuals, families or limited ethnic groups is in stark contrast to universal screening. Until recently there was little overlap between the two approaches but this has changed with screening for sickle-cell disease. The current technology of electrophoresis, which separates hemoglobin species, identifies both homozygotes (for which it was designed) **and heterozygotes**. For the first time a universal, mandated, newborn test identifies asymptomatic carriers of an ethnically sensitive disease trait. This raises fierce political and socioethical issues which must be addressed by any program in which sickle-cell screening is done, and which, for the most part, have not been resolved in any state.

At present, although this technology is available to do widespread screening for specific mutations in heterozygotes on filter paper samples (HbS, PKU, cystic fibrosis), none is being deployed for this purpose. Thus it is only the hemoglobin screening programs which are currently, serendipitously, detecting heterozygotes and which have highlighted the difficulties of doing this and handling the abnormal results. Three different disorders exemplify the present situation.

(a) Carrier detection for Tay–Sachs disease

This disorder occurs in about 1:3500 Ashkenazim, which indicates that about 1:27 of this ethnic group is a carrier. There has been a vast international collaborative effort to identify carriers through well-publicized voluntary programs designed to identify individuals and couples at risk before they have married or conceived. This testing is not done on filter paper but on serum and is based upon an enzyme assay for hexosaminidase under extremely stringent conditions. Pregnancy and systemic diseases invalidate the serum test, which must then be performed on leukocytes. Both methods are costly and cumbersome and neither is a screening test in the same genre as newborn screening. Screening for the Tay–Sachs gene is now widely accepted and it is now standard of care to offer this testing to all Ashkenazim. However, as of 1992, only about one million people have yet been tested around the world. It is pertinent to ask why more people have not chosen to be tested. Cost, ignorance, availability of the test and disinterest all contribute their share.

(b) Sickle-cell disease

The current situation in regard to screening for carriers of sickle-cell disease could not be more different. The homozygous condition occurs in about 1:400 Afro-Americans. This corresponds to a carrier incidence of about 1:10.

Since standard filter paper methods for newborn screening detect HbS, it follows that heterozygotes will be identified even though the test was not designed to do this. It therefore becomes critical to have policy decisions about how this information should be processed since all genetic testing should be pre-informed and voluntary. What should be done if the laboratory possesses information, which, while having no direct bearing on this individual's health, may be detrimental or of value to them in their own or other people's family planning? Just one issue is the non-paternity rate which, in the general population is around 8–10%; in certain segments of the population it can exceed 40%. What responsibility does the screening program have to inform such heterozygotes? One thing is clear and it is that information without considerable counseling and follow-up is likely to be detrimental. Thus a decision to inform individuals of their probable carrier status entails major decisions regarding follow-up, and greatly expanded costs for doing so. The situation is not analogous to the surplus information which is provided by multichannel chemical panel testing in which the tests are all designed to explore an individual's health. If a physician orders a 'chem-screen' to determine renal function, for example, and an abnormal cholesterol or a suspicious transaminase result which could impact upon an individual's health were ignored, this could be construed as malpractice.

(c) Cystic fibrosis

This disorder is one of the most common of the severe autosomal recessive traits, with an incidence of around 1:2500 Caucasians; the gene is very infrequent in other races. The screening test, based on serum immuno-reactive trypsin, is only valid in neonatal infants and cannot detect heterozygotes. In the decade since its introduction there has been a storm of controversy over the value of early detection of the disease and the cost:benefit ratios to families and to society. This is still unresolved, with convinced advocates and implacable opponents both defending their views [16]. During this time, the gene has been identified and it has been shown

that about a dozen mutations account for the majority of the cases.

This information has led to interest in some areas to start widespread, voluntary, but not universal, screening for cystic fibrosis carriers (about 1:25 of the population). There has been heated debate on this, with certain proponents already pushing to start the testing. However, even using a battery of available DNA probes, only about 85% of carriers can be firmly identified and about 10% of couples at risk would be missed. The cost for this kind of selective voluntary family based study is around $200 per individual. Such testing is usually welcomed and is entirely appropriate for individuals. Apart from the laboratory testing, it requires an extensive support system for genetic counseling and, indeed, it remains to be validated that such a program is desirable and effective in achieving its goals. Clearly, it is totally unacceptable to consider universal or even widespread screening for carriers of cystic fibrosis or any other disease at this time.

References

1. Editorial (1991) Phenylketonuria grows up. *Lancet*, 337, 1256–57.
2. Waggoner, D.D., Buist, N.R.M. and Donnell, G.N. (1990) Longterm prognosis in galactosemia: results of a survey of 350 cases. *J. Inherited Metab. Dis.*, 13, 802–18.
3. World Health Organization (1972) Genetic Disorders: Preventions, Treatment and Rehabilitation. *WHO Tech. Rep. Ser. 497*.
4. Andrews, B.L. (1985) *State Laws and Regulations Governing Newborn Screening*, American Bar Association, Chicago.
5. Faden, R., Chwalow, A.J. Holtzman, N.A. and Horn, S.D. (1982) A survey to evaluate parental consent as public policy for neonatal screening. *Am. J. Public Health*, 72, 1347–52.
6. Knoppers, B.M. and Laberge, C.M. (eds) (1990) *Genetic Screening*, Experta Medica, Amsterdam.
7. Congress of the United States, Office of Technology Assistance (1988) *Healthy Children, Investing in the Future*, Government Printing Office, Washington, DC.
8. Hannon, W.H., Aziz, K.J., Collier, F.C. *et al.* (1989) *Approved Standard: Blood Collection on Filter Paper for Neonatal Screening Programs*, National Committee for Clinical Laboratory Standards, LA-4-1A, Villanova, PA, pp. 163–82.
9. Tuerck, J.M., Buist, N.R.M., Skeels, M.R. *et al.* (1989) Computerized surveillance of errors in newborn screening practice. *Am. J. Public Health*, 77, 1528–31.
10. Smerdely, P., Lim, A., Boyages, S.C. *et al.* (1989) Topical iodine-containing antiseptics and neonatal hypothyroidism in very low birthweight infants. *Lancet*, ii, 661–64.
11. Holtzman, C., Slazyk, W.E., Cordero, J.F. *et al.* (1986) Descriptive epidemiology of missed cases of phenylketonuria and congenital hypothyroidism. *Pediatrics*, 78, 553–58.
12. LaFranchi, S.H., Hanna, C.E., Krainz, P.L. *et al.* (1985) Screening for congenital hypothyroidism with specimen collection at two time periods: results of the Northwest regional screening program. *Pediatrics*, 76, 734–38.
13. Redus, M.A., Wasser, S., Hennon, W.H. *et al.* (1991) *Estimates from the National HIV Survey in Childbearing Women*. Presented at the 8th National Neonatal Screening Symposium, January 29–February 2, 1991, Saratoga Springs, NY (abstract – unpublished data).
14. Naito, H., Sasaki, M., Yamashiso, K., *et al.* (1990) Improvement in prognosis of neuroblastoma through mass population screening. *J. Pediatr. Surg.*, 25, 245–48.
15. Zhang, Y.H. and McCabe, E.R.B. (1992) What's new in DNA/RNA? in *Neonatal Screening in the Nineties* (Eds B. Wilcken and D.R. Webster), Kelvin Press, New South Wales, pp. 219–21.
16. Dankert-Roelse, J., te Meerman, G.J., Martign, A. *et al.* (1989) Survival and clinical outcome in patients with cystic fibrosis with or without neonatal screening. *J. Pediatr.*, 114, 362–67.

64 PREIMPLANTATION GENETIC DIAGNOSIS

E. Pergament

64.1 Introduction

The past quarter of a century has been witness to a series of remarkable advances in the prenatal diagnosis of genetic disorders. Obstetrical procedures such as mid-trimester amniocentesis, introduced in the 1960s, and first trimester chorionic villus sampling (CVS), developed in the 1980s, are now considered standards of care for high-risk pregnancies. For the prenatal identification of congenital malformations, there are a number of complementing diagnostic and screening techniques, including maternal serum α-fetoprotein screening, ultrasonography, percutaneous umbilical blood sampling and fetal skin biopsy. These techniques do share one feature in common, namely, all are applicable many weeks after conception, during the postimplantation period of gestation. With rare exceptions, there are no satisfactory treatments or cures available for the thousands of genetic diseases that occur in humans. Therefore, when prenatal testing identifies a genetically abnormal fetus, prospective parents have only two options: either to terminate the pregnancy electively or to continue the pregnancy and give birth to an affected newborn. With postimplantation diagnosis, families at significant risk of a conception with a genetic disease must continuously face the prospect of repeated pregnancy termination accompanied by considerable psychological stress.

Diagnosing genetic diseases in embryos prior to implantation was proposed as a possible alternative to avoid these two options. Preimplantation genetic diagnosis became possible with the development of three technical advances: first, the development of *in vitro* fertilization (IVF), an artificial reproductive technology to serve the infertile; second, the development of micromanipulation techniques enabling the biopsy of single cells with minimal trauma; and, third, the development of ultramicrobiochemical methods for the analysis of gene mutations. A new dimension in the prevention of genetic diseases will be achieved if gene mutations can be routinely diagnosed prior to the formal initiation of a pregnancy. With preimplantation genetic diagnosis, only embryos determined to be unaffected would be transferred to the prospective maternal parent. High-risk families would be able to undertake a pregnancy free of the fear about the possibility of having to undergo an abortion because of a genetically abnormal conception and free of the concern about the obstetrical safety of such procedures as CVS and amniocentesis.

64.2 Approaches to preimplantation genetic diagnosis

Preimplantation genetic diagnosis can be approached either preconceptually or postconceptually. In preconceptual diagnosis, genetic analyses could theoretically be conducted on gametes, either oocytes or spermatozoa, and on the first polar body. In postconceptual diagnosis, genetic analyses could be conducted on the second polar body, on blastomeres after cleavage of the zygote, on cells of the inner cell mass, and on trophectoderm cells at the blastula stage of embryogenesis.

64.2.1 GENOTYPING HUMAN GAMETES

Despite a considerable body of literature describing a seemingly endless variety of methods for separating X and Y spermatozoa, claims of success have not been confirmed but rather are the subject of considerable and strenuous criticism. For female carriers of X-linked mutations, the possibility of such a separation would circumvent the high reproductive risk of conceiving affected males. It is possible to conduct genetic analyses of the DNA from individual human sperm using the polymerase chain reaction (PCR) [1]; however, the loss of viability in preparing the spermatozoa for genotyping negates its application to the preconceptual diagnosis of any heritable disorder. At the present time,

Diseases of the Fetus and Newborn, 2nd edn, Edited by G.B. Reed, A.E. Claireaux and F. Cockburn. Published in 1995 by Chapman & Hall, London. ISBN 0 412 39160 0

therefore, this approach cannot be considered a realistic option to prevent the conception of males affected with X-linked mutations.

Genetic studies have been successfully performed on fertilized oocytes, including determination of chromosome constitution, enzyme activity and the presence of DNA mutations [2,3], but the technical methods used in these analyses are also unsuitable for conducting preimplantation diagnosis because of the loss of viability. An alternative approach to determining the genotype of an oocyte without compromising its viability is the biopsy and genetic analysis of the polar body [3,4]. In the absence of crossing over, the genotype of the first polar body of a heterozygous carrier of a mutant gene is the complement to that of the secondary oocyte. Thus, if the polar body contains the mutant gene, the normal gene is present in the oocyte, and vice versa. There are considerable limitations to this approach, however; crossing over between the gene locus and the centromere significantly reduces the number of suitable oocytes available for transfer, as does amplification failure, and the diagnostic error rate of polar body biopsy was estimated to be as high as 15–29%, significantly greater than other approaches to preimplantation diagnosis [5].

64.2.2 EMBRYONIC BIOPSY DURING EARLY CLEAVAGE

The genetic analysis of one or more embryonic cells or blastomeres obtained by biopsy at the four- and eight-cell stage has been successfully applied to the preimplantation diagnosis of a series of X-linked, recessively-inherited disorders [6]. The sex of embryos was determined by amplification of a repeated sequence of a Y-specific probe using recombinant DNA technology in conjunction with PCR [7]. The preimplantation genetic diagnosis of cystic fibrosis resulting in the birth of an unaffected newborn has also been accomplished by PCR analysis of a single blastomere biopsied at the four- to eight-cell stage [8]. Despite the small number of pregnancies that have occurred following embryonic biopsy for preimplantation diagnosis, there have been at least two laboratory errors in genotyping, for sex and resulting in elective termination following prenatal testing [9] and for cystic fibrosis, resulting in the birth of an affected infant [10]. The sources of error include failure of placement of the blastomere into the reaction tube, failure of amplification with PCR and contamination with foreign DNA [5]. The probabilities of errors for preimplantation genetic diagnoses for dominant, recessive and X-linked disorders using PCR to amplify the target sequence in blastomeres have been calculated assuming a realistic range in the magnitude of PCR efficiency, cell transfer and contamination. Genetic analyses based on a single blastomere have an esti-

mated unacceptable error rate as high as 1.8% for autosomal recessive genes, 15% for autosomal dominant genes, and 7.4% for X-linked recessive genes [5]. Other approaches have focused on the possibility of analyzing single blastomeres with a 'cocktail' of chromosome probes to detect the most common aneuploidies (trisomies 13, 18 and 21) by fluorescent *in situ* hybridization [11]; on measuring activities of enzymes associated with inborn errors of metabolism [12]; and on chromosome analysis at the metaphase stage of mitosis [13]. Similar to PCR, each of these approaches has inherent technical limitations, particularly in reliability and reproducibility, such that their error rates preclude their clinical application at the present time.

The possibility of damage to the human embryo as a consequence of biopsy will not be resolved until a substantial number of pregnancies following preimplantation diagnosis have been shown conclusively to have developed normally. Cell loss occurring with cryopreservation has not been associated with an untoward outcome; despite the loss of more than one blastomere at the eight-cell stage during the freeze–thaw process, normal pregnancies have resulted [14]. In addition, programmed cell death appears to be part of normal embryogenesis [15], suggesting that abnormal embryonic development is unlikely to occur because of the removal of one or more cells. Nevertheless, ascertaining that the process of embryonic biopsy is safe and does not alter normal embryogenesis is critically important if preimplantation diagnosis is to become a clinically useful approach to the prevention of genetic disease.

64.2.3 EMBRYONIC BIOPSY AT THE BLASTOCYST STAGE

The first preimplantation genetic diagnosis was conducted almost 25 years ago with the determination of the X-chromatin pattern in trophectoderm of rabbit blastocysts [16]. A biopsy of the trophectoderm is technically easy to perform and the resulting sample of 10–20 cells not only permits direct assay by recombinant DNA technology but can also be cultured *in vitro* so as to make possible a range of genetic analyses. The problem is that only 20–30% of preimplantation embryos reach the blastocyst stage *in vitro*, reducing the number of embryos available for transfer. Another potential problem is that the accuracy of the genetic diagnosis based on this approach may be questionable because of possible discrepancies between the genotype of the trophectoderm and inner cell mass.

As an alternative method to obtaining blastocysts by IVF, flushing of the uterus prior to implantation has been proposed. This approach has consistently failed to obtain a sufficient number of embryos for biopsy.

Moreover, there is an increased risk of ectopic implantation [17].

64.3 Patient perspectives

It is uncertain as to whether or not testing embryos prior to implantation will in time be applied clinically on a wide scale. The responses of prospective parents at high reproductive risk for a genetic disorder have highlighted several practical problems [18]. When asked to consider preimplantation diagnosis as an alternative to CVS or amniocentesis, their major concerns were cost (US$5000–10 000), possible damage to the embryo following biopsy (unknown), and the low rate of successful pregnancy outcomes (approximately 12–15%). Three-quarters of the prospective parents found that these disadvantages significantly outweighed the singular advantage of preimplantation diagnosis of not having to undergo a pregnancy termination of a genetically abnormal conception. There should be substantial concern about the potential misuses of IVF and molecular techniques by entrepreneurial interests. One obvious example of misuse is sex selection of a conception for non-medical reasons.

64.4 The future of preimplantation diagnosis

Despite its recent introduction and limited application, the current practice of preimplantation genetic diagnosis has already raised a number of serious clinical and laboratory problems. There is the practical issue of cost, affordability and who should pay for such services, the family, insurance or the government; there are unresolved concerns about damage to embryos undergoing biopsy by micromanipulation, the low rates of completed pregnancies with IVF in general and whether women undergoing stimulated IVF cycles will have any unforeseen consequences, e.g. higher risk of ovarian cancer [19]; and, because errors in the genetic analyses have already occurred, there are doubts about the accuracy, reproducibility and consistency of diagnoses based on preimplantation embryos. The aftermath of an incorrect diagnosis and a genetically abnormal pregnancy is the complete negation of the original reason for at-risk parents undertaking preimplantation diagnosis, avoiding the need for pregnancy termination and its associated emotional stresses. A review of experimental studies investigating the sources and the magnitude of errors in preimplantation diagnosis based on human oocytes, polar bodies and embryos is not reassuring at the present time: the error rate has been reported to be as high as 70% in oocytes and 36% in polar bodies [3] and to range from 3% [20] to 45% [21] for single blastomeres. Additional

technical improvements are certainly required to eliminate diagnostic errors due to embryonic cell placement failure, failed amplification and DNA contamination. Concerns that the risks to prospective parents outweigh its benefits have led one respected investigator to propose that 'research on preimplantation genetic analysis should continue with human embryonic cells that are not transferred to patients until confidence is gained on the accuracy and efficiency of these techniques before clinical services are offered widely for preimplantation embryo diagnosis' [22]. It would also seem appropriate to establish forthwith international guidelines and standards as well as administrative bodies to monitor objectively the development, implementation and outcomes of preimplantation diagnosis programs.

References

1. Li, H., Gyllensten, U.B., Cui, X. et al. (1988) Amplification and analysis of DNA sequences in single human sperm and diploid cells. Nature, 335, 414–17.
2. Coutelle, C., Williams, C., Handyside, A.H. et al. (1989) Genetic analysis of DNA from single human oocytes: a model for preimplantation diagnosis of cystic fibrosis. BMJ, 299, 22–24.
3. Monk, M. and Holding, C. (1990) Amplification of a beta-haemoglobin sequence in individual human oocytes and polar bodies. Lancet, 335, 985–88.
4. McLaren, A. (1985) Prenatal diagnosis before implantation: opportunities and problems. Prenat. Diagn., 5, 85–90.
5. Navidi W. and Arnheim, N. (1991) Using PCR in preimplantation genetic disease diagnosis. Hum. Reprod., 6, 836–49.
6. Handyside, A.H., Penketh, R.J.A., Winston, R.M.L. et al. (1989) Biopsy of human preimplantation embryos and sexing by DNA amplification. Lancet, i, 347–49.
7. Handyside, A.H., Kontogianni, E.H., Hardy, K. et al. (1990) Pregnancies from biopsied human preimplantation embryos sexed by Y-specific DNA amplification. Nature, 344, 768–70.
8. Handyside, A.H., Lesko, J.G., Tarin, J.J. et al. (1992) Birth of a normal girl after in vitro fertilization and preimplantation diagnostic testing for cystic fibrosis. N. Engl. J. Med., 327, 905–909.
9. Handyside, A.H. and Delhanty, D.A. (1992) Cleavage stage biopsy of human embryos and diagnosis of X-linked recessive disease, Preimplantation Diagnosis of Human Genetic Disease (ed. R.G. Edwards), Cambridge University Press, Cambridge, pp. 239–70.
10. Strom, C.M. and Rechitsky, S. (1993) DNA analysis of polar bodies and preembryos, in Preimplantation Diagnosis of Genetic Diseases (eds Y. Verlinsky and A.M Kuliev), Wiley–Liss, NY, pp. 69–90.
11. Lichter, P.L., Jauch, A., Cremer, T. and Ward, D.C. (1990) Detection of Down syndrome by in situ hybridization with chromosome 21 specific DNA probes, in Molecular Genetics of Chromosome 21 and Down Syndrome (ed. D. Patterson), Wiley–Liss, NY, pp. 69–78
12. Monk, M., Handyside, A.H., Buggleton-Harris, A. et al. (1990) Preimplantation sexing and diagnosis of hypoxanthine phosphoribosyltransferase deficiency in mice by biochemical microassay. Am. J. Med. Genet., 35, 201–205.
13. Angell, R.R., Templeton, A.A. and Aitken, R.J. (1986) Chromosome studies in human in vitro fertilization. Hum. Genet., 72, 333–39.
14. Hartshorne, A.M., Wick, K., Elder, K. and Dyson, H. (1990) Effect of cell number at freezing upon survival and viability of cleaving embryos generated from stimulated IVF cycles. Hum. Reprod., 5, 587–61.
15. Hardy, K., Handyside, A.H. and Winston, R.M.L. (1989) The human blastocyst: cell number, death and allocation during late preimplantation development in vitro. Development, 107, 597–604.
16. Gardner, R.L. and Edwards, R.G. (1968) Control of the sex ratio at full term in the rabbit by transferring sexed blastocysts. Nature, 218, 346–48.
17. Brambati, B. and Tului, L. (1990) Preimplantation genetic diagnosis: a new simple uterine washing technique. Hum. Reprod., 5, 448–50.
18. Pergament, E. (1992) Preimplantation diagnosis: patient perspectives. Prenat. Diagn., 11, 493–500.
19. Whittemore, A.S., Harris, R., Itnyre, J., Halpern, J. and the Collaborative

Ovarian Cancer Group (1992) Characteristics relating to ovarian risk: collaborative analysis of twelve US case-control studies. I, II, III, IV. *Am. J. Epidemiol.*, **136**, 1176–83, 1184–1203, 1204–11, 1212–20.

20. Grifo, J.A., Tang, Y.X., Cohen, J. *et al.* (1992) Pregnancy after embryo biopsy and coamplification of DNA from X and Y chromosomes. *JAMA* **268**, 727–29.

21. Pickering, S.J., McConnell, J.M., Johnson, M.H. and Braude, P.R. (1992) Reliability of detection by polymerase chain reaction of the sickle cell-containing region of the beta-globin gene in single human blastomeres. *Hum. Reprod.*, 7, 630–36.

22. Trounson, A.L. (1992) Preimplantation genetic diagnosis – counting chickens before they hatch? *Hum. Reprod.*, 7, 583–84.

65 FETAL CELL ISOLATION FROM MATERNAL BLOOD

D.W. Bianchi

65.1 Introduction

The currently accepted techniques of prenatal genetic diagnosis, amniocentesis, cordocentesis and chorionic villus sampling have two inherent disadvantages. First, they are invasive and pose a small but significant risk of miscarriage to the pregnancy. Second, they are only offered to the small percentage of pregnant women with clinical indications for the procedure. Despite the availability of prenatal genetic diagnosis, there has been little impact on the birth rate of infants with Down syndrome in the UK [1]. In the USA, 80% of the infants with Down syndrome are born to women under the age of 35 [2]; these women are not considered candidates for invasive prenatal diagnosis. Consequently, there is great interest in the development of non-invasive methods for prenatal diagnosis. One approach, discussed elsewhere in this text, has been the measurement of specific proteins in maternal serum that originate in the fetus or placenta. The absolute values of these proteins are subsequently compared with population norms, and a recalculated risk for fetal aneuploidy is provided. Although non-invasive, this is a screening assay, not a diagnostic test, and as many as 50% of cases of Down syndrome are undetected [3]. Our approach has been to isolate the rare fetal nucleated cells circulating in maternal peripheral blood as these cells are a source of fetal chromosomes and DNA.

65.2 Historical aspects

The existence of fetal cells in maternal blood has been known for over 100 years. Schmorl, in 1893, demonstrated trophoblasts in the pulmonary circulation of women who died of eclampsia [4]. Douglas *et al.* [5] and Goodfellow and Taylor [6] documented circulating trophoblast cells in peripheral venous blood samples from living pregnant women. In 1969, Walknowska, Conte and Grumbach found occasional cells with an XY karyotype in cultured lymphocytes derived from the peripheral blood of 30 pregnant women [7]. The presence of a male karyotype was highly correlated with the birth of a male infant. The passage of fetal erythrocytes into the maternal circulation has been long appreciated as the initial step in the pathogenesis of erythroblastosis fetalis [8].

65.3 Challenges of current research

Fetal cell isolation represents an enormous technical challenge due to the rare numbers present in maternal blood samples. Estimates of the frequency of fetal cells in maternal blood range from 1 in 10^5 to 1 in 10^8 [9,10]. Recent efforts to isolate fetal cells from maternal blood have been aided by a variety of cell separation and genetic amplification techniques. Although it is possible to demonstrate fetal gene sequences in unpurified maternal DNA [11], most investigators agree that for the purpose of clinical diagnosis some degree of enrichment of the proportion of fetal cells present is necessary. Some of the variables in fetal cell isolation studies are summarized in Table 65.1.

65.4 Selection of target cell type

The three fetal cell types presently being investigated are the nucleated erythrocyte, trophoblast and lymphocyte.

65.4.1 'TROPHOBLAST CELLS'

'Trophoblast cells' are particularly attractive candidates for fetal isolation because they are uniquely fetal and

Table 65.1 Variables in fetal cell isolation studies

Selection of target cell type
Choice of monoclonal antibody
Cell separation methods
Means of genetic analysis

Diseases of the Fetus and Newborn, 2nd edn, Edited by G.B. Reed, A.E. Claireaux and F. Cockburn. Published in 1995 by Chapman & Hall, London. ISBN 0 412 39160 0

are in intimate contact with maternal blood. Syncytio-trophoblast is a syncytia. The 'cells' are exfoliated blebs or fragments of cytoplasm plus nuclei derived from the syncytia. They have both a distinctive morphology and specific immunophenotype. Initially, the monoclonal antibody H315 was described as specific for the recognition of trophoblast cell surface antigens. Covone et al. [12] described the binding of H315 to three types of cells in 46 maternal blood samples taken at different times in gestation. The frequency of H315+ cells in mononuclear cell suspensions was 1–8 per 1000. In subsequent studies, both Covone et al. [13] and Bertero et al. [14] physically isolated H315+ cells from maternal blood but neither could demonstrate the presence of fetal DNA sequences. Covone concluded that the H315 antigen was adsorbed on to maternal leukocytes.

More recently, Mueller and colleagues [15] generated 6800 monoclonal antibodies, two of which (FD066Q and FD0338P) were determined to be specific for trophoblast membrane surface proteins. These antibodies were used to isolate fetal trophoblast cells from the blood of 13 pregnant women. The polymerase chain reaction (PCR) was utilized to amplify and detect Y chromosomal DNA sequences originating in male fetuses. A correct prediction of fetal sex was made in 12 of 13 cases. There was one false-positive prediction of a male fetus.

Bruch et al. [16] employed three antitrophoblast antibodies, GB17, GB21 and GB25, to separate 'trophoblast-like' cells from maternal blood. The incidence of cells binding antibody was, on average, 700 ± 200 per 1×10^6 maternal cells. After flow sorting, the antibody positive cells were analyzed by transmission electron microscopy and consisted of lymphocytes (45%), monocytes (30%), and polymorphonuclear leukocytes (20%). No definitive intact trophoblast cells were visualized. Despite the negative morphologic results, male DNA was detected in the trophoblast-like cells in 2 out of 3 women carrying male fetuses.

Using a variety of monoclonal antibodies to trophoblast, Chua et al. [17] studied the deportation of syncytiotrophoblast cells into the maternal circulation and documented that in pre-eclamptic women trophoblast cells were detected at a frequency of 0.5–51.5 cells/ml. In normal pregnancies, however, the transport of trophoblastic cells into the maternal circulation occurs at a much lower frequency [18].

At the present time there is still no general consensus as to whether trophoblast cells persist in the maternal circulation in normal pregnancies long enough to permit fetal genetic analysis [19]. Many of the trophoblast antibodies crossreact with maternal lymphocytes. Other promising antibodies, notably HLA-G [20] and the anticytokeratin antibody Cam 5.2 [21], await further clinical testing.

65.4.2 LYMPHOCYTES

Lymphocytes were the first fetal tissue to be isolated for the purpose of genetic testing. Both cultured and uncultured fetal lymphocytes were the source of unbanded and quinacrine-banded studies of the Y chromosome in maternal blood [22–24]. The difficulty with the lymphocyte studies was that the visual inspection of thousands of maternal cells to find occasional evidence of a male fetal cell was time consuming. In 1979, Herzenberg and collaborators [25] reported on the application of fluorescence activated cell sorting to increase the proportion of fetal cells available for analysis. In a study of 138 pregnant women, antibody to human lymphocyte antigen (HLA) A2 was used to sort putative fetal lymphocytes, which were then analyzed for the presence of interphase Y chromatin. The results of the study demonstrated a highly statistically significant correlation between the detection of the quinacrine-positive Y body in sorted cells and the presence of both male gender and HLA-A2 at birth ($P = 0.0000058$) [26]. The novel combination of cell surface antigens and nuclear markers provided two independent means of confirming fetal origin of the cells. Unfortunately, the cell sorting experiments resulted in few cells for subsequent analysis. The proliferative capability of the sorted cells was determined to be zero. Metaphase karyotype analysis was therefore impossible. A decade later, Yeoh et al. [27] again used HLA-A2 antibody to sort fetal lymphocytes from a woman at 28 weeks of gestation whose own lymphocytes did not express this antigen. The fetal cells were identified by PCR amplification of paternally inherited HLA-DR4 sequences.

Lymphocytes have several disadvantages as a target cell for fetal cell separation. These include: the lack of generic fetal-specific cell surface markers; the need to obtain paternal tissue for identification of paternal HLA loci; and the potential problem of persistence of fetal lymphocytes in the maternal circulation for as long as 5 years postpartum [28,29].

65.4.3 NUCLEATED ERYTHROCYTES (NRBCs)

Our research efforts have focused on immature erythrocytes (erythroblasts and nucleated erythrocytes) because they are a cell type found abundantly in fetal blood [30,31] but rarely in adult blood. Because the majority of pregnancies are blood-group compatible, our hypothesis has been that small numbers of fetal erythrocytes can circulate in the mother, unchallenged by her immune system. In any fetomaternal transfusion, no matter how small, a thousandfold more red cells than white cells are available for analysis. NRBCs have a full complement of nuclear genes. Importantly, because NRBCs are nearly completely differentiated and have a life span of only about 3 months, isolated fetal NRBCs represent the current pregnancy being studied. This is especially important if non-invasive prenatal diagnosis is attempted on a woman with a prior aneuploid fetus.

Initially, we selected the transferrin receptor antigen (CD71) as a fetal marker because erythroblasts express this cell surface antigen from the burst-forming unit, erythroid stage up until the reticulocyte stage [32]. The CD71 antigen alone is not fetal specific. It is expressed on any cell incorporating iron, which is a characteristic of dividing cells. We used the fluorescence-activated cell sorter (FACS, section 65.5.1) to analyze histograms depicting fluorescence intensity (as a measure of CD71 binding) versus light scatter in six non-pregnant adults, six pregnant women (10–33 weeks of gestation), and three newborn umbilical cord bloods. CD71+ cells were sorted on to microscope slides for morphologic studies and detection of fetal hemoglobin. The non-pregnant adults had lymphocytes, monocytes and platelets in the CD71+ fraction. No cells containing fetal hemoglobin were visualized. In contrast, the CD71+ cells from the newborn umbilical cord blood contained many NRBCs and reticulocytes that stained positively for fetal hemoglobin. The samples from the pregnant women revealed the small but consistent presence of a CD71+ population of cells. Upon microscopic analysis, these cells were demonstrated to be predominantly maternal reticulocytes, but NRBCs containing fetal hemoglobin, monocytes and lymphocytes were also seen [33]. To show that the isolated NRBCs were fetal, we used PCR to amplify Y chromosome specific sequences in the CD71+ sorted cells. There was a statistically significant correlation between the detection of amplified male DNA and the presence of a male fetus. These results demonstrated that fetal DNA sequences could be detected in flow-sorted NRBCs found in maternal blood. Our subsequent experiments were directed towards defining a 'biologic window' for the fetomaternal transfer of NRBCs. Preliminary data obtained from 12 pregnant women bearing males have suggested that maximal transfer occurs between 8 and 17 weeks of gestation [34,35].

Other investigators have also concluded that NRBCs are the target cell of choice for fetal cell separation. Simpson and Elias [36] have cited that the spontaneously dividing cells in newborn umbilical cord blood are erythroblasts [37]. Ganshirt-Ahlert, Burschyk and Garritsen [38] have stated that 'the number of nucleated erythrocytes as a source of fetal deoxyribonucleic acid is assumed to be higher [than trophoblast]'. Adinolfi, while writing that 'erythroblasts seem to be the best candidates for the introduction of new, non-invasive prenatal diagnostic test', is concerned about maternal cell contamination, lack of data on the frequency of fetal cell detection at different gestational ages in the same pregnancy, and the effect of maternal–fetal blood group incompatibility [39].

We, as well as others, have reasoned that although NRBCs are preferable for fetal cell studies, CD71 alone is not the most effective monoclonal antibody for physical isolation. We have recently summarized an analysis of the percentage of mononuclear cells expressing the transferrin receptor in blood samples obtained from 139 pregnant women who were between 7 and 26 weeks of gestation [40]. The interpatient variability was pronounced. For example, at 11 weeks of gestation, the range of CD71+ was 0.2 to 8.5%. The differences reflect variation in the maternal reticulocyte count as well as medical complications known to increase fetomaternal hemorrhage, such as placental abruption.

Wachtel and collaborators [41] added the monoclonal antibody to glycophorin A, a red cell sialoglycoprotein, to anti-CD71 to more specifically target immature erythrocytes in a dual color immunofluorescence protocol. They reported that with a multiparametric approach, sorting fetal NRBCs on the basis of cell size, cell granularity, green fluorescence and orange fluorescence resulted in a 94% accurate prediction of fetal gender. Using the same protocol, Price et al. [10] were able to diagnose fetal aneuploidy in sorted fetal NRBCs by interphase analysis of nuclei (section 65.6.2)

The ideal reagent for fetal NRBC separation will not react with maternal cells. Such reagents are currently under development. In the meantime, other commercially available monoclonal antibodies hold promise for the unique recognition of fetal NRBCs. As an example, we have described the combination of CD36 and glycophorin A (GPA) to label erythroblasts [42]. CD36, the thrombospondin receptor, is a marker of early erythroid differentiation, but it is also expressed on lymphocytes. Only the erythrocyte series will bind both monoclonal antibodies when used with glycophorin A. Protocols comparing CD36 and GPA to CD71 and GPA are currently under investigation in our laboratory.

65.5 Cell separation methods

The tremendous excess in the copies of the maternal genome relative to the fetal genome in maternal blood would seem to make purification, or enrichment, of fetal cells a necessity. Lo et al. [11,43], however, took maternal DNA prepared from unpurified maternal nucleated cells and subjected it to two separate rounds of PCR amplification using a 'nested' primer technique. He was able to demonstrate the presence of a Y chromosome in the women who were carrying male fetuses. Camaschella and colleagues [44] studied couples with different β-globin mutations to facilitate prenatal diagnosis of fetal hemoglobin (Hb) Lepore–Boston disease from maternal blood. In each of the three couples studied, the father carried Hb Lepore–Boston trait and the mother carried a β-thalassemia mutation. DNA was prepared from maternal peripheral blood buffy coats at 8–10 weeks of gestation. PCR primers were selected to amplify only the paternal mutation. Two of the three fetuses were shown to be carriers of the Hb Lepore–Boston by detection of amplified sequence in maternal blood; results were concordant with pure fetal DNA studies obtained by chorionic villus sampling. These three papers demonstrated that it was possible to detect fetal DNA sequences in unenriched maternal blood, but only if the sequence was absent in the mother's DNA.

65.5.1   FLUORESCENCE-ACTIVATED CELL SORTER (FACS)

The FACS is a complex and sophisticated instrument designed to acquire simultaneously many pieces of information regarding a single living cell as it is passes through a laser beam. Certain criteria or 'gates' may be established so that only cells with desired characteristics are physically isolated. These criteria may include: light-scattering properties (as indications of cell volume and nuclear complexity) and fluorescence in multiple wavelengths (facilitating selection on the presence or absence of multiple antigens). An example of a FACS histogram depicting candidate fetal cells is shown in Figure 65.1.

Many of the studies already presented have employed the FACS; examples include the work of Herzenberg *et al.* [25], Iverson *et al.* [26], Yeoh *et al.* [27], Wachtel *et al.* [41], Price *et al.* [10], Chueh and Golbus [21,45], Bruch *et al.* [16], Covone *et al.* [12,13], and Bianchi *et al.* [33,34,35,40,42,46]. The FACS is considered the 'gold standard' for fetal cell isolation, enabling enrichment of fetal cells on the order of 10^4–10^5-fold. The disadvantages of FACS are that the equipment is costly, the operators need special training, and only one sample can be processed at a time. The advantages of FACS are purity and reproducibility, and that the cells can remain alive while being flow sorted.

65.5.2   MAGNETIC-ACTIVATED CELL SORTER (MACS)

The MACS represents an alternative form of cell separation that is less expensive and simpler to perform than the FACS. With the MACS, the maternal–fetal cell suspension is mixed with monoclonal antibodies and antibody-conjugated magnetic beads and then passed over a separation column attached to a strong magnetic field [47]. Unbound (negative) cells pass through the column, leaving the bound (positive) cells complexed to the magnetic beads. A subsequent elution step removes the bound candidate fetal cells. Ganshirt-Ahlert, Burs-

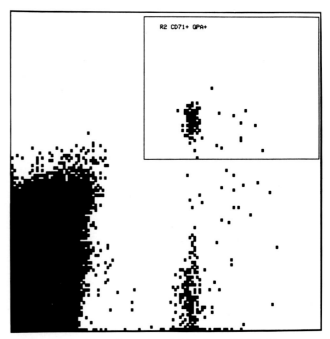

Figure 65.1 Two-dimensional bivariate FACS histogram, depicting physical isolation of the candidate fetal cells from maternal mononuclear cells. On the *x* axis is red fluorescence, an indication of binding to glycophorin A (GPA). On the *y* axis is green fluorescence, demonstrating binding to CD71. The box defines the nucleated erythrocytes, which express both CD71 and GPA.

chyk and Garritsen [38] have described the use of the MACS with antibody to CD71 to identify nucleated erythrocytes in umbilical cord blood samples.

Holzgreve and colleagues have further refined their separation techniques to include a multiple density gradient centrifugation prior to the MACS [48]. With this method, they were able to diagnose fetal aneuploidy by fluorescence *in situ* hybridization using chromosome-specific probes [49].

65.5.3   IMMUNOMAGNETIC BEADS

Immunomagnetic beads, specifically, polystyrene beads coated with sheep antibody to mouse IgG, have been used successfully in the isolation of trophoblast cells from maternal blood [15]. In Mueller's paper, the immunomagnetic beads were used for a positive (fetal cell) selection. In Camaschella's work on detection of fetal Hb Lepore–Boston sequences in maternal blood, immunomagnetic beads were used to deplete CD3+ cells (mature lymphocytes) from the cell suspension [44]. This is an example of a negative selection designed to reduce the ratio of maternal to fetal cells present.

While immunomagnetic beads, MACS, and a number of other cell separation devices appear favorable for fetal cell isolation, they have not yet been tested in large scale clinical studies. They do, however, have several advantages over FACS including lower cost, disposability, ease of use, and the ability to process many samples in a rapid manner.

65.6 Genetic analysis

Because many of the candidate fetal cell types currently being studied do not have unique morphology or cell surface markers, the diagnosis of 'fetal cell' relies upon the demonstration of fetal gene sequences in isolated material. Historically, the first and most easily documented fetal genes have derived from the Y chromosome. Since normal fertile females do not carry the Y chromosome, the presence of the Y has been assumed to originate in a male fetus. Originally, evidence of the Y was sought in metaphase and interphase karotypes prepared from maternal blood. The more recently developed genetic amplification techniques have been applied to fetal cell isolation studies with successful outcomes.

65.6.1 POLYMERASE CHAIN REACTION (PCR)

The PCR is of great importance in fetal cell separation from maternal blood because of the anticipated low numbers of fetal cells present. PCR enables many thousands of copies of a rare target gene sequence to be made, removing the limitations of working with small numbers of cells [50,51].

The overwhelming majority of studies published thus far have described PCR amplification of Y chromosomal sequences to identify fetal material. As already discussed, the advantages of detecting the Y is that it is absent in maternal cells and could serve to identify male gender in families at risk for X-linked conditions. The disadvantage of the Y is that it is non-specific and prone to the phenomenon of 'false-positive' amplification [52].

Theoretically, any paternally-inherited DNA polymorphism can be amplified and detected in fetal cells. Two published examples of fetal autosomal DNA sequences demonstrated in maternal blood include Hb Lepore–Boston [44] and HLA-DR4 [27]. Ultimately, to diagnose autosomal recessive conditions in fetal cells derived from maternal blood, the final purity of the isolated cells will need to be at least 90% to prevent preferential amplification of the maternal genome.

65.6.2 FLUORESCENCE IN SITU HYBRIDIZATION (FISH)

A major goal of prenatal cytogenetic diagnosis is the detection of aneuploidy. Under normal circumstances, each cell should have two copies of each autosome and a total of two sex chromosomes. If more or fewer than two copies of each chromosome or pair of sex chromosomes exist, the fetus would be expected to demonstrate clinical manifestations. The development of techniques of FISH has already facilitated the rapid detection of aneuploidies in uncultured amniocytes [53].

Chromosome-specific DNA probe sets currently exist for all of the human chromosomes. When the probes are coupled to a fluorescent dye, hybridization to the probe can identify an individual chromosome of interest. The beauty of the technique, however, is that it can be applied to interphase nuclei as well as metaphase spreads. Thus, for the individual fetal cell isolated from maternal blood, detection of aneuploidy can be performed whether or not the cell has the capability of further division. After hybridization to the fluorescently-labeled chromosome-specific DNA probe, each chromosome will be detected as a colored dot. The number of dots will correlate with the number of copies of that chromosome.

Several groups have already demonstrated that fetal aneuploidy can be diagnosed in fetal NRBCs isolated from maternal blood. We have described the existence of fetal cells, as defined by hybridization to a Y chromosomal probe and three copies of a chromosome 21 probe, in the CD71+ population flow sorted from a woman carrying a male fetus with trisomy 21 [46]. Price et al. [10] have diagnosed trisomy 21, 18 and Kleinfelter syndrome in CD71+ glycophorin A+ flow-sorted maternal cells. Gänshirt-Ahlert et al. [49] and Simpson and Elias [54] have further validated the potential for aneuploidy detection in fetal NRBCs.

Although the preceding studies were all performed by FISH detection of a single chromosome, the possibility of simultaneous multiple chromosomal probe detection has already been achieved in uncultured amniotic fluid cells [55]. Given that aneuploidies involving chromosomes 13, 18, 21, X and Y account for 95% of all liveborn chromosome abnormalities, the exciting role of multiprobe FISH in non-invasive prenatal screening becomes rapidly apparent (Chapter 73).

65.7 Conclusion

While the goal of detecting fetal chromosome aneuploidy in fetal cells obtained non-invasively from maternal blood has already been accomplished, many questions remain to be answered. The practical matters of the best target fetal cell type, cell separation techniques and analytic methods are all being explored in active research groups around the world. The reproducible finding by many investigators of fetal nucleated cells in maternal blood seems to indicate that fetomaternal transfer is a universal or nearly universal phenomenon. What implications, if any, do these cells have for the immunobiology of pregnancy and the mother's subsequent immune status and health? What is the life span of the fetal cells in the maternal circulation? Do the cells proliferate in maternal blood? Will the ability to perform accurate fetal genetic diagnosis by maternal venipuncture seriously affect reproductive decisions? Hopefully, as a result of some of the research advances presented in this chapter, the answers will be forthcoming.

References

1. Nicolaides, K.H. and Campbell, S. (1992) Ultrasound diagnosis of congenital abnormalities, in *Genetic Disorders and the Fetus*, 3rd edn (ed. A. Milunsky), Johns Hopkins University Press, Baltimore, pp. 616–17.
2. Holmes, L.B. (1978) Genetic counseling for the older pregnant woman: new data and questions. *N. Engl. J. Med.*, 298, 1419–21.
3. MacDonald, M.L., Wagner, R.M. and Slotnick, R.N. (1991) Sensitivity and specificity of screening for Down syndrome with α-fetoprotein, hCG, unconjugated estriol, and maternal age. *Obstet. Gynecol.*, 77, 63–68.
4. Schmorl, G. (1893) *Pathologisch-anatomische Undersuchungen über puerperal-Eklampsie*, Vogel, Leipzig.
5. Douglas, G.W., Thomas, L., Carr, M. et al. (1959) Trophoblast in the circulating blood during pregnancy. *Am. J. Obstet. Gynecol.*, 78, 960–73.
6. Goodfellow, C.F. and Taylor, P.V. (1982) Extraction and identification of trophoblast cells circulating in peripheral blood during pregnancy. *Br. J. Obstet. Gynaecol.*, 89, 65–68.
7. Walknowska, J., Conte, F.A. and Grumbach M.M. (1969) Practical and theoretical implications of fetal/maternal lymphocyte transfer. *Lancet*, i, 1119–22.
8. Creger, W.P. and Steele, M.R. (1957) Human fetomaternal passage of erythrocytes. *N. Engl. J. Med.*, 256, 158–61.
9. Ganshirt-Ahlert, D., Basak, N., Aidynli, K. and Holzgrave, W. (1992) Fetal DNA in uterine vein blood. *Obstet. Gynecol.*, 80, 1–3.
10. Price, J.O., Elias, S., Wachtel, S.S. et al. (1991) Prenatal diagnosis using fetal cells isolated from maternal blood by multiparameter flow cytometry. *Am. J. Obstet. Gynecol.*, 165, 1731–37.
11. Lo, Y.-M., Patel, P., Wainscoat, J.S. et al. (1989) Prenatal sex determination by DNA amplification from maternal peripheral blood. *Lancet*, ii, 1363–65.
12. Covone, A.E., Johnson, P.M., Mutton, D. and Adinolfi, M. (1984) Trophoblast cells in peripheral blood from pregnant women. *Lancet*, ii, 841–43.
13. Covone, A.E., Kozma, R. Johnson, P.M. et al. (1988) Analysis of peripheral maternal blood samples for the presence of placenta-derived cells using Y-specific probes and McAb H315. *Prenat. Diagn.*, 8, 591–607.
14. Bertero, M.T., Camaschella, C., Serra, A. et al. (1988) Circulating 'trophoblast' cells in pregnancy have maternal genetic markers. *Prenat. Diagn.*, 8, 585–90.
15. Mueller, U.W., Hawes, C.S., Wright, A.E. et al. (1990) Isolation of fetal trophoblast cells from peripheral blood of pregnant women. *Lancet*, 336, 197–200.
16. Bruch, J.F., Metezeau, P., Garcia-Fonknechten, N. et al. (1991) Trophoblast-like cells sorted from peripheral maternal blood using flow cytometry: a multiparametric study involving transmission electron microscopy and fetal DNA amplification. *Prenat. Diagn.*, 11, 787–98.
17. Chua, S., Wilkins, T., Sargent, I. and Redman, C. (1991) Trophoblast deportation in pre-eclamptic pregnancy. *Br. J. Obstet. Gynaecol.*, 98, 973–79.
18. Wagner, D. (1968) Trophoblastic cells in the blood stream in normal and abnormal pregnancy. *Acta Cytol.*, 12, 137–39.
19. Adinolfi, M. (1991) On a non-invasive approach to prenatal diagnosis based on the detection of fetal nucleated cells in maternal blood samples. *Prenat. Diagn.*, 11, 799–804.
20. Kovats, S., Main, E.K., Librach, C. et al. (1990) A class I antigen, HLA-G, expressed in human trophoblasts. *Science*, 248, 220–23.
21. Chueh, J. and Golbus, M.S. (1990) Prenatal diagnosis using fetal cells in the maternal circulation. *Semin. Perinatol.*, 14, 471–82.
22. Grosset, L., Barrelet, V. and Odartchenko, N. (1974) Antenatal fetal sex determination from maternal blood during early pregnancy. *Am. J. Obstet. Gynecol.*, 120, 60–63.
23. Zimmerman, A. and Schmickel, R. (1971) Fluorescent bodies in maternal ciruclation. *Lancet*, i, 1305.
24. Polani, P. and Mutton, D.E. (1971) Y fluorescence of interphase nuclei, especially circulating lymphocytes. *BMJ*, i, 138–42.
25. Herzenberg, L.A., Bianchi, D.W., Schröder, J. et al. (1979) Fetal cells in the blood of pregnant women: detection and enrichment by fluorescence-activated cell sorting. *Proc. Natl Acad. Sci. USA*, 76, 1453–55.
26. Iverson, G.M., Bianchi, D.W., Cann, H.M. and Herzenberg, L.A. (1981) Detection and isolation of fetal cells from maternal blood using the fluorescence-activated cell sorter (FACS). *Prenat. Diagn.*, 1, 61–73.
27. Yeoh, S.C., Sargent, I.L., Redman, C.W.G. et al. (1991) Detection of fetal cells in maternal blood. *Prenat. Diagn.*, 11, 117–23.
28. Ciaranfi, A., Curchod, A. and Odartchenko, N. (1977) Survie de lymphocytes foetaux dans le sang maternal post-partum. *Schweiz. Med. Wochenschr.*, 107, 134–38.
29. Schröder, J., Tiilikainen, A. and de la Chapelle, A. (1974) Fetal leukocytes in the maternal circulation after delivery. *Transplantation*, 17, 346–54.
30. Thomas, D.B. and Yoffey, J.M. (1962) Human fetal haemopoiesis. I. The cellular composition of foetal blood. *Br. J. Haematol.*, 8, 290–95.
31. Millar, D.S., Davis, L.R., Rodeck, C.H. et al. (1985) Normal blood cell values in the early mid-trimester fetus. *Prenat. Diagn.*, 5, 367–73.
32. Loken, M.R., Shah, V.O., Dattilio, K.L. and Civin, C.I. (1987) Flow cytometric analysis of human bone marrow. I. Normal erythroid development. *Blood*, 69, 255–63.
33. Bianchi, D.W., Flint, A.F., Pizzimenti, M.F. et al. (1990) Isolation of fetal DNA from nucleated erythrocytes in maternal blood. *Proc. Natl Acad. Sci. USA*, 87, 3279–83.
34. Bianchi, D.W., Stewart, J.E., Garber, M.F. et al. (1991) Possible effect of gestational age on the detection of fetal nucleated erythrocytes in maternal blood. *Prenat. Diagn.*, 11, 523–28.
35. Bianchi, D.W., Stewart, J.E., Ladoulis, M. et al. (1992) Detection of fetal nucleated erythrocytes in first trimester blood samples, in *Early Fetal Diagnosis: Recent Progress and Public Health Implications* (eds M. Macek, M.A. Ferguson-Smith and M. Spala), Karolinum-Charles University Press, Prague, pp. 431–34.
36. Simpson, J.L. and Elias, S. (1992) Isolating and analyzing fetal cells in maternal blood: current status (1992), in *Early Fetal Diagnosis: Recent Progress and Public Health Implications* (eds M. Macek, M.A. Ferguson-Smith and M. Spala), Karolinum-Charles University Press, Prague, pp. 424–30.
37. Tipton, R.E., Tharapel, A.T., Chang, H-H.T. et al. (1989) Rapid chromsome analysis with the use of spontaneously dividing cells derived from umbilical cord blood (fetal and neonatal). *Am. J. Obstet. Gynecol.*, 161, 1546–48.
38. Gänshirt-Ahlert, D., Burschyk, M., Garritsen, H.S.P. et al. (1992) Magnetic cell sorting and the transferrin receptor as potential means of prenatal diagnosis from maternal blood. *Am. J. Obstet. Gynecol.*, 166, 1350–55.
39. Adinolfi, M. (1992) Breaking the blood barrier. *Nature Genet.*, 1, 316–18.
40. Bianchi, D.W., Yih, M.C., Zickwolf, G.K. and Flint, A.F. (1994) Transferrin receptor (CD71) expression on circulating mononuclear cells during pregnancy. *Am. J. Obstet. Gynecol.*, 170, 202–206.
41. Wachtel, S., Elias, S., Price, J. et al. (1991) Fetal cells in the maternal circulation: isolation by multiparameter flow cytometry and confirmation by polymerase chain reaction. *Hum. Reprod.*, 6, 1466–69.
42. Bianchi, D.W., Zickwolf, G.K., Yih, M.C. et al. (1993) Erythroid-specific antibodies enhance detection of fetal nucleated erythrocytes in maternal blood. *Prenat. Diagn.*, 13, 293–300.
43. Lo, Y.-M.D., Patel, P., Sampietro, M. et al. (1990) Detection of single-copy fetal DNA sequence from maternal blood. *Lancet*, 335, 1463–64.
44. Camaschella, C., Alfarano, A., Gottardi, E. et al. (1990) Prenatal diagnosis of fetal hemoglobin Lepore–Boston disease on maternal peripheral blood. *Blood*, 75, 2102–106.
45. Chueh, J. and Golbus, M.S. (1991) The search for fetal cells in the maternal circulation. *J. Perinat. Med.*, 19, 411–20.
46. Bianchi, D.W., Mahr, A., Zickwolf, G.K. et al. (1992) Detection of fetal cells with 47, XY, +21 karyotype in maternal peripheral blood. *Hum. Genet.*, 90, 368–70.
47. Miltenyi, S., Müller, W., Weichel, W. and Radbruch, A. (1990) High gradient magnetic cell separation with MACS. *Cytometry*, 11, 231–38.
48. Bhat, M.M., Bieber, M.M. and Teng, N.N.H. (1990) One step separaton of human fetal lymphocytes from nucleated red blood cells. *J. Immunol. Methods*, 131, 147–49.
49. Gänshirt-Ahlert, D., Börjesson-Stoll, R., Burschyk, M. et al. (1993) Detection of fetal trisomies 21 and 18 from maternal blood using triple gradient and magnetic cell sorting. *A. J. Reprod. Immunol.*, 30, 194–201.
50. Erlich, H.A., Gelfand, D. and Sninsky, J.J. (1991) Recent advances in the polymerase chain reaction. *Science*, 252, 1643–51.
51. Wright, P.A. and Wynford-Thomas, D. (1990) The polymerase chain reaction: miracle or mirage? A critical review of its uses and limitations in diagnosis and research. *J. Pathol.*, 162, 99–117.
52. Kwok, S. and Higuchi, R. (1989) Avoiding false positives with PCR. *Nature*, 339, 237–38.
53. Klinger K., Landes G., Shook, D. et al. (1992) Rapid detection of chromosome aneuploidies in uncultured amniocytes by using fluorescence *in situ* hybridization (FISH). *Am. J. Hum. Genet.*, 51, 55–65.
54. Simpson, J.L. and Elias, S. (1993) Isolating fetal cells from maternal blood. Advances in prenatal diagnosis through molecular technology. *J. Am. Med. Assoc.*, 270, 2357–61.
55. Ried, T., Landes, G., Dackowski, W. et al. (1992) Multicolor fluorescence *in situ* hybridization for the simultaneous detection of probe sets for chromosomes 13, 18, 21, X and Y in uncultured amniotic fluid cells. *Hum. Mol. Genet.*, 1, 307–13.

66 EMBRYOSCOPY AND FIRST TRIMESTER PRENATAL DIAGNOSIS

Y. Dumez, J.-F. Oury, M. Dommergues and L. Mandelbrot

66.1 Introduction

Over the last decade, an objective of fetal medicine has been to offer increasingly earlier prenatal diagnosis. Chorionic villus sampling allowed for first trimester diagnosis of genetic disorders, and vaginal ultrasound imaging permitted early diagnosis of some major morphological abnormalities. The availability of first trimester diagnosis may encourage couples at risk for transmitting dominant or recessive disorders to attempt pregnancy. For this reason, 10 years ago we developed the technique of embryoscopy, which allows for endoscopic observation of inherited abnormalities of the face and extremities as early as 9 menstrual weeks. Embryoscopy also has potential applications for fetal therapy by opening access to the embryonic circulation at an early stage in development.

66.2 Technique

66.2.1 PRINCIPLES

Embryoscopy consists of observing the embryo through the intact amniotic membrane via an endoscope introduced across the chorion into the extraembryonic coelom [1]. The chorion is opaque and flimsy, while the amniotic membrane is transparent and strong. These anatomical features allow introduction of the endoscopic device across the chorion without damaging the amnion. Because of the relatively large size of the extraembryonic coelom, it is possible to move the tip of the endoscope without tearing the amnion.

Embryoscopy should be performed after the major features of the embryo's external body form are established (i.e. after 9 menstrual weeks), but before the extraembryonic coelom is obliterated by the growth of the amniotic cavity, which brings the amnion in contact with the inner aspect of the chorion (i.e. before 11 menstrual weeks). Moreover, we believe that endoscopic lighting of the amniotic cavity should be avoided until the development of the embryo's eyelids is accomplished (9 menstrual weeks) in order to prevent potential eye damage due to excessive exposure to light. In addition, the maximal size of the extraembryonic coelom is achieved at 9 weeks and this period is the ideal gestational age for performing embryoscopy.

66.2.2 MATERIALS

We use a rigid fiberoptic endoscope with a 0° wide-angle lens (Needlescope, Olympus) measuring 17 cm in length and 1.7 mm in diameter and introduced through a 2 mm outer diameter cannula. The cannula is equipped with a side channel, allowing for the injection of normal saline. Ultrasound guidance is achieved using a 5 MHz sector probe (Kretz, Combison 330, Austria).

66.2.3 METHODS

Embryoscopy is an outpatient procedure that can be carried out either by a transcervical or a transabdominal approach. Preoperative ultrasound is required to rule out a multiple gestation and to check the size of the embryo and the extraembryonic coelom, as well as fetal viability. Preoperative ultrasound is also needed to guide the endoscope directly into the coelom, to avoid the trophoblast, and to orient the tip of the device towards the desired part of the embryo.

(a) Transcervical embryoscopy (Figure 66.1)

The original technique of embryoscopy was based on a transcervical approach [2], which can be used unless the thickest part of the trophoblast is located in direct contact with the internal cervical os. Anesthesia or

Diseases of the Fetus and Newborn, 2nd edn, Edited by G.B. Reed, A.E. Claireaux and F. Cockburn. Published in 1995 by Chapman & Hall, London. ISBN 0 412 39160 0

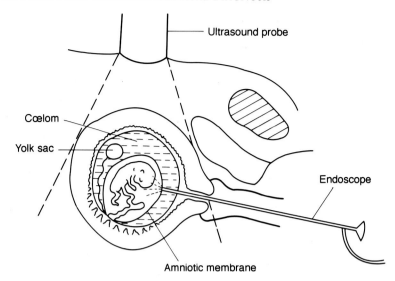

Figure 66.1 Transcervical embryoscopy.

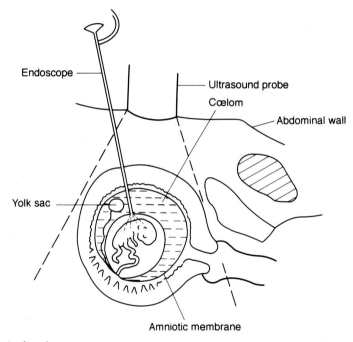

Figure 66.2 Transabdominal embryoscopy.

sedation is not required. The cervix is exposed by a single valve speculum and carefully cleaned. The endoscope and the cannula are gently introduced through the cervix, under ultrasound guidance, towards the lowest part of the sac in contact with the chorion. The device is then briskly pushed forward in order to cross the chorion and enter the coelom. The smooth and relatively large tip of the endoscope may reach the amnion but will not damage it. Endoscopic vision of the extraembryonic coelom confirms whether or not the location of the endoscope is appropriate. If needed, the cavity is flushed with 1–2 ml of physiological saline to remove blood and particles. The tip of the device is then brought in contact with the amniotic sac, through

which the embryo is observed. The initial observation is made directly through the endoscope. A video-camera is then attached to the endoscope, allowing the mother to view the embryo on a television monitor and to document the presence of fetal malformations. In normal pregnancies the duration of the procedure should be as short as possible to minimize the risk of miscarriage.

(b) Transabdominal embryoscopy (Figure 6.6.2)

A transabdominal approach can be used when the thickest trophoblastic area is not located in the anterior aspect of the uterus.

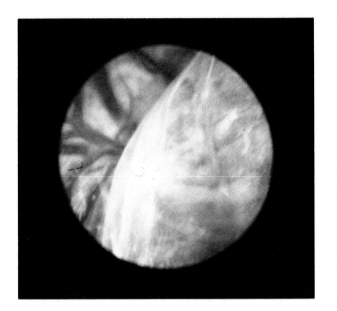

Figure 66.3 Extraembryonic coelom.

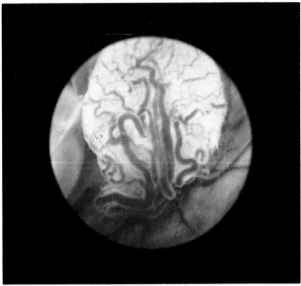

Figure 66.4 Yolk sac.

After local anesthesia with 1% lidocaine (lignocaine) solution, the cannula is introduced into the coelom with a trocar with a sharp end. The trocar is removed and replaced by the endoscope. The integrity of the amniotic sac is checked and the tip is placed in contact with the transparent amniotic membrane.

Following embryoscopy, the patient is discharged from the hospital the next morning after a follow-up ultrasound scan. Antibiotics are given after a transcervical procedure. If indicated, termination of pregnancy is achieved by suction and curettage.

66.3 Results

66.3.1 NORMAL PREGNANCY

(a) Extraembryonic coelom and yolk sac

The extraembryonic coelom appears as a clear space (Figure 66.3) in which thin trabeculae may sometimes be observed. Numerous vessels run on the inner aspect of the chorion, which is easily identified by its red color. The embryo can be seen through the whitish amniotic sac that limits the coelom opposite to the chorionic plate. The two vessels of the vitelline duct can be identified at the insertion of the amnion around the umbilical cord. The vitelline duct runs freely in the coelom and connects the yolk sac to the fetal circulation. The yolk sac appears as a yellowish sphere, with a rich vascular network connected to the vitelline duct vascular pedicle (Figure 66.4). Later in gestation the vascular network of the yolk sac decreases. By following the vitelline duct upward from the yolk sac the

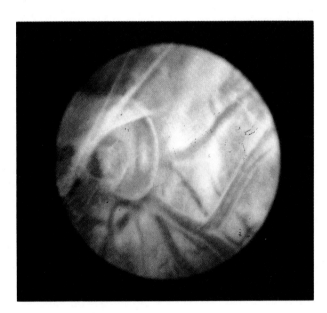

Figure 66.5 Cord insertion.

endoscope reaches the cord insertion on the chorionic plate (Figure 66.5). At 9 menstrual weeks the umbilical cord next to the chorionic plate is located in the coelom and outside the amniotic cavity. The umbilical vein appears deep blue in color, while the umbilical arteries appear bright red.

(b) Embryo

After observing the coelom, the tip of the endoscope is moved in contact with the amnion. A nearly complete

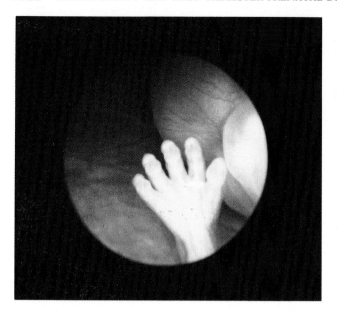

Figure 66.6 Hand at 9 weeks.

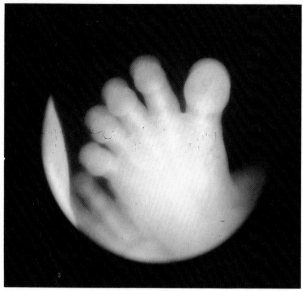

Figure 66.7 Foot at 9 weeks.

wide-angle view of the embryo can be obtained up to a 35-mm crown–rump length. The four extremities and the face are approached with the endoscope, allowing for detailed examination within a few seconds.

Extremities

When the device is brought near an embryonic hand or foot, the region studied occupies the whole endoscopic field and morphological details can be studied with great accuracy.

At 9 weeks the hands are found in a symmetrical position in front of the embryonic face (Figure 66.6), with the radial border being directed cranially. Minor spontaneous movements of the fingers, forearm and arm can be observed. The number of fingers can be easily counted and the phalanges can be clearly identified. The thumb has a typical two phalangeal structure and is opposed by the other digits. The size of each entire limb as well as the relative dimensions of each region can be assessed. Both preaxial and postaxial aspects of the hand and forearm can be observed in detail. Later in gestation, at 10 weeks, the primary nail fields can be identified. Earlier, at 7 weeks, the fingers are normally fused at the distal end of the upper limb bud, but the outlines of the future five digits are clearly visible.

The feet have a different appearance. At 9 weeks the plantar surfaces of the feet oppose each other and the tibial border of the leg is directed cranially. The heel can be visualized and the foot, oriented perpendicular to the leg, forms a right angle in the region of the ankle. The toes are also clearly identifiable and their size and shape can be assessed (Figure 66.7). The preaxial and

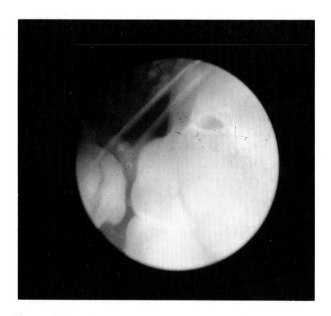

Figure 66.8 Face at 9 weeks.

postaxial borders of the leg can be observed. Earlier in gestation, at 7 weeks, the distal end of the hindlimb bud has a grossly triangular shape with the future toes still appearing as united rays.

Face

The face can be thoroughly examined. At 9 weeks the eyes are located in the anterior aspect of the face and the eyelids are fused, completely covering the eyes. The

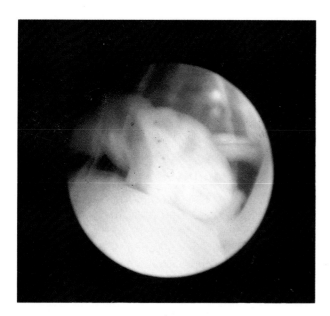

Figure 66.9 Physiological umbilical hernia.

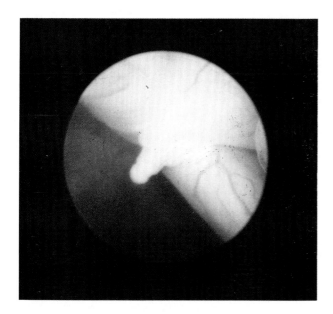

Figure 66.10 Genital tubercle at 9 weeks.

nose and nostrils are well established, the upper lip is fused, and the mouth and the ears are also formed. The chin is prominent. Earlier, at 8 weeks, the eyelids are not established and deep blue eyes can be observed on the lateral aspect of the face. The eyes appear like convex discs covered by a thin transparent membrane corresponding to the corneal ectoderm (Figure 66.8).

Abdomen and external genitalia

At 9 weeks the midgut normally herniates at the embryonic insertion of the umbilical cord. The small intestine can be observed through the transparent wall of the physiological umbilical hernia (Figure 66.9). At 11 weeks the hernia has usually, but not always, completely disappeared. The abdominal wall is then completely closed. At 10 weeks, during the process of reduction of the physiological hernia, a vestigial sac may persist adjacent to the umbilical cord.

The external genitalia are not yet differentiated and exist in a genital turbercle with two labioscrotal swellings (Figure 66.10). At 9 weeks, the embryonic sex cannot be phenotypically diagnosed.

Skull and back

The skull is round and covered by a thin skin, through which can be seen subcutaneous blood vessels as well as a large sagittal suture. The neural tube is closed and can be observed through the skin. Earlier in gestation (less than 4 weeks) the neural tube is still open in the cranial and caudal regions.

66.3.2 MALFORMED EMBRYOS

Although any external malformation can be theoretically diagnosed by embryoscopy, this technique is clinically relevant only for anomalies of the face and extremities that are considered to be inherited with a high genetic risk. These anomalies may be either isolated or part of the phenotypic expression of a complex genetic syndrome. In selected cases, the risk of having a fetus affected by a face or limb defect may reach 25–50%, thereby justifying early invasive prenatal diagnosis.

(a) Extremities

The quality of embryoscopic imaging allows prenatal diagnosis of any congenital defect of the foot or hand at 9 weeks.

Gross anomalies such as ectrodactyly, monodactyly and adactyly are easily observed the first time. However, because the expression of the disease may differ from one extremity to the other, all four extremities must always be studied. Hexadactyly is also easy to diagnose. The sixth digit is usually found on the ulnar border of the hand but it can also be located on the radial border.

Syndactyly is more difficult to diagnose. However, in the case of syndactyly the appearance of the entire hand is abnormal. The hand appears wide but does not look flat like the distal end of the limb found earlier in pregnancy.

Subtle anomalies can be diagnosed by embryoscopy, including hypoplasia of one digit, nail hypoplasia and a short phalanx.

(b) Face

The face may be more difficult to observe than the extremities. A cleft lip can be unequivocally diagnosed based on a divided upper lip at 9 weeks. Anophthalmia has not as yet been diagnosed by embryoscopy; the fusion of the eyelids is a potential limitation for such a diagnosis. Ear hypoplasia or aplasia can be diagnosed. In the absence of a well-defined malformation, facial dysmorphy cannot be demonstrated at embryoscopy.

66.4 Indications

Prenatal diagnosis by embryoscopy should be offered only to patients with a high genetic risk of limb or face malformations. Genetic counselling is crucial to identify the index case and to assess the risk of recurrence in the couple. Four types of indication can be considered.

- Isolated abnormalities of the extremities with likely dominant inheritance, e.g. ectrodactyly, syndactyly, adactyly and acromesomelia.
- Isolated cleft lip with suspected dominant inheritance.
- Complex syndromes with anomalies of the face with probable hereditary transmission [3]. This includes autosomal recessive diseases such as Carpenter or Mohr syndromes and syndromes with syndactyly and cleft face. Autosomal dominant syndromes can also be involved, such as Nager syndrome (radial ray agenesia and cleft lip) and EEC syndrome (ectrodactyly, ectodermal dysplasia and cleft palate).
- Malformation syndromes with anomalies of the extremities with probable hereditary transmission. This includes autosomal recessive syndromes (Baller–Gerold, Saldino–Noonan, Bardet–Biedl, Rothmund–Thomson, Meckel, Quazi, Ellis–van Creveld, Smith–Lemli–Opitz) and X-linked disorders with hexadactyly, such as the Golaby–Rosen syndrome [4].

66.5 Diagnostic value and obstetric risk

Due to the low frequency of occurrence of malformation syndromes, our clinical experience is limited to 57 cases, although data have been collected over a 10-year period [5].

The diagnostic value of embryoscopy appears excellent [6]. All positive diagnoses were confirmed by postmortem examinations and there were no false-negative diagnoses.

Six miscarriages occurred following embryoscopy; all procedures were performed after 10 weeks' gestation. Postnatal follow-up did not suggest any pediatric morbidity associated with embryoscopy.

66.6 Future prospects

Embryoscopy may have considerable importance for future developments in fetal diagnosis and therapy. It may open the way to the sampling of fetal blood and the yolk sack [7] and the injection of cells in the early embryo. This latter approach has potential applications for early therapy of genetic disorders in the embryo, including hematologic, metabolic and immune deficiencies.

66.7 Conclusions

Embryoscopy allows prenatal diagnosis of face and limb defects as early as 9 weeks. Although invasive, this approach has clinical application in couples with a high risk of transmitting a severe congenital disorder that can be identified in the embryo by a minor morphological marker.

References

1. Cullen, M., Reesce, A., Whetham, J. and Hobbins, A. (1990) Embryoscopy: description and utility of a new technique. *Am. J. Obstet. Gynecol.*, **162**, 82–86.
2. Reece, A., Rotmenschs, S., Whethman, J. *et al.* (1992) Embryoscopy: a closer look at first-trimester diagnosis and treatment. *Am. J. Obstet. Gynecol.*, **166**, 775–80.
3. Gorlin, R., Cohen, M. and Levin, S. (1990) *Syndromes of the Head and Neck*, 3rd edn, Oxford University Press, Oxford.
4. Smith, D.W. and Jones, K. (eds)(1988) *Recognizable Patterns of Human Malformation: Genetic, Embryologic, and Clinical Aspects*, W.B. Saunders, Philadelphia.
5. Dumez, Y., Oury, J.F. and Dommergues, M. (1992) Diagnostic embryoscopy: 50 cases of early diagnosis. International Symposium: From Gametes to Embryo (May 18–20, 1992, Milan, Italy (abstract) *Prenat. Diagn.* (suppl.), **12**, 10.
6. Cullen, M., Whetham, J., Viscarello, R. *et al.* (1991) Transcervical endoscopic verification of congenital anomalies in the second trimester of pregnancy. *Am. J. Obstet. Gynecol.*, **165**, 95–97.
7. Dumez, Y., Dommergues, M. and Beuzard, Y. (1990) Study of a method for early first trimester fetal blood sampling intravascular injection. *Symposium on Fetal Therapy and Development: Outlook for the 21st Century*, November 27–30, 1988, Chicago, p. 12 (abstract).

67 CORDOCENTESIS (PERCUTANEOUS UMBILICAL BLOOD SAMPLING AND FETAL BLOOD SAMPLING)

P. Johnson and D.J. Maxwell

67.1 Introduction

Advances in modern technology, particularly that of high-resolution ultrasound, have allowed access to the fetus *in utero* for invasive investigation. Antepartum fetal blood sampling is now an established part of prenatal diagnosis, with wide application.

67.2 Methods

Early attempts to obtain fetal blood involved blind aspiration of blood from the placenta (placentocentesis), with high rates of maternal contamination. Access to the fetal circulation was initially gained at hysterotomy during early attempts at intrauterine transfusion for rhesus haemolytic disease [1]. The development of fetoscopy followed, allowing fetal blood sampling from the umbilical cord under direct vision with the fetus intact *in utero* [2]. Ultrasound-guided access to the fetal circulation was first described during selective fetocide by Aberg *et al.* in 1978 [3], and later for diagnostic and therapeutic purposes by Bang, Bock and Trolle in 1982 [4].

The first report of the technique of ultrasound guided fetal blood sampling from the umbilical cord came from Daffos, Capella Pavlovsky and Forestier in 1983 [5]. This account described the basic technique which has now been widely adopted. Ultrasound examination is performed to identify the placental insertion of the umbilical cord. The maternal skin is then cleansed with a suitable antiseptic, the abdomen draped and local anaesthetic infiltrated into the maternal skin and subcuticular tissues. Under continuous ultrasound visualization, a 20- or 22-gauge single use spinal needle is then inserted into the umbilical vessel and blood aspirated into a heparinized syringe. The approach can be transplacental or transamniotic. Other sites available for venepuncture are the fetal insertion of the cord, a free loop, the intrahepatic vein [4,6] and the fetal heart [7,8].

The initial technique described by Bang, Bock and Trolle [4] involved inserting a guide needle into the fetal body, through which the sampling needle was advanced into the intrahepatic vein. This technique has been adapted for sampling from the umbilical cord [9] but does not appear to have any great advantage over the single needle technique.

The technique can either be free hand or involve the use of a needle guide on the ultrasound transducer. We employ the free hand technique, feeling that this provides the greatest flexibility, particularly with an active fetus. Maternal and fetal sedation can be administered [6,10,11], but in our experience this is rarely necessary. Throughout and following the procedure the fetal heart rate is observed, and the site of puncture is observed at the end of the sampling to ascertain whether there is any blood leakage. We do not administer any drugs, other than anti-D if indicated, after the procedure, although some do advocate antibiotics [12].

Technically, fetal blood sampling is easiest to perform between 18 and 26 weeks gestation. Prior to 18 weeks, imaging the cord insertion may be difficult, particularly in obese patients. The cord itself is smaller in diameter and may be more easily traumatized. Orlandi *et al.* have documented their experience with early cordocentesis, confirming a higher rate of pregnancy loss at gestations less than 18 weeks [13]. We have sampled successfully at 15 weeks gestation, but would only do so in exceptional circumstances. At later gestations, particularly after 26 weeks, the fetus itself may prove obstructive, interposing its body between the scanner or the intended line of entry and the target

Diseases of the Fetus and Newborn, 2nd edn, Edited by G.B. Reed, A.E. Claireaux and F. Cockburn. Published in 1995 by Chapman & Hall, London. ISBN 0 412 39160 0

area. This is the case more frequently with posterior placentas. Patience and care are necessary, and the fetus will normally move sufficiently to allow unhindered access if patience is exercised. External manipulation of the fetus by gentle pushing may be successful. However, in some cases it may be necessary to sample from an alternative site (for example the intrahepatic vein, a free loop of cord, or the fetal heart).

The choice of ultrasound transducer depends on what is available. A curvilinear probe provides the best compromise for most, with the combination of the large visual field of a sector scanner and the advantage of a linear scanner which allows visualization of the needle along the full length of its course [14].

It is essential that the sample is confirmed to be of pure fetal origin [15]. A Coulter counter will assess the size of the erythrocytes, and a graphic display of red and white cell counts will demonstrate single peaks in the fetal range for an uncontaminated sample. Alternatively, the Kleihauer–Betke stain will demonstrate the presence of maternal cells. It is important that the confirmation of fetal blood is rapid, so that the sampling can be repeated if necessary without needing to bring the mother back on another occasion.

The maternal blood group must be known. If she is rhesus-negative, a quantitative Kleihauer–Betke test should be performed after the procedure and anti-D given, usually 500 iu.

67.3 Indications

Invasive fetal investigation has been available since the advent of amniocentesis. There is a limit to the information that can be obtained from analysis of liquor and, as our knowledge of fetal physiology and pathophysiology has increased, it has become increasingly desirable to have access to fetal blood in order to maximize the information available and thus optimize management. Not only does fetal blood lend itself to an increasingly wide range of investigations, but it also allows for rapid provision of results. The simplicity of the technique has led to a dramatic increase in the number of cases where invasive fetal investigation is performed. However, as the risk:benefit ratio is examined, it may be that there will be a reduction in the indications for fetal blood sampling in the future.

7.3.1 RAPID KARYOTYPE

The ability to obtain an accurate fetal karyotype in 24–48 hours accounts for a large proportion of fetal blood samples performed today. As our knowledge of the association between structural abnormalities and chromosomal anomalies has increased, so has the necessity to obtain an accurate karyotype quickly. Only with such information can the parents make informed decisions about their pregnancy, and antenatal and postnatal management can then be optimized for outcome and appropriate application of resources. The rapid provision of such information, particularly in the investigation of structural anomalies detected by ultrasound in the mid-trimester, allows management options to be discussed fully, often while the possibility of therapeutic termination of pregnancy is still available under local legislation.

Fetal chromosomal analysis can be performed on liquor and chorionic villi as well as blood [16]. However, in addition to the wide range of complementary investigations that can be performed on blood, with subsequent advancement of our knowledge of fetal pathophysiology [17], culture of lymphocytes from a pure fetal blood sample provides an accurate karyotype and therefore minimizes the potential problems of maternal contamination and mosaicism. This is of great importance in the investigation of mosaicism discovered in chorionic villous samples and amniocentesis [18], although dilemmas in management can still exist [19].

67.3.2 RHESUS IMMUNIZATION

The investigation and management of rhesus haemolytic disease has been greatly advanced by direct access to the fetal circulation [20], both for assessment of the fetal haematocrit and also for intrauterine intravascular transfusion. The outcome of affected pregnancies has improved dramatically with modern invasive management. However, concern has been voiced regarding the potential for increasing maternal levels of anti-D as a result of fetal blood sampling. There is an increase in maternal anti-D following fetal blood sampling, probably due to placental trauma, but this is thought to occur principally at the first sampling [21], and the advantages of the technique, with resultant improvement in perinatal morbidity and mortality, would appear to outweigh this disadvantage [22].

67.3.3 HAEMATOLOGY

The investigation of haematological disorders has been transformed by access to the fetal circulation [23]. Indications for fetal blood sampling include autoimmune idiopathic thrombocytopenia [24] and the haemoglobinopathies, particularly thalassaemia [8]. First trimester fetal blood sampling has been performed in this diagnostic group [13].

67.3.4 INTRAUTERINE GROWTH RETARDATION

Failure to fulfil growth potential has numerous associations, including chromosomal anomalies and intrauterine infection. In addition, measurement of blood gases in severe intrauterine growth retardation may help the clinician to optimize management and delivery options [25]. However, it is important to realize that biochemical information so obtained only provides a 'snapshot' of the fetal state. In order to optimize management in the long term, repeated investigations would be of more value, but may not be clinically or ethically desirable.

The analysis of blood taken in growth retarded fetuses has allowed the development of a database of endocrinological and physiological data which has increased our knowledge of the pathogenesis of this condition [25–30]. This in turn will help in the development of prenatal therapeutic options in some cases, with, hopefully, improved outcome.

67.3.5 FETAL PHYSIOLOGY

Access to fetal blood has permitted researchers to gain insight into many aspects of human fetal physiology, with normative data available for many physiological variables [31–33]. The changes in many metabolic processes have been investigated in fetuses with growth retardation. Investigation of blood gas status and its correlation with Doppler blood flow studies has at times provided conflicting and confusing data, but nevertheless has helped to increase our understanding of fetal pathophysiology [25,34]. In addition, the fetal effects of maternal illness have been investigated, particularly thyroid disease [35–37], as a preliminary to fetal therapy.

67.3.6 INFECTIONS

Intrauterine infection is associated with a number of structural and functional abnormalities. The ability to diagnose intrauterine infection has improved with fetal blood sampling, although other tissues may be used for this purpose. However, in many cases a combined approach, sampling liquor, chorionic villi and fetal blood, is feasible and may allow the most accurate information [38]. Other pathophysiological details can be gained from blood, e.g. abnormal liver function in association with cytomegalovirus infection [39]. Investigation of fetal toxoplasma status was the principal reason for fetal blood sampling in Daffos' first large series. The technique has also been used for investigation of rubella, cytomegalovirus and parvovirus [38,40].

67.3.7 NON-IMMUNE HYDROPS FETALIS

This condition, with its high fetal loss rate, has been poorly understood. The advent of fetal blood sampling, together with strict protocols for investigation, has led to an improvement in the diagnostic accuracy, with fewer than 15% of cases remaining unexplained [41].

We are firmly of the belief that fetal blood sampling is an essential part of the investigation of the majority of cases of non-immune hydrops.

67.3.8 PHARMACOLOGY

The passage of drugs across the placenta, and the possible effects on the fetus, has been difficult to study in the human fetus. This is of particular importance in the development of new drugs which may be indicated to treat maternal problems during pregnancy, e.g. azathiothymidine, low molecular weight heparin [42,43], as well as the study of older preparations, e.g. morphine [44]. Not only are potential adverse effects important to assess, but it is also necessary to study the efficiency with which drugs given to the mother for fetal therapy cross into the fetal circulation, e.g. placental transfer of digoxin [45].

In this area of study, the paths of research and clinical practice run very close and it is important to remain aware of the real value of results obtained in such an invasive investigation which carries an inherent risk to the pregnancy.

67.4 Risks of the procedure

The exact estimation of the procedure-related loss rate of fetal blood sampling is very difficult to establish and procedure-related loss has never been precisely defined. Most would agree that a loss within 24 hours of an invasive procedure should be described as procedure related but later losses, particularly in the presence of chorioamnionitis, may be a direct consequence of performing the procedure. It is our policy to describe a loss as related to the procedure if it occurs within 2 weeks of the fetal blood sampling as this should include all immediate losses and any cases of chorioamnionitis. The risk of pregnancy loss associated with percutaneous umbilical blood sampling has been estimated at 1–2% [46]. There have, however, been references to increased loss rates in 'high-risk' pregnancies [14,35,47]. There exists in the literature a large number of individual case reports of complications of fetal blood sampling [48,49], and loss rates varying from 0.15% to 25% [50] are reported in series of varying sizes. In an attempt to address this problem, we performed a retrospective study of the procedures performed in our unit, and examined the pregnancy losses in relation to the indication for fetal blood sampling [51].

The patients were divided into four groups for the purpose of analysis:

1. prenatal diagnosis of genetic disorders;
2. investigation of fetuses with structural anomaly;
3. fetal assessment (e.g. acid–base status);
4. non-immune hydrops.

Table 67.1 Fetal blood sampling and total pregnancy losses

	Group[a]				
	1	2	3	4	Total
Total procedures	116	163	36	48	363
Total patients	113	156	35	40	344
Failed procedures	4	7	3	–	14
Repeat samples	3	7	1	8	19
Termination	21	39	2	8	70
Desired pregnancy	92	117	33	32	274
Losses within 2 weeks	1	9	5	10	25
(percentage of desired ongoing pregnancies)[b]	(1.1)	(7.3)	(14.7)	(25)	(8.5)

[a] See text.
[b] Percentage of desired ongoing pregnancies = losses within 2 weeks ÷ (total procedures − terminations).

We reviewed 363 procedures performed between 16 and 38 weeks' gestation. Ten were cardiac punctures, five were taken from the intrahepatic vein and all others were cord samples. There were 13 failed samplings but repeat procedures were not always performed, amniocentesis, chorion villus sampling or fetoscopic blood sampling being employed as alternative procedures in five cases. There was a significant difference between the rates of pregnancy loss between the groups. In a structurally normal fetus the risk of pregnancy loss was 1%, but this increased to 25% in the group with non-immune hydrops (Table 67.1). The aim of our data analysis was to provide information that might be helpful in prospective counselling prior to the procedure of fetal blood sampling.

The four groups of patients studied were representative of common clinical situations where information from a fetal blood sample would be deemed helpful in obstetric management. There were no control groups in which no procedure was performed for comparison. Therefore, a precise procedure-related risk cannot be established for any of the groups in the study. Inevitably, bias is introduced into such an analysis by the fact that, of those pregnancies terminated, some would have been destined to miscarry. In addition, the clinician's freedom on whether or not to deliver a 'sick' hypoxic or acidotic fetus makes estimation of risk at later gestations more difficult.

This analysis confirmed an inherent risk related to the procedure of ultrasound guided fetal blood sampling. In an uncomplicated pregnancy a realistic estimate is 1–2%. However, if a fetus is known to be structurally, or suspected of being metabolically, abnormal the pregnancy losses are higher. How much of the increased loss in the more complicated pregnancies is due to the procedure or to the natural history of the disease in utero remains uncertain. Loss rates rose from 1.3% in the prenatal diagnosis group to 25% in the group with non-immune hydrops, reflecting the severity of underlying clinical disease within the groups.

When pregnancy losses for sites other than the umbilical cord are considered, only one occurred within 2 weeks following cardiac puncture in a severely anaemic, hypoxic and acidotic fetus with hydrops secondary to infection with parvovirus. Other workers have found little difference in procedure-related loss when alternative sampling sites are employed [5,47].

67.5 Informed consent

With modern investigative techniques, particularly those involving the fetus, there are problems with the concept of informed consent. The *Oxford English Dictionary* defines consent as: 'voluntary agreement to, or acquiescence in, what another proposes or desires'.

Informed consent implies that the patient has received all the information necessary to enable him or her to give consent. However, in many branches of modern medical care it is often impossible to give this information in full. Informed consent must therefore be a relative term. In the case of a pregnant woman, her consent applies to the fetus as well as herself [52].

The information required for a patient to give informed consent includes accurate estimation of the risk of the procedure and assessment of the value and implications of the results. Investigations performed during pregnancy carry a risk of pregnancy loss over and above the risk to the pregnancy inherent in the indication for the investigation, and this is often very difficult to establish.

67.6 Conclusions

In less than a decade, our ability to investigate the human fetus *in utero* using invasive procedures has changed from a few units employing fetoscopy to the present situation where most fetal medicine units offer fetal blood sampling. The indications for this procedure appear to be ever increasing, but it may well be that the number of such indications reduce with time. However, we are firmly of the belief that fetal investigations, particularly chromosomal studies, are best performed prenatally. Apart from their value when assisting with prognosis and management choice, knowledge of fetal karyotype is important in counselling with respect to possible recurrence in future pregnancies. Post-mortem samples are not infrequently lost or forgotten following delivery, and it is the experience of our laboratory and others that culture of such samples is less reliable. Even in cases where the ultrasound findings alone mitigate in favour of termination, we will recommend karyotyping beforehand to ensure that an adequate sample is obtained and reaches the laboratory.

Although access to fetal blood has allowed a greater understanding of fetal physiology, particularly in the presence of intrauterine growth retardation, the value of blood results remains difficult to establish and many now feel the other non-invasive investigations such as Doppler blood flow studies of the fetal circulation may be of more merit, and carry no risk to the fetus. In addition, many laboratories, including our own, have improved cell culture techniques, and amniocentesis results for karyotype can now be made available in 14 days rather than 28–35 as previously. In the investigation of 'soft ultrasound markers' of chromosomal anomaly, e.g. renal pelvis dilation, patients and doctors alike may feel happier with amniocentesis than fetal blood sampling.

We have heard of instances where resistance has been encountered, or indeed invasive investigation withheld, either where the pregnancy is beyond the gestational limit for termination, or where the patients have indicated that they would not wish to terminate a pregnancy following an abnormal result. We believe that this is ethically and professionally incorrect. The results of fetal blood tests may be reassuring, and to deny the patients this knowledge is unacceptable. In the presence of abnormal results, particularly chromosomal anomalies, the prognosis and thus parents' expectations can be clarified. This can sometimes lead to parents changing their minds with regard to the continuation of the pregnancy. In cases where fetal blood sampling is clinically appropriate, and the risk:benefit ratio for a particular case has been assessed and discussed, we believe the procedure should be offered to women. If the offer is accepted, it should be performed irrespective of initial thoughts regarding the future of the pregnancy.

We feel that ultrasound guided fetal blood sampling will continue to be an important tool in the armamentarium of the prenatal diagnostician, although in the future the indications for the procedure may reduce.

References

1. Freda, V.J. and Adamsons Jr, K. (1964) Exchange transfusion *in utero*. *Am. J. Obstet. Gynecol.*, **89**, 17–21.
2. Valenti, C. (1973) Antenatal detection of haemoglobinopathies. *Am. J. Obstet. Gynecol.*, **115**, 851–53.
3. Aberg, A., Mitelman, F., Cantz, M. and Gehler, J. (1978) Cardiac puncture of a fetus with Hurler's disease avoiding abortion of unaffected co-twin. *Lancet*, **ii**, 990–91.
4. Bang, J., Bock, J.E. and Trolle, D. (1982) Ultrasound guided fetal intravenous transfusion for severe rhesus haemolytic disease. *BMJ*, **284**, 373–74.
5. Daffos, F., Capella Pavlovsky, M. and Forestier, F. (1983) A new procedure for fetal blood sampling *in utero*: preliminary results of fifty-three cases. *Am. J. Obstet. Gynecol.*, **146**, 985–86.
6. Nicolini, U., Santolaya, J., Ojo, O.E. *et al.* (1988) The fetal intrahepatic umbilical vein as an alternative to cord needling for prenatal diagnosis and therapy. *Prenat. Diag.* **3**, 665–71.
7. Westgren, M., Selbing, A. and Stangenberg, M. (1988) Fetal intracardiac transfusions in patients with severe rhesus isoimmunisation. *BMJ*, **296**, 885–86.
8. Antsaklis, A.I., Papantoniou, N.E., Mesogitis, S.A. *et al.* (1992) Cardio-

9. Bovicelli, L., Orsini, L.F., Grannum, P.A.T. *et al.* (1989) A new funipuncture technique: two-needle ultrasound and needle biopsy-guided procedure. *Obstet. Gynecol.*, **73**, 428–31.
10. Hobbins, J.C., Grannum, P.A., Romero, R. *et al.* (1985) Percutaneous umbilical blood sampling. *Am. J. Obstet. Gynecol.* **152**, 1–6.
11. Weiner, C.P. (1987) Cordocentesis for diagnostic indications: two years experience. *Obstet. Gynecol.* **70**, 664–68.
12. Ludomirsky, A. and Weiner, S. (1988) Percutaneous fetal umbilical blood sampling. *Clin. Obstet. Gynecol.* **31**, 19–26.
13. Orlandi, F., Damiani, G., Jakil, C. *et al.* (1990) The risks of early cordocentesis (12–21 weeks): analysis of 500 procedures. *Prenat. Diag.*, **10**, 425–28.
14. Nicolaides, K. (1988) Cordocentesis. *Clin. Obstet. Gynecol.* **31**, 123–35.
15. Forestier, F., Cox, W.L., Daffos, F. and Rainaut, M. (1988) The assessment of fetal blood samples. *Am. J. Obstet. Gynecol.*, **158**, 1184–88.
16. Bald, R., Chatterjee, M.S., Gembruch, U. *et al.* (1991) Antepartum fetal blood sampling with cordocentesis. Comparison with chorionic villus sampling and amniocentesis in diagnosing karyotype anomalies. *J. Reprod. Med.*, **36**, 655–58.
17. Tannirandorn, Y., Nicolini, U., Nicolaidis, P.C. *et al.* (1990) Fetal cystic hygromata; insights gained from fetal blood sampling. *Prenat. Diag.*, **10**, 189–93.
18. Gosden, C., Nicolaides, K.H. and Rodeck, C.H. (1988) Fetal blood sampling in the investigation of chromosome mosaicism in amniotic fluid culture. *Lancet*, **i**, 613–17.
19. Fejgin, M., Barnes, I., Lipnick, N. *et al.* (1992) The dilemma of a low rate of chromosomal mosaicism found in fetal blood sampling. *Prenat. Diag.*, **12**, 129–31.
20. Swinhoe, D.J., Gilmore, D.H., McNay, M.B. and Whittle, M.J. (1990) Rhesus haemolytic disease: continuing problem of management. *Arch. Dis. Child.* **65**, 365–68.
21. Bowell, P.J., Selinger, M., Ferguson, J. *et al.* (1988) Antenatal fetal blood sampling for the management of alloimmunized pregnancies: effect upon maternal anti-D potency levels. *Br. J. Obstet. Gynaecol.*, **95**, 759–64.
22. MacGregor, S.N., Silver, R.K. and Sholl, J.S. (1991) Enhanced sensitization after cordocentesis in a rhesus-isoimmunized pregnancy. *Am. J. Obstet. Gynecol.*, **165**, 382–83.
23. Daffos, F., Forestier, F., Kaplan, C. and Cox, W. (1988) Prenatal diagnosis and management of bleeding disorders with fetal blood sampling. *Am. J. Obstet. Gynecol.* **158**, 939–46.
24. Scioscia, A.L., Grannum, P.A.T., Copel, J.A. and Hobbins, J.C. (1988) The use of percutaneous umbilical blood sampling in immune thrombocytopenic purpura. *Am. J. Obstet. Gynecol.*, **159**, 1066–68.
25. Soothill, P.W. (1989) Cordocentesis: role in the assessment of fetal condition. *Clin. Perinatol.*, **16**, 755–70.
26. Pardi, G., Buscaglia, M., Ferrazzi, E. *et al.* (1987) Cord sampling for the evaluation of oxygenation and acid–base balance in growth retarded human fetuses. *Am. J. Obstet. Gynecol.*, **157**, 1221–28.
27. Cox, W.L., Daffos, F., Forestier, F. *et al.* (1988) Physiology and management of intrauterine growth retardation: a biologic approach with fetal blood sampling. *Am. J. Obstet. Gynecol.*, **159**, 36–41.
28. Economides, D.L., Nicolaides, K.H., Gahl, W.A. *et al.* (1989) Cordocentesis in the diagnosis of intrauterine starvation. *Am. J. Obstet. Gynecol.*, **161**, 1004–1008.
29. Nicolini, U., Hubinont, C., Santolaya, J. *et al.* (1989) Maternal–fetal glucose gradient in normal pregnancies and pregnancies complicated by alloimmunization and fetal growth retardation. *Am. J. Obstet. Gynecol.*, **161**, 924–27.
30. Weiner, C.P. and Williamson, R.A. (1989) Evaluation of severe growth retardation using cordocentesis – hematologic and metabolic alterations by etiology. *Obstet. Gynecol.*, **73**, 225–29.
31. Ludomirsky, A., Weiner, S., Ashmead, G.G. *et al.* (1988) Percutaneous fetal umbilical blood sampling: procedure safety and normal fetal hematological indices. *Am. J. Perinatol.*, **5**, 264–66.
32. Khoury, A.D., Moretti, M.L., Barton, J.R. *et al.* (1991) Fetal blood sampling in patients undergoing elective cesarean section: a correlation with cord blood gas values obtained at delivery. *Am. J. Obstet. Gynecol.*, **165**, 1026–29.
33. Thorpe Beeston, J.G., Nicolaides, K.H., Felton, C.V. *et al.* (1991) Maturation of the secretion of thyroid hormone and thyroid stimulating hormone in the fetus. *N. Engl. J. Med.*, **324**, 532–36.
34. Weiner, C.P. (1990) The relationship between the umbilical artery systolic/ diastolic ratio and umbilical blood gas measurements in specimens obtained by cordocentesis. *Am. J. Obstet. Gynecol.*, **162**, 1198–202.
35. Perelman, A.H., Johnson, R.L., Clemons, R.D. *et al.* (1990) Intrauterine diagnosis and treatment of fetal goitrous hyperthyroidism. *J. Clin. Endocrinol. Metab.*, **71**, 618–21.
36. Porreco, R.P. and Bloch, C.A. (1990) Fetal blood sampling in the management of intrauterine thyrotoxicosis. *Obstet. Gynecol.*, **76**, 509–12.

37. Wenstrom, K.D., Weiner, C.P., Williamson, R.A. and Grant, S.S. (1990) Prenatal diagnosis of fetal hyperthyroidism by funipuncture. *Obstet. Gynecol.*, **76**, 513–17.

38. Lynch, L., Daffos, F., Emanuel, D. *et al.* (1991) Prenatal diagnosis of fetal cytomegalovirus infection. *Am J. Obstet. Gynecol.*, **165**, 714–18.

39. Hohlfield, P., Maillard-Brignon, C., Vaudaux, B. and Farver, C-L. (1991) Cytomegalovirus fetal infection: prenatal diagnosis. *Obstet. Gynecol.*, **78**, 615–18.

40. Peters, M. and Nicolaides, K.H. (1990) Cordocentesis for the diagnosis and treatment of human fetal parvovirus infection. *Obstet. Gynecol.*, **75**, 501–504.

41. Johnson, P. and Maxwell, D.J. (1992) Non-immune hydrops. *Contemp. Rev. Obstet. Gynaecol.*, **4**, 71–76.

42. Pons, J.C., Taburet, A.M. Singlas, E. *et al.* (1991) Placental passage of azathiothymidine (AZT) during second trimester of pregnancy: study by direct fetal blood sampling under ultrasound. *Eur. J. Obstet. Gynecol. Reprod. Biol.*, **40**, 229–31.

43. Forestier, F., Daffos, F. and Capella-Pavlovsky, M. (1984) Low molecular weight heparin (PK10169) does not cross the placenta during the second trimester of pregnancy: study by direct fetal blood sampling under ultrasound. *Thromb. Res.*, **34**, 557–560.

44. Gerdin, E., Rane, A. and Lindberg, B. (1990) Transplacental transfer of morphine in man. *J. Perinat. Med.*, **18**, 305–12.

45. Kanhai, H.H., van Kamp, I.L., Moolenaar, A.J. and Gravenhorst, J.B. (1990) Transplacental passage of digoxin in severe rhesus immunization. *J. Perinat. Med.*, **18**, 339–43.

46. Daffos, F., Capella Pavlovsky, M. and Forestier, F. (1985) Fetal blood sampling during pregnancy with use of a needle guided by ultrasound: a study of 606 consecutive cases. *Am. J. Obstet. Gynecol.*, **153**, 655–60.

47. Nicolini, U., Nicolaidis, P., Fisk, N.M. *et al.* (1990) Fetal blood sampling from the intrahepatic vein: analysis of safety and clinical experience with 214 procedures. *Obstet. Gynecol.*, **76**, 47–53.

48. Benacerraf, B.R., Barss, V.A., Saltzman, D.H. *et al.* (1987) Acute fetal distress associated with percutaneous umbilical blood sampling. *Am. J. Obstet. Gynecol.*, **156**, 1218–20.

49. Feinkind, L., Nanda, D., Delke, I. and Minkoff, H. (1990) Abruptio placentae after percutaneous umbilical cord sampling: a case report. *Am. J. Obstet. Gynecol.*, **162**, 1203–204.

50. Weiner, C.P. (1988) The role of cordocentesis in fetal diagnosis. *Clin. Obstet. Gynecol.*, **32**, 285–92.

51. Maxwell, D.J., Johnson, P., Hurley, P. *et al.* (1991) Fetal blood sampling and pregnancy loss in relation to indication. *Br. J. Obstet. Gynaecol.*, **98**, 892–97.

52. Wilkinson, A.M. (1981) Consent, in *Dictionary of Medical Ethics* (eds A.S. Duncan, G.R. Dunstan and R.B. Welbourn), Darton Longman and Todd, London, pp. 113–17.

68 CHORIONIC VILLUS SAMPLING (EARLY AND LATE)

B. Brambati

68.1 Acceptability and benefits of first trimester testing

Chorionic villus sampling (CVS) has opened the first trimester to scientific investigation and replaced mid-trimester amniocentesis for fetal genetic diagnosis. CVS is safe and effective and provides diagnosis much earlier in pregnancy, thereby allowing selective termination at a safer time. Prenatal diagnosis in the first trimester, when a physical awareness of the conceptus may not yet be present, was expected to have less distressing effects on the mother. Psychological studies on patients after amniocentesis and CVS found that a high percentage of women would accept a significantly higher risk of fetal loss in order to benefit from an earlier first trimester diagnosis [1–3]. Moreover, several of the legal and religious obstacles to selective abortion have been overcome by the precocity of the procedure.

All these social and medical advantages may explain the rapidly expanding worldwide experience that can be assumed from some 200 000 cases in 1992 [4].

68.2 Sampling methods

Technology for obtaining chorionic tissue has advanced over less than 10 years experience. Until recently most centers have used ultrasound guided transcervical aspiration, but the current trend shows a growing number of investigators are preferring the transabdominal route, using either a single or a double needle technique [5]. Transvaginal needling under vaginal ultrasound probe guidance has also been evaluated [6,7]. The experience is still very limited, however it could in theory be used in cases where the transcervical and transabdominal approaches are felt to be too risky (Figure 68.1).

CVS is an outpatient procedure and no preoperative or postoperative care is required. A full bladder may be advantageous only in specific cases, either to straighten the angle of a pronounced anteflexion of the uterus or to push intestinal loops away from the anterior uterine wall in patients with retroflexed uterus. Generally, a retroflexed uterus can be rotated and maintained in a more favorable position by manual replacement at the time of sampling.

Accurate ultrasound examination should precede sampling to evaluate uterine anatomy, placental location and gestational age, to document fetal viability and to detect multiple pregnancy and fetal malformations. Extraovular echo-free areas should also be evaluated to differentiate between a vanishing twin and a fluid-filled space (e.g. hematoma). Permanent fetal bradycardia [8], a significantly low value of either crown–rump length or gestational sac volume [9,10] and too large a yolk sac [11] are all signs of pending fetal demise, therefore it is wise to postpone sampling and suggest ultrasound monitoring.

Transcervical sampling is more frequently performed with a polypropylene cannula, 1.45 mm outer diameter and 26 cm long, provided with a fashionable metallic obturator (Trophocan, Portex Ltd, UK) [12,13]. The system is appropriately bent after an accurate evaluation of the sampling route and gently introduced along the cervical canal and the uterine cavity under continuous ultrasound surveillance. Prior to any sampling maneuver, the external genitalia, the vagina and the cervix should be cleaned using antiseptic solution. In cases of clinical vaginal infection the transabdominal sampling route should be considered.

Transabdominal sampling can be performed either by inserting a 20-gauge 9-cm spinal needle free-hand [14] or by inserting a double coaxial needle system through a needle guide fixed to the ultrasound probe [15]. In the latter approach an 18-gauge 15-cm guide needle is first introduced; a 20–22-gauge 20-cm needle is then repeatedly inserted for adequate chorionic tissue aspiration. The ultrasound probe should be sterilized or protected by a sterile bag and sterile gel should maintain a suitable contact with the maternal surface.

Transvaginal needling requires the same preliminary

Diseases of the Fetus and Newborn, 2nd edn, Edited by G.B. Reed, A.E. Claireaux and F. Cockburn. Published in 1995 by Chapman & Hall, London. ISBN 0 412 39160 0

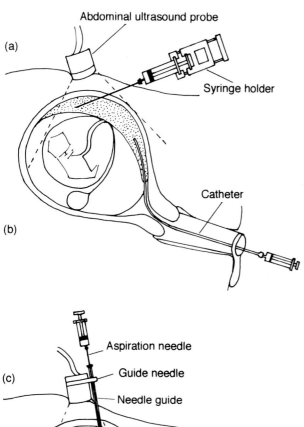

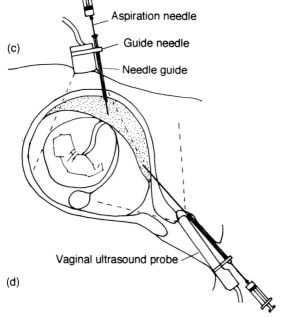

Figure 68.1 The main sampling techniques: (a) transabdominal needling by free-hand needle insertion; (b) transcervical aspiration by thin plastic catheter; (c) transabdominal aspiration by a double needle system and guide needle; (d) transvaginal needling by needle guide affixed to the vaginal ultrasound probe.

preparation of the external genitalia, vagina and cervix as transcervical sampling. A vaginal 5–7.5-MHz ultrasound probe, covered with a sterile rubber sheath and provided with a sterile needle guide, is inserted into the vagina [6,7]. Chorionic tissue may be aspirated by a 20-gauge needle with stylet, 30 cm long, or by a double needle system.

No more than two sampling insertions in the same session should be attempted because of a significant increase in the complication rate if three or more insertions are made [16–19]. In cases of potential fetomaternal rhesus incompatibility Coombs' test should be performed before CVS and, if antibodies are absent, a dose of 50 μg or more of anti-D immune globulin administered. Studies of the increase in maternal serum α-fetoprotein (MSAFP) levels before and after CVS suggest fetomaternal hemorrhage frequently occurs [20–23], therefore the potential risk of worsening maternal immunization by CVS should be discussed with the immunized patient before sampling. Recently, rhesus typing on a small (as little as 2 mg) aliquot of the chorionic tissue specimen in cases at potential risk of immunization has been suggested to avoid unnecessary rhesus immunoglobulin prophylaxis [24].

68.3 Multiple pregnancy

Multiple pregnancy is not a contraindication to CVS; transabdominal sampling has proved to be highly successful, but in some instances the combined use of transabdominal and transcervical or transvaginal routes may be most profitable [25,26].

Concerns on sampling reliability may arise in cases of fused placentas and dichorionic sacs: the main criterion for a reliable biopsy of each placenta is to guide the extremity of the sampling device next to the umbilical cord insertions and avoid passing through any adjacent placenta. Nevertheless, if like-sex dichorionic twins and no difference on the basis of chromosome and/or DNA polymorphisms are found, the patient should be counselled to wait for confirmation by amniocentesis. Genetic investigations prior to first trimester fetal reduction in multiple pregnancies induced by superovulation and artificial fertilization techniques do not apparently change clinical outcome and must be recommended to avoid the disastrous eventuality of saving fetuses with chromosomal abnormalities [27,28].

68.4 Timing

CVS is usually performed between 9 and 12 weeks, however the transabdominal route has also proved to be a valuable approach for sampling chorionic tissue in earlier or later gestational periods. Transabdominal CVS may be used after 12 weeks as an alternative to early or mid-trimester amniocentesis, and later on for rapid karyotyping in late booking cases or those with suspicious ultrasound findings [29–30]. Transabdominal sampling has also been offered at 6–7 weeks gestation in high genetic risk pregnancies [31]. The very early conclusion of the diagnostic process (before 9 weeks) proved to reduce greatly the psychological sequelae of genetic abortion and clearly to increase the pregnancy rate, and offered the opportunity for the use of the pill RU486 for clinical abortion instead of the traditional surgical evacuation. Although early transabdominal sampling was sucessfully performed in 100% of cases, the study supports the potential risk of severe vascular damage of the chorionic plate and therefore the opportunity to shift to transvaginal needling under high resolution ultrasound visualization for a more reliable and safer needle guidance [32].

68.5   Indications

CVS has greatly contributed to the expansion of prenatal diagnosis of genetic disorders by DNA analysis. Chorionic tissue is well established as the optimal substrate for molecular diagnosis: the major advantage is the large yield of DNA, while it is quite easy to avoid any maternal contamination by accurate selection of the material [32]. Usually one obtains about 20–50 μg of DNA by a single aspiration, although karyotyping can easily be carried out together with enzymatic or DNA analysis. Cystic fibrosis investigation has recently been added to chromosome analysis as a routine screening test in first trimester prenatal diagnosis, and it is realistic to expect, in the future, a battery of genomic probes for screening the most frequent hereditary disorders. Inborn errors of metabolism may also be easily and reliably investigated on fresh or cultured chorionic tissue, and in very few conditions has enzymatic activity been found too low for a reliable diagnostic conclusion [33].

Cytogenetic analysis may be carried out either by direct or culture methods: the former avoids any maternal cell contamination problem and provides results in a few hours or days, while the latter provides high standard metaphase banding for detecting small structural changes. No false-negative results have so far been reported when chorionic tissue has been processed by both analytical methods [34]. False-positive cytogenetic results are no longer a matter of error: in cases of placental mosaicism or pure non-viable trisomy, the patient is counselled to wait for further investigation on

amniotic fluid or fetal blood. A relationship between poor fetal outcome and cytogenetic abnormality confined to the placenta has been documented, therefore patients must be informed about this potential event and the pregnancy monitored to detect abnormal fetal development [35,36].

Two diagnostic issues have become available recently through first trimester CVS and DNA analysis and should be mentioned because of their practical interest. First, cDNA probes complementary to the DNA of infectious agents of obstetrical interest (e.g. toxoplasma, rubella, varicella) have been developed [37–39]: if the new approach is proved reliable in predicting fetal conditions, diagnostic conclusions of fetal involvement in cases of maternal infection will be greatly anticipated in regard to the actual evaluation of the immunological response in fetal blood at 20–22 weeks gestation. Moreover, the recent discovery and characterization of hypervariable, repetitive human DNA sequences have made it possible to do prenatal paternity testing [40]. Definitive identification or exclusion of paternity on fetal DNA from chorionic tissue is a powerful diagnostic tool for selected cases which can provide help to women who have had extramarital relationships in avoiding unnecessary termination of pregnancy.

68.6   Transabdominal versus transcervical CVS

The randomized trials have demonstrated that transabdominal and transcervical techniques are equally efficient and safe (Table 68.1) [41–43]. Although the overall success rate after two insertions is virtually 100% for both techniques, a higher failure rate at the first insertion has been reported for transcervical CVS (9.7 versus 3.7%), and this may be largely explained by more frequent difficult or contraindicated conditions met by the transcervical approach [41]. Tissue weight distribution of chorionic tissue specimens obtained by transabdominal needling appears significantly shifted

Table 68.1 Safety and efficacy of the transabdominal (TA) and transcervical (TC) routes in randomized trials

Study	No. of cases		Mean tissue weight (mg)		Failure rate (%)		Fetal loss rate (%)	
	TA	TC	TA	TC	TA	TC	TA	TC
Italian [41]	575	581	24.0	30.6[a]	0.2	0.2	16.5	15.5
Danish [43]	1191	1175	NA	NA	1.8	3.4	6.2	10.1[a]
American [42]	1944	1929	20	25[a]	1.4	2.4	2.6	2.6

NA = not available.
[a] Statistically significant.

towards lighter values [41,42], but no statistical difference has been found between techniques when considering samples of less than 10 mg (5.9 versus 5.0%) [41].

Which sampling techniques should be used in clinical practice, transabdominal or transcervical? Although randomized trials have been unable to demonstrate a clear-cut difference between techniques, from my experience, starting with transcervical catheter aspiration, free-hand transabdominal needling became the method of choice for a number of practical reasons. In fact, with the transabdominal route many fewer cases need to be postponed or shifted to the alternative technique (3.1 versus 15.8%), the learning curve is shorter (less than 100 versus 200–300 experimental cases), the procedure take less time (5–10 versus 20–30 min), the sampling device is cheaper, and the fear of ascending infection to the uterine cavity is definitely avoided [41,44]. Nevertheless, the safety and efficacy of the routine sampling activity would improve with the availability of both techniques, choosing the appropriate sampling route as indicated and possible.

68.7 Complications

Vaginal spotting has been the most frequent early complication of both transabdominal (1.5–4.4%) and transcervical (19.2–32.2%) CVS [42,45,46]. Light to moderate bleeding occurs less frequently: it has been reported in 6.0–7.3% and 0.5% of cases after transcervical and transabdominal sampling, respectively [42,46]. Although no relationship has been demonstrated between bleeding and fetal loss [13], this complication was suggested in some transcervical CVS cases as the first clinical feature of a sequence of events, including fluid leakage and chorioamnionitis, leading to fetal loss [47,48]. Mild localized peritonitis has been observed rarely (0.1%) after transabdominal CVS [49], while chorioamnionitis and septic abortion have been documented after transcervical sampling in fewer than 0.5% of cases [44,47,50–52]. Fetomaternal hemorrhage following CVS has been demonstrated in 40–72% of cases by a significant increase of MSAFP levels, and the volume of fetal hemorrhage exceeded 0.1 ml in 6–18% of cases [20–24]. Although this complication appears unlikely to harm fetal well-being, an association between MSAFP increase and fetal demise early after CVS was suspected in cases with the highest AFP level increase [21].

Complications of the second half of pregnancy, including hypertension and pre-eclampsia (1.3–1.4%), abruptio placentae and placenta previa (0.4–1.0%), preterm birth (4.9–8.1%), intrauterine growth retardation (1.0–5.3%) and malformations (1.0–2.6%), did not show any significant increase in clinical studies and trials comparing CVS and amniocentesis [41,42,44, 45,

Table 68.2 Limb defects reported in the WHO-CVS Registry and the British Columbia Registry

Registry	Total no. of registered cases	Cases with limb reductions	Incidence (per 10 000)
WHO-CVS Registry [4]	75 592	40*	5.29
WHO-CVS Registry [60]	130 819	76*	5.81
British Columbia Registry [59]	1 213 913	659	5.43

* This number includes both cases observed at birth and detected during pregnancy by ultrasound and aborted.

47,53,54]. Recently, clusters of severe limb reduction abnormalities (before 9 completed weeks) have been reported in small experiences and one claimed the possible role of CVS [32,55,56]. However, a number of reports from large series of cases performed between 8 and 12 weeks showed no statistical increase [55]. This is also the conclusion of an extensive review in seven Eurocat birth defects registries including over 600 000 births and 336 cases of limb reduction anomalies, four of which were exposed to CVS [58]. In addition, more recently, the comparison between the frequency of limb reduction defects following CVS, from over 75 thousand cases reported in the WHO–CVS Registry [4] by centers with series of 700 CVS or more and the incidence reported in the British Columbia Registry [59], including 1213 913 livebirths, did not show any statistically significant difference (Table 68.2). The results have been more recently confirmed by comparing the actual total number of consecutive cases with complete follow-up reported in the WHO-CVS Registry by all the participating centers [60]. However, by the present evidence, a causal relationship between CVS and the three clusters of limb defects previously reported [32,55,56] very likely exists, and trauma and gestational age seem to play the most important role in the causation of fetal abnormalities. Limb defect cases mostly followed CVS undertaken before 9 weeks, when limb organogenesis makes tissue more sensitive to teratogenic agents. Moreover, poor control of needle tip movements may cause vascular disruption of the chorionic plate and hypoxic tissue damage as a result of severe hemorrhage [32]. Therefore, the consensus of opinion has recently been [4,61] that CVS is extremely unlikely to cause developmental abnormalities when performed by expert hands, at 9–10 weeks or more, and fundamental methodological prerequisites are respected, namely clear visualization of the uterine anatomy, precise definition of the placental limits and absolute control of the needle path [31].

Table 68.3 Safety and efficacy of CVS and amniocentesis (A) in controlled trials

Study	No. of centers	No. of cases sampled		Sampling failures (%)		Total fetal losses (%)		Perinatal mortality (%)	
		CVS	A	CVS	A	CVS	A	CVS	A
Canadian [62]	11	1169	1174	6.3	NA	7.5	7.0	0.5	0.1
American [46]	7	2235	671	1.8	NA	7.2	5.7	0.6	0.7
Danish [43]									
TA-CVS	2	1180	1003	1.8	None	6.2	6.3	0.6	0.7
TC-CVS		1164		3.4		10.1[a]		0.4	
European [53]	31	1609	1594	4.8	1.8	13.6[a]	9.0	1.0	0.7

TA = transabdominal; TC = transcervical; NA = not available.
[a] Statistically significant.

68.8 Risk evaluation of CVS versus amniocentesis

There are now four reports comparing CVS and amniocentesis (Table 68.3) [43,46,53,62]. The Canadian study [62] was the first randomized trial and included 2787 women of more than 34 years of age. Sampling was performed by transcervical aspiration in 11 centers with a recent and limited experience, and the operators were admitted when they had performed at least 30 CVSs and achieved a successful sampling in 23 out of 25 consecutive cases. A second randomized study was planned in the USA [46], but because of a too low acceptance rate it was changed to a control study comparing a total of 2272 cases of transcervical CVS with 671 cases of amniocentesis matched for age and several other variables. Women entered the study in the first trimester, at which time fetal viability and gestational age were monitored by ultrasound. The majority of the seven American centers already had considerable experience at the time the trial started. In the Medical Research Council European Collaborative Study [53], 3248 patients were randomized in 31 centers, two of which contributed more than 35% of the total number of cases, while an average of 67 cases was the contribution of the remaining centers over a 4-year study period. Catheter aspiration, biopsy forceps and transabdominal needling were the sampling techniques used in the study. Interestingly, the success rate at the first insertion was 69% and 94% for CVS and amniocentesis, respectively, thereby suggesting a poor average operator's skill in both sampling approaches. More ambitious was the Danish trial [43] randomizing 2183 women of under 35 years of age to transabdominal CVS, transcervical CVS and amniocentesis. The study was carried out by only one operator in each of the two centers. No statistically significant difference in fetal loss rate was found in the Canadian, American and Danish studies, whereas a higher value for the CVS series was reported in the European trial. By the critical analysis of the studies the most plausible explanation of the discrepancy seems to be the low technical level of the operators of the European trial centers, except for the largest one, which interestingly did not report any fetal loss rate difference between techniques [53].

In conclusion: (1) CVS should be considered a more difficult sampling approach than mid-trimester amniocentesis; therefore (2) it should be confined to the centers where adequate resources are available and considerable training and routine sampling may be done; and (3) no obvious differences in safety and efficiency should be expected between techniques when high levels of experience and expertise are present.

References

1. McCormick, M.J., Rylance, W.E. and Newton, J. (1990) Patients' attitudes following chorionic villus sampling. *Prenat. Diagn.*, 10, 253–55.
2. Abramsky, L. and Rodeck, C.H. (1991) Women's choices for fetal chromosome analysis. *Prenat. Diagn.*, 11, 23–28.
3. Cao, A., Cossu, P., Monni, G. and Rosatelli, M.C. (1987) Chorionic villus sampling and acceptance rate of prenatal diagnosis. *Prenat. Diagn.*, 7, 531–33.
4. Kuliev, A.M., Modell, B., Jackson, L. *et al.* (1993) Risk evaluation of CVS. *Prenat. Diagn.*, 13, 197–209.
5. Jackson, L. (1991) CVS Newsletter, Philadelphia, Jan. 28.
6. Sidransky, E., Black, S.H., Soenksen, D.M. *et al.* (1990) Transvaginal chorionic villus sampling. *Prenat. Diagn.*, 10, 583–86.
7. Ghirardini, G., Popp, W.L., Camurri, L. and Stoeckenius, M. (1986) Vaginosonographic guided chorionic villi needle biopsy (transvaginal chorionic villi sampling). *Eur. J. Obstet. Gynecol. Reprod. Biol.*, 23, 315–19.
8. Laboda, L.A., Estroff, J.A. and Benacerraf, B.R. (1989) First trimester bradycardia: a sign of impending fetal loss. *J. Ultrasound Med.*, 8, 561–63.
9. Brambati, B. and Lanzani, A. (1987) A clinical look at early post-implantation pregnancy failure. *Hum. Reprod.*, 2, 401–05.
10. Bromley, B., Harlow, B.L., Laboda, L.A. and Benacerraf, B.R. (1991) Small sac size in the first trimester: a predictor of poor fetal outcome. *Radiology*, 178, 375–79.
11. Ferrazzi, E., Brambati, B., Lanzani, A. *et al.* (1988) The yolk sac in early pregnancy failure. *Am. J. Obstet. Gynecol.*, 158, 137–42.
12. Ward, R.H.T., Modell, B., Petrou, M. *et al.* (1983) Method of sampling chorionic villi in first trimester of pregnancy under guidance of real time ultrasound. *BMJ*, 286, 1542–44.
13. Brambati, B., Simoni, G., Danesino, C. *et al.* (1985) First trimester fetal diagnosis of genetic disorders: clinical evaluation of 250 cases. *J. Med. Genet.*, 22, 92–99.
14. Brambati, B., Oldrini, A. and Lanzani, A. (1987) Transabdominal chorionic villus sampling: a freehand ultrasound-guided technique. *Am. J. Obstet. Gynecol.*, 157, 134–37.
15. Smidt-Jensen, S. and Hahnemann, N. (1984) Transabdominal fine needle biopsy from chorionic villi in the first trimester. *Prenat. Diagn.*, 4, 163–69.
16. WHO Consultation on First Trimester Fetal Diagnosis (1986) Risk evaluation in chorion villus sampling. *Prenat. Diagn.*, 6, 451–56.
17. Brambati, B., Oldrini, A., Ferrazzi, E. and Lanzani, A. (1987) Chorionic villus sampling: an analysis of the obstetric experience of 1000 cases. *Prenat. Diagn.*, 7, 157–69.
18. Wade, R.V. and Young, S.R. (1989) Analysis of fetal loss after transcervi-

cal chorionic villus sampling: a review of 719 patients. *Am. J. Obstet. Gynecol.*, **161**, 513–19.

19. Jackson, L.G. and Wapner, R.J. (1987) Risk of chorion villus sampling. *Baillière's Clin. Obstet. Gynaecol.*, **1**, 513–31.

20. Blackemore, K.J., Baumgarten, A., Schoenfeld-Dimaio, A.M. et al. (1986) Rise in maternal serum alpha-fetoprotein concentration after chorionic villus sampling and the possibility of isoimmunization. *Am. J. Obstet. Gynecol.*, **155**, 988–93.

21. Fuhrman, W., Altland, K., Kohler, A. et al. (1988) Fetomaternal transfusion after chorionic villi sampling. *Hum. Genet*, **78**, 83–85.

22. Brambati, B., Guercilena, S., Bonacchi, I. et al. (1986) Fetomaternal transfusion after chorionic villus sampling: Clinical implications. *Hum. Reprod.*, **1**, 37–39.

23. Perry, T.B., Vekemans, M.J.J., Lippman, A. et al. (1985) Chorionic villus sampling: clinical experience, immediate complications and patients' attitudes. *Am. J. Obstet. Gynecol.*, **151**, 61–66.

24. Kickler, T.S., Blakemore, K., Shirey, R.S. et al. (1992) Chorionic villus sampling for fetal Rh typing: clinical implications. *Am. J. Obstet. Gynecol.*, **166**, 1407–11.

25. Brambati, B., Tului, L., Lanzani, A. et al. (1991) First trimester genetic diagnosis in multiple pregnancy: principles and potential pitfalls. *Prenat. Diagn.*, **11**, 767–74.

26. Pergament, E., Schulman, J.D. Copeland, K. et al. (1992) The risk and efficacy of chorionic villus sampling in multiple gestations. *Prenat. Diagn.*, **12**, 377–84.

27. Brambati, B., Formigli, L., Tului, L. and Simoni, G. (1990) Selective reduction of quadruplet pregnancy at risk of beta-thalassemia. *Lancet*, **336**, 1325–26.

28. Wapner, R.J., Davis, G.H., Johnson, A. et al. (1991) Selective termination of multifetal pregnancies. *Lancet*, **335**, 90–93.

29. Holzgreve, W., Miney, P., Schloo, R. and Participants of the 'Late CVS Registry' (1990) Late CVS International Registry. Compilation of data from 24 centres. *Prenat. Diagn.* **20**, 159–67.

30. Jahoda, M.G.J., Pijpers, L., Reuss, A. et al. (1990) Transabdominal villus sampling in early second trimester: a safe sampling method for women of advanced age. *Prenat. Diagn.*, **10**, 307–11.

31. Brambati, B., Tului, L., Simoni, G., Travi, M. et al. (1991) Genetic diagnosis before the eighth gestational week. *Obstet. Gynecol.*, **77**, 318–21.

32. Brambati, B., Simoni, G., Travi, M. et al. (1992) Genetic diagnosis by chorionic villus sampling before 8 gestational weeks: efficiency, reliability, and risks on 317 completed pregnancies. *Prenat. Diagn.*, **12**, 789–99.

33. Desnik, R.J., Schuette, J.L., Golbus, M.S. et al. (1992) First trimester biochemical and molecular diagnoses using chorionic villi: high accuracy in the US Collaborative Study. *Prenat. Diagn.*, **12**, 357–72.

34. Ledbetter, D.H., Zachary, J.M., Simpson, J.L. et al. (1992) Cytogenetic results from the US Collaborative Study on CVS. *Prenat. Diagn.*, **12**, 317–45.

35. Johnson, A., Wapner, R.J., Davis, G.H. and Jackson L.G. (1990) Mosaicism in chorionic villus sampling: an association with poor perinatal outcome. *Obstet. Gynecol.*, **75**, 573–77.

36. Wapner, R.J., Simpson, J.L., Golbus, M.S. et al. (1992) Chorionic mosaicism: association with fetal loss but not with adverse perinatal outcome. *Prenat. Diagn.*, **12**, 347–55.

37. Grover, G.M., Thulliez, P., Remington, J.S. and Boothroyd, J.C. (1990) Rapid prenatal diagnosis of congenital toxoplasma infection by using polymerase chain reaction and amniotic fluid. *J. Clin. Microbiol.*, **28**, 2297–301.

38. Isada, N.B., Paar, D.P., Johnson, M.P. et al. (1991) *In utero* diagnosis of congenital varicella zoster virus infection by CVS and polymerase chain reaction. *Am. J. Obstet. Gynecol.*, **165**, 1727–30.

39. Cradock-Watson, J.E., Miller, E., Ridehalch, M.K.S. et al. (1989) Detection of rubella virus in fetal and placental tissues and in the throats of neonates after serologically confirmed rubella in pregnancy. *Prenat. Diagn.*, **9**, 91–96.

40. Lobbiani, A., Nocco, A., Vedrietti, P. et al. (1991) Prenatal paternity testing by DNA analysis. *Prenat. Diagn.*, **11**, 343–46.

41. Brambati, B., Terzian, E. and Tognoni, G. (1991) Randomized clinical trial of transabdominal versus transcervical chorionic villus sampling methods. *Prenat. Diagn.*, **11**, 285–94.

42. Jackson, L. and the USNICHD Collaborative CVS Study Group (1990) Transcervical and transabdominal chorionic villus sampling are comparably safe procedures for first trimester prenatal diagnosis: preliminary analysis (abstract). *Am. J. Hum. Genet.*, **4** (suppl.); A278

43. Smidt-Jensen, S., Permin, M. and Philip, J. (1991) Sampling success and risk by transabdominal chorionic villus sampling, transcervical chorionic villus sampling and amniocentesis: a randomized study. *Ultrasound Obstet. Gynecol.* **1**, 86–90.

44. Brambati, B., Lanzani, A. and Tului, L. (1990) Transabdominal and transcervical chorionic villus sampling: effciciency and risk evaluation of 2411 cases. *Am. J. Med. Genet.*, **35**, 160–64.

45. Bovicelli, L., Rizzo, N., Montacuti, V. et al. (1988) Transabdominal chorionic villus sampling: analysis of 350 consecutive cases. *Prenat. Diagn.* **8**, 495–500.

46. Rhoads, G.G., Jackson, L.G., Schlesselman, S.E. et al. (1989) The safety and efficacy of chorionic villus sampling for early prenatal diagnosis of cytogenetic anomalies. *N. Engl. J. Med.*, **320**, 610–17.

47. Wapner, R.J. (1989) Transcervical CVS, in Proceedings of the 12th World Congress of Gynecology and Obstetrics, vol. 2 *Fetal Physiology and Pathology* (eds P. Berfort, J.A. Pinotti and T.K.A.B. Eskes), Parthenon, London, pp. 39–43.

48. Goldberg, J.D., Porter, A.E. and Golbus, M.S. (1990) Current assessment of fetal losses as a direct consequence of chorionic villus sampling. *Am. J. Med. Genet.*, **35**, 174–77.

49. Brambati, B., Oldrini, A. and Lanzani, A. (1988) Tranaabdominal chorionic villus sampling: clinical experience of 1159 cases. *Prenat. Diagn.*, **8**, 609–17.

50. Hogge, W.A., Schonberg, S.A. and Golbus, M.S. (1986) Chorion villus sampling: experience of the first 1000 cases. *Am. J. Obstet. Gynecol.*, **154**, 1249–52.

51. Green, J.E., Dorfmann, A., Jones, S.L. et al. (1988) Chorionic villus sampling: experience with an initial 940 cases. *Obstet. Gynecol.*, **71**, 208–12.

52. Leschot, N.J., Wolf, H., Van Prooijen-Knegt, A.C. et al. (1989) Cytogenetic findings in 1250 chorionic villus samples obtained in the first trimester with clinical follow-up of the first 1000 pregnancies. *Br. J. Obstet. Gynaecol.*, **96**, 663–70.

53. Medical Research Council Working Party on the Evaluation of Chorionic Villus Sampling (1991) Medical Research Council European trial of chorion villus sampling and amniocentesis. *Lancet*, **377**, 1491–99.

54. Jahoda, M.G.J., Pijpers, L., Reuss, A. et al. (1989) Evaluation of transcervical villus sampling with a completed follow-up of 1550 consecutive pregnancies. *Prenat. Diagn.*, **9**, 621–28.

55. Firth, H.V., Boyd, P.A., Chamberlain, P. et al. (1991) Severe limb abnormalities after chorion villus sampling at 56–66 days' gestation. *Lancet*, **337**, 762–63.

56. Burton, B.K., Schulz, C.J. and Burd, L.I. (1992) Limb anomalies associated with chorionic villus sampling. *Obstet. Gynecol.*, **79**, 726–30.

57. Fetoscopy Working Group (1991) XIII Annual Meeting, Sept. 23–24, Hong Kong.

58. Dolk, H., Bertrand, F. and Lechat, M.F. (1992) Chorionic villus sampling and limb abnormalities. *Lancet*, **339**, 876–77.

59. Froster-Iskenius, U.G. and Baird, P.A. (1989) Limb reduction defects in over one million consecutive livebirths. *Teratology*, **39**, 127–35.

60. Jackson, L. (1992) *CVS Late(st) News*, Philadelphia, 31 Mar. no. 32.

61. Rodeck, C.H. (1993) Prenatal diagnosis. Fetal development after chorionic villus sampling. *Lancet*, **341**, 468–69.

62. Canadian Collaborative CVS–Amniocentesis Clinical Trial Group (1989) Multicentre randomized clinical trial of chorion villus sampling and amniocentesis. *Lancet*, **i**, 1–6.

69 AMNIOCENTESIS (EARLY AND LATE)

G.G. Ashmead and M.A. Krew

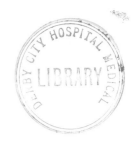

69.1 Introduction

Amniocentesis is one of the most frequently performed invasive methods of evaluating the fetus. Once restricted to symptomatic relief of hydramnios [1], amniocentesis came into widespread use in the early 1960s for the diagnosis and management of erythroblastosis fetalis [2]. The development of reliable cytogenetic and biochemical techniques later in that decade made prenatal detection of genetic defects the most common indication for amniocentesis in the first half of pregnancy. In the mid-1980s widespread use of maternal serum α-fetoprotein screening for neural tube defects also increased utilization of mid-trimester amniocentesis [3]; however in many cases high resolution ultrasound may obviate the need for amniotic fluid analysis [4]. In the third trimester confirmation of fetal lung maturity is the most common indication. Other third trimester indications include cytogenetics, the diagnosis of chorioamnionitis and treatment for hydramnios.

In the USA, amniocentesis for cytogenetic analysis is offered to women aged 35 and above. Unfortunately 70–80% of infants with trisomy 21 are born to women under the age of 35. Several fetal ultrasound measurements and ratios have been proposed as a screening tool for trisomy 21 [5]. The simultaneous evaluation of maternal serum α-fetoprotein, unconjugated estriol and chorionic gonadotropin, also known as the 'triple screen', can detect two-thirds of fetuses with trisomy 21 but may result in 5–7% of screened women being offered mid-trimester amniocentesis [6].

69.2 Mid-trimester amniocentesis

69.2.1 TECHNIQUE AND SAFETY

Amniocentesis was a blind procedure until the advent of ultrasound. Initially it was difficult to demonstrate a clear-cut advantage to the use of ultrasound [7]; however, ultrasound guidance did decrease the incidence of bloody and multiple insertions [8]. Static ultrasound was initially used to select the site of amniocentesis but the needle was still inserted blindly. The introduction of real-time ultrasound allowed continuous monitoring of the fetus and amniocentesis needle. Amniocentesis under continuous ultrasound guidance is an accepted technique, with many variations [9]. After performing an ultrasound examination, a wide field is prepared with an antiseptic and draped. A sterile coupling agent is applied to the skin. Gel is placed inside a sterile transducer cover. Although several commercial covers are available, plastic sandwich bags are inexpensive, readily available, easily sterilized and make an excellent transducer cover. A sterile glove may also be used as a transducer cover. A 22-gauge needle can be used. Higher gauge needles do not offer the necessary stiffness for midcourse manipulation and larger needles, 18 gauge and lower, have been associated with a higher complication rate [10]. Needle insertion and withdrawal of fluid is carried out under continuous guidance, using a sector scanner to demonstrate the path of the needle [11]. If possible, myometrial contractures and the placenta should be avoided. If a transplacental approach is necessary, the needle should be guided through the thinnest portion of the placenta and away from the umbilical cord insertion. Special needle guides are available which can be attached to the transducer and can be useful when the amniotic fluid pocket is small, when a long needle path is required in an obese patient and when the operators are inexperienced. Rh immune globulin, 300 μg, should be given to all unsensitized rhesus-negative women [12].

69.2.2 COMPLICATIONS

The American [13], Canadian [10], British [14] and Danish [15] collaborative studies suggest an increased fetal loss rate of 0.4 to 1% after amniocentesis. Transplacental amniocentesis as a cause of an increased loss

Diseases of the Fetus and Newborn, 2nd edn, Edited by G.B. Reed, A.E. Claireaux and F. Cockburn. Published in 1995 by Chapman & Hall, London. ISBN 0 412 39160 0

rate is controversial; however, obtaining green or brown fluid, which may represent old intra-amniotic blood indicates a high risk of poor outcome. A slightly increased risk of respiratory difficulties and orthopedic deformities in infants whose mothers had a genetic amniocentesis has been suggested but not consistently demonstrated. Continuous ultrasound guidance should make direct fetal injury a less likely possibility. Amniotic fluid leakage after the procedure may occur in 1% of patients but conservative management of these cases is warranted as amniotic fluid often reaccumulates within 7 days without other adverse sequelae [16].

69.2.3 MULTIPLE GESTATION

Genetic amniocentesis in a twin pregnancy requires special care to ensure that the same sac is not tapped twice. Between 1 and 5 ml of 0.08% indigo carmine dye can be injected into the first sac after the sample is obtained. Obtaining clear fluid from the second sac ensures that the second sac has been sampled [17]. Methylene blue should not be used as a marker dye because it has been associated with intestinal obstruction [18] and hemolytic anemia due to methemoglobinemia [19] in neonates. An alternative technique has been reported in which the first sac is tapped, the sample is withdrawn, the needle stylet replaced and, under ultrasound guidance, advanced through the intra-amniotic membrane into the second sac [20]. Membrane disruption and cord entanglement has been reported when the dividing membrane has been punctured during a funipuncture [21]. The single needle insertion technique may be helpful when the second sac can only be reached through the first, as in the case of overlying twins. When accessible pockets of fluid can be visualized simultaneously on either side of the separating membrane, the second sac can be tapped with the first needle still in place. Thus, both needles can be documented to be in separate sacs, and the need for dye injection eliminated [22]. Regardless of the technique used, it is essential that the location and differentiating features of the twins at the time of amniocentesis should be described in case it later becomes necessary to identify a twin with an abnormal test result. Although the twins' relative position can easily change, their cord insertions and placentation should remain constant. The major collaborative studies of amniocentesis either do not include multiple gestations or include them in insufficient numbers to calculate the procedure-associated fetal loss rate. Two recent retrospective series of 339 and 529 cases of genetic amniocentesis in multiple gestation suggest that the increased natural fetal loss rate in multiple gestations may account for the higher fetal loss rate seen with amniocentesis in twins [23,24].

69.3 'Early' amniocentesis

As early as 1967, genetic amniocentesis and successful cell cultures were reported as soon as 8 weeks in women undergoing elective termination of pregnancy [24]. In women with ongoing pregnancies the procedure was carried out as early as 13 weeks; however, the ease and safety of amniocentesis were felt to be optimal at 16 weeks [25]. Beginning in 1987, several groups reported first trimester amniocentesis for prenatal diagnosis [26–28].

69.3.1 TECHNIQUE AND SAFETY

In first trimester or 'early' amniocentesis (14 weeks gestation or less), ultrasound guidance is essential. If the uterus is extremely retroverted or if bowel is observed in the needle path, chorionic villus sampling (CVS) or a later routine amniocentesis should be considered. The same basic technique can be used with first trimester as with mid-trimester amniocentesis; however membrane tenting is more likely at early gestational ages due to incomplete fusion of the amnion and chorion. An insertion site near the placental margin may decrease tenting. It is also important to not be tentative with the needle. The amniotic cavity should be entered with a quick thrust across the membranes after advancing the needle into the myometrium and confirming its position. One milliliter of amniotic fluid per week of completed gestation is removed because higher fetal loss rates have been reported when larger volumes of fluid are removed [29]. It is because of this limitation that the procedure is usually not performed before 11 weeks. Concern over the volume of fluid needed for successful cell culture has led some investigators to propose closed loop amniofiltration and reinfusion systems [30,31]. Rh immune globulin, 300 μg, should administered to all unsensitized rhesus-negative women after early amniocentesis.

No large collaborative prospective trial (similar to those which exist for mid-trimester amniocentesis and CVS) which rigorously examines the safety and reliability of first trimester amniocentesis has been published, but several individual series suggest that the complication rate is relatively low and that there is no increase in the incidence of pseudomosaicism or maternal cell contamination compared with amniocentesis after 14 weeks [32–36].

69.3.2 ALTERNATIVE OR COMPLEMENT TO CVS?

Although CVS is well established and amniocentesis is beyond the investigational stage, early amniocentesis can be offered when transcervical CVS is anticipated to be difficult due to uterine and placental position or contraindicated as in the case of active herpes. A single center randomized trial of early amniocentesis versus transabdominal CVS in 650 women showed that the procedures were similar in sampling and cell culture success, as well the interval from successful sampling culture results, but no fetal loss data were given [37]. Initial experience in CVS is usually acquired with patients undergoing elective termination. Learning the technique for early amniocentesis for the practitioner already experienced in the mid-trimester procedure can be accomplished by working down in gestational age, and thus the procedure has the potential to become more widely available. Unlike CVS, early amniocentesis can screen for fetal anomalies by measuring amniotic fluid α-fetoprotein. Enough data exists at some centers to allow interpretation of α-fetoprotein levels earlier than 15 weeks but the reliability of acetylcholinesterase testing this early is still questioned [38,39]. In multiple gestations with a single fused placenta, it may be difficult to determine which twin was sampled with CVS. In this situation early amniocentesis may be advantageous and has been reported with twin and triplet gestations using a dye technique similar to the second trimester procedure [40]. CVS may be advantageous when testing requires large amounts of DNA. Early amniocentesis and CVS are likely to remain complementary techniques. Controlled trials are under way comparing the techniques [41].

69.4 Amniocentesis after fetal viability

The most frequent indication for third trimester amniocentesis is assessment of fetal lung maturity [42]. Amniocentesis may also be considered when late cytogenetics is indicated. Cytogenetic results are often available within 9 days. Although quicker results are available with umbilical blood sampling, this technique is not always available or possible. When anomalies are diagnosed, the presence of a chromosomal abnormality not compatible with life may prevent aggressive intervention. When fetal death is diagnosed, expedient amniocentesis may represent the best chance of obtaining cytogenetic studies [43] on still viable fetal cells.

When clinical presentation, preterm labor or premature rupture of the membranes lead to suspected chorioamnionitis, amniocentesis may confirm the diagnosis. While culture of amniotic fluid may be definitive, results may take days. Other more rapid amniotic fluid studies such as Gram stain, the presence of meconium [44], decreased glucose level [45] or the presence of leukocyte esterase [46] may be useful in the diagnosis of infection.

69.5 Therapeutic amniocentesis

69.5.1 HYDRAMNIOS

Hydramnios is possibly the oldest indication for amniocentesis, which should be considered when hydramnios

results in premature labor or maternal respiratory compromise. A fetal karyotype is indicated when ultrasound identifies fetal anomalies. Carefully monitored indomethacin therapy can be used to prevent rapid reaccumulation of the fluid [47]. Slow decompression amniocentesis may be indicated in laboring patients with hydramnios to improve uterine contractility and prevent rapid uterine decompression at membrane rupture.

69.5.2 THE 'STUCK TWIN' SYNDROME

The 'stuck twin' syndrome, in which one twin rapidly develops acute hydramnios and the 'stuck twin' has severe oligohydramnios, may be a severe form of twin–twin transfusion. Fetal salvage without intervention approaches zero. Recent reports have suggested that repeated aggressive amniocentesis improves outcome, with perinatal survival rates of 60% (48–50). The volume of fluid removed has been reported to be as high as 5 liters per therapeutic amniocentesis. Often fluid reaccumulates in the 'stuck twin' sac and hydrops, if present, resolves in the twin with hydramnios. Best results are obtained if diagnosis and initiation of therapy occur prior to the onset of premature labor. These events have been interpreted to indicate that amniocentesis causes a beneficial alteration of the physiology of the twin–twin transfusion, although no effect could be demonstrated with umbilical blood sampling [51].

69.5.3 AMNIOINFUSION

In the presence of oligohydramnios, a second trimester transabdominal saline infusion will allow confirmation of membrane status and allow better ultrasonographic visualization of the fetus. Bladder filling after amnioinfusion can confirm renal function. If amniotic fluid cannot be obtained prior to the amnioinfusion for cytogenetic studies, amniocentesis for cytogenetics can be performed immediately or hours to days after the infusion. Using serial therapeutic amnioinfusion to prevent pulmonary hypoplasia is controversial and should be considered experimental [52,53]. Amnioinfusion can be used for drug delivery to the fetus but little is known about fetal absorption. This route would seem to offer little advantage to the transplacental one via maternal administration of drugs. An exception is thyroxine which does not cross the placenta and which has been administered via amnioinfusion to treat congenital hypothyroidism [54].

69.6 Isoimmunization

Prior to the availability of prenatal cytogenetic investigations anti-D immunization was the major indication for amniocentesis. The availability of Rh immune globulin has fortunately caused a drastic reduction in the number of pregnancies complicated by anti-D sensitization, leading to a relative increase in the importance of isoimmunization to the other antigens such as C, c, E, e, Kell, Duffy and Kidd. Amniotic fluid change in absorbance (optical density) at 450 mm ($\Delta A450$) analysis remains an accepted method of initially evaluating the fetus of the isoimmunized mother with significant antibody titers. Abnormal elevations of $\Delta A450$ in amniotic fluid may indicate delivery or cordocentesis to assess fetal anemia and transfusion therapy of the severely affected fetus. Umbilical blood sampling may be initially indicated for the fetus at high risk of severe disease prior to 27 weeks [55] and in cases of Kell sensitization [56]. In these situations $\Delta A450$ determinations may not be reliable indicators of fetal anemia. Determination of fetal antigen status when the father is likely to be heterozygous for the antigen in question can be done with umbilical blood sampling. Theoretically such a determination could be done on amniocytes if the appropriate DNA probes are developed.

69.7   Conclusion

The desire to relieve parental anxiety over a potentially aborted pregnancy or to allow an earlier and less traumatic termination of pregnancy when an abnormality is found has pushed the horizon for prenatal diagnosis of chromosomal abnormalities to an even earlier gestational age. Despite the advent of techniques such as embryoscopy, chorionic villus sampling, cordocentesis and prenatal diagnosis using fetal cells in the maternal circulation [57], mid-trimester amniocentesis is still the standard method of prenatal diagnosis of karyotypic abnormalities and inborn errors of metabolism. Amniocentesis throughout gestation continues to be a major and valuable technique in prenatal diagnosis and therapy.

References

1. DeLee, J.B. (1918) *Principles and Practice of Obstetrics*, 3rd edn, W.B. Saunders, Philadelphia, p. 580.
2. Gerbie, A.B., Nadler, H.L. and Gerbie, M.V. (1971) Amniocentesis in genetic counseling. *Am. J. Obstet. Gynecol.*, 109, 765–70.
3. Milunsky, A. (1986) The prenatal diagnosis of neural tube and other congenital defects, in *Genetic Disorders and the Fetus: Diagnosis, Prevention and Treatment*, 2nd edn (ed. A. Milunsky), Plenum Press, NY, pp. 453–519.
4. Nadel, A.S., Green, J.K., Holmes, L.B. *et al.* (1990) Absence of need for amniocentesis in patients with elevated levels of maternal serum alpha-fetoprotein and normal ultrasonographic examinations. *N. Engl. J. Med.*, 323, 557–61.
5. Benacerraf, B.R. (1991) Prenatal diagnosis of autosomal trisomies. *Ultrasound Obstet. Gynecol.*, 1, 66–75.
6. Cheng, E.Y., Luthy, D.A., Hickok, D.E. *et al.* (1992) A prospective evaluation of triple marker maternal serum screening for trisomy-21 (abstract). *Am. J. Obstet. Gynecol.*, 166 (suppl.), 283.
7. Golbus, M.S., Loughman, W.D. and Epstein, C.J. (1979) Prenatal diagnosis in 3000 amniocenteses. *N. Engl. J. Med.*, 300, 157–63.
8. Romero R., Jeanty, P., Reece, E.A. *et al.* (1985) Sonographically monitored amniocentesis to decrease intraoperative complications. *Obstet. Gyencol.*, 65, 426–29.
9. Jeanty P., Rodesch F., Romero, R. *et al.* (1983) How to improve your amniocentesis technique. *Am. J. Obstet. Gynecol.*, 146, 593–96.
10. Simpson, N.E., Dallaire, L., Miller, J.R. *et al.* (1976) Prenatal diagnosis of genetic disease in Canada: report of a collaborative study. *Can. Med. Assoc. J.*, 115, 739–48.
11. Benacerraf, B.R. and Frigoletto, F.D. (1983) Amniocentesis under continuous ultrasound guidance: a series of 232 cases. *Obstet. Gynecol.*, 62, 760–63.
12. American College of Obstetricians and Gynecologists (1990) Prevention of D isoimmunization, *ACOG Tech. Bull.* 147, ACOG, Washington, DC.
13. NICHHD (1976) National Registry for Amniocentesis Study Group. *JAMA*, 236, 1471–76.
14. Report to the Medical Research Council by their Working Party on Amniocentesis (1978) An assessment of the hazards of amniocentesis. *Br. J. Obstet. Gynecol.*, 85(suppl. 2), 1–41.
15. Tabor, A., Madsen, M., Obel, E.B. *et al.* (1986) Randomized controlled trial of genetic amniocentesis in 4606 low-risk women. *Lancet*, i, 1287–93.
16. Gold, R.B., Goyert, G.L., Schwartz, D.B. *et al.* (1989) Conservative management of second-trimester post-amniocentesis fluid leakage. *Obstet. Gynecol.*, 74, 745–47.
17. Elias, S., Gerbie, A.B. and Simpson, J.L. (1980) Genetic amniocentesis in term gestation. *Am. J. Obstet Gynecol.*, 138, 169–74.
18. Nicolini, U. and Monni, G. (1990) Intestinal obstruction in babies exposed *in utero* to methylene blue (letter). *Lancet*, 336, 1258–59.
19. Vincer, M.J., Allen, A.C., Evans, J.R. *et al.* (1987) Methylene-blue induced hemolytic anemia in a neonate. *Can. Med. Assoc. J.*, 136, 503–504.
20. Jeanty, P., Shah, D. and Roussis, P. (1990) Single needle insertion in twin amniocentesis. *J. Ultrasound Med.*, 9, 511–17.
21. Megory, E., Weiner, E., Shalev, E. and Ohel, G. (1991) Pseudoamniotic twins with cord entanglement following genetic funipuncture. *Obstet. Gynecol.*, 78, 915–17.
22. Bahado-Singh, R., Schmitt, R. and Hobbins, J.C. (1992) New technique for genetic amniocentesis in twins. *Obstet. Gynecol.*, 79, 304–307.
23. Anderson, R.L., Goldberg, J.D. and Golbus, M.D. (1991) Prenatal diagnosis in multiple gestation: 20 years' experience with amniocentesis. *Prenat. Diagn.*, 11, 263–70.
24. Jacobsen, C.B. and Barter, R.H. (1967) Intrauterine diagnosis and management of genetic defects. *Am. J. Obstet. Gynecol.*, 99, 796–807.
25. Nadler, H. (1968) Antenatal detection of hereditary disorders. *Pediatrics*, 42, 912–17.
26. Hanson, F.W., Zorn, E.M., Tennant, F.R. *et al.* (1987) Amniocentesis before 15 weeks gestation: outcome, risks and technical problems. *Am. J. Obstet. Gynecol.*, 156, 1524–31.
27. Evans, M.I., Koppich, F.C., Nemitz, B. and Zador, I.E. (1988) Early genetic amniocentesis and chorionic villus sampling. Expanding the opportunities for early prenatal diagnosis. *J. Reprod. Med.*, 33, 450–52.
28. Benacerraf, B.R., Green, M.F., Saltzman, D.H. *et al.* (1988) Early amniocentesis for prenatal cytogenetic evaluation. *Radiology*, 169, 709–10.
29. Hanson, F.W., Happ, R.L., Tennant, F.R., *et al.* (1990) Ultrasonography-guided early amniocentesis in singleton pregnancies. *Am. J. Obstet. Gynecol.*, 162, 1376–81.
30. Sundberg, K., Smidt-Jenson, S. and Philip, J. (1991) Amniocentesis with increased cell yield, obtained by filtration and reinjection of the amniotic fluid. *Ultrasound Obstet. Gynecol.*, 1, 91–94.
31. Byrne, D.L., Marks, K., Braude, P.R. and Nicolaides, K. (1991) Amniofiltration in the first trimester: feasibility, technical aspects and cytological outcome. *Ultrasound Obstet. Gynecol.*, 320–24.
32. Evans, M.I., Drugan, A., Koppitch, F.C. *et al.* (1989) Genetic diagnosis in the first trimester; the norm for the 1990s. *Am. J. Obstet. Gynecol.*, 160, 1332–36.
33. Penso, C.A., Sandstrom, M.M., Garber, M.F. *et al.* (1990) Early amniocentesis: report of 407 cases with neonatal follow-up. *Obstet. Gynecol.*, 76, 1032–36.
34. Nevin, J., Nevin, N.C., Dornan, J.C. *et al.* (1990) Early amniocentesis experience of 222 consecutive patients, 1987–1988. *Prenat. Diagn.*, 10, 79–83.
35. Elejalde, B.R., de Elejalde, M.M., Acuna J.M. *et al.* (1990) Prospective study of amniocentesis performed between weeks 9 and 16 of gestation: its feasibility, risks, complications and use in early genetic prenatal diagnosis. *Am. J. Med. Genet.*, 35, 188–96.
36. Hacket, G.A., Smith, J.H., Rebello, M.T. *et al.* (1991) Early amniocentesis at 11–14 weeks gestation for the diagnosis of fetal chromosomal abnormality – a clinical evaluation. *Prenat. Diagn.*, 11, 311–15.
37. Byrne, D., Marks, K., Azar, G. and Nicolaides, K. (1991) Randomized study of early amniocentesis versus chorionic villus sampling: a technical and cytogenetic comparison of 650 patients. *Ultrasound Obstet. Gynecol.*, 1, 235–42.
38. Penso, C.A. and Frigoletto, F.D. (1990) Early amniocentesis. *Semin. Perinatol.*, 14, 465–70.
39. Drugan, A., Syner, F.N., Greb, A. and Evans, M.I. (1988) Amniotic fluid

alpha-fetoprotein and acetylcholinesterase in early genetic amniocentesis. *Obstet. Gynecol.,* **72**, 35–38.

40. Drugan, A., Johnson, M.P. and Evans, M.I. (1992) Amniocentesis, in *Reproductive Risks and Prenatal Diagnosis* (ed. M.I. Evans), Appleton & Lange, Norwalk, CT, pp. 191–200.

41. Choo, V. (1991) Early amniocentesis. *Lancet,* **ii** 751–52.

42. Rome, R.M., Glover, J.J. and Simmons, S.C. (1975) The benefits of amniocentesis for the assessment of fetal lung maturitity. *Br. J. Obstet. Gynecol.,* **82**, 662–68.

43. Saal, H.M., Rodis, J., Weinbaum, P.J. *et al.* (1987) Cytogenetic evaluation of fetal death: the role of amniocentesis. *Obstet. Gynecol.,* **70**, 601–603.

44. Romero, R., Hanaoka, S., Mazor, M. *et al.* (1991) Meconium stained amniotic fluid: a risk factor for microbial invasion of the amniotic cavity. *Am. J. Obstet. Gynecol.,* **164**, 859–62.

45. Kirshon, B., Rosenfeld, B., Mari, G. and Belfort, M. (1991) Amniotic fluid glucose and intraamniotic infection. *Am. J. Obstet. Gynecol.,* **164**, 818–20.

46. Hoskins, I.A., Marks, F., Ordorica, S.A. and Young, B.K. (1990) Leukocyte esterase activity in amniotic fluid: normal values during pregnancy. *Am. J. Perinatol.,* **7**, 130–32.

47. Moise, K.J. (1991) Indomethacin therapy in the treatment of symptomatic polyhydramnios. *Clin. Obstet. Gynecol.* **34**, 310–18.

48. Mahoney, B.S., Petty, C.N., Nyberg, D.A. *et al.* (1990) The 'stuck twin' phenomenon: ultrasonographic findings, pregnancy outcome and management with serial amniocentesis. *Am. J. Obstet. Gynecol.,* **163**, 1513–22.

49. Urig, M.A., Clewell, W.H. and Elliott, J.P. (1990), Twin–twin transfusion syndrome, *Am. J. Obstet. Gynecol.,* **163**, 1522–26.

50. Elliott, J.P., Urig, M.A. and Clewell, W.H. (1991) Aggressive therapeutic amniocentesis for treatment of twin–twin transfusion syndrome. *Obstet. Gynecol.,* **77**, 537–40.

51. Weiner, C. and Ludomirsky, A. (1992) Diagnosis and treatment of twin to twin transfusion syndrome (abstract). *Am. J. Obstet. Gynecol.,* **166** (suppl.), 284.

52. Gembruch, U. and Hansmann, M. (1988) Artificial instillation of amniotic fluid as a new technique for the diagnostic evaluation of cases of oligohydramnios. *Prenat. Diagn.,* **8**, 33–45.

53. Fisk, N.W., Ronderos-Dumit, D., Soliani, A. *et al.* (1991) Diagnostic and therapeutic transabdominal amnioinfusion in oligohydramnios. *Obstet. Gynecol.,* **78**, 270–78.

54. Hirsch, M., Josefsberg, Z., Schoenfeld, A. *et al.* (1990) Congenital hereditary hypothroidism: prenatal diagnosis and treatment. *Prenat. Diagn.,* **10**, 491–96.

55. Nicolaides, K.H., Rodeck, C.H., Mibahan, R.H. and Kemp, J.R. (1986) Have Liley charts outlived their usefulness? *Am. J. Obstet. Gynecol.,* **155**, 90–94.

56. Caine, M.H. and Mueller-Heubach, E. (1986) Kell sensitization in pregnancy. *Am. J. Obstet. Gynecol.,* **154**, 85–90.

57. Selypes, A. and Lorencz, R. (1988) A noninvasive method for determination of the sex and karyotype of the fetus from the maternal blood. *Hum. Genet.,* **79**, 357–59.

70 HISTOPATHOLOGICAL INVESTIGATION OF PRENATAL TISSUE SAMPLES (EXCLUDING SKIN)

B.D. Lake

70.1 Introduction

There have been many attempts to correlate placental/chorionic villous morphological changes with chromosome abnormalities, spontaneous abortions and genetic factors [1–4] and environmental factors [5], with variable and sometimes conflicting results. Consequently the morphological approach in these areas is unsuitable for prenatal diagnosis. This chapter is concerned with the morphological examination of prenatal tissue samples and deals with metabolic disease where morphological changes are present in the term infant and child.

The results of individual disorders are culled from the literature and from personal experience of cases verified by enzymological studies performed mainly at the Institute of Child Health, London.

70.2 Requirements for prenatal diagnosis

(a) Definite diagnosis in proband or within family

Before embarking on prenatal diagnosis it is important to have a firm diagnosis to search for. This usually means that there is a family history of a particular disorder with an affected child on whom the diagnosis has been made. The diagnosis is usually enzymatic, but may in exceptional circumstances be a morphological one.

(b) Centre undertaking prenatal diagnosis to have experience in the disorder

Most of the metabolic disorders, and especially those of the lysosomal enzymes, have well-defined morphologic criteria. Increasingly an undiagnosed-in-life disorder is revealed by microscopic investigation. It is on that evidence alone that some biochemical prenatal diagnoses are undertaken, and it is imperative that the morphological diagnosis is made by someone who has experience of that group of disorders. Careful counselling will of course be necessary in these circumstances.

(c) A thorough working knowledge of the normal and abnormal morphology of the tissue to be studied

Some of the metabolic diagnoses have been reached by microscopic examination of the term placenta. The morphology of the placenta and of fetal tissues obtained after termination following a definitive prenatal diagnosis on biochemical assay is known for a large number of conditions, but now that chorionic villus sampling is used more often than amniocentesis, such fetal material is less available for morphological study. There appears to have been very little use of the morphological approach, apart from the demonstration of peroxisomes in chorionic villus samples in Zellweger syndrome [6,7]. Indeed there must be very few centres which would even consider microscopy of a chorionic villus sample for metabolic disorders, and the reliance on biochemical assay is almost universal.

These requirements are similar to those applied by the geneticists and biochemists for their prenatal diagnoses. The same strictness is necessary for any morphological assessment.

70.3 Microscopic assessment

70.3.1 CHORIONIC VILLUS SAMPLES

Pathological changes in the placenta have been observed in a number of metabolic storage disorders [8–16], and in some cases the observations have been the only clue to diagnosis [17,18]. Study of the placenta

Diseases of the Fetus and Newborn, 2nd edn, Edited by G.B. Reed, A.E. Claireaux and F. Cockburn. Published in 1995 by Chapman & Hall, London. ISBN 0 412 39160 0

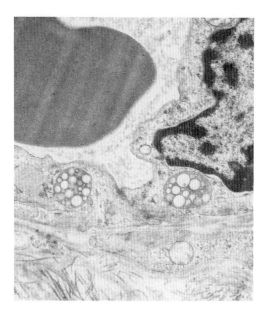

Figure 70.1 Wolman's disease, term placenta. Electron photomicrograph showing membrane bound lipid inclusions in endothelial cells in a capillary (15 500X).

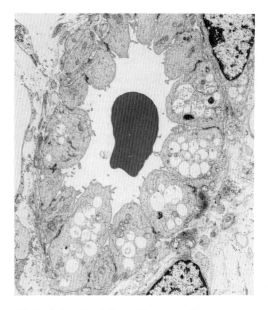

Figure 70.2 Infantile sialic acid storage disease, placenta 20 weeks. Electron photomicrograph showing numerous membrane bound vacuoles in endothelial cells of a larger vessel (3500X).

from abortions performed because an enzyme defect had been found on prenatal testing (Figures 70.1 and 70.2) has provided useful information which can be applied to chorionic villus samples. The use of morphological examination of chorionic villus in pre-natal diagnosis was anticipated by Powell *et al.* in 1976 [17]. In sampling for morphology it should be noted that the younger more terminal villous sprouts [19]

may not be old enough to have acquired evidence of disease in all cell types, and for this reason the thicker villous profiles (trunk of the tree) should be taken for examination. For the changes to be of diagnostic value they should be clear cut, relatively frequent, preferably occurring in the expected cell type, and if there is a particular ultrastructural appearance in the disease the appearance in the chorionic villus sample should be identical.

Plastic sections of the tissue sample will show the morphology of the trophoblast, and vacuolation of the syncytiotrophoblast in sialic acid storage disease [20], G_{M1}-gangliosidosis [12,21] and I-cell disease (mucolipidosis II) [8] is readily seen by light microscopy. (Figures 70.3 and 70.4). Each sample should be examined for involvement of fibroblasts, endothelial cells, syncytiotrophoblast and cytotrophoblast. Calcium deposits at or just under the basement membrane of the tropho-blast layer are not uncommon in the normal chorionic villus sample.

The changes in the trophoblast, fibroblasts and endothelial cells in the various disorders are listed in Table 70.1.

It is important to note that at the time of chorionic villus sampling there is, in the normal unaffected placenta, a prominent population of Hofbauer cells. These vacuolated macrophages look very like storage cells and have membrane bound vacuoles and it would be tempting to use their presence and appearance as evidence of a storage disorder. Since they are frequent in normal chorionic villus, **for the purposes of prenatal diagnosis Hofbauer cells should be ignored.** However in the mature placenta an abundance of Hofbauer cells is an indication of metabolic storage disease [18]. Careful examination of the whole range of cell types present in a chorionic villus sample is necessary. In many disorders the expected changes are found, but in others the changes may be patchy or absent [14]. The patchiness may be related to the relative ages of the cell types and the time taken for a particular cell type to acquire evidence of storage of a morphologically recognizable structure. Thus for ultrastructural examin-ation, several grids at different levels should be viewed and any abnormal findings recorded.

Note also that there is a subpopulation in the chorion laeve only of trophoblast cells which are normally vacuolated. Yeh, O'Connor and Kurman [22] describe the vacuolated cytotrophoblast which has numerous non-membrane bound lipid droplets, and suggest the cells are involved in maternal/fetal transport.

70.3.2 CULTURED CHORIONIC VILLUS SAMPLES AND AMNIOCYTES

Electron microscopic examination of cultured fibro-blasts from examples of lysosomal storage disorders

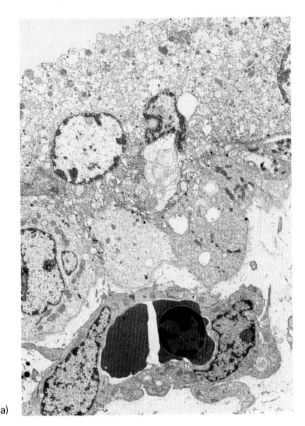
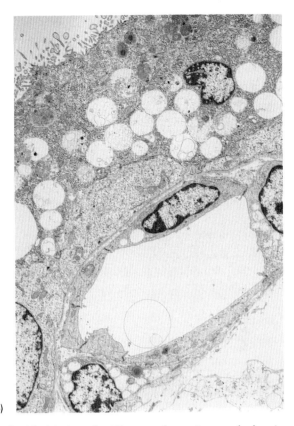

(a)   (b)

Figure 70.3   (a) Normal chorion villus sample (at risk for G_{M1} gangliosidosis), 9 weeks. Electron photomicrograph showing trophoblast layers and a capillary in the stroma. Abnormal inclusions are not present (3400X). (b) Chorionic villus sample, sialic acid storage disease, 10 weeks. Electron photomicrograph showing numerous membrane bound vacuoles in the syncytiotrophoblast and in the endothelial cells and pericytes of a capillary (3400X). Compare with (a).

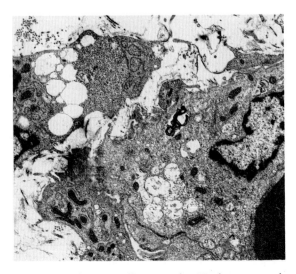

Figure 70.4   Chorion villus sample, Hurler mucopolysaccharidosis I, 9 weeks. Electron photomicrograph showing membrane bound vacuoles in endothelial cells of a capillary, and in a fibroblast (6600X).

usually shows the characteristic changes of enlarged membrane bound lysosomes in which the storage material accumulates. This is generally true for disorders in which there is visceral systemic involvement and fibroblasts *in vivo* show morphological changes (Table 70.1). Cultured chorionic villus samples and amniocytes tend to display fibroblast-like characteristics and may be used in conjunction with a biochemical assay. In mucolipidosis IV, morphological studies of cultured amniocytes have been used as the sole diagnostic test [23], but more recently the biochemical study of accumulation of phospholipids and gangliosides and pulse chase experiments [24,25] have proved informative and thus may offer additional support until an enzyme defect can be detected [26]. Ultrastructural examination of chorionic villus samples at 8 weeks was unhelpful [27]. In mucolipidosis IV, membrane bound lipid lamellae are prominent in cultured fibroblasts and in cultured amniocytes. Care should be taken to discount any effects of antibiotic or antifungal agents added to the culture medium producing pseudo storage bodies [28].

Table 70.1 Involvement of various cell types revealed by light and electron microscopy

Disease	Trophoblast	Fibroblast	Endothelial cell	Other comments
Sialic acid storage disease	+ (syn and cyto)	+	+	
G_{M1} gangliosidosis	+ (syn and cyto)	+	+	
β-Glucuronidase deficiency	+ (patchy)	+	+	
Neuraminidase deficiency	+ (syn and cyto)	+	+	
I-cell disease	+ (syn)	+	+	
Mucopolysaccharidosis I and II	−	+	+	
Aspartylglucosaminuria	+ (cyto but rare)	+	+	
Pompe's disease (glycogen storage disease)	+ (cyto)	+	+	
Wolman's disease	−	+	+	Lipid-laden macrophages are present but patchy
Niemann–Pick A	+ (patchy and not seen in one CVS)	+ (in cord)	?	Sphingomyelin in macrophages
Niemann–Pick C	−	−	−	
Fabry's disease	−	−	−	No changes seen in CVS or umbilical cord
Mucolipidosis IV	−	−	+	No changes seen in CVS
Gaucher's disease	−	−	−	
Batten's (late infantile)	−	−	−	Endothelial cells expected to show change, but do not
Batten's (infantile)	−	−	+	DNA probe also available for prenatal diagnosis
Batten's (juvenile)	−	−	−	Reported trophoblast changes dubious. DNA probe available for prenatal diagnosis
Krabbe's leucodystrophy	−	−	−	No change expected
Zellweger's (cerebrohepatorenal) syndrome	Absent peroxisomes	−	−	
Cystinosis	−	−	−	
Tay–Sachs disease	−	−	−	No change expected

+ = Present; − = absent; syn = syncytiotrophoblast; cyto = cytotrophoblast; CVS = chorionic villus sample.

70.3.3 UNCULTURED AMNIOCYTES

Ultrastructural examination of uncultured amniocytes may be used for the prenatal diagnosis of late infantile Batten's disease [29–31]. An affected pregnancy shows curvilinear bodies in a proportion of cells (Figure 70.5), which are probably derived from periderm (section 70.3.5). Membrane-bound glycogen deposits have been reported in uncultured amniocytes in Pompe's disease [32,33]. In culture the membrane bound glycogen deposits were not evident.

70.3.4 FETAL BLOOD SAMPLING

Fetal hydrops, detected on scanning at around 18 weeks, may arise from one of a number of metabolic storage disorders. It is important to consider a metabolic cause once the hydrops is established as 'non-immune'. Simple screening by light microscopy of a fetal blood film stained by any standard haematological method can eliminate some disorders or can indicate which is the most likely diagnosis (Figure 70.6). Table 70.2 lists storage disorders in which fetal hydrops has

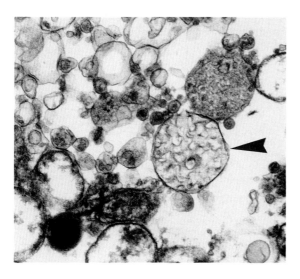

Figure 70.5 Uncultured amniotic fluid cell, late infantile Batten's disease, 17 weeks. Electron photomicrograph showing a membrane bound curvilinear body (arrow) (38 500X).

been reported, and disorders in which fetal blood shows or is predicted to show significant changes. One of the conditions most commonly causing fetal hydrops is β-glucuronidase deficiency and in this disorder prominent Alder granulation is readily detected in neutrophils. Microscopy is at present the only means for prenatal diagnosis of Chediak–Higashi syndrome [34,35]. In this disorder the characteristic large granules can be found in fetal neutrophils at 17 weeks gestation. Diukman *et al.* [34] also indicated that staining cultured chorionic villus samples for lysosomal enzyme activity to highlight the larger than normal lysosomes present in Chediak–Higashi syndrome might be a useful and earlier alternative. Durandy *et al.* [35] have used fetal hair (obtained by fetal scalp skin biopsy) examination at 21 weeks for diagnosis of Chediak–Higashi syndrome and Griscelli's syndrome. In both conditions the hair shaft contains large irregularly dispersed melanin granules.

The presence of curvilinear bodies, characteristic of late infantile Batten's disease, in fetal lymphocytes in an affected fetus [31] indicates that fetal blood sampling for preparation of a buffy coat for electron microscopy may be a useful adjunct to the ultrastructural study of uncultured amniotic fluid cells for this diagnosis. Care should be taken to distinguish lymphocytes from normoblasts which do not contain any diagnostically useful cytoplasmic ultrastructural features.

70.3.5 FETAL SKIN, LIVER AND MUSCLE

The use of fetal skin biopsies in diagnosis of genodermatoses is covered in Chapter 41. In addition to the disorders mentioned there, the use of fetal skin biopsy for the diagnosis of late infantile Batten's disease has been suggested [31]. Chow and his colleagues [31] reported curvilinear bodies in the periderm of an affected fetus diagnosed on the basis of ultrastructural examination of uncultured amniocytes. They felt that the amniocytes containing curvilinear bodies were probably mostly periderm cells and confirmed their suspicions by examination of fetal skin from the abortus.

Fetal liver biopsies, formerly used in the diagnosis of ornithine carbamoyl transferase or carbamoyl phosphate synthase deficiency, are now rarely needed because a DNA probe is usually informative. The role of microscopy, where liver biopsy is performed, is merely to confirm that the tissue (usually received as a suspension because of the friable nature of fetal liver) is indeed liver. This is best achieved by a squash preparation stained by haematoxylin and eosin.

Fetal muscle biopsies are of potential value where no deletion can be detected in the dystrophin gene in a proband affected with morphologically and immuno-

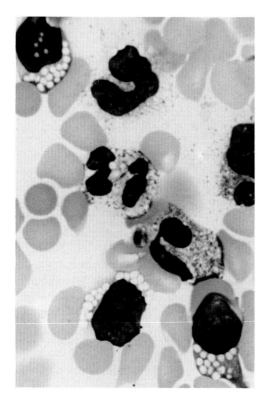

Figure 70.6 Fetal blood film, G_{M1} gangliosidosis with hydrops. Lymphocytes with numerous discrete cytoplasmic vacuoles are present (May–Grünwald–Giemsa 1250X).

Table 70.2   Fetal blood changes known or expected in metabolic diseases

Disorder	Congenital ascites or fetal hydrops reported	Fetal blood changes
Gaucher	+ (Refs 12,36)	E; no changes
Sialic acid storage disease	+ (Ref. 12)	K; lymphocytes with large abundant vacuoles
G$_{M1}$ gangliosidosis	+ (Refs 12,21,37)	K; lymphocytes with large abundant vacuoles
β-Glucuronidase deficiency	+ (Refs 37–39)	K; Alder granulation of neutrophils
Neuraminidase deficiency	+ (Ref. 40)	E; vacuolation of lymphocytes
Galactosialidosis	+ (Ref. 41)	E; vacuolation of lymphocytes
I-cell disease	?	E; lymphocytes with vacuoles
Morquio (MPS IV)	+ (Refs 42,43)	E; possible vacuolation of some lymphocytes
Maroteaux–Lamy (MPS VI)	–	K; Alder granulation of neutrophils
Pompe's disease (glycogen storage disease II)	–	K (Ref. 47); lymphocytes with small vacuoles containing glycogen
Wolman's disease	+ (Ref. 44)	E; lymphocytes with small vacuoles
Niemann–Pick A (unproven)	+ (Ref. 45)	E; lymphocytes with small vacuoles
Niemann–Pick C	+ (Ref. 45)	K; no changes
Batten's disease (late-infantile)	–	K; lymphocytes with curvilinear bodies on electron microscopy
Batten's disease (juvenile)	–	E; vacuolation of lymphocytes
Chediak–Higashi syndrome	–	K; abnormal large coarse granules in neutrophils (Refs 34,35)

E = expected; K = known; MPS = mucopolysaccharidosis

histochemically proven Duchenne muscular dystrophy [48]. Cryostat sections of a frozen sample could be immunostained for dystrophin (using the same antibody as that used in the initial diagnosis), which is known to be present from around 9–10 weeks' gestation, and immunoblotting performed.

70.4   Value of investigation

70.4.1   SOLE DIAGNOSTIC TEST

In a few disorders a morphological approach may be the only means of diagnosis but, with the current rate of advance in the knowledge of metabolic disorders and genetic probing, the need to rely on morphology alone is diminishing. For example, the prenatal diagnosis of

infantile Batten's disease, initially a morphological diagnosis on chorionic villus sample [49], has been supplemented by the application of a DNA probe giving concordant results [50]. The potential of a morphological prenatal diagnosis in juvenile Batten's disease by chorionic villus sample – never quite realized [51,52] – has been supplanted by a DNA probe diagnosis [53]. In the late infantile form of Batten's disease the morphological approach is, to date, the only means of prenatal diagnosis, and samples of fetal skin, amniotic fluid cells (mainly periderm) and/or fetal blood are of diagnostic value [31].

In Chediak–Higashi syndrome fetal blood sampling or culture of a chorionic villus sample or amniotic fluid cells are the only means of prenatal diagnosis, although fetal hair has also been used [35].

70.4.2 CONFIRMATORY TEST FOR BIOCHEMICAL DIAGNOSIS

The application of a morphological diagnostic approach is quite independent of the enzyme or metabolite assay, giving two separate means of diagnosis. This is of particular help where the initial diagnosis may not have been unequivocally established.

70.4.3 BACK-UP FOR UNCERTAIN BIOCHEMISTRY

In a number of cases, and particularly where the samples have come from a distance (arriving up to 24 hours after being taken), the biochemical results may be less clear cut than is needed for a definitive result. Morphological studies in these cases often reveal that the integrity of the tissue is less than perfect. The changes range from mild (mitochondrial degeneration), to moderate (a general fuzziness of membranes and cellular detail) and severe, where there has been almost complete autolysis. These changes can be attributed to differences in the culture medium in which the samples are despatched, and to the temperature at which they have been kept. In the few cases where autolysis had occurred the biochemical results were (almost) uninterpretable, with very low activities of several enzymes, including the specific index enzyme sought. No structural detail was apparent and only collagen fibrils could be identified in the worst sample.

The absence of morphological change, where change is expected in an affected case, in samples where the enzyme activity is low but not quite into the affected range can be taken as evidence of carrier status [54]. The presence of characteristic ultrastructural change would be evidence for an affected fetus in these circumstances.

70.5 Turnaround time

It is usually imagined that ultrastructural study takes several days or even weeks to produce an answer. Much will depend on the urgency for diagnosis, and on the availability of a pathologist experienced in the particular groups of diseases. It is possible to receive, fix, process into resin, cut ultrathin sections, view and photograph the results within 24 hours. However it is not always necessary to proceed at such speed, since it causes disruption to the routine laboratory work, but should it be needed, a turnaround time of 24 hours can be achieved provided the sample is received before noon.

70.6 Techniques used

70.6.1 CHORIONIC VILLUS SAMPLE

A small portion (2–3 mm) of the chorionic villus sample, probably best taken from the more proximal part (i.e. the thickest end) and including several villus cores, is taken from the sample received in tissue culture medium and placed in electronmicroscopy fixative. The exact composition of the fixative is immaterial and any that is in routine use may be used. In our practice 2.5% glutaraldehyde in 0.1 mol/l cacodylate buffer pH 7.4 containing 2.4 mmol/l Ca^{2+} is kept frozen in 5 ml aliquots, thawed and **used at room temperature** for fixation. Fix for 2 hours (or for any length of time greater than 2 hours), follow by a quick wash in 0.1 mol/l cacodylate buffer pH 7.4 before postfixation in 1% osmium tetroxide for 1 hour at 4°C. Wash in buffer, transfer to 70% alcohol, dehydrate in acidified dimethoxypropane [55] for 2–5 minutes and transfer to araldite for impregnation for 2 hours before blocking out in a coffin mould to allow correct orientation. Polymerize overnight at 60°C. Ultrathin sections are contrasted with uranyl acetate and lead citrate before viewing. Photographs are taken at low power (say 2000×) for orientation, as well as at high power (say 5000–10 000×) to illustrate the fine detail. It is important to know in which cell the abnormal inclusion is found, and extreme high power pictures (above 20 000×) are generally unhelpful. Diagnostic features should be recognizable within the range 2000–10 000×. Magnifications refer to those on the film, usually 8 × 10 cm.

70.6.2 CULTURED (AND UNCULTURED) AMNIOCYTES

Loose pellets of cells are resuspended in 10% bovine serum albumin in phosphate-buffered saline and centrifuged at 1000–2000 rev./min. The supernatant is decanted and replaced with fixative (as defined above). The albumin in the pellet is crosslinked by the glutaraldehyde and allows the pellet to be processed as a solid piece of tissue. Without crosslinking there is a danger of the cell pellet falling apart during processing. The schedule is the same as for chorionic villus samples.

70.6.3 FETAL BLOOD

Standard blood films are made from an anticoagulated sample obtained by cordocentesis, and stained by any of the standard haematological methods (May–Grünwald–Giemsa, Leishman, Wright, etc.). If electron microscopy is necessary the sample is centrifuged (1000–2000 rev./min. for 10 minutes), the plasma gently pipetted off and replaced with glutaraldehyde fixative (as above). The fixative is changed twice over the next 10 minutes (to allow fresh fixative to be in contact with the small surface area and minimize fixative depletion). The buffy coat is eased from the sides of the tube using a histological needle and lifted out complete, leaving the red cells behind, and placed in fresh fixative. Processing of blocks of buffy coat cut from the fixed disc of white cells is as for tissue samples. Blocks are orientated before embedding to allow sections to be cut vertically through the buffy coat to show layers of platelets, lymphocytes, normoblasts, neutrophils and red cells. The plasma albumin in the buffy coat crosslinks with the glutaraldehyde and holds the sample together. This process can be performed with as little as 300 μl of fetal blood, but 1-ml samples are easier to handle.

References

1. Rehder, H., Coerdt, W., Eggers, R. et al. (1989) Is there a correlation between morphological and cytogenetic findings in placental tissue from early missed abortions? Hum. Genet., 82, 377–85.
2. Ruschoff, J., Kohler, A., Chudoba, I. and Steuber, E.D. (1989) Investigations of chorionic villi after chorionic villus sampling (CVS). Correlation of morphological with clinical and laboratory data. Hum. Genet. 81, 329–34.
3. Minguillon, C., Eiben, B., Bahr-Porsch, S. et al. (1989) The predictive value of chorionic villus histology for identifying chromosomally normal and abnormal spontaneous abortions. Hum. Genet., 82, 373–76.
4. Jauniaux, E. and Hustin, J. (1992) Histological examination of first trimester spontaneous abortions: the impact of materno-embryonic interface features. Histopathology, 21, 409–14.
5. Jauniaux, E. and Burton, G.J. (1992) The effect of smoking in pregnancy on early placental morphology. Obstet. Gynecol., 79, 645–48
6. Roels,F., Verdonck,V., Pauwels, M. et al. (1987) Vizualization of peroxisomes and plasmalogens in first trimester chorionic villus. J. Inherited Metab. Dis., 10 (suppl. 2), 349–54.
7. Wanders, R.J.A., Wiemer, E.A.C., Brul, S. et al. (1989) Prenatal diagnosis of Zellweger syndrome by direct visualization of peroxisomes in chorionic villus fibroblasts by immunofluorescence microscopy. J. Inherited Metab. Dis., 12 (suppl. 2), 301–304.
8. Rapola, J. and Aula,P. (1977) Morphology of the placenta in fetal I-cell disease. Clin. Genet., 11, 107–13.
9. Sekeles, E., Ornoy, A. and Cohen, G. (1978) Mucolipidosis IV. Fetal and placental pathology. Monogr. Hum. Genet., 10, 47–50.
10. Aula, P., Rapola, J., von Koskull, H. and Ammala, A. (1984) Prenatal diagnosis and fetal pathology of aspartylglucosaminuria. Am. J. Med. Genet., 19, 359–67.
11. Beck, M., Bender, S.W., Reiter, H-L. et al. (1984) Neuraminidase deficiency presenting as a non-immune hydrops fetalis. Eur. J. Pediatr. 143, 135–39.
12. Gillan, J.E., Lowden, J.A., Gaskin, K. and Cutz, E. (1984) Congenital ascites as a presenting sign of lysosomal storage disease. J. Pediatr., 104, 225–31
13. Bendon, W. and Hug, G. (1985) Morphologic characteristics of the placenta in glycogen storage disease type II (α-1,4-glucosidase deficiency). Am. J. Obstet. Gynecol., 152, 1021–26
14. Schoenfeld, A., Abramovici, A., Klibanski, C. and Ovadia, J. (1985) Placental ultrasonographic biochemical and histochemical studies in human fetuses affected with Niemann–Pick disease type A. Placenta, 6, 33–44.
15. Jauniaux, E., Vamos, E., Libert, J. et al. (1987) Placental electron microscopy and histochemistry in a case of sialic acid storage disorder. Placenta, 8, 433–42.
16. Rapola, J., Santavuori, P. and Heiskala, H. (1988) Placental pathology and prenatal diagnosis of infantile type of neuronal ceroid-lipofuscinosis. Am. J. Med. Genet., Suppl. 5, 99–103.
17. Powell, H.C., Benirschke, K., Favara, B.E. and Pflueger, O.H. (1976) Foamy changes of placental cells in fetal storage disorders. Virchows Arch. [A], 369, 191–96.
18. Roberts, D.J., Ampola, M.G. and Lage, J.M. (1991) Diagnosis of unsuspected fetal metabolic storage disease by routine placental examination. Pediatr. Pathol., 11, 647–56.
19. Castellucci, M., Scheper, M., Scheffen, I. et al. (1990) The development of the human placental villous tree. Anat. Embryol. (Berl.), 181, 117–28.
20. Lake, B.D., Young, E.P. and Nicolaides, K. (1989) Prenatal diagnosis of infantile sialic acid storage disease in a twin pregnancy. J. Inherited Metab. Dis., 12, 152–56.
21. Lowden, J.A., Cutz, E., Conen, P.E. et al. (1973) Prenatal diagnosis of G_{M1}-gangliosidosis. N. Engl. J. Med., 288, 225–28.
22. Yeh, I.T., O'Connor, D.M. and Kurman, R.J. (1989) Vacuolated cytotrophoblast: a subpopulation of trophoblast in the chorion laeve. Placenta, 10, 429–38.
23. Kohn, G., Sekeles, E., Arnon, J. and Ornoy, A. (1982) Mucolipidosis IV: prenatal diagnosis by electron microscopy. Prenat. Diagn., 2, 301–307.
24. Bach, G., Cohen, M.M. and Kohn, G. (1975) Abnormal ganglioside accumulation in cultured fibroblasts from patients with mucolipidosis IV. Biochem. Biophys. Res. Commun., 66, 1583–1590.
25. Bargal, R. and Bach, G. (1988) Phospholipids accumulation in mucolipidosis IV cultured fibroblasts. J. Inherited Metab. Dis., 11, 144–50.
26. Zeigler, M., Bargal, R., Suri, V. et al. (1992) Mucolipidosis type IV. Accumulation of phospholipids and gangliosides in cultured amniotic fluid cells. A tool for prenatal diagnosis. Prenat. Diagn., 12, 1037–42.
27. Ornoy, A., Arnon, J., Grebner, E.E. et al. (1987) Early prenatal diagnosis of mucolipidosis IV. Am. J. Med. Genet., 27, 983–85.
28. D'Amico, D.J., Kenyon, K.R., Albert, D.M. and Hanninen, L. (1982) Lipid inclusions in human ocular tissues in vitro induced by aminoglycoside antibiotics. Birth Defects, 18, 411–20.
29. MacLeod, P.M., Dolman, C.L., Nickel, R.E. et al. (1984) Prenatal diagnosis of neuronal ceroid-lipofuscinosis. Am. J. Med. Genet., 22, 781–89.
30. MacLeod, P.M., Nag, S. and Berry, C. (1988) Ultrastructural studies as a method of prenatal diagnosis of neuronal ceroid-lipofuscinosis. Am. J. Med. Genet. Suppl., 5, 93–97.
31. Chow, C.W., Borg, J., Billson, V. and Lake, B.D. (1993) Fetal tissue involvement in the late infantile type of neuronal ceroid lipofuscinosis. Prenat. Diagn., 13, 833–41.
32. Hug, G. (1974) Enzyme therapy and prenatal diagnosis in glycogenosis type II. Am. J. Dis. Child., 128, 607–09.
33. Hug, G., Soukup, S., Ryan, M. and Chuck, G. (1984) Rapid prenatal diagnosis of glycogen storage disease type II by electron microscopy of uncultured amniotic fluid cells. N. Engl. J. Med., 310, 1018–22.
34. Diukman, R., Tanigawara, S., Cowan, M.J. and Golbus, M.S. (1992) Prenatal diagnosis of Chediak–Higashi syndrome. Prenat. Diagn., 12, 877–85.
35. Durandy, A., Breton-Gorius, J., Guy-Grand, D. et al. (1993) Prenatal diagnosis of syndromes associating albinism and immune deficiencies (Chediak–Higashi syndrome and variant). Prenat. Diagn., 13, 13–20.
36. Ginsberg, S. and Groll, M. (1973) Hydrops fetalis due to infantile Gaucher's disease. J. Pediatr., 82, 1046–48.
37. Bonduelle, M., Lissens, W., Goossens, A. et al. (1991) Lysosomal storage diseases presenting as transient or persistent hydrops fetalis. Genet. Couns., 2, 227–32.
38. Nelson, A., Peterson, L., Frampton, B. and Sly, W.S. (1982) Mucopolysaccharidosis VII (β-glucuronidase deficiency) presenting as non-immune hydrops fetalis. J. Pediatr., 101, 574–76.
39. Irani, D., Kim, H–S., El-Hibri, H. et al. (1983) Post mortem observations on β-glucuronidase deficiency presenting as hydrops fetalis. Ann. Neurol., 14, 486–90.
40. Aylsworth, A.S., Thomas, G.H., Hood, J.L. et al. (1980) A severe infantile sialidosis. Clinical, biochemical and microscopic features. J. Pediatr., 96, 662–68.
41. Sewell, A.C., Pontz, B.F., Weitzel, D. and Humburg, C. (1987) Clinical heterogeneity in infantile galactosialidosis. Eur. J. Pediatr., 146, 528–31.
42. Applegarth, D.A., Toone, J.R., Wilson, R.D. et al. (1987) Morquio disease presenting as hydrops fetalis and enzyme analysis of chorionic villus tissue in a subsequent pregnancy. Pediatr. Pathol., 7, 593–99.
43. Beck, M., Braun, S., Coerdt, W. et al. (1992) Fetal presentation of Morquio disease type A. Prenat. Diagn., 12, 1019–29.
44. Uno, Y., Taniguchi, A. and Tanaka, E. (1973) Histochemical studies in Wolman's disease. Report of an autopsy case accompanied with a large amount of milky ascites. Acta Pathol. Jpn., 23, 779–90.
45. Meizner, I., Levy, A., Carmi, R. and Robinsin, C. (1990) Niemann–Pick disease associated with non-immune hydrops fetalis. Am. J. Obstet. Gynecol., 163, 128–29.
46. Maconochie, I.E., Chong, S., Mieli-Vergani, G. et al. (1989) Fetal ascites: an unusual presentation of Niemann–Pick disease type C. Arch. Dis. Child., 64, 1391–93.
47. Sutherland, G.R. and Henderson, D.W. (1992) Prenatal diagnosis of genetic disease by electron microscopy, in Diagnostic Ultrastructure of Non-neoplastic Diseases (eds J.M. Papadimitriou, D.W. Henderson, and D.V. Spagnolo), Churchill Livingstone, Edinburgh, chap. 7.
48. Evans, M.I., Greb, A., Kunkel, L.M. et al. (1991) In utero fetal muscle biopsy for the prenatal diagnosis of Duchenne muscular dystrophy. Am. J. Obstet. Gynecol., 165, 728–32.
49. Rapola, J., Salonen, R., Ämmälä, P. and Santavuori, P. (1990) Prenatal diagnosis of the infantile type of neuronal ceroid lipofuscinosis by electron microscopic investigation of human chorionic villi. Prenat. Diagn., 10, 553–59.
50. Järvelä, I., Rapola, J., Peltonen, L. et al. (1991) DNA-based prenatal diagnosis of the infantile form of neuronal ceroid lipofuscinosis (INCL, CLN1). Prenat. Diagn., 11, 323–28.
51. Conradi, N.G., Uvebrandt, P., Hökegård, K-H. et al. (1989) First-trimester diagnosis of juvenile neuronal ceroid lipofuscinosis by demonstration of fingerprint inclusions in chorionic villi. Prenat. Diagn., 9, 283–87.

52. Kohlschütter, A., Rauskolb, R., Goebel, H.H. *et al.* (1989) Probable exclusion of juvenile neuronal ceroid lipofuscinosis in a fetus at risk. An interim report. *Prenat. Diagn.*, **9**, 289–92.

53. Uvebrandt, P., Bjorck, E., Conradi, N. *et al.*(1992) Successful DNA-based prenatal exclusion of juvenile neuronal ceroid lipofuscinosis. *Clin. Neurol.*, **11**, 165.

54. Cooper, A., Thornley, M. and Wraith, J.E. (1991) First-trimester diagnosis of Hunter syndrome: very low iduronate sulphatase activity in chorionic villi from a heterozygous female fetus. *Prenat. Diagn.*, **11**, 731–35.

55. Muller, L.L. and Jacks, T.J. (1975) Rapid chemical dehydration of samples for electron microscopic examinations. *J. Histochem. Cytochem.*, **23**, 107–10.

71 CHROMOSOMAL MOSAICISM

C.M. Gosden, K. Harrison and
D.K. Kalousek

71.1 Introduction

71.1.1 DEFINITION OF MOSAICISM

By definition, constitutional chromosomal mosaicism means the presence of two or more cell lines with different chromosomal complements in one individual derived from a single zygote. During development an individual consists of an embryo/fetus and its placenta. Mosaicism in the embryo/fetus and placenta will be discussed separately, since they are not always congruent or equally involved in mosaicism.

71.1.2 ORIGIN OF MOSAICISM

Constitutional mosaicism originates as a mutational event in early embryonic development resulting in non-disjunction, anaphase lag or structural rearrangement, and can occur in both trisomic or diploid conceptions (Figure 71.1) as well as in polyploid ones. The resultant mosaic pattern in the conceptus depends on many factors, such as the number of blastomeres at the time of mutational event, the cell lineage affected by the mutational event, and the viability of mutant cells [1]. Generally, better viability is expected for mutant trisomic cell lines than monosomic ones unless monosomy involves the X chromosome.

High levels of mosaicism (15–30%) among preimplantation human embryos have been documented [2–4]. Although the majority of mosaic embryos are eliminated prior to implantation, it has been shown that among trisomic specimens of early spontaneous abortions 10% of gestational sacs are mosaic [5]. Among viable gestations at 9–12 gestational weeks, 1–2% show mosaicism [6,7].

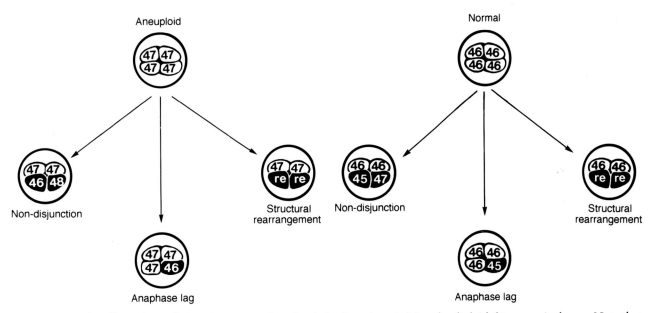

Figure 71.1 The effect of non-disjunction or anaphase lag in both a trisomic (a) and a diploid (b) zygote is shown. Note that in a diploid conceptus they produce monosomic cell lines, while the same event in a trisomic conceptus is likely to produce diploid cell lines.

Diseases of the Fetus and Newborn, 2nd edn, Edited by G.B. Reed, A.E. Claireaux and F. Cockburn. Published in 1995 by Chapman & Hall, London. ISBN 0 412 39160 0

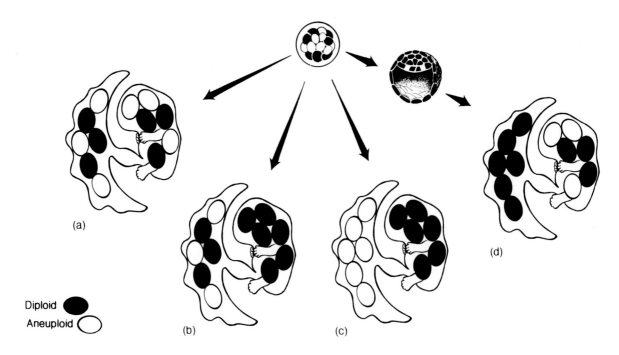

Figure 71.2   The different types of mosaicism originating in the preimplantation period: (a) generalized; (b) and (c) confined to the placenta; (d) confined to the embryo.

71.1.3   TYPES OF MOSAICISM AND THEIR FREQUENCIES

Depending on the timing of the mutational event, cell lineage involvement and mutant cell viability, the postzygotic mutational event can result in several different types of mosaicism. The mosaicism can be generalized, affecting both placental tissue and embryo/ fetus, or confined to a specific cell lineage. The confined mosaicism may be limited either to placenta or to the embryo/fetus itself (Figure 71.2). Within the embryo/ fetus mosaicism may be preferentially expressed in specific tissues.

(a)   Generalized mosaicism

Generalized mosaicism originates from an early mutational event, most likely in the first or second postzygotic division (Figure 71.2a). All tissues of the whole conceptus, specifically both embryonic and extraembryonic ones, are affected. This type of mosaicism has been described for most autosomal trisomies and for both monosomy and trisomy of the sex chromosomes. It is most commonly detected in cultured amniotic fluids. Based on the data obtained from second trimester amniocentesis for cytogenetic prenatal diagnosis, its frequency is estimated to be 0.1–0.3% in a general population [8].

(b)   Confined mosaicism

The mosaicism may be confined either to the placenta or to the embryo/fetus (Figure 71.2b–d). Significant confined placental mosaicism results from viable mutations occurring in progenitor cells of either trophoblast or extraembryonic mesoderm or both (Figure 71.2b,c), while significant confined embryonic mosaicism originates after the initiation of development of the embryo proper (Figure 71.2d) from a designated small number of embryoblasts in the inner cell mass [9]. Confined placental mosaicism is usually detected prenatally by chorionic villus sampling (CVS). Its frequency is estimated to be about 2% among pregnancies exposed to CVS and prenatal diagnosis [6,7,10]. There are no available figures for frequencies of confined embryonic or fetal mosaicism.

(c)   Tissue specific or preferentially expressed in certain tissues

Perhaps the best known example of tissue specific mosaicism is Pallister–Killian syndrome involving tetrasomy or isochromosome for the short arm of chromosome 12. In this syndrome, the chromosomal abnormality is expressed preferentially in fibroblastic cell lines but not in lymphoid cell lines. It is important to identify this as a potential source of false-negative results if pregnancies at risk for such disorders were only karyotyped using tissues in which the chromosomal abnormalities were not expressed. At a practical level this can be illustrated in pregnancies where abnormalities such as diaphragmatic hernia or polyhydramnios are detected. The most frequent chromosomal anomalies seen in association with these abnormalities are trisomy 18 or Pallister–Killian syndrome. Detailed ultrasound scanning for fetal anomalies is usually undertaken at about 18–20 weeks gestation, and at such advanced gestations there is a need for very rapid karyotyping [11]. The most rapid methods of karyotyping are those of direct CVS preparations and fetal blood cultures. Direct CVS preparations would have a substantial risk of showing a normal karyotype and thus of giving false-negative results in many cases of trisomy 18 but fetal blood sampling would be expected to have a high degree of accuracy. However, for Pallister–Killian syndrome the fetal blood sample would have a high risk of yielding a false-negative result because the anomaly is rarely observed in lymphoid cell lines.

71.2 Mosaicism in the fetus

Mosaicism in prenatal diagnosis is not rare. For amniotic fluid cultures where the mosaicism is encountered less frequently than in CVS, if cases of single abnormal cells (described as type I mosaicism) are excluded, then types II (multiple cells with the same abnormality in a single flask or colony) and type III mosaicism (multiple cells in multiple flasks or colonies) occur in 0.7% and 0.2% of all amniotic fluid samples [12–14]. In early second trimester amniotic fluid samples, over 60% of the cells are derived from extra-embryonic membrane, amnion, rather than from fetal surfaces [15]. Thus a number of cases of mosaicism in cultured amniotic fluid cells obtained by early amniocentesis may arise.

The principal problem in prenatal diagnosis in cases of mosaicism, either in CVS or amniocentesis, is to distinguish those cases due to confined placental mosaicism, culture artefact or unrecognized twin pregnancy, from those involving true mosaicism in the fetus. A corollary of this is of course trying to predict the possible phenotype from a mosaic karyotype and this is covered in section 71.2.1.

71.2.1 KARYOTYPE–PHENOTYPE CORRELATIONS: IMPLICATIONS OF MOSAICISM

A number of different factors influence the phenotype in mosaic individuals. One of the most important is the proportion of normal to abnormal cells in each tissue. The abnormal cell lines have duplications or deletions of chromosomal regions, most of which lead to genetic imbalance. Complex factors such as the number and types of genes involved, gene dosage, chromosomal imprinting and transcriptional regulation may all interact in a complex fashion so that phenotypic consistency is by no means certain. The genes involved affect critical target organs and tissues and some of the major influences may occur very early in development.

Monozygotic twin studies have been of fundamental importance in understanding the way in which mosaicism affects the phenotype, even in individuals sharing an identical genetic background. Whilst the occurrence of monozygotic twins who are also mosaic is relatively rare (although more frequent than would be predicted on the basis of the independent events of twinning and mosaicism, since the same error which leads to monozygotic twinning may predispose to mitotic nondisjunction), such cases can illustrate fundamental principles of how the phenotype relates to the karyotype. As an example, the Edinburgh Medical Research Council Human Cytogenetic Registry has details of monozygotic twins who have 45,X/46,XY mosaicism, originally identified in a newborn survey. Blood chromosome studies of the twins at birth showed them to have very similar proportions of 45,X cells in their blood, but one was phenotypically female while the other twin was male. All genotyping studies showed the twins to be monozygotic. Subsequent follow-up showed the female twin to have Turner syndrome, whilst the male grew and developed within the normal range for males. Skin biopsies from the twins showed that the female twin with Turner syndrome had a considerably greater proportion of 45,X cells than her monozygotic twin brother.

The proportion of cells with an abnormal karyotype (and thus genotype) in brain, gonads and other organs influences the development, differentiation and metabolism of the whole conceptus. Since the nature of the exact chromosomal region and the genes involved differs according to the type of anomaly, the principal types of mosaicism will be considered separately.

(a) Mosaicism involving autosomes

Much of the information about the modifying effects of the presence of a normal cell line in a karyotype with a mosaic abnormality has come from studies of individuals with trisomy 21 mosaicism as this is probably the most common form of mosaic abnormality. Some 2–3% of all cases of Down syndrome show mosaicism. Use of chromosomal polymorphisms and latterly DNA markers has shown that although the majority of cases occur as a result of postzygotic non-disjunctional errors occurring in a karyotypically normal early zygote, a proportion arise by loss of a chromosome 21 in a trisomic conceptus [16]. It is not yet clear whether the parental origin of the abnormal chromosome influences the phenotype in any way. The phenotype can be influenced either by an imprinting effect (see below) or by the level of mosaicism for a specific trisomy.

The presence of normal cells in an individual with Down syndrome mosaicism tends to have an effect of 'diluting' many of the syndromal features. The characteristic facial features, including the width of the nasal bridge, brachycephaly, epicanthic folds and macroglossia, tend to become less pronounced and the mean IQ tends to be higher than in non-mosaic Down syndrome. It has always been assumed that this is due to the presence of normal cells in the brain ameliorating the effects of the trisomy 21 cells. When identification of mosaicism relied on karyotyping dividing cells, the ability to classify trisomic and normal neurones was not possible, but the availability of chromosome specific probes which can be used in interphase cells should lead to much greater understanding of the influence of cells with different karyotypes in brain development and differentiation and to the intellectual consequences of abnormal gene expression. Presenile dementia of the Alzheimer type occurs in individuals with both mosaic and non-mosaic Down syndrome. Expression and gene dosage of the APP gene on chromosome 21 makes this a very interesting system for the study of the effects of mosaicism in brain.

Many autosomal trisomies such as trisomies 7, 8, 9, 13, 14 and 18 are generally lethal in pure non-mosaic form, but individuals who are mosaic for these abnormalities may survive. Prediction of the phenotype is difficult: catalogues of human chromosomal abnormalities [17] suggest that most cases are associated with mental handicap and many with disturbances of growth and dysmorphic features.

(b) Mosaicism for sex chromosome abnormalities

A number of studies have shown that mosaicism for sex chromosome abnormalities and in particular mosaicism for 45,X may involve false-positive results in CVS or amniotic fluid because of some form of preferential loss of X or Y chromosomes. The Canadian and European randomized trials of CVS versus amniocentesis [18,19] showed that 45,X mosaicism occurred at quite a high frequency in amniotic fluid, and at an even higher frequency in CVS. The European collaborative study of mosaicism [20] indicated that over 50% of cases with apparent 45,X mosaicism were actually false-positive results. Thus when confronted with a 45,X mosaic karyotype in CVS or amniotic fluid culture this poses complex questions about the need for confirmatory karyotyping and presents parents with difficult decisions about the fate of the pregnancy. Although a substantial proportion of cases involve false-positive results, others reflect true mosaicism in the fetus [21]. The spectrum of abnormality for true mosaics varies from that of normal fertile females to those with a full Turner syndrome phenotype [22].

Prediction of the phenotype when a mosaic karyotype is involved is difficult for both 45,X/46,XX and 45,X/46,XY. For 45,X/46,XX mosaicism the phenotype may be either normal female or Turner female; the proportion of cells is not always an absolute indicator but when over 75% of blood cells are 45,X then a Turner phenotype is more probable. Possible phenotypes for 45,X/46,XY include Turner syndrome female, intersex or normal male. The pathway which is followed seems to depend on the proportion of cells with 45,X and the partition of these cells in the different organs and tissues, especially gonads, brain and endocrine organs. In the case of the monozygotic twins with 45,X/46,XY mosaicism, where one was a male and the other a Turner syndrome female, there is a suggestion that a critical number or proportion of Y-bearing cells are necessary in the primitive gonads and other organs for development of male characteristics, and similarly the proportion of cells with 45,X in the germ cell of the developing ovary and possibly developing endocrine organs which determine a Turner-like phenotype.

Other sex chromosome anomalies such as XY/XXY, XY/XYY and XX/XXX follow the same trends as other mosaics. The phenotype depends upon the proportion of abnormal cells and their distribution in critical target tissues and organs. There are interesting data from the prospective longitudinal follow-up studies of newborns with sex chromosomal anomalies on the IQ, growth, behavioural and endocrinological characteristics of these individuals in comparison with those with non-mosaic sex chromosome abnormalities and with normal controls. These show that most of the mosaics (with the exception of 45,X mosaics) tend towards the norm. Most were indistinguishable from the normal controls for the majority of parameters studied, including IQ and behaviour [23]. Many fertile men with Klinefelter syndrome are thought to be mosaic, with a normal cell line influencing testicular development and endocrine control.

(c) Mosaicism for polyploidy

Triploidy

The phenotype in pure triploidy varies according to the parental origin of the extra set of chromosomes because of parental chromosomal imprinting effects. A paternal (androgenetic) origin is associated with hydatidiform degeneration of the placenta (and potential choriocarcinoma in the mother is associated with this in a small proportion of cases). In some cases, there is growth retardation in utero. When the extra chromosomal set is derived from the mother (digynic triploidy), affected fetuses tend to have severe intrauterine growth retardation and neural tube defects, including spina bifida [24,25]. Whether mosaic triploids follow these patterns remains to be clarified, especially with respect to the risk of choriocarcinoma. It is possible that in future, the prediction of the possible phenotype from the karyotype will depend not only in trying to establish whether there is true mosaicism in the fetus and the proportion of cells affected, but also on the parental origin of the abnormality.

It is not yet clear what proportion of cases involving mosaicism for triploidy seen in prenatal diagnosis are due to unrecognized twin pregnancy with death of the affected co-twin but persistence of the trophoblast and how many involve mutations in the early developing embryo. The development of new molecular genetic techniques including the use of polymorphic probes to identify the parental origin in such cases may help to shed light on this.

Tetraploidy

Major diagnostic problems are encountered in prenatal diagnosis because of the very high proportion of tetraploid cells seen in some amniotic fluid, CVS and fetal blood samples. There appears to be considerable doubt as to whether or not polyploid cells are a feature of normal development stages in certain embryonic tissues and organs and whether *in vitro* culture methods (such as culture conditions, media, sera or growth factors) affect the proportions of polyploid cells seen.

Endoreduplication and other mechanisms of producing polyploid cells rather than errors of mitotic nondisjunction in the early embryo may be a particular problem of fetal cells, especially those in culture. Certain culture media or conditions may exacerbate the tendency to undergo nuclear division without cytokinesis. An understanding of which cases of diploid/tetraploid mosaicism are due to true mosaicism, which to confined placental abnormalities and which to culture artefact is fundamental to trying to predict the potential phenotype.

There are some interesting data from experiments on diploid/tetraploid chimaeric mice [26] which suggest that the distribution of the tetraploid cells within the different tissues of the mouse embryos and extra-embryonic membranes is not random and that there is preferential distribution to certain tissues. In 12.5-day diploid/tetraploid mouse chimaeras, tetraploid cells were commonly found in derivatives of primitive endoderm (yolk sac and parietal endoderm) and were found less often and with uneven distribution in trophectoderm (placenta). Derivatives of primitive ectoderm (fetus, amnion, yolk sac mesoderm) rarely contained tetraploid cells. If this were also true for mosaic human embryos, it would be very important for the prediction of the phenotype.

(d) Mosaicism involving chromosomal rearrangements

Mosaicism involving supernumerary marker chromosomes is important because this type of mosaicism is encountered relatively frequently and the clinical effects of marker chromosomes, even in mosaic form, may be severe. Some are inherited from a parent, but most markers, particularly larger ones, tend to occur *de novo*. There is a very strong association between advanced maternal age and marker chromosome formation. As with ring chromosomes, the behaviour of markers and their effect on phenotype depends on the chromosomal bands from which they are derived. In some cases of mosaicism there may be different cell lines with more than one marker chromosome present. Cell cycle times for cells containing marker chromosomes differ according to the tissue, culture conditions for *in vitro* studies and the type and number of markers.

Ring chromosomes occur relatively rarely (in about 1 in 50 000 newborns [27]), but tend to involve chromosomes where the risks of both generalized mosaicism and confined placental mosaicism are very high, such as 13, 18, 21, 22 and 15 [17]. Ring chromosomes may sometimes be inherited from a parent, but most arise *de novo*. In the formation of a ring chromosome, deletion of chromosomal material usually occurs and ring chromosomes are often unstable at mitosis because of the breakage–fusion–bridge cycle occurring during division. The instability is related to the breakpoints, whether or not there are dicentric derivatives, and structure of the segments involved.

Mosaicism may occur as a result of this mitotic instability; the ring chromosome may be lost in some cell lines resulting in monosomy, may be duplicated so that some cell lines have two, or even three rings and therefore show partial trisomy, or produce centric or acentric fragments. There may also be differences in the levels of mosaicism in different tissues and studies in cultured stimulated peripheral blood cultures show that there are different proportions of cells with rings and fragments after 48, 72, and 96 hours in culture. Fibroblast cultures also differ according to the media and culture conditions and the type of ring chromosome involved. This makes prediction of the possible phenotype very difficult. Among problem cases for the prediction of the phenotype in cases of mosaicism are those where a parent has a ring chromosome in mosaic form at a low level in peripheral blood but the fetus shows very high levels in cultured amniotic fluid cells.

Prediction of the phenotype from the karyotype in the case of rearrangements is more complex because this depends on the chromosomal regions involved and the stability of the rearrangement at mitosis, as well as cell cycle times for the normal and abnormal cell lines. Prediction is also difficult because most cases involve *de novo* rearrangements, where the chromosomal abnormality may be unique or there will only be a very few similar cases in the literature. The most difficult problem in prenatal diagnosis is that the proportion of abnormal cells in the critical organs is difficult to predict from the proportion of cells seen in CVS, amniocentesis or fetal blood. This is partly because the first two involve cells largely derived from extraembryonic tissues and trophoblast and also because the effects of culture *in vitro* influence the proportion of normal and abnormal cells.

71.2.2 MOSAICISM IN DIFFERENT TISSUES

Until molecular cytogenetic techniques such as fluorescence *in situ* hybridization (FISH) became available for the analysis of the chromosomal constitution of interphase nuclei, information about the karyotype of an individual (i.e. the *in vivo* state) was derived by analysis of metaphase from dividing cells, and thus mainly from *in vitro* studies using cell cultures. There has thus been a tendency to extrapolate the results from such *in vitro* studies to derive conclusions about the state of mosaicism *in vivo*. The two tissues used most frequently in studies of mosaicism are blood and skin because these are the most readily available. Other tissues can only be obtained at operation or post mortem.

Blood culture has provided the most information about mosaic individuals. However, even the most elementary culture and analysis of mosaic individuals highlights the problems of studying mosaicism *in vitro*. Each different culture medium will tend to favour the growth of one of the cell lines at the expense of the other (or others) but whether the normal or abnormal line is favoured will vary from case to case. Often, too, there is a time dependency. One medium may give better growth of the normal cell line after 72 hours culture, but the reverse might be true after 48 hours culture. As a general rule, cell lines with high levels of genetic imbalance or abnormalities such as ring chromosomes tend to have their highest levels of expression after 48 hours in culture when the cells are in the first division after stimulation with mitogen because some abnormal cell lines are unable to replicate further *in vitro*. Attempts to synchronize the cells (so that all the cell lines present should perhaps have a more equal chance of being represented among the metaphases obtained) may be useful in some cases.

Skin cells too have similar problems to those of blood cells in culture. The method of establishing the cultures (such as explant, enzyme digestion or collagen methods) may favour either normal or abnormal cell lines. Once primary cultures have been established, then different culture media, sera, growth factors, culture conditions, frequency of subculture, clonability and harvesting methods may all affect the proportion of abnormal cells, and thus estimates of the degree of mosaicism. Almost every tissue obtained will have problems of cell selection *in vitro*, but it is impossible to predict, even for mosaicism involving cell lines with the same apparent karyotype, whether the normal or abnormal cell line will predominate under any given culture conditions.

Tissues critical in determining the phenotype (and thus those upon which information about the degree of mosaicism is sought) are often those which are not easy to obtain and in which substantial proportions of cells do not divide, or only non-representative cells (e.g. fibroblasts from gonads or glial cells from brain) can be induced to divide in culture for karyotyping and investigation of mosaicism. These studies of brain, gonads and other organs suffered severe limitations until methods which are not dependent on dividing cells (such as recombinant DNA methods using chromosome specific probes and FISH) became available.

(a) Cell cycle in normal and abnormal cells

Studies of cell cycle times of the abnormal and normal cell lines in mosaic individuals for the same chromosomal abnormality have appeared to be at minimum at rather equivocal and at maximum totally conflicting. However, this might be expected since cell cycle times probably depend most fundamentally on the genotype rather than the karyotype and even then be critically dependent on the tissue or organ involved. Not only might karyotypically abnormal cells respond diferently to developmental influences and growth factors, but programmed cell death might be very different in mosaicism and affect the proportions of surviving normal and abnormal cells.

71.2.3 CELL SELECTION AND PROPORTIONS OF ABNORMAL CELLS *IN VIVO* AND *IN VITRO*

Individuals who are chromosomal mosaics may not exhibit constancy in the proportion of abnormal cells with time, especially for blood cell lines. In the majority of people the proportions of normal to abnormal cells probably remain reasonably constant, but some individuals may show a decreasing proportion of abnormal cells with time, whereas in others the proportion of abnormal cells may actually increase. There are a number of clinically important factors involved in prenatal diagnosis which can perhaps be best illustrated by two cases of Down syndrome mosaicism. Both were diagnosed by the detection of mosaicism in cultured amniotic fluid cells and in both cases the parents elected to continue the pregnancy, based on the fact that the mosaicism involved only a relatively small proportion of cells with trisomy 21. The first baby showed a greater proportion of trisomic cells in cord blood than had been predicted from the amniotic fluid cells and showed a number of characteristic features of Down syndrome. His development and IQ were intermediate between the means for Down syndrome children and normals. Sequential blood karyotype analysis showed an increase in the proportion of trisomy 21 cells with time. In the second case, the baby looked almost normal, with only very slight indications of mosaic Down syndrome being present; these became less with time. The proportion of trisomy 21 cells in blood at birth was only 5% and follow-up studies at the age of 5 years revealed no trisomy 21 cells in 100 metaphases analysed. His development and IQ were within the normal range. The question of whether or not he would have any significant risks of having children with trisomy 21 because of germ cell mosaicism were discussed with his parents and it was suggested that he should have genetic counselling when he reached reproductive age.

Cell proliferation rates for normal and abnormal cell lines are not the same in all individuals. In some the abnormal cell line increases, whilst in others the normal cell line has a selective advantage and the abnormal cell line can in some cases be difficult to detect in later life. This is probably why the results of cell cycle time studies in Down syndrome have been equivocal because there is so much heterogeneity.

In vivo selection is also affected by the number of divisions which occur from the original non-disjunctional error and this will differ according to the tissue or organ concerned. This can be very important in critical tissues, e.g. brain, where all the neurons are laid down by the time of birth, and in other tissues, e.g. blood, which is a tissue with rapid turnover throughout life and where even small differences in cell cycle times are likely to have a major effect. There may also be preferential selection in different tissues, for example because of cellular receptors for growth factors or differences in intracellular intermediaries.

71.2.4 TISSUES FOR DIAGNOSIS: SAMPLING, RISKS AND KARYOTYPING METHODS

The choice of method for fetal karyotyping is a complex balance between a number of different factors which include the safety of the method, the accuracy and the time in pregnancy at which the test can be carried out. Safety is difficult to assess because it includes miscarriages after testing, which must be balanced against a high background rate of fetal loss (especially in older mothers), later losses and perinatal deaths, low birth weight, prematurity and other hazards to the fetus, which include possible fetal anomalies occurring as a result of the test. Accuracy is not just a function of the proportion of false-positive and false-negative results associated with each testing method, but also the success rates for each test and the number of cases which require further invasive sampling, with the attendant risks. The gestational age at which testing can be carried out is an important factor in uptake rates for prenatal diagnosis as parents are anxious to have

testing as early in pregnancy as possible on account of the advantages this has with respect to privacy and in avoiding the problems of late termination of pregnancy if the fetus is found to be affected.

Amniocentesis and amniotic fluid culture appears to be the safest and most established technique and it is with this method that most of our knowledge has been gained of the frequency, types and problems of mosaicism in prenatal diagnosis. The new methods of FISH using chromosomal probes for interphase nuclei, which can be used in problems cases of mosaicism, may help to resolve some of the diagnostic difficulties which are encountered in amniotic fluid cultures. CVS allows the option of early sampling, but the risks of the procedure and the problems of accuracy (particularly those of confined placental mosaicism) seem to be greater than those of amniotic fluid cultures. Fetal blood sampling seems to offer the greatest accuracy as the cells obtained are known to be fetal in origin and are closest to the true fetal karyotype, thus avoiding the difficulties of cells derived from trophoblast and extraembryonic membrane which give rise to problems such as those of confined placental mosaicism in CVS, and to a lesser extent in AF cultures. It is particularly useful in helping to resolve problems of mosaicism occurring in either amniocentesis or CVS and offers the advantage of rapid karyotyping with control of cell cycle times and culture conditions (although one should be alert to the rare cases where there might be problems of tissue specific expression in fibroblasts rather than lymphoid cell lines, e.g. Pallister–Killian syndrome). However, this a specialized sampling technique, only available in a limited number of centres and probably carries the greatest risk of fetal loss and problems of premature delivery.

The problems caused by mosaicism in prenatal diagnosis require further research so that methods can be developed for the rapid resolution of the difficulties with the least risk to the pregnancy. It is important that there is recognition of the amount of parental anxiety engendered in these cases. The cost, too, is not inconsiderable and includes the time spent on analysing large numbers of cells in the original sample, and resampling, karyotyping and counselling. Failure to address these problems satisfactorily leads to major effects on the safety, accuracy and efficacy of prenatal karyotyping and screening programmes.

71.3 Mosaicism in the placenta

Confined placental mosaicism (CPM), defined as a dichotomy between the chromosomal constitution of placental tissues (both cytotrophoblast and villus stroma) and embryonic/fetal tissues, is usually detected on chorionic villus sampling at 9–12 weeks of gestation. It has been reported in 2% of pregnancies studied

Table 71.1 Types of confined placental mosaicism

	Type I	Type II	Type III
Cytotrophoblast	+	–	+
Chorionic stroma	–	+	+
Fetus	–	–	–

+ Second cell line present.

by CVS [6,7]. Although chorion confined mosaicism has previously been designated in the literature as cytogenetic discordance or pseudomosaicism [28,29], it exemplifies true constitutional mosaicism confined to the placenta. The existence of this mosaicism has been demonstrated not only in first trimester chorionic villi, but also in term placentas [30,31]. It can assume three different forms, as shown in Table 71.1. Each type of CPM affects different placental cell lineage(s) and has specific chromosomal involvement and specific clinical consequences.

71.3.1 MOSAICISM CONFINED TO TROPHOBLAST (TYPE I CPM)

Mosaicism confined to trophoblast is designated in Table 71.1 as type I mosaicism. Type I is the most common form of CPM. It occurs in pregnancies with both diploid and aneuploid fetuses. In pregnancies with a diploid fetus, the aneuploid line in the cytotrophoblast detected on CVS has been shown to persist throughout the entire gestation in the same proportion [30]. Certain autosomal trisomies occur frequently in type I CPM, while others are rarely seen in this type (Table 71.2a,b). The most common trisomies are those for chromosomes 3, 7, 11, 13, 16 and 18. Rare trisomies involve chromosomes 5, 10, 14, 17 and 19. No trisomies 1, 4 or 6 have been described. Among sex chromosome aneuploidies, the monosomy in its complete or mosaic form is the most frequent finding. It is interesting to note that triploidy confined to cytotrophoblast has not been described, while tetraploidy is relatively common. It supports the idea that type I CPM originates from postzygotic non-disjunction, anaphase lag or abnormal cell division affecting specifically trophoblastic progenitors only. The clinical effect of this type of mosaicism is not well documented, although some clinical studies have reported no effect at the time of delivery [99].

Type I CPM can also occur in aneuploid gestations. In these gestations, placental stroma, amnion and fetus show non-mosaic trisomy and a diploid cell line is present in the cytotrophoblast (Figure 71.3). This type of mosaicism has been most commonly described for viable trisomy 18 and 13 pregnancies [100,101], but has also been described for other viable trisomies [102,103].

The presence of the diploid cell line confined to the cytotrophoblast in otherwise non-mosaic aneuploid conceptions appears to provide a protective effect and facilitates their intrauterine survival. It has been shown that all studied placentas from trisomic live newborns and from terminated viable pregnancies around 20 weeks of gestation with trisomies 13 and 18 have type I CPM involving the diploid cell line [100]. This finding has been confirmed by so-called false-negative CVS reports in the literature [103,104].

71.3.2 MOSAICISM CONFINED TO CHORIONIC STROMA (TYPE II CPM)

Chromosomal mosaicism confined to chorionic villus stroma represents type II CPM. It is equally common as mosaicism confined to the cytotrophoblast. Although many pregnancies with this type of confined placental mosaicism progress to term uneventfully and result in the birth of a normal live infant, some are associated with unexplained intrauterine fetal death, intrauterine growth restriction or perinatal morbidity [30,47]. A mosaic placenta may result in abnormal placental function that interferes with normal fetal development and may be the cause of these complications (Table 71.2). Trisomies commonly seen in this type of mosaicism involve chromosomes 2, 7, 8, 9, 12, 16, 18 and 21. Trisomies 1, 4, 6 and 19 have not been reported. Trisomies for chromosomes 3, 5, 10, 11, 13, 14, 15, 17, 20 and 22 are rare. Sex chromosome aneuploidy seen in this type of CPM involves mainly monosomy of the X chromosome. Mosaicism involving triploidy and tetraploidy have also been reported.

71.3.3 MOSAICISM INVOLVING BOTH TROPHOBLAST AND STROMA (TYPE III CPM)

Type III CPM, representing involvement of both trophoblast and chorionic stroma, is the least commonly documented. Aneuploidy is present in both cytotrophoblast and villus stroma but absent in embryo/fetus. The pregnancies with this type of CPM are frequently complicated by intrauterine growth restriction or intrauterine death [74,76]. There are specific chromosomes such as 7, 15 and 16 which are commonly found in this type of mosaicism (Table 71.2), while other chromosomal aneuploidies do not occur [1,3,4,5,6,8,10,11,13, 14,17,19]. The remaining chromosomes [2,9,12,18, 20,21,22] are observed occasionally.

71.3.4 ASSOCIATION OF CONFINED PLACENTAL MOSAICISM WITH FETAL UNIPARENTAL DISOMY

The occurrence of a diploid fetus with either non-mosaic or high level mosaic trisomy in both placental lineages (type III CPM) at the time of CVS most likely

Table 71.2(a) Summary of 384 first trimester CVS cases reported to have a mosaic or non-mosaic trisomy cell line confined to the cytotrophoblast (I), villous stroma (II) or both (III)

Chromosome	n	I	II	III	References
+2	15	1	13	1	7,30–36[a]
+3	22	21	1	0	7,28,29,36,37–49
+5	6	5	1	0	7,32,41,50–52
+7	40	20	16	4	7,29,30,32,34,36,43–45,49,53,55,56,59,60,90[a]
+8	17	7	10	0	7,30–32,40,47,61–63
+9	12	1	10	1	7,31,32,43,45,57[a]
+10	7	1	6	0	7,30,90[a]
+11	7	5	2	0	7,29–31,40,54[a]
+12	17	3	13	1	7,30,31,34,50,57,64,90[a]
+13	21	14	7	0	7,29–32,48,61,64–66,90[a]
+14	3	1	2	0	7,43,64
+15	16	8	5	3	7,29–31,39,42,58,62,67–70[a]
+16	43	13	19	11	7,28–30,34,35,37,38,45,47,49,57,58,62,66,71–80[a]
+17	2	1	1	0	64,90
+18	33	20	11	2	7,28–32,38–40,42,49,62,66,68,82,83[a]
+19	3	3	0	0	7,40,54
+20	12	4	6	2	7,32,38,41,58,63,84,85[a]
+21	14	3	10	1	7,29–32,51,52,66,86[a]
+22	7	3	3	1	7,45,90[a]
Sex chromosome aneuploidies					
45,X	8	7	1	0	31,48,49,62,68,69,81,87
45,X/46,XX	27	15	10	2	7,30–32,36,39,40,42,54,58,62,64,65,67,88,90[a]
45,X/46,XY	22	8	13	1	7,28,30–32,36,38,41,62,90[a]
46,XX/47,XXX	7	2	5	0	7,38,39,42,61,65
46,XX/47,XXY	4	4	0	0	7,32,65,85
45,X/46,XX/47,XXX	1	1	0	0	7
46,XY/47,XYY	1	1	0	0	32
45,X/46,XY/47,XXY	1	1	0	0	30
Polyploidy					
Triploidy	1	0	1	0	[a]
Tetraploidy	15	2	7	6	7,30,31,36,41,45,52,54,66,81,89,90[a]
Total	384	175	173	36	

[a] And D.K. Kalousek, unpublished data.
See footnote to Table 71.2(b).

Table 71.2(b) Summary of ten second and third trimester CVS cases reported to have a mosaic or non-mosaic trisomy cell line confined to the cytotrophoblast (I), villus stroma (II) or both (III)

| Chromosome | n | Confined placental mosaicism type | | | References |
		I	II	III	
+2	1	0	0	1	91
+3	2	2	0	0	92
+9	1	0	1	0	93
+16	4	1	1	2	94–96
Polyploidy					
Triploidy	1	0	0	1	97
Tetraploidy	1	1	0	0	98

Eight of ten pregnancies exhibited intrauterine growth retardation or intrauterine death.

This literature survey documents diploid pregnancies reported with CPM involving chromosomal trisomies or sex chromosome aneuploidies. All included cases were defined to have CPM if there were discrepancies between the chromosomal constitution of the fetus/neonate and the placenta. Pregnancies reported to have CPM involving structural chromosome abnormalities, marker chromosomes or aneuploidy of more than one chromosome were not included. Placental mosaicism was further categorized as being confined to the cytotrophoblast (direct preparations) or villus stroma (cultured preparations). If the method of CVS preparation (direct or culture) was not specified, these cases were excluded from the literature survey. Cases with inadequate follow-up by amniocentesis, fetal blood sampling or neonatal karyotyping were also excluded from the survey as generalized mosaicism could not be ruled out. Pregnancies with CPM, detected by first trimester CVS, are summarized in Table 71.2(a). Second and third trimester pregnancies diagnosed with CPM by CVS are summarized in Table 71.2(b).

results from postzygotic loss of one of the three chromosomes in the embryonic/fetal progenitor cells. In one third of cases, a loss of the extra chromosome will result in uniparental disomy (Figure 71.4) in which both chromosomes originate from the same parent [105,106]. Uniparental disomy may or may not affect the embryonic/fetal development. An effect may be observed if the involved chromosomal pair carries imprinted DNA segment(s). Genomic imprinting is a phenomenon whereby a specific DNA segment is differentially modified and functions differently, depending on the parental origin of the chromosome. It has been well documented in both mouse experimental work and clinical observations in man.

In the mouse, both maternal and paternal sets of chromosomes are necessary for complete and undisturbed development [107]. Neither androgenic (diploid paternal) nor gynogenic (diploid maternal) embryos survive intrauterine development. Experiments support the concept that duplication of certain chromosomes from one parent with loss of the homologue from the

other parent, or uniparental disomy, causes embryonic lethality and disturbed growth and viability [108]. This has allowed the assignment of 'imprinted' and 'non-imprinted' regions of the mouse genome. Similar effects of uniparental disomy have been described in man for specific chromosomal regions as well as for the whole maternal and paternal sets of chromosomes [105].

When one considers all three possible consequences (biparental disomy, uniparental disomy with no genomic imprinting and uniparental disomy with genomic imprinting) arising from the loss of a trisomic chromosome in the embryonic progenitors of a developing trisomic embryo, it is not surprising that there is little agreement on the effect of type III CPM on intrauterine fetal development. There are reports describing a significant increase in prenatal and perinatal complications [47,88], while other reports describe the absence of any such complications in pregnancies which seemingly had identical types of placental mosaicism [41,109].

In the literature, 73 well-documented pregnancies with CPM involving chromosomes 2, 3, 7, 8, 15, 16, 18 and 45,X/46,XX were reported to have intrauterine growth restriction or be complicated by intrauterine fetal death. These cases are summarized in Tables 71.3, 71.4 and 71.5. The role of uniparental disomy in these pregnancy complications remains to be established [74].

71.3.5 CONCEPT OF TRISOMIC ZYGOTE 'RESCUE'

In humans, high frequency of aneuploid gametes resulting in frequent non-viable aneuploid conceptions has been well recognized [113]. The fact that the viability of some of these aneuploid embryos is achieved through postzygotic mutation in either placental or embryonic progenitors, giving rise to generalized or lineage confined mosaicism in placenta, is less appreciated.

Specific lineage confined mosaicism is seen in viable trisomies 18 and 13, where a normal diploid cell line is found in the cytotrophoblast, while the chorionic stroma, amnion and all tissues of the fetus/newborn are non-mosaic trisomy 18 or 13 [47,82,100].

Placental mosaicism involving both placental cell lineages is observed in 0.04% of pregnancies undergoing CVS. In these pregnancies both cytotrophoblast and chorionic stroma show chromosomal aneuploidy, usually trisomy, while the fetus is diploid [34,74]. The frequency with which various chromosomes are involved in placental aneuploidy seems to correspond to the frequency with which specific chromosomal trisomies are observed in spontaneous abortions. The most common placental trisomy is trisomy 16. Other reported aneuploidies are trisomies 15, 7, 22, 2 and 9. It is likely that trisomies for chromosome 13, 18 and 21

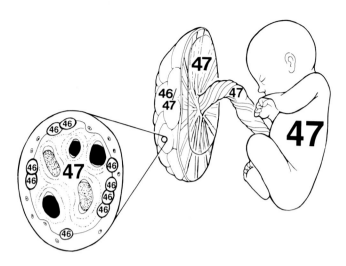

Figure 71.3   Aneuploid gestation with type I CPM. Note that the fetus shows non-mosaic trisomy.

Table 71.3   Seventy-three reported cases associated with pregnancy complications:
42 pregnancy losses and 31 fetal intrauterine growth restrictions (IUGR)

Chromosome involved in CPM	Total cases of CPM	Pregnancy complication		References
		Loss	IUGR	
Autosomes				
2	22	2	3	7,30,35,91,110
3	24	5	1	7,46,47,92
7	42	1	3	30,59[a]
8	7	1	0	91
9	15	4	0	42,61,91
13	21	1	0	49
14	4	2	0	7,91
15	17	2	2	30,42,70
16	55	13	19	35,47,53,71–77,79,80, 94,95,110,111[a]
18	34	4	1	7,60,81,112
22	7	0	1	36
Sex chromosomes				
X/XX	28	5	0	7,41,60,87
Polyploidy				
XY/XXYY	39	2	0	40,55
XX/XXY	2	0	1	29

[a] And D.K. Kalousek, unpublished data.

confined to placenta are under-reported as such pregnancies will generally be terminated and the placental tissue would be used for the confirmation of prenatal iagnosis. Therefore, the likelihood of detecting diploidy in the fetus is low in these rare mosaic pregnancies.

The concept of trisomic zygote rescue is diagramatically summarized in Figure 71.5. The diagram shows

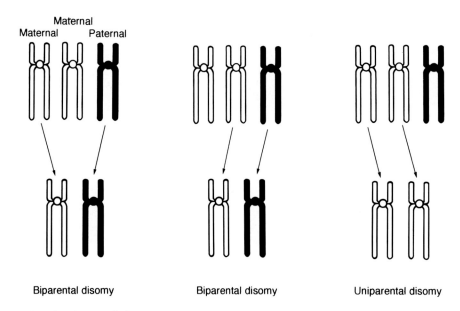

Figure 71.4 The origin of uniparental disomy in a trisomic conceptus.

Table 71.4 Forty-two reported cases of confined placental mosaicism associated with intrauterine death and pregnancy loss

Chromosome involved in CPM	Total reported cases of CPM	Total reported loss	CPM type			Gestational age[a] (weeks)[a]		References
			I	II	III	11–20	20–40	
Autosomes								
2	22	2	1	1	–	1	1	7,91
3	24	5	5	–	–	4	1	7,47,92
7	42	1	–	1	–	1	–	59
8	7	1	1	–	–	–	1	91
9	15	4	3	–	1	4	–	42,61,91
13	21	1	1	–	–	1	–	49
14	4	2	1	1	–	1	–	7,91
15	17	2	1	–	1	–	–	42
16	55	13	6	5	2	5	5	47,54,73,74,76, 80,110–112[a]
18	34	4	3	1	–	–	3	7,61,113
Sex chromosomes								
X/XX	28	5	4	1	–	3	–	7,42,61,88
Tetraploidy								
XY/XXYY	39	2	2	–	–	1	–	41,56

[a] Gestational age available only for 32 cases.

that the outcome of postzygotic mutation is dependent on the mutant cell lineage. When the trisomic chromosome is lost in the trophoblast, a viable trisomic infant is delivered (Figure 71.5a). When a similar mutation occurs in the embryonic progenitor cell, a diploid fetus newborn develops, supported by trisomic placenta (Figure 71.5b). There is an increased rate of pregnancy complications, including intrauterine fetal growth restriction, pregnancy associated hypertension and intrauterine fetal death, in these pregnancies. It remains to be established whether the pregnancy complications are chromosome specific and whether some of the complications are related to the presence of fetal uniparental disomy for the specific chromosome. In the case of

Table 71.5 Seventeen cases of confined placental mosaicism involving trisomy 16 with analysis available on both cytotrophoblast and stroma

	CPM type	
Pregnancy outcome	I	III
Pregnancy loss	4	1
Intrauterine growth restriction	1	8
Normal newborn	0	3
Total	5[a]	12

[a] Gestational ages 13, 21, 37 and 38 (×2) weeks.

trisomy 16 zygote rescue among nine studied pregnancies, six showed complications, and uniparental disomy was detected in four of them [74].

71.4 Technical aspects

Any time tissue is cultured a potential *in vitro* artefact is introduced on the basis of selective cell survival in culture. When all cell types of that particular tissue are represented in the culture, the duration of the culture becomes important as increased time in culture increases the likelihood of developing clonal artefacts [114,115]. The role of various culturing techniques in producing culture artefacts needs to be considered [8]. Use of *in situ* harvest techniques and subsequent colony analysis is advantageous over flask culture and trypsinization [116]. Studies of non-dividing cells using various DNA probes represent a major advance in studying chromosomal mosaicism. Interphase nucleus studies are a particularly good method of choice for confirmation of prenatally diagnosed mosaicism in various tissues of the placenta and cord blood [117,118].

The second important aspect of mosaicism is its selective presence in certain cell lineages and its absence in others. Therefore, for mosaicism studies, selection of appropriate tissues is very important.

The number of cells studied and analysis of multiple sites within an organ or body also represent significant factors in chromosomal mosaicism studies [119].

The entire conceptus (placenta and embryo/fetus) must be studied to document various types of mosaicism, such as generalized, confined and tissue specific.

71.5 Future directions

The entire spectrum of chromosomal mosaicism has recently been amplified by recent discoveries such as those of high levels of mosaicism in preimplantation embryos and findings of confined placental mosaicism and fetal uniparental disomy. Even in cases where there is apparent karyotypic normality, phenomena such as uniparental disomy or chromosomal imprinting may lead to mosaic genetic status. These new discoveries are having a great impact on ideas about the way in which mosaicism might affect human development and growth. The new recombinant DNA techniques have provided a number of tools which have given entirely new perspectives for the study of mosaicism; these include polymorphisms within introns and exons of genes so that underlying factors such as parental origin or parental imprinting can now be studied. New probes including DNA, cDNA, mRNA and chromosome specific probes for chromosomal painting in both metaphase and interphase cells have revolutionized the approaches to studying mosaicism and this can now be done in a variety of different cell types and different tissues.

Until recently the demonstration of chromosomal mosaicism was dependent on identifying two or more karyotypically distinct cell lines in dividing (i.e. mitotic) cells. Few cells have sufficient mitotic activity *in vivo* for direct karyotypes to be prepared, so that virtually all investigations of mosaicism were dependent on tissue culture. The problems which accompany any *in vitro* transformation include the selection of predominantly unspecialized cells which can be induced to dedifferentiate and divide *in vitro*. Furthermore, the range of tissues which can be sampled for an investigation of mosaicism in a living individual is effectively limited to skin and blood and prenatal samples such as amniotic fluid and CVS; post-mortem samples give access to a wider range of tissues but the problem of obtaining mitotic cells becomes much greater; for certain tissues, such as neurones (in contrast with the less specialized glial cells, which will sometimes divide in culture) this may be impossible.

Recognition that mosaicism seems to be associated with a number of different, clinically important conditions has increased interest in the subject and is beginning to change the way in which investigations are carried out. Abnormalities of fetal growth and development and adverse pregnancy outcome, and their association with factors such as confined placental mosaicism or uniparental disomy, will certainly intensify investigations on the placenta as well as the fetus. The possibility of using chromosome painting techniques [120] to look at cells in interphase, such as neurones, germ cells and other cell types which were previously refractory to studies of mosaicism (because dividing cells could not be obtained), will now enable studies to be undertaken on the possible contribution of mosaicism in a wide variety of conditions, including intersexuality and neurological impairment.

71.6 Summary

Chromosomal mosaicism is the presence of two or more cell lines with different chromosomal comple-

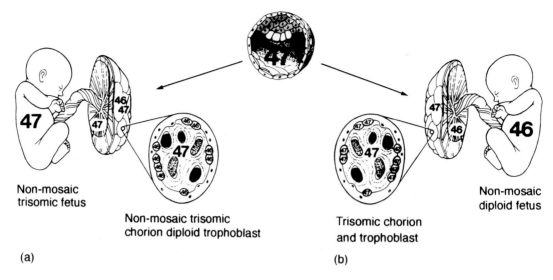

Figure 71.5 The outcome of trisomic zygote rescue through postzygotic loss of the trisomic chromosome. (a) The intrauterine survival of a trisomic fetus correlates with the presence of a diploid cell line in the cytotrophoblast. (b) The mitotic mutation in the embryonic progenitors results in complete dichotomy between diploid fetus and trisomic placenta.

ments in an individual derived from a single zygote (distinguished from chimaerism in which individuals are derived from more than one zygote). Mosaicism may involve a number of different karyotypic abnormalities, including those for whole sets of chromosomes (polyploidy, including triploidy and tetraploidy), trisomies, sex chromosomal anomalies and chromosomal rearrangements.

Mosaicism itself may be present in all the tissues of the body but, depending upon the stage of development at which it originated, the tissue layers to which the abnormal cell lines were distributed and the cell cycle times of both the normal and abnormal cells, mosaicism may only be seen in certain tissues or may be restricted to only the placenta and extraembryonic membranes.

The phenotypic effects or consequences of chromosomal mosaicism may be dramatic. High levels of mosaicism are seen in early abnormal preimplantation embryos, spontaneous abortions, growth retardation (both prenatal and postnatal), intersexuality and mental handicap. However, not all cases of mosaicism are serious and the presence of a normal cell line may dilute the effects of an abnormal cell line to such an extent that many cases of mosaicism will remain undetected because the consequences are not severe.

Investigations of chromosomal mosaicism were, until recently, restricted to those cells from an individual which could be induced to divide and karyotyped from metaphase analysis. Advances in molecular genetics and cytogenetics have made possible the identification of abnormal cells and thus mosaicism in interphase cells; the identification of abnormalities such as confined placental mosaicism and uniparental disomy has led to the recognition that chromosomal mosaicism plays a

major role in abnormal human development and dysmorphology. An understanding of mosaicism, and the role of the placenta during development, including trisomic zygote rescue, is helping to cast light on problems in prenatal diagnosis many of which involve mosaicism or confined placental mosaicism.

Acknowledgement

Support by Clinical Research Grant no. FY93-300 from the March of Dimes Birth Defect Foundation in collection of the data is gratefully acknowledged.

References

1. Kalousek, D.K. and Dill, F.J. (1983) Chromosomal mosaicism confined to the placenta in human conceptions, *Science*, **221**, 665–67.
2. Plachot, M., Mandelbaum, J., Junca, A.M. *et al.* (1989) Cytogenetic analysis and developmental capacity of normal and abnormal embryos of the IVF. *Hum. Reprod.*, **4** (suppl.), 99–103.
3. Bongso, A., Ng, C.S., Lim, J. *et al.* (1991) Preimplantation genetics: chromosomes of fragmented human embryos. *Fertil. Steril.*, **56**, 66–70.
4. Pieters, M.H., Dumoulin, J.C., Ignone-Vanvuchelen, R.C. *et al.* (1992) Triploidy after *in vitro* fertilization. Cytogenetic analysis of human zygotes and embryos. *J. Assist. Reprod. Genet.*, **9**, 68–76.
5. Warburton, D., Yu, C-Y, Kline, J. *et al.* (1978) Mosaic autosomal trisomy in cultures from spontaneous abortions. *Am. J. Hum. Genet.*, **30**, 609–17.
6. Mikkelsen, A. and Ayme, S. (1987) Chromosomal findings in chorionic villi: a collaborative study, in *Human Genetics* (eds F. Vogel and K. Sperling), Springer, Berlin, pp. 597–606.
7. Ledbetter, D.H., Zachery, J.M., Simpson, J.L. *et al.* (1992) Cytogenetic results from the US collaborative study on CVS. *Prenat. Diagn.*, **12**, 317–54.
8. Hsu, L. (1992) Chromosomal disorders, in *Medicine of the Fetus and Mother* (eds A.E. Reece, J.C. Hobbins, M.J. Mahoney *et al.*), Lippincott, Philadelphia, pp. 426–54.
9. Markert, C.L. and Peters, R.M. (1978) Manufactured hexaparental mice show that adults are derived from three embryonic cells. *Science*, **202**, 56–58.
10. Kalousek, D.K. (1990) Confined placental mosaicism and intrauterine development. *Pediatr. Pathol.*, **10**, 69–77.
11. Thorpe-Beeston, J.G., Gosden, C.M. and Nicolaides, K.H. (1989) Prenatal diagnosis of congenital diaphragmatic hernia: associated malformations and chromosomal defects. *Fetal Ther.*, **4**, 21–28.

12. Bui, T.H., Iselius, L. and Lindstein, J. (1984) European collaborative study on prenatal diagnosis: mosaicism, pseudomosaicism and single abnormal cells in amniotic fluid cell cultures. *Prenat. Diagn.*, 4, 145–62.

13. Hsu, L.Y.F. and Perlis, T.E. (1984) United States survey on chromosome mosaicism and pseudomosaicism in prenatal diagnosis. *Prenat. Diagn.*, 4, 97–130.

14. Worton, R.G. and Stern, R.A. (1984) A Canadian collaborative study of mosaicism in amniotic fluid cell cultures. *Prenat. Diagn.*, 4, 131–44.

15. Gosden, C.M. (1983) Amniotic fluid cell types and culture. *Br. Med. Bull.*, 39, 348–54.

16. Nisani, R., Chemke, J., Voss, R. *et al.* (1989) The dilemma of chromosomal mosaicism in chorionic villus sampling – 'direct' versus long-term cultures. *Prenat. Diag.*, 9, 223–26.

17. Borgaonkor, D.S. (1992) *Chromosomal Variation in Man*, 5th edn, Alan R. Liss, NY.

18. Canadian Collaborative CVS–Amniocentesis Clinical Trial Group (1989) Multicentre randomised trial of chorionic villus sampling and amniocentesis. *Lancet*, i, 1–6.

19. Medical Research Council European Trial of Chorion Villus Sampling (1991) *Lancet*, 337, 1491–99.

20. Vejerslev, L.O. and Mikkelsen, M. (1989) European collaborative study on mosaicism in chorionic villus sampling; data from 1986–1987. *Prenat. Diagn.*, 9, 575–88.

21. Gosden, C.M., Nicolaides, K.H. and Rodeck, C.H. (1988) Fetal blood sampling in investigation of chromosome mosaicism in amniotic fluid cell culture. *Lancet*, i, 613–17.

22. Hsu, L.Y.F. (1989) Prenatal diagnosis of 45,X/46,XY mosaicism. A review and update. *Prenat. Diagn.*, 9, 31–48.

23. Netley, C.T. (1986) Summary overview of behavioural development in individuals with neonatally identified X and Y aneuploidy. *Birth Defects*, 22, 293–306.

24. Nicolaides, K.H., Rodeck, C.H. and Gosden, C.M. (1986) Rapid karyotyping in non-lethal malformations. *Lancet*, i, 283–87.

25. Nicolaides, K.H., Snijders, R.J.M., Thorpe-Beeston, J.G. *et al.* (1989) Mean red cell volume in normal, anaemic, small, trisomic and triploid fetuses. *Fetal Ther.* 4, 1–13.

26. James, R.M. and West, J.D. (1994) A chimaeric animal model for confined placental mosaicism (in press).

27. Hook, E. and Hamerton, J.L. (1977) The frequency of chromosomal abnormalities detected in consecutive newborn series – differences between studies – results by sex and severity of phenotypic involvement, in *Population Cytogenetics – Studies in Humans* (eds E.B. Hook and I.H. Porter), Academic Press, NY, pp. 63–79.

28. Simoni, G., Gimelli, G., Cuoco, C. *et al.* (1985) Discordance between prenatal cytogenetic diagnosis after chorionic villi sampling and chromosomal constitution of the fetus, in *First Trimester Fetal Diagnosis* (eds M. Fraccaro, G. Simoni and G. Brambati), Springer, Berlin, pp. 137–43.

29. Callen, D.F., Korban, G., Dawson, G. *et al.* (1988) Extra embryonic/fetal karyotypic discordance during diagnostic chorionic villus sampling. *Prenat. Diagn.*, 8, 453–60

30. Kalousek, D.K., Howard-Peebles, P.N., Olson, S.B. *et al.* (1991) Confirmation of CVS mosaicism in term placentae and high frequency of intrauterine growth retardation association with confined placental mosaicism. *Prenat. Diagn.*, 11, 743–50.

31. Miny, P., Hammer, P., Gerlach, B. *et al.* (1991) Mosaicism and accuracy of prenatal cytogenetic diagnosis after chorionic villus sampling and placental biopsies. *Prenat. Diagn.*, 11, 581–89.

32. Wang, B.T., Rubin, C.H. and Williams III, J. (1993) Mosaicism in chorionic villus sampling: an analysis of incidence and chromosomes involved in 2612 consecutive cases. *Prenat. Diagn.*, 13, 179–84.

33. Chudoba, I., Kleinart-Skopnick, C., Steuber, E. *et al.* (1989) Mosaicism in chorionic villi samples: two additional cases and a review of the literature, in *Chorionic Villus Sampling and Early Prenatal Diagnosis* (eds A. Antsaklis and C. Metaxotou), BETA Medical Arts, Athens, pp. 153–61.

34. Dorfmann, A.D., Perszyk, J., Robinson, P. *et al.* (1992) Rare, non-mosaic trisomies in chorionic villus tissue not confirmed in amniocentesis. *Prenat. Diagn.*, 12, 889–902.

35. Fryburg, J.S., DiMaio, M.S. and Mahoney, M.J. (1991) Non-mosaic trisomy 2 and high level mosaicism for trisomy 16 detected at chorionic villus sampling. *Prenat. Diagn.*, 12, 157–62.

36. Nocera, G., Dalpra, L., Tibiletti, M.G. *et al.* (1989). Prenatal chromosome mosaicism in the first trimester, in *Chorionic Villus Sampling and Early Prenatal Diagnosis* (eds A. Antsaklis and C. Metaxotou), BETA Medical Arts, Athens, pp. 181–82.

37. Brambati, B., Simoni, G., Danesino, C. *et al.* (1985) First trimester fetal diagnosis of genetic disorders. Clinical evaluation of 250 cases. *J. Med. Genet.*, 22, 92–99.

38. Mikkelsen, M. (1985) Cytogenetic findings in first trimester chrionic villi biopsies: a collaborative study, in *First Trimester Fetal Diagnosis* (eds M. Fraccaro, G. Simoni and B. Brambati), Springer, Berlin, pp. 109–29.

39. Schulze, B. and Miller, K. (1986) Chromosomal mosaicism and maternal cell contamination in chorionic villi cultures. *Clin. Genet.*, 30, 239.

40. Green, J.E., Dorfmann, A., Jones, S.L. *et al.* (1988) Chorionic villus sampling: experience with an initial 940 cases. *Obstet.Gynecol.*, 71, 208–12.

41. Schwinger, E., Seidl, E., Klink, F. *et al.* (1989) Chromosome mosaicism of the placenta: a cause of developmental failure of the fetus? *Prenat. Diagn.*, 9, 639–47.

42. Miller, K., Schlesinger, C., Schulze, B. *et al.* (1989) Cytogenetic experience in 500 diagnostic CVS cases, in *Chorionic Villus Sampling and Early Prenatal Diagnosis* (eds A. Antsaklis and C. Metaxotou), BETA Medical Arts, Athens, pp. 58–62.

43. Brambati, B. (1992) Genetic diagnosis by chorionic villus sampling before 8 gestational weeks: efficiency, reliability and risks on 317 completed pregnancies. *Prenat. Diagn.*, 12, 789–99.

44. Sachs, E.S., Los, F.J., Pijpers, L. *et al.* (1989) Chromosomal mosaicism in chorionic villi cells, in *Chorionic Villus Sampling and Early Prenatal Diagnosis* (eds A. Antsaklis and C. Metaxotou), BETA Medical Arts, Athens, pp. 162–63.

45. Longy, M., Grison, O., Saura, R. *et al.* (1992) Fetoplacental discrepancies on direct chromosomal analysis after CVS: 9 cases out of 1300 diagnoses, in *Early Fetal Diagnosis* (eds M. Macek, M.A. Ferguson-Smith and M. Spala), Karolinum-Charles University Press, Prague, E1.32.

46. Guerneri, S., Fortuna, R., Romitti, L. *et al.* (1989) Seven cases of trisomy 3 mosaicism in chorionic villi. *Prenat. Diagn.*, 9, 691–95.

47. Johnson, A., Wapner, R.J., Davis, G.H. and Jackson, L.G. (1990) Mosaicism in chorionic villus sampling: an association with poor perinatal outcome. *Obstet. Gynecol.*, 75, 573–77.

48. May, K.M., Saxe, D.F., and Priest, J. (1992) Confirmation of CVS mosaicism. *Prenat. Diagn.*, 12, 626–27.

49. Sachs, E.S., Jahoda, M.G., Los, F.J. *et al.* (1990) Interpretation of chromosome mosaicism and discrepancies in chorionic villi studies. *Am. J. Med. Genet.*, 37, 268–71.

50. Verjaal, M., Leshot, N.J., Wolf, H. *et al.* (1987) Karyotypic differences between cells from placenta and other fetal tissues. *Prenat. Diagn.*, 7, 343–48.

51. Copeland, K.L., Hanna, G.J., Elder, F.F.B. *et al.* (1989) Is CVS mosaicism really different than amniocentesis? in *Chorionic Villus Sampling and Early Prenatal Diagnosis* (eds A. Antsaklis and C. Metaxotou), BETA Medical Arts, Athens, pp. 167–70.

52. Wright, D.J., Brindley, B.A., Koppitch, F.C. *et al.* (1989) Interpretation of chorionic villus sampling laboratory results as just as reliable as amniocentesis. *Obstet. Gynecol.*, 74, 739–44.

53. Bartels, I., Rauskolb, R. and Hansmann, I. *et al.* (1986) Chromosomal mosaicism of trisomy 7 restricted to chorionic villi. *Am. J. Med. Genet.*, 25, 161–2.

54. Leschot, N., Wolf, H. and Verjaal, M., *et al.* (1987) Chorionic villi sampling: cytogenetic and clinical findings in 500 pregnancies. *BMJ*, 295, 407–10.

55. Delozier-Blanchet, C.D., Engel, E. and Extermann, P. *et al.* (1988) Trisomy 7 in chorionic villi: follow-up studies of pregnancy, normal child and placental anomalies. *Prenat. Diagn.*, 8, 281–86.

56. Vamos, E., Ogur, G. and Rodesch, F. (1989) First trimester chromosome diagnosis on chorionic villi: report of 219 cases, in *Chorionic Villus Sampling and Early Prenatal Diagnosis* (eds A. Antsaklis and C. Metaxotou) BETA Medical Arts, Athens, pp. 41–45.

57. Murer-Orlando, M., Llerena Jr, J. and Zahed, L. *et al.* (1989) Evaluating descrepant results in CVS cytogenetic studies, in *Chorionic Villus Sampling and Early Prenatal Diagnosis* (eds A. Antsaklis and C. Metaxotou), BETA Medical Arts, Athens, pp. 213–17.

58. Marguerat, P.H., Klinke, S. and Pescia, G. *et al.* (1989) Current issues in the methodological assessment of CVS, in *Chorionic Villus Sampling and Early Prenatal Diagnosis* (eds A. Antsaklis and C. Metaxotou), BETA Medical Arts, Athens, pp. 203–206.

59. Reddy, K.S., Stetton, G. and Corson, V.L. *et al.* (1988) Interpreting chromosomal mosaicism in chorionic villus sample (CVS). *Am. J. Med. Genet.*, 43S, A267.

60. Watt, A.J., Devereux, F.J. and Monk, N. *et al.* (1991) The phenotype in placental trisomy 7. *Aust. NZ J. Obstet. Gynaecol.*, 31, 246–48.

61. Wapner, R., Jackson, L. and Davis, G. *et al.* (1985) Cytogenetic discrepancies found at chorionic villus sampling (CVS). *Am. J. Med. Genet.*, 37, A122.

62. Hogge, W.A., Schonberg, S.A. and Golbus, M.S. *et al.* (1986) Chorionic villus sampling: experience of the first 1000 cases. *Am. J. Obstet. Gynecol.*, 154, 1249–52.

63. Schreck, R.R., Falik-Borenstein, Z. and Hirata, G. (1990) Chromosomal mosaicism in chorionic villus sampling. *Clin. Perinatol.* 17, 867–88.

64. Kalousek, D.K., Dill, F.J. and Pantzar, T. *et al.* (1987) Confined chorionic mosaicism in prenatal diagnosis. *Hum. Genet.*, 77, 163–67.

65. Cheung, S.W., Crane, J.P. and Beaver, H.A. *et al.* (1987) Chromosome mosaicism and maternal cell contamination in chorionic villi. *Prenat. Diagn.*, 7, 535–42.

66. Cuoco, C., Glimelli, G., Bicocchi, M.P. et al. (1989) Cytogenetic findings in 911 CVS, in *Chorionic Villus Sampling and Early Prenatal Diagnosis* (eds A. Antsaklis and C. Metaxotou), BETA Medical Arts, Athens, pp. 190–92.

67. Martin, A.O., Simpson, J.L., Rosinsky, B. *et al.* (1986) Chorionic villus

sampling in continuing pregnancies. II. Cytogenetic reliability. *Am. J. Obstet. Gynecol.*, **154**, 1353–62.

68. Breed, A.S.P.M., Mantingh, A., Beekhuis, J.R. *et al.* (1990) The predictive value of cytogenetic diagnosis after CVS: 1500 cases. *Prenat. Diagn.*, **10**, 101–10.

69. Smidt-Jensen, S., Christensen, B. and Lind, A.-M. (1989) Chorionic villus culture for prenatal diagnosis of chromosome defects: reduction of the long-term cultivation time. *Prenat. Diagn.*, **9**, 309–19.

70. Morichon-Delvallez, N., Mussat, P., Dumez, Y. *et al.* (1992) Trisomy 15 in chorionic villi and Prader–Willi syndrome at birth. *Prenat. Diagn.*, **12**, S125.

71. Tharapel, A.T., Elias, S., Shulman, L.P. *et al.* (1989) Resorbed co-twin as an explanation for discrepant chorionic villus results: non-mosaic 47,XX, +16 in villi (direct and culture) with normal (46,XX) amniotic fluid and neonatal blood. *Prenat. Diagn.*, **9**, 467–72.

72. Verp, M.S., Rosinsky, B., Sheikh, Z. *et al.* (1989) Non-mosaic trisomy 16 confined to villi. *Lancet*, **ii**, 915–16.

73. Wang, B.T. and William, J. (1992) Effect of confined placental mosaicism for trisomy 16 on fetal growth. *Appl. Cytogenet.*, **18**, 197–99.

74. Kalousek, D.K., Langlois, S., Barrett, I. *et al.* (1993) Uniparental disomy for chromosome 16 in humans. *Am. J. Hum. Genet.*, **52**, 8–16.

75. Post, J.G. and Nijhuis, J.G. (1992) Trisomy 16 confined to the placenta. *Prenat. Diagn.*, **12**, 1001–1007.

76. Simoni, G., Brambati, B., Maggi, F. *et al.* (1992) Trisomy 16 confined to chorionic villi and unfavourable outcome of pregnancy. *Ann. Genet.*, **35**, 110–12.

77. Mayger, W.A., Anderson, J.M. and Pertile, M.D. (1992) Nonmosaic trisomy 16 detected at chorionic villus sampling associated with a karyotypically normal (46,XX) growth retarded infant. 16th Annual Meeting of Human Genetics Society of Australia. *Bull. Hum. Genet. Soc. Aust.*, p. 39.

78. Sumdberg, K. and Smidt-Jensen, S. (1991) Non-mosaic trisomy 16 on chorionic villus sampling but normal placenta and fetus after termination. *Lancet*, **337**, 1233–34.

79. Dworniczak, B., Koppers, B., Kurlemann, G. *et al.* (1992) Maternal origin of both chromosomes 16 in a phenotypically normal newborn. *Am. J. Hum. Genet.*, **51**, A11.

80. Kalousek, D.K., Langlois, S., Barrett, I. *et al.* (1993) Intrauterine development and confined placental mosaicism. *Mod. Pathol.*, **6**, 5P.

81. Stengel-Rutkowski, S. and Nimmerman, C.H. (1992) West-German collaborative study on prenatal diagnosis after chorionic villus sampling (BMFT-Study), in *Early Fetal Diagnosis* (ed: M. Macek, M.A. Ferguson-Smith and M. Spala), Karolinum-Charles University Press, Prague, pp. 135–39.

82. Wirtz, A., Gloning, K.P.H. and Murken, J. (1991) Trisomy 18 in chorionic villus sampling: problems and consequences. *Prenat. Diagn.*, **11**, 563–67.

83. Bommer, C., Korner, H. and Wegner, R.-D. (1992) False negative findings in short term cultures of chorionic villi. *Prenat. Diag.*, **12**, S53.

84. Ward, B.E., Boswell, A.F. and Watson, J.D. (1988) Confined chorionic mosaicism for structural and numerical chromosomal abnormalities in CVS. *Am. J. Hum. Genet.*, **43**, A252.

85. Chieri, P. and Aldini, A. (1989) Cytogenetic diagnosis after transabdominal CVS in the first trimester, in *Chorionic Villus Sampling and Early Prenatal Diagnosis* (eds. A. Antsaklis and C. Metaxotou), BETA Medical Arts, Athens, pp. 46–47.

86. Penketh, R., Davis, G. and Rodek, C. (1990) Mosaicism confined to the cytotrophoblast: near misdiagnosis of trisomy 21 after the first trimester CVS. *5th International Congress on Early Pediatric Diagnosis*, July, 1990 Prague, E1. 33

87. Qumsiyeh, M.B., Tharapel, A.T., Shulman, L.P. *et al.* (1990) Anaphase lag as the most likely mechanism for monosomy X in direct cytotrophoblasts but not in mesenchymal core cells from the same villi. *J. Med. Genet.*, **27**, 780–1.

88. Breed, A.S.P.M., Mantingh, A., Vosters, R. *et al.* (1991) Follow up and pregnancy outcome after a diagnosis of mosaicism CVS. *Prenat. Diagn.*, **11**, 577–80.

89. Heim, S., Kristoffersson, U., Mandahl, N. *et al.* (1985) Chromosome analysis in 100 cases of first trimester trophoblast sampling. *Clin. Genet.*, **27**, 451–57.

90. Teshima, L.E., Kalousek, D.K., Vekemans, M.J.J. *et al.* (1992) Chromosome mosaicism in CVS and amniocentesis samples. *Prenat. Diagn.*, **12**, 443–66.

91. De Andreis, C., Pariani, S., Maggi, F. *et al.* (1992) Trisomy 2 confined to the placenta in 2 cases with intrauterine growth delay. *Acta Med. Auxol.*, **24**, 21–24.

92. Guerneri, S., Fortuna, R., Romitti, L. *et al.* (1989) Seven cases of trisomy 3 mosaicism in chorionic villi. *Prenat. Diagn.*, **9**, 691–95.

93. Appelman, Z., Rosensaft, J., Chemke, J. *et al.* (1991) Trisomy 9 confined to the placenta: prenatal diagnosis and neonatal follow-up. *Am. J. Med. Genet.*, **40**, 464–66.

94. Kennerknecht, I. and Terinde, R. (1990) Intrauterine growth retardation associated with chromosomal aneuploidy confined to the placenta. Three observations: triple trisomy 6, 21, 22; trisomy 16; and trisomy 18. *Prenat. Diagn.*, **10**, 539–44.

95. Bennett, P., Vaughan, J., Henderson, D. *et al.* (1992) The association between confined placental trisomy, fetal uniparental disomy and early intrauterine growth retardation. *Lancet*, **340**, 1284–85.

96. Szabo, J., Gellen, J. and Szemere, G. (1992) Transabdominal amnio- and choriocentesis a combined procedure, in *Early Fetal Diagnosis* (M. Macek, M.A. Ferguson-Smith and M. Spala), Karolinum-Charles University Press, Prague, pp. 182–84.

97. Callen, D.F., Fernandez, H., Hull, Y.J. *et al.* (1991) A normal 46,XX infant with a 46,XX/69,XXY placenta; a major contribution to the placenta is from a resorbed twin. *Prenat. Diagn.*, **11**, 437–42.

98. Wolstenholme, J., Hoogwerf, A.M., Sheridan, H. *et al.* (1980) Practical experience using transabdominal chorionic villus biopsies taken after 16 weeks gestation for rapid prenatal diagnosis of chromosomal aneuploidies. *Prenat. Diagn.*, **9**, 357–59.

99. Brandenburg, H., Jahoda, M.G.S., Los, F.J. and Wladimiroff, J.W. (1991) Acceptance of chorionic villus sampling in the southwest region of the Netherlands: a 5 year evaluation. *Am. J. Med. Genet.*, **41**, 236–38.

100. Kalousek, D.K., Barrett, I.J. and McGillivray, B.C. (1989) Placental mosaicism and intrauterine survival of trisomies 13 and 18. *Am. J. Hum. Genet.*, **44**, 338–43.

101. Pindar, L., Whitehouse, M. and Ocraft, K. (1992) A rare case of a false negative finding in both direct and culture of a chorionic villus sample. *Prenat. Diagn.*, **12**, 523–27.

102. Lilford, R.J., Caine, A., Linton, B. *et al.* (1991) Short-term culture and false-negative results for Down syndrome on chorionic villus sampling. *Lancet*, **337**, 861.

103. Bartels, I., Hansmann, I., Holland, U. *et al.* (1989) Down syndrome at birth not detected by first trimester chorionic villus sampling. *Am. J. Med. Genet.*, **34**, 606–607.

104. Simoni, G., Fraccaro, M., Gimelli, G. *et al.* (1987) False positive and false negative findings on chorionic villus sampling. *Prenat. Diagn.* 7, 671–72.

105. Hall, J.G. (1990) Genomic imprinting: review and relevance to human diseases. *Am. J. Hum. Genet.*, **46**, 857–73.

106. Engel, E. and Delozier-Blanchet, C.D. (1991) Uniparental disomy, isodisomy, and imprinting: probable effects in man and strategies for their detection. *Am. J. Med. Genet.*, **40**, 432–39.

107. Solter, D.A. (1988) Differential imprinting and expression of maternal and paternal genomes. *Ann. Rev. Genet.* 22, 127–46.

108. Searle, A.G., Peters, J., Lyon, M.F. *et al.* (1989) Chromosome maps of men and mouse. *Ann. Hum. Genet.*, **53**, 89–140.

109. Leschot, N.J. and Wolf, H. (1991) Is placental mosaicism associated with poor perinatal outcome? *Prenat. Diagn.* 11, 403–404.

110. Holzgreve, B., Exeler, R., Holzgreve, W. *et al.* (1992) Non-viable trisomies confined to the placenta leading to poor pregnancy outcome. *Prenat. Diagn.*, **12S**, S95.

111. Knoll, W., Seidlitz, G., Schutz, M. *et al.* (1992) Rapid karyotyping in the first trimester by placental biopsy and early amniocentesis, in *Early Fetal Diagnosis* (M. Macek, M.A. Ferguson-Smith and M. Spala), Karolinum-Charles University Press, Prague, p. 275.

112. Hashish, A.A., Monk, N., Levell-Smith, M.P. *et al.* (1989) Trisomy 16 detected at chorionic villus sampling. *Prenat. Diagn.* 9, 427–32.

113. Jacobs, P. and Hassold, T. (1987) Chromosome abnormalities: origin and etiology in abortions and livebirths, in *Human Genetics* (eds F. Vogel and K. Sperling), Springer, Berlin, pp. 233–44.

114. Hunt, P.A. and Jacobs, P.A. (1985) *In vitro* growth and chromosomal constitution of placental cells. I. Spontaneous and elective abortions *Cytogenet. Cell Genet.*, **39**, 1–6.

115. Hunt, P.A. and Jacobs, P.A. (1985) *In vitro* growth and chromosomal constitution of placental cells, II. Hydatidiform moles. *Cytogenet. Cell Genet.*, **39**, 7–13.

116. Crane, J.P. and Cheung, S.W. (1988) An embryonic model to explain cytogenetic inconsistencies observed in chorionic villus versus fetal tissue. *Prenat. Diagn.*, **8**, 119–29.

117. Lomax, B.L., Kalousek, D.K., Kuchinka, B.D. *et al.* The utilization of fluorescence in situ hybridization for the detection of mosaicism in interphase nuclei. *Hum. Genet.* (in press).

118. Eastwood, D.A., and Pinkel, D. (1989) Aneuploidy detection by analysis of interphase nuclei using fluorescence *in situ* hybridization with chromosome-specific probes, in *Mechanisms of Chromosome Distribution and Aneuploidy* (eds M.A. Resnick and B.K. Vig), Alan R. Liss, NY, pp. 277–84.

119. Hook, E.B. (1977) Exclusion of chromosomal mosaicism. Tables of 90%, 95% and 99% confidence limits and comments on use. *Am. J. Hum. Genet.*, **29**, 94–97.

120. Tkachuk, D.C., Pinkel, D., Kuo, W.-L. *et al.* (1991) Clinical applications of fluorescence *in situ* hybridization. *Genet. Anal. Tech. Appl.*, 8(2), 67–74.

72 FRAGILE X SYNDROME

G.R. Sutherland and R.I. Richards

72.1 Introduction

Fragile X syndrome is the most common familial form of mental handicap and one of the most common genetic diseases. It is found in all ethnic groups exposed to Western medicine. Many reviews of the clinical, cytogenetic and epidemiological aspects of fragile X [1–4] and more recently its molecular genetics [5–7] have been published. Molecular genetic characterization of the fragile X has shed much light on its genetics, dramatically improved diagnosis, provided a candidate gene (*FMR1*) for the syndrome and revealed a new genetic mechanism which is also responsible for some other genetic diseases [5,6].

72.2 The syndrome

The main feature of fragile X syndrome which makes it of medical importance is mental handicap, which is usually accompanied by a variety of subtle dysmorphic features. It can affect both males and females variably and, apart from consideration in the differential diagnosis of any retarded child, can be difficult to diagnose clinically. In addition to the main features listed in Table 72.1 a number of other anomalies have been described as part of the fragile X syndrome. In the newborn, often the only feature of note may be muscle hypotonia.

Autism, especially in males, has been a frequent primary diagnosis prior to detection of the fragile X and there is some controversy about whether the fragile X is a significant cause of autism [8]. Certainly many fragile X syndrome individuals have autistic and other abnormal features to their behaviour.

Macro-orchidism has been used as a diagnostic sign for fragile X syndrome. While this can be helpful, very few prepubertal boys with fragile X syndrome have

Table 72.1 Features of males with fragile X syndrome

Birth weight	Normal but usually greater than sibs; mean at about 70th percentile
Height	Mostly between 50th and 97th percentiles in infancy and childhood; mostly below the 50th percentile in adulthood
Head circumference	Slightly increased in childhood; usually above the 50th percentile in adulthood
Forehead	Prominent, especially in older children and adults
Jaw	Prominent, especially in adults
Ears	Prominent and mildly dysmorphic; long ears
Eyes	Myopia and strabismus
Genitalia	Macro-orchidism usually seen in adults, occasionally in children; penis usually normal length; scrotal skin sometimes thickened; possibly increased incidence of hypospadias, cryptorchidism, and other genitourinary problems
Connective tissue	Hyperextensibility of joints, particularly fingers; fine velvety skin with striae; high arched or cleft palate; mitral valve prolapse and dilatation of ascending aorta; torticollis and kyphoscoliosis; flat feet; inguinal hernia; pectus excavatum
Other features	Epilepsy; hyper-reflexia of lower limbs; gynaecomastia
Behaviour	Stereotyped with odd mannerisms, especially hand flapping and biting; autistic; hyperactive; excessive shyness (poor eye contact); mild self-mutilation (biting)
Speech	Litany speech; perseveration; echolalia; better language form than content
Cognitive defects	Better verbal than spatial abilities; deficit in digit span; deficient in verbal abstractions; no specific verbal versus performance difference; possible specific left hemisphere defect

Diseases of the Fetus and Newborn, 2nd edn, Edited by G.B. Reed, A.E. Claireaux and F. Cockburn. Published in 1995 by Chapman & Hall, London. ISBN 0 412 39160 0

macro-orchidism and, postpubertally, not all macro-orchid males have the fragile X.

Females with the fragile X syndrome are usually less severely affected than males. The degree of mental impairment is less, the behaviour problems are milder and fewer and the dysmorphic features less obvious. In fragile X carrier females of normal intelligence there is an increase in psychiatric symptoms, particularly schizophrenia spectrum disorders [9,10].

72.3 Molecular genetics

Fragile X syndrome is a dynamic mutation disorder [11]. At the fragile site there is a section of DNA composed only of the triplet CCG repeated many times. Normal X chromosomes have from six to about 60 copies of this triplet. Normal carrier males (sometimes called transmitting males) have approximately 60–230 copies and fragile X syndrome males have more than 230 copies (up to about 1000 copies) [12–14]. For females, probably because they have two X chromosomes and one of these is inactived, the situation is a little more complex. Those carriers with about 60–230 copies are all normal but about half of those with more than 230 copies are mentally impaired. Once there are more than 230 copies of the repeat the DNA surrounding the repeat becomes 'hypermethylated', that is methyl groups are added to many of the C (cytosine) bases in the DNA molecule. This methylation is associated with inactivation of the gene (FMR1) containing the repeat sequence and protection of the DNA from the action of some restriction enzymes.

The CCG repeat sequence is unstable because it can change in copy number when transmitted from parent to child, hence the term **dynamic mutation** since the initial change to the DNA sequence alters the chance of further changes to it. This instability is manifested by carriers only, and not by the polymorphic sequence present on normal X chromosomes. When women transmit the sequence it usually increases in size (although decreases have also been seen). When a male transmits the sequence it usually changes only marginally. A male never gives his child more than 230 copies, consequently all fragile X syndrome children receive their fragile X, with more than 230 copies of the repeat, from their mothers.

The fragile site DNA is viewed on a Southern blot. Figure 72.1 shows the patterns seen in various types of individual and demonstrates the instability in a family. The normal X chromosome gives a band of approximately 1.0 kb when DNA is digested with the enzyme PstI and probed with pfxa3. This 1.0-kb band represents about 900 bp of DNA flanking the repeat plus 18–180 bp (6–60 copies) of the CCG repeat unit. The

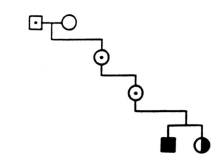

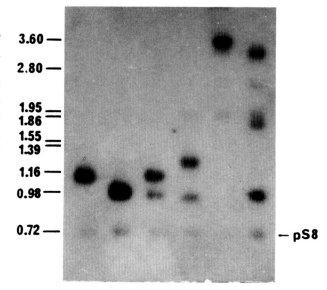

Figure 72.1 Inheritance of the fragile X unstable element in a four-generation lineage from a large affected pedigree. Chromosomal DNA was digested with PstI and probed with pfxa3. Pedigree symbols: normal carrier male (dot in square); normal carrier female not expressing the fragile X (dot in circle); normal carrier female expressing the fragile X (half-shaded circle); affected fragile X syndrome male expressing the fragile X (shaded square); normal female (open circle). The carrier male in the first lane has no normal 1-kb band but an ~1.15-kb band; his wife in the second lane has a 1-kb band. The daughter in the third lane has an ~1.15-kb band on her fragile X from her father and a 1-kb band from her mother. When this daughter has transmitted this band to her daughter the fragile X band has increased to about 1.3 kb in size. This band has increased dramatically in size to about 3.5 kb in the fragile X syndrome band, and appears as a somatically unstable smear in the carrier girl who expresses the fragile X (last lane). She has major bands of about 3.2 kb and 1.9 kb and a 1.0-kb band from her normal X chromosome.

fragile X chromosome gives a larger DNA band. The size, in kilobases, is increased by three times the number of copies of the repeat: hence for 230 copies the band is 1.6 kb in size.

The mechanism by which the CCG repeat leads to fragile X syndrome is not yet fully clarified, however the repeat is located within the non-coding portion of a gene called FMR1, the product of which is a protein of unknown function [15]. But, when more than 230 copies of the repeat are present the DNA in this area is hypermethylated and the gene ceases to function [16].

This dynamic mutation at a trinucleotide repeat is also responsible for Kennedy's spinal and bulbar muscular atrophy and for myotonic dystrophy where the amplified DNA is unstable [6,11]. The behaviour of the unstable DNA in fragile X syndrome and myotonic dystrophy is very similar and provides the mechanism by which these two diseases show anticipation (a progressive increase in severity of the disease in successive generations).

72.4 Genetics

Originally it was presumed that the fragile X syndrome followed standard X-linked inheritance. However, it was soon realized that the inheritance of the disorder was atypical. The proportion of females with fragile X chromosomes who exhibited features of the syndrome was high (in the order of 35%) and, amazingly, there were normal male carriers. These carrier males had completely normal phenotypes and usually did not express the fragile site on their X chromosome.

Segregation patterns of the fragile X syndrome were examined in the mid-1980s [17,18] when only cytogenetic testing in families was available. A number of rather remarkable conclusions were drawn.

- Mutation only occurs in sperm and the mutation rate was estimated to be 7.3×10^{-4}, the highest estimate ever made for a single human gene.
- All mothers of fragile X syndrome children are carriers.
- The penetrance of the fragile X in children is determined by the clinical status (normal or mentally impaired) of their mothers.
- The incidence of fragile X syndrome is higher in the offspring of daughters of normal carrier males than in the offspring of mothers of these males. (This became known as the Sherman paradox.)

Studies of the transmission of the unstable sequence in many fragile X families [19–23] have now provided a preliminary clarification of the inheritance of the fragile X. A number of points have emerged.

1. No new mutation has been observed. The mothers of all fragile X syndrome individuals are carriers and, where study has been possible, so is a grandparent. The rate of new mutation would thus appear to be very **low**, so low in fact that evidence of founder chromosomes has not been observed.

2. When the unstable sequence is transmitted by males it usually does not increase in size.
3. When the unstable sequence is transmitted by females it usually increases in size. The women with small copy numbers, however, show less increase in size than women with larger copy numbers. For example, women with about 30 extra copies mostly have offspring with less than 230 copies (normal carrier sons and daughters), whereas women with 100–200 copies mostly have offspring with much larger numbers of copies, i.e. all their sons who inherit the fragile X have the syndrome.
4. The Sherman paradox was an example of anticipation in which the mothers of transmitting males had far fewer handicapped sons than did the daughters of these males. It is now clear that, on average, the copy number of these two groups of women is different, the mothers having smaller copy numbers than their grand-daughters. Since the risk of a retarded son is a function of copy number, the paradox is explained [19,20,24].

72.5 Cytogenetics

The fragile X chromosome has a characteristic appearance (Figure 72.2). The fragile site is not spontaneously expressed on the X chromosome when most standard cytogenetics methods are used. It must be induced. There are various methods of induction and these have been outlined in detail [25]. These methods all lead to a relative deficiency of either thymidine or deoxycytidine at the time of DNA synthesis. Either of these conditions appear to be a requirement for expression of the fragile X.

The fragile X is only expressed cytogenetically in a relatively small proportion of cells (10–40% in most fragile X syndrome males) after the cells have been appropriately cultured. Individuals with copy numbers of less than 230 do not express the fragile X cytogenetically; most of those with higher copy numbers do.

72.6 Diagnosis

The postnatal diagnosis of fragile X syndrome by cytogenetic methods is reasonably efficient, especially as that technology also detects other significant chromosomal causes of mental handicap. All individuals with mental handicap merit chromosome study. Once an index case has been diagnosed, further family studies by molecular methods are needed to detect carriers reliably and to predict phenotype at prenatal diagnosis.

Caution is required in the cytogenetics laboratory. There are two other fragile sites close to the fragile X which can lead to misdiagnosis [26]. One, in band Xq27.2, can be found in most individuals but usually

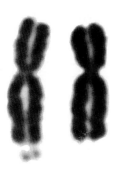 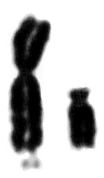

Figure 72.2 Sex chromosome complements from individuals expressing the fragile site at Xq27.3. A female (left) showing the fragile X and a normal X chromosome, and a male (right) showing the fragile X and a normal Y chromosome

only in a very low (1–4%) proportion of cells. The other, in band Xq28, is rare but cytogenetically indistinguishable from the fragile X. DNA analysis will ensure that the true fragile X is present or confirm that one of the other fragile sites is intruding. Only the fragile X is presently detected by molecular analysis.

Detection of the amplified (CCG) is best carried out by Southern blot analysis. Various probe/enzyme systems have been described [5,23,27] but these all essentially determine the size of the CCG repeat; some also assess the methylation status of the DNA adjacent to the repeat. The results are usually unequivocal. Although polymerase chain rection (PCR) analysis of the p [CCG]$_n$ repeat has been demonstrated in fragile X pedigrees, the preferential amplification of the smallest allele renders results for carrier females and males with multiple bands difficult at best. In isolation, PCR may be an inaccurate means of predicting phenotype and until extensive experience with it has been documented it should be used in conjunction with Southern analysis.

72.7 Prenatal diagnosis

Cytogenetics no longer has a place in prenatal diagnosis of fragile X syndrome. Prenatal diagnosis can be accomplished by analysis of DNA obtained from chorion villus samples (CVS) [28–30] by Southern blot using probes which detect the number of copies of the CCG repeat. Fetuses with copy numbers in the normal range (6–60) do not have the fragile X genotype. Male fetuses with 60–230 copies of the repeat should be asymptomatic carriers and those with more than 230 copies will have fragile X syndrome. For female fetuses the situation is a little less certain. Fetuses with 60–230 copies will be asymptomatic. For those with more than

230 copies there is a high (50–60%) risk of mental impairment.

At the cut-off point of 230 copies there is a 'grey area' which could be difficult to interpret; fortunately very few individuals with the fragile X appear to fall into this grey area. In this situation additional studies such as looking for hypermethylation of the DNA around the repeat, and possibly cord blood chromosome studies, might help [20]. If the DNA was hypermethylated the prognosis would be poor but the absence of methylation would be unhelpful in predicting the phenotype since hypermethylation is not always present in DNA extracted from CVS. If the fragile X chromosome was seen in a fetal blood sample, again prognosis would be poor but failure to see the fragile X would be unhelpful. It should however be stressed that in spite of this grey area, for more than 95% of pregnancies prenatal diagnosis is unequivocal, with the exception that phenotype cannot be accurately predicted in those female carrier fetuses with more than 200 copies of the repeat.

References

1. Sutherland, G.R. (1983) The fragile X chromosome. *Int. Rev. Cytol.*, **81**, 107–43.
2. Turner, G. and Jacobs, P. (1983) Marker (X) linked mental retardation. *Adv. Hum. Genet.*, **13**, 83–112.
3. Nussbaum, R.L. and Ledbetter, D.H. (1986) Fragile X syndrome: a unique mutation in man. *Ann. Rev. Genet.*, **20**, 109–45.
4. Hagerman, R. and Silverman, A.C. (1991) *Fragile X Syndrome: Diagnosis, Treatment and Research*, Johns Hopkins University Press, Baltimore.
5. Richards, R.I. and Sutherland, G.R. (1992) Fragile X syndrome: the molecular picture comes into focus. *Trends Genet.*, **8**, 249–55.
6. Caskey, C.T., Pizzuti, A., Fu, Y.H. *et al.* (1992) Triplet repeat mutations in human disease. *Science*, **256**, 784–89.
7. Sutherland, G.R. and Richards, R.I. (1993) The fragile X syndrome. *Baillières Clinical Paediatrics*, **1**, 477–503.
8. Einfeld, S. and Hall, W. (1992) Behaviour phenotype of the fragile X syndrome. *Am. J. Med. Genet.*, **43**, 56–60.

9. Reiss, A.L., Hagerman, R.J., Vinogradov, S. *et al.* (1988) Psychiatric disability in female carriers of the fragile X chromosome. *Arch. Gen. Psychiatry*, **45**, 25–30.

10. Hagerman, R.J. and Sobesky, W.E. (1989) Psychopathology in fragile X syndrome. *Am. J. Orthopsychiatry*, **59**, 142–52.

11. Richards, R.I. and Sutherland, G.R. (1992) Dynamic mutations. A new class of mutations causing human disease. *Cell*, **70**, 709–12.

12. Kremer, E.J., Pritchard, M., Lynch, M. *et al.* (1991) DNA instability at the fragile X maps to a trinucleotide repeat sequence p(CCG)n. *Science*, **252**, 1711–14.

13. Yu, S., Pritchard, M., Kremer, E. *et al.* (1991) Fragile X genotype characterized by an unstable region of DNA. *Science*, **252**, 1179–81.

14. Oberlé, I., Rousseau, F., Heitz, D. *et al.* (1991) Instability of a 550-base pair DNA segment and abnormal methylation in fragile X syndrome. *Science*, **252**, 1097–102.

15. Verkerk, A.J.M.H., Pieretti, M., Sutcliffe, J.S. *et al.* (1991) Identification of a gene (FMR-1) containing a CGG repeat coincident with a breakpoint cluster region exhibiting length variation in fragile X syndrome. *Cell*, **65**, 905–14.

16. Pieretti, M., Zhang, F., Fu, Y.-H. *et al.* (1991) Absence of expression of the *FMR-1* gene in fragile X syndrome. *Cell*, **66**, 817–22.

17. Sherman, S.L., Morton, N.E., Jacobs, P.A. and Turner, G. (1984) The marker (X) syndrome: a cytogenetic and genetic analysis. *Ann. Hum. Genet.*, **48**, 21–37.

18. Sherman, S.L., Jacobs, P.A., Morton, N.E. *et al.* (1985) Further segregation analysis of the fragile X syndrome with special reference to transmitting males. *Hum. Genet.*, **69**, 289–99.

19. Yu, S., Mulley, J., Loesch, D. *et al.* (1992) Fragile X syndrome: unique genetics of the heritable unstable element. *Am. J. Hum. Genet.*, **50**, 968–80.

20. Rousseau, F., Heitz, D., Biancalana, V. *et al.* (1991) Direct diagnosis by DNA analysis of the fragile X syndrome of mental retardation. *N. Engl. J. Med.*, **325**, 1673–81.

21. Verkerk, A.J.M.H., deVries, B.B.A., and Niermeijer, M.F. *et al.* (1992) Intragenic probe used for diagnostics in fragile X families. *Am. J. Med. Genet.*, **43**, 192–96.

22. Knight, S.J.L., Hirst, M.C., and Roche, A. *et al.* (1992) Molecular studies of the fragile X syndrome. *Am. J. Med. Genet.*, **43**, 217–23.

23. Mulley, J.C., Yu, S., and Gedeon, A.K. *et al.* (1992) Experience with direct molecular diagnosis of fragile X. *J. Med. Genet.*, **29**, 368–74.

24. Fu, Y.-H., Kuhl, D.P.A., and Pizzuti, A. *et al.* (1991) Variation of the CGG repeat at the fragile X site results in genetic instability: resolution of the Sherman paradox. *Cell*, **67**, 1047–58.

25. Sutherland, G.R. (1991) The detection of fragile sites on human chromosomes, in *Advanced Techniques in Chromosome Research* (ed. K.W. Adolph), Marcel Dekker, NY, pp. 203–22.

26. Sutherland, G.R. and Baker, E. (1992) Characterisation of a new rare fragile site easily confused with the fragile X. *Hum. Mol. Genet.*, **1**, 111–13.

27. Rousseau, F., Heitz, D., and Biancalana, V. *et al.* (1992) On some technical aspects of direct DNA diagnosis of the fragile X syndrome. *Am. J. Med. Genet.*, **43**, 197–207.

28. Sutherland, G.R., Gedeon, A., and Kornman, L. *et al.* (1991) Prenatal diagnosis of fragile X syndrome by direct detection of the unstable DNA sequence. *N. Engl. J. Med.*, **325**, 1720–22.

29. Dobkin, C.S., Ding, X.-H., and Jenkins, E.C. *et al.* (1991) Prenatal diagnosis of fragile X syndrome (letter). *Lancet*, **338**, 957–58.

30. Hirst, M., Knight, S., and Davies, K. *et al.* (1991) Prenatal diagnosis of fragile X syndrome (letter). *Lancet*, **338**, 956–57.

73 MOLECULAR CYTOGENETICS

B.A. Clark and S. Schwartz

73.1 Introduction

Women are referred for prenatal diagnosis because of an age-related risk of chromosome abnormality or an abnormal value on a triple analyte screen. They may also be referred for abnormalities on ultrasound or a positive family history. For many reasons, advances in the field of genetics have insinuated themselves into modern obstetric care in the form of prenatal diagnosis.

73.1.1 ADVANCES IN HUMAN CYTOGENETICS

The history of human cytogenetics has been one of advances in the laboratory with clinical correlation soon following in practice. In 1956 Tijo and Levan established the human chromosome complement at 46. Penrose had initially recognized the maternal age effect for Down syndrome in 1938. In the early 1960s the chromosomal basis for this syndrome was demonstrated. This association of advanced maternal age with chromosome anomalies kindled interest in the field of prenatal diagnosis. In the late 1960s chromosome banding was developed with the evolution of Q and G banding. Individual chromosomes could be identified by a distinct pattern and abnormalities of chromosome structure and number were characterized. Work on spontaneous abortions and recurrent pregnancy loss established aneuploidy and structural abnormalities as significant factors in human genetic morbidity.

With G banding came prometaphase analysis (high resolution chromosome banding) and chromosomal duplications and deletions were further characterized. Several genetic conditions were recognized as microdeletions and the concept of microdeletion syndrome or contiguous gene syndrome was proposed by Schmickel [1]. More recently advances in molecular biology, gene cloning and *in situ* hybridization have clarified the concept of the 'critical region' in cytogenetics and identified the phenomena of genomic imprinting and uniparental disomy, new and unanticipated forms of non-traditional, non-mendelian inheritance. Molecular cytogenetics has now evolved as a powerful tool for syndrome analysis, syndrome identification and prenatal diagnosis. It has also played a significant role in expanding our understanding of basic genetics.

73.2 Molecular cytogenetics

As the tools and techniques of molecular biology are applied to the field of human cytogenetics, the impact has been immediate and profound. Molecular cytogenetics is the application of labeled DNA probes to cells, whether *in situ* on chromosomes or directly to native DNA on gels, for the analysis of chromosome number, delineation of chromosome structure or the detection of the presence or absence of specific genes or gene sequences. In a cytologic preparation, its fine structure analysis can detect changes down to 10 to 100 kb or less. Molecular cytogenetics uses the principle of heat or chemical denaturation of double stranded DNA to single strands, specific hybridization of a probe to the single stranded DNA, and recognition of the hybridization sequence by a reporter or labeling molecule.

Advances in the use of DNA probes for fine structure analysis of chromosomes have been complemented by advances in the technology of probe labeling. These advances away from autoradiographic techniques to fluorescent technology have extended the realm of cytogenetic analysis from metaphase cells to interphase cells in prepared specimens and even *in situ* analysis of tissue specimens.

73.2.1 *IN SITU* HYBRIDIZATION

The first attempts at using labeled DNA on metaphase chromosome preparations were reported by Pardue, Gall and colleagues [2,3]. Metaphase chromosomes were treated with heat or alkali and labeled with 'satellite' DNA probes which had been obtained by density gradient centrifugation of genomic DNA. They found that the DNA probes hybridized to the heterochromatic centromeric regions of chromosomes. In

Diseases of the Fetus and Newborn, 2nd edn, Edited by G.B. Reed, A.E. Claireaux and F. Cockburn. Published in 1995 by Chapman & Hall, London. ISBN 0 412 39160 0

similar fashion human ribosomal genes were localized to the short arms of chromosomes 13, 14, 15, 21 and 22 [4]. Initial attempts at using this *in situ* hybridization methodology for single gene mapping were not encouraging. However, with the advent of DNA cloning using restriction endonucleases and plasmid vectors, it became possible to produce large amounts of specific DNA for hybridization. Still, the techniques relied on using radioactive nucleotides and autoradiography, a tedious procedure. There was no way for signal amplification and accurate detection of silver grains over a target locus had to rely on statistical methods for accurate interpretation.

73.2.2 FLUORESCENCE *IN SITU* HYBRIDIZATION

The use of radioactive isotopes for probe labeling could require weeks for photographic exposure and alternative reporter molecules were sought. Fluorescence *in situ* hybridization (FISH) is the use of non-isotopically labeled DNA probes for cytologic and molecular analysis of chromosomes at metaphase or interphase. Non-isotopic labeling is accomplished by incorporating a modified nucleotide that can be detected by a reporter molecule, such as one that has been fluorescently tagged. For DNA probes with FISH, DNA polymerase is used to 'nick-translate' a native DNA strand, for example, where biotin-dUTP or digoxigenin-dUTP replaces thymine in the probe strand. The labeled probe is then denatured and hybridized to the denatured native DNA of the cytologic preparation by incubation at 37°C. The probe will then anneal to the complementary DNA sequences in the native DNA. Avidin, tagged with a fluorescent marker, binds to biotin which has been incorporated into the probe DNA. Antiavidin (or an antibody) which has also been biotinylated can then be added to further amplify the signal.

Other reporter compounds in addition to avidin can be used. For example, digoxigenin can be substituted for biotin, and antidigoxigenin which has been labeled with a different flurochrome can be substituted for avidin for amplification of the signal. Therefore, it is possible to use simultaneously two or more DNA probes labeled with different reporter molecules for detection of multiple chromosome anomalies. Using three haptens and three reporter molecules to label probes with combinations of one, two and three reporter molecules along with digital imaging microscopy, Reid *et al.* [5] have simultaneously visualized seven distinct probes. Most recently some probes have been labeled directly with fluorochromes that can be detected without using a reporter molecule. Using this technique along with digital imaging microscopy multiple probes and colors can be detected in a single hybridization.

73.2.3 CLONED GENES

Advances in molecular biology have permitted the cloning of DNA. This has been facilitated by the use of restriction endonucleases, enzymes that cut DNA at a specific base sequence in an asymmetric fashion, such that 'sticky ends' are produced. Restriction enzyme sites are located throughout the human genome. Therefore by using different restriction enzymes specific pieces of human genomic DNA can be cut and inserted into a cloning vector such as a plasmid, cosmid or yeast artificial chromosome (YAC). Plasmids can hold DNA inserts with up to 20 kb, cosmids approximately 40–50 kb and YACs have been used as cloning vectors for DNA inserts up to 1000 kb.

Three general types of DNA probes have been used with FISH, each with a specific application. Single gene probes having from 2 kb to tens of kilobases are used to target a specific locus. Chromosome specific centromere probes are derived from and hybridize to specific centromeric regions. Chromosome paints or libraries are multiple probe 'cocktails' derived from many regions of a particular chromosome which hybridize to an entire chromosome.

73.2.4 SINGLE GENE PROBES

Single gene probes range from 2 kb to hundreds of kilobases and can be used for hybridization to a specific chromosome region, a specific gene, to characterize the chromosomes involved in complex chromosome rearrangements, or for detection of aneuploidy, such as in Down syndrome. These probes have been produced after a gene has been identified, sequenced, cloned and mapped to a chromosome. Or, they may represent single copy genes or anonymous DNA sequences not yet understood.

In addition to directly labeling probes, the polymerase chain reaction (PCR) has also been used to simultaneously amplify and label a probe. PCR uses heat to denature double-stranded DNA into single-stranded DNA, cooling to anneal short segments of primers to the DNA that flank the region of interest to be amplified, and then a heat stable DNA polymerase to elongate the desired sequence. This sequence of denaturing, annealing and elongation can be cycled many times for amplifying DNA. One technique known as inter-Alu-PCR utilizes Alu sequences as primers. Alu sequences are repetitive sequences of about 300 bp in length that are found interspersed throughout the human genome about 500 000 times.

73.2.5 CENTROMERIC PROBES

The DNA associated with the centromeric regions of human chromosomes has been found to contain highly repetitive sequences arranged in a tandem fashion [6]. These α-satellite DNA repetitive sequences are highly chromosome specific and have been used for the detection of aneuploidy, both trisomy and monosomy [7]. They can be used either for sex chromosome or autosome identification. When used in interphase cells, these probes produce discrete dot-like signals that are easy to recognize and score. By using different fluorochromes for the identification of different centromeric probes, it is possible to do simultaneous multicolor FISH interphase analysis. However, these probes are not available for the centromeric regions of all chromosomes and some are more chromosome specific than others.

73.2.6 CHROMOSOME PAINTING

Chromosome paints (libraries) are a mixture of locus specific DNA, some moderately and highly repetitive, all derived from a specific chromosome, usually isolated by flow cytometry or chromosome specific mouse–human cell hybrids. These chromosome specific 'libraries' will 'paint' the whole length of a chromosome [8]. Chromosome painting has been most useful in characterizing unknown 'marker' chromosomes and in identifying complex chromosome rearrangements.

73.3 Fluorescence *in situ* hybridization methodology

Protocols for FISH involve a number of common steps. The material used can be metaphase chromosomes harvested from actively dividing cells or interphase nuclei from tissue not actively dividing. The slides are initially treated with RNAse to remove RNA that may cross-hybridize with the probe, followed by proteinase or heat treatment for removal of chromatin and protein.

The hybridization procedure begins with heat treatment of the slide in formamide to denature the DNA. Cold ethanol is then used to fix the preparation in the denatured state until hybridization with the DNA probe. The probe is denatured for hybridization by heating in a water bath. The probe and chromosome preparation are then mixed, sealed with a coverslip, and incubated at 37°C for 5–24 hours for the hybridization.

The precise conditions of the hybridization can be altered for different probes and specific results. The incubation temperature of the hybridization should be below the melting temperature of the probe and native DNA. The stringency or the selectivity of the binding can be increased and the non-selective background labeling reduced by varying the incubation temperature or the salt composition of the hybridization solution.

73.4 Applications

In cytogenetics, the technique of *in situ* hybridization first proved useful as a means for localizing genes to chromosomes. With the development of fluorescence labeling, *in situ* hybridization was then used to study chromosome abnormalities in cases where traditional chromosome banding had failed. FISH played an indispensible role in the understanding of one of the most unusual discoveries of modern genetics, that of human genomic imprinting. FISH and interphase genetics have also begun to have a broad impact on clinical medicine, and prenatal diagnosis in particular.

73.4.1 PRENATAL DIAGNOSIS

Most women are referred for prenatal diagnosis because of advanced maternal age and its risk of chromosome abnormalities. Amniocentesis and standard karyotype analysis take about 7–14 days for results. For traditional cytogenetic analysis, amniocytes must be cultured, arrested in cell division, stained, and the chromosomes analyzed. This process is one of anxiety for the patient and physician alike. This explains in part the growth of new technologies such as chorionic villus sampling (CVS) and early amniocentesis as faster and earlier diagnoses are sought. For similar reasons, FISH technology has been promoted by some within the prenatal community; FISH and its power to do interphase genetics can expedite preliminary results and enhance standard analysis, if not obviate the need for traditional cell culture and metaphase analysis.

(a) Aneuploidy detection – interphase genetics

For obstetricians, the clinical application of FISH to prenatal diagnosis holds the allure of rapid aneuploidy detection, minimizing the anxiety associated with traditional cytogenetic analysis. For cytogeneticists, however, FISH permits microscopic visualization of targeted DNA sequences, increasing the resolution of cytogenetics beyond the level of banded chromosomes. Specific gene sequences and copy number can be analyzed by FISH in both metaphase chromosomes and interphase cells. This ability makes FISH a powerful technique for detection of autosomal and sex chromosomal aneuploidies as well as fetal sex determination (e.g. for use in preimplantation genetic diagnosis).

The most common chromosome abnormalities detected at CVS and amniocentesis are trisomy 21, 18 and 13 and the sex chromosome aneuploidies (45,X, XXY, XYY and XXX). Trisomy 21, 18 and 13 show the strongest correlation with advanced maternal age, XXY and XXX less so. Turner syndrome, 45,X and XYY do not show an association with advanced maternal age but are represented significantly in the

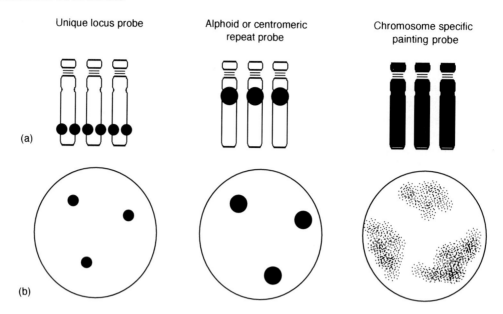

Unique locus probe   Alphoid or centromeric   Chromosome specific
                                repeat probe   painting probe

(a)

(b)

Figure 73.1 (a) The hypothetical appearance of chromosome 21 in a metaphase spread when hybridized with each of the appropriate probe types. Black indicates probe-specific fluorescent signal. Thus, a locus specific probe gives a sharp, discrete signal at its relevant position. An alphoid or centromeric repeat probe gives a large, more diffuse signal near the centromere. A painting probe decorates the entire chromosome. The copy number of the specific chromosome can be determined with any of the probe types. (b) The appearance of G_1 interphase nuclei after hybridization with each of the probe types. The locus-specific probe gives the best resolution and also would detect duplication of the Down syndrome critical region as a result of translocation. The alphoid repeat probe gives a bright and discrete signal but would not necessarily detect a translocation. Because of the diffuse nature of the chromosomal domain in interphase, overlapping domains visualized with the painting probe can make chromosome enumeration more difficult. (Reproduced with permission from Emanuel, B. (1993). The use of fluorescence *in situ* hybridization to identify human chromosomal anomalies. *Growth Genet. Horm.*, 1993; 9: 6–12.)

abnormalities found at prenatal diagnosis. Therefore, any prenatal program using interphase FISH analysis must use probes that can reliably detect chromosomes 21, 18, 13, X and Y.

Three strategies have been developed for use of probes in FISH: single copy or unique sequence probes, chromosome specific repetitive centromeric probes and whole chromosome paints. These strategies produce characteristic signals in metaphase chromosomes and interphase nuclei (Figure 73.1). Each probe type must balance the need for a strong discrete signal with the necessity of preventing signal or domain convergence in interphase nuclei.

Centrometric (α-satellite) probes are relatively chromosome specific and have been the most widely used in the application of interphase genetics [9,10]. They produce a signal of adequate strength giving discrete dots in interphase nuclei without significant overlapping of their domains (Figure 73.2). However, because of sequence similarity between α-satellite DNA in chromosome 21 and chromosome 13 no chromosome specificity can be detected. Therefore, five signals from the use of chromosome 13 and 21 α-satellite probes would identify a trisomic fetus, but would not differentiate a trisomy 21 from a trisomy 13 [11]. Additionally, all D and G group chromosomes tend to

coalesce in the region of the nucleolus organizer in interphase cells, exacerbating the problem of overlapping domains and reducing the likelihood that trisomic nuclei will show three discrete signals in trisomies.

Use of single copy probes avoids the problem of cross-hybridization between similar sequences and gives a discrete signal. Single copy or locus specific probes can detect copy number and the critical cytogenetic regions associated with syndromes, which can be important for detecting trisomies associated with translocations. Multiple single copy probes can be combined into a chromosome specific set (a cosmid contig) to cover a chromosome region. These regions covered by the probe are consistently found in an aneuploid syndrome, and they are called the 'critical region' of that syndrome [12]. Klinger *et al.* [12] developed cosmid contigs for specific regions of each of chromosomes 13, 18, 21, X and Y. These single copy probes covered between 60 and 109 kb of contiguous DNA. Using a prospective blinded FISH protocol on 526 amniotic fluid samples, 21 aneuploid abnormalities were identified, with no false positives or false negatives identified after conventional cytogenetic analysis. However, a false-positive diagnosis of 45,X was reported later from this study in a normal 46,XY male confirmed at routine cytogenetic analysis [13].

A large clinical experience with FISH for rapid prenatal diagnosis has now been reported [14]. FISH was performed as an adjunct to routine cytogenetic analysis. A sample was considered normal when a euploid autosomal and sex-chromosomal pattern was seen in 80% of hybridized nuclei, and aneuploid when 70% of nuclei appeared aneuploid with a specific probe. With this protocol, 10% of samples did not meet criteria for analysis. The authors reported an accuracy of all FISH results at 99.8%, and a specificity of 99.9%. However, the detection rate for aneuploidies was only 73%, as there were seven false-negative reports but no false positives. The finding of false-negative reports is not of significant concern because parents are not likely to act upon the information and the aneuploidies would be identified with routine cytogenetic confirmation. It has been pointed out that in a prenatal population with a risk of aneuploidy of 1/270 or higher, a sensitivity of 97–98% can be obtained with an assumption of normal results for all samples, and that the real accuracy rate is the ability to detect aneuploidies, not normals, and that rate was only 73% [15]. Additionally, aneuploidies account only for 50–70% of the anomalies detected at prenatal diagnosis [16]. Structural chromosome rearrangements have been found with high resolution chromosome banding in as many as 0.9% in an advanced maternal age population, with 70% of these familial and unknown to families at the time of prenatal diagnosis. Although this risk is higher than the risk of aneuploidy for a 35-year-old woman, the consequences of a structural chromosome rearrangement are not equal to the consequences of aneuploidy; but the standard of care has not been to ignore them.

Whole chromosome paints have not proved as useful for prenatal aneuploidy detection. Kuo *et al.* [17] constructed whole chromosome paints from chromosome specific libraries in plasmids for chromosome 13, 18 and 21. The chromosome number was correctly identified in 20 of 20 metaphase samples, and in 43 of 43 interphase samples of cultured amniocytes. However, the acrocentric chromosomes of 13, 18 and 21 showed significant satellite association in the region of the nucleolus and as a result only about 50% of trisomic cells had three discrete signals.

A clinical role for FISH in prenatal diagnosis is probably not in debate. It has been shown to be a rapid and relatively accurate technique for aneuploidy detection. Fundamentally, the issue is not whether, but how, to adopt a diagnostic test with less accuracy because of rapid results and patient anxiety. There is precedence for this approach, as similar findings were seen with the use of CVS and direct villus preparations. These studies showed a mosaic rate, false-positive rate and false-negative rate higher than traditional cytogenetics [11]. There will be a role for FISH as an adjunctive tool for prioritizing samples in the laboratory and as a screening tool in pregnancies at very high risk for aneuploidy by virtue of age, triple analyte screen or ultrasound findings [15]. How and when these results should be transmitted to the patient or physician remains a troubling issue.

73.4.2 MICRODELETION SYNDROMES

Contiguous gene syndromes, also referred to as microdeletion syndromes or segmental aneusomy, were first described by Schmickel in 1986 [1]. These syndromes involve a deletion of a continuous stretch of DNA on a chromosome and usually include the deletion of multiple genes. These syndromes have been better defined over the last several years because of the application of molecular cytogenetics. Many of these syndromes, most of which are sporadic, were clinically recognized prior to the determination of their cytogenetic or molecular basis.

(a)   Critical regions

The deletion in some patients can be detected utilizing high resolution chromosomes; however, many can only be detected with FISH or by detecting submicroscopic deletions with Southern blots and DNA probes. The critical region is the smallest deleted region consistently associated with the syndrome or phenotype. At least 18 syndromes that fall into this category have now been described [18,19]. The more common syndromes include: aniridia–Wilms' tumor association (AWTA), Miller–Dieker syndrome (MDS), Prader–Willi syndrome (PWS), Angelman's syndrome (AS) and DiGeorge's syndrome (DGS). AWTA is a syndrome which involves a deletion in the short arm of chromosome 11 (11p 13). Findings in this disorder encompass several different and unrelated organ systems including: kidney (Wilms' tumor), eye (aniridia), genitalia and urinary system (genitourinary dysplasia), along with mental handicap. The DiGeorge syndrome involves abnormalities in the development of the third and fourth branchial arches, leading to thymic hypoplasia, parathyroid hypoplasia and conotruncal heart defects. Additionally, facial dysmorphology and hypocalcemia can be found. Approximately 30% of the cases show a cytogenetic deletion in chromosome 22 (22q11). However, with the use of both FISH and molecular techniques 83% of these patients can be shown to have a deletion. Molecular techniques have also demonstrated a deletion in 22q11 in 68% of the patients with the velocardiofacial syndrome (which has some overlapping features of the DiGeorge syndrome) and surprisingly in 29% of the isolated (non-syndromic) cases of patients with conotruncal heart defects [20,21]. In Miller–Dieker syndrome, a syndrome involving mental

1126

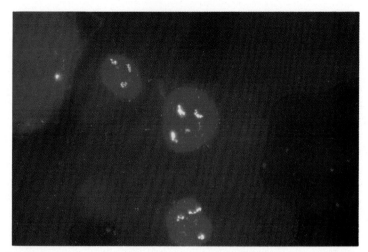

Figure 73.2 Interphase cells from an amniotic fluid sample using FISH. Cells have been labeled with an α-satellite probe from Oncor Inc D18Z1 and digoxigenin. This fetus had trisomy 18 and demonstrates three discrete signals.

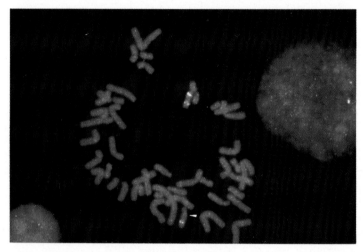

Figure 73.3 A metaphase preparation of a patient with Prader–Willi syndrome. Probe D15S11 for the critical region of Prader–Willi/Angelman syndrome (15q11-q13) was used in this FISH preparation. The probe does not hybridize to the chromosome with the paternally inherited deletion (arrow) on the long arm of chromosome 15. The second pair of signals are from the PML chromosome 15 control probe (15q22) which hybridized to both chromosome 15s. Both probes are from Oncor Inc.

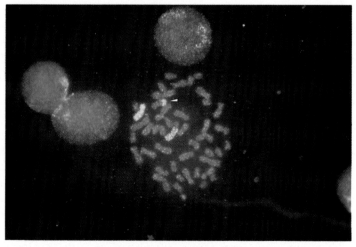

Figure 73.4 A metaphase preparation from an infant with multiple congenital abnormalities. The traditional karyotype showed additional material had been translocated on to the long arm of chromosome 11 (46,XY,11q+). Using FISH with probe WCP^{TM}4 the additional material was identified as a duplication from chromosome 4.

handicap, facial dysmorphology and lissencephaly, a deletion in 17p13 has been detected. Using FISH, deletions have been detected in 92% of the patients with this syndrome, whereas a deletion using FISH has been seen in 20% of the patients with isolated lissencephaly [22]. All of these studies indicate the involvement of multiple genes in these syndromes and the utility of FISH in diagnosing the deletions.

(b) Uniparental disomy and imprinting

Prader–Willi syndrome and Angelman syndrome are two contiguous gene syndromes which exemplify the complexity of these disorders. Both involve a similar deletion in the proximal long arm of chromosome 15 (15q11–q13); however, if the deletion is paternally inherited the child will have PWS, whereas if the deletion is maternally inherited the child will have AS. This phenomenon is called imprinting. Imprinting is the diferential transcription of DNA segments in the fetus depending on whether it has been inherited from the mother or the father. Approximately 72% of the patients with PWS and 74% of the patients with AS demonstrate deletions (from the paternal or maternal chromosome 15, respectively) [23]. Many of these deletions can be detected with high resolution chromosome banding; however, some can only be detected with FISH, using the appropriate critical region probes from the proximal long arm of chromosome 15 (Figure 73.3). Molecular genetic studies of DNA polymorphisms eventually explained why some of the PWS and AS patients failed to show deletions. Approximately 23% of the patients with PWS demonstrate uniparental disomy, an unusual form of inheritance where both copies of chromosome 15 were inherited from the mother and no copy of chromosome 15 from the father. Therefore, even though this individual has two normal no. 15 chromosomes, no paternal specific product for genes in the PWS/AS region have been produced and they demonstrate Prader–Willi syndrome. Similarly, 4% of the AS patients also appear to have uniparental disomy (with two paternally derived no. 15 chromosomes). In one unusual case, trisomy 15 was detected at CVS and a follow-up amniocentesis revealed a normal karyotype. After birth, the child was diagnosed with PWS and subsequent molecular testing demonstrated uniparental disomy with two maternal no. 15 chromosomes [24]. Thus the cells in the villus sample contained two maternally derived no. 15 chromosomes and one paternally derived no. 15, whereas the cells in the amniotic fluid contained only the two maternally derived no. 15 chromosomes (losing the one paternally derived no. 15).

73.4.3 STRUCTURAL REARRANGEMENT

With the advent of chromosome banding, many unusual chromosome rearrangements could be identified and characterized. These rearrangements, however, tended to be large and obvious. Small complex rearrangements and small duplications and deletions often went unrecognized. FISH has significantly expanded the ability of cytogeneticists to analyze complex chromosome rearrangements.

(a) Cryptic and complex rearrangements

Fluorescence in situ hybridization with both unique sequence probes and chromosome specific DNA libraries provides an excellent method of characterizing karyotypic abnormalities (Figure 73.4). Plasmid libraries [25] specific for the 24 human chromosomes are now available, as are multiple specific unique sequence probes, and both have been used to identify chromosomes involved in subtle translocations [26] and to clarify complex karyotypes in solid tumours [27]. In addition, there have been several examples of complex rearrangements that have only been delineated after utilization of FISH. Most have involved three chromosome rearrangements, where the involvement of one of the chromosomes could only be detected with FISH. In addition, these libraries by themselves or in conjunction with cosmid probes have been used to identify cryptic translocations [22]. These cryptic translocations are usually initially identified as a deletion; however, with the use of the appropriate cosmid probes or chromosomal libraries, they have been delineated as unbalanced (or cryptic) translocations. This has been found for several cases involving 17p (in conjunction with Miller–Dieker syndrome) and others involving 4p (in conjunction with Wolf–Hirschhorn syndrome) [22].

(b) Marker chromosomes

Small accessory, or 'marker', chromosomes are estimated to occur in 0.05% of livebirths [28]. Occasionally, marker chromosomes are identified in clinically normal individuals but, more typically, they are found in individuals with multiple congenital abnormalities, including mental handicap. Little is known concerning the exact structure or the precise phenotypic–karyotypic correlations for most of these markers. Studies to elucidate their genetic significance are hindered by the fact that, although cytogenetically indistinguishable, they may indeed derive from different sources. Identifying the origin of this chromosomal material, which cannot be determined using conventional banding techniques, remains one of the major difficulties of clinical cytogenetics. Classification of such marker chromosomes is important for establishing phenotype–karyotype correlations.

One of the most obvious examples of this is in

patients with 45,X/46,X,+mar. These patients are at an increased risk for gonadal malignancy when the marker is derived from the Y chromosome. FISH is the easiest, most reliable and most effective technique for identifying marker chromosomes. A total of 51 sex chromosome markers studied with FISH have been reported [for a review see reference 29]. Approximately half of the patients (24/51; 47%) studied with FISH were ascertained because they had phenotypes suggestive of Turner syndrome. Although a 45,X karyotype is the most frequent cytogenetic finding in patients with Turner syndrome, it is estimated that 40–50% of patients with Turner syndrome demonstrate sex chromosomal mosaicism and 3–15% possess a second cell line containing an unidentified marker (or ring) chromosome. Of the 24 markers from patients with Turner syndrome which have been analyzed using FISH, 19 were X-derived (13 with a ring X and six with a marker X), and five were Y-derived (four with dicentric Y chromosome and one with a ring Y chromosome).

FISH has also been used to identify over 150 supernumerary autosomal marker chromosomes of unknown origin. These included over 75 cases with a satellited marker chromosome and more than 75 cases with a non-satellited marker chromosome. The results from these studies show that the majority of our non-satellited autosomal markers originate from chromosome 18 (50%) and that most of the satellite markers are derived from chromosome 15 (57%) [30].

73.5   Conclusion

The application of molecular cytogenetic techniques to clinical practice has broadened the scope of cytogenetic diagnoses. FISH has proven indispensable in the evaluation of subtle or cryptic chromosome rearrangements and previously unidentified marker chromosomes. With the identification of additional microdeletion syndromes and their 'critical regions' that are consistently associated with the syndrome, FISH is becoming the standard of care for syndrome diagnosis. Uniparental disomy and genomic imprinting have been shown to cause significant genetic morbidity and represent a new form of non-mendelian inheritance. Now that FISH has been clinically applied in prenatal programs for routine aneuploidy, the time required for diagnosis has been significantly shortened.

The extent to which molecular cytogenetic techniques and FISH become part of routine cytogenetics remains to be seen. A recent survey by the American College of Pathologists and the American Society of Human Genetics shows that only 45% of the cytogenetic laboratories surveyed are using FISH [15]. However, there is no question that FISH will have a significant impact on cytogenetic testing and prenatal diagnosis. Newer technologies of diagnosis such as preimplantation genetic diagnosis and the isolation of fetal cells from the maternal circulation are now possible because of these advances in molecular cytogenetics.

References

1. Schimckel, R.D. (1986) Contiguous gene syndromes: a component of recognizable syndromes. *J. Pediatr.*, **109**, 231–41.
2. Pardue, M.L. and Gall, J.G. (1970) Chromosomal localization of mouse satellite DNA. *Science*, **168**, 1356–58.
3. Pardue, M.L., Gerbie, S.A., Eckhardt, R.A. and Gall, J.G. (1970) Cytological localization of DNA complementary to ribosomal RNA in polytene chromosomes in Diptera. *Chromosoma*, **29**, 268–69.
4. Henderson, A.S., Warburton, D. and Atwood, K.C. (1972) Location of rDNA in the human chromosome complement. *Proc. Natl Acad. Sci. USA*, **69**, 3394–98.
5. Ried, T., Landes, G., Dackowski, W. *et al.* (1992) Multicolor fluorescence *in situ* hybridization for the simultaneous detection of probe sets for chromosomes 13, 18, 21, X, and Y in uncultured amniotic fluid cells. *Hum. Mol. Genet.*, **1**, 307–13.
6. Willard, H.F. (1985) Chromosome-specific organization of human alpha satellite DNA. *Am. J. Hum. Genet.*, **37**, 524–32.
7. Devilee, P., Cremer, T., Slagboom, P. *et al.* (1986) Two subsets of human alphoid repetitive DNA show distinct preferential localization in the pericentromeric regions of chromosome 13, 18, and 21. *Cytogenet. Cell Genet.*, **41**, 193–201.
8. Pinkel, D., Landegent, J., Collins, C. *et al.* (1988) Fluorescence *in situ* hybridization with human chromosome-specific libraries: detection of trisomy 21 and translocation of chromosome 4. *Proc. Natl Acad. Sci. USA*, **8**, 9138–42.
9. Manuelidis, L. (1985) Individual interphase chromosome domains revealed by *in situ* hybridization. *Hum. Genet.*, **71**, 288–93.
10. Pinkel, D., Straume, T. and Gray, J.W. (1986) Cytogenetic analysis using quantitative, high-sensitivity, fluorescence hybridization. *Proc. Natl Acad. Sci. USA*, **85**, 2934–38.
11. Ledbetter, D.H. (1992) The 'colorizing' of cytogenetics: is it ready for prime time? *Hum. Mol. Genet.*, **1**, 297–99.
12. Klinger, K., Landes, G., Shook, D. *et al.* (1992) Rapid detection of chromosome aneuploidies in uncultured amniocytes by using fluorescence *in situ* hybridization (FISH). *Am. J. Hum. Genet.*, **51**, 55–65.
13. Benn, P., Ciarleglio, L., Lettieri, L. *et al.* (1992) A rapid (but wrong) prenatal diagnosis. *N. Engl. J. Med.*, **326**, 1638–40.
14. Ward, B., Gersen, S.L., Carelli, M.P. *et al.* (1993) Rapid prenatal diagnosis of chromosomal aneuploidies by fluorescence *in situ* hybridization: clinical experience with 4500 specimens. *Am. J. Hum. Genet.*, **52**, 854–56.
15. Schwartz, S. (1993) Efficacy and applicability of interphase fluorescence *in situ* hybridization for prenatal diagnosis. *Am. J. Hum. Genet.*, **52**, 851–53.
16. Clark, B., Kennedy, K. and Olson, S. (1993) The need to reevaluate trisomy screening for advanced maternal age in prenatal diagnosis. *Am. J. Obstet. Gynecol.*, **168**, 812–16.
17. Kuo, W.-L., Tenjin, H., Segraves, R. *et al.* (1991). Detection of aneuploidy involving chromosomes 13, 18, or 21, by fluorescence *in situ* hybridization (FISH) to interphase and metaphase amniocytes. *Am. J. Hum. Genet.*, **49**, 112–19.
18. Greenberg, F. (1993) Contiguous gene syndromes. *Growth Genet. Horm.*, **9**, 5–10.
19. Ballabio, A. (1991) Contiguous deletion syndromes. *Curr. Opin. Genet. Dev.*, **1**, 25–29.
20. Hall, J. (1993) Catch 22. *J. Med. Genet.*, **30**, 801–802.
21. Greenberg, F. (1993) DiGeorge syndrome: an historical review of clinical and cytogenetic features. *J. Med. Genet.*, **30**, 803–806.
22. Kuwano, A., Ledbetter, S.A., Dobyns, W.B. *et al.* (1991) Detection of deletions and cryptic translocations in Miller–Dieker syndrome by *in situ* hybridization. *Am. J. Hum. Genet.*, **49**, 707–14.
23. Nichols, R.D. (1993) Genomic imprinting and candidate genes in the Prader–Willi and Angelman syndromes. *Curr. Opin. Genet. Dev.*, **3**, 445–56.
24. Cassidy, S.B., Lai, L.W., Erickson, R.P. *et al.* (1992) Trisomy 15 with loss of the paternal 15 as a cause of Prader–Willi syndrome due to maternal disomy. *Am. J. Hum. Genet.*, **51**, 701–708.
25. Collins, C., Kuo, W.-L., Segraves, R. *et al.* (1991) Construction and characterization of plasmid libraries enriched in sequences from single human chromosomes. *Genomics*, **11**, 997–1006.
26. Sullivan, B., Leana-Cox, J., Belt, M. and Schwartz, S. (1993) Characterization of reciprocal translocations using chromosome-specific DNA libraries. *Am. J. Med. Genet.*, **47**, 223–30.

27. Smit, V.T., Wessels, J.W., Mollevanger, P. *et al.* (1990) Combined GTG-banding and nonradioactive *in situ* hybridization improves characterization of complex karyotypes. *Cytogenet. Cell Genet.*, **54**, 20–23.

28. Buckton, K.E., O'Riordan, M.L., Ratcliffe, S. *et al.* (1980) A G-band study of chromosomes in liveborn infants. *Ann. Hum. Genet.*, **43**, 227–39.

29. Schwartz, S., Depinet, T.W., Leana-Cox, J. *et al.* (1993) Sex chromosome markers: characterization using fluorescance *in situ* hybridization and review of the literature. *Am. J. Med. Genet.* (in press).

30. Schwartz, S., Leana-Cox, J., Depinet, T.W. *et al.* (1993) Identification of supernumary autosomal chromosomes and unbalanced *de novo* rearrangements with FISH; experience with 78 cases. *Am. J. Hum. Genet.* **53** (suppl. 3) 257.

74 BIOCHEMICAL AND MOLECULAR GENETICS

D.A. Applegarth, G.T.N. Besley and L.A. Clarke

74.1 Introduction

Approximately 6000 inherited mendelian phenotypes are recognized in humans [1] and over 200 genes have been causally related to a specific disease-producing biochemical defect. Most of the phenotypes are inherited in an autosomal dominant manner, where the biochemical defect may be only partial (single gene dose), and in most of these diseases the underlying metabolic or expressed defect is not yet recognized. However, of the 800 or so recessive disorders the primary biochemical defect has now been identified in some 300 disorders. For these diseases, specific diagnostic tests are now available and in many instances treatment can also be provided. The mutant gene product may be a protein having one of a variety of functions. In this chapter we are concerned particularly with those disorders in which the defect is an inherited enzyme deficiency.

The clinical expression of metabolic disorders may be remarkably varied, and, even for specific diseases, phenotypic heterogeneity is common. In the fetus or newborn, features may be particularly difficult to recognize and selection of suitable diagnostic tests may often be difficult.

When a specific enzyme deficiency gives rise to accumulation of metabolites which are permeable and of low molecular weight, these may leak to the extracellular space and be measurable. If they are of high molecular weight they may accumulate within tissues as storage products, leading to cellular vacuolation and organomegaly. Low molecular weight metabolites in plasma or urine can be identified by many techniques, including bacterial growth inhibition [2], thin-layer or paper chromatography [3], and gas chromatography, often coupled to mass spectrometry [4]. The biochemical investigation of these disorders is discussed in section 74.3. Large molecule disorders are discussed in sections dealing with lysosomal storage diseases and glycogenoses. Space does not allow us to discuss all the various inherited metabolic disorders but most are listed in the Appendix 74.A. For further information the reader is referred to a number of useful reference works [1,5–7].

Because there is often the possibility of subsequent prenatal diagnosis, a skin biopsy should usually be taken to establish a culture not only from the proband but also from the parents. These fibroblasts are then available for future investigations and to provide intrafamily controls during prenatal studies. This is particularly important in those families where low enzyme activities in heterozygotes may give rise to difficulties in interpreting results. Because viable cells may be maintained for many years (at least 17, in our experience) in liquid nitrogen, it may also be possible to establish retrospective diagnoses in the light of subsequent research. Even if the metabolic defect is not expressed in cultured cells, these may still be useful in providing a ready source of genomic DNA (Chapters 76 and 77). However, establishing a fibroblast culture is costly and some form of selectivity must operate, such as by storing biopsies [8] until results of other tests are available, especially in cases of unexplained death.

Careful consideration should always be given to the type of sample that is required for enzyme assay. Tissue or subcellular distribution of an enzyme, its stability and the presence of isoenzymes under separate genetic control may all influence the choice and handling of samples. Some enzymes are tissue specific. For example ornithine carbamoyl transferase may only be measured in liver; myophosphorylase, as the name implies, only in skeletal muscle; histidase in skin and liver; and testosterone 5α-reductase in genital skin. Some enzymes associated with cellular or mitochondrial membranes may be highly labile or sensitive to freeze–thawing, such as the liver translocases deficient in glycogenosis types Ib and Ic [9]. Where artificial substrates are used, enzyme activities not specific for the diagnosis may interfere with assays; for example the appearance of hexosaminidase B during pregnancy may compromise

Diseases of the Fetus and Newborn, 2nd edn, Edited by G.B. Reed, A.E. Claireaux and F. Cockburn. Published in 1995 by Chapman & Hall, London. ISBN 0 412 39160 0

carrier detection of Tay–Sachs disease [10], or the 'renal' α-glucosidase in granulocytes may mask the underlying deficiency in Pompe disease (glycogenosis type II) [11,12]. For these and other reasons the laboratory should be consulted before samples are obtained for assay.

It is often a good idea to collect a tissue sample for DNA analysis for future assays and potential family studies. Frozen blood or blood on blood spot screening cards may be sufficient but for some diseases one may need blood from family members. There are ethical and legal issues concerning banking of DNA samples so local and national guidelines must be observed.

74.2 Biochemical investigation of small molecule diseases

Small molecule diseases often present with an acute life-threatening episode and may, if not diagnosed and treated, lead to unexplained death or a death which is mistakenly attributed to some other cause.

74.2.1 GENERAL BIOCHEMICAL TESTS

A list of general biochemical tests that will lead to the diagnosis of many perinatal metabolic diseases is shown in Table 74.1 These tests are all likely to be available in most large hospitals. A brief discussion of each of the tests follows but specific diseases will be covered later in separate sections. For a general reference to the principles involved see Applegarth, Dimmick and Toone [13].

(a) Plasma amino acids

Plasma amino acids should be measured on fasting blood (just before a feed in the case of an infant). Primary disorders of amino acid metabolism such as

Table 74.1 Tests needed to detect an acute metabolic disease

Blood	Urine
Blood glucose	Reducing substances by a non-specific reducing sugar assay (alkaline copper method)
Plasma amino acids	Glucose (specific test for glucose only)
Blood ammonia	Organic acids
Some measure of metabolic acidosis (serum electrolytes or blood base excess)	
Plasma lactate	

phenylketonuria and maple syrup urine disease can be diagnosed immediately but in addition there are useful non-specific secondary changes in the amino acid pattern which indicate the presence of other disease. For instance, increased plasma glycine heightens suspicion of a disorder of organic acid metabolism, and increased tyrosine and/or methionine suggest liver disease. An increase in plasma glutamine should suggest an ammonia assay. Increases in many amino acids together suggest, among other causes, mitochondrial dysfunction (including Reye syndrome or 'shock') [14]. Many laboratories measure urine amino acids and while this can be a useful screen it will not detect modest, but diagnostically important, increases in glycine, glutamine or alanine, etc.

(b) Blood ammonia

Children with a urea cycle disorder may present with an acute life-threatening episode. The finding of high blood ammonia should always be followed by plasma amino acid analysis. Specific diseases of the urea cycle may be recognizable by characteristic amino acid patterns (see below).

(c) Blood gases and electrolytes

Evidence of metabolic acidosis could come from plasma electrolyte or arterial blood gas determinations. In sick infants, the anion gap should be determined. Those with an increased anion gap should have blood gas determinations done to confirm an increased (negative) base excess. The most common cause of metabolic acidosis is lactic acidosis, often secondary to conditions such as liver disease or 'shock'. It is always advisable to measure blood lactate when metabolic acidosis is encountered. In the absence of a high lactate concentration we suggest identifying the acids by examining the urinary organic acid pattern. Some disorders of organic acids cause an appreciable odour from the urine but not all smells can be related to organic acids. One cause of foul smelling urine is trimethylamine and this is probably a benign entity [15]. Hyperammonaemia can present as primary respiratory alkalosis caused by the effect of ammonia on the respiratory centre. Therefore unexplained respiratory alkalosis indicates the need for blood ammonia measurement.

(d) Urinary reducing substances

The ultimate aim of this test is to diagnose galactosaemia and one way to diagnose this disease is to look for urine-reducing substances. If the urine does not then react with a glucose-specific test, galactosaemia is suspected. The presence of galactose in the urine can be confirmed later by sugar chromatography. Unfortunately infants with this disease are often receiving only dextrose/water infusions and the diagnostic test depends on the child being fed milk. If the child is not on milk, galactose is not excreted. This topic is dealt with more fully in section 74.2.4(c).

74.2.2 DISORDERS OF ORGANIC ACID METABOLISM

The organic acidaemias are disorders of amino acid metabolism. The metabolic block in the catabolism of amino acids or pyruvate is due to a primary enzymopathy or is secondary to co-factor disturbances. The metabolites in these disorders are short chain acids (up to approximately 12–14 carbon atoms) formed after the amino group has been removed. They are non-reactive with ninhydrin and are not detected by amino acid screening. Gas–liquid chromatography and gas chromatography/mass spectrophotometry are required for diagnosis. Some diseases such as maple syrup urine disease may be classified as either an amino acidopathy or an organic acidopathy.

The organic acidaemias may present in the newborn as acute fulminant disorder, or later in infancy or childhood. In the neonate, severe central nervous system dysfunction including seizures, disordered tonicity and coma can occur, coupled with vomiting sometimes mimicking pyloric stenosis. Older infants may fail to thrive [16,17]. Odours can be a feature of some of the organic acidaemias. Accumulated metabolites can suppress bone marrow precursor cells, resulting in neutropenia, thrombocytopenia and sometimes anaemia [18].

In this chapter we shall discuss only representative examples of organic acid diseases. We have chosen to discuss propionic and methylmalonic acidaemias because they are relatively common, and isovaleric acidaemia as an example of a disease which causes a distinctive odour. Our discussion of the rest of the organic acid disorders, with the exception of pyruvic and lactic acids, will be rather sparse and we recommend review articles [4,19], but we will try to comment on how to interpret some of the more difficult organic acid reports that might be received from a laboratory.

(a) Propionic acidaemia and methylmalonic acidaemia

Propionic acidaemia and methylmalonic acidaemia are clinically similar disorders resulting from defects in the catabolic pathway of isoleucine [20]. In the newborn infant both disorders produce an acute fulminant disease with vomiting, hypotonia, respiratory distress, seizures, coma and death. Modest hepatomegaly is often recorded. Biochemically, affected infants are severely acidotic, usually ketotic and have variably elevated levels of ammonia (due to suppression of carbamoyl-phosphate synthetase, probably by interference in N-acetylglutamate synthesis). Hypoglycaemia, due to interference of gluconeogenesis, also occurs and hyperglycinaemia is usually present. Propionic acid and its derivatives accumulate in urine and plasma of patients with propionic acidaemia and methylmalonic acid and its derivatives are found in methylmalonic acidaemia. Ketone bodies may be long chain (butanone) or the conventional acetoacetate and acetone. Patients with either disease may have thrombocytopenia, neutropenia or anaemia.

Both entities can be caused by problems associated with co-factors (biotin or cobalamin). Both are inherited in an autosomal recessive fashion and can be diagnosed by enzyme analysis using leucocytes or cultured fibroblasts [20]. Prenatal diagnosis is possible for these diseases but, unfortunately, there is much heterogeneity in the specific enzyme defects. In the case of propionic acidaemia (propionyl-CoA carboxylase deficiency), patients can be classified into at least two complementation groups, A or C. Cell lines are said to be in different complementation groups if their metabolic defect is corrected by cell fusion with a cell line from another patient with the same metabolic disease. This demonstrates that the pathogenesis underlying the disease is actually different in the two cell lines. Carriers of the group C trait have completely normal enzyme activity and carrier detection is not possible. In methylmalonic acidaemia there are several enzyme defects, usually involving methylmalonyl-CoA mutase. Since the enzyme propionyl-CoA carboxylase requires biotin as its cofactor and methylmalonyl-CoA mutase requires deoxyadenosylcobalamin, there is also a series of disorders involving metabolism of both of these cofactors and their interaction with the apoenzymes involved. The elucidation of specific defects is important because vitamin therapy using biotin or cobalamin is possible for some of these patients [19,20]. The genes for the apoenzymes propionyl-CoA carboxylase and methylmalonyl-CoA carboxylase have been identified. Two mutations in the B-subunit of propionyl-Co-A carboxylase have been found to account for a significant number of alleles in the C complementation group. These mutations are a three base pair deletion and a 14 base pair deletion with 12 added bases [21,22]. A mutation of the leader sequence of the apoenzyme methylmalonyl-Co-A mutase has been described, as have many informative polymorphisms of the gene [23–25].

Multiple carboxylase deficiency results from errors in biotin metabolism resulting in deficient activites of at least three carboxylases, namely pyruvate, propionyl-CoA and 3-methylcrotonoyl-CoA. The respective organic acid metabolites are found in urine. This defect is the cause of one form of propionic acidaemia. In the neonatal form of multiple carboxylase deficiency, acidosis, ketosis, hyperammonaemia, hypoglycaemia, hyperglycinaemia, coma, seizures and an erythematous rash occur. A tom-cat odour to the urine (methylcrotonic acid) may be noted. In fibroblast culture the carboxylase enzyme activities are low but enhanced in the presence of increased concentrations of biotin [26,27] in culture medium. Accordingly, leucocyte assay may be preferred. One of the causes of this group of diseases is a deficiency of biotinidase, an enzyme involved in 'recycling' of biotin for metabolic needs [28]. Similar symptoms have been seen, in a less severe form, when biotin deficiency was inadvertently caused by parenteral alimentation [27].

(b) Isovaleric acidaemia

Deficiency of isovaleryl-CoA dehydrogenase, an enzyme in the catabolism of leucine, accounts for this organic acidaemia. Clinical presentation, like that of propionic and methylmalonic acidaemia, includes an acute fulminant form in the newborn. The presentation may be identical but there is the significant additional finding of an odour of sweaty feet on the infant's breath or urine. In the acute attack, isovaleric acid levels increase in plasma, and metabolites of isovaleryl-CoA accumulate. Definitive diagnosis requires demonstration of the enzyme deficiency in fibroblast culture or leucocytes [29].

(c) Dicarboxylic aciduria and glutaric aciduria

A common problem is interpretation of dicarboxylic aciduria which can often be found when a patient is acutely ill. It is a non-specific consequence of defective mitochondrial β-oxidation [19] and arises from the fact that any fatty acids not oxidized by mitochondria will be metabolized by the microsomal P450 system from the omega (far end of the chain from the carboxylic acid) end of the fatty acid. This omega oxidation produces dicarboxylic acids such as adipic (six carbons), suberic (eight carbons) and sebacic (ten carbons) acids.

An excretion pattern which shows $C_6 > C_8 > C_{10}$ is typical for patients with medium and long chain acyl-CoA dehydrogenase (MCAD and LCAD) deficiencies. These can present with a Reye-like syndrome, myopathy or cardiomyopathy. MCAD deficiency is discussed below. Patients fed a diet rich in medium chain triglyceride oil also have dicarboxylic aciduria but one in which $C_{10} > C_8 > C_6$.

The presence of glutaric acid in a dicarboxylic aciduria pattern usually suggests some form of multiple acyl-CoA dehydrogenase deficiency (so-called glutaric aciduria type II). The milder forms of these conditions are called ethylmalonic–adipic aciduria. If the patient excretes glutaric acid and metabolites other than dicarboxylic acids, glutaric aciduria type I (a deficiency of glutaryl-CoA dehydrogenase) may be suspected.

Glutaric aciduria type II can present in the newborn infant. This disease may result from more than one biochemical defect and can have a fulminant course [30]. Affected infants have liver dysfunction with elevated transaminases, hyperbilirubinaemia, hyperammonaemia, acidosis, hypoglycaemia and an odour of sweaty feet. The phenotype may be similar to the cerebrohepatorenal syndrome of Zellweger [31–33] (section 74.2.5).

Glutaric aciduria type I is a separate disease involving mitochondrial glutaryl-CoA dehydrogenase but enzyme systems for glutaric acid oxidation occur in both mitochondria and peroxisomes [34]. This link with peroxisomal metabolism may account for dysmorphism reported in children with diseases of glutaric acid metabolism (section 74.2.5). Because glutaric acid is so readily excreted in urine, patients with these disorders will not necessarily demonstrate a metabolic acidosis and, in addition, the excretion of glutaric acid is quite variable.

Other disorders of fatty acid oxidation which can present with dicarboxylic aciduria have recently attracted much interest [35–37] as a cause of hypoketotic hypoglycaemia giving rise to a familial Reye-like syndrome and sudden unexplained death. Characteristic dicarboxylic acids as well as conjugates such as suberylglycine and octanoylcarnitine may be excreted in the urine. Usually the liver shows marked microvesicular fatty change and a proliferation of peroxisomes. Cultured fibroblasts have a reduced capacity to oxidize fatty acids of short, medium or long chain length, depending on which mitochondrial acyl-CoA dehydrogenase is deficient. The enzyme involved in the dehydrogenation of medium chain fatty acids, MCAD, has been shown to be a dimer of identical subunits. The full length cDNA has been sequenced and one mutation, which creats an NcoI restriction site within the coding region, has been identified to account for over 85% of mutant alleles in the Caucasian population [38,39].

MCAD deficiency is an especially interesting disease from the point of view of DNA diagnosis because over 80% of cases can be identified by looking for one characteristic nucleotide mutation, which is fairly easily diagnosed by using polymerase chain reaction techniques on small amounts of blood or tissue, and it is a good idea to consider this assay whenever the clinical situation is of an unexplained death with steatosis reported at autopsy.

When the organic acid pattern shows increased amounts of ketone bodies one should consider that this could be as a result of ketothiolase deficiency. Such patients excrete β-hydroxybutyric acid and acetoacetic acid but the diagnostic feature of this disease will be the presence of 2-methylacetoacetic acid and 2-methyl-succinic acid [35].

Occasionally some children have an acidosis and an organic acid pattern which is hard to interpret. Often the measurement of acyl carnitines in blood or urine can help. The reason for this is that if there is a defect of fatty acid oxidation, levels of acyl-CoA esters rise consequent to the block in their metabolism and are converted by carnitine acyltransferases to acyl carnitines. These are excreted in the urine and this can even cause a secondary carnitine deficiency syndrome. One can identify many defects of fatty acid oxidation by measuring both esterified and free carnitine in plasma or urine and by identifying the acyl carnitines present [40].

(d) Disorders of pyruvate metabolism

Disorders of pyruvate metabolism have broad phenotypic expression varying from acute severe lactic acidosis in the newborn infant (when this is not caused by perfusion problems or anoxia), to a more long-term metabolic acidosis with psychomotor retardation [41]. Lactic acidosis in the neonate has multiple aetiologies (see also section 74.2.6). Biochemical abnormalities of amino acid, carbohydrate and urea cycle metabolism secondary to the deficiency in pyruvate metabolism complicate the diagnosis [41].

Primary defects of pyruvate oxidation are caused by either pyruvate carboxylase or pyruvate dehydrogenase deficiency. Pyruvate carboxylase is an enzyme necessary for gluconeogenesis. Pyruvate dehydrogenase produces the acetyl-CoA used by the citric acid cycle and the enzyme is necessary for complete oxidation of glucose.

Clinical deterioration may be precipitous in patients with pyruvate dehydrogenase deficiency who are fed a high carbohydrate diet. Deterioration can also occur in pyruvate carboxylase-deficient infants fed a high fat diet. Both enzyme deficiencies may be diagnosed by enzyme assay using cultured skin fibroblasts or lymphocytes [41,42].

Pyruvate carboxylase deficiency is an autosomal recessive disorder with an acute severe neonatal and a milder infantile form. In the former there is no detectable enzyme protein [43]. Pyruvate carboxylase requires biotin and, as discussed earlier, deficiencies may occur with primary or secondary defects of biotin metabolism (multiple carboxylase deficiency or nutritional biotin deficiency). Infants with the fulminant neonatal form have respiratory distress, depressed central nervous system function, seizures, a bleeding diathesis and jaundice. Severe lactic acidosis occurs conjointly with hyperammonaemia, ketosis, hypoglycaemia and elevated levels of citrulline, alanine and lysine. Lactate and ketones appear in the urine. The broader biochemical impact of the neonatal versus the infantile form may be attributed to the inability to produce oxaloacetate directly from pyruvate in the neonatal type, resulting in a compromised urea cycle and redox state [43].

Deficiencies in the pyruvate dehydrogenase complex can also produce a spectrum of clinical presentations, ranging from a fulminant disorder in the newborn infant to less severe lactic acidosis and variable central nervous system dysfunction in the older infant and child. The most common identified cause of pyruvate dehydrogenase deficiency is a deficiency of the E1α subunit of the enzyme. The gene for this subunit has been localized to the X chromosome. Females with this deficiency have extreme variation in phenotype, probably due to lyonization. It is felt that a complete deficiency of this subunit in males is lethal *in utero*. Therefore infant males with E1α defects invariably have partial activity [44–46].

Pyruvate oxidation is affected by many forms of mitochondrial dysfunction and there has been speculation concerning the relationship of Leigh's disease to lactic acidosis. Two groups of authors [47,48] have reported no relationship between Leigh's disease and pyruvate carboxylase deficiency, but Leigh's disease and lactic acidosis may occur in mitochondrial disorders such as cytochrome c oxidase deficiency [49].

74.2.3 DISORDERS OF AMINO ACID METABOLISM

(a) Urea cycle disorders

The urea cycle converts ammonia to urea. The first two enzymes of the cycle occur in the mitochondrion and the rest are in the cytosol. In the first step of the cycle (Figure 74.1) carbamoyl phosphate is formed from ammonia and bicarbonate through the action of carbamoyl-phosphate synthetase I. N-Acetylglutamate (formed from glutamate and acetyl-CoA) is mandatory for proper enzyme function. Hyperammonaemia in the organic acidaemias may be due to interference with N-acetylglutamate formation. Carbamoyl phosphate is also the substrate for carbamoyl-phosphate synthetase II, a cytosol enzyme (which does not require N-acetylglutamate) which is involved in pyrimidine synthesis. Orotic acid is the pre-eminent urinary metabolite from this series of reactions. Any defect resulting in elevated carbamoyl phosphate will shift the substrate to the cytosol pathway and cause an orotic aciduria.

In the second reaction of the urea cycle, ornithine carbamoyltransferase catalyses the formation of citrulline from carbamoyl phosphate and ornithine. Citrulline, transposed to the cytosol, is converted to argininosuccinate and then to arginine. The last enzyme in the sequence, arginase, acts to generate urea and ornithine, which enters the mitochondrion to begin the cycle again. Thus, there are two mitochondrial enzymes and

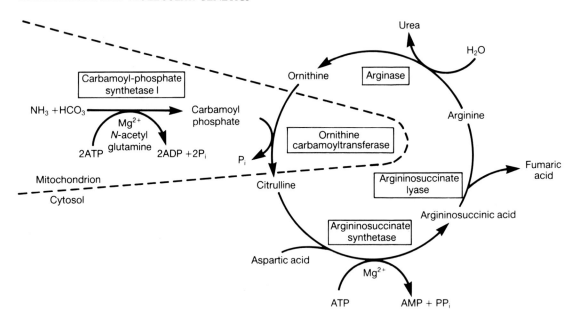

Figure 74.1 Urea cycle showing enzymes involved in inherited defects.

three cytosol enzymes involved in the urea cycle. Deficiency of all but the last, arginase, can result in an acute metabolic disease in the newborn infant [50].

As with other inherited metabolic diseases, varied clinical expressions exist, the most severe forms occurring in the neonate and the less severe chronic or relapsing forms in the older infant. Probably the most severe expression of disease is related to the greatest degree of enzyme deficiency. In the newborn infant, inborn errors of the urea cycle cause hypotonia, lethargy, poor feeding and, more severely, seizures, coma and death. Infants frequently vomit and have respiratory disease. Marked hyperammonaemia is characteristic of all inherited urea cycle disorders presenting in the neonatal period.

Generally the urea cycle disorders are not associated with hypoglycaemia, ketosis, metabolic acidosis or organic aciduria. Respiratory alkalosis should suggest a urea cycle disorder (see earlier). Some brief comments on the specific diseases follow. For specific details of any of the urea cycle disorders a specialized review should be consulted [50].

The genes for each enzyme in the urea cycle have been identified and multiple mutations are described in each. The vast number of possible mutations preclude a direct mutation analysis for prenatal diagnosis but many intragenic markers are described for each locus, thus providing information to families who have already had an affected infant.

Carbamoyl-phosphate synthetase deficiency

Carbamoyl-phosphate synthetase deficiency is an autosomal recessive disorder presenting in the newborn

period. Marked hyperammonaemia is usually associated with diminished plasma citrulline and arginine. Orotic acid in urine is not elevated. There is no organic aciduria. Definitive diagnosis requires enzyme assay on liver tissue. Prenatal diagnosis is feasible through fetal liver biopsy [51] or DNA assay of aminocytes [52]. Although no mutations in the gene have been described to date, prenatal diagnosis by linkage analysis to linked markers close to the gene is possible in families with a previously affected child.

Ornithine carbamoyltransferase deficiency

Ornithine carbamoyltransferase deficiency is an X-linked disorder in which hemizygotic male infants suffer a fulminant neonatal disease. Heterozygotic females may have variable expression of the disease at a later age. Severe hyperammonaemia and marked orotic aciduria occur and there is often a low plasma citrulline level. Enzyme assay on liver biopsy may be done for confirmation. Prenatal dignosis requires fetal liver biopsy [51,53] or DNA analysis of amniocytes [54–56].

Citrullinaemia

Citrullinaemia is due to a deficiency of argininosuccinate synthetase. This is an autosomal recessive disorder which in its neonatal form has a clinical behaviour similar to the other urea cycle disorders. Marked hyperammonaemia with low arginine and very high plasma citrulline occur. There is no argininosuccinic acid present in the urine or plasma and orotic acid output may be mildly increased. Enzyme assays can be carried out on fibroblast culture or amniocytes [57,58] but care should be exercised due to differences in enzyme activity in epitheloid and fibroblastic cultures [59]. Mutations have been described in the gene and linkage studies can be useful in some families [60–62].

Argininosuccinic aciduria

Argininosuccinic aciduria is due to an autosomal recessive deficiency of argininosuccinate lyase. Neonatal, subacute and delayed onset forms occur. Presentation in the newborn is similar to other urea cycle disorders and usually occurs in the first week of life. Arginino-succinic acid can co-elute with isoleucine on many amino acid analysers so the presence of an apparent isoleucinaemia should heighten suspicion of this disease. Older infants may have abnormalities of hair. In the newborn hyperammonaemia coexists with elevated argininosuccinic acid in plasma and urine; plasma citrulline is moderately elevated. Infants may have hepatomegaly and increased transaminase levels. Enzyme assay may be done on fibroblast culture, liver or erythrocytes [50,63,64]. Many mutations and linked markers have been described for this gene.

(b) Tyrosinaemia (type 1, hepatorenal)

Tyrosinaemia is an autosomal recessive error involving fumarylacetoacetate hydrolase, the last enzyme in the degradative pathway of tyrosine [65]. Acute and chronic forms exist; the former is more common and clinically commences soon after birth. Infants fail to thrive, develop hepatomegaly early in the course, with liver dysfunction, jaundice, diarrhoea, vomiting, fever, and may be hypertensive. Most infants die within the acute phase and a few convert to chronic tyrosinaemia. Tyrosinaemia is uncommon in most populations (1 per 100 000–200 000) except in Quebec where the incidence rises to 1 per 685 livebirths [66].

The presence of succinylacetoacetate and succinyl-acetone in these patients provides a useful diagnostic test. Succinylacetone can be detected in urine of patients with this disease by gas–liquid chromatography and mass spectrometry. The succinylaceto-acetate can be converted to succinylacetone by heating the urine samples in a boiling waterbath for 30 minutes. This process greatly increases the size of the succinylacetone peak, making gas chromatographic detection much easier [67,68]. The presence of succinylacetone in amniotic fluid has been used for prenatal diagnosis of the disease and this has been extensively done by the Quebec group in Canada [69, 70]. Neonatal diagnosis by measurement of fumaryl-acetoacetate hydrolase activity in blood spots is possible.

(c) Maple syrup urine disease (branched chain ketoaciduria)

Maple syrup urine disease, initially described by Menkes, Hurst and Craig in 1954 [71], is an autosomal recessive disorder of the catabolism of branched chain amino acids, leucine, isoleucine and valine. Several variants of the disease exist: the most common is a severe disorder of the newborn infant associated with markedly deficient branched chain ketoacid decarboxy-lase activity [72].

Beginning in the latter part of the first week of life the affected infant becomes irritable, fails to feed, vomits, develops alternating hypo- and hypertonicity, may have a high-pitched cry and, as the disease progresses, develops seizures, and ultimately coma and death follow. Severe mental handicap follows if the infant survives. An odour of maple syrup from urine or sweat is present. Diagnosis may be established by studying the decarboxylation by leucocytes or fibro-blasts of branched chain ketoacids, usually by trapping the carbon dioxide produced from radioactive leucine [72]. The enzyme keto acid decarboxylase is complex and contains multiple subunits. The E1α gene has been cloned and sequenced. A specific mutation has been identified in a Mennonite population with thiamine-unresponsive maple syrup urine disease [73]. Other thiamine responsive patients have not shown mutations in the E1α subunit [74].

(d) Non-ketotic hyperglycinaemia

Non-ketotic hyperglycinaemia is an autosomal recess-ive condition in which glycine accumulates in blood, cerebrospinal fluid and brain. It was first described in 1965 [75], and occurs at a frequency of 1:55 000 in both Finland and British Columbia [76]. It can be distinguished from other diseases with secondary hyperglycinaemia (for example, methylmalonic acid-aemia and propionic acidaemia) by the absence of both ketosis and abnormal organic acid excretion. Biochemi-cal diagnosis of the disease is usually made initially by measurement of plasma glycine, but this may be only minimally elevated; cerebrospinal fluid glycine is at least 10 and often 15–30 times elevated [77]. Non-ketotic hyperglycinaemia results in severe mental handi-cap and seizures. It is life threatening in the neonatal period. The disease is heterogeneous and some later-onset patients with mild handicap have been reported. The disorder is characterized by a defective glycine cleavage system in the brain and liver [77,78]. In brain, the glycine cleavage enzyme system is apparently a major degradative pathway for glycine. It is located in mitochondria and has four protein components (P, H, T, L proteins). The enzyme is not expressed in fibroblasts but it can be measured in lymphoblasts [79]. The DNA mutations have now been reported for the

Finnish mutation [80]. However, prenatal diagnosis has been successfully made [81] by measurement of glycine cleavage activity in chorionic villus biopsy tissue. The disease is essentially untreatable, although many attempts have been made. cDNAs have been isolated for the H protein component and one patient has been identified with a significant deletion of a portion of the gene on one allele [82] but the mutations reported are heterogeneous and DNA diagnosis continues to be difficult for this disease.

Various other amino acid disorders, including phenyl-ketonuria, do not present diagnostic problems in the perinatal period and are therefore not discussed here. Many of these are however included in Appendix 74.A.

74.2.4 DISORDERS OF CARBOHYDRATE METABOLISM – FRUCTOSE METABOLISM

Disorders of fructose metabolism in the newborn infant include, foremost, hereditary fructose intolerance, and also, essential fructosuria and fructose-1,6-bisphosph-atase deficiency.

(a) Hereditary fructose intolerance

Hereditary fructose intolerance is inherited in an autosomal recessive manner and is caused by a deficiency of fructose-1-phosphate aldolase B in liver, kidney and intestinal mucosa [83]. Clinical presentation and severity of disease correspond to the introduction of fructose in the diet. Older infants may be difficult to wean from breast milk or thrive poorly and have hepatomegaly. The affected infant, introduced to dietary fructose, develops hepatomegaly, ascites, hepatic failure, jaundice, coagulopathy and vomiting, and may become septic and develop rickets [84–87]. Disseminated intravascular coagulopathy may also occur. The diagnosis in early infancy may be particularly difficult: the florid presentation mimics other acute metabolic diseases such as galactosaemia or tyrosinaemia and can simulate sepsis, which may also be present.

The pathogenesis of hereditary fructose intolerance is well understood. Ingested fructose passes to the liver where it is phosphorylated by ATP to fructose 1-phosphate which is normally converted to dihydroxy-acetone phosphate and glyceraldehyde by fructose-1-phosphate aldolase. This enzyme is deficient in hereditary fructose intolerance. In hereditary fructose intolerance the fructose 1-phosphate level increases, and plasma phosphate levels and cellular (liver) ATP levels fall (even in normal control patients given fructose liver ATP falls following a fructose load [88]). Most of the results of fructose ingestion can be traced to the accumulation of fructose 1-phosphate and decreased levels of ATP and phosphate. The chemical findings, following oral fructose, consist of decreased levels of

plasma phosphate, glucose and potassium, and increased plasma uric acid, lactate, methionine and magnesium. The gene for fructose aldolase has been identified and two mutations, A174P and A149P, are the most common in the Caucasian population and may be useful for early diagnosis of a child with a positive family history [89–92].

(b) Fructose-1,6-bisphosphatase deficiency

Infants with a deficiency of this enzyme also become symptomatic when fructose is introduced into the diet. The enzyme catalyses conversion of fructose-1,6-bisphosphate to fructose 6-phosphate. The disease is also characterized by hypoglycaemia, hepatomegaly and metabolic acidosis. Lactic acidosis and concomitant increases in plasma alanine occur; glycerol levels in plasma and urine may also be increased. The infant may or may not be jaundiced and other liver function tests may be normal [92,93].

(c) Galactosaemia

Classic galactosaemia is an autosomal recessive disorder occurring with a frequency reportedly varying between 1 per 35 000 and 1 per 150 000 births. The enzyme galactose-1-phosphate uridyltransferase is deficient, causing an accumulation of galactose, galactose 1-phosphate and galactitol. These compounds are presumed to be responsible for most aspects of the disease. Galactitol and galactose 1-phosphate in the eye can induce an osmotic effect, ultimately causing cataracts. Galactokinase deficiency, in which no galactose 1-phosphate can be formed directly from galactose, may cause no disease other than cataracts. Variants of galactosaemia exist but classic galactosaemia is the one of major concern in the newborn infant. Defects in galactose metabolism have been reviewed [95] and first trimester diagnosis has been reported [96]. The gene for galactose-1-phosphate uridyltransferase has been isolated and mutations have been identified for some classical patients. The early data would suggest that there are many different mutations for classical deficiency [97,98].

On exposure to lactose, enzyme-deficient newborn infants fail to thrive, develop vomiting and diarrhoea and quickly show evidence of severe liver injury. Sepsis, particularly with *Escherichia coli*, is common and in part is attributed to depressed neutrophil function by galactose. Infants may also develop a haemorrhagic diathesis, haemolysis, acidosis, aminoaciduria, proteinuria and, if recently exposed to lactose, will have galactosuria, as indicated by a positive Benedict test.

Comments on the diagnosis of galactosaemia by using urine-reducing sugar tests have been made in the first part of this chapter. Cases of unexplained severe neonatal jaundice in whom galactosaemia is suspected may however be diagnosed rapidly by sending a blood spot card to a screening programme which is doing the galactosaemia test. If the normal phenylketonuria card has been sent to such a programme this will be all that is needed. If there is no convenient screening laboratory carrying out the galactosaemia test, a test-tube assay for red cell galactose-1-phosphate uridyltransferase should be done. Neither blood test is reliable if the child has received a packed red blood cell transfusion during the previous 6 months. In our experience galactosaemic infants present with unexplained unconjugated hyperbilirubinaemia and in these children urine tests would not have been reliable because the infants were not receiving milk and therefore would not have been excreting galactose. A newborn screening programme is invaluable in diagnosing these patients. Newborn screening programmes often measure galactose phosphate on the blood spot card and our experience suggests that this metabolite remains in high concentration in red blood cells after the urine galactose has (relatively soon after cessation of milk feeding) become undetectable.

74.2.5 DISORDERS OF PEROXISOMAL FUNCTION

Much current interest is focused on the involvement of peroxisomes in a variety of metabolic disorders. These cellular organelles, primarily involved in various oxidative functions, were originally implicated in human disease when they were found to be deficient in patients with Zellweger syndrome [99]. Patients present at birth with characteristic craniofacial dysmorphism, profound hypotonia and other neurological and ocular manifestations. These infants also have hepatomegaly, renal cysts and a variety of other features [100,101], which generally lead to death in the first year. Biochemical abnormalities include accumulations of very long chain fatty acids, bile acid intermediates, phytanic acid, pipecolic acid and dicarboxylic acids, all normally oxidized in the peroxisome. There is also a lack of plasmalogen biosynthesis due to deficiencies of two key peroxisomal enzymes [102,103]. Patients with Zellweger syndrome, neonatal (autosomal recessive) adrenoleucodystrophy, infantile Refsum disease and hyperpipecolic acidaemia are all deficient in peroxisomes and exhibit many similar clinical features. The genetic relationship of these disorders is not yet understood. Nevertheless, diagnosis of this group of diseases may be accomplished by plasma or fibroblast very long (usually 26 carbons) chain fatty acid analysis, as well as dihydroxyacetone-phosphate acyltransferase (DHAP-AT) assay and the demonstration of increased levels in plasma of the various metabolites mentioned above. It is felt that this group of disorders is caused by

Table 74.2 Peroxisomal disorders

Group	Electron microscopic assessment of peroxisomes	Enzymopathy
1. Failed peroxisomal biogenesis		
Cerebrohepatorenal syndrome	Deficient	Multiple
Neonatal adrenoleucodystrophy	Deficient	Multiple
Infantile Refsum disease	Deficient	Multiple
Hyperpipecolic acidaemia	Deficient	Multiple
2. Multiple enzyme deficiencies		
Rhizomelic chondrodysplasia punctata	Irregular hepatic distribution/normal	Multiple
Zellweger-like syndrome	Normal	Multiple
3. Single enzyme deficiencies		
X-linked adrenoleucodystrophy	Normal	Very long chain fatty acyl-CoA synthetase/transporter
Pseudo-Zellweger syndrome	Enlarged	Thiolase
Pseudo-neonatal adrenoleucodystrophy	Enlarged	Acyl-CoA oxidase
Bifunctional protein deficiency	Normal	Bifunctional protein
Acatalasaemia	Normal	Catalase
Hyperoxaluria type 1	?Normal	Alanine:glycosylate aminotransferase
Glutaric oxidase deficiency	?Normal	Glutaric acid oxidase
Isolated dihydroxyacetone phosphate acyl transferase deficiency	?Normal	Dihydroxyacetone phosphate acyl transferase

defects of peroxisomal assembly. One such gene, peroxisome assembly factor 1, has been isolated and a homozygous non-sense mutation in this integral membrane protein gene has been identified as a cause of Zellweger syndrome in an individual patient [104].

Patients with the rhizomelic form of chondrodysplasia punctata are also deficient in DHAP-AT activity as well as phytanic acid oxidase. As a result patients have low levels of tissue plasmalogens but increased plasma phytanic acid [105]. Patients have characteristic skeletal dysplasias (which may be identified in the fetus by ultrasound) as well as cataracts and a failure to thrive. This disorder is genetically distinct from those mentioned above [106].

The classical form of adrenoleucodystrophy results from a single peroxisomal defect [107]. Patients with adult Refsum disease have a defect in mitochondrial phytanic acid oxidation [108]. Prenatal diagnosis of these disorders and the generalized peroxisomal defects discussed above can now be undertaken on cultured amniotic fluid cells or chorionic villus biopsy. The gene causing X-linked adrenoleucodystrophy has recently been isolated [109]. Linked markers in the Xq28 region are very useful for both carrier detection and prenatal diagnosis in families [110]. A classification of these diseases is given in Table 74.2.

74.2.6 MITOCHONDRIAL DISORDERS

The mitochondrion is a cellular organelle that is involved in multiple areas of metabolism, although its key function is that of energy production. The term 'mitochondrial disorder' relates to disorders associated with dysfunction of mitochondrial energy production. More specifically these disorders are secondary to defects in the mitochondrial respiratory chain. The 'mitochondrial diseases' are a heterogeneous group of disorders that are associated with defects in the mitochondrial production of ATP. By combining clinical phenotype, inheritance pattern, biochemical and pathological information, these diseases can be classified into specific syndrome categories. Since energy production is vital for cell survival, it is likely that a complete block in energy production in all cells would be lethal to the embryo. Therefore by their very nature these metabolic defects must either lead to only partial loss of activity or be expressed in only certain cell lines. Consequently the diagnosis can prove difficult. As one would expect, the phenotypes of these disorders relate to their effect on vital tissues like brain, muscle, heart, liver and kidney. Although the diseases are discussed with respect to the predominant organ system involved, the multisystem nature of the disorders should be kept in mind. In addition, the evolution of the specific syndrome may develop over considerable time and therefore the diagnosis may become clearer in time.

The majority of patients with mitochondrial dysfunction present in infancy or adulthood. In the perinatal period severe lactic acidosis is the most common presentation. In addition, multisystem organ dysfunction with renal, cardiac and liver involvement is not uncommon in the affected neonate.

Diagnosis of these disorders relies on showing increased plasma lactate. It is often helpful also to consider cerebrospinal fluid lactate as its level is less likely to be influenced by systemic factors such as hypoperfusion. Plasma amino acid determination may show hyperalaninaemia. Confirmation of diagnosis can be done by direct analysis of the activity of the electron transport complexes in mitochondria isolated from tissue, i.e. skin fibroblast or muscle. Electron microscopy of muscle can also be helpful in showing pleotrophic changes in the mitochondria.

Mitochondrial disorders presenting in the perinatal period may be due to either autosomal gene defects of the electron transport chain or mitochondrial DNA-based mutations. The sequence of the mitochondrial chromosome is now completely known and specific disease phenotypes have been associated with specific alterations in the mitochondrial DNA. Point mutations involving the mitochondrial tRNA *lys* gene have been associated with myoclonic epilepsy and ragged red fibre disease (MERRF) [111]. Multiple point mutations have been found to account for patients with mitochondrial encephalomyopathy, lactic acidosis and stroke-like episodes (MELAS) [112]. Nevertheless, a significant number of mitochondrial disorders involve alterations of nuclear genes. No specific electron transport genes have been mapped in humans. Further information may be found in recent reviews [113–115].

74.2.7 DISORDERS OF PURINE AND PYRIMIDINE METABOLISM

These are rare conditions, particularly in the newborn period. Some ten disorders of purine metabolism are recognized, as well as three disorders of pyrimidine metabolism [116]. The conditions are heterogeneous both in terms of clinical presentation as well as degree of enzyme deficiency. Common symptoms include: renal failure, nephrolithiasis, mental handicap, immunodeficiency and anaemia [5].

One of the most severe conditions that presents in the neonatal period is that of adenosine deaminase deficiency. This leads to severe combined immunodeficiency (SCID) due to marked lymphopenia with loss of T-cell and B-cell immune function. Most patients die of overwhelming infections. Diagnosis is by enzyme assay of erythrocytes, so long as these have not been transfused. Purine nucleoside phosphorylase deficiency may present in a similar way but here the defect is primarily one of cellular immunity due to the marked lack of T cells. Diagnosis is by enzyme assay of erythrocytes. Patients with these conditions are currently being considered for bone marrow transplantation as well as somatic gene therapy [117]. Prenatal diagnosis is possible.

Disorders of purine salvage pathways are well known, particularly the deficiency of hypoxanthine phosphoribosyltransferase activity in Lesch–Nyhan disease. Patients may present at around 6 months of age and develop choreoathetosis, ataxia and self-mutilation. This disorder is X-linked and many different mutations from point mutations to complete gene deletion have been identified [118–122].

Patients with disorders of pyrimidine metabolism rarely present in the neonatal period but severe forms of orotic aciduria with congenital malformations have been reported, and a severe case of dihydropyrimidine dehydrogenase deficiency with neuromuscular and hepatic involvement.

74.3 Biochemical investigation of large molecule diseases

Most of these diseases involve storage of large molecules in specific tissues. This chapter is written for pathologists and clinical biochemists who are likely to be asked to investigate patients with ill-defined symptoms. We have found it helpful to suggest investigations which are based on biochemistry targeted towards diseases in which specific tissues are involved. For instance, if the liver is enlarged one can ask if there is hypoglycaemia. If so, tests may be chosen for glycogen storage disease. If these are negative and if the child has dysmorphic features these may result from storage of mucopolysaccharides in growing bone. We may then ask whether there is evidence of storage in bone (by looking for radiological evidence of dysostosis multiplex), liver or spleen. By asking such questions it should be possible to tailor investigations towards diseases with specific patterns of tissue involvement.

74.3.1 GLYCOGEN STORAGE DISEASES (GSDs)

There are presently at least 12 disorders (enzyme deficiencies) resulting in the abnormal accumulation of glycogen or a structurally related form of this important polysaccharide [123]. Apart from phosphorylase kinase deficiency, which is generally inherited in an X-linked manner, all are autosomal recessive diseases. The more severe hepatic types have recently been reviewed [124]. Although not strictly a GSD, the deficiency of glycogen synthetase activity in GSD type 0 leads to a reduction in total liver glycogen, present as a highly branched polysaccharide which is not readily broken down. Patients therefore have marked hypoglycaemia, high ketone levels and no response to glucagon stimu-

lation. The enzyme deficiency appears only to be expressed in liver.

(a) Glycogenosis type I (von Gierke disease)

Deficiency of glucose-6-phosphatase in GSD type I may lead to early and marked hypoglycaemia with lactic acidosis and increased uric acid levels. Patients may have stunted growth and hepatomegaly. On glucose loading there may be a marked reduction in lactate levels [125,126] and patients are unable to convert galactose or fructose to blood glucose. These responses and those to glucagon stimulation provide useful initial diagnoses for the hepatic glycogenoses (Table 74.3). Since the deficient enzyme is only expressed in liver, kidney and intestinal mucosa, diagnosis should be established by liver biopsy, but care should be taken due to bleeding difficulties in these patients. To diagnose patients with variant types GSD Ib and Ic, which are deficient in specific microsomal translocases [9], fresh liver must be taken and analysed without freezing.

(b) Glycogenosis type II (Pompe disease)

Pompe disease (GSD type II) is the only lysosomal glycogen storage disease. It was the first lysosomal disorder in which the primary enzyme defect, acid α-glucosidase or acid maltase, was recognized, as well as the first metabolic disease to be diagnosed prenatally by enzyme assay [127]. Patients suffer hepatomegaly, cardiomegaly and hypotonia, but there is also a milder adult form which is primarily myopathic. The genetic relationship between these two types is unclear, especially since the two may coexist in the same family [128] and biosynthetic studies have revealed a high degree of enzyme heterogeneity in phenotypically similar patients [129]. Periodic acid–Schiff (PAS) positive granules may be found in peripheral lymphocytes and, in this disorder, because glycogen accumulation is within lysosomes, high levels are retained *post mortem*. The presence of electron microscopic changes, even in uncultured amniotic fluid cells, may assist in diagnosis [130]. Postnatal diagnosis is best made by enzyme assay on fibroblasts; leucocytes may be used but care should be taken due to interfering activity [11,12]; lymphocytes are preferred. The gene for α-glucosidase has been characterized and many different point mutations have been described [131,132].

(c) Glycogenosis type III (limit dextrinosis)

Type III GSD may exist in several different subgroups, reflecting the tissues affected and the nature of the mutation affecting the deficient debrancher enzyme [133]. Patients have hepatomegaly, stunted growth and

Table 74.3 Useful tests for tentative diagnosis of hepatic glycogen storage diseases

Tests	GSD Ia	GSD Ib	GSD III	GSD VI	GSD VIII
Blood chemistry					
Fasting hypoglycaemia	++	++	+	±	±
Lactic acidosis	+	+	−	−	−
Ketosis	−	±	+	±	±
Hyperlipidaemia	++	+	+	±	±
Uricacidaemia	+	−	−	−	−
Functional tests					
Glucose tolerance	Lactate ↓	Lactate ↓	Lactate ↑	Lactate ↑	Lactate ↑
Galactose/fructose load	No conversion to glucose	No conversion to glucose	Glucose ↑	Glucose ↑	Glucose ↑
Glucagon stimulation					
Fasting: Glucose	Variable	↓	No increase	No increase	Normal rise
Lactose	↑	↑	No increase	No increase or small rise	No increase
Postprandial: Glucose	Variable rise	↓	Normal rise	No increase	Normal rise
Lactose	↑	↑	No increase	No increase or small rise	No increase

Note: Not all patients will respond as predicted and diagnosis should always be confirmed by appropriate enzyme studies.

often some muscle involvement. There is accumulation of highly branched glycogen (limit dextrin) which is not broken down by phosphorylase. Consequently, hypoglycaemia is common after an overnight fast when no response may be elicited by glucagon stimulation [125, 126]. Diagnosis can be made by amylo-1,6-glucosidase assay in erythrocytes or leucocytes [134,135]. Biopsy may be necessary to establish the involvement of muscle in these patients. The accumulating polysaccharide has a characteristic iodine-stained spectrum, but due to its increased solubility it is easily lost from histochemical sections. When the defect is also expressed in peripheral cells, such as cultured fibroblasts, prenatal diagnosis may be feasible [136,137] but this is generally not warranted. However, if undertaken, care should be exercised due to the action of α-glucosidase activity [138] and the pattern of expression in different cell types [139]. Immunoblot analysis may help with the diagnosis in some patients [140].

(d)   Glycogenosis type IV (amylopectinosis)

Deficiency of branching enzyme activity [141] is a rare but generalized and severe form of GSD. Patients display hepatosplenomegaly, muscle wasting and ascites. Serum transaminases may be raised and there is generally a liver cirrhosis in reaction to the relatively insoluble storage product, which resembles amylopectin in structure, giving a blue reaction with iodine. Although glycogen has abnormal structure, glycogen levels may not be raised in tissue. Branching enzyme activity can be measured on a variety of sources, and for diagnostic purposes leucocytes, fibroblasts or liver

may be used [141,142]. Prenatal diagnosis of this condition has been successfully carried out.

(e)   Glycogenosis type V (McArdle disease) and type VII (Tarui disease)

These disorders are unlikely to present in infancy, however forms with severe early presentation have been reported [143,144]. Both disorders primarily affect muscle, leading to lethargy and cramps. The failure of venous lactate levels to rise after ischaemic exercise provides a useful initial diagnostic test for each condition. Diagnosis is established by demonstration of the appropriate enzyme deficiency in muscle, phosphorylase in GSD type V [143] and phosphofructokinase in GSD type VII [144]. These enzyme deficiencies are not expressed in blood cells or fibroblasts, and prenatal diagnosis is generally not warranted. The phosphofructose kinase gene has been isolated and a 14 base pair deletion has been described in one allele from a patient [145].

(f)   Glycogenosis type VI and type VIII

Defects in the hepatic phosphorylase system are found in GSD types VI and VIII. Primary deficiency of this enzyme in liver is rare [146] and most patients with a partial deficiency have been found on further studies to have a defect in the activating enzyme, phosphorylase *b* kinase [147]. This disorder is probably the most common form of GSD but is rarely severe. It is usually inherited in an X-linked manner [148] and may be conveniently diagnosed by enzyme studies on erythrocytes [149,150], which may also be used for heterozygote detection. The enzymes involved with the phosphorylase system are highly labile and great care should be exercised in the handling of these specimens in order that a true assessment of total phosphorylase activity and its active 'a' component may be quantified. Preliminary tests for hepatic GSD (Table 74.3) are generally not very informative for patients with defects of the phosphorylase system [124]. Numerous genes responsible for the phosphorylase kinase complex have been localized to Xq12–q13, 16q12–q13 and chromosome 14 [151,152].

Patients with fructose-1,6-bisphosphatase deficiency may also present with symptoms similar to those seen in hepatic glycogenoses, including increased levels of glycogen. Diagnosis is established by enzyme assay on liver biopsy or leucocytes [153].

74.3.2 LYSOSOMAL STORAGE DISEASES

Lysosomes are membrane bound cellular organelles, rich in hydrolytic enzymes which degrade often complex macromolecules in an acid environment. Much has been learned in recent years of the biosynthesis of these enzymes and the various mutations that give rise to lysosomal storage disorders. Storage of specific metabolites may result from any one of a number of defects. These include failure to synthesize a specific enzyme or polypeptide, synthesis of a catalytically inactive or unstable enzyme, post-translational defects which prevent normal maturation or location of the enzyme, defects in stabilizing proteins or activator proteins, or mutations affecting transport proteins in the lysosomal membrane. Examples of defects in each of these are to be found in the lysosomal storage diseases.

At present around 30 distinct lysosomal diseases are known and, apart from Fabry's and Hunter's diseases which are X-linked, all are inherited in an autosomal recessive manner. Presentation may be early as hydrops fetalis [154–157], or late in adulthood. Even within single families variation may exist [128,158]. Depending on the nature of the primary storage product, the disorders may be divided into four major groups: sphingolipidoses, glycoproteinoses, mucolipidoses and mucopolysaccharidoses. Two disorders of lysosomal transport, cystinosis and Salla disease, result in the accumulation of low molecular weight but impermeable products (cystine and sialic acid respectively). Lysosomal enzymes appear to be expressed early in fetal development and in all cells apart from mature erythrocytes. For practical purposes enzyme diagnosis is best made on blood leucocytes (mixed population or lymphocytes) or cultured cells (skin fibroblasts or amniotic fluid cells), although for prenatal diagnosis chorionic villus biopsy, taken in the first trimester, may be assayed directly or after culture.

Prenatal diagnosis has been successfully carried out for most of these disorders. Some 15 different lysosomal disorders have already been successfully identified in the first trimester following chorionic villus sampling. Enzyme activities in fresh villus samples vary considerably. For example α-fucosidase is high whereas α-neuraminidase and α-iduronidase activities are normally low [159,160]. False-negative diagnoses have been reported in the diagnosis of Hurler disease using fresh villus [161], however, with adequate and good quality samples, diagnosis should now be reliable [162]. A different problem concerns the diagnosis of metachromatic leucodystrophy and Maroteaux–Lamy disease on fresh villus samples, due to the normally high activity in this tissue of arylsulphatase C (deficient as steroid sulphatase in X-linked ichthyosis). To prevent false-negative diagnosis, it is necessary that steps are taken to avoid this interference in villous tissue.

(a) Lipidoses and sphingolipidoses

These disorders characteristically present in the first months of life, with psychomotor deterioration, visceromegaly and at least one of the following manifestations: vacuolated lymphocytes, foamy histiocytes in the bone marrow, macular cherry-red spot in the eye and delayed nerve conduction velocity. Diagnosis is generally established by enzyme assay of blood leucocytes or cultured fibroblasts, although for Tay–Sachs and Sandhoff diseases serum may be preferred, particularly for carrier detection. Identification of storage material in body fluids [163–165] may help to confirm diagnosis or point to an unusual variant. The various degradative pathways involved in these disorders are illustrated in Figure 74.2.

Gangliosidoses

Patients present in the first months of life with degeneration of grey matter leading progressively to blindness (cherry-red spot), deafness, spasticity and decerebrate rigidity. Visceromegaly, bone involvement and vacuolated lymphocytes are common in G_{M1} gangliosidosis, whereas macular degeneration is more prominent in G_{M2} gangliosidosis.

Diagnosis of these conditions is straightforward, usually by direct enzyme assay of leucocyctes or cultured fibroblasts. A deficiency of β-galactosidase activity is associated with G_{M1} gangliosidosis but the same enzyme deficiency is also found in two other conditions, Morquio's disease (mucopolysaccharidosis IV) type B and in galactosialidosis. Each results from different mutations [166].

G_{M2} gangliosidosis may be divided into three major types [164]. In Sandhoff disease (type O) there is a total deficiency of hexosaminidase activity, whereas in Tay–Sachs disease (type B) hexosaminidase A isoenzyme is

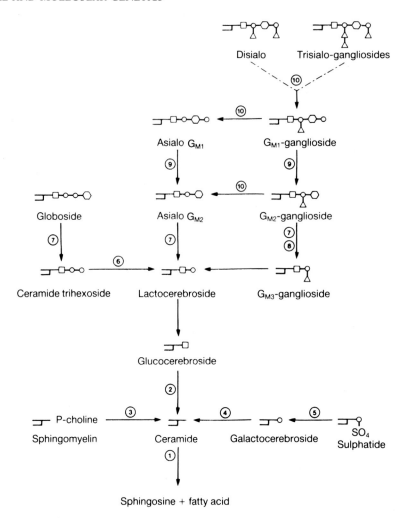

Figure 74.2 Ganglioside and sphingolipid degradation, showing sites of metabolic blocks. Disease (enzyme): 1 = Farber (ceramidase); 2 = Gaucher (glucocerebrosidase); 3 = Niemann–Pick (sphingomyelinase); 4 = Krabbe (galactocerebrosidase); 5 = metachromatic leucodystrophy (arylsulphatase A); 6 = Fabry (α-galactosidase); 7 = Sandhoff (total hexosaminidase); 8 = Tay–Sachs (hexosaminidase A); 9 = G_{M1} gangliosidosis (β-galactosidase); 10 = mucolipidosis IV (ganglioside sialidase). ⊐ = ceramide; □ = glucose; ○ = galactose; ⬡ = N-acetylgalactosamine; △ = N-acetylneuraminic acid (sialic acid).

deficient. This latter disorder is common in Ashkenazi Jews, with an estimated gene frequency of approximately 1:30. Carrier detection programmes have significantly reduced the incidence of this disease. It should be noted that serum assay for carrier detection may be unreliable when the subject is pregnant, due to pregnancy-associated enzyme activity [10]. A sulphated substrate specific for hexosaminidase A activity does not appear to be so useful for carrier detection but is useful for patients with α-subunit mutation leading to the B1 variant of Tay–Sachs disease [168]. Patients with the AB variant, G_{M2} activator defect, require complex studies with the natural substrate to identify this defect.

Numerous mutations have been identified in the hexosaminidase α-subunit and mutations in this gene are responsible for Tay–Sachs disease. In the Ashkenazi Jewish population three mutations are common but sufficient additional mutations are present so that DNA based carrier detection is not practical [169–172].

A patient has been described with a point mutation in the G_{M2} activator gene as the primary cause of the Tay–Sachs AB variant [173]. Numerous β-subunit mutations have been found in patients with Sandhoff disease [174–176].

Fabry disease

In this X-linked disorder widespread deposition of glycosphingolipids leads to the characteristic features of painful extremities, angiokeratoma in skin, corneal opacities and renal and cardiovascular impairment. Increased levels of ceramide trihexoside may be found in plasma and urine [163]. When the deficient enzyme, α-galactosidase A, is measured with artificial substrates it may be necessary to confirm the deficiency by kinetic and heat stability studies, since residual activity may be due to the high K_m more stable B isoenzyme [177]. The disease does not generally present in infancy but some clinical expression of the disease may be found in female carriers. The α-galactosidase gene is located on the X chromosome and numerous mutations have been described in patients. Carrier detection can be performed using linked DNA markers [178,179].

Krabbe disease and metachromatic leucodystrophy

These two diseases result in a loss of myelin with attendant problems. The enzyme substrates involved in these diseases, galactocerebroside and sulphatide, are each structural elements of the myelin sheath. Onset of Krabbe disease is generally in the first 3–6 months of life, with irritability leading to mental and motor deterioration, hypertonia and spastic quadriparesis. Levels of cerebrospinal fluid protein are usually raised and nerve conduction velocity slow. Patients become blind, deaf and profoundly hypotonic. Most succumb by 18 months. Multinucleate PAS-positive globoid cells are found in the white matter of brain, but in the affected fetus, where myelination would be limited, these cells are only found in spinal cord. The deficient enzyme, galactocerebroside β-galactosidase [180,181], is specific in its substrate requirements and should only be assayed with the appropriate galactolipid and detergent mixture, otherwise non-specific β-galactosidase (deficient in G_{M1} gangliosidosis) will be measured. The most reliable substrate is the natural galactocerebroside, radiolabelled in the galactose moiety. Some recently developed analogues containing coloured or fluorescent fatty acids may also be used [182].

At least three variants of metachromatic leucodystrophy are recognized: late infantile (classic), juvenile and adult. Although all patients are profoundly deficient in *in vitro* arylsulphatase A activity, there may however be differences in *in vivo* activity [183] as a result of different molecular mutations [184–186]. Onset of the classical form is usually in the second year of life, with gait disturbance and peripheral neuropathy. In the adult form, dementia may be the prevailing feature. As with Krabbe disease, cerebrospinal fluid protein is raised and nerve conduction delayed. There is no specific organomegaly despite widespread deposition of undegraded substrates. Accumulation in kidney may be marked and the presence of metachromatic material in urinary cells has long been a hallmark of the disease. Excessive excretion of galactosyl- and lactosyl-sulphatides in urine may provide a useful confirmatory test [164]. Enzymatic diagnosis is generally straightforward but a common pseudodeficient mutation has been identified [184], with an allele frequency up to 15% in the general population. This may lead to difficulties in enzyme interpretation, especially when one of the metachromatic leucodystrophy alleles is also present [187]. Loading studies in cultured cells using radiolabelled sulphatide

have proved helpful in the past [188] but DNA studies may now prove more informative [189]. Patients with multiple sulphatase deficiency have features of metachromatic leucodystrophy as well as mucopolysaccharidosis due to deficiencies of several sulphatases. The disorder is rare and may arise from defective post-translational modification of sulphatases [190].

Gaucher disease and Niemann–Pick disease

In these disorders patients have marked hepatosplenomegaly with characteristic foam cells in the marrow. In Gaucher disease there may be marked infiltration into bone, whereas in Niemann–Pick disease pulmonary infiltration is more common.

There are three variants of Gaucher disease: type 1, adult non-neuronopathic form common in Ashkenazi Jews; type 2, acute infantile neuronopathic form; and type 3, subacute neuronopathic form, commonly found in the Norbottnian region of Sweden. All patients accumulate excessive glucocerebroside, especially in the reticuloendothelial system. Brain involvement (Gaucher cells and substrate accumulation) is generally only found in the neuronopathic forms [191]. All patients are deficient in acid β-glucosidase activity but recent studies point to subtle changes in enzyme behaviour which may reflect phenotype expression [192]. These are now being defined by DNA mutation analysis [193–197]. Many specific mutations have been identified, some of which enable the prediction of phenotype when in the homozygous state.

Several variants of Niemann–Pick disease have been recognized: type A, acute neuronopathic; type B, chronic non-neuronopathic; type C, subacute neuronopathic group; and type D, a Nova Scotian variant similar to type C disease. All patients accumulate excessive amounts of sphingomyelin in the reticuloendothelial system, especially the spleen [198,199]; foam cells or sea-blue histiocytes are seen in bone marrow. Only in type A disease is sphingomyelin accumulation evident in brain [199]; however, in both types A and B disease there is a deficiency of sphingomyelinase activity in all tissues studied. Recent work has shown mutations in the sphingomyelinase gene in both type A and B patients [200,201]. Patients with the type C variant may be difficult to diagnose. Neonatal jaundice and hepatosplenomegaly may give way to neurological symptoms, including vertical ophthalmoplegia [202,203]. There is a complex lipid storage pattern including sphingomyelin, cholesterol, glucocerebroside and bis(monoacylglyceryl)phosphate in spleen. A similar pattern is found [204] in the type D variant. A partial deficiency of sphingomyelinase and β-glucosidase activities is commonly found in type C disease fibroblasts but not leucocytes or tissues [205]. Recent studies point to a defect in cholesterol esterification [206], which allows prenatal diagnosis to be undertaken [207].

Farber disease

The final product of sphingolipid breakdown is ceramide, which itself is hydrolysed by ceramidase, the enzyme deficient in Farber disease. In this rare disorder, patients have painful and deformed joints [208]. Onset is in the first weeks of life and patients usually succumb by 4 years of age. Diagnosis is by enzyme assay [209].

Wolman disease

This condition has been mistaken for Niemann–Pick or Gaucher disease [210]. Patients have hepatosplenomegaly with vacuolated lymphocytes and foamy histiocytes. There is also a marked failure to thrive, with diarrhoea and vomiting. The presence of bilateral adrenal calcification is however pathognomonic for Wolman disease and not usually seen in the milder variant, cholesterol ester storage disease. In both variants patients accumulate excessive amounts of cholesterol esters due to the deficiency of acid lipase activity [211,212].

(b) Glycoproteinoses and mucolipidoses

These are relatively rare lysosomal disorders of glycoprotein and mucolipid metabolism, and the initial presentation may be confused with a mucopolysaccharidosis. Patients have hepatomegaly, coarse facies, dysostosis multiplex and psychomotor deterioration. Vacuolated lymphocytes are commonly found, as well as corneal opacities. Angiokeratoma (as in Fabry disease) are reported in some cases. Patients excrete excessive amounts of structurally complex oligosaccharides, or aspartylglucosamine, which may be identified by thin-layer [213] or liquid chromatography [214]. However, these patterns may not always be easy to interpret and final diagnosis must rest on appropriate enzyme assays.

In mannosidosis [215], fucosidosis [216] and aspartylglucosaminuria [217], enzyme assay may be performed on leucocytes, serum or fibroblasts. Owing to the presence of α-mannosidases under separate genetic control [218] and a polymorphism giving rise to low α-fucosidase activity [219], care should be exercised in interpretation of results. Deficient activities of β-mannosidase [220] and α-N-acetylgalactosaminidase [221] have recently been found, but the few families identified do not allow phenotypes to be predicted.

Patients with Salla disease excrete excessive amounts of free sialic acid [222]; the primary defect is located to a lysosomal transport protein [223]. A severe infantile form of the disease is recognized [224].

In the sialidoses and mucolipidoses, patients accumulate excessive amounts of bound sialic acid, as well as other oligosaccharides. Mucolipidosis I, resulting from sialidase deficiency, may be clinically severe (type II) with somatic involvement, or less pronounced but with myoclonus (type I), although in each a cherry-red spot may be seen in the eye [225]. Because the enzyme is highly labile, α-neuraminidase assay should only be carried out on fresh cells which have been disrupted with great care; fibroblasts are recommended.

Cellular inclusions are prominent in mucolipidoses II and III and may be observed in cultured fibroblasts under phase microscopy [226]. In these disorders there is a primary defect in post-translational modification of lysosomal enzymes, the most common being a deficiency of N-acetylglucosaminylphosphotransferase activity [227]. This prevents normal phosphorylation of precursor enzymes and their failure to be recognized by receptors necessary for lysosomal uptake. Since assay of this transferase is relatively complex, identification of increased amounts of extracellular (precursor) activity in serum, amniotic fluid or cell culture medium, or the finding of low activites of several lysosomal enzyme in cultured cells, provide the most practical methods of diagnosis [228,229]. First trimester diagnosis of mucolipidoses II and III is possible by enzyme assay of amniotic fluid [230]. The pathogenesis of mucolipidosis IV is still not known [231].

(c) Mucopolysaccharidoses (MPS)

Patients with these disorders present with a number of characteristic features which include bone dysplasia, coarse facies, joint contractures, growth retardation, psychomotor deterioration, hepatomegaly, corneal opacities and hirsutism [232]. Although Hurler patients (mucopolysaccharidosis (MPS) IH) may have all these manifestations, all features are not necessarily found in each type of MPS. Patients with Sanfilippo syndrome may have severe neurological features, whereas these may not be found in Morquio or Maroteaux–Lamy diseases. Corneal opacities found in MPS I, IV and VI are generally not present in MPS II and III. However, as with other lysosomal storage disorders, there is a wide spectrum of clinical phenotypes found in each disease. Widespread accumulation of incompletely degraded mucopolysaccharides (glycosaminoglycans) within lysosomes of the parenchymal and mesenchymal tissues leads to the characteristic pathology. Hepatosplenomegaly is common and abnormal urinary excretion and amniotic fluid patterns provide useful markers of the primary enzyme deficiency. Both total glycosaminoglycan excretion (high especially in MPS I and II) and qualitative separation by electrophoresis should be carried out to identify abnormal patterns [233]. Although total glycosaminoglycan excretion can generally be quantified by uronic acid determination, this test is not suitable for Morquio disease since the keratan sulphate excreted does not contain uronic acids.

Enzymatic diagnosis is now possible for all the mucopolysaccharidoses but some of the assays are complex and only available in a few laboratories. Leucocytes or serum may be used for most enzymes but, where there is doubt as to the diagnosis or samples have to be sent some distance, it may be more practical to use cultured fibroblasts.

Deficiency of α-iduronidase activity in MPS I is easily demonstrated in leucocytes or fibroblasts, but care is required in case the synthetic substrate contains a glucuronide contaminant [234]. Synthetic substrate is not available for MPS II diagnosis and a radiolabelled disulphated disaccharide [235] derived from heparin is required. A number of enzyme sources may be used for diagnosis but carrier detection appears most convenient by serum assay. During pregnancy, serum iduronate sulphatase activity may increase, unless the fetus is affected with MPS II [236]. This finding may be a useful indicator of fetal genotype, which should be confirmed by direct fetal diagnosis.

Female carriers may exhibit remarkably low enzyme activities, depending on the degree of lyonization. At prenatal diagnosis this may lead to difficulties in interpretation unless the sex of the fetus is known [237]. Extreme lyonization may even lead to females manifesting the full Hunter phenotype [238]. The Hunter syndrome gene has been isolated and sequenced in patients. Many point mutations and deletions are described [239–241].

Four types of Sanfilippo disease are recognized, all phenotypically similar and each excreting excessive amounts of heparan sulphate. Because these patients may have only mild somatic manifestations but severe neurological defect [242], some may escape early diagnosis. Generally, the most common form is MPS IIIA due to heparan N-sulphatase deficiency [242,243]. This enzyme may be assayed with $^{35}SO_4$-labelled heparin as substrate, but the short half-life of this isotope may impose difficulties if only used infrequently. A tritium-labelled tetrasaccharide derived from heparin has been found to be a more convenient substrate [244].

Morquio disease type A is more common than the rather mild B variant. Both types have severe skeletal abnormalities with dwarfism and kyphosis and excessive excretion of keratan sulphate. N-Acetylgalactosamine-6-sulphatase is deficient in type A and β-galactosidase deficient in type B. Each enzyme can be assayed by simple fluorimetric procedures [245]. The gene responsible for type A has been isolated and point mutations are described in patients [246].

Maroteaux–Lamy patients may be spared neurological involvement but skeletal changes are usually marked, similar to Hurler syndrome patients. The metachromatic inclusions in lymphocytes may be particularly prominent in this MPS. There is excessive excretion of dermatan sulphate and deficiency of arylsulphatase B activity provides the diagnosis [247].

Deficiency of β-glucuronidase activity is probably one of the rarest of the mucopolysaccharidoses but it is also one of the easiest to diagnose enzymatically. Few cases have been described but the defect may be severe (hydrops fetalis) [157] or mild and almost asymptomatic [248,249].

74.4 Conclusions and general considerations

We have discussed examples of various metabolic diseases, many of which will present clinically in the first year of life but, of course, biochemically these defects are present from the time of conception. Thus, theoretically, it should be possible to achieve diagnosis at a very early stage. Enzyme diagnosis has the advantage of uncovering many different mutations but unfortunately early fetal samples may not express certain enzyme activities, nor may there be sufficient sample available for assay. For these reasons early preimplantation diagnosis will require DNA analysis but the specific mutations must be clearly defined in each family being investigated.

Nineteen subsets of disorders are listed in Appendix 74.A. These were not all discussed in the text. There are around 120 inherited metabolic disorders in which the identity of the primary gene product (enzyme or protein defect) has been established with reasonable certainty. The affected metabolites, identification of which will assist in diagnosis, are listed, together with the type of sample recommended for primary diagnosis. Where positive prenatal diagnoses have been successfully made, these are indicated. When the deficient enzyme or mutant protein is expressed in cultured fibroblasts and this activity or protein is normally present in cultured amniotic fluid cells or chorionic villus biopsy, prenatal diagnosis is considered 'possible'. Where these proteins are not expressed in readily available fetal material, prenatal diagnosis is considered 'not practical'. However, the prenatal diagnosis of ornithine carbamoyltransferase deficiency by fetal liver biopsy [51,53] indicates that even for disorders previously thought to be not practical, prenatal diagnosis may soon be available, even if this is restricted to specialized centres. In the appendix, 'not practical' means not currently or presently possible.

Appendix 74.A Inherited metabolic disorders

DISORDERS OF CARBOHYDRATE METABOLISM – GLYCOGENOSES

Disease/disorder McKusick No./Inheritance	Enzyme or protein defect	Affected metabolites	Diagnostic sample	Prenatal diagnosis
Glycogenosis type 0 240600 AR	Hepatic glycogen synthetase	Glycogen	Liver	Not practical
Glycogenosis type Ia (von Gierke) 232200 AR	Glucose-6-phosphatase	Glycogen	Liver	Not practical
Glycogenosis type Ib 232220 AR	Glucose-6-phosphate translocase	Glycogen	Fresh liver	Not practical
Glycogenosis type Ic 232240 AR	Phosphate/pyrophosphate translocase	Glycogen	Fresh liver	Not practical
Glycogenosis type II (Pompe) 232300 AR	Acid α-glucosidase (acid maltase)	Glycogen	Fibroblasts, liver, muscle, leucocytes	Made
Glycogenosis type III (Forbes) 232400 AR	Amylo-1,6-glucosidase (debrancher enzyme)	Limit dextrin–glycogen	Liver, muscle, erythrocytes, leucocytes	Made
Glycogenosis type IV (Anderson) 232500 AR	α-1,4-Glucan:α-1,4-glucan-6-glucosyltransferase (brancher enzyme)	Amylopectin–glycogen	Fibroblasts, liver, leucocytes	Made
Glycogenosis type V (McArdle) 232600 AR	Muscle phosphorylase	Glycogen	Muscle	Not practical
Glycogenosis type VI (Hers) 232700 AR	Hepatic phosphorylase	Glycogen	Liver	Not practical
Glycogenosis type VII (Tarui) 232800 AR	Phosphofructokinase	Glycogen	Muscle, erythrocytes	Not practical
Glycogenosis type III 306000 XLR or 261750 AR	Hepatic phosphorylase b kinase	Glycogen	Liver, erythrocytes (or muscle)	Not practical
Hereditary fructose intolerance 229600 AR	Fructose-1-phosphate aldolase B	Fructose-1-phosphate	Liver	Not practical
Fructose-1,6-bisphosphatase deficiency 229700 AR	Fructose-1,6-bisphosphatase	Lactate, ketones, glucose	Liver, leucocytes	Not practical
Galactosaemia 230400 AR	Galactose-1-phosphate uridyl transferase	Galactose, gal-1-phosphate	Erythrocytes (fibroblasts)	Made
Galactosaemia 230200 AR	Galactokinase	Galactose	Erythrocytes (fibroblasts)	Possible
Uridine diphosphate galactose-4-epimerase deficiency 230350 AR	Epimerase	Gal-1-phosphate	Erythrocytes	Not practical

DISORDERS OF AMINO ACID AND ORGANIC ACID METABOLISM

Phenylalanine and tyrosine disorders

Disorder	Enzyme defect	Metabolites	Tissue	Prenatal diagnosis
Phenylketonuria (PKU I) 261600 AR	Phenylalanine hydroxylase	Phenylalanine, phenylpyruvate	Liver	Made by DNA analysis
Phenylketonuria (PKU II) 261630 AR	Dihydropteridine reductase	Phenylalanine, tetrahydrobiopterin	Fibroblasts, leucocytes	Made
Phenylketonuria (PKU III) 261640 AR	'Dihydrobiopterin synthesis', phosphate eliminating enzyme	Total biopterin ↓	Liver, erythrocytes	Made
Phenylketonuria (PKU IV) 233910 AR	GTP-cyclohydrolase	Neopterin ↓ Biopterin ↓	Liver	Possible
Tyrosinaemia II (Richner–Hanhart) 276600 AR	? Tyrosine aminotransferase (cytosol)	Tyrosine, p-hydroxyphenyl pyruvate	Liver	Not practical
Tyrosinaemia I 276700 AR	Fumarylacetoacetate hydrolase	Tyrosine, p-hydroxyphenyllactate, succinylacetone	Fibroblasts, lymphocytes, liver	Made
Alkaptonuria 203500 AR	Homogentisic acid oxidase	Homogentisic acid	Liver	Not practical
Oculocutaneous albinism 203100 AR	Tyrosinase (hair bulbs)	Melanins	Hair bulb	Made

Urea cycle disorders

Disorder	Enzyme defect	Metabolites	Tissue	Prenatal diagnosis
N-Acetylglutamate synthase deficiency 237310 AR	N-Acetylglutamate synthase	Amminia, glutamine	Liver	Not practical
Carbamoyl-phosphate synthetase deficiency 237300 AR	Carbamoyl-phosphate synthetase I	Ammonia, glutamine	Liver	Made
Ornithine carbamoyltransferase deficiency 311250 XLD	Ornithine carbamoyltransferase	Ammonia, orotic acid, glutamine	Liver	Made
Citrullinaemia 215700 AR	Argininosuccinate synthetase	Citrulline, ammonia	Fibroblasts	Made
Argininosuccinic aciduria 207900 AR	Argininosuccinate lyase	Argininosuccinic acid	Erythrocytes, fibroblasts	Made
Argininaemia 207800 AR	Arginase	Arginine	Erythrocytes	Possible

Appendix 74.A *continued*

Disease/disorder McKusick No./Inheritance	Enzyme or protein defect	Affected metabolites	Diagnostic sample	Prenatal diagnosis
Disorders of ornithine and lysine metabolism				
Gyrate atrophy 258870 AR	Ornithine-δ-aminotransferase	Ornithine	Fibroblasts	Possible
Hyperornithinaemia (HHH syndrome) 238970 AR	? Mitochondrial ornithine transport	Ornithine, ammonia, homocitrulline	Fibroblasts	Made
Glutaric aciduria type I 231970 AR	Glutaryl-CoA dehydrogenase	Glutaric acid	Fibroblasts	Made
Glutaric aciduria type II and ethyl–malonic–adipic aciduria 231680 AR	Electron transfer flavoprotein (ETF) or ETF ubiquinone oxidoreductase	Glutaric, dicarboxylic and other organic acids	Fibroblasts	Made
Disorders of sulphur amino acids				
Cystinosis 219800 AR	Lysosomal cystine transport protein	Cystine	Fibroblasts, leucocytes	Made
Homocystinuria 236200 AR	Cystathionine β-synthase	Homocysteine, methionine	Fibroblasts	Made
Methylene tetrahydrofolate reductase deficiency 236250 AR	Methylene tetrahydrofolate reductase	Homocysteine	Fibroblasts, leucocytes	Made
β-Cystathionase deficiency 219500 AR	β-Cystathionase	Cystathionine	Fibroblasts, liver	Not indicated
Other amino acid disorders				
Histidinaemia 235800 AR	Histidase	Histidine	Skin	Not practical
Canavan 271900 AR	Aspartoacylase	N-Acetylaspartate	Urine, fibroblasts	Made
Prolidase deficiency 170100	Prolidase	Proline-rich iminodipeptides	Erythrocytes, fibroblasts	Possible
Non-ketotic hyperglycinaemia 238300 AR	Glycine cleavage	Glycine	Cerebrospinal fluid, plasma, liver, brain	Made

1151

Branched chain organic acid disorders

Disorder	Enzyme	Metabolite(s)	Tissue	Prenatal diagnosis
Maple syrup urine disease 248600 AR	Branched chain ketoacid decarboxylase	Leucine, isoleucine, valine	Leucocytes, fibroblasts	Made
Isovaleric acidaemia 243500 AR	Isovaleryl-CoA dehydrogenase	Isovaleric acid	Leucocytes, fibroblasts	Made
3-Methylcrotonyl-glycinuria 210200 AR	3-Methylcrotonyl-CoA carboxylase	3-Methylcrotonylglycine, 3-hydroxyisovaleric acid	Leucocytes, fibroblasts	Possible
3-Methylglutaconic aciduria I 250950 AR	3-Methylglutaconyl-CoA hydratase	3-Methylglutaconate, 3-hydroxyisovalerate	Fibroblasts	Possible
3-Methylglutaconic aciduria II 250950 AR	Not known	3-Methylglutaconate, 3-methylglutarate	–	Not possible at present
3-Hydroxy-3-methylglutaryl-CoA-lyase deficiency 246450 AR	3-Hydroxy-3-methylglutaryl-CoA lyase	3-Hydroxy-3-methylglutarate, 3-methylglutaconate and other related organic acids	Leucocytes, fibroblasts	Made
Mevalonic aciduria 251170 AR	Mevalonate kinase	Mevalonate	Fibroblasts	Made
2-Methylacetoacetic aciduria 203750 AR	2-Methylacetoacetyl-CoA thiolase (β-ketothiolase)	2-Methyl-3-hydroxybutyrate, 2-methylacetoacetate	Fibroblasts	Possible

Other organic acid disorders

Disorder	Enzyme	Metabolite(s)	Tissue	Prenatal diagnosis
Medium chain dicarboxylic aciduria, β-oxidation defect 201450 AR	Medium chain acyl-CoA dehydrogenase	C_6–C_{10} dicarboxylic acids, suberyl-glycine, octanoyl carnitine	Fibroblasts, urine, DNA	Made
Long chain β-oxidation defect 201460 AR	Long chain acyl-CoA dehydrogenase	C_6–C_{14} dicarboxylic acids	Fibroblasts, urine	Possible
Long chain hydroxyacyl-CoA dehydrogenase deficiency 143450 AR	Long chain hydroxyacyl-CoA dehydrogenase	Hydroxydicarboxylic acids	Fibroblasts	Made
Primary hyperoxaluria type I 259900 AR	Alanine:glyoxylate aminotransferase	Oxalate, glycolate	Liver	Made
Primary hyperoxaluria type II 260000 AR	D-Glycerate dehydrogenase	Oxalate, glycerate	Leucocytes	Not practical
4-Hydroxybutyric aciduria 271980 AR	Succinic semialdehyde dehydrogenase	4-Hydroxybutyrate	Lymphocytes	Made
Pyroglutamic aciduria 266130 AR	Glutathione synthetase	Pyroglutamate	Erythrocytes, fibroblasts	Possible
Glycerol kinase 307030 XLR	Glycerol kinase	Glycerol	Fibroblasts	Made

Appendix 74.A *continued*

Disease/disorder McKusick No./Inheritance	Enzyme or protein defect	Affected metabolites	Diagnostic sample	Prenatal diagnosis
Disorders of propionate and methylmalonate metabolism				
Propionic acidaemia 232000 AR	Propionyl-CoA carboxylase	Propionate, methylcitrate	Leucocytes, fibroblasts	Made
Multiple carboxylase deficiency (early onset) 253270 AR	Holocarboxylase synthase	3-Methylcrotonylglycine, 3-hydroxyisovaleric acid	Leucocytes, fibroblasts	Made
Multiple carboxylase deficiency (later onset) 253260 AR	Biotinidase	3-Methylcrotonylglycine, 3-hydroxyisovaleric acid	Serum, fibroblasts	Possible but treatable
Methylmalonic aciduria 251000 AR	Methylmalonyl-CoA mutase	Methylmalonate	Fibroblasts, leucocytes	Made
Methylmalonic aciduria 251100 AR	Adenosylcobalamin synthesis	Methylmalonate	Fibroblasts	Made
Lactic acidaemia and mitochondrial disorders				
Pyruvate dehydrogenase deficiency 208800 AR 312170 XLR	Pyruvate dehydrogenase complex E1 α-subunit	Lactate, pyruvate	Fibroblasts	Made
Pyruvate carboxylase deficiency 266150 AR	Pyruvate carboxylase	Lactate, pyruvate	Fibroblasts, leucocytes	Made
Fumarase deficiency 136850 AR	Fumarase	Fumarate	Fibroblasts	Possible
Electron transport defects				
Complex I deficiency 252010	NADH-CoQ reductase	Lactate	Muscle	Not possible at present
Complex II deficiency 252011	Succinate-CoQ reductase	Lactate	Muscle	Not possible at present
Complex III deficiency 124000	Ubiquinone cytochrome *c* oxidoreductase	Lactate	Muscle	Not possible at present
Complex IV deficiency 220110	Cytochrome *c* oxidase	Lactate	Muscle, fibroblasts	Made
Complex V deficiency	ATP synthetase	Lactate	Muscle	Not possible at present
DISORDERS OF PURINE AND PYRIMIDINE METABOLISM				
Gout 311850 XLR	Increased phosphoribosyl pyrophosphate synthetase	Uric acid, phosphoribosylpyrophosphate	Erythrocytes	Not possible at present

1153

Disorder	Enzyme/Protein	Metabolite	Tissue	Diagnosis
Lesch–Nyhan 308000 XLR	Hypoxanthine:guanine phosphoribosyl transferase	Uric acid, phosphoribosylpyrophosphate	Fibroblasts, erythrocytes	Made
Adenine phosphoribosyl transferase deficiency 102600 AR	Adenine phosphoribosyl transferase	2,8-Dihydroxyadenine	Fibroblasts, erythrocytes	Possible
Hereditary xanthinuria 278300 AR	Xanthine oxidase	Xanthine, uric acid ↓	Jejunum, liver	Not possible at present
Severe combined immunodeficiency 102700 AD or AR	Adenosine deaminase	Adenosine, deoxyadenosine	Erythrocytes, fibroblasts	Made
T-cell immunodeficiency 164050 AD or AR	Purine nucleoside phosphorylase	Inosine, guanosine	Erythrocytes, fibroblasts	Made
Hereditary orotic aciduria type I 258900 AR	UMP synthase	Orotic acid	Erythrocytes, fibroblasts	Possible
Pyrimidine 5-nucleotidase deficiency 266120	Pyrimidine 5'-nucleotidase	Pyrimidine nucleotides	Erythrocytes	Possible
Dihydropyrimidine dehydrogenase deficiency 274270 AR	Dehydropyrimidine dehydrogenase	Uracil and thyamine	Urine	Made

DISORDERS OF LIPOPROTEINS AND NEUTRAL LIPIDS

Disorder	Enzyme/Protein	Metabolite	Tissue	Diagnosis
Familial lipoprotein deficiency (abetalipoproteinaemia) 200100 AR	Apolipoprotein B	Low plasma cholesterol and triglycerides	Plasma, erythrocytes	Not possible at present
Tangier 205400 AR	High-density lipoprotein	Tissue cholesterol esters	Plasma	Not possible at present
Lipoprotein lipase deficiency 238600 AR	Lipoprotein lipase	Plasma triglycerides	Postheparin plasma, adipose tissue	Not possible at present
Apolipoprotein CII deficiency 207750 AR	Apolipoprotein CII	Lipoproteins, triglycerides	Plasma	Not possible at present
Hyperlipoproteinaemia type III polygenic co-dominant 107741	Apolipoprotein E	Plasma cholesterol and triglycerides	Plasma	Not possible at present
Hypercholesterolaemia 143890 AD	Plasma membrane low-density lipoprotein receptor	Cholesterol	Plasma, fibroblasts	Made
Lecithin:cholesterol acyl transferase deficiency 245900 AR	Lecithin:cholesterol acyl transferase	Cholesterol, phosphatidylcholine	Plasma	Possible
Refsum 266500 AR	Phytanic acid α-hydroxylase	Phytanic acid	Fibroblasts	Made
Cerebrotendinous xanthomatosis 213700 AR	C_{27}-steroid 26-hydroxylase	Tissue cholesterol and cholestanol	Fibroblasts, liver, (plasma)	Possible
Smith–Lemli–Opitz syndrome 270400 AR	?7-Dehydrocholesterol reductase	Cholesterol, 7-dehydrocholesterol	Plasma	Made

Appendix 74.A *continued*

Disease/disorder McKusick No./Inheritance	Enzyme or protein defect	Affected metabolites	Diagnostic sample	Prenatal diagnosis
DISORDERS OF PORPHYRIN AND HAEM METABOLISM				
Congenital erythropoietic porphyria 263700 AR	Uroporphyrinogen III synthase	Porphyrins	Erythrocytes, fibroblasts	Made
Erythropoietic protoporphyria 177000 AD	Ferrochelatase	Protoporphyrin	Erythrocytes, fibroblasts	Possible
Acute intermittent porphyria 176000 AD	Porphobilinogen deaminase (uroporphyrinogen I synthase)	δ-Aminolaevulinic acid, porphobilinogen	Erythrocytes, fibroblasts	Made
Hereditary coproporphyria 121300 AD	Coproporphyrinogen III oxidase	Coproporphyrin	Fibroblasts lymphocytes	Possible
Variagate porphyria 176200 AD	Protoporphyrinogen oxidase	Protoporphyrin	Fibroblasts	Possible
Familial porphyria cutanea tarda 176100 AD	Uroporphyrinogen III decarboxylase	Uroporphyrin	Liver	Not practical
DISORDERS OF METAL METABOLISM				
Menkes 309400 XLR	Copper-binding ATPase	Copper	Fibroblasts	Made
Wilson 277900 AR	Copper-binding ATPase	Copper (ceruloplasmin)	Serum	Not possible at present
Xanthine oxidase/sulphite oxidase deficiency 252150 AR	Molybdenum cofactor	Sulphite, xanthine, S-sulphocysteine	Fibroblasts, urine	Made
LYSOSOMAL STORAGE DISEASE – LIPIDOSES				
Farber 228000 AR	Ceramidase	Ceramide	Leucocytes, fibroblasts	Made
(Anderson) Fabry 301500 XLR	α-Galactosidase A	Ceramide–trihexoside	Leucocytes, plasma, fibroblasts	Made

Disorder	Enzyme/defect	Storage substrate	Tissue	Prenatal diagnosis
Gaucher				
Type 1 230800 AR	Acid β-glucosidase	Glucocerebroside	Leucocytes, fibroblasts	Made
Type 2 230900 AR	Acid β-glucosidase	Glucocerebroside	Leucocytes, fibroblasts	Made
Type 3 231000 AR	Acid β-glucosidase	Glucocerebroside	Leucocytes, fibroblasts	Made
Krabbe 245200 AR	Galactocerebroside β-galactosidase	Galactocerebroside	Leucocytes, fibroblasts	Made
G_{M1} gangliosidosis				
Infantile 230500 AR	G_{M1} ganglioside β-galactosidase	G_{M1} ganglioside	Leucocytes, fibroblasts	Made
Juvenile 230600 AR	G_{M1} ganglioside β-galactosidase	G_{M1} ganglioside	Leucocytes, fibroblasts	Made
Adult 230650 AR	G_{M1} ganglioside β-galactosidase	G_{M1} ganglioside	Leucocytes, fibroblasts	Possible
G_{M2} gangliosidosis				
Tay–Sachs (B variant) 272800 AR	β-Hexosaminidase A	G_{M2} ganglioside	Leucocytes, serum, fibroblasts	Made
Sandhoff (O variant) 268800 AR	β-Hexosaminidase A + B	G_{M2} ganglioside, asialo G_{M2} and globoside	Leucocytes, serum, fibroblasts	Made
AB variant 272750 AR	G_{M2} ganglioside activator protein	G_{M2} ganglioside	Fibroblasts	Possible
Mucolipidosis IV 252650 AR	?	Gangliosides (G_{M3} and G_{D3})	Fibroblasts	Made
Niemann–Pick				
Type A 257200 AR	Sphingomyelinase	Sphingomyelin	Leucocytes, fibroblasts	Made
Type B 257200 AR	Sphingomyelinase	Sphingomyelin	Leucocytes, fibroblasts	Made
Type C 257220 AR	Cholesterol esterification	Sphingomyelin, cholesterol, lysobisphosphatidic acid, glucocerebroside	Fibroblasts	Made
Type D 257250 AR	Cholesterol esterification	Sphingomyelin, cholesterol, lysobisphosphatidic acid	Fibroblasts	Possible
Metachromatic leucodystrophy 250100 AR	Arylsulphatase A	Galactosyl sulphatide	Leucocytes, fibroblasts	Made
Metachromatic leucodystrophy (ASA variant) 249900 AR	Cerebroside sulphatase activator	Galactosyl sulphatide	Fibroblasts	Possible
Multiple sulphatase deficiency 272200 AR	Various sulphatases	Sulpholipids, mucopolysaccharides, steroids	Fibroblasts, leucocytes	Made
Wolman and cholesterol storage disease 278000 AR	Acid esterase	Cholesterol esters, triglycerides	Leucocytes, fibroblasts	Made

Appendix 74.A continued

Disease/disorder McKusick No./Inheritance	Enzyme or protein defect	Affected metabolites	Diagnostic sample	Prenatal diagnosis
GLYCOPROTEIN AND MUCOLIPID STORAGE DISEASES				
Mucolipidosis I (sialidosis) 256550 AR	α-Neuraminidase	Sialyloligosaccharides	Fibroblasts	Made
Galactosialidosis 256540 AR	β-Galactosidase + α-neuraminidase – 'protective protein'	Sialyloligosaccharides	Fibroblasts	Made
Aspartylglucosaminuria 208400 AR	N-Aspartyl-β-glucosaminidase	Aspartylglucosamine	Plasma, leucocytes, fibroblasts	Made
Fucosidosis 230000 AR	α-Fucosidase	Fucolipid, fuco-oligosaccharides	Leucocytes, fibroblasts	Made
α-Mannosidosis 248500 AR	α-Mannosidase	Manno-oligosaccharides	Leucocytes, fibroblasts	Made
β-Mannosidosis 248510 AR	β-Mannosidase	Oligosaccharides	Leucocytes, fibroblasts	Possible
Salla/infantile variant 268740 AR	Lysosomal transport protein	Sialic acid	Urine, fibroblasts	Made
Mucolipidosis II (I-cell disease) 252500 AR	UDP-GlcNAc:lysosomal enzyme GlcNAc-1-phosphotransferase	Oligosaccharides	Serum, fibroblasts	Made
Mucolipidosis III (pseudo-Hurler polydystrophy) 252600 AR	UDP-GlcNAc:lysosomal enzyme GlcNAc-1-phosphotransferase	Oligosaccharides	Serum, fibroblasts	Possible
MUCOPOLYSACCHARIDOSES				
Hurler/Scheie (MPS IH) 252800 AR	α-L-Iduronidase	Dermatan sulphate, heparan sulphate	Leucocytes, fibroblasts	Made
Hunter (MPS II) 309900 XLR	Iduronate sulphate sulphatase	Heparan sulphate, dermatan sulphate	Serum, leucocytes, fibroblasts	Made
Sanfilippo A (MPS III) 252900 AR	Heparan N-sulphatase	Heparan sulphate	Leucocytes, fibroblasts	Made
Sanfilippo B (MPS IIIB) 252920 AR	N-Acetyl-α-glucosaminidase	Heparan sulphate	Serum, leucocytes, fibroblasts	Made
Sanfilippo C (MPS IIIC) 252930 AR	Acetyl CoA:α-glucosaminide N-acetyltransferase	Heparan sulphate	Fibroblasts, leucocytes	Made

Disorder	Enzyme/defect	Accumulated substance	Diagnostic tissue	Prenatal diagnosis
Sanfilippo D (MPS IIID) 252940 AR	N-Acetyl-α-glucosaminide-6-sulphatase	Heparan sulphate	Fibroblasts, leucocytes	Possible
Morquio type A (MPS IVA) 243000 AR	N-Acetyl-galactosamine-6-sulphate sulphatase	Keratan sulphate	Fibroblasts, leucocytes	Made
Morquio type B (MPS IVB) 253010 AR	β-Galactosidase	Keratan sulphate	Leucocytes, fibroblasts	Possible
Maroteaux–Lamy (MPS VI) 253200 AR	Arylsulphatase B (N-acetylgalactosamine-4-sulphate sulphatase)	Dermatan sulphate	Leucocytes, fibroblasts	Made
Sly (MPS VII) 253220 AR	β-Glucuronidase	Dermatan sulphate, heparan sulphate	Leucocytes	Made

PEROXISOMAL DISORDERS

Disorder	Enzyme/defect	Accumulated substance	Diagnostic tissue	Prenatal diagnosis
Zellweger 214100 AR including: Neonatal adrenoleucodystrophy 202370 AR; Infantile Refsum 266510 AR	Disorders of peroxisome biogenesis. Several peroxisomal enzyme activities deficient including dihydroxyacetone phosphate acyl transferase (DHAP-AT)	Very long chain fatty acids, plasmalogens, bile acids (phytanic acid, pipecolic acid)	Thrombocytes, fibroblasts, plasma	Made
Zellweger-like syndrome	?Peroxisome import defect	Plasmalogens, very long chain fatty acids	Plasma, thrombocytes, fibroblasts	Possible
Rhizomelic chondrodysplasia punctata 215100 AR	Disorder of some peroxisomal functions (DHAP-AT, phytanic acid oxidase, thiolase)	Plasmalogens, phytanic acid	Plasma, thrombocytes, fibroblasts	Made
DHAP-DT deficiency	Dihydroxyacetone phosphate acyltransferase	Plasmalogens	Thrombocytes, fibroblasts	Possible
Pseudoneonatal adrenoleucodystrophy 264470 AR	Peroxisomal oxidase	Very long chain fatty acids	Plasma, fibroblasts	Made
Bifunctional enzyme deficiency	Bifunctional enzyme	Very long chain fatty acids	Plasma, fibroblasts	Possible
Pseudo-Zellweger 261510 AR	Peroxisomal thiolase	Very long chain fatty acids, bile acids	Plasma, fibroblasts	Possible
Adrenoleucodystrophy/adrenomyeloneuropathy 300100 XLR	Very long chain fatty acyl-CoA synthase or transporter	Very long chain fatty acids	Plasma, fibroblasts	Made
Glutaric aciduria type III 231690 AR	Glutaryl-CoA oxidase	Glutaric acid	Fibroblasts	Possible

Appendix 74.A *continued*

Disease/disorder McKusick No./Inheritance	Enzyme or protein defect	Affected metabolites	Diagnostic sample	Prenatal diagnosis
DISORDERS OF STEROID METABOLISM				
X-linked ichthyosis 308100 XLR	Steroid sulphatase	Dihydroepiandrosterone sulphate	Fibroblasts	Made
Congenital adrenal hyperplasia type III 209910 AR	21-Hydroxylase	17-Hydroxyprogesterone	(Adrenal), urine	Made
Congenital adrenal hyperplasia type IV 202010 AR	11-β-Hydroxylase	Deoxycorticosterone, 11-deoxycortisol	(Adrenal), urine	Made
Pseudohermaphroditism 264600 AR	Testosterone 4α-reductase	Testosterone	Genital skin, fibroblasts	Not possible at present
OTHER DISORDERS				
α₁-Antitrypsin deficiency 107400 AD	α₁-Antitrypsin	Proteases	Serum	Made by DNA analysis
Carbohydrate deficient glycoprotein disorder 212065 AR		Glycoproteins, especially transferrins	Serum	Not possible at present
Hypophosphatasia 241500 AR	Alkaline phosphatase (bone/liver forms)	Phosphoethanolamine pyrophosphate	Fibroblasts, serum	Made
Sjögren–Larsson 270200 AR	Fatty alcohol:NAD oxidoreductase	Fatty alcohols	Fibroblasts	Possible
Carbonic anhydrase deficiency 259730 AR	Carbonic anhydrase	Bicarbonate	Erythrocytes	Not possible at present
Ceroid lipofuscinosis 204200 AR	Not known	Motochondrial ATP synthase subunit c	Muscle	Made

AD = autosomal dominant; AR = autosomal recessive; XLR = X-linked recessive; ASA = arylsulphatase A deficiency; MPS = mucopolysaccharidosis.

References

1. McKusick, V. (1992) *Mendelian Inheritance in Man*, 19th edn, Johns Hopkins University Press, Baltimore.
2. Guthrie, R. (1961) Blood screening for phenylketonuria. *JAMA*, **178**, 863.
3. Smith, I. and Seakins, J. (1976) *Chromatographic and Electrophoretic Techniques*, 4th edn, Heinemann, London.
4. Chalmers, R. and Lawson, A. (1982) *Organic Acids in Man*, Chapman & Hall, London.
5. Scriver, C., Beaudet, A., Sly, W. *et al.* (1989) *The Metabolic Basis of Inherited Disease*, 6th edn, McGraw-Hill, NY.
6. Galjaard, H. (1970) *Genetic Metabolic Diseases: Early Diagnosis and Prenatal Analysis*, Elsevier North-Holland, Amsterdam.
7. Benson, P. and Fensom, A. (1985) *Genetic Biochemical Disorders*, Oxford University Press, Oxford.
8. Fowler, K. (1984) Storage of skin biopsies at −70°C for fibroblast culture. *J. Clin. Pathol.*, **37**, 1191–93.
9. Nordlie, R. and Sukalski, K. (1986) Multiple forms of type 1 glycogen storage disease: underlying mechanisms. *Trends Biochem. Sci.* **11**, 85–88.
10. Lowden, J. (1979) Serum β-hexosaminidases in pregnancy. *Clin. Chim. Acta*, **93**, 409–17.
11. Broadhead, D. and Butterworth, J. (1978) Pompe's disease: diagnosis in kidney and leucocytes using 4-methylumbellifery-α-D-glucopyranoside. *Clin. Genet.*, **13**, 504–10.
12. Potter, J., Robinson, H., Kramer, J. *et al.* (1980) Apparent normal leukocyte acid maltase activity in glycogen storage disease type II (Pompe's disease). *Clin. Chem.*, **26**, 1914–15.
13. Applegarth, D., Dimmick J. and Toone, J. (1989) Laboratory detection of metabolic disease. *Pediatr. Clin. North Am.*, **36**, 49–66.
14. Romsche, C., Hilty, M., McClung, H. *et al.* (1981) Amino acid pattern in Reye syndrome: comparison with clinically similar entities. *J. Pediatr.*, **98**, 788–90.
15. Todd, W. (1979) Psychosocial problems as the major complication of an adolescent with trimethylaminuria. *J. Pediatr.*, **94**, 936–37.
16. Ampula, M. (1982) *Metabolic Diseases in Pediatric Practice*, Little, Brown, Boston, pp. 119–40.
17. Mahoney, M. (1976) Organic acidemias. *Clin. Perinatol.*, **3**, 61–78.
18. Hutchinson, R., Bunnell, K. and Thoene, J. (1985) Suppression of granulopoietic progenitor cell proliferation by metabolites of the branched chain amino acids. *J. Pediatr.*, **106**, 62–65.
19. Symposium on Organic Acidurias (1984) *J. Inherited Metab. Dis.*, **7** (suppl. 1), 1–99.
20. Rosenberg, L. and Fenton W. (1989) Disorders of propionate and methylmalonate metabolism, in *The Metabolic Basis of Inherited Disease*, 6th edn (eds C.R. Scriver, A.I. Beaudet, W.S. Sly and D. Valle), McGraw-Hill, NY, pp. 821–44.
21. Lamhonwah, A., Troxel, C., Schuster, S. and Gravel, R. (1990) Two distinct mutations at the same site in the PCCB gene in propionic acidemia. *Genomics*, **8**, 249–54.
22. Tahara, T., Eto, Y. and Kraus, J. *et al.* (1990) Molecular basis of organic acidemia – propionic acidemia. *Human Cell*, **3**, 311–7.
23. Ledley, F. (1990) Perspectives on methylmalonic acidemia resulting from molecular cloning of methylmalonyl CoA mutase. *Bioessays*, **12**, 335–40.
24. Ledley, F., Jansen, R., Nham, S. *et al.* (1990) Mutation eliminating mitochondrial leader sequence of methylmalonyl CoA mutase causes methylmalonic acidemia. *Proc. Natl Acad. Sci. USA*, **87**, 3147–50.
25. Ledley, F., Crane A. and Lumetta, M. (1990) Heterogeneous alleles and expression of methylmalonyl CoA mutase in methylmalonic acidemia. *Am. J. Hum. Genet.*, **46**, 539–47
26. Wolf, B., Hsia, Y., Sweetman, L. *et al.* (1981) Multiple carboxylase deficiency: clinical and biochemical improvement following neonatal biotin treatment. *Pediatrics*, **68**, 113–18.
27. Ampola, M. (1981) Multiple carboxylase deficiency: clinical and biochemical improvement following neonatal biotin treatment. *Pediatrics*, **68**, 113–18.
28. Wolf, B., Hard, G., Jefferson, L. *et al.* (1985) Clinical findings in four children with biotinidase deficiency detected through a statewide neonatal program. *N. Engl. J. Med.*, **313**, 16–19.
29. Sweetman, L. (1989) Branched chain organic acidurias, in *The Metabolic Basis of Inherited Disease*, 6th edn (eds C.R. Scriver, A.I. Beaudet, W.S. Sly and D. Valle), McGraw-Hill, NY, pp. 791–820.
30. Goodman, S., Norenberg, M., Shikes, R. *et al.* (1977) Glutaric aciduria: biochemical and morphologic considerations. *J. Pediatr.*, **90**, 746–50.
31. Sweetman, L., Nyhan, W., Trauner, D. *et al.* (1980) Glutaric aciduria type II. *J. Pediatr.* **96**, 1020–26.
32. Frerman, F. and Goodman, S. (1989) Glutaric acidemia type II and defects of the mitochondrial respiratory chain, in *The Metabolic Basis of Inherited Disease*, 6th edn (eds C.R. Scriver, A.J. Beaudet, W.S. Sly and D. Valle), McGraw-Hill, NY, pp. 915–32.
33. Gregersen, N. (1985) Riboflavin-responsive defects of beta oxidation. *J. Inherited Metab. Dis*, **8** (suppl. 1), 65–69.
34. Bennett, M., Pollit, R., Goodman, S. *et al.* (1991) Atypical riboflavin-responsive glutaric aciduria and deficient peroxisomal glutaryl CoA-oxidase activity: a new peroxisomal disorder. *J. Inherited Metab. Dis.* **14**, 165–73.
35. Fukao, T. and Yamaguchi, S. (1992) Identification of three mutant alleles of the gene for mitochondrial acetoacetyl-coenzyme A thiolase. *J. Clin. Invest.*, **89**, 474–79.
36. Hale, D. and Bennett, M. (1992) Fatty acid oxidation disorders: new class of metabolic diseases. *J. Pediatr.*, **121**, 1–11.
37. Coates, P. and Tanaka, K. (1992) Molecular basis of mitochondrial fatty acid oxidation defects. *J. Lipid Res.*, **33**, 1099–110.
38. Miller, M., Brooks, J., Forbes, N. *et al.* (1992) Frequency of medium-chain acyl-CoA dehydrogenase deficiency G-985 mutation in sudden infant death syndrome. *Pediatr. Res.*, **31**, 305–307.
39. Gregersen, N., Blakemore, A., Winter, V. *et al.* (1991) Specific diagnosis of medium-chain acyl-CoA dehydrogenase (MCAD) deficiency in dried blood spots by a polymerase chain reaction (PCR) assay detecting a point-mutation (G985) in the MCAD gene. *Clin. Chim. Acta*, **203**, 23–34.
40. Millington, D., Kodo, N., Norwool, D. *et al.* (1990) Tandem mass spectrometry: a new method for acylcarnitine profiling with potential for neonatal screening for inborn errors of metabolism. *J. Inherited Metab. Dis.*, **13**, 321–24.
41. Robinson, B. (1989) Lactic acidemia, in *The Metabolic Basis of Inherited Disease*, 6th edn (eds C.R. Scriver, A.I. Beaudet, W.S. Sly and D. Valle), McGraw-Hill, NY, pp. 915–32.
42. Robinson, B., Oei, J., Sherwood, W. *et al.* (1984) The molecular basis for the two different clinical presentations of classical pyruvate carboxylase deficiency. *Am. J. Hum. Genet.*, **36**, 283–94.
43. Wong, L., Davidson, A., Applegarth, D. *et al.* (1986) Biochemical and histologic pathology in an infant with CRM (negative) pyruvate carboxylase deficiency. *Pediatr. Res.*, **20**, 274–79.
44. Chun, K., Mackay, N., Willard, H. *et al.* (1990) Isolation, characterization and chromosomal localization of cDNA clones for the E1 beta subunit of the pyruvate dehydrogenase complex. *Eur. J. Biochem.*, **194**, 587–92.
45. Hansen, L., Brown, G., Kirby, D. *et al.* (1991) Characterization of the mutations in three patients with pyruvate dehydrogenase E1 alpha deficiency. *J. Inherited Metab. Dis.*, **14**, 140–51.
46. Wexler, I., Hemalatha, S., Liu, T. *et al.* (1992) A mutation in the E1 alpha subunit of pyruvate dehydrogenase associated with variable expression of pyruvate dehydrogenase complex deficiency. *Pediatr. Res.*, **32**, 169–74.
47. Murphy, J., Isohashi, F., Weinberg, B. *et al.* (1981) Pyruvate carboxylase deficiency: an alleged biochemical cause of Leigh's disease. *Pediatrics*, **68**, 401–404.
48. Sander, J., Packman, S., Berg, B. *et al.* (1984) Pyruvate carboxylase activity in subacute necrotizing encephalopathy (Leigh's disease). *Neurology*, **34**, 515–16.
49. Miyabashi, S., Ito, T., Narisawa, K. *et al.* (1985) Biochemical study in 28 children with lactic acidosis in relation to Leigh's encephalomyelopathy. *Eur. J. Pediatr.*, **143**, 278–83.
50. Brusilow S. and Horwich A. (1989) Urea cycle enzymes in *The Metabolic Basis of Inherited Disease*, 6th edn (eds C.R. Scriver, A.I. Beaudet, W.S. Sly and D. Valle), McGraw-Hill, NY, pp. 629–63.
51. Holzgreve, W. and Golbus, M. (1984) Prenatal diagnosis of ornithine transcarbamylase deficiency using fetal liver biopsy. *Am. J. Hum. Genet.*, **36**, 320–28.
52. Fearon, E., Mallonee, R., Phillips III, J. *et al.* (1985) Genetic analysis of carbamyl phosphate synthetase I deficiency. *Hum. Genet.*, **70**, 207–10.
53. Rodeck, C., Patrick, A., Pembrey, M. *et al.* (1982) Fetal liver biopsy for prenatal diagnosis of ornithine carbamoyl transferase deficiency. *Lancet*, **ii**, 297–99.
54. Horwich, A., Fenton, W., Williams, K. *et al* (1984) Structure and expression of a complementary DNA for the nuclear coded precursor of human mitochondrial ornithine transcarbamylase. *Science*, **224**, 1068–74.
55. Old, J., Briand, P., Purvis-Smith, S. *et al.* (1985) Prenatal exclusion of ornithine transcarbamylase deficiency by direct gene analysis. *Lancet*, **i**, 73–75.
56. Pembrey, M., Old, J., Leonard, J. *et al.* (1985) Prenatal diagnosis of ornithine carbamoyltransferase deficiency using a gene specific probe. *J. Med. Genet.*, **22**, 462–65.
57. Hill, H. and Goodman, S. (1974) Detection of inborn errors of metabolism. III. Defects in urea cycle metabolism. *Clin. Genet.*, **6**, 7–81.
58. Schimke, R. (1964) Enzymes of arginine metabolism in cell culture. *J. Biol. Chem.*, **239**, 136–45.
59. Fleischer, L., Harris, C., Mitchell, D. *et al.* (1983) Citrullinaemia: prenatal diagnosis of an affected fetus. *Am. J. Hum. Genet.*, **35**, 85–90.
60. Beaudet, A., O'Brien, W., Bock, H. *et al.* (1986) The human argininosuccinate synthetase locus and citrullinemia. *Adv. Hum. Genet.*, **15**, 161–96, 291–92.

61. Su, T. and Lin, L. (1990) Analysis of a splice acceptor site mutation which produces multiple splicing abnormalities in the human argininosuccinate synthetase locus. *J. Bio. Chem.*, **265**, 19716–20.

62. Kobayashi, K., Rosenbloom, C., Beaudet, A. *et al.* (1991) Additional mutations in argininosuccinate synthetase causing citrullinemia. *Mol. Biol. Med.*, **8**, 95–100.

63. Goodman, S. (1981) Antenatal diagnosis of defects of ureagenesis. *Pediatrics*, **68**, 446–47.

64. Margalith, D., Crichton, J., Wong, L. *et al.* (1983) Argininosuccinic aciduria: a developmental and biochemical study. *J. Neurol. Sci.*, **60**, 217–33.

65. Kvittingen, E., Jellum, E. and Stokke, O. (1981) Assay of fumaryl acetoacetate-fumaryl hydrolase in human liver – deficient activity in a case of hereditary tyrosinemia. *Clin. Chim. Acta*, **115**, 311–19.

66. Bergeron, P., Laberge, C. and Grenier, A. (1974) Hereditary tyrosinemia in the Province of Quebec: prevalence at birth and geographic distribution. *Clin. Genet.*, **5**, 157–62.

67. Grenier, A., Lescault, L., Laberge, C. *et al.* (1982) Detection of succinyl acetone and the use of its measurement in massive screening for hereditary tyrosinemia. *Clin. Chim. Acta*, **123**, 93–9.

68. Lindblad, G. and Sten, G. (1982) Identification of 4,6-dioxoheptanoic acid (succinyl acetone), 3,5-dioxooctanedioic (succinyl acetoacetate) and 4-oxo-6-hydroxyheptanoic acid in the urine from patients with hereditary tyrosinaemia. *Biomed. Mass Spectrom.*, **9**, 419–24.

69. Gagne, R., Lescault, A., Grenier, A. *et al.* (1982) Prenatal diagnosis of hereditary tyrosinemia: measurement of succylacetone in amniotic fluid. *Prenat. Diagn.*, **2**, 185–88.

70. Goldsmith, L. and La Berge, C. (1989) Tyrosinemia and related disorders, in *The Metabolic Basis of Inherited Disease*, 6th edn (eds C.R. Scriver, A.I. Beaudet, W.S. Sly and D. Valle), McGraw-Hill, NY, pp. 547–62.

71. Menkes, J., Hurst, P. and Craig, J. (1954) A new syndrome: progressive familial infantile cerebral dysfunction associated with an unusual urinary substance. *Pediatrics*, **14**, 462–67.

72. Snyderman, S. (1974) Maple syrup urine disease, in *Heritable Disorders of Amino Acid Metabolism* (ed. W.L. Nyhan), Wiley, NY, pp. 17–31.

73. Zhang, B., Wappner, R., Brandt, I. *et al.* (1990) Sequence of the E1 alpha subunit of branched-chain alpha-ketoacid dehydrogenase in two patients with thiamine-responsive maple syrup urine disease. *Am. J. Hum. Genet.*, **46**, 843–46.

74. Fisher, C., Fisher, C., Chuang, D. *et al.* (1991) Occurrence of a Tyr393-Asn (Y393N) mutation in the E1 alpha gene of the branched-chain alpha-keto acid dehydrogenase complex in maple syrup urine disease patients from a Mennonite population. *Am. J. Hum. Genet.*, **49**, 429–34.

75. Gerritson, T., Kaveggia, E. and Waisman, H. (1965) A new type of idiopathic hyperglycinemia with hypo-oxaluria. *Pediatrics*, **36**, 882–91.

76. Toone, J. and Applegarth, D. (1989) Use of placental enzyme analysis in assessment of the newborn at risk for non-ketotic-hyperglycinemia (NKH). *J. Inherited Metab. Dis.*, **12**, 281–85.

77. Perry, T., Urquhart, N., MacLean, J. *et al.* (1975) Nonketotic hyperglycaemia. Glycine accumulation due to absence of glycine cleavage in brain. *N. Engl. J. Med.*, **292**, 1269–73.

78. Tada, K., Narisawa, K., Yoshida, T. *et al.* (1969) Hyperglycinemia: a defect in glycine cleavage reaction. *Tohoku J. Exp. Med.*, **98**, 289–96.

79. Kure, S., Narisawa, K. and Tada K. (1992) Enzymatic diagnosis of non-ketotic hyperglycinemia with lymphoblasts. *J. Pediatr.*, **120**, 95–98.

80. Kure, S., Takayanagi, M., Narisawa, K. *et al.* (1992) Identification of a common mutation in Finnish patients with NKH. *J. Clin. Invest.*, **90**, 160–64.

81. Toone, J., Applegarth, D. and Levy H. (1992) Prenatal diagnosis of non-ketotic hyperglycinemia: experience in 50 at-risk pregnancies. *J. Inherited Metab. Dis.*, **17**, in press.

82. Hiraga, K., Koyata, H., Sakakibara, T. *et al.* (1991) Non-ketotic hyperglycinemia: an aim of the second generation of studies on pathogenesis. *Mol. Biol. Med.* **8**, 65–79.

83. Gitzelmann, R. Steinmann, B. and Van den Berghe, G. (1983) Essential fructosuria, hereditary fructose intolerance and fructose 1,6-diphosphatase deficiency, in *The Metabolic Basis of Inherited Disease*, 5th edn (eds J.B. Stanbury, J.B. Wyngaarden, D.S. Fredrickson *et al.*). McGraw-Hill, NY, pp. 118–40.

84. Odievre, M., Gentil, C., Gautier, M. *et al.* (1978) Hereditary fructose intolerance in childhood. *Am. J. Dis. Child.*, **132**, 605–608.

85. Odievre, M. (1969) Les difficultés du diagnostic de l'intolérance héréditaire au fructose. *Arch. Fr. Pediatr.*, **26**, 5–19.

86. Baerlocher, K., Gitzelmann, R., Steinmann, B. et al. (1978) Hereditary fructose intolerance in early childhood: a major diagnostic challenge. *Helv. Paediatr. Acta*, **33**, 465–87.

87. Bender, S., Vieweg, B., Posselt, H. *et al.* (1982) Hereditaire fructose Intoleranz. *Monatsschr. Kinderheilkd.*, **130**, 21–26.

88. Bode, C., Schumacher, H., Goebell, H. *et al.* (1971) Fructose induced depletion of liver adenine nucleotides in man. *Horm. Metab. Res.*, **3**, 289–90.

89. Kaiser, U. and Hegele, R. (1991) Case report: heterogeneity of aldolase B in hereditary fructose intolerance. *Am. J. Med. Sci.*, **302**, 364–68.

90. Gregori, C., Besmond, C., Odievre, M. *et al.* (1984) DNA analysis in patients with hereditary fructose intolerance. *Ann. Hum. Genet.*, **48**, 291–96.

91. Cross, N., Tolan, D. and Cox, T. (1988) Catalytic deficiency of human aldolase B in hereditary fructose intolerance caused by a common missense mutation. *Cell*, **53**, 881–85.

92. Sebastio, G., de Franchis, R., Strisciuglio, P. *et al.* (1991) Aldolase B mutations in Italian families affected by hereditary fructose intolerance. *J. Med. Genet.*, **28**, 241–43.

93. Rallison, M., Meikle, A. and Zigrang, W. (1979) Hypoglycemia and lactic acidosis associated with fructose 1,6 diphosphatase deficiency. *J. Pediatr.*, **94**, 933–36.

94. Saudubray, J., Dreyfus, J. and Cepanec, C. (1973) Acidose lactique hypoglycémie et hépatomegalie par deficit héréditaire et fructose 1.6 diphosphatase hépatique. *Arch. Fr. Pediatr.*, **30**, 609–32.

95. Gitzelmann, R. and Hansen, R. (1980) Galactose metabolism, hereditary defects and their clinical significance, in *Inherited Disorders of Carbohydrate Metabolism* (eds D. Burman, J.B. Holton and C.A. Pennock), MTP Press, Lancaster, 61–101.

96. Kleijer, W., Janse, H., van Diggelen, O. *et al.* (1986) First trimester diagnosis of galactosaemia. *Lancet*, i, 748.

97. Reichardt, J. and Woo, S. (1991) Molecular basis of galactosemia: mutations and polymorphisms in the gene encoding human galactose-1-phosphate uridylyltransferase *Proc. Natl Acad. Sci. USA*, **88**, 2633–37.

98. Reichardt, J., Packman, S. and Woo, S. (1991) Molecular characterization of two galactosemia mutations: correlation of mutations with highly conserved domains in galactose-1-phosphate uridyl transferase. *Am. J. Hum. Genet.* **9**, 860–67.

99. Goldfischer, S., Moore, C., Johnson, A. *et al.* (1973) Peroxisomal and mitochondrial defects in the cerebro–hepato–renal syndrome. *Science*, **182**, 62–4.

100. Schutgens, R., Heymans, H., Wanders, R. *et al.* (1986) Peroxisomal disorders: a newly recognised group of genetic diseases. *Eur. J. Pediatr.*, **144**, 430–40.

101. Wilson, G., Holmes, R. and Custer, J. (1986) Zellweger syndrome: diagnostic assays, syndrome delineation, and potential therapy. *Am. J. Med. Genet.*, **24**, 69–82.

102. Schutgens, R., Romeyn, G., Wanders, R. *et al.* (1984) Deficiency of acyl-CoA: dihydroxyacetone phosphate acyltransferase in patients with Zellweger (cerebro-hepato-renal) syndrome. *Biochem. Biophys. Res. Commun.*, **120**, 179–84.

103. Datta, N., Wilson, G. and Hajra, A. (1984) Deficiency of enzymes catalyzing the biosynthesis of glycerol-ether lipids in Zellweger syndrome. *N. Engl. J. Med.*, **311**, 1080–83.

104. Shimozawa, N., Tsukamoto, T., Suzuki, Y. *et al.* (1992) A human gene responsible for Zellweger syndrome that affects peroxisome assembly. *Science*, **255**, 1132–34.

105. Hoefler, G., Hoefler, S., Watkins, P. *et al.* (1988) Biochemical abnormalities in rhizomelic chondrodysplasia punctata. *J. Pediatr.*, **112**, 726–33.

106. Wanders, R., Saelman, D., Heymans, H. *et al.* (1986) Genetic relation between the Zellweger syndrome, infantile Refsum's disease, and rhizomelic chondrodysplasia punctata. *N. Engl. J. Med.*, **314**, 787–88.

107. Hashmi, M., Stanley, W. and Singh, I. (1986) Lignoceroyl-CoASH ligase: enzyme defect in fatty acid β-oxidation system in X-linked childhood adrenoleukodystrophy. *FEBS Lett.*, **196**, 247–50.

108. Watkins, P., Mihalik, S. and Skjeldad O. (1990) Mitochondrial oxidation of phytanic acid in human and monkey liver. Implication that Refsum's disease is not a peroxisomal disorder. *Biochem. Biophys. Res. Commun.*, **167**, 580–86.

109. Mosser, J., Lutz, Y., Stoeckel, M. *et al.* (1994) The gene responsible for adrenoleukodystrophy encodes a peroxisomal membrane protein. *Hum. Mol. Genet.*, **3**, 265–71.

110. Del Mastro, R., Bundey, S. and Kilpatrick, M. (1990) Adrenoleucodystrophy: a molecular genetic study in five families. *J. Med. Genet.*, **27**, 670–75.

111. Shoffner, J., Lott, M., Lezzal, M.S. *et al.* (1991) Myoclonic epilepsy and ragged-red fiber disease is associated with a mitochondrial DNA tRNA-lys mutation. *Cell*, **61**, 931.

112. Tanaka, M., Ino, H., Ohno K. *et al.* (1991) Mitochondrial DNA mutations in mitochondrial myopathy, encephalopathy, lactic acidosis, and stroke like episodes (MELAS). *Biochem. Biophy. Res. Commun.*, **174**, 861–68.

113. Shoffner IV, J. and Wallace, D. (1990) Oxidative phosphorylation diseases. *Adv. Hum. Genet.*, **19**, 267–330.

114. Tulinius, M., Holme, E., Kristiansson, B. *et al.* (1991) Mitochondrial encephalomyopathies in childhood. I. Biochemical and morphologic investigations. *J. Pediatr.*, **119**, 242–59.

115. Munnich, A., Rustin, P., Rötig *et al.* (1992) Clinical aspects of mitochondrial disorders. *J. Inherited Metab. Dis.*, **15**, 448–55.

116. Simmonds, H., Duley, J. and Davies, P. (1991) Analysis of purines and pyrimidines in blood, urine and other physiological fluids, in *Techniques in Diagnostic Human Biochemical Genetics* (ed. F.A. Hommes), Wiley–Liss, NY, pp. 397–424.

117. Miller, A., Kaleko, M., Garcia, J. et al. (1991) Gene transfer into haematopoietic and skin cells, in Treatment of Genetic Diseases (ed. R.J. Desnick), Churchill Livingstone, NY, pp. 261–71.

118. Igarashi, T., Minami, M. and Nishida, Y. (1989) Molecular analysis of hypoxanthine–guanine phosphoribosyltransferase mutations in five unrelated Japanese patients. Acta Paediatr. Jpn, 31, 303–13.

119. Yamada, Y., Goto, H. and Ogasawara, N. (1991) Identification of two independent Japanese mutant HPRT genes using the PCR technique. Adv. Exp. Med. Biol., 309B, 121–24.

120. Singh, S., Willers, I., Held, K. et al. (1989) Lesch–Nyhan syndrome and HPRT variants: study of heterogeneity at the gene level. Adv. Exp. Med. Biol., 253A, 145–50.

121. Fujimori, S., Davidson, B., Kelley, W. et al. (1989) Lesch–Nyhan syndrome due to a single nucleotide change in the hypoxanthine–guanine phosphoribosyltransferase gene (HPRTYale). Adv. Exp. Med. Biol., 253A, 135–38.

122. Gordon, R., Emmerson, B., Stout, J. et al. (1987) Molecular studies of hypoxanthine–guanine phosphoribosyltransferase mutations in six Australian families. Aust. N. Z. J. Med., 17, 424–29.

123. Hug, G. (1980) Pre- and postnatal diagnosis of glycogen storage disease, in Inherited Disorders of Carbohydrate Metabolism (eds D. Burnam, J.B. Holton and C.A. Pennock), MTP Press, Lancaster, pp. 327–67.

124. Maire, I., Baussan, C., Moatti, N. et al. (1991) Biochemical diagnosis of hepatic glycogen storage diseases: 20 years French experience. Clin. Biochem., 24, 169–78.

125. Dunger, D. and Leonard, J. (1982) Value of the glucagon test in screening for hepatic glycogen storage disease. Arch. Dis. Child., 57, 384–89.

126. Fernandes, J., Huijing, F. and Van de Kamer, J. (1969) A screening method for liver glycogen storage diseases. Arch. Dis. Child., 44, 311–17.

127. Nadler, H. and Messina, A. (1969) In utero detection of type II glycogenosis (Pompe's disease). Lancet, ii, 1277–78.

128. Loonen, M., Busch, H., Koster, J. et al. (1981) A family with different clinical forms of acid maltase deficiency (glycogenosis type II): biochemical and genetic studies. Neurology, 31, 1209–16.

129. Reuser, A., Kross, M., Oude Elferink, R. et al. (1985) Defects in synthesis, phosphorylation and maturation of acid α-glucosidase in glycogenosis type II. J. Biol. Chem., 260, 8336–41.

130. Hug, G., Soukup, S., Ryan, M. et al. (1984) Rapid prenatal diagnosis of glycogen storage disease type II by electron microscopy of uncultured amniotic fluid cells. N. Engl. J. Med., 310, 1018–22.

131. Van der Ploeg, A., Hoefsloot, L., Hoogeveen-Westerveld, M. et al. (1989) Glycogenosis type II: protein and DNA analysis in five South African families from various ethnic origins. Am. J. Hum. Genet., 44, 787–93.

132. Hermans, M., de Graaff, E., Kroos, M. et al. (1991) Identification of a point mutation in the human lysosomal alpha-glucosidase gene causing infantile glycogenosis type II. Biochem. Biophys. Res. Commun., 179, 919–26.

133. Van Hoof, F. and Hers, H. (1967) The sub-groups of type III glycogenosis. Eur. J. Biochem., 2, 265–70.

134. Van Hoof, F. (1967) Amylo-1,6-glucosidase activity and glycogen content of the erythrocytes of normal subjects, patients with glycogen storage disease and heterozygotes. Eur. J. Biochem., 2, 271–74.

135. Steinitz, K., Bodur, H. and Annan, T. (1963) Amylo-1,6-glucosidase activity in leucocytes of patients with glycogen storage disease. Clin. Chim. Acta, 8, 807–809.

136. Besley, G., Cohen, P., Faed, M. et al. (1983) Amylo-1,6-glucosidase activity in cultured cells: a deficiency in type III glycogenosis with prenatal studies. Prenat. Diagn., 3, 13–9.

137. Maire, I. and Mathieu, M. (1986) Possible prenatal diagnosis of type III glycogenosis. J. Inherited Metab. Dis., 9, 89–91.

138. Van Diggelen, O., Janse, H. and Smit, G. (1985) Debranching enzyme in fibroblasts, amniotic fluid cells and chorionic villi: pre- and postnatal diagnosis of glycogenosis type III. Clin. Chim. Acta, 149, 129–34.

139. Gutman, A., Barash, V., Schramm, H. et al. (1985) Incorporation of [14C] glucose into α-1,4 bonds of glycogen by leukocytes and fibroblasts of patients-with type III glycogen storage disease. Pediatr. Res., 19, 28–32.

140. Ding, J., de Barsy, T., Brown, B. et al. (1990) Immunoblot analyses of glycogen debranching enzyme in different subtypes of glycogen storage disease type III. J. Pediatr., 116, 95–100.

141. Brown, B. and Brown, D. (1966) Lack of an α-1,4-glucan:α-1,4-glucan 6-glycosyl transferase in a case of type IV glycogenosis. Proc. Natl Acad. Sci. USA, 96, 725–29.

142. Howell, R., Kaback, M. and Brown, B. (1971) Type IV glycogen storage disease: branching enzyme activity in skin fibroblasts and possible heterozygote detection. J. Pediatr., 78, 638–42.

143. DiMauro, S. and Hartlage, P. (1978) Fatal infantile form of muscle phosphorylase deficiency. Neurology, 28, 1124–29.

144. Danon, M., Carpenter, S., Manaligod, J. et al. (1981) Fatal infantile glycogen storage disease: deficiency of phosphofructokinase and phosphorylase b kinase. Neurology, 31, 1303–307.

145. Nakajima, H., Kono, N., Yamasaki, T. et al. (1990) Genetic defect in muscle phosphofructokinase deficiency. Abnormal splicing of the muscle phosphofructokinase gene due to a point mutation at the 5'-splice site. J. Biol. Chem., 265, 9392–95.

146. Hug, G., Chuck, G., Walling, L. et al. (1974) Liver phosphorylase deficiency in glycogenosis type VI: documentation by biochemical analysis of hepatic biopsy specimens. J. Lab. Clin. Med., 84, 26–35.

147. Hug, G., Schubert, W. and Chuck, G. (1966) Phosphorylase kinase of the liver; deficiency in a girl with increased hepatic glycogen. Science, 153, 1534–35.

148. Huijing, F. and Fernandes, J. (1969) X-chromosomal inheritance of liver glycogenosis with phosphorylase kinase deficiency. Am. J. Med. Genet., 21, 278–84.

149. Lederer, B., Van Hoof, F., Van den Berghe, G. et al. (1975) Glycogen phosphorylase and its converter enzymes in haemolysates of normal human subjects and of patients with type VI glycogen storage disease. A study of phosphorylase kinase deficiency. Biochem. J., 147, 23–25.

150. Lederer, B., van der Werve, G., de Barsy, Th. et al. (1980) The autosomal form of phosphorylase kinase deficiency in man: reduced activity of the muscle enzyme. Biochem. Biophys. Res. Commun., 92, 169–74.

151. Newgard, C., Fletterick, R., Anderson, L. et al. (1987) The polymorphic locus for glycogen storage disease VI (liver glycogen phosphorylase) maps to chromosome 14. Am. J. Hum. Genet., 40, 351–64.

152. Kilimann, M. (1990) Molecular genetics of phosphorylase kinase: cDNA cloning, chromosomal mapping and isoform structure. J. Inherited Metab. Dis., 13, 435–41.

153. Alexander, D., Assaf, M., Khudr, A. et al. (1985) Fructose-1,6-diphosphatase deficiency: diagnosis using leucocytes and detection of heterozygotes with radiochemical and spectrophotometric methods. J. Inherited Metab. Dis., 8, 174–77.

154. Abu-Dalu, K., Tamary, H., Livoni, N. et al. (1982) G$_{M1}$-gangliosidosis presenting as neonatal ascites. J. Pediatr., 100, 940–43.

155. Sun, C., Panny, S., Combs, J. et al. (1984) Hydrops fetalis associated with Gaucher disease. Pathol. Res. Pract., 179, 101–104.

156. Beck, M., Bender, S., Reiter, H. et al. (1984) Neuraminidase deficiency presenting as non-immune hydrops fetalis. Eur. J. Pediatr., 14, 135–39.

157. Irani, D., Kim, H., El-Hibri, H. et al. (1983) Postmortem observations on β-glucuronidase deficiency presenting as hydrops fetalis. Ann. Neurol., 14, 486–90.

158. Farrell, D. and Ochs, U. (1981) GM$_1$-gangliosidosis: phenotypic variation in a single family. Ann. Neurol., 9, 225–31.

159. Poenaru, L., Kaplan, L., Dumez, J. et al. (1984) Evaluation of possible first trimester prenatal diagnosis in lysosomal diseases by trophoblast biopsy. Pediatr. Res., 18, 1032–34.

160. Gatti, R., Lombardo, C., Filocamo, M. et al. (1985) Comparison of the activities of 15 lysosomal enzymes in chorionic villi and cultured amniotic fluid cells, in First Trimester Fetal Diagnosis (eds M. Fraccaro, G. Simoni, and B. Bambati), Springer, Berlin, pp. 238–41.

161. Galjaard, H. (1985) Biochemical analysis of chorionic villi in a worldwide survey of first trimester fetal diagnosis of inborn errors of metabolism, in First Trimester Fetal Diagnosis (eds M. Fraccaro, G. Simoni and B. Bambati), Springer, Berlin, pp. 209–17.

162. Young, E. (1992) Prenatal diagnosis of Hurler disease by analysis of α-iduronidase in chorionic villi. J. Inherited Metab. Dis., 15, 224–30.

163. Desnick, R. (1989) Fabry's disease: α-galactosidase A deficiency, in The Metabolic Basis of Inherited Disease, 6th edn (eds C.R. Scriver, A.I. Beaudet, W.S. Sly and D. Valle), McGraw-Hill, NY, pp. 1751–80.

164. Strasberg, P., Warren, I., Skomorowski, M. et al. (1985) HPLC analysis of urinary sulfatide: an aid in the diagnosis of metachromatic leukodystrophy. Clin. Biochem., 18, 92–97.

165. Warner, T., Robertson, A., Mock, A. et al. (1983) Prenatal diagnosis of G$_{M1}$-gangliosidosis by detection of galactosyloligosaccharides in amniotic fluid by high-performance liquid chromatography. Am. J. Hum. Genet., 35, 1034–41.

166. O'Brien, J. (1989) β-Galactosidase deficiency; ganglioside sialidase deficiency, in The Metabolic Basis of Inherited Disease, 6th edn (eds C.R. Scriver, A.I. Beaudet, W.S. Sly and D. Valle), McGraw-Hill, NY, pp. 1797–1806.

167. Sandhoff, K., Conzelmann, E., Neufeld, E. et al. (1989) The G$_{M2}$ gangliosidoses, in The Metabolic Basis of Inherited Disease, 6th edn (eds C.R. Scriver, A.I. Beaudet, W.S. Sly and D. Valle), McGraw-Hill, NY, pp. 1807–42.

168. Fuchs, W., Navon, R., Kaback, M. et al. (1983) Tay–Sachs disease: one-step assay of β-N-acetylhexosaminidase in serum with a sulphated chromogenic substrate. Clin. Chim. Acta, 113, 253–61.

169. Triggs-Raine, B., Akerman, B., Clarke, J. et al. (1991) Sequence of DNA flanking the exons of the HEXA gene, and identification of mutations in Tay–Sachs disease. Am. J. Hum. Genet., 49, 1041–54.

170. Grebner, E. and Tomczak, J. (1991) Distribution of three alpha-chain beta-hexosaminidase A mutations among Tay–Sachs carriers. Am. J. Hum. Genet., 48, 604–607.

171. Mules, E., Dowling, C., Petersen, M. et al. (1991) A novel mutation in the invariant AG of the acceptor splice site of intron 4 of the beta-hexosaminidase alpha-subunit gene in two unrelated American black GM2-gangliosidosis (Tay–Sachs disease) patients. Am. J. Hum. Genet., 48, 1181–85.

172. Paw, B., Tieu, P., Kaback, M. et al. (1990) Frequency of three Hex A

mutant alleles among Jewish and non-Jewish carriers identified in a Tay–Sachs screening program. *Am. J. Hum. Genet.*, 47, 698–705.

173. Schroder, M., Schnabel, D., Suzuki, K. *et al.* (1991) A mutation in the gene of a glycolipid-binding protein (GM2 activator) that causes GM2-gangliosidosis variant AB. *FEBS Lett.*, 290, 1–3.

174. Bikker, H., van den Berg, F., Wolterman, R. *et al.* (1989) Demonstration of a Sandhoff disease-associated autosomal 50-kb deletion by field inversion gel electrophoresis. *Hum. Genet.*, 81, 287–88.

175. Wakamatsu, N., Kobayashi, H., Miyatake T. *et al.* (1992) A novel exon mutation in the human beta- hexosaminidase beta subunit gene affects 3′ splice site selection. *J. Biol. Chem.*, 267, 2406–13.

176. O'Dowd, B., Klavins, M., Willard, H. *et al.* (1986) Molecular heterogeneity in the infantile and juvenile forms of Sandhoff disease (O-variant GM2 gangliosidosis). *J. Biol. Chem.*, 261, 12680–85.

177. Schram, A. and Tager, J. (1981) The specificity of lysosomal hydrolases: human α-galactosidase isoenzymes. *Trends Biochem. Sci.*, 6, 328–30.

178. Sakuraba, H., Oshima, A., Fukuhara, Y. *et al.* (1990) Identification of point mutations in the alpha-galactosidase A gene in classical and atypical hemizygotes with Fabry disease. *Am. J. Hum. Genet.*, 47, 784–89.

179. Fukuhara, Y., Sakuraba, H., Oshima, A. *et al.* (1990) Partial deletion of human alpha-galactosidase A gene in Fabry disease: direct repeat sequences as a possible cause of slipped mispairing. *Biochem. Biophys. Res. Commun.*, 170, 296–300.

180. Suzuki, Y. and Suzuki, K. (1971) Krabbe's globoid cell leucodystrophy: deficiency of galactocerebrosidase in serum, leucocytes and fibroblasts. *Science*, 17, 73–75.

181. Besley, G. and Bain, A. (1976) Krabbe's globoid cell leucodystrophy. Studies on galactosylceramide β-galactosidase and non-specific β-galactosidase of leucocytes, cultured skin fibroblasts and amniotic fluid cells. *J. Med. Genet.*, 13, 195–99.

182. Besley, G. and Gatt, S. (1981) Spectrophotometric and fluorimetric assays of galactocerebrosidase activity: their use in the diagnosis of Krabbe's disease. *Clin. Chim. Acta*, 110, 19–26.

183. Kihara, H. (1982) Genetic heterogeneity in metachromatic leukodystrophy. *Am. J. Hum. Genet.*, 34, 171–81.

184. Polten, A., Fluharty, A., Fluharty, C. *et al.* (1991) Molecular basis of different forms of metachromatic leukodystrophy. *N. Engl. J. Med.*, 324, 18–22.

185. Gieselmann, V. and von Figura, K. (1990) Advances in the molecular genetics of metachromatic leukodystrophy. *J. Inherited Metab. Dis.*, 13, 560–71.

186. Zhang, X., Rafi, M., DeGala, G. *et al.* (1990) Insertion in the mRNA of a metachromatic leukodystrophy patient with sphingolipid activator protein-1 deficiency. *Proc. Natl Acad. Sci. USA*, 87, 1426–30.

187. Gieselmann, V. (1991) An assay for the rapid detection of the arylsulfatase A pseudodeficiency allele facilitates diagnosis and genetic counseling for metachromatic leukodystrophy. *Hum. Genet.*, 86, 251–55.

188. Hreidarsson, S., Thomas, G., Kihara, H. *et al.* (1983) Impaired cerebroside sulfate hydrolysis in fibroblasts of sibs with 'pseudo' arylsulfatase A deficiency without metachromatic leukodystrophy. *Pediatr. Res.*, 17, 701–704.

189. Gieselmann, V., Fluharty A., Tonnesen, T. *et al.* (1991) Mutations in the arylsulfatase A pseudodeficiency allele causing metachromatic leukodystrophy. *Am. J. Hum. Genet.*, 49, 403–407.

190. Rommerskirch, W. and Von Figura, K. (1992) Multiple sulfatase deficiency: catalytically inactive sulfatases are expressed from retrovirally introduced sulfatase cDNAs. *Proc. Natl Acad. Sci. USA*, 89, 2561–65.

191. Nilsson, O. and Svennerholm, L. (1982) Accumulation of glucosylceramide and glucosylsphingosine (psychosine) in cerebrum and cerebellum in infantile and juvenile Gaucher disease. *J. Neurochem.*, 39, 709–26.

192. Van Weely, S., van Leeuwen, M., Jansen, I. *et al.* (1991) Clinical phenotype of Gaucher disease in relation to properties of mutant glucocerebrosidase in cultured fibroblasts. *Biochim. Biophys. Acta*, 1096, 301–11.

193. Mistry, P., Smith, S., Ali, M. *et al.* (1992) Genetic diagnosis of Gaucher's disease. *Lancet*, 339, 889–92.

194. Zimran, A., Gelbart, T. and Beutler, E. (1990) Linkage of the *PvuII* polymorphism with the common Jewish mutation for Gaucher disease. *Am. J. Hum. Genet.*, 46, 902–905.

195. Theophilus, B., Latham, T., Grabowski, G. *et al.* (1989) Gaucher disease: molecular heterogeneity and phenotype–genotype correlations. *Am. J. Hum. Genet.*, 45, 212–25.

196. Dahl, N., Lagerstrom, M., Erikson, A. *et al.* (1990) Gaucher disease type III (Norrbottnian type) is caused by a single mutation in exon 10 of the glucocerebrosidase gene. *Am. J. Hum. Genet.*, 47, 275–78.

197. Choy, F., Woo, M. and Der Kaloustian, V. (1991) Molecular analysis of Gaucher disease: screening of patients in the Montreal/Quebec region. *Am. J. Med. Genet.*, 41, 469–74.

198. Vanier, M. (1983) Biochemical studies in Niemann–Pick disease. I. Major sphingolipids of liver and spleen. *Biochim. Biophys. Acta*, 75, 178–84.

199. Besley, G. and Elleder, M. (1986) Enzyme activities and phospholipid storage patterns in brain and spleen samples from Niemann–Pick disease variants: a comparison of neuropathic and non-neuropathic forms. *J. Inherited Metab. Dis.*, 9, 59–71.

200. Ferlinz, K., Hurwitz, R. and Sandhoff K. (1991) Molecular basis of acid sphingomyelinase deficiency in a patient with Niemann–Pick disease type A. *Biochem. Biophys. Res. Commun.*, 179, 1187–91.

201. Takahashi, T., Suchi, M., Desnick, R. *et al.* (1992) Identification and expression of five mutations in the human acid sphingomyelinase gene causing types A and B Niemann–Pick disease. Molecular evidence for genetic heterogeneity in the neuronopathic and non-neuronopathic forms. *J. Biol. Chem.*, 267, 12552–58.

202. Neville, B., Lake, B., Stephens, R. *et al.* (1973) A neurovisceral storage disease with vertical supranuclear ophthalmoplegia and its relationship to Niemann–Pick disease. *Brain*, 96, 97–120.

203. Fink, J., Filling-Katz, M. Sokol, J. *et al.* (1992) Clinical spectrum of Niemann–Pick disease type C. *Neurology*, 39, 1040–49.

204. Rao, B. and Spence, M. (1977) Niemann–Pick disease type D: lipid analyses and studies on sphingomyelinases. *Ann. Neurol.*, 1, 385–92.

205. Besley, G. and Moss, S. (1983) Studies on sphingomyelinase and β-glucosidase activities in Niemann–Pick disease variants. Phosphodiesterase activities measured with natural and artificial substrates. *Biochim. Biophys. Acta*, 752, 54–64.

206. Vanier, M., Wenger, D., Comly, M. *et al.* (1988) Niemann–Pick disease group C: clinical variability and diagnosis based on defective cholesterol esterification. A collaborative study of 70 patients. *Clin. Genet.*, 33, 331–48.

207. Vanier, M., Rodriguez–Lafrasse, C. Rousson, R. *et al.* (1992) Prenatal diagnosis of Niemann–Pick type C disease: current strategy from an experience of 37 pregnancies at risk. *Am. J. Hum. Genet.*, 51, 111–22.

208. Toppet, M., Vamos–Hurwitz, E. Jonniaux, G. *et al.* (1978) Farber's disease as a ceramidosis: clinical, radiological and biochemical aspects. *Acta Pediatr. Scand.*, 67, 113–19.

209. Dulaney, J., Milunsky, A. Sidbury, J. *et al.* (1976) Diagnosis of lipogranulomatosis (Farber disease) by use of cultured fibroblasts. *J. Pediatr.*, 89, 59–61.

210. Schaub, J., Janka, G., Christomanou, H. *et al.* (1980) Wolman's disease: clinical, biochemical and ultrastructural studies in an unusual case without striking adrenal calcification. *Eur. J. Pediatr.*, 135, 45–53.

211. Patrick, A. and Lake, B. (1969) Deficiency of an acid lipase in Wolman's disease. *Nature*, 222, 1067–68.

212. Besley, G., Broadhead, D. Lawlor, E. *et al.* (1984) Cholesterol ester storage disease in an adult presenting with sea-blue histiocytosis. *Clin. Genet.*, 26, 195–203.

213. Sewell, A. (1980) Urinary oligosaccharide excretion in disorders of glycolipid, glycoprotein and glycogen metabolism. A review of screening for differential diagnosis. *Eur. J. Pediatr.*, 134, 183–94.

214. Mononen, T., Parviainen, M. Penttila, I. *et al.* (1986) Liquid-chromatographic detection of aspartylglycosaminuria. *Clin. Chem.*, 32, 501–2.

215. Ockerman, P. (1967) A generalised storage disorder resembling Hurler's syndrome. *Lancet*, ii, 239–41.

216. Durand, P., Borrone, C. and Della Cella, G. (1966) A new mucopolysaccharide lipid-storage disease? *Lancet*, ii, 1313.

217. Pollitt, R., Jenner, F. and Mersky, H. (1968) Aspartylglucosaminuria. An inborn error of metabolism associated with mental defect. *Lancet*, ii, 253–55.

218. Pohlmann, R., Hasilik, A. and Cheng, S. (1983) Synthesis of lysosomal α-mannosidase in normal and mannosidosis fibroblasts. *Biochem. Biophys. Res. Commun.*, 115, 1083–89.

219. Turner, B., Turner, V., Beratis, N. *et al.* (1975) Polymorphism of human α-fucosidase. *Am. J. Hum. Genet.*, 27, 651–61.

220. Cooper, A., Wraith, J., Savage, W. *et al.* (1991) β-Mannosidase deficiency in a female infant with epileptic encephalopathy. *J. Inherited Metab. Dis.*, 14, 18–22.

221. Desnick, R. and Wang A. (1990) Schindler disease: an inherited neuroaxonal dystrophy due to α-acetylgalactosaminidase deficiency. *J. Inherited Metab. Dis.*, 13, 549–59.

222. Renlund, M., Aula, P., Raivio, K. *et al.* (1983) Salla disease: a new lysosomal storage disorder with disturbed sialic acid metabolism. *Neurology*, 33, 57–66.

223. Jonas, A. (1986) Studies of lysosomal sialic acid metabolism: retention of sialic acid by Salla disease lysosomes. *Biochem. Biophys. Res. Commun.*, 137, 175–81.

224. Stevenson, R., Lubinsky, M., Taylor, H. *et al.* (1983) Sialic acid storage disease with sialuria: clinical and biochemical features in the severe infantile type. *Pediatrics*, 72, 441–9.

225. Lowden, J. and O'Brien, J. (1979) Sialidosis: a review of human neuraminidase deficiency. *Am. J. Hum. Genet.*, 31, 1–18.

226. Leroy, J. and DeMars, R. (1967) Mutant enzymatic and cytological phenotypes in cultured human fibroblasts. *Science*, 157, 804–806.

227. Reitman, M., Varki, A. and Kornfeld, S. (1981) Fibroblasts from patients with I-cell disease and pseudo-Hurler polydystrophy are deficient in uridine 5-diphosphate-N-acetylglucosamine: glycoprotein N-acetyl glucosaminylphosphotransferase activity. *J. Clin. Invest.*, 67, 1574–79.

228. Wiesmann, U., Vasella, F. and Herschkowitz, N. (1971) I-cell disease: leakage of lysosomal enzymes into extracellular fluids. *N. Engl. J. Med.*, 285, 1090–91.

229. Gehler, J., Cantz, M., Stoeckenius, M. *et al.* (1976) Prenatal diagnosis of mucolipidosis II (I-cell disease). *Eur. J. Pediatr.*, **122**, 201–206.

230. Besley, G., Broadhead, D., Nevin, N. *et al.* (1990) Prenatal diagnosis of mucolipidosis II by early amniocentesis. *Lancet*, **335**, 1164–65.

231. Chityat, D., Mevnier, C., Hodgkinson, K. *et al.* (1991) Mucolipidosis type IV: clinical manifestations and natural history. *Am. J. Med. Genet.*, **41**, 313–18.

232. Kresse, H., Cantz, M., von Figura, K. *et al.* (1981) The mucopolysaccharidoses: biochemistry and clinical symptoms. *Klin. Wochenschr.*, **59**, 867–76.

233. Mossman, J. and Patrick, A. (1982) Prenatal diagnosis of mucopolysaccharidosis by two-dimensional electrophoresis of amniotic fluid glycosaminoglycans. *Prenat. Diagn.*, **2**, 169–76.

234. Stirling, J., Robinson, D., Fensom, A. *et al.* (1979) Prenatal diagnosis of two Hurler fetuses using an improved assay for methylumbelliferyl-α-L-iduronidase. *Lancet*, **ii**, 37.

235. Lim, T., Leder, I., Bach, G. *et al.* (1974) An assay for iduronate sulfatase (Hunter corrective factor). *Carbohydr. Res.*, **37**, 103–109.

236. Zlotogora, J. and Bach, G. (1986) Hunter syndrome: prenatal diagnosis in maternal serum. *Am. J. Hum. Genet.*, **38**, 253–60.

237. Besley, G., Broadhead, D. and Ellis, P. (1992) First trimester diagnosis of Hunter syndrome (MPS II). *Prenat. Diagn.*, **12**, 72–73.

238. Broadhead, D., Kirk, J., Burt, A. *et al.* (1986) Full expression of Hunter's disease in a female with an X-chromosome deletion leading to non-random inactivation. *Clin. Genet.*, **30**, 392–98.

239. Clarke, J., Wilson, P., Morris, C. *et al.* (1992) Characterization of a deletion at Xq27-q28 associated with unbalanced inactivation of the nonmutant X chromosome. *Am. J. Hum. Genet.*, **51**, 316–22.

240. Flomen, R., Green, P., Bentley D. *et al.* (1992) Detection of point mutations and a gross deletion in six Hunter syndrome patients. *Genomics*, **13**, 543–50.

241. Clements, P. and Hopwood J. (1990) Hunter syndrome: isolation of an iduronate-2-sulfatase cDNA clone and analysis of patient DNA. *Proc. Natl Acad. Sci. USA*, **87**, 8531–35.

242. Van de Kamp, J., Niermeijer, M., von Figura, K. *et al.* (1981) Genetic heterogeneity and clinical variability in the Sanfilippo syndrome (type A, B and C). *Clin. Genet.*, **20**, 152–60.

243. Whiteman, P. and Young, E. (1977) The laboratory diagnosis of Sanfilippo disease. *Clin. Chim. Acta*, **76**, 139–47.

244. Hopwood, J. and Elliot, H. (1981) Radiolabelled oligosaccharides as substrates for the estimation of sulfamidase and the detection of the Sanfilippo Type A syndrome. *Clin. Chim. Acta*, **112**, 55–66.

245. Zhao, H., Van Diggelen, O., Thoomes, R. *et al.* (1990) Prenatal diagnosis of Morquio disease type A using a simple fluorometric enzyme assay. *Prenat. Diagn.*, **10**, 85–91.

246. Tomatsu, S., Fukuda, S., Masue, M. *et al.* (1991) Morquio disease: isolation, characterization and expression of full-length cDNA for human N-acetylgalactosamine-6-sulfate sulfatase. *Biochem. Biophys. Res. Commun.*, **181**, 677–83.

247. Stumpf, D., Austin, J., Crocker, A. *et al.* (1973) Mucopolysaccharidosis type VI (Maroteaux–Lamy syndrome): 1. Sulfatase B deficiency in tissues. *Am. J. Dis. Child.*, **126**, 747–55.

248. Beaudet, A., DiFerrante, N., Ferry, G. *et al.* (1975) Variation in the phenotypic expression of β-glucuronidase deficiency. *J. Pediatr.*, **86**, 388–94.

249. Gitzelmann, R., Wiesmann, U., Spycher, M. *et al.* (1978) Unusually mild course of β-glucuronidase deficiency in two brothers (mucopolysaccharidosis VII). *Helv. Paediatr. Acta*, **33**, 413–28.

75 HEMOGLOBINOPATHIES

A. Cao, M.C. Rosatelli, G.B. Leoni and R. Sardu

75.1 Introduction

The thalassemias are a heterogeneous group of genetic disorders characterized by the defective production of one of the globin chains of the hemoglobin tetramer (α_2–β_2). According to the type of globin chain involved, we distinguish α-thalassemias, resulting from the defective output of α-globin chains, and β-thalassemias characterized by reduced synthesis of β-chains. $\delta\beta$ and $\gamma\delta\beta$-thalassemias are rarer forms, in which the production of either δ- and β-chains or γ-, δ- and β-globin chains are reduced. Considered together the thalassemias are the most common autosomal recessive disorders affecting human beings [1–3].

75.2 α-Thalassemias

75.2.1 CLINICAL ASPECTS

The α-globin chains are coded by two α-globin gene loci on the short arm of chromosome 16 in the order $5'$-α_2-α_1-$3'$ [1,3]. In addition to the α-globin genes, the α-globin gene cluster contains a ζ-globin gene which codes for the embryonic ζ-globin chains, a number of

pseudogenes ($\psi\zeta$, $\psi\alpha_2$, $\psi\alpha_1$) and a gene of undetermined function (ϑ_1) (Figure 75.1). The α-globin chain output of the α_2-globin gene is two to three times greater than that of the α_1 gene [4]. In relation to the number of defective α-globin genes, four clinical states with increasing severity are recognized (Table 75.1) [3,4]. The silent carrier state is a result of the defective function of one of the α-globin genes. This condition is manifested clinically in the newborn period with an increased percentage (2%) of Hb Bart's, a tetramer composed of γ-chains (γ_4) which is produced in the presence of an excess of γ-chains in relation to α-chains. In adult life the silent carrier state is either completely silent or shows a modest thalassemia-like hematological picture (reduced mean corpuscular volume and hemoglobin, normal Hb A_2 and F). However, the α/β-globin chain synthesis ratio is constantly reduced, in the order of 0.9. The defective function of two globin genes either in *cis* or in *trans* results in the α-thalassemia carrier state, characterized in the neonatal period by a more markedly increased level (5–6%) of Hb Bart's and, in adulthood, by thalassemia-like red cell indices, normal Hb pattern, and reduced α-globin chain synthesis (α/β ratio of $\sim$ 0.7). When three α-globin genes are involved

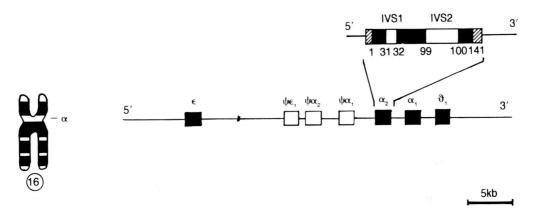

Figure 75.1 The chromosomal localization and genomic organization of the α-globin genes. Upper part: structure of an α-globin gene. Coding regions are represented by solid boxes, introns (IVS) by open boxes, and $3'$ and $5'$ untranslated regions by hatched boxes. Lower part: α-globin gene cluster. Genes are represented by solid boxes and pseudogenes by open boxes.

Diseases of the Fetus and Newborn, 2nd edn, Edited by G.B. Reed, A.E. Claireaux and F. Cockburn. Published in 1995 by Chapman & Hall, London. ISBN 0 412 39160 0

Table 75.1 Summary of hematologic findings in individuals with α-thalassemia

Phenotype	Equivalent number of functional α-genes	Level of Hb Bart's at birth (%)	MCV	MCH	α/β-Globin chain synthesis ratio
α-Thalassemia (silent carrier)	3	0–2	75–85	≈26	≈0.9
α-Thalassemia (carrier state)	2	2–8	65–75	≈22	≈0.7
Hb H disease	1	10–40	60–70	≈20	≈0.4
Hb Bart's hydrops fetalis	0	≈80	110–120	Reduced	0.0

MCV = mean corpuscular volume; MCH = mean corpuscular hemoglobin.

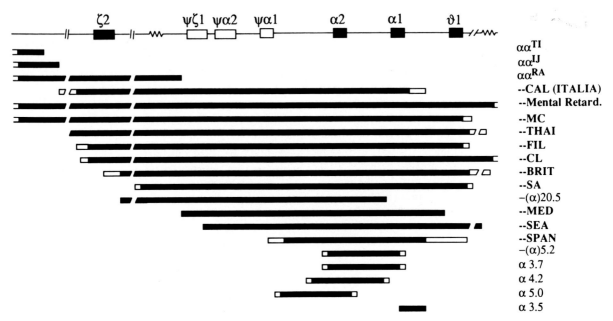

Figure 75.2 Deletions in the α-globin gene cluster. Upper line: the α-globin gene cluster; genes are represented by solid boxes, pseudogenes by open boxes and hypervariable regions (HVR) by zig-zag lines. Lower lines: the extent of each deletion is represented as a solid box, and the uncertainty of breakpoints is indicated by open boxes.

the resulting phenotype is Hb H disease. This is a moderately severe microcytic anemia characterized by microcytosis, the presence of Hb H (a tetramer of β-chains produced when there is an excess of β-chains over α-chains) in the order of 2–25%, numerous red blood cells in the peripheral blood containing inclusion bodies formed by precipitated β-chains, and marked reduction of the α/β-chain synthesis ratio (~ 0.4). In the neonatal period Hb Bart's is consistently elevated (25%). Hydrops fetalis is the most severe clinical condition and is caused by the defective function of all four α-globin genes. This condition is generally not compatible with postnatal life and all affected individuals are stillborn or die shortly after birth. A few infants have been treated with intrauterine transfusions and are surviving. Infants with fetal hydrops have severe microcytic anemia, marked spleen–liver enlargement and anasarca. The Hb electrophoretic pattern

shows solely Hb Bart's and Hb Portland ($\zeta_2 \gamma_2$), which is the only functional Hb of these patients.

75.2.2 MOLECULAR PATHOLOGY

The vast majority (95%) of α-thalassemias result from deletion of either one or both α-globin genes on chromosome 16. Two common types of single α-globin gene deletion are recognized; the rightward type, which includes 3.7 kb of DNA; and the leftward type, which deletes 4.2 kb of DNA. Rarer forms of single α-globin gene deletion have been described (Figure 75.2) [3,4].

A large number of deletions of different extents involving both α-globin genes have been reported [4–8]. As we shall see later on for β-thalassemia, there are a number of deletions located upstream of the α-like globin gene cluster which leave the α-globin genes intact but silence their expression, indicating the

Table 75.2 Non-deletional α-thalassemia mutations

Mutant class	Affected gene	Affected sequence	Mutation	Geographical distribution
RNA processing	α2	IVS-1 donor site	GAGGTGAGG→GAGG----	Mediterranean
	α2	Poly(A) signal	AATAAA→AATAAG	Middle East, Mediterranean
RNA translation	α2	Initiation codon	CCACCATGG→CCACCACGG	Mediterranean
	α1	Initiation codon	CCACCATGG→CCACCGTGG	Mediterranean
	−α	Initiation codon	CCACCATGG→CCACCGTGG	Black
	−α3.7	Initiation codon	CCACCATGG→CC--CATGG	North African, Mediterranean
	α2	Exon III	α116:GAC→UAG	Black
	α2	Termination codon	α142:TAA→CAA	South-East Asian
	α2	Termination codon	α142:TAA→AAA	Mediterranean
	α2	Termination codon	α142:TAA→TCA	Indian
	α2	Termination codon	α142:TAA→GAA	Black
	−α	Exon I	α30/31:GAGAGG→GAG--G	Black
Post-translational instability	α2	Exon III	α125:Leu→Pro	South-East Asian
	α2	Exon III	α109:Leu→Arg	South-East Asian
	α	Exon III	α110:Ala→Asp	Middle Eastern
	−α	Exon I	α14:Trp→Arg	Black
Uncharacterized	α	Unknown	Not determined	Black
	α	Unknown	Not determined	Greek

presence in the deleted region of a locus controlling the function of the cluster [9]. In South-East Asia, because both the single (−α/αα) and the two α-globin gene deletions (−−/αα) are very common, Hb H disease and fetal hydrops are frequently encountered. By contrast, in black populations, while the single α-globin gene deletion is rather frequent (30%), the deletion of two α-globin genes is very uncommon. The clinical forms of α-thalassemia seen in black populations are, therefore, the silent carrier state and the α-thalassemia trait. Hb H disease occurs very rarely and fetal hydrops has never been reported. In the Mediterranean population, while the single α-globin gene deletion is common, the two α-globin gene deletion is rare, but not exceptional. Hb H disease therefore is not uncommon and rare cases of fetal hydrops have been described [10]. Less commonly α-thalassemias may be produced by non-deletion lesions which are summarized in Table 75.2. The most common of the non-deletion mutations is Hb Constant Spring which occurs frequently in South-East Asia. Defects of the α-globin gene have greater clinical impact because the α2-gene codes 2–3 times as many α-globin chains compared with the α1-globin gene. Because of the very mild defect of α-globin output resulting from deletion lesions of the α1-globin gene, these defects may escape detection, explaining why only a few have so far been described. Hb H disease resulting from the compound heterozygous state for deletion of the two α-globin genes and non-deletion defect affecting the α2-globin gene, has a more severe clinical course compared with the deletion variety (−α/−−) [4].

75.3 β-Thalassemia and complex β-thalassemia

75.3.1 CLINICAL ASPECTS

β-Thalassemias are very heterogeneous at the clinical level. Heterozygous β-thalassemia produces the β-thalassemia carrier state which is characterized by microcytosis (MCV), reduced Hb content per cell (MCH), increased percentage of Hb A_2 (>3.5%) and, in a limited proportion, the increase of fetal hemoglobin (in the order of 2–5%). The α/β-globin chain synthesis ratio is definitively increased (2.12 + 0.44) [1]. The β-thalassemia trait is compatible with a normal life span. Individuals with two defective β-globin genes (homozygous β-thalassemia) usually have thalassemia major. The severe anemia characteristic of this disease is caused by the defective production of β-chains and, to a greater extent, by ineffective erythropoiesis resulting from excess α-globin chain synthesis leading to α-chain precipitation and damage to the membrane. Thalassemia major is characterized clinically by dependence on continuous blood transfusions. The excess of iron accumulated through the transfusions can be eliminated by subcutaneous desferrioxamine administered by means of a portable pump. Managed in this way, life span may be greatly pro-

Table 75.3 Mutations causing β-thalassemia [After Ref. 12]

Mutation	Type	Ethnic group
Transcriptional mutants		
−101 (C→T)	β⁺	Turkish, Bulgarian, Italian
−92 (C→T)	β⁺	Mediterranean
−90 (C→T)	β⁺	Portuguese
−88 (C→T)	β⁺	Black American, Asian Indian
−88 (C→A)	β⁺	Kurdish
−87 (C→G)	β⁺	Mediterranean
−87 (C→T)	β⁺	German/Italian
−87 (C→A)	β⁺	Yugoslavian, black American
−86 (C→G)	β⁺	Lebanese
−86 (C→A)	β⁺	Italian
−32 (C→A)	β⁺	Taiwanese
−31 (A→G)	β⁺	Japanese
−30 (T→A)	β⁺	Turkish, Bulgarian
−30 (T→C)	β⁺	Chinese
−29 (A→G)	β⁺	Black American, Chinese
−28 (A→C)	β⁺	Kurdish
−28 (A→G)	β⁺	Chinese
+22 (G→A)	β⁺	Turkish, Bulgarian, Italian
+43 to +40 (−AAAC)	β⁺	Chinese
RNA Processing mutants		
1. Splice junction		
IVS-I-1(G→A)	β°	Mediterranean
IVS-I-1 (G→T)	β°	Asian Indian, Chinese
IVS-II-1 (G→A)	β°	Mediterranean, Tunisian, black American
IVS-I-2 (T→G)	β°	Tunisian
IVS-I-2 (T→C)	β°	Black American
IVS-I-2 (T→A)	β°	Algerian
IVS-I, 17 nt del.(3′ end)	β°	Kuwaiti
IVS-I, 25 nt del.(3′ end)	β°	Asian Indian
IVS-I-130 (G→C)	β°	Turkish, Japanese
IVS-I-130 (G→A)	β°	Egyptian
IVS-II-849 (A→G)	β°	Black American
IVS-II-849 (A→C)	β°	Black American
2. Consensus sequence		
IVS-I-5 (G→C)	β⁺	Asian Indian, Chinese, Melanesian
IVS-I-5 (G→T)	β⁺	Mediterranean, black American
IVS-I-5 (G→A)	β⁺	Algerian, Mediterranean
IVS-I-6 (T→C)	β⁺	Mediterranean
IVS-I-1 (G→C) (CD 30)	β⁺	Tunisian, black American
IVS-I-1 (G→A) (CD 30)	?	Bulgarian
IVS-I-3 (C→T) (CD 29)	?	Lebanese
IVS-I-128 (T→G)	β⁺	Saudi Arabian
IVS-II-837 (T→G)	β?	Asian Indian
IVS-II-843 (T→G)	β⁺	Algerian
IVS-II-844 (C→G)	β⁺	Italian
IVS-II-848 (C→A)	β⁺	Black American, Egyptian, Iranian
IVS-II-848 (C→G)	β⁺	Japanese
IVS-II-850 (G→C)	β°	Yugoslavian
IVS-II-850 (−G)	β°	Italian

Table 75.3 *continued*

Mutation	Type	Ethnic group
3. IVS changes		
IVS-I-110 (G→A)	β$^+$	Mediterranean
IVS-I-116 (T→G)	β°	Mediterranean
IVS-II-4,5 (−AG)	β$^+$	Portuguese
IVS-II-654 (C→T)	β$^+$	Chinese
IVS-II-705 (T→C)	β$^+$	Mediterranean
IVS-II-745 (C→G)	β$^+$	Mediterranean
4. Cryptic splice activation		
CD 19 (A→G) (Asn→Ser) (Hb Malay)	β$^+$	Malaysian
CD 24 (T→A)	β$^+$	Black American, Japanese
CD 26 (G→A) (Glu→Lys) (Hb E)	β$^+$	South-East Asian
CD 27 (G→T) (Ala→Ser) (Hb Knossos)	β$^+$	Mediterranean
Nonsense and frameshift		
1. Nonsense		
CD 15 (TGG→TAG)	β°	Asian Indian
CD 15 (TGG→TGA	β°	Portuguese
CD 17 (A→T)	β°	Chinese
CD 22 (G→T)	β°	Reunion Islander
CD 26 (G→T)	β°	Thai
CD 35 (C→A)	β°	Thai
CD 37 (G→A)	β°	Saudi Arabian
CD 39 (C→T)	β°	Mediterranean
CD 43 (G→T)	β°	Chinese
CD 61 (A→T)	β°	Black
CD 90 (G→T)	β°	Japanese
CD 121 (G→T)	β°	Polish, French Swiss, Japanese
CD 127 (C→T)	β°	English
2. Frameshift		
CD 1 (−G)	β°	Mediterranean
CD 5 (−CT)	β°	Mediterranean
CD 6 (−A)	β°	Mediterranean, black American
CD 8 (−AA)	β°	Mediterranean
CDs 8/9 (+G)	β°	Asian Indian
CDs 9/10 (+C)	β°	Turkish
CD 11 (−T)	β°	Mexican
CDs 14/15 (+G)	β°	Chinese
CD 15 (−T)	β°	Asian Indian, Thai
CD 16 (−C)	β°	Asian Indian
CD 24 (−G, +CAC)	β°	Egyptian
CDs 25/26 (+T)	β°	Tunisian
CDs 27/28 (+C)	β°	Chinese
CD 35 (−C)	β°	Malaysian
CDs 36/37 (−T)	β°	Iranian, Kurdish
CDs 37/38/39 (−GACCCAG)	β°	Turkish
CDs 38/39 (−C)	β°	Czechoslovakian
CD 41 (−C)	β°	Thai
CDs 41/42 (−TTCT)	β°	Chinese

1170

Table 75.3 *continued*

Mutation	Type	Ethnic group
CD 44 (−C)	β^0	Kurdish
CD 47 (+A)	β^0	Surinamese
CD 54 (+G)	β^0	Japanese
CD 64 (−G)	β^0	Swiss
CD 71 (+T)	β^0	Chinese
CDs 71/72 (+A)	β^0	Chinese
CDs 74/75 (−C)	β^0	Turkish
CD 76 (−C)	β^0	Italian
CDs 82/83 (−G)	β^0	Azerbaijani, Czechoslovakian
CD 88 (+T)	β^0	Asian Indian
CD 95 (+A)	β^0	Thai
CDs 106/107 (+G)	β^0	Black American
CDs 109/110 (−G)	β^+	Lithuanian
RNA cleavage and polyadenylation		
AATAAA→AACAAA	β^+	Black American
AATAAA→AATAAG	β^+	Kurdish
AATAAA→AATGAA	β^+	Mediterranean
AATAAA→AATAGA	β^+	Malaysian
AATAAA→A (−AATAA)	β^+	Arabian
AATAAA→AAAA (−AT)	β^+	French
Cap site		
+1 (A→C)	β^+	Asian Indian
3′ UTR (+1570 bp, T→C, relative to the CAP site)	β^+	Irish
3′ UTR (term. CD +6, C→G)	β^+	Greek
Initiation codon		
ATG→ACG	β^0	Yugoslavian
ATG→AGG	β^0	Chinese, Japanese, Korean
ATG→GTG	β^0	Japanese
Hyperunstable globins		
CD 60 (GTG→GAG) (Val→Glu)	β	Italian
CD 94 (+TG) frameshift; extended β chain (Hb Agnana)	β	Italian
CD 110 (T→C) (Hb Showa–Yakushiji)	β	Japanese
CD 114 (−CT,+G) frameshift; extended β chain (Hb Geneva)	β	French Swiss
CD 123 (−A) frameshift; extended β chain (Hb Makabe)	β	Japanese
CDs 123–125 (−ACCCCACC)	β^0	Thai
CD 126 (−T) frameshift; extended β chain (Hb Vercelli)	β	Italian
CD 127 (Gln→Pro) (Hb Houston)	β	British
CD 127 (CAG→CGG)	β	French
CDs 127/128 (−AGG) (Hb Gunma)	β	Japanese
CDs 128/129 (−4,+5) (−GCTG,+CCACA) and CDs 132–135 (−11) (−AAAGTGGTGGC)	β^0	Irish
CDs 134–137 (−10+4)	β^0	Portuguese
Thalassemic hemoglobinopathies		
CD 28 (CTG→CGG)	β^0	Hb Chesterfield
CDs 32/34 (−GGT)	β^0	Hb Corea
CD 69 (GGT→AGT)	β^+	Hb City of Hope
CD 114 (T→C)	?	Hb Brescia
CD 126 (GTG→GGG)	β^0	Hb Neapolis

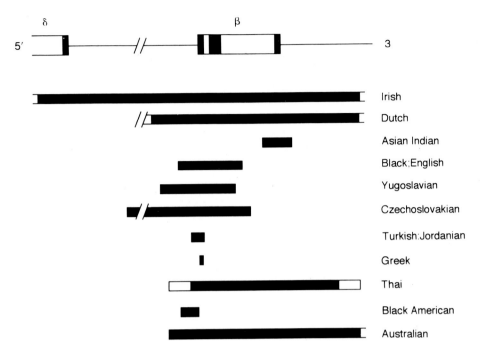

Figure 75.3 Deletions causing β-thalassemia. Upper line: β-globin gene. Lower lines: the extent of each deletion is represented as a solid box, and the uncertainty of breakpoints is indicated by open boxes.

longed. Oral chelating agents are being developed and may be available in the near future. An alternative to transfusional management is bone marrow transplantation from HLA identical siblings which has been widely used with considerable success. However, mortality is still very high (18%) and chronic graft-versus-host disease may occur. Long-term prospective agents are those that boost fetal hemoglobin production and gene therapy.

A number of clinical conditions ranging in severity between the β-thalassemia carrier state and thalassemia major are relatively common. These forms of β-thalassemia of intermediate severity are known as thalassemia intermedia. The clinical picture is characterized by a mild microcytic anemia not requiring continuous transfusions. The molecular bases of these mild forms will be described in the next section.

β-Thalassemia is very common in the Mediterranean basin, the Middle East, the Indian subcontinent and South-East Asia [2]. World distribution of β-thalassemia, as well as that of α-thalassemia reported above, is related to the reduced mortality of carriers of both α and β-thalassemia *vis-à-vis* malaria compared with normal individuals. This phenomenon produced a positive selection and thus, in the long term, an increase in the gene frequency of these disorders.

75.3.2 MOLECULAR PATHOLOGY OF β-THALASSEMIA

The vast majority of the β-thalassemias are produced by a single nucleotide substitution, small addition or deletion affecting the coding region or critical areas for the function of the β-globin gene [11,12]. These molecular defects include non-sense and frameshift mutations, resulting in non-functional mRNA, RNA processing mutations, transcriptional mutants, RNA cleavage plus polyadenylation and CAP site mutants and mutations resulting in the production of hyper-unstable globins (Table 75.3) [12]. By contrast, β-thalassemia very rarely results from the mechanism of gross deletion (Figure 75.3).

β-Thalassemia mutations may silence the function of the β-globin gene and thus result in the phenotype of β°-thalassemia or only reduce the β-globin chain output, producing the phenotype of β⁺-thalassemia. The group of β⁺-thalassemias includes both mutations which severely curtail the output of the β-globin chains from the affected locus, and mutations associated with a consistent residual output of β-globin chains. While homozygosity for severe mutations generally results in thalassemia major, homozygosity for mild mutations or compound heterozygosity for severe and mild mutations usually produce thalassemia intermedia (see below) [13]. For many mutations, however, scarce

Table 75.4 Frequencies of different β-thalassemia mutations in Mediterranean populations

Mutation	Sardinia	Italy	France	Spain	Portugal	Greece	Cyprus	Turkey	Tunisia	Egypt	Lebanon	Yugoslavia	Bulgaria	Germany
−101	–	–	–	–	–	–	–	0.96	–	–	–	–	0.78	–
−87	0.20	1.1	–	–	–	1.72	–	0.38	–	–	–	0.92	3.91	–
−30	–	–	–	–	–	0.29	–	3.08	–	–	–	–	–	–
−28	–	–	–	–	–	–	–	0.38	–	–	–	–	–	–
Codon 1 (−1 bp)	0.10	–	–	–	–	–	–	–	–	–	–	–	–	–
Codon 5 (−2 bp)	–	–	–	–	–	1.15	–	1.15	–	–	–	0.92	4.69	–
Codon 6 (−1 bp)	2.10	1.9	–	5.0	–	2.87	–	0.19	16.0	4.2	–	1.39	4.69	–
Codon 8 (−2 bp)	–	–	–	1.7	–	0.57	–	6.75	–	–	6	0.46	5.46	–
Codon 8/9 (+1 bp)	–	–	–	–	–	0.29	–	0.96	–	–	–	–	5.46	–
Codon 29	–	–	–	–	–	–	–	–	–	–	6	0.92	0.92	–
Codon 39	95.70	41.2	41.9	64.0	53.57	16.95	1.5	4.63	19.0	2.1	4	3.70	21.88	50.0
Codon 76 (−1 bp)	0.70	–	–	–	–	–	–	–	–	–	–	–	–	–
IVS-I-1	0.03	10.7	10.5	3.5	32.90	13.22	11.7	2.50	1.5	10.4	–	10.65	3.14	2.5
IVS-I-5	–	–	–	–	–	0.86	–	2.30	–	–	4	–	–	–
IVS-I-6	0.10	10.3	8.6	15.5	–	7.18	8.7	18.14	10.5	18.8	8	23.15	10.15	–
IVS-I-110	0.50	23.2	25.7	8.5	10.71	42.55	69.9	39.96	7.5	27.1	62	43.05	24.21	7.5
IVS-II-1	0.03	3.6	1.0	–	–	2.01	–	11.77	–	4.2	4	0.92	1.56	5.0
IVS-II-705	–	–	–	1.7	–	–	–	–	–	–	–	–	–	–
IVS-II-745	0.40	5.8	2.8	–	–	6.90	5.6	2.89	7.5	8.3	4	1.39	10.15	–
Others	0.00	2.2	9.5	0.1	2.82	3.44	2.6	3.96	38.0	25.0	–	12.53	3.92	35.0

Table 75.5 Frequencies of different β-thalassemia mutations in Asians

Mutation	Thailand	China	India	Malaysia	Indonesia
−88	−	−	2.0	−	−
−29	−	−	−	−	−
−28	10.3	6.5	−	−	−
Codon 8/9 (+1 bp)	−	−	19.6	−	−
Codon 14/15 (+1 bp)	−	0.6	−	−	−
Codon 15	−	−	4.9	−	5.55
Codon 16 (−1 bp)	−	−	1.0	−	−
Codon 17	10.3	11.8	−	2.4	1.39
Codon 19	1.7	−	−	14.6	−
Codon 26	−	−	−	−	18.05
Codon 35 (−1 bp)	−	−	−	4.8	1.39
Codon 35	2.6	−	−	−	−
Codon 41/42 (−4 bp)	50.9	31.8	11.8	12.2	1.39
Codon 43	−	−	−	−	−
Codon 71/72 (+1 bp)	0.8	14.1	−	−	-
IVS-I-1	1.7	0.6	13.7	7.3	9.7
IVS-I-5	5.2	5.3	22.5	48.8	44.44
IVS-II-654	11.2	17.0	−	7.3	9.72
619 bp deletion	−	−	20.5	−	−
Others	4.2	12.3	4.0	2.4	8.35

information on genotype–phenotype correlations is presently available. As a general rule each of these mutations is contained in a specific chromosomal haplotype (set of polymorphic sites at the β-globin gene cluster) [14]. The association between specific haplotypes and specific mutations is, however, very high, but not absolute. A number of β-thalassemia mutations, for instance the codon 39 non-sense mutation, have in fact been detected in different chromosomal haplotypes [15]. The association of the same mutation with several distinct haplotypes may be explained by meiotic recombination, gene conversion or recurrent mutation.

As shown in Table 75.3 and Figure 75.3, β-thalassemia seems to be highly heterogeneous at the molecular level. More than 100 different β-thalassemia mutations have been described [12]. Notwithstanding this marked heterogeneity, in each population at risk a limited number of β-thalassemia mutations have been detected and among these mutations only a few account for the vast majority of the molecular defects. Tables 75.4 and 75.5 summarize the available data on the distribution and frequency of the different β-thalassemia mutations in each population at risk. The analysis of these tables indicates that a limited number of allelic specific probes or primers specific for each population may allow detection of most of the β-thalassemia mutations.

75.3.3 CLINICAL AND MOLECULAR ASPECTS OF COMPLEX β-THALASSEMIAS

δβ and γδβ-thalassemias are uncommon mutations. Heterozygous δβ-thalassemia is characterized hemato-logically by thalassemia-like hematological features, normal or reduced Hb A_2 levels, markedly increased (15%) Hb F levels and unbalanced α/β-globin chain synthesis. Homozygosity for δβ-thalassemia or compound heterozygosity for δβ-thalassemia and typical β-thalassemia may result in a mild clinical picture (thalassemia intermedia) [1]. Heterozygous γδβ-thalassemia may manifest in the neonatal period with a mild microcytic anemia. In adulthood γδβ-thalassemia heterozygotes show thalassemia-like hematological features associated with normal Hb A_2 and F levels. Both δβ and γδβ-thalassemias usually result from the deletion of a variable extent of the DNA in the β-like globin gene cluster (Figure 75.4). In addition to δβ-thalassemias, other deletions of the β-globin gene cluster result in the phenotype of hereditary persistence of fetal hemoglobin (HPFH) [16,17]. In contrast to δβ-thalassemia in HPFH mutations, however, the reduced output of β-globin chains is fully compensated by the increased production of γ-chains. The hematological features and globin chain synthesis in this condition are thus within the normal range. δβ-thalassemia may, however, be produced very occasionally by a non-deletion mechanism. An example of this mechanism is Sardinian δβ-thalassemia in which the β-globin gene is silenced by the codon 39 non-sense mutation, while a mutation in *cis* to the Aγ promoter (−196 C→T) results in increased output of Aγ chains, partially compensating for the shortage of β-chains [18]. A very interesting group of deletions in the β-like globin gene cluster leaves the β-globin gene intact and yet silences its expression. This effect is related to the deletion of the DNA region lying 6–20 kb 5′ to the ε-globin gene

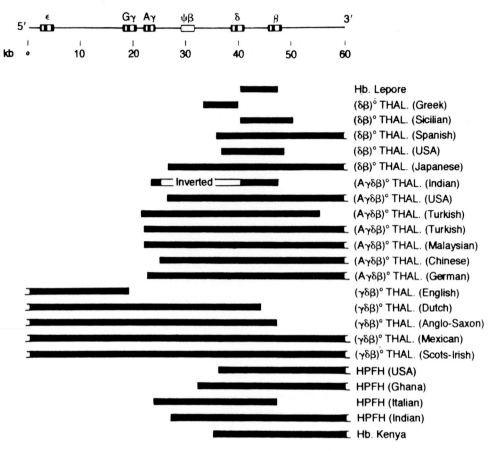

Figure 75.4 Complex deletions in the β-globin gene cluster: the extent of each deletion is represented as a solid box.

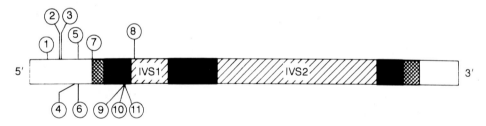

Figure 75.5 Common mild β-thalassemia mutations. 1 = −101 C→T (Mediterranean); 2 = −88 C→T (black American); 3 = −87 C→G (Mediterranean); 4 = −31 A→G (Japanese); 5 = −29 A→G (black American); 6 = −28 A→G (Chinese); 7 = CAP +1 A→G; (Asian Indian); 8 = IVS-I-6 T→C (Mediterranean); 9 = β 24 (T→A) (black American); 10 = β 28 (G→A) (South-East Asian); 11 = β 27 (G→T; Hb Knossos) (Mediterranean).

which controls the function of all the β-like globin gene cluster and contains a powerful enhancer (locus control region) [19,20].

75.3.4 HETEROGENEITY OF β-THALASSEMIA: IMPLICATION FOR CARRIER SCREENING

The different β-thalassemia alleles vary widely in their phenotypic expression. At one extreme there are mutations such as the distal CACCC promoter mutation (−101 C→T), which results in the β-thalassemia silent carrier phenotype characterized hematologically by normal red cell indices and hemoglobin pattern and defined only by slightly unbalanced globin chain synthesis [21,22]. At the other extreme a group of mutations resulting in the production of hyperunstable globin is associated in the heterozygous state with the phenotype of thalassemia intermedia [23]. Between these two extremes a spectrum of variation may be recognized. Broadly speaking, we can distinguish severe alleles which in the homozygous state result in thalassemia major and mild mutations, homozygosity for which produces thalassemia intermedia [24–26]. Severe alleles include non-sense and frameshift mutations, splice junction changes and some nucleotide substitutions activating cryptic splice sites. Mild mutations, which are given in Figure 75.5, are those that affect transcription, alter the CAP site or the polyadenylation signal, and some of those activating cryptic splice sites or disrupting the consensus sequence for splicing. Compound heterozygosity for mild and severe alleles has an unpredictable phenotype ranging from mild thalassemia intermedia to thalassemia major. In addition to the inheritance of a mild β-thalassemia mutation, thalassemia intermedia may result from a number of other molecular mechanisms [24,26]. Coinheritance with homozygous β-thalassemia of α-thalassemia, either in the form of the deletion of two α-globin genes or as a non-deletion defect affecting the α_2-globin gene, may produce a mild clinical picture [27,28]. Likewise the presence of an up-promoter mutation (C→T) at position −158 to the Gγ-gene, by increasing the production of Gγ-chains and then compensating the reduced output of β-chains, may also improve the clinical picture [29]. However, of the mechanisms for thalassemia intermedia discussed above, only homozygosity for mild β-thalassemia alleles has an outcome consistent enough to be used in genetic counselling.

Double heterozygosity for β-thalassemia and the triple α-globin gene arrangement may also result in mild clinical features [30,31].

75.3.5 β-THALASSEMIA DUE TO UNKNOWN MUTATIONS

Over the past few years, we and others have found typical β-thalassemia heterozygotes in which sequencing of the β-globin gene from 600 nucleotides (nt) 5′ to the CAP site to 200 nt 3′ to the end of the gene failed to reveal causative mutations [32,33]. These β-thalassemias may arise from mutations in the locus activating region 5′ to the ε-globin gene or in other genes coding for DNA binding protein(s) crucial for the function of the β-globin gene.

75.4 Prenatal diagnosis

Methodologies for prenatal diagnosis of thalassemia have evolved over time. In the 1970s prenatal diagnosis was accomplished by globin chain synthesis analysis on fetal blood obtained by placental aspiration or fetoscopy [34]. In the early 1980s identification of β-thalassemia was carried out indirectly by polymorphism haplotype analysis [35], while α-thalassemia was defined directly by molecular hybridization [36]. Later, β-thalassemia mutations were directly defined by oligonucleotide hybridization on electrophoretically separated DNA fragments [37,38]. Nowadays, prenatal diagnosis of thalassemia is obtained by a number of different procedures detecting the mutation directly on enzymatically amplified fetal DNA by the polymerase chain reaction (PCR) [39].

75.4.1 FETAL SAMPLING

Fetal DNA is obtained either by amniocentesis or from chorionic villi [40,41]. With chorionic villús sampling, carried out by the vaginal route or transabdominally, there is a definite, slightly higher risk of fetal mortality compared with amniocentesis [42,43]. However, because chorionic villus biopsy may be carried out at 9–10 weeks gestation, thus allowing diagnosis during the first trimester, it is most commonly preferred by couples undergoing genetic counselling [44].

75.4.2 β-THALASSEMIAS

A number of different procedures may be used to detect β-thalassemia mutations directly. When the mutation is known, non-denaturing gel electrophoresis, restriction endonuclease analysis, allele specific probes, allele specific primers or the ligase chain reaction may be used. For unknown mutations, the methods available are denaturing gradient gel electrophoresis, chemical mismatch cleavage analysis, single strand conformation polymorphism analysis and direct sequencing.

(a) Known mutations

Restriction endonuclease analysis

Restriction endonuclease analysis may be used for those mutations which are caused by the gross structural rearrangement of DNA or affect a restriction recognition site. The method consists of the digestion of an amplified DNA sample with the appropriate restriction enzyme, followed by gel electrophoresis to separate the restricted DNA fragments and direct visualization of the electrophoretic pattern by ethidium bromide or silver nitrate staining [45,46]. An example of the use of this procedure to detect the sickle mutation is shown in Figure 75.6. This procedure is very fast and has the advantage of not relying on the use of radioactive material. However, it can only be applied to define a limited number of β-thalassemia mutations. By inducing the formation of a restriction site with an appropriate design of the primers, the application of this procedure can be greatly extended [47]. At the present time restriction endonuclease analysis is the method of choice to detect the S mutation.

Non-denaturing gel electrophoresis

Deletion and addition of two nucleotides may also be detected directly because of the different migration of the β-globin gene fragment in which the mutation

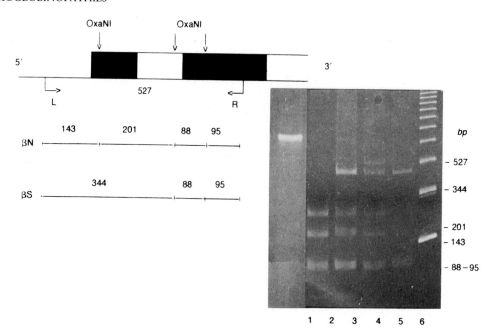

Figure 75.6 Detection of β^s mutation by restriction endonuclease digestion of amplified DNA. Top left: the *Oxa*NI sites in the amplified region are shown. The 5' site is removed by the sickle mutation. Bottom left: schematic diagram of the DNA fragments resulting from *Oxa*NI digestion of normal and β^s amplified DNA. On the right: ethidium bromide-stained polyacrylamide gel after electrophoresis of *Oxa*NI digested amplified DNA. Lane 1 = undigested amplified DNA; lane 2 = normal subject; lanes 3, 4 = subjects heterozygous for the β^s mutation; lane 5 = subject homozygous for the β^s mutation; lane 6 = molecular weight marker.

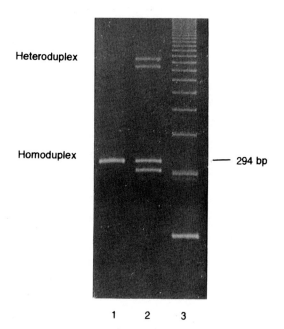

Figure 75.7 Detection of a small deletion by polyacrylamide gel electrophoresis of amplified DNA. Lane 1 = normal control; lane 2 = subject heterozygous for a 25-bp deletion in the 3' end of IVS-I of the β-globin gene; lane 3 = molecular weight marker.

resides, using the very simple procedure of non-denaturing polyacrylamide gel electrophoresis [48–50]. In Figure 75.7 the detection by this procedure of a mutation resulting from the deletion of 25 bp is depicted. The generation of heteroduplexes obtained by mixing the PCR products from different mutated DNA as well as with wild-type product may allow the use of polyacrylamide gel electrophoresis to detect even single base substitutions. In this condition, in fact, heteroduplexes migrate more slowly than the corresponding homoduplexes and identification of the mutation is straightforward [51,52].

Dot-blot analysis

The most widely used procedure to detect a mutation directly is dot-blot analysis with allele-specific oligonucleotide probes. With this method, the DNA is spotted on a nylon filter, to which two ^{32}P-labelled oligonucleotide probes, either complementary to the mutation (β-thalassemia probe) to be detected or homologous to normal DNA sequences at the same position (normal probe), are hybridized successively [53,54]. Normal DNA hybridizes only to the normal probe; DNA from affected individuals hybridizes only to the β-thalassemia probe; and DNA from heterozygotes hybridizes to both probes (Figure 75.8). The high

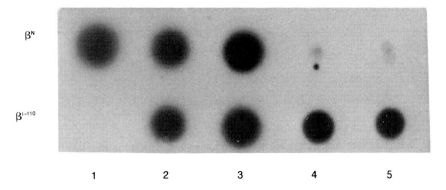

β^N

β^{I-110}

1   2   3   4   5

Figure 75.8 Dot-blot analysis on amplified DNA using allele specific probes complementary to the β IVS-I-110 mutation or normal DNA at the same position. Control DNA from a normal individual (1) and a patient homozygous for the β IVS-I-110 mutation (5). Mother (2) and father (3) heterozygous and fetus (4) homozygous for the β IVS-I-110 mutation.

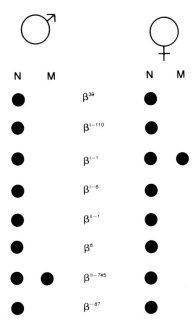

Figure 75.9 Screening for the most common β-thalassemia mutants by reverse oligonucleotide hybridization in a couple at risk for β-thalassemia. ♂ = Father heterozygous for IVS-I-1; ♀ = mother heterozygous for β IVS-II-745.

specificity of DNA amplification makes it possible to use non-radioactively labelled probes, such as, horseradish peroxidase labelled oligonucleotides [55].

Reverse oligonucleotide hybridization

The procedure outlined above has recently been simplified by using a reverse approach (reverse oligonucleotide hybridization) (Figure 75.9) [56]. According to this procedure, allele-specific oligonucleotide probes with an NH₂ 5′ terminal group, either complementary to the mutation to be detected or to normal DNA at the corresponding position, are covalently linked to a negatively charged nylon membrane. Biotinylated dUTP

is incorporated in place of thymine by PCR in the amplification of the DNA segment containing the mutation to be investigated (F.F. Chehab, personal communication). After hybridization of the DNA fragment to the nylon filter, streptavidin–alkaline phosphatase conjugate is added. Positive hybridization is detected by using a chromogenic substrate for alkaline phosphatase. The main advantages of this procedure are its extreme rapidity and simplicity, because it allows the analysis of a large number of mutations in just one step and the possibility of full automation.

Primer specific amplification

With this method, DNA amplification is obtained using a common primer and either of two different primers, one which has the 3′-nucleotide homologous to the mutation to be detected, the other having a sequence complementary to the normal DNA at the same position. The normal primer amplifies only normal DNA and the primer homologous to the mutation amplifies only the affected DNA, whereas both primers amplify heterozygous DNA (Figure 75.10) [57,58]. In order to control this reaction another polymorphic sequence is usually co-amplified. This methodology may be simplified and automated by labelling the two specific primers with two different fluorescent dyes [59]. In this procedure, oligonucleotides homologous to the normal or to the mutant DNA sequences are labelled with fluorescein and rhodamine, respectively, and used to prime the PCR together with a common primer corresponding to normal sequences of the opposite strand. When normal DNA is amplified, the primer homologous to the normal sequence is extended. Since the primer is labelled with fluorescein, the amplified DNA emits a green colour under ultraviolet light. When DNA from a patient homozygous for a mutation is amplified only the rhodamine conjugated primer homologous to the mutation is extended and the amplified

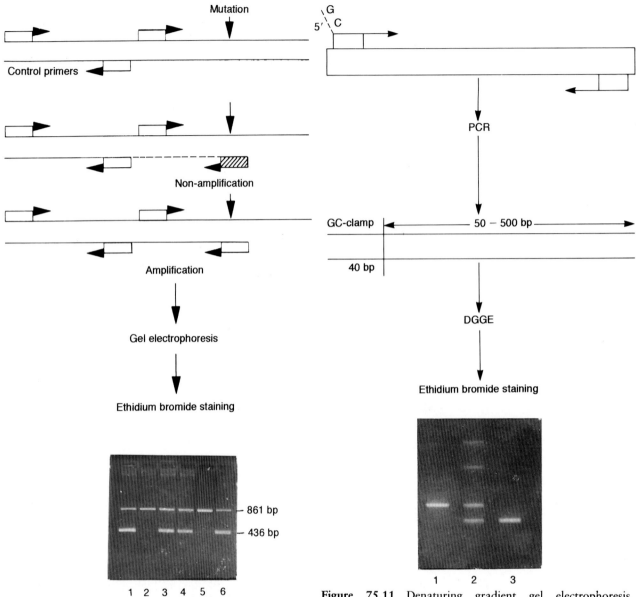

Figure 75.10 Procedure of amplification refractory mutation system (ARMS) (top; ▨ = normal primer; □ = mutant primer) and gel electrophoresis of amplified DNA fragments (bottom). The 861-bp fragment represents the DNA amplified by the control primers, which is used to monitor the amplification procedure. Lanes 1, 3, 5 = amplification with normal primer; Lanes 2, 4, 6 = amplification with mutant primer. DNA from normal (1,2), heterozygous (3,4) and homozygous (5,6) individuals for the codon 39 non-sense mutation (β° 39).

Figure 75.11 Denaturing gradient gel electrophoresis (DGGE). Detection of a β IVS-I-6 mutation: normal (1), heterozygous (2) and homozygous (3) individuals for the β IVS-I-6.

of the amplified product can also be analyzed by gel electrophoresis.

(b)   Unknown mutations

Denaturing gradient gel electrophoresis

Denaturing gradient gel electrophoresis is a gel system which separates amplified DNA fragments in relation to their melting temperature, i.e. the temperature at which the two constitutive DNA strands separate from each other [60]. A DNA fragment migrates in the gel until it reaches the concentration of the denaturing agent corresponding to the melting temperature of its low-melting domain. Denaturation of DNA, i.e. sepa-

amplified product fluoresces red. When DNA from a heterozygous individual is amplified both the fluorescein-labelled and rhodamine-labelled primers are extended and the amplified product is yellow as a result of the complementary fluorescence of the two dyes. After removing the unincorporated primer by centrifugation the colour of the amplified product can be seen and, if necessary, confirmed by fluorimetry. The colour

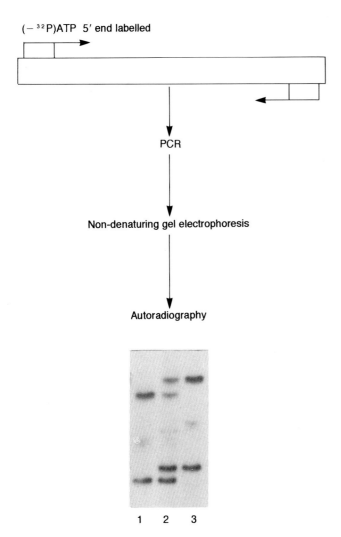

Figure 75.12 Single strand conformation polymorphism (SSCP). Detection of codon 39 non-sense mutation (β° 39): normal (1), heterozygous (2) and homozygous (3) individuals for the β° 39 mutation.

ration of the constitutive DNA strands of a low-melting domain, determines a rapid reduction of the migration of the fragment. DNA fragments differing by one base pair in the low-melting domain may have a different melting temperature and may thus be separated by this system. However, only those fragments having two different melting domains are separated. This is due to the fact that when a fragment having only a single melting domain reaches the melting temperature the two strands separate completely and mutation–migration differences are lost. During the amplification step, by adding a GC-rich sequence (GC-clamp) with high melting temperature to the fragment to be analyzed, practically all fragments containing specific mutations may be converted into two different melting domain fragments and can hence be defined in this system [61].

Amplified β-globin gene fragments suitable for analysis by this system may be selected either by computer analysis of the melting domains or empirically. DNA from normals or homozygotes for β-thalassemia mutation produces a specific DNA fragment consisting of the homoduplexes of the normal or mutated allelic segment respectively. DNA from heterozygotes, however, results in the production of four fragments, of which two are the homoduplexes of the normal and mutated allele respectively and two are heteroduplexes resulting from annealing the strands from the normal allele to those of the mutated allele (Figure 75.11) [62,63].

Single strand conformation polymorphism analysis

This method is based on the finding that two single stranded DNA fragments in which the DNA sequences differ at only one position can be separated by neutral polyacrylamide gel electrophoresis [64]. As the mobility shift caused by nucleotide substitutions might be due to conformational changes in single stranded DNAs, this method has been designated single strand conformation polymorphism analysis (SSCP). Amplified single strand DNA fragments may be visualized on the gel directly, or following hybridization with specific probes (Figure 75.12). This method has not been extensively used to detect β-thalassemia mutations. We do not know, therefore, whether nucleotide substitution at any position in a β-globin fragment can be detected by SSCP analysis.

Chemical mismatch cleavage analysis

This procedure is based on the knowledge that DNA heteroduplexes containing mismatched base pairs may be modified either by osmium tetroxide, which reacts with mismatched thymine (T), or by hydroxylamine, which reacts with mismatched cytosine (C) (Figure 75.13). Piperidine may then cleave the DNA heteroduplexes at the modified mismatched base. The cleaved DNA fragments are then detected by gel electrophoresis. The heteroduplexes to be analyzed are formed by annealing the DNA fragment to be investigated to ^{32}P-labelled wild-type DNA. By using sense and antisense probes, all single base pair mismatches may be identified [65]. The main advantage of this procedure is that, by comparison with the Maxam–Gilbert sequencing ladder of limited cleavage of heteroduplexes, it allows rapid and ready identification of the position and type of mismatch. This method has recently been successfully applied to detect β-thalassemia mutations [66].

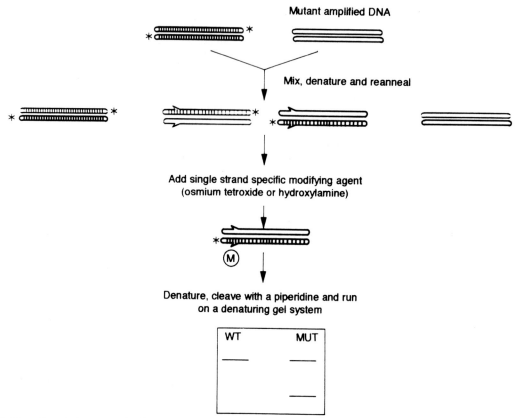

Figure 75.13 Chemical mismatch cleavage analysis.

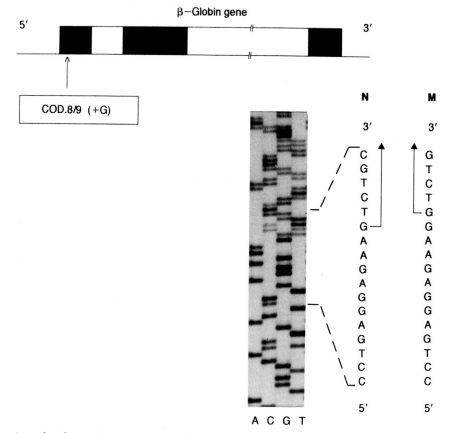

Figure 75.14 Detection of codons 8/9 (+G) mutation by direct sequencing of amplified DNA. Top: β-globin gene. Bottom: sequence analysis. N and M are sequences corresponding to the normal and mutated allele respectively.

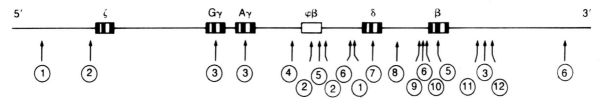

Figure 75.15   Restriction polymorphic sites in the β-globin gene cluster. 1 = *Taq*I; 2 = *Hinc*II; 3 = *Hind*III; 4 = *Pvu*II; 5 = *Ava*II; 6 = *Rsa*I; 7 = *Pst*I; 8 = *Nco*I; 9 = *Hin*fI; 10 = *Hgi*AI; 11 = *Hpa*I; 12 = *Bam*HI.

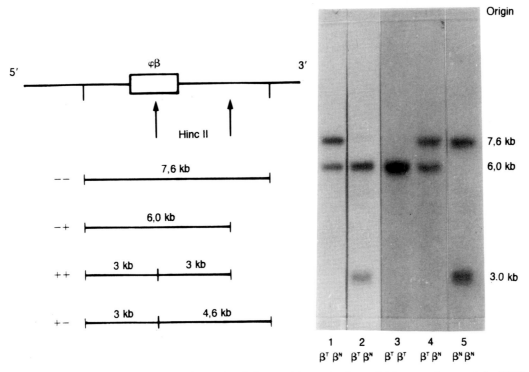

Figure 75.16   Prenatal diagnosis by linkage analysis. Top left: *Hinc*II map in the β globin gene. Bottom left: DNA fragments produced by *Hinc*II digestion in the absence (−) or presence (+) of the polymorphic *Hinc*II sites. Right: Southern blot of *Hinc*II-digested DNA hybridized to a β-globin specific probe. Lanes 1,2 = father and mother heterozygous for β-thalassemia and for the presence/absence of the polymorphic *Hinc*II sites. Lanes 3,4 = previous affected children homozygous (3) and heterozygous (4) for β-thalassemia. Lane 5 = normal fetus.

Sequence analysis

Identification of a mutation in the β-globin gene by one of the previously outlined procedures is followed by its definition by DNA sequencing, which may be carried out manually or automatically (Figure 75.14) [67,68].

(c)   Polymorphism analysis

A number of restriction polymorphic sites lie in the β-globin gene cluster (Figure 75.15) [14,69,70]. These polymorphisms were largely used in the early 1980s to make prenatal diagnosis of β-thalassemia indirectly by linkage analysis [35]. An example of this procedure is outlined in Figure 75.16. More recently, short tandem repeats (STRs) or microsatellites consisting in a $(CA)_n$ repeat, and a $(ATTTT)_n$ repeat, have been detected at

position 2643 nt and 1390 nt 5′ to the β-globin gene respectively [71–73]. These two STRs showed extensive polymorphism with five different alleles for the $(CA)_n$ repeat and three for the $(ATTT)_n$ repeat. The resulting heterozygosity is 62.3 for the $(CA)_n$ and 36.5 for the $(ATTT)_n$ repeat. Polymorphism analysis now has a limited place in prenatal diagnosis of β-thalassemia, being used only for those couples presenting at advanced gestation and carrying rare mutations not detected by the commonly used procedures to define known mutations.

75.4.3   α-THALASSEMIA

Indications for prenatal diagnosis of α-thalassemia are limited to the hydrops fetalis syndrome because Hb H disease is a mild microcytic anemia compatible with a

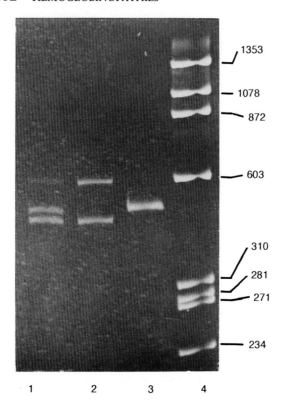

Figure 75.17 Variable number of tandem repeat (VNTR) analysis to control the presence of maternal contamination. Lane 1 = fetus; lane 2 = mother; lane 3 = father; lane 4 = molecular weight marker (*Hind*III digested φX174). The fetus shows both maternal bands, one very tiny, indicating maternal contamination.

normal lifespan. The most common mutation responsible for the severe form of α-thalassemia, homozygosity for which results in hydrops fetalis, is a deletion of 23 kb of DNA within the α-globin gene cluster [3]. This mutation, as well as other less common deletions, may be detected directly as discrete fragments by agarose or polyacrylamide gel electrophoresis followed by ethidium bromide or silver nitrate staining. According to this procedure, DNA synthesis is primed in the PCR with a pair of oligonucleotides homologous to the DNA sequence flanking the deletion. A PCR product is obtained only in the presence of the deletion. When the deletion is absent, in fact, the distance between the primers is too large to obtain an amplified product. Simultaneously the DNA is amplified by using one of the primers complementary to a DNA region deleted by the mutation and one of the primers flanking the deletion, which allows an amplified product to be obtained only if DNA is normal [74]. A very simple fluorescent assay to detect the fetal hydrops syndrome has recently been developed [59]. A pair of α-globin specific primers are labelled with rhodamine (red), while a pair of β-globin specific primers which amplify a β-globin specific segment, are labelled with fluorescein (green). In normal DNA both the red and green

amplified bands can be seen after gel electrophoresis, while in hydrops DNA only the green amplified band is seen. After removing most of the unincorporated primers by centrifugation the color of the amplified DNA can be visualized directly. Thus yellow (green plus red) indicates a normal DNA sample, while green is diagnostic of α-globin gene deletion. This method is very quick, easy and non-radioactive and is amenable to complete automation.

75.4.4   PITFALLS IN PRENATAL DIAGNOSIS

A potential pitfall which can occur with all procedures based on DNA amplification is the coamplification of maternal sequences, which may confuse the diagnosis. In a large series consisting of 3533 cases, we have made one misdiagnosis because of maternal contamination. This pitfall may be avoided by a more careful dissection of maternal decidua from fetal DNA, by requesting a minimal amount of chorionic villi, of the order of 5–10 mg, a quantity which dilutes the possible maternal contamination, and by cutting down the amplification cycles to no more than 20, thus reducing the chances of amplifying the small amount of maternal sequences present in the original sample. In any case, in order to check for the presence of contaminating maternal sequences it seems wise to co-amplify a suitable polymorphic DNA sequence, as is illustrated in Figure 75.17 [75]. This approach may also allow us to avoid misdiagnosis due to mispaternity [63]. Another potential danger is the failure to amplify the target segment of the DNA. This may be avoided by the simultaneous amplification of another DNA fragment, containing the mutation to be analyzed, by a set of specific primers. Finally, of course, all the precautions in use to avoid false-positive diagnosis due to a contaminating PCR product should be carefully followed.

75.5   Control of β-thalassemia

Prenatal diagnosis, in combination with carrier screening of individuals at child-bearing age following education of the population, is used to prevent β-thalassemia major in several populations 'at risk' in the Mediterranean area, namely Italians, Greeks and Greek and Turkish Cypriots. These programmes have produced a consistent reduction in the incidence of thalassemia major. The results obtained in the Sardinian population are shown in Figure 75.18 [44].

75.6   Future prospects

From the technical point of view it is realistic to predict further simplification and full automation of the procedures for detection of the β-thalassemia mutations to be used for carrier screening and prenatal diagnosis. Primer specific amplification and reverse oligonucleo-

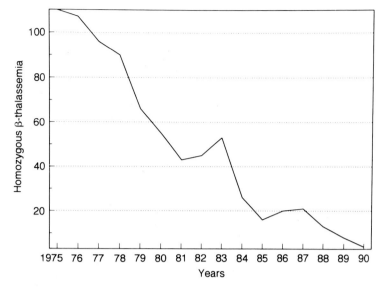

Figure 75.18   Fall in the birth rate of babies with homozygous β-thalassemia in Sardinia. Ordinate gives absolute number of children affected by thalassemia major. The carrier screening programme began in 1975.

tide hybridization, for instance, may easily be fully automated. The forseeable progressive reduction of the cost of DNA analysis may lead in the future to the use of mutation detection as a screening method, thus skipping all the steps in the carrier detection methods based on hematologic analysis.

The advent of DNA amplification has made it possible to analyze the genotype of a single cell. This development has paved the way for preimplantation or even preconception diagnosis. Preimplantation diagnosis is carried out by biopsy of the blastula, obtained by uterine cavity washing following *in vivo* fertilization, or by the analysis of a single blastomere from an eight-cell embryo following *in vitro* fertilization [76]. Preconception diagnosis is based on the analysis of the first polar body, which gives an indication of the genetic constitution of the relative ovum [77]. By fertilizing *in vitro* only those eggs without the defect and replacing these in the mother, a successful pregnancy with a normal fetus may be obtained. Of course the genotype of the fetus will be further checked by chorion villus biopsy.

Successful pregnancies following the transfer of human embryos which had been sexed *in vitro* by amplification of a specific repeat sequence [78], or in which the cystic fibrosis transregulator has been molecularly defined, have been reported (A.M. Handyside, personal communication) (Chapter 64).

However, before preimplantation and preconception gamete diagnosis by DNA analysis can be offered to couples at risk, the safety of these procedures should be demonstrated and the serious problems arising from PCR contamination must be overcome.

The most important challenge for the future is to organize preventive genetic programmes, such as those ongoing in the Mediterranean area, in the parts of the world, namely the Middle East, the Indian subcontinent and the Far East, where β-thalassemia is prevalent. However the resources for population education and the present state of technical development would seem to preclude such a program materializing.

References

1. Weatherall, S.J. and Clegg, J.B. (1981) *The Thalassaemia Syndromes*, 3rd edn, Blackwell, Oxford.
2. Kazazian Jr, H.H. (1990) The thalassemia syndromes: molecular basis and prenatal diagnosis in 1990. *Semin. Hematol.*, **27**, 209–28.
3. Higgs, D.R., Vickers, M.A., Wilkie, A.O.M. *et al.* (1989) A review of the molecular genetics of the human α-globin gene cluster. *Blood*, **73**, 1031–104.
4. Liebhaber, S.A. (1989) α-Thalassemia. *Hemoglobin*, **13**, 685–731.
5. Liebhaber, S.A., Griese, E.U., Weiss, I. *et al.* (1990) Inactivation of human α-globin gene expression by a *de novo* deletion located upstream of the α-globin gene cluster. *Proc. Natl Acad. Sci. USA*, **87**, 9431–35.
6. Wilkie, A.O.M., Lamb, J., Harris, P.C. *et al.* (1990) A truncated human chromosome 16 associated with a thalassemia is stabilized by addition of telomeric repeat (TTAGGG)$_n$. *Nature*, **346**, 868–71.
7. Fortina, P., Dianzani, I., Serra, A. *et al.* (1991) A newly-characterized α-thalassemia-1 deletion removes the entire α-like globin gene cluster in an Italian family. *Br. J. Haematol.*, **78**, 529–34.
8. Hatton, C.S.R., Wilkie, A.O.M., Drysdale, H.C. *et al.* (1990) α-Thalassemia caused by a large (62 kb) deletion upstream of the human α-globin gene cluster. *Blood*, **76**, 221–27.
9. Higgs, D.R., Wood, W.G., Jarman, A.P. *et al.* (1990) A major positive regulatory region is located far upstream of the human α-globin gene locus. *Genes Dev.*, **4**, 1588–601.
10. Galanello, R., Sanna, M.A., Maccioni, L. *et al.* (1990) Fetal hydrops in Sardinia: implications for genetic counselling. *Clin. Genet.*, **27**, 209–28.
11. Chang, J.C. and Kan, Y.W. (1979) β°-thalassemia, a nonsense mutation in man. *Proc. Natl Acad. Sci. USA*, **76**, 2886–89.
12. Huisman, T.H.J. (1992) The β- and δ-thalassemia repository. *Hemoglobin*, **16**, 237.
13. Huisman, T.H.J. (1990) Frequencies of common β-thalassemia alleles among different populations: variability in clinical severity. *Br. J. Haematol.*, **75**, 454–57.
14. Orkin, S.H., Kazazian Jr, H.H., Antonorakis, S.E. *et al.* (1982) Linkage of β-thalassemia mutation and β-globin gene polymorphisms with DNA polymorphisms in human β-globin gene cluster. *Nature*, **296**, 627–31.

15. Pirastu, M., Galanello, R., Doherty, M. *et al.* (1987) The same β-globin gene mutation is present on nine different β-thalassemia chromosomes in a Sardinian population. *Proc. Natl Acad. Sci. USA*, **84**, 2882–84.

16. Stamatoyannopoulos, G. and Nienhuis, A.W. (1987) Hemoglobin switching, in *The Molecular Basis of Blood Disease* (eds G. Stamatoyannopoulos, A.W. Nienhuis, P. Leder and P.W. Majerus), W.B. Saunders, Philadelphia, pp. 66–105.

17. Bunn, H.F. and Forget, B.F. (1985) *Hemoglobin: Molecular Genetic and Clinical Aspects*, W.B. Saunders, Philadelphia.

18. Pirastu, M., Kan Y.W., Galanello, R. and Cao, A. (1984) Multiple mutations produce δβ-thalassemia in Sardinia. *Science*, **223**, 924–30.

19. Townes, T.M. and Behringer, R.R. (1990) Human globin locus activation region (LAR): role in temporal control. *Trends Genet.*, **6**, 219–23.

20. Orkin, S.E. (1990) Globin gene regulation and switching: circa 1990. *Cell*, **63**, 665–72.

21. Gonzalez-Redondo, J.M., Stoming, T.A., Kutlar, A. *et al.* (1989) ACT substitution at nt −101 in a conserved DNA sequence of the promoter region of the β-globin gene is associated with 'silent' β-thalassemia. *Blood*, **73**, 1705–11.

22. Ristaldi, M.S., Murru, S., Loudianos, G. *et al.* (1990) The CT substitution in the distal CACCC box is a common cause of silent β-thalassemia in the Italian population. *Br. J. Haematol.*, **74**, 480–86.

23. Thein, S.L. (1992) Dominant β-thalassemia: molecular basis and pathophysiology. *Br. J. Haematol.*, **80**, 273–77.

24. Wainscoat, J.S., Thein, S.L. and Weatherall, D.J. (1987) Thalassemia intermedia. *Blood Rev.*, **1**, 273–79.

25. Rosatelli, M.C., Oggiano, L., Leoni, G.B. *et al.* (1989) Thalassemia intermedia resulting from a mild thalassemia mutation. *Blood*, **73**, 601–605.

26. Cao A., Gasperini D., Podda A. and Galanello, R. (1990) Molecular pathology of thalassemia intermedia. *Eur. J. Intern. Med.*, **1**, 227–36.

27. Wainscoat, J.S., Kanavakis, E., Wood, W.G. *et al.* (1983) Thalassemia intermedia: the interaction of α and β thalassemia. *Br. J. Haematol.*, **53**, 411–27.

28. Galanello, R., Dessì, E., Melis, M.A. *et al.* (1989) Molecular analysis of β⁰-thalassemia intermedia in Sardinia. *Blood*, **74**, 823–27.

29. Gilman, J.G. and Huisman, T.H.J. (1985) DNA sequence variation associated with elevated fetal Gγ production. *Blood*, **66**, 783.

30. Galanello, R., Ruggeri, R., Paglietti, E. *et al.* (1983) A family with segregating triplicated alpha globin loci and beta thalassemia. *Blood*, **62**, 1035–40.

31. Kulozik, A.E., Thein, S.L., Wainscoat, J.S. *et al.* (1987) Thalassemia intermedia: interaction of the triple α-globin gene arrangement and heterozygous β-thalassemia. *Br. J. Haematol.*, **66**, 109–12.

32. Murru, S., Loudianos, G., Vaccargiu, S. *et al.* (1990) A β-thalassemia carrier with normal sequences within the β-globin gene. *Blood*, **76**, 2164–65.

33. Murru, S., Loudianos, G., Porcu, S. *et al.* (1992) A β-thalassaemia phenotype not linked to the β-globin cluster in an Italian family. *Br. J. Haematol.*, **81**, 283–87.

34. Kan, Y.W., Golbus, M.S., Klein, P. and Dozy, A.M. (1975) Successful application of prenatal diagnosis in a pregnancy at risk for homozygous β-thalassemia. *N. Engl. J. Med.*, **292**, 1096–99.

35. Boehm, C.D., Antonarakis, S.E., Phillips, A. *et al.* (1983) Prenatal diagnosis using DNA polymorphisms. Report on 95 pregnancies at risk for sickle cell disease or β-thalassemia. *N. Engl. J. Med.*, **308**, 1054–58.

36. Kan, Y.W., Golbus, M.S. and Dozy, A.M. (1976) Prenatal diagnosis of α-thalassemia: clinical application of molecular hybridization. *N. Engl. J. Med.*, **295**, 1165–67.

37. Pirastu, M., Kan, Y.W., Cao, A. *et al.* (1983) Prenatal diagnosis of β-thalassemia. Detection of a single nucleotide mutation on DNA. *N. Engl. J. Med.*, **309**, 284–87.

38. Rosatelli, C., Falchi, A.M. and Tuveri, T. (1985) Prenatal diagnosis of β-thalassemia with the synthetic-oligomer technique. *Lancet*, **i**, 241–43.

39. Saiki, R.K., Gelfand, D.H., Stoffel, S. *et al.* (1988) Primer direct enzymatic amplification of DNA with a thermostable DNA polymerase. *Science*, **239**, 487–91.

40. Hogge, W.A., Schonberg, S.A. and Golbus, M.S. (1986) Chorionic villus sampling: experience of the first 1000 cases. *Am. J. Obstet. Gynecol.*, **154**, 1249–52.

41. Brambati, B., Lanzani, A. and Oldrini, A. (1988) Transabdominal chorionic villus sampling, clinical experience of 1159 cases. *Prenat. Diagn.*, **8**, 609–13.

42. Canadian Collaborative CVS–Amniocentesis Clinical Trial Group (1989) Multicentre randomized clinical trial of chorionic villus sampling and amniocentesis. *Lancet*, **i**, 1–6.

43. MRC Working Party on the Evaluation of Chorion Villus Sampling (1991) Medical Research Council European Trial of chorion villus sampling. *Lancet*, **337**, 1491–99.

44. Cao, A. (1987) Results of programmes for antenatal detection of thalassemia in reducing the incidence of the disorder. *Blood Rev.*, **1**, 169–76.

45. Chehab, F.F., Doherty, M., Cai, S.P. *et al.* (1987) Detection of sickle cell anemia and thalassemia. *Nature*, **329**, 293–94.

46. Pirastu, M., Ristaldi, M.S. and Cao, A. (1989) Prenatal diagnosis of β-thalassemia based on restriction endonuclease analysis of amplified fetal DNA. *J. Med. Genet.*, **26**, 363–67.

47. Sorcher, E.G. and Huang, Z. (1991) Diagnosis of genetic disease by primer-specified restriction map modification, with application to cystic fibrosis and retinitis pigmentosa. *Lancet*, **337**, 1115–58.

48. Cai, S.P., Eng, B., Chui, D.H.K. and Kan, Y.W. (1990) A rapid and simple electrophoretic method for the detection of small insertions and deletions: application to β-thalassemia (abstract). *Blood*, **76** (suppl.), A216.

49. Gonzalez-Redondo, J.M., Kattamis, C. and Huisman, T.H.J. (1989) Characterization of three types of β-thalassemia resulting from a partial deletion of the β-globin gene. *Hemoglobin*, **13**, 377–92.

50. Faà, V., Rosatelli, C. and Sardu, R. *et al.* (1992) A simple electrophoretic procedure for fetal diagnosis of β-thalassemia due to short deletions. *Prenat. Diagn.* **12**, 903–908.

51. Triggs-Raine, B.L. and Gravel, R.A. (1990) Diagnostic heteroduplexes: single detection of carriers of a 4 bp insertion mutation in Tay–Sachs disease. *Am. J. Hum. Genet.*, **46**, 183–4.

52. White, M.B., Carvalho, M. and Derse, D. *et al.* (1992) Detecting single base substitutions as heteroduplex polymorphisms. *Genomics*, **12**, 301–306.

53. Saiki, R.K., Bugawan, T.L. and Horn, G.T. *et al.* (1986) Analysis of enzymatically amplified β-globin and HLA-DQα DNA with allele-specific oligonucleotide probes. *Nature*, **324**, 163–66.

54. Ristaldi, M.S., Pirastu, M. and Rosatelli, C. *et al.* (1989) Prenatal diagnosis of β-thalassemia in Mediterranean populations by dot-blot analysis with DNA amplification and allele specific oligonucleotide probes. *Prenat. Diagn.*, **9**, 629–38.

55. Saiki, R.K., Chang, C.A. and Levenson, C.H. *et al.* (1988) Diagnosis of sickle cell anemia and β-thalassemia with enzymatically amplified DNA and nonradioactive allele-specific oligonucleotide probes. *N. Engl. J. Med.*, **319**, 537–41.

56. Saiki, R.K., Walsh, P.S., Levenson, C.H. and Erlich, H.A. (1989) Genetic analysis of amplified DNA with immobilized sequence specific oligonucleotide probes. *Proc. Natl Acad. Sci. USA*, **86**, 6230–34.

57. Newton, C.R., Graham, A. and Heptinstall, L.E. *et al.* (1989) Analysis of any point mutation in DNA. The Amplification Refractory Mutation System (ARMS). *Nucleic Acids Res.*, **17**, 2503–16.

58. Old J.M., Varawalla, N.Y. and Weatherall, D.J. (1990) Rapid detection and prenatal diagnosis of β-thalassemia: studies in Indian and Cypriot population in the UK. *Lancet*, **336**, 834–37.

59. Chehab, F.F. and Kan, Y.W. (1989) Detection of specific DNA sequences by fluorescence amplification: a color complementation assay. *Proc. Natl Acad. Sci. USA*, **86**, 9178–82.

60. Myers, R.M., Maniatis, T. and Lerman, L.S. (1987) Detection and localization of single base changes by denaturing gradient gel electrophoresis. *Methods Enzymol.*, **155**, 501–27.

61. Myers, R.M., Fisher, S.G., Lerman, L.S. and Maniatis, T. (1985) Nearly all single base substitution in DNA fragments joined to a GC-clamp can be detected by denaturing gradient gel electrophoresis. *Nucleic Acids Res.*, **13**, 3131–45.

62. Cai, S.P. and Kan, Y.W. (1990) Identification of the multiple β-thalassemia mutation by denaturing gradient gel electrophoresis. *J. Clin. Invest.*, **85**, 550–53.

63. Rosatelli, M.C., Tuveri, T., and Scalas, M.T. *et al.* (1992) Molecular screening and fetal diagnosis of β-thalassemia in the Italian population. *Hum. Genet.*, **89**, 585–89.

64. Orita, M., Suzuki, Y., Sexiya, T. and Hayashi, K. (1989) Rapid and sensitive detection of any point mutation and DNA polymorphism using the polymerase chain reaction. *Genomics*, **5**, 874–79.

65. Cotton, R.G.H., Rodrigues, N.R. and Campbell, R.D. (1988) Reactivity of cytosine and thimine in single-base-pair mismatches with hydroxylamine and osmium tetroxide and its application to the study of mutations. *Proc. Natl Acad. Sci. USA*, **85**, 4397–401.

66. Dianzani, I., Camaschella, C., and Saglio, G. *et al.* (1991) Simultaneous screening for β-thalassemia mutations by chemical cleavage of mismatch. *Genomics*, **11**, 48–53.

67. Gyllenstein, U.B. and Erlich, H.A. (1988) Generation of single stranded DNA by the polymerase chain reaction and its application to direct sequencing of the HLA-DQa locus. *Proc. Natl Acad. Sci. USA*, **85**, 7652–56.

68. Ansorge, W., Sproat, B.S., Stegemann, J. and Schwager, C. (1986) A nonradioactive automated method for DNA sequencing determination. *J. Biochem. Biophys. Methods*, **13**, 315–23.

69. Kan, Y.W. and Dozy, A. (1978) Polymorphism of DNA sequence adjacent to the human β-globin structural gene: relationship to sickle mutation. *Proc. Natl Acad. Sci. USA*, **75**, 5631–35.

70. Kan, Y.W., Lee, K.W. and Furbetta, M. *et al.* (1980) Polymorphism of DNA sequence in the β-globin gene region: application to prenatal diagnosis of β⁰-thalassemia in Sardinia. *N. Engl. J. Med.*, **302**, 185–88.

71. Miesfeld, R., Krystal, M. and Arnheim, N. (1981) A member of a new

repeated sequence which is conserved throughout eucaryotic evolution is found between the human δ and β-globin genes. *Nucleic Acids Res.*, 9, 5931–47.

72. Spritz, R.A. (1981) Duplication/deletion polymorphism 5 to the human β-globin gene. *Nucleic Acids Res.*, 9, 5038–46.

73. Loudianos, G., Cao, A. and Pirastu, M. (1992) Feasibility of prenatal diagnosis of β-thalassemia using two highly polymorphic microsatellites 5 to the β-globin gene. *Haematologica*, 77, 361–62.

74. Bowden, D.K., Vickers, M.A. and Higgs, D.R. (1992) A PCR-based strategy to detect the common severe determinants of α-thalassemia. *Br. J. Haematol.*, 81, 104–108.

75. Decorte, R., Cuppens, H., Marynen, P. and Cassiman, J.J. (1990) Laboratory Methods. Rapid detection of hypervariable regions by the polymerase chain reaction technique. *DNA Cell Biol.*, 9, 461–69.

76. Buster, J.E. and Carson, S.A. (1989) Genetic diagnosis of the preimplantation embryo. *Am. J. Med. Genet.*, 34, 211–16.

77. Monk, M. and Holding, C. (1990) Amplification of a β-hemoglobin sequence in individual human oocytes and polar bodies. *Lancet*, 335, 985–85.

78. Handyside, A.M., Penceth, R.J.A. and Wiston, R.M.L. (1989) Biopsy of human preimplantation embryos and sexing by DNA amplification. *Lancet*, i, 347–49.

J.M. Connor

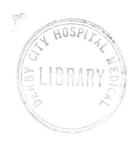

76.1 Nucleic acid structure and function

There are an estimated 100 000 human structural genes encoded in the DNA of every nucleated cell. These genes carry information for the direction of protein synthesis and are regulated so that at any one time only about 1% of the total are active in a particular cell type. With the important exception of genes on the sex chromosomes, the genes are paired and occupy the same location (**locus**) on a pair of chromosomes. During normal cell division (**mitosis**) every gene is normally accurately duplicated so that each cell has an identical genetic composition (**genotype**). In contrast, in the production of gametes (**meiosis**) each mature sperm or egg receives only one of each pair of genes and children thus receive one half of their genes from each parent.

DNA consists of a double helix with the two strands bound together by hydrogen bonds between projecting nitrogenous bases which are attached to a deoxyribose–phosphate backbone. The nitrogenous bases are attached to the 1′ position of deoxyribose and phosphate links the 3′- and 5′-hydroxyl groups of adjacent deoxyribose residues (-5′-deoxyribose-3′–phosphate–5′-deoxyribose-3′–phosphate–5′-deoxyribose-3′–phosphate–). These 5′ to 3′ links allow DNA molecules to be orientated and within a double helix the two DNA strands run in opposite directions (i.e. one is 5′ to 3′ whereas the other is 3′ to 5′). There are four types of nitrogenous bases: adenine (A), cytosine (C), guanine (G) and thymine (T). A pairs specifically with T, and G with C, and so the parallel strands of DNA must be complementary to one another. Thus for example if one strand reads ATGA the complementary strand must read TACT. This **complementarity** of base pairing is the key to understanding normal DNA replication and approaches to DNA diagnosis and manipulation.

The unit of length of DNA is the base pair (bp) with 1000 bp in a kilobase (kb) and 1000 000 bp in a megabase (Mb). The total length of DNA in a half set of human chromosomes is 3000 Mb and, of this, one half represents the structural genes which occur singly or in clusters with intervening DNA (**intergenic DNA**), which is involved in gene regulation or has no known function. Much of the intergenic DNA consists of repetitive DNA, which may be moderately repetitive with several hundred copies or highly repetitive with many thousands of copies, and may be dispersed or occur in clusters. Three families of highly repetitive DNA are particularly frequent as each accounts for about 4% of the total DNA. One of these families (alphoid repeats) is clustered, whereas the other two (Alu and LINE 1 or L1 families) are interspersed throughout the genome. The alphoid repeats occur as short tandem repeats near the centromeres of all chromosomes and are especially abundant in chromosomes 1, 9, 16 and the Y chromosome. The Alu family consists of about 500 000 copies of a 300 bp sequence which share a recognition site for the restriction enzyme *Alu*I (see below). The L1 family consists of 50 000–100 000 copies which are found on average every 8 kb. In contrast to the alphoid family, some members of the Alu and L1 families may be transferred (transposed) to different chromosomal locations and if the new location is a functional gene sequence this transposition can cause genetic disease (e.g. some patients with haemophilia A or neurofibromatosis type I).

Proteins, whether structural components, enzymes, carrier molecules, hormones or receptors, are all composed of a series of amino acids whose sequence determines the form and function of the resulting protein. Within a structural gene each set of three DNA base pairs, or triplet, codes for an amino acid. As each base in the triplet may be any of the four types this results in 4^3 or 64 possible combinations or codons. This exceeds the number (20) of known amino acids and so, except for methionine and tryptophan, all amino acids are coded by more than one codon (Table 76.1). Three codons designate termination of protein synthesis and one (AUG which also codes for methionine) acts as a start signal for protein synthesis. By

Diseases of the Fetus and Newborn, 2nd edn, Edited by G.B. Reed, A.E. Claireaux and F. Cockburn. Published in 1995 by Chapman & Hall, London. ISBN 0 412 39160 0

Table 76.1 The genetic code with codons shown as messenger RNA. The corresponding DNA codons are complementary

First base	Second base				Third base
	U	C	A	G	
U	UUU Phe	UCU Ser	UAU Tyr	UGU Cys	U
	UUC Phe	UCC Ser	UAC Tyr	UGC Cys	C
	UUA Leu	UCA Ser	UUA STOP	UGA STOP	A
	UUG Leu	UCG Ser	UAG STOP	UGG Trp	G
C	CUU Leu	CCU Pro	CAU His	CGU Arg	U
	CUC Leu	CCC Pro	CAC His	CGC Arg	C
	CUA Leu	CCA Pro	CAA Gln	CGA Arg	A
	CUC Leu	CCG Pro	CAG Gln	CGG Arg	G
A	AUU Ile	ACU Thr	AAU Asn	AGU Ser	U
	AUC Ile	ACC Thr	AAC Asn	AGC Ser	C
	AUA Ile	ACA Thr	AAA Lys	AGA Arg	A
	*AUG Met	ACG Thr	AAG Lys	AGG Arg	G
C	GUU Val	GCU Ala	GAU Asp	GGU Gly	U
	GUC Val	GCC Ala	GAC Asp	GGC Gly	C
	GUA Val	GCA Ala	GAA Glu	GGA Gly	A
	GUG Val	GCG Ala	GAG Glu	GGG Gly	G

Abbreviations for amino acids (short code): Ala = alanine (A); Arg = arginine (R); Asn = asparagine (N); Asp = aspartic acid (D); Cys = cysteine (C); Gln = glutamine (Q); Glu = glutamic acid (E); Gly = glycine (G); His = histidine (H); Ile = isoleucine (I); Leu = leucine (L); Lys = lysine (K); Met = methionine (M); Phe = phenylalanine (F); Pro = proline (P); Ser = serine (S); Thr = threonine (T); Trp = tryptophan (W); Tyr = tyrosine (Y); Val = valine (V).
STOP = chain terminators (X); * start codon for protein synthesis.

convention in Table 76.1 the codons are shown in terms of the messenger RNA (mRNA) which is complementary to the coding strand of the structural gene. mRNA has three bases in common with DNA (A,C and G) but uracil (U) replaces thymine and also pairs with A, and ribose replaces deoxyribose.

The first stage in protein synthesis is transcription. The two strands of DNA separate in the area of the gene to be transcribed. One strand (the template strand – this strand is consistent for a given gene but varies from one gene to another) functions as a template and is read 3′ to 5′ and mRNA is formed 5′ to 3′ with a complementary sequence under the influence of the enzyme RNA polymerase II. Transcription proceeds at about 30 bases per second until a transcription terminator is reached. After some processing and modification the mRNA molecule diffuses to the cytoplasm and the DNA strands reassociate. The next stage of protein synthesis occurs in the cytoplasm and is called translation. Each mRNA molecule becomes attached to one or more ribosomes. As the ribosome moves along the mRNA each codon is recognized by a matching transfer RNA which contributes its amino acid to the end of a new growing protein chain (Figure 76.1). Many pro-teins are not in their final form after ribosomal translation and post-translational processing (e.g. cleavage, formation of disulphide bonds or glycosylation) may be required to allow the protein to achieve its final functional form.

The average protein contains about 300 amino acids which could be coded by 900 base pairs. It was thus a surprise to discover that human genes are much larger than expected (Table 76.2). Some of this excess is due to regulatory sequences and to processing of the initial protein product but the majority is due to the presence of intervening sequences (or introns). Nearly all structural genes have been found to consist of alternating protein coding segments (or exons) and non-protein coding intervening sequences of 50 to over 10 000 bp. The initial mRNA transcript is a complete complementary copy of the coding strand of the gene (including exons, intervening sequences and flanking sequences) but prior to its entry to the cytoplasm the segments corresponding to the intervening sequences are removed by splicing. The sequences at the boundaries of each intervening sequence (commonly GT at the beginning and AG at the end) are important for such

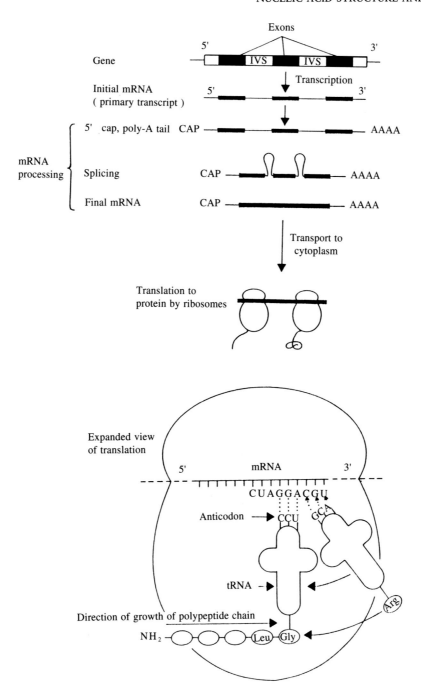

Figure 76.1 Diagram of transcription, messenger RNA processing and translation.

splicing, and mutations in these sequences can result in defective splicing and consequent disease.

All nucleated cells of an individual have an identical genome, yet at any one time in a cell only about 1% of the total is being expressed and the relative pattern of expression varies widely not only for the differentiation of cells and tissues but also to meet fluctuating demands for synthesis of different proteins in each cell. In addition to the start and chain terminator codons, areas of each gene and of the neighbouring DNA seem to play an important role in regulating transcription and hence synthesis of each protein. Mutations within a gene's regulatory sequences can occur and may result in no gene product (e.g. some patients with β-thalassaemia), abnormal persistence of a fetal gene product (e.g. hereditary persistence of α-fetoprotein or haemoglobin F) or anomalous patterns of gene expression (e.g. ectopic expression of creatine kinase).

Table 76.2 Examples of genes and their protein products

Protein	No. of amino acids in final protein	Chromosomal location of gene	Approximate gene size (bp)	No. of coding regions in each gene
α-Globin	141	16	850	3
α₁-Antitrypsin	394	14	10 000	5
β-Globin	146	11	1 600	3
Coagulation factor VIII	2332	X	186 000	26
Cystic fibrosis transmembrane regulator protein	1480	7	250 000	24
Dystrophin	3700	X	2400 000	80
Glucose-6-phosphate dehydrogenase	515	X	18 000	13
Hypoxanthine–guanine phosphoribosyltransferase	217	X	44 000	9
Insulin	51	11	1 430	3
Low-density lipoprotein receptor	839	19	45 000	18
Phenylalanine hydroxylase	451	12	90 000	13

Table 76.3 Examples of DNA mutation

DNA base sequence	mRNA sequence	Amino acid sequence	Comment
CAA TTC CGA CGA	GUU AAG GCU GCU	Val-Lys-Ala-Ala	Normal sequence
CAA TTT CGA CGA	GUU AAA GCU GCU	Val-Lys-Ala-Ala	Point mutation with unchanged AA sequence
CAA CTC CGA CGA	GUU GAG GCU GCU	Val-Glu-Ala-Ala	Point mutation with AA substitution (Mis-sense mutation)
CAA ATC CGA CGA	GUU UAG GCU GCU	Val-stop	Point mutation with premature chain termination (Non-sense mutation)
CAA—TCC GAC GA	GUU AGG CUG CU	Val-Arg-Leu	Base deletion with frame shift (Non-sense mutation)
CAA TTT CCG ACG A	GUU AAA GGC UGC	Val-Lys-Gly-Cys	Base insertion with frame shift (Non-sense mutation)

76.2 Nucleic acid pathology

Normally DNA replication at mitosis or meiosis is completely accurate but errors or mutations can occur. These are divisible into length mutations, with gain or loss of DNA, and point mutations, with alteration of the codon but no change in the amount of DNA.

76.2.1 LENGTH MUTATIONS

Length mutations include deletions, trinucleotide amplifications, duplications and insertions of DNA. Deletions can arise from chromosomal breakage, as a result of a parental translocation or inversion (which is itself caused by chromosomal breakage), as a result of slipped mispairing with excision of the single-stranded loop, or by unequal crossing over. The spontaneous rate of chromosomal breakage is markedly increased by ionizing radiation and by some mutagenic chemicals. Deletions can vary in size from one base pair to many megabases. Very large deletions (over 4 Mb) will be visible at chromosomal analysis but smaller deletions are submicroscopic and need DNA analysis for their diagnosis. Removal of all of a gene directly prevents transcription but smaller deletions of more or less than three (or a multiple of three) base pairs can be equally serious by altering the reading frame of the mRNA (frameshift/ non-sense mutations; Table 76.3). Duplications can also affect the reading frame and in some patients the structural gene is disrupted by insertion of an L1 or Alu sequence.

These length mutations are normally stably inherited but unstable length mutations have also been described due to trinucleotide amplifications. For example, mental handicap due to the fragile X syndrome occurs when the normal number of 6–54 CGG repeats in the first exon of this gene is exceeded and the repeat number tends to increase at subsequent cell divisions, with a parallel increase in disease severity.

Table 76.4 Examples of DNA mutations using standardized nomenclature

Gene	Mutation	Description
β-Globin	E6V	Substitution of valine for glutamic acid at position 6 (sickle-cell disease)
Cystic fibrosis	ΔF508	Deletion of codon for phenylalanine at position 508
Cystic fibrosis	G551D	Substitution of aspartic acid for glycine at position 551
Cystic fibrosis	R542X	Premature termination codon in place of arginine at position 542

76.2.2 POINT MUTATIONS

Alteration of a single base may (25%) lead to no change in the amino acid coded by that triplet due to overlap of coding, may result in the substitution of a different amino acid (70%, mis-sense mutations) or alteration to a chain terminator (5%, non-sense mutation). These mutations can be described using a standardized nomenclature which is based upon the type of mutation, the amino acid short code (Table 76.1) and the amino acid position within the protein (Table 76.4). Most point mutations are spontaneous and unexplained but certain factors, particularly mutaganic chemicals, can increase the spontaneous mutation rate.

Substitution of T for C is a particularly common point mutation and accounts for 35–50% of all point mutations. In contrast to other types of deamination which can be identified and repaired, deamination of methylated cytosine produces thymidine (with substitution of adenine for guanine on the complementary strand): changes which are not recognized by the DNA repair mechanisms.

76.2.3 MOLECULAR PATHOLOGY OF SINGLE GENE DISORDERS

Determination of the molecular lesion in a single gene disorder is not just of academic interest because it allows the mutation to be tracked within a family in order to provide accurate genetic counselling. As more conditions are studied, two generalizations are possible. Lesions can occur at any stage in the protein biosynthetic pathway and most conditions show a diversity of molecular pathology (**molecular heterogeneity**).

The β-globin gene is currently the best documented gene in respect of molecular pathology. In patients with β-thalassaemia over 100 different molecular defects have now been described and can result in reduced output of the normal gene product (β°, i.e. reduction in protein function proportionate to level) or synthesis of an abnormal gene product (β⁺, i.e. reduction in protein function disproportionate to level). In general, mutations affecting transcription (16% of the total), mRNA processing (33%) or translation (33%) result in β°

thalassaemia, whereas mis-sense mutations, fusion genes and in-frame small deletions or insertions result in β⁺-thalassaemia. Both length and point mutations are observed, with the latter predominating.

In contrast, in conditions such as α-thalassaemia and Duchenne muscular dystrophy, length mutations, particularly deletions, are far more frequent than point mutations, and in sickle-cell anaemia all patients have the same point mutation (E6V).

76.2.4 DNA POLYMORPHISMS

Most, but not all, mutations in protein coding DNA result in an altered protein which may or may not cause disease. In contrast, mutations in non-protein coding DNA (intervening sequences and intergenic DNA) usually do not cause disease. Many of these mutations which are not associated with disease are found at relatively high frequencies within the population and, by definition, if 1 in 50 or more have the variant it is called a **DNA polymorphism**.

Length or point mutations can be involved in DNA polymorphisms. The length polymorphisms are usually associated with multiple repeats of a dinucleotide (microsatellite repeats), tetranucleotide or larger repeat unit (commonly 10–15, minisatellite repeats). Dinucleotide repeats, especially CA and CT, are very frequent, with an estimated total of 50 000 dispersed throughout the genome. This abundance coupled with the fact that most (about 70%) individuals generate different sized fragments (i.e. **heterozygous**) from each member of a chromosome pair has meant that this type of polymorphism is very useful for tracking mutant genes within affected families and for gene mapping studies. The minisatellite repeats also show marked variability in the number of repeats and again most (about 70%) individuals are heterozygous. This type of polymorphism is also useful for gene mapping studies but this has been limited by their uneven distribution, with many close to the ends of the chromosomes.

Polymorphisms due to point mutations occur every 200–500 bp and, as only two alternative sequences (normal and altered) are found, most individuals have identical sequences (**homozygous**) and relatively few (up to 35%) are heterozygous. This type of polymorphism is usually demonstrated by loss (or gain) of a cutting site for a DNA cleavage enzyme (**restriction enzyme**) and thus they are usually called restriction fragment length polymorphisms (RFLPs).

All of these DNA polymorphisms are normally stably inherited and will cosegregate with neighbouring genes. This cosegregation is known as **linkage** and allows mutant genes to be tracked within families.

76.3 Nucleic acid analysis

DNA can be extracted from any nucleated tissue, and lymphocytes from a 10-ml venous blood sample yield about 300 µg which is sufficient for many DNA analyses. At post mortem a sample of spleen or liver can be taken into a dry sterile tube or snap-frozen in liquid nitrogen and stored at −20°C pending DNA extraction.

DNA **probes** are labelled (radioactive or non-radioactive) sections of DNA, from tens of base pairs to several kilobases in size, which are used to identify fragments with a complementary sequence amongst a mixture of DNA fragments. The probe and target DNA are first rendered single stranded (by heating or exposure to alkali) and complementary fragments hybridize to form labelled double standed DNA fragments which can be visualized. For visualization a large number of labelled hybrid DNA fragments need to be formed and this is achieved by either starting with a relatively large amount of target DNA (**Southern analysis**) or by selectively amplifying the target sequence(s) from an initial tiny sample of DNA (**polymerase chain reaction analysis, PCR analysis**). In general, Southern analysis uses 5–10 µg of DNA for each analysis and takes 5–7 days to produce a result. Each Southern analysis needs target DNA which is fragmented with the appropriate restiction enzyme, separated according to fragment size by gel electrophoresis and then transferred to a DNA binding filter. The appropriate DNA probe will then identify the complementary sequence(s) and the labelled hybrid molecules are identified by autoradiography (for radio-labelled probes, e.g. Figure 76.2). Each PCR reaction needs target DNA, a pair of primers which are complementary to DNA sequences flanking the target sequence and an enzyme (Taq polymerase) which directs repeated rounds of localized DNA replication. Theoretically amplification will increase exponentially to 2^n (where n is the number of cycles) and amplification of more than a million-fold can be routinely obtained from 30 or so cycles, which takes a couple of hours in an automated procedure. The amplified DNA segment can then be digested, if required, with the appropriate restriction enzyme and the resulting frag-

ment(s) separated according to size by gel electrophoresis and visualized directly when stained with ethidium bromide and viewed under ultraviolet light (Figure 76.3). Direct visualization in this fashion gives white target DNA bands on a dark background, as compared with autoradiography in Southern analysis which gives black target DNA bands on a light background. Each PCR analysis can start with considerably less than 1 µg of target DNA and produces a result in a matter of hours. Its speed and sensitivity are key advantages over Southern analysis but it can only be applied for DNA sequences where flanking primer sequence is available and its extreme sensitivity means that meticulous care to avoid exogenous DNA contamination (and hence a false result) is required. As PCR analysis can use tiny starting quantities of impure genomic DNA, it has proved possible to use PCR amplification to provide a DNA analysis on buccal mucosal cells from a mouth rinse, single hairs, single cells (sperm, ova, preimplantation embryo biopsies, etc.), fixed pathological specimens and dried blood spots, including stored Guthrie neonatal screening cards.

For these experiments DNA is cleaved using **restriction enzymes**. Restriction enzymes (restriction endonucleases) are widespread in bacteria where they function as a defence mechanism against the incorporation of foreign DNA. More than 400 different restriction enzymes have been described, which have over 100 different recognition sites. Each is named after the organism from which it was first isolated, and each will only cleave at a specific DNA sequence – the **recognition site**, which is commonly four or six bases in length – to produce fragments with flush (blunt) or staggered (sticky or cohesive) ends (Figure 76.4). The enzyme *Taq*I will cut DNA at each point where the sequence TCGA occurs. Human DNA contains about one million *Taq* I recognition sites and so cleavage (digestion) with this enzyme yields about one million fragments of DNA. These fragments would be of variable length but each would have the same base order at their staggered

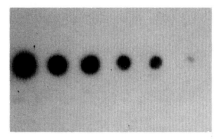

Figure 76.2 Autoradiograph of Southern DNA analysis with detection of a target sequence in serial dilutions of a DNA sample.

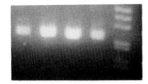

Figure 76.3 Direct visualization of a PCR amplified specific DNA fragment in four DNA samples (with size controls in the right-hand lane).

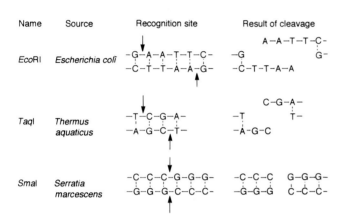

Figure 76.4 Examples of restriction enzymes with their recognition sites (shown 5' to 3' on the upper DNA strand) and their cleavage products.

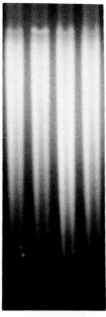

Figure 76.5 Smear of DNA fragments after total DNA digestion with a restriction enzyme.

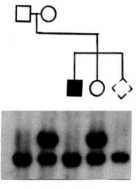

Figure 76.6 Pedigree and results of Southern DNA analysis for a family with Duchenne muscular dystrophy (see text for interpretation).

ends. As these fragments differ in length they can be separated by gel electrophoresis. These DNA fragments can be visualized by viewing the gel under ultraviolet light and at this stage appear as a smear of overlapping fragments (Figure 76.5). Subsequently a DNA probe would be used to identify specific fragments from this complex mixture.

76.3.1 INDIRECT MUTANT GENE TRACKING

DNA polymorphisms can be used to follow or track the inheritance of a part of a chromosome through a family. Figure 76.6 shows a family with X-linked Duchenne muscular dystrophy. The mother is a carrier as she had an affected brother and now has an affected child. The mother is heterozygous for a DNA polymorphism and the affected son has inherited the lower maternal DNA band with the disease. The male pregnancy has also inherited the lower band from the mother and is thus predicted to be affected, whereas the daughter has inherited the lower band from the father and the upper band from the mother and is thus predicted to not be a carrier. This DNA marker is outside the gene for Duchenne muscular dystrophy (i.e.

extragenic) and there is thus a small possibility that at meiosis a recombination could occur between the mutant gene and the DNA polymorphism. This error rate due to recombination increases as more distant polymorphic markers are used and hence intragenic or very tightly linked extragenic polymorphisms should be used wherever possible.

Indirect mutant gene tracking has the advantage of being applicable in the absence of knowledge of the precise molecular defect but has the disadvantages of potential error if the polymorphic site is at some distance from the mutant gene or if genetic hetero-

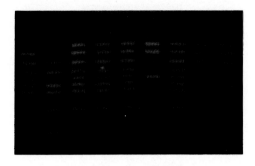

Figure 76.7 Simultaneous PCR amplification of nine segments of the gene for Duchenne muscular dystrophy.

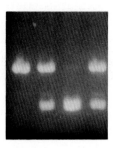

Figure 76.9 PCR amplification of a segment of the gene for cystic fibrosis which contains the point mutation G551D. This causes loss of a restriction site for *Hinc*II and thus lane 1 is homozygous mutant, lanes 2 and 4 are heterozygous and lane 3 is homozygous normal.

Figure 76.8 PCR amplification of a segment of the cystic fibrosis gene containing the common 3 bp deletion mutation. Lane 1, homozygous normal; lane 2, heterozygous; and lane 3, homozygous mutant.

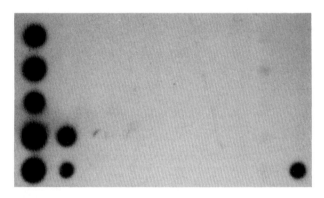

Figure 76.10 Application of normal (left panel) and mutant (right panel) allele specific oligonucleotide probes to seven PCR amplified DNA samples.

geneity exists with different genes causing a similar clinical picture in different families. Mutant gene tracking also requires DNA samples from several family members in order to distinguish the mutant and normal genes and may not be applicable if few samples are available or if key individuals are homozygous for the polymorphic site. Direct mutation detection circumvents many of these difficulties as demonstration of the molecular lesion confirms the diagnosis and allows direct demonstration of other family members who carry each mutant gene. The disadvantage of this approach is the need to define the mutation(s) for each family.

76.3.2 DIRECT MUTATION DETECTION

Large length mutations may be visible at cytogenetic analysis but if less than 4 Mb in size then DNA analysis is required. Figure 76.7 shows simultaneous PCR analysis of nine regions of the gene for Duchenne muscular dystrophy in nine affected patients. In the patients in lanes 1, 6 and 8, bands are missing due to partial gene deletions.

Even small deletions can be revealed by DNA analysis. The single most common mutation in cystic

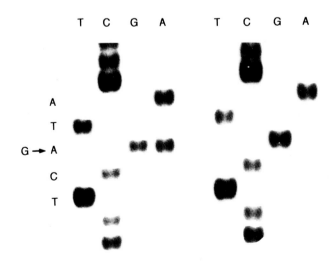

Figure 76.11 DNA sequencing with normal sequence in the right-hand set of lanes (TCGA) and mutant sequence showing replacement of a G with an A in a patient with acute intermittent porphyria.

fibrosis is a 3-bp deletion which removes the codon for phenylalanine at position 508 (ΔF508). Figure 76.8 demonstrates this mutation with a normal homozygote in lane 1, a heterozygote in lane 2 and a homozygote for ΔF508 in lane 3. The PCR product from the mutant gene is 3 bp smaller and hence migrates further in the gel than the normal fragment (the additional pair of slowly migrating bands in the heterozygote represent heteroduplexes between the normal and mutant PCR products).

Point mutations can be detected by several approaches, including loss or gain of a cutting site for a restriction enzyme and by allele specific oligonucleotide probes. Figure 76.9 shows an example of a point mutation which can be detected by loss of a cutting site for a restriction enzyme. The mutation G551D in the gene for cystic fibrosis results in loss of a site for the restriction enzyme *Hinc*II and hence a larger-sized fragment than normal. Lanes 2 and 4 show heterozygotes and lanes 1 and 3 are homozygous mutant and normal respectively.

Allele specific oligonucleotide (ASO) probes are short (17–30 nucleotide) probes which have the complementary sequence to either the normal DNA or mutant DNA sequence at the point of interest. Under appropriate experimental conditions the presence or absence of hybridization with these probes will distinguish normal homozygotes from heterozygotes and homozygous affected individuals. Figure 76.10 illustrates an application of this approach for a rare point mutation for cystic fibrosis. Seven DNA samples are hybridized to the normal sequence ASO in the left panel of the figure and to the mutant ASO in the right-hand panel. Six samples show only a signal with the normal ASO and are thus homozygous normal, but the seventh gives a signal with both the normal and mutant ASOs and thus identifies a heterozygote.

If the mutation is unknown in a family then a variety of approaches can be used to delineate the molecular lesion. Screening for length mutations can be performed by Southern analysis or PCR analysis with absence of specific hybridization or an altered length of the specific DNA fragment. Screening for point mutations is more difficult and several approaches are under active development. Heteroduplexes between PCR amplified single stranded normal and mutant DNA may show altered electrophoretic mobility in special gels (e.g. hydrolink gel electrophoresis and denaturing gradient gel electrophoresis) or the point mismatches may be identified by susceptibility to chemical cleavage (amplification and mismatch detection). The mobility of PCR amplified single stranded DNA depends upon both its size and sequence and single base changes may be detected as mobility shifts (single stranded conformation polymorphism analysis). Confirmation of the suspected point mutation then requires DNA sequencing. Figure 76.11 illustrates normal DNA sequence and mutant sequence in a patient with autosomal dominant acute intermittent porphyria. The disease in this patient is due to a point mutation with substitution of A for G in the gene for porphobilinogen deaminase. This information can then be used to identify other family members carrying the mutation by ASOs or gain or loss of an RFLP.

Further reading

Antonarakis, S.E.(1989) Diagnosis of genetic disorders at the DNA level. *N. Engl. J. Med.*, **320**, 153–63.
Connor, J.M. and Ferguson-Smith, M.A.(1993). *Essential Medical Genetics*, 4th edn, Blackwell, Oxford.
Cotton, R.G.H.(1989) Detection of single base changes in nucleic acids. *Biochem. J.* **263**, 1–10.
Eisenstein, B.I.(1990) The polymerase chain reaction. A new method using molecular genetics for medical diagnosis. *N. Engl. J. Med.*, **322**, 178–83.
Hearne, C.M., Ghosh, S. and Todd, J.A. (1992) Microsatellites for linkage analysis of genetic traits. *Trends Genet.*, **8**, 288–93.
Human Gene Mapping 11 (1992) Eleventh International Workshop on Human Gene Mapping. *Cytogenet. Ceil Genet.*, **58**, 1–2184.
Miles, J.S. and Wolf, C.R. (1989) Principles of DNA cloning. *BMJ* 299, 1019–22.
Weatherall, D.J. (1991) *The New Genetics and Clinical Medicine*, 3rd edn, Oxford University Press, Oxford.

77 COMPENDIUM OF PRENATALLY DIAGNOSABLE DISEASES

J.M. Connor

This chapter aims to provide in tabular form (Table 77.1) details of conditions which have been prenatally diagnosed. Entries have an MIM number, where available from the current edition of McKusick's *Mendelian Inheritance in Man* (McKusick, 1990). This has advantages in providing consistency of nosology and in allowing direct access to a summary and bibliography but does have the potentially confusing limitation that inclusion of the MIM does not mean that the condition is always or even usually inherited as a single gene disorder. Hence the table should be used as a guide to the prenatal diagnostic situation for the condition and other data will be required to determine appropriate recurrence risks for genetic counselling. Furthermore the inclusion of a condition in the table does not mean that prenatal diagnosis is necessarily indicated or desirable in each affected family.

Table 77.1 contains some 600 entries, and approaches to prenatal diagnosis are divided into 'imaging,' 'biochemistry', 'DNA' and 'other'. Imaging is further subdivided into ultrasound and other (which includes fetoscopy, radiography, magnetic resonance imaging and fetal echocardiography). Biochemistry is subdivided into amniotic fluid cells (AFC), amniotic fluid supernatant (AFS), chorionic villus samples (CVS) and other. (Mucolipidosis IV and neuronal ceroid lipofuscinosis are also included in the biochemical section even though electron microscopy of cultured cells is employed for prenatal diagnosis rather than biochemical analysis.) DNA is subdivided into gene tracking using linked probes, which may be either intragenic (ILP) or extragenic (ELP), and direct detection of molecular pathology (MP). The 'other' category is subdivided into fetal blood sampling (FBS), fetal liver biopsy (FLB), fetal skin biopsy (FSKB) and chromosomal analysis (CHR). These approaches and the general

pitfalls in relation to prenatal diagnosis are discussed elsewhere in this volume.

The current status of prenatal diagnosis is indicated under each subheading using +, (+), (−) or −. The symbol + indicates that successful prenatal diagnosis has been widely reported with a high degree of reliability in the second trimester or earlier. The symbol (+) indicates that prenatal diagnosis has been reported but with a limitation: (+)E = limited world experience (under 5–10 cases); (+)R = known reduced sensitivity or specificity or suspected limited reliability (see cited references); (+)P = only applicable in a proportion of cases; and (+)L = diagnosis may not be possible until the third trimester. The symbol (−) indicates that the appropriate technology exists but that prenatal diagnosis has not yet been reported and the symbol − indicates that prenatal diagnosis using that particular approach is impossible.

For each entry up to four references are cited. These aim to be recent, easily accessible and to give good cover of the relevant previously published work. Currently there are over 500 publications per annum in the field of prenatal diagnosis and hence the selection of a limited number of key references is bound to generate some controversy. I look to the generosity of the user to accept this limitation and also to help identify misconceptions and omissions.

Acknowledgements

I wish to thank Dr Guy Besley, Mr Gordon Graham, Miss Marion Hoggan, Dr Margaret McNay and Professor Martin Whittle for their invaluable assistance in compiling and updating the Glasgow database of prenatally diagnosable conditions.

Diseases of the Fetus and Newborn, 2nd edn, Edited by G.B. Reed, A.E. Claireaux and F. Cockburn. Published in 1995 by Chapman & Hall, London. ISBN 0 412 39160 0

Table 77.1 Compendium of prenatally diagnosable diseases

Disease	MIM	Imaging	Biochemistry	DNA	Other	References
Abruption, placental	–	US (+)R	–	–	–	Gottesfeld (1978)
Absent cerebellum	–	US +	–	–	–	Campbell and Pearce (1983) (see also Joubert syndrome)
Absent pulmonary valve	121000	US (+)E	–	–	–	Kleinman et al. (1982)
Acardius	–	US +	–	–	–	Wexler et al. (1985), Zanke (1986)
Acatalasia (Takahara disease)	115500	–	AFC (–), AFS –	ILP (–), MP (–)	–	Quan et al. (1986)
Acetylgalactosaminidase deficiency (Schindler disease)	104170	–	AFC (–), CVS (–)	–	–	Schindler et al. (1989)
Achondrogenesis type IA (Parenti–Fraccaro syndrome)	200600	US (+)E	–	–	–	Benaceraf et al. (1984), Mahoney et al. (1984a), Glenn and Teng (1985)
Achondrogenesis type IB (Langer–Saldino syndrome)	200610	US (+)E	–	–	–	Wenstrom et al. (1989)
Achondroplasia	100800	US (+)L	–	–	–	Kurtz et al. (1986)
Acid phosphatase deficiency	200950	–	AFC +, AFS –	–	–	Nadler and Egan (1970)
Acrorenal syndrome	102520	US (+)E	–	–	–	Meizner et al. (1986a)
Acute intermittent porphyria	176000	–	–	–	–	See Porphyria, acute intermittent
Acyl-CoA oxidase deficiency (pseudoneonatal adrenoleucodystrophy)	264470	–	AFC (+)E, CVS (+)E	–	–	Wanders et al. (1990)
Adenine phosphoribosyl transferase deficiency	102600	–	AFC (–), AFS –	MP (–)	FBS (–)	Linch et al. (1984), Berkvens et al. (1987), Dooley et al. (1987)
Adenosine deaminase deficiency	102700	–	AFC (+)E, AFC (+)E, CVS (+)E	ILP (–), MP (–)	FBS (+)E	–
Adrenal haemorrhage	–	US (+)E	–	–	–	Gotoh et al. (1989), Marino et al. (1990)
Adrenogenital syndrome (11-beta-hydroxylase deficiency)	202010	–	AFC –, AFS +, CVS –	–	–	Rosler et al. (1979), Schumert et al. (1980), Keller et al. (1991)
Adrenogenital syndrome (congenital adrenal hyperplasia, 21-hydroxylase deficiency)	201910	–	AFC –, AFC (+)R, CVS –	ILP +, ELP +, MP (+)P	FBS (+)E	Hughes et al. (1987), Speiser et al. (1990)
Adrenoleucodystrophy (Schilder disease)	300100	–	AFC +, AFS –, CVS +	ELP(+)	–	Boue et al. (1985)
Adrenoleucodystrophy, autosomal neonatal form	202370	–	AFC +, AFS –, AFC +, CVS (+)E	–	–	Schutgens et al. (1989)
Adrenoleucodystrophy, pseudoneonatal form	–	–	–	–	–	Schutgens et al. (1989); See Acyl-CoA oxidase deficiency
Adult polycystic kidney disease	173900	US (+)E	–	ELP (+)P	–	Ceccherini et al. (1989), Journel et al. (1989), Novelli et al. (1989)
Agammaglobulinaemia, X-linked	300300	–	–	ELP (+)P	FBS +	Durandy et al. (1982b), Lau et al. (1988)
Agenesis of corpus callosum	217990	–	–	–	–	See Corpus callosum, agenesis

Disorder	OMIM	US	AFC/AFS	CVS	ILP/ELP	MP	FBS	FSKB	References
Agnathia–holoprosencephaly syndrome	202650	US (+)E	—	—	—	—	—	—	Persutte et al. (1990), Rolland et al. (1991)
Agnathia–microstomia–synotia syndrome	—	US (+)E	—	—	—	—	—	—	Cayea et al. (1985)
Albinism, oculocutaneous (tyrosinase negative)	203100	—	AFC — AFS —	CVS —	—	MP (—)	—	FSKB (+)E	Haynes and Robertson (1981), Eady et al. (1983), Spritz et al. (1990)
Allantoic cyst	—	US (+)E	—	—	—	—	—	—	Fink and Filly (1983)
Alpha-1-antitrypsin deficiency	107400	—	—	—	ILP +	MP (+)P	FBS +	—	Corney et al. (1987), Hejtmancik et al. (1989)
Alport syndrome	301050	—	—	—	ELP (—)	MP (—)	—	—	Barker et al. (1990)
Ambiguous genitalia	—	US (+)E	—	—	—	—	—	—	Cooper et al. (1985)
Amelia	104400	US +	—	—	—	—	—	—	Campbell and Pearce (1983)
Amniotic bands	104400	US +	—	—	—	—	—	—	Herbert et al. (1985), Mahony et al. (1985a), Hill et al. (1988)
Amyloidosis I (Portuguese type of familial amyloid neuropathy)	176300	—	AFS (+)R	—	—	MP +	—	—	Nichols et al. (1989), Morris et al. (1991), Almeida et al. (1990)
Amyloidosis II (Indiana/Swiss type, familial amyloidotic polyneuropathy type II)	176300	—	—	—	—	MP (+)E	—	—	Nichols et al. (1989), Nichols and Benson (1990)
Anal atresia (imperforate anus)	207500	US (+)R	—	—	—	—	—	—	Shalev (1983)
Anderson disease	232500	—	—	—	—	—	—	—	See Glycogen storage disease IV
Androgen insensitivity syndrome (testicular feminization)	313700	US (+)E	—	—	ILP (—) ELP (—)	MP (—)	—	—	Stephens (1984), Wieacker et al. (1987), Brown et al. (1988)
Anencephaly	182940	US +	—	—	—	—	—	—	Goldstein et al. (1989)
Aneurysm, left ventricular	—	US (+)E	—	—	—	—	—	—	Gembruch et al. (1990c)
Aneurysm, vein of Galen	—	US (+)E	—	—	—	—	—	—	Jeanty et al. (1990a), Ordorica et al. (1990)
Angiokeratoma corporis diffusum (Fabry disease)	301500	—	AFC + AFC —	CVS +	ILP (—) ELP (—)	MP (—)	—	—	Kleijer (1987), Macdermot et al. (1987)
Angioneurotic oedema	106100	—	—	—	ELP (+)E	—	—	—	See Hereditary angioedema
Anhidrotic (hypohidrotic) ectodermal dysplasia (Christ–Siemens–Touraine syndrome)	305100	—	—	—	—	—	—	FSKB (+)E	Arnold et al. (1984), Zonana et al. (1990)
Annular pancreas	—	US (+)E	—	—	—	—	—	—	Boomsa et al. (1982)
Anophthalmia	206900	US (+)E	—	—	—	—	—	—	Pilu et al. (1986a)
Antithrombin III deficiency	107300	—	—	—	ILP (—) ELP (—)	MP (—)	—	—	Bock and Prochownik (1987)
Antley–Bixler syndrome	207410	US (+)E	—	—	—	—	—	—	Savoldelli and Schinzel (1983), Schinzel et al. (1983)
Aortic atresia	121000	US (+)E	—	—	—	—	—	—	Silverman et al. (1984), Allan et al. (1985), Gembruch et al. (1990b)
Aortic stenosis	121000	US (+)E	—	—	—	—	—	—	Allan et al. (1985)
Apert syndrome (acrocephalosyndactyly type I)	101200	US (+)E Other (+)E	—	—	—	—	—	—	Hill et al. (1987), Narayan and Scott (1991)

Table 77.1 *continued*

Disease	MIM	Imaging	Biochemistry	DNA	Other	References
Aplasia cutis congenita	107600	-	Other (+)E	-	-	Bick et al. (1987)
Arachnoid cyst	-	US (+)E	-	-	-	Chervenak et al. (1983)
Argininaemia	207800	-	AFC -, AFS -, CVS -	MP (-)	FBS (-)	Spector et al. (1980)
Argininosuccinicaciduria	207900	-	AFC +, AFS +, CVS +	-	-	Fleisher et al. (1979), Vimal et al. (1984), Chadefaux et al. (1990)
Arnold–Chiari malformation	207950	US +	-	-	-	Johnson et al. (1980)
Arterial calcification, idiopathic infantile	208000	US (+)E	-	-	-	Juul et al. (1990), Spear et al. (1990)
Arteriovenous fistula (brain)	-	US (+)E	-	-	-	Mao and Adams (1983)
Arteriovenous fistula (lung)	-	US (+)E	-	-	-	Kalugdan et al. (1989)
Arteriovenous malformation of the vein of Galen	-	US (+)E	-	-	-	Reiter et al. (1986)
Arthrogryposis	108110	US (+)E	-	-	-	Baty et al. (1988), Gorczyca et al. (1989)
Aspartylglucosaminuria	208400	-	AFC +, AFS +, CVS +	ILP (-), MP (-)	-	Aula et al. (1989)
Asphyxiating thoracic dysplasia (Jeune syndrome)	208500	US (+)E	-	-	-	Elejalde et al. (1985), Schinzel (1985)
Asplenia syndrome	208530	-	-	-	-	See Ivemark syndrome
Asymmetric septal hypertrophy (hypertrophic obstructive cardiomyopathy)	192600	US (+)E	-	ELP (-)	-	Allan et al. (1985), Stewart et al. (1986)
Ataxia telangiectasia	208900	-	-	ELP (-)	CHR +	Schwartz et al. (1985), Gatti et al. (1988), Jaspers et al. (1990)
Atelencephalic microcephaly	-	US (+)E	-	-	-	Siebert et al. (1986)
Atelosteogenesis	108720	US (+)E	-	-	-	Chervenak et al. (1986)
Atrial bigeminal rhythm	-	US (+)E	-	-	-	Steinfeld et al. (1986)
Atrial flutter	-	US (+)E	-	-	-	Kleinman et al. (1983)
Atrial haemangioma	-	US (+)E	-	-	-	Leitheser et al. (1986)
Atrial septal defect	108800	US (+)E	-	-	-	Allan et al. (1985)
Atrioventricular canal defect	-	US (+)E	-	-	-	Kleinman et al. (1983), Gembruch et al. (1990a)
Bare lymphocyte syndrome	209920	-	-	-	FBS (+)E	Durandy et al. (1982b, 1987), Schuurman et al. (1985)
Bartter syndrome	241200	US (+)E	-	-	-	Sieck and Ohlsson (1984)
Becker muscular dystrophy	310200	-	-	ILP +, ELP +, MP (+)P	-	Wood et al. (1987) (see also Duchenne muscular dystrophy)
Beckwith–Wiedemann syndrome (EMG syndrome)	130650	US (+)E	-	-	-	Cobellis (1988), Shah and Metlay (1990)
Bernard–Soulier syndrome (giant platelet syndrome)	231200	-	-	-	FBS (+)E	Gruel et al. (1986)
Beta mannosidosis	248510	-	AFC +, AFS -, CVS +	ILP +, MP (+)P	-	see Mannosidosis, beta
Beta-glucosidase deficiency (Gaucher disease, types I, II and III)	230800, 230900	-	-	-	-	Besley et al. (1988)

Disorder	No.						References
Beta-methylcrotonyl glycinuria I (3-methylcrotonyl-CoA-carboxylase deficiency)	210200	–	AFC (–) AFS (–)	CVS (–)	–	–	Benson and Fensom (1985)
Blackfan–Diamond syndrome	205900	US (+)E	–	–	–	–	Visser et al. (1988)
Bladder exstrophy	–	US (+)E	–	–	–	–	Barth et al. (1990), Jaffe et al. (1990)
Blagowidow syndrome	–	US (+)E	–	–	–	–	Blagowidow et al. (1986)
Blighted ovum	–	US +	–	–	–	–	Kurjak and Latin (1979)
Blood grouping	110300	–	–	–	FBS +	–	Teichler-Zallen and Doherty (1983)
Bloom syndrome	111700	–	–	–	–	CHR +	Rudiger et al. (1980)
Body stalk anomaly	201900	US +	–	–	–	–	Abu-Yousef et al. (1987), Jauniaux et al. (1990)
Bar syndrome (branchio-oto-renal dysplasia)	113650	US (+)E	–	–	–	–	Greenberg et al. (1988)
Bradycardia, sinus	–	US +	–	–	–	–	Kleinman et al. (1983)
Bronchial atresia	–	US (+)E	–	–	–	–	McAlister et al. (1987)
Bronchogenic cyst	–	US (+)E	–	–	–	–	Young et al. (1989) (see also Pulmonary cyst)
Bullous erythroderma ichthyosiformis congenita of Brocq (bullous ichthyosiform erythroderma, epidermolytic hyperkeratosis)	113800	–	–	–	–	FSKB +	Golbus et al. (1980), Anton-Lamprecht (1981), Eady et al. (1986)
Calcification, ectopic	–	US (+)E	–	–	–	–	Corson et al. (1983)
Calcification, intracranial	–	–	–	–	–	–	See Intracranial calcification
Campomelic dysplasia	211970	US (+)E	–	–	–	–	Cordone et al. (1989)
Canavan's disease (aspartoacylase deficiency)	271900	–	AFC + AFS +	CVS +	–	–	Matalon et al. (1992)
Carbamoyl-phosphate synthetase deficiency	237300	–	–	–	–	–	See Hyperammonaemia II
Cardiac rhabdomyoma	–	US (+)E	–	–	–	–	Schaffer et al. (1986), Stanford et al. (1987) (see also Tuberous sclerosis)
Cardiomyopathy	–	US (+)E	–	–	–	–	Schmidt et al. (1989)
Caudal regression syndrome	–	US (+)E	–	–	–	–	Loewy et al. (1987), Baxi et al. (1990)
Cerebrocostomandibular dysplasia	117650	US (+)E	–	–	–	–	Merlob et al. (1987)
Cerebrohepatorenal syndrome (Zellweger syndrome)	214100	–	AFC + AFS (+)E	CVS +	–	–	Stellaard et al. (1988), Schutgens et al. (1989)
Cerebrotendinous xanthomatosis	213700	–	AFC (–)	–	–	–	Skrede et al. (1986)
Charcot–Marie–Tooth disease	118200	–	–	–	–	–	See Hereditary motor and sensory neuropathy type I
Chediak–Higashi syndrome	214500	–	–	–	FBS (+)E	–	–
Choledochal cyst	–	US (+)E	–	–	–	–	Elrad et al. (1985), Schroeder et al. (1989)
Cholesterol ester storage disease (Wolman disease)	278000	–	AFC +	CVS +	–	–	Gatti et al. (1985), Iavarone et al. (1989)
Chondrodysplasia punctata (Conradi Hunermann type)	118650	US (+)E	–	–	–	–	Tuck et al. (1990)

Table 77.1 *continued*

Disease	MIM	Imaging	Biochemistry	DNA	Other	References
Chondrodysplasia punctata (rhizomelic type)	215100	US (+)E	AFC + / CVS +	–	–	Connor et al. (1985), Holmes et al. (1987), Schutgens et al. (1989), Duff et al. (1990)
Chondroectodermal dysplasia (Ellis–van Creveld syndrome)	225500	US (+)E / Other (+)E	–	–	–	Mahoney and Hobbins (1977) Bui et al. (1984)
Chordae tendinae, thickening	–	US (+)E	–	–	–	Schecter (1987)
Chorioangioma of placenta	–	–	–	–	–	see Placental tumour
Choroid plexus cyst	–	US +	–	–	–	Gabrielli et al. (1989), Khouzam and Hooker (1989)
Choroid plexus haemorrhage	–	US (+)E	–	–	–	Chambers et al. (1988)
Choroideraemia	303100	–	–	ILP (–) / ELP (+)E / MP (–)	–	Cremers et al. (1987, 1990)
Chromosomal aneuploidy	–	–	–	–	CHR +	Hsu (1986)
Chromosomal deletion/duplication	–	–	–	–	CHR +	Hsu (1986)
Chronic granulomatous disease	306400	–	CVS (–)	ELP (+)E / MP (–)	FBS (+)E	Levinsky et al. (1986), Huu et al. (1987), Lindlof et al. (1987), Nakamura et al. (1990)
Chylothorax	–	US (+)E	–	–	–	Petres et al. (1982), Schmidt et al. (1985), Meizner et al. (1986b)
Citrullinaemia	215700	–	AFC + / AFS + / CVS +	ILP (+)E	–	Northrup et al. (1990)
Cleft lip/palate	119530	US (+)E	–	–	–	Chervenak et al. (1984b), Saltzman et al. (1986)
Cleidocranial dysostosis	119600	US (+)E	–	–	–	Campbell and Pearce (1983)
Cloacal dysgenesis	–	US (+)E	Other +	–	–	Petrikovsky et al. (1988)
Cloverleaf skull (Kleeblattschädel anomaly)	148800	US (+)E	–	–	–	Salvo (1981), Stamm et al. (1987) (see also Thanatophoric dysplasia with cloverleaf skull)
Coarctation of the aorta	120000	US (+)E	–	–	–	Benacerraf et al. (1989a)
Cobalamin E disease	251100	–	–	–	–	See Methylmalonic acidaemia
Cockayne syndrome type I	261400	–	–	–	CHR +	Sugita et al. (1982), Lehmann et al. (1985)
Coffin–Lowry syndrome	303600	–	–	ELP (–)	–	Hanauer et al. (1988)
Congenital adrenal hyperplasia	201910	–	–	–	–	See Adrenogenital syndrome
Congenital adrenal hypoplasia (autosomal recessive variant)	240200	–	Other +	–	–	Hensleigh et al. (1978)
Congenital adrenal hypoplasia (X-linked variant)	300200	–	Other +	ELP (–)	–	Hensleigh et al. (1978), Yates et al. (1987)
Congenital amegakaryocytic thrombocytopenia	–	–	–	–	FBS +	Mibashan and Rodeck (1984)
Congenital bowing, isolated	–	US (+)E	–	–	–	Kapur and Van Vloten (1986)
Congenital chloridorrhoea (congenital chloride diarrhoea)	214700	US (+)E	–	–	–	Patel et al. (1989)
Congenital coxa vara	122750	US (+)E	–	–	–	Russell (1973)

Disorder	No.	US	AF	CVS	LP	MP	FBS	Other	Reference
Congenital dislocation of the knee	–	–	–	–	–	–	–	Other (+)E	McFarland (1929)
Congenital dyserythropoietic anaemia type II	224100	–	–	–	–	–	FBS (+)E	–	Fukuda et al. (1987)
Congenital heart block	140400	US (+)E	–	–	–	–	–	–	Moodley et al. (1986)
Congenital ichthyosiform erythroderma	242100	–	–	–	–	–	–	FSKB +	Holbrook et al. (1988)
Congenital ichthyosiform erythroderma, bullous type (epidermolytic hyperkeratosis)	113800	–	–	–	–	–	–	–	See Bullous erythroderma ichthyosiformis congenita of Brocq
Congenital muscular dystrophy with arthrogryposis	158810	US (+)E	–	–	–	–	–	–	Socol et al. (1985)
Congenital short femur (proximal focal femoral deficiency)	–	US (+)E	–	–	–	–	–	–	Graham (1985), Jeanty and Kleinman (1989)
Conjoined twins		US +	–	–	–	–	–	–	Apuzzio et al. (1988), Lituania et al. (1988), Filly et al. (1990)
Conradi disease	215100	–	–	–	–	–	–	–	see Chondrodysplasia punctata
Convulsions, benign familial neonatal	121200	–	–	–	ELP (–)	–	–	–	Leppert et al. (1989)
Copper deficiency (Menkes disease)	309400	–	AFC +, AFS –	CVS +	–	–	–	–	Tonnensen and Horn (1989)
Coproporphyria	121300	–	AFC (–), AFS –	–	–	–	–	–	Elder et al. (1976)
Cori disease	232400	–	–	–	–	–	–	–	see Glycogen storage disease III
Cornelia de Lange syndrome	122470	Other (+)E	–	Other (+)E	–	–	–	–	Westgergaard et al. (1983)
Coronal cleft vertebra	–	–	–	–	–	–	–	–	Rowley (1955)
Corpus callosum, agenesis	217900	US (+)E	–	–	–	–	–	–	Meizner et al. (1987), Mulligan and Meier (1989), Hilpert and Kurtz (1990)
Corpus callosum, lipoma	–	US (+)E	–	–	–	–	–	–	Mulligan and Meier (1989)
Craniopharyngioma	–	US (+)E	–	–	–	–	–	–	Snyder et al. (1986), Bailey et al. (1990)
Craniosynostosis, sagittal suture	123100	US (+)E	–	–	–	–	–	–	Campbell and Pearce (1983)
Cranium bifidum	–	US (+)E	–	–	–	–	–	–	Barr et al. (1986)
Crossed renal ectopia	–	US (+)E	–	–	–	–	–	–	Greenblatt et al. (1985)
Crouzon craniofacial dysostosis	123500	US (+)E	–	–	–	–	–	–	Menashe et al. (1989)
Cryptophthalmia syndrome	219000	US (+)E	–	–	–	–	–	–	Feldman et al. (1985)
Cyctochrome b5 reductase deficiency	250800	–	–	–	–	–	–	–	See Methaemoglobinaemia
Cystic adenomatoid malformation	–	US (+)E	–	–	–	–	–	–	Fitzgerald and Toi (1986), Rempen et al. (1987)
Cystic fibrosis (mucoviscidosis)	219700	–	AFS (+)R	–	ILP +, ELP +	MP (+)P	–	–	Brock et al. (1988), Feldman et al. (1989), Lemna et al. (1990)
Cystic hygroma	257350	US +	–	–	–	–	–	–	Macken et al. (1989)
Cystinosis	219800	–	AFC +, AFS –	CVS +	–	–	–	–	Schneider et al. (1974), Steinherz (1985), Patrick et al. (1987)
Cystinuria	220100	–	AFS (+)E	–	–	–	–	–	Komrower (1974)
Cytochrome c oxidase deficiency	220110	–	AFC (+)E	CVS (+)E	–	–	–	–	Ruitenbeek et al. (1988)
Dandy–Walker syndrome	220200	US (+)E	–	–	–	–	–	–	Russ et al. (1989)
De la Chapelle dysplasia (neonatal osseous dysplasia I)	256050	US (+)E	–	–	–	–	–	–	Whitley et al. (1986)

Table 77.1 *continued*

Disease	MIM	Imaging	Biochemistry	DNA	Other	References
Diaphragmatic hernia/eventration	222400	US (+)E	–	–	–	Comstock (1986), Benaceraff and Adzick (1987), Thiagarajah et al. (1990)
Diastematomyelia	222500	US (+)E	–	–	–	Winter et al. (1989), Caspi et al. (1990)
Diastrophic dysplasia	222600	US (+)E	–	ELP (–)	–	Gembruch (1988), Hastbacka et al. (1990)
DiGeorge syndrome	188400	–	–	MP (+)E	CHR (+)E	Driscoll et al. (1991)
Dihydropteridine reductase deficiency	261630	–	–	–	–	See Phenylketonuria type II
Dihydropyrimidine dehydrogenase deficiency	274270	–	AFS (+)E	–	–	Jakobs et al. (1991)
Diverticulum, left ventricular	–	US (+)E	–	–	–	Kitchiner et al. (1990)
Double outlet right ventricle	121000	US (+)E	–	–	–	Stewart et al. (1985)
Duchenne muscular dystrophy	310200	–	Other (+)E	ILP +, ELP +, MP (+)P	–	Bakker et al. (1989), Ward et al. (1989), Evans et al. (1991) (see also Becker muscular dystrophy)
Duodenal atresia	223400	US +	–	–	–	Miro and Bard (1988)
Dyskeratosis congenita	305000	–	–	ILP (–)	–	Connor et al. (1986)
Dyssegmental dwarfism	224400	US (+)E	–	–	–	Andersen et al. (1988), Izquierdo et al. (1990)
Ebstein's anomaly	224700	US (+)E	–	–	–	Allan et al. (1982), Roberson and Silverman (1989)
Ectodermal dysplasia	305100	–	–	–	–	See Anhidrotic (hypohidrotic) ectodermal dysplasia
Ectopia cordis	–	US (+)E, US +, Other +	–	–	–	Klingensmith et al. (1988)
Ectopic beat	–	–	–	–	–	Steinfeld et al. (1986)
Ectopic fetal liver	–	US (+)E	–	–	–	Mack et al. (1978)
Ectopic pregnancy	–	US (+)R	–	–	–	Smith et al. (1981)
Ectrodactyly	183600, 225300	US (+)E	–	–	–	Henrion et al. (1980)
Ectrodactyly, ectodermal dysplasia, cleft palate (EEC) syndrome	129900	US (+)E	–	–	–	Kohler et al. (1989), Anneren et al. (1991)
Ehlers–Danlos syndrome type IV	225350	–	AFC (–)	MP (–)	–	Pope et al. (1989)
Ehlers–Danlos syndrome type V	130050	–	AFC (–), AFS –	–	–	Di Ferrante et al. (1975)
Ehlers–Danlos syndrome Type VI	305200	–	CVS –	–	–	Dembure et al. (1984)
Ehlers–Danlos syndrome Type VII	225400	–	AFC (+)E	–	–	Dherny et al. (1987)
Elliptocytosis type I (rhesus-linked type, protein 4.1 of erythrocyte membrane defect)	130500	–	–	MP (–)	FBS (+)E	Dherny et al. (1987)
Elliptocytosis type II (rhesus-unlinked type)	130600	–	–	–	FBS (+)E	Dherny et al. (1987)
Ellis–van Creveld syndrome	225500	–	–	–	–	See Chondroectodermal dysplasia

Disease	OMIM	US	AFC/AFS	ELP/ILP	MP	FBS	FSKB/other	References
Emery–Dreifuss muscular dystrophy	310300	US +	–	ELP (–)	–	–	–	Yates *et al.* (1986)
Encephalocoele	182940	–	–	–	–	–	–	Chatterjee *et al.* (1985), Cullen *et al.* (1990)
Endocardial fibroelastosis	226000 305300	US (+)E	–	–	–	–	–	Ben Ami *et al.* (1986), Achiron *et al.* (1988)
Epidermolysis bullosa dystrophica (Hallopeau–Siemens type)	226600	–	–	–	–	–	FSKB +	Anton-Lamprecht *et al.* (1981), Heagerty *et al.* (1986), Bakharev *et al.* (1990)
Epidermolysis bullosa dystrophica	131700	–	–	–	–	–	FSKB +	Fine *et al.* (1988)
Epidermolysis bullosa dystrophica inversa	226450	–	–	–	–	–	FSKB +	Anton-Lamprecht (1981)
Epidermolysis bullosa lethalis (junctional Herlitz–Pearson type)	226700	–	–	–	–	–	FSKB +	Heagerty *et al.* (1986), Eady *et al.* (1989), Bakharev *et al.* (1990), Fine *et al.* (1990)
Epidermolysis bullosa with pyloric atresia	226730	–	–	–	–	–	FSKB (+)E	Nazzaro *et al.* (1990)
Exencephaly	–	US (+)E	–	–	–	–	–	Hendricks *et al.* (1988), Kennedy *et al.* (1990)
Exomphalos	164750	US +	–	–	–	–	–	Brown *et al.* (1989), Gray *et al.* (1989), Pagliano *et al.* (1990)
Extralobar pulmonary sequestration	–	US (+)E	–	–	–	–	–	Mariona *et al.* (1986), Thomas (1986)
Fabry disease	301500	–	–	–	–	–	–	See Angiokeratoma corporis diffusum
Facioscapulohumeral muscular dystrophy	158900	–	–	ELP (–)	–	–	–	Wijmenga *et al.* (1990)
Familial hypercholesterolaemia	143890	–	AFC +	ILP (+)E	MP (–)	FBS +	–	Martini *et al.* (1986), Taylor *et al.* (1988)
Familial polyposis coli	175100	–	–	–	–	–	–	See Intestinal polyposis type I
Fanconi's pancytopenia type I	227650	–	–	–	–	–	CHR +	Dallapiccola *et al.* (1985), Auerbach *et al.* (1986)
Farber disease	228000	–	–	–	–	–	–	See Lipogranulomatosis
Femoral hypoplasia – unusual facies syndrome	134780	US (+)E	–	–	–	–	–	Gamble *et al.* (1990)
Femur, congenital short (proximal focal femoral deficiency)	–	–	–	–	–	–	–	See Congenital short femur
Femur–fibula–ulna (FFU) syndrome	228200	US (+)E	–	–	–	–	–	Hirose (1988)
Fetal cytomegalovirus infection	–	US (+)R	AFS +	–	–	FBS +	–	Hohlfeld *et al.* (1991), Lynch *et al.* (1991), Lamy *et al.* (1992)
Fetal HIV infection	–	–	–	–	–	FBS +	–	Daffos *et al.* (1989)
Fetal hydantoin syndrome	–	–	AFC (–)	–	–	–	–	Buehler *et al.* (1990)
Fetal listeriosis	–	–	AFS (+)E	–	–	FBS +	–	Boucher and Yonekura (1986), Liner (1990)
Fetal parvovirus infection	–	–	–	–	–	FBS +	–	Naides and Weiner (1989), Peters and Nicolaides (1990)
Fetal rubella infection	–	–	–	–	–	FBS +	–	Morgan-Capner *et al.* (1985), Terry *et al.* (1986)
Fetal toxoplasmosis infection	–	US (+)R	–	–	–	FBS +	–	Blaakaer (1986), Daffos *et al.* (1988), Foulon *et al.* (1990)

Table 77.1 *continued*

Disease	MIM	Imaging	Biochemistry	DNA		Other	References
Fetal varicella infection	-	US (+)R	-	-	-	FBS +	Cutherbertson et al. (1987), Byrne et al. (1990)
Fetofetal transfusion syndrome	-	US (+)E	-	-	-	-	Brennan et al. (1982), Pretorius et al. (1988), Filly et al. (1990) (see also Twin embolization syndrome)
Fetus *in fetu*	-	US (+)E	-	-	-	-	Sada et al. (1986)
Fetus papyraceous	-	US (+)E	-	-	-	-	Kurjak and Latin (1979)
Foramen ovale, premature closure	-	US (+)E	-	-	-	-	Buis-Liem et al. (1987), Fraser et al. (1989)
Forbe disease	232400	-	-	-	-	-	See Glycogen storage disease III
Fragile X syndrome	309550	-	-	ILP (+) ELP (+)	MP (+)	CHR +	Shapiro et al. (1988), Webb et al. (1989), Richards et al. (1991), Verkerk et al. (1991)
Fraser syndrome (cryptophthalmos with other malformations)	219000	US (+)E	-	-	-	-	Ramsing et al. (1990), Schauer et al. (1990)
Friedreich's ataxia	229300	-	-	ELP (+)E	-	-	Wallis et al. (1989)
Fryns syndrome	229850	US (+)E	-	-	-	-	Samueloff et al. (1987)
Fucosidosis	230000	-	AFC + AFS - CVS (-)	MP (-)	-	-	Gatti et al. (1985), Lissens et al. (1987)
Fumarase deficiency (fumarate hydratase deficiency)	136850	-	AFC (-)	MP (-)	-	-	Petrova-Benedict et al. (1987)
Galactokinase deficiency	230200	-	AFC (-) AFS (-)	-	FBS (-)	-	Holton et al. (1989)
Galactosaemia	230400	-	AFC + AFS + CVS +	-	-	-	Holton et al. (1989)
Galactose epimerase deficiency	230350	-	AFC (-)	-	-	-	Gillet et al. (1983)
Galactosialidosis (neuraminidase deficiency with β-galactosidase deficiency)	256540	-	AFC (+)E CVS (-)	-	FBS (-)	-	Sewell and Pontz (1988)
Gallstones (fetal)	-	US (+)E	-	-	-	-	Heijne et al. (1985), Abbitt and McIlhenny (1990)
Gangliosidosis, generalized G$_{M1}$, types I and II	230500	-	AFC + AFS + CVS +	-	-	-	Lowden et al. (1973), Warner et al. (1983)
Gangliosidosis, G$_{M2}$ type I (Tay–Sachs disease)	272800	-	AFC +AFS (+)E CVS +	ILP (-)	MP (+)P	-	Grebner and Jackson (1979, 1985), Triggs-Raine et al. (1990)
Gangliosidosis, G$_{M2}$ type II (Sandhoff disease)	268800	-	AFC + AFS (+)E CVS +	ILP (-)	MP (-)	-	Giles et al. (1988)
Gangliosidosis, G$_{M2}$ type III (juvenile-onset variant)	230700	-	AFC (-)	-	-	-	Zerfowski and Sandhoff (1974)
Gangliosidosis, G$_{M2}$ (adult-onset variant)	272800	-	AFC +	-	-	-	Navon et al. (1986)

Disorder	No.	US	AFC/AFS	CVS/Other	ILP/ELP	MP	FBS/FLB	Reference
Gardner syndrome	175300	–	–	–	–	–	–	see Intestinal polyposis type III
Gastric obstruction	–	US (+)E	–	–	–	–	–	Zimmerman (1978)
Gastroenteric cyst	–	US (+)E	–	–	–	–	–	Newnham et al. (1984)
Gastroschisis	230750	US +	–	–	–	–	–	Bair et al. (1986), Lindfors et al. (1986), Guzman (1990), Kushnir et al. (1990)
Gaucher disease	230800	–	–	–	–	–	–	See Beta-glucosidase deficiency
Gerstmann–Straussler disease	137440	–	–	–	–	MP (–)P	–	Collinge et al. (1989)
Glanzmann thrombasthenia	187800	–	–	–	–	–	FBS +	Kaplan et al. (1985), Seligsohn et al. (1985)
	273800	–	–	–	–	–	–	Geraghty et al. (1989)
Glioblastoma	137800	US (+)E	–	–	–	–	–	Dallapiccola et al. (1986)
Glucose phosphate isomerase deficiency (phosphohexose isomerase deficiency)	172400	–	AFC +, AFS –	CVS +	–	–	FBS (–)	Martini et al. (1986), de Vita et al. (1989)
Glucose-6-phosphate dehydrogenase deficiency	305900	–	–	–	ILP (–), ELP (–)	MP (–)P	FBS (–)	Poenaru (1987), Holme et al. (1989)
Glutaricaciduria type I (glutaryl-CoA dehydrogenase deficiency)	231670	–	AFS –, AFC +, AFS +	CVS (–)	–	–	–	Mitchell et al. (1983)
Glutaricaciduria type IIA (neonatal form of type II)	305950	–	AFC (+)E, AFS (+)E, AFS (+)E	–	–	–	–	Jakobs et al. (1984), Sakuma et al. (1991)
Glutaricaciduria type IIB (electron transfer flavoprotein dehydrogenase deficiency)	231680	–	–	Other (+)E	–	–	–	Golbus et al. (1988)
Glycogen storage disease IA (von Gierke disease)	232200	–	AFC –, AFS –	CVS –	–	–	FLB (+)E	Shin et al. (1989)
Glycogen storage disease II (Pompe disease)	232300	–	AFC +	CVS +	–	–	–	Maire et al. (1989), Shin et al. (1989), Yang et al. (1990)
Glycogen storage disease III (Forbe or Cori disease)	232400	–	AFC +	CVS (+)E	–	–	–	Brown and Brown (1989)
Glycogen storage disease IV (Anderson disease)	232500	–	AFC +	CVS +	–	–	–	Newgard et al. (1987)
Glycogen storage disease VI (Hers disease)	232700	–	–	–	ILP (–)	MP (–)	–	Vora et al. (1987)
Glycogen storage disease VII (muscle phosphofructokinase deficiency)	232800	–	–	–	–	MP (–)	–	Kourides et al. (1984)
Goitre	274600	US (+)E	–	–	–	–	–	See Hemifacial microsomia
Goldenhar syndrome	164210	–	–	–	–	–	–	See Thyrotoxicosis
Graves disease	–	–	–	–	–	–	–	Phillips et al. (1981)
Growth hormone deficiency (one type)	262400	–	–	–	ILP (–)	MP (–)	–	Bruinse et al. (1989), Deter et al. (1989)
Growth retardation	–	US (+)R	–	–	–	–	–	Dhondt et al. (1990)
GTP cyclohydrolase I deficiency	233910	–	AFS (+)E	–	ILP (–)	MP (–)	–	Mitchell et al. (1989)
Gyrate atrophy	258870	–	–	–	–	–	–	Sabbagha et al. (1980), Trecet et al. (1984), Grundy et al. (1985), McGahan and Schneider (1986), Pennel and Baltarowich (1986)
Haemangioma/teratoma	–	US (+)E	–	–	–	–	–	

Table 77.1 *continued*

Disease	MIM	Imaging	Biochemistry	DNA	Other	References
Haematoma, extracranial	–	US (+)E	–	–	–	Harper et al. (1989)
Haematoma, retroplacental	–	US (+)R	–	–	–	Spirt et al. (1987)
Haemoglobin O Arab	141900	–	–	ILP +	–	Weatherall et al. (1985)
Haemoglobin Lepore	141900	–	–	ILP + MP +	–	Weatherall et al. (1985)
Haemoglobin S (sickle-cell disease)	142300	–	–	ILP + ELP + MP +	FBS +	Kazazian et al. (1988)
Haemoglobin S-O Arab	141900	–	–	ILP +	–	Kazazian et al. (1978)
Haemoglobinopathies	142300	–	–	ILP + ELP + MP (+)P	FBS +	Alter (1984), Kazazian et al. (1985), Old et al. (1986)
Haemophilia A (factor VIII deficiency)	306700	–	–	ILP + ELP + MP (+)P	FBS +	Mibashan et al. (1979), Forestier et al. (1986), Brocker-Vriends et al. (1988)
Haemophilia B (factor IX deficiency)	306900	–	–	ILP + ELP + MP (+)P	FBS +	Mibashan et al. (1979), Zeng et al. (1987)
Hair–brain syndrome (Pibids syndrome)	234050	–	AFC (+)E	–	–	Savary et al. (1991)
Harlequin ichthyosis	242500	–	–	–	–	See Ichthyosis congenita, harlequin fetus type Benacerraf and Frigoletto (1988)
Hemifacial microsomia (Goldenhar syndrome)	164210 257700 257700	US (+)E –	–	–	–	Abrams and Filly (1985), Benacerraf et al. (1986a)
Hemivertebra	–	US (+)E	–	–	–	Marks et al. (1990)
Hepatic adenoma	–	US (+)E	–	–	–	Chung (1986)
Hepatic cyst	–	US (+)E	–	–	–	Foucar et al. (1983)
Hepatic hamartoma	–	US (+)E	–	–	–	Nakamoto et al. (1983)
Hepatic haemangioma	–	US (+)E	–	–	–	Nguyen and Leonard (1986)
Hepatic necrosis	–	US (+)E	–	–	–	
Hereditary angioedema (C1 esterase inhibitor deficiency)	106100	–	–	ILP (–) MP (–)	–	Cicardi et al. (1987)
Hereditary enlarged parietal foramina	168500	US (+)E	–	–	–	Rasore-Quartino et al. (1985)
Hereditary motor and sensory neuropathy type I (Charcot–Marie–Tooth disease)	118200	–	–	ELP (–)P MP (–)	–	Middleton-Price et al. (1990)
Hereditary motor and sensory neuropathy, X-linked	302800	–	–	ELP (–) MP (–)	–	Rozear et al. (1987)
Herrmann–Opitz syndrome	–	US (+)E	–	–	–	Anyane-Yeboa et al. (1987)
Hirschsprung disease	249200	US (+)E	–	–	–	Vermesh et al. (1986)
Holoprosencephaly	236100	US (+)E Other (+)E	–	–	–	McGahan et al. (1990), Toma et al. (1990), Wenstrom et al. (1991)
Holoprosencephaly with hypokinesia	306990	US (+)E	–	–	–	Morse et al. (1987b)
Holt–Oram syndrome	142900	US (+)E	–	–	–	Brons et al. (1988a)
Homocystinuria I	236200	–	AFC +	ILP (–) ELP (–) MP (–)	CVS + FBS (–)	Fowler et al. (1982), Fensom et al. (1983)

Disorder	MIM No.	US	AF	CVS	ELP/ILP	MP	FLB	References
Homocystinuria II (methyltetrahydrofolate reductase deficiency)	236250	–	AFC +	–	–	–	–	Wendel et al. (1983), Christensen and Brandt (1985)
Horseshoe kidney	–	US (+)E	–	–	–	–	–	Sherer et al. (1990)
Hunter syndrome	309900	–	–	–	–	–	–	See Mucopolysaccharidosis type II
Huntington's disease	143100	–	–	–	ELP +	MP+	–	Hayden et al. (1987), Quarrell et al. (1987)
Hurler syndrome	252800	–	–	–	–	–	–	See Mucopolysaccharidosis type IH, IS
Hydatidiform mole	236500	US +	–	–	–	–	–	Spirt et al. (1987)
Hydranencephaly	236500	US (+)E; Other (+)E	–	–	–	–	–	Hadi et al. (1986), Wenstrom et al. (1991)
Hydrocoele	–	US +; Other (+)E	–	–	–	–	–	Cacchio et al. (1983)
Hydrocephalus	236600	US (+)L; Other (+)E	–	–	–	–	–	Benacerraf and Birnholz (1987), Dreazen et al. (1989), Wenstrom et al. (1991)
Hydrocephalus and cystic renal disease	–	US (+)E	–	–	–	–	–	Reuss et al. (1989)
Hydrocephalus, X-linked	307000	US (+)L	–	–	ELP (–)	MP (–)	–	Van Egmond-Linden et al. (1983), Friedman and Santos-Ramos (1983)
Hydrolethalus syndrome	236680	US (+)E	–	–	–	–	–	Hartikainen-Sorri et al. (1983), Siffring et al. (1991)
Hydrometrocolpos	–	US (+)E	–	–	–	–	–	Hill and Hirsch (1985)
Hydrometrocolpos, postaxial polydactyly, congenital heart malformation syndrome (Kaufman–McKusick syndrome)	236700	US (+)E	–	–	–	–	–	Chitayat et al. (1987)
Hydronephrosis	143400	US +	–	–	–	–	–	Grignon et al. (1986a), Quinlan et al. (1986), Mahony et al. (1984b), Barss et al. (1985)
Hydrops fetalis	–	US +	–	–	–	–	–	Toma et al. (1991)
Hydrosyringomyelia	–	US (+)E	–	–	–	–	–	–
Hydrothorax	–	US (+)E	–	–	–	–	–	Bovicelli et al. (1981), Peleg et al. (1985)
Hydroureter	–	US (+)E	–	–	–	–	–	Grignon et al. (1986b)
Hydroxy-3-methylglutaryl-CoA lyase deficiency (3-hydroxy-3-methylglutaricaciduria)	246450	–	AFC (+)E; AFS (+)E	CVS (+)E; Other (+)L	ILP +; ELP +	MP (–)	FLB +	Duran et al. (1979), Chalmers et al. (1989)
Hyperammonaemia I (ornithine transcarbamylase deficiency)	311250	–	AFC –; AFS –	CVS –	ILP (–)	MP (–)	FLB +	Rodeck et al. (1982), Spence et al. (1989)
Hyperammonaemia II (carbamoyl-phosphate synthetase deficiency)	237300	–	AFC –; AFS –	CVS –	–	–	FLB +	Serini et al. (1988)
Hyperammonaemia III (N-acetylglutamate synthetase deficiency)	237310	–	AFC –; AFS –	CVS –	–	–	FLB +	Bachmann et al. (1981)
Hypercholesterolaemia, familial	143890	–	–	–	–	–	–	See Familial hypercholesterolaemia

Table 77.1 *continued*

Disease	MIM	Imaging	Biochemistry	DNA	Other	References
Hyperglycerolaemia	307030	–	AFC (+)E AFS (–)	MP (+)E	–	McCabe et al. (1982), Borresen et al. (1987)
Hyperglycinaemia, ketotic	232000	–	–	–	–	See Propionic acidaemia
Hyperglycinaemia (isolated), non-ketotic type I	238300	–	AFS (+)R CVS (+)E	–	–	Garcia-Munoz et al. (1989), Hawasaka et al. (1990), Parvy et al. (1990)
Hyperornithinaemia, hyperammonaemia and homocitrullinuria syndrome	238970	–	AFC (+)E AFS (+)E CVS (+)E	–	–	Chadefaux et al. (1989)
Hyperoxaluria type I	259900	–	–	–	FLB +	Danpure et al. (1987, 1989)
Hyperphenylalaninaemia	261600	–	–	–	–	See Phenylketonuria types I and II
Hypertelorism	145400	US (+)E	–	–	–	Pilu et al. (1986a) (see also Opitz G syndrome)
Hypertrophic obstructive cardiomyopathy	192600	–	–	–	–	See Asymmetric septal hypertrophy
Hypertrophic pyloric stenosis	179010	–	–	–	–	See Pyloric stenosis
Hypochondrogenesis	–	US (+)E	–	–	–	Donnenfeld et al. (1986)
Hypochondroplasia	146000	US (+)E	–	–	–	Stoll et al. (1985), Jones et al. (1990)
Hypophosphatasia (severe autosomal recessive variant)	241500	US (+)E	AFC (+)E CVS (+)E	ILP (+)E MP (–)	–	De Lange and Rouse (1990), Brock and Barron (1991), Kishi et al. (1991), Sahn et al. (1982), Allan et al. (1985), Yagel et al. (1986)
Hypoplastic left heart	241550	US +	–	–	–	
Hypoplastic right ventricle	121000	US (+)E	–	–	–	De Vore and Hobbins (1979)
Hypotelorism	–	US (+)E	–	–	–	Pilu et al. (1986a)
Hypothyroidism	274600	–	AFS +	–	–	Kourides et al. (1984), Hirsch et al. (1990), Perelman et al. (1990) (see also Goitre)
Hypoxanthine guanine phosphoribosyltransferase deficiency (Lesch–Nyhan syndrome)	308000	–	AFC + CVS +	ILP (+)E MP (+)P	FBS (–)	Gibbs et al. (1986), Zoref-Shani et al. (1989)
I-cell disease	252500	–	–	–	–	See Mucolipidosis type II
Ichthyosis congenita (congenital ichthyosiform erythroderma, lamellar exfoliation of the newborn, collodion fetus)	242300	–	–	–	FKSB +	Perry et al. (1987)
Ichthyosis congenita, harlequin fetus type (congenital ichthyosiform erythroderma)	242500	–	–	–	FKSB +	Blanchet-Bardon and Dumez (1984), Suzumori and Kanzaki (1991)

Disorder	MIM No.	US	AFC/AFS	CVS	ILP	MP	FBS		References
Ichthyosis, X-linked (steroid sulphatase deficiency)	308100	–	AFC + AFS (+)E	CVS (+)E	ILP (–)	MP (–)	–	–	Braunstein et al. (1976), Hahnel et al. (1982), Honour et al. (1985), Ballabio et al. (1989)
Ileal atresia	–	US (+)E	–	–	–	–	–	–	Filkins et al. (1984), Kjoller et al. (1985)
Immunodeficiency disease (T-cell)	164050	–	–	–	–	–	–	–	See Nucleoside phosphorylase deficiency
Immunodeficiency disease, severe combined	102700	–	–	–	–	–	FBS +	–	Durandy et al. (1982a,b, 1987) (see also Adenosine deaminase deficiency)
Immunodeficiency disease, severe combined X-linked variant	300400	–	–	–	ELP (+)	–	FBS (+)E	–	Goodship et al. (1989), Puck et al. (1990)
Immunodeficiency with increased IgM	308230	–	–	–	ELP (–)	–	–	–	Mensink et al. (1987)
Immunodeficiency, X-linked progressive combined variable (Duncan disease, X-linked lymphoproliferative disease)	308240	–	–	–	ELP (–)	–	–	–	Skare et al. (1987)
Imperforate anus	207500	–	–	–	–	–	–	–	See Anal atresia
Infantile cortical hyperostosis (Caffey disease)	114000	US (+)E	–	–	–	–	–	–	Langer and Kaufmann (1986)
Infantile hereditary agranulocytosis (Kostmann disease)	202700	–	–	–	–	–	FBS (+)E	–	Cividalli et al. (1983)
Infantile polycystic disease	263200	US +	AFS (+)R	–	–	–	–	–	Morin (1981), Romero et al. (1984), Argubright and Wicks (1987), Zerres et al. (1988), Reuss et al. (1990)
Iniencephaly	–	US +	–	–	–	–	–	–	Foderaro et al. (1987), Meizner and Bar-Ziv (1987)
Interrupted aortic arch	107550	US (+)E	–	–	–	–	–	–	Allan et al. (1985)
Intestinal duplication	–	US (+)E	–	–	–	–	–	–	Van Dam et al. (1984)
Intestinal perforation	–	US (+)E	–	–	–	–	–	–	Shalev et al. (1982), Glick et al. (1983)
Intestinal polyposis type I (familial polyposis coli, adenomatous polyposis of the colon)	175100	–	–	–	ELP (–)	MP (–)	–	–	Bodmer et al. (1987)
Intestinal polyposis type III (Gardner syndrome)	175300	–	–	–	ELP –	MP (–)	–	–	Bodmer et al. (1987)
Intestinal volvulus	–	US (+)E	–	–	–	–	–	–	Witter and Molteni (1986)
Intracerebral haemorrhage	–	US (+)E	–	–	–	–	–	–	Mintz et al. (1985)
Intracranial arteriovenous fistula	–	US (+)E	–	–	–	–	–	–	See Arteriovenous fistula (brain)
Intracranial calcification	–	US (+)E	–	–	–	–	–	–	Ghidini et al. (1989), Koga et al. (1990)
Intracranial haemorrhage (including subdural haematoma)	–	US (+)E Other (+)E	–	–	–	–	–	–	Fogarty et al. (1989), Rotmensch et al. (1991)
Intracranial teratoma	–	US (+)E	–	–	–	–	–	–	Vintners et al. (1982)
Intrauterine fetal death	–	US +	–	–	–	–	–	–	Bass et al. (1986)
Intrauterine growth retardation	–	US (+)R	–	–	–	–	–	–	Rizzo et al. (1987)

Table 77.1 *continued*

Disease	MIM	Imaging	Biochemistry	DNA	Other	References
Intrauterine membranous cyst	–	US (+)E	–	–	–	Kirkinen and Jouppila (1986)
Intraventricular haemorrhage	–	US (+)E	–	–	–	McGahan et al. (1984)
Isoimmune thrombocytopenia	–	–	–	–	FBS +	Lynch et al. (1988)
Isovaleric acidaemia	243500	–	AFC (+)E, AFS +	–	–	Hine et al. (1986)
Ivemark syndrome (asplenia syndrome)	208530	US (+)E	–	–	–	Chitayat et al. (1988a)
Jarcho–Levin syndrome	277300	US (+)E	–	–	–	Apuzzio et al. (1987), Tolmie et al. (1987a), Romero et al. (1988)
Jejunal atresia	–	US (+)E	–	–	–	Filkins et al. (1984)
Jejunal atresia (apple-peel type)	243600	US (+)E	–	–	–	Fletman et al. (1980)
Jeune syndrome	208500	–	–	–	–	See Asphyxiating thoracic dysplasia
Joubert syndrome	243910	US (+)E	–	–	–	Campbell et al. (1984)
Kennedy disease	313200	–	–	–	–	See Spinal and bulbar muscular atrophy
Kleeblattschädel anomaly	148800	–	–	–	–	See Cloverleaf skull
Klippel–Trenaunay–Weber syndrome	149000	US (+)E	–	–	–	Hatjis et al. (1981), Lewis et al. (1986), Shalev et al. (1988)
Krabbe disease	245200	–	AFC +, CVS +	ELP (–)	–	Giles et al. (1987), Harzer et al. (1987), Zlotogora et al. (1990)
Lacrimal duct cysts	–	US (+)E	–	–	–	Davis et al. (1987)
Langer–Saldino syndrome	200610	–	–	–	–	See Achondrogenesis type IB
Larsen-like syndrome, lethal type	245650	US (+)E	–	–	–	Mostello et al. (1991)
Laryngeal atresia	–	US (+)E	–	–	–	Arizawa et al. (1989)
Laurence–Moon–Biedl syndrome	245800	US (+)E	–	–	–	Ritchie et al. (1988)
Leigh disease	–	–	–	–	–	See Mitochondrial complex deficiencies
Leprechaunism	246200	–	AFC (+)E	–	–	Maasen et al. (1990)
Lesch–Nyhan syndrome	308000	–	–	–	–	See Hypoxanthine guanine phosphoribosyl transferase deficiency
Leucocyte adhesion deficiency	116920	–	–	MP (–)	FBS (+)E	Liskowska-Grospierre et al. (1986), Kishimoto et al. (1989), Weening et al. (1991)
Leukaemia	–	–	–	–	FBS (+)E	Zerres et al. (1990)
Lipogranulomatosis (Farber disease)	228000	–	AFC +, AFS –, CVS (–)	–	–	Fensom et al. (1979)
Lipomyelomeningocele	–	US (+)E	–	–	–	Seed and Powers (1988)
Lissencephaly (Miller–Dieker syndrome)	247200	US (+)L	–	–	–	Saltzman et al. (1991)
Long chain acyl-CoA dehydrogenase deficiency	201460	–	AFC (–), CVS (–)	–	–	Wanders and Ijlst (1992)
Lowe oculocerebrorenal syndrome	309000	–	–	ELP (–)	–	Silver et al. (1987), Gazit et al. (1990)
Lymphangiomatosis	–	US (+)E	–	–	–	Haeusler et al. (1990)

Disorder	MIM	US	AFC/AFS	CVS	ELP/ILP	MP/FBS	Reference
Lymphoedema	153100	US (+)E	—	—	—	—	Adam et al. (1979)
Macrocephaly, benign familial	153470	US (+)E	—	—	—	—	Derosa et al. (1989)
Majewski syndrome	263520	—	—	—	—	—	See Short rib–polydactyly syndrome type II
Mandibulofacial dysostosis (Treacher Collins syndrome)	154500	US (+)E / Other (+) E	—	—	ELP(−)	—	Nicolaides et al. (1984), Crane and Beaver (1986)
Mannosidosis, alpha	248500		AFC +	CVS +	—	—	Poenaru et al. (1979), Jones et al. (1984)
Mannosidosis, beta	248510	—	AFC (−)	CVS (−)	—	—	Dahl et al. (1986)
Maple syrup urine disease	248600	—	AFC + / AFS −	CVS +	—	MP (−)	Fensom et al. (1978), Wendel and Claussen (1979), Poenaru (1987)
Marfan syndrome	154700		AFC (−)	—	ILP (−) / ELP (−)	MP (−)	Godfrey et al. (1990), Kainulainen et al. (1990), Dietz et al. (1991)
Maroteaux–Lamy disease	253200	—	—	—	—	—	See Mucopolysaccharidosis type VI
Meckel–Gruber syndrome	249000	US +	—	—	—	—	Pachi et al. (1984), Nyberg et al. (1987)
Meconium ileus	–	US (+)E	—	—	—	—	Denholm et al. (1984), Nyberg et al. (1987)
Meconium peritonitis	–	US (+)E	—	—	—	—	McGahan and Hanson (1983), Nancarrow et al. (1985)
Meconium plug syndrome	–	US (+)E	—	—	—	—	Samuel (1986)
Median cleft face syndrome	136760	US (+)E	—	—	—	—	Chervenak et al. (1984b)
Medium chain acyl-CoA dehydrogenase deficiency	201450	–	AFC +	CVS (+)E	—	MP (−)	Bennett et al. (1987), Pollitt (1989), Yokota et al. (1990)
Megacystis–microcolon–intestinal hypoperistalsis syndrome	249210	US (+)E	—	—	—	—	Garber et al. (1990), Stamm et al. (1991)
Megalourethra	–	US (+)E	—	—	—	—	Fisk et al. (1990)
Megaureters	–	US (+)E	—	—	—	—	Dunn and Glasier (1985)
Menkes' disease	309400	–	—	—	—	—	See Copper deficiency
Mesoblastic nephroma	–	US (+)E	—	—	—	—	Apuzzio et al. (1986)
Mesomelic dwarfism, Langer type	249700	US (+)E	—	—	—	—	Quigg et al. (1985), Evans et al. (1988)
Metachromatic leucodystrophy	250100		AFC +	CVS +	—	MP (−), FBS (−)	Poenaru et al. (1988)
Methaemoglobinaemia (NADH cytochrome b_5 reductase deficiency)	250800		AFC +	CVS +	—	MP (−)	Junien et al. (1981)
Methylacetoaceticaciduria (beta-ketothiolase deficiency)	203750	–	AFC (−) / AFS (−)	—	—	—	Hiyama et al. (1986)
Methylglutaconicaciduria (3-methylglutaconyl-CoA hydratase deficiency)	250950	–	AFC (−) / AFS (−)	CVS (−)	—	—	Narisawa et al. (1986)
Methylmalonic acidaemia (B12 non-responsive)	251000	–	AFC + / AFS +	CVS +	—	—	Fowler et al. (1988)
Methylmalonic acidaemia (B12 responsive) (cobalamin E disease)	251100	–	AFC + / AFS +	CVS (−)	—	—	Ampola et al. (1975), Rosenblatt et al. (1985)
Mevalonic acidaemia	251170	–	AFC (+)E / AFS (+)E	—	—	—	Hoffmann et al. (1986)
Microcephaly	251200	US (+)L	—	—	—	—	Chervenak et al. (1984a), Tolmie et al. (1987b)
Microcephaly–micromelia syndrome	251230	US (+)E	—	—	—	—	Ives and Houston (1980)

Table 77.1 *continued*

Disease	MIM	Imaging	Biochemistry	DNA	Other	References
Micrognathia	–	US (+)E	–	–	–	–	Pilu et al. (1986a), Majoor-Krakauer et al. (1987)
Microphthalmia	251600	US (+)E	–	–	–	–	Feldman et al. (1985)
Mitochondrial complex I deficiency	–	–	CVS (+)E	–	–	–	Ruitenbeek et al. (1992)
Mitochondrial complex IV deficiency	–	–	CVS (+)E	–	–	–	Ruitenbeek et al. (1992)
Mitochondrial complex I and IV deficiency	–	–	CVS (+)E	–	–	–	Ruitenbeek et al. (1992)
Mitral atresia	121000	US (+)E	–	–	–	–	Allan (1987)
Molybdenum co-factor deficiency (combined xanthine and sulphite oxidase deficiencies)	252150	–	AFC (+)E AFS (+)E	CVS (+)E	–	–	Ogier et al. (1983), Gray et al. (1990)
Morquio disease	253000	–	–	–	–	–	See Mucopolysaccharidosis type IVA
Mucoid degeneration of cord	–	US (+)E	–	–	–	–	Iaccarino et al. (1986)
Mucolipidosis type I (sialidosis)	252400	–	AFC +	–	–	–	Kleijer et al. (1979), Steinman et al. (1980)
Mucolipidosis type II (I-cell disease)	252500	–	AFC + AFS +	CVS +	–	–	Ben-Yoseph et al. (1988), Poenaru et al. (1990)
Mucolipidosis type III (pseudo-Hurler polydystrophy)	252600	–	AFC (–)	CVS (–)	–	–	Ben-Yoseph et al. (1988)
Mucolipidosis type IV	252650	–	AFC (+)E	CVS (+)E	–	–	Orney et al. (1987)
Mucopolysaccharidosis type IH, IS (Hurler syndrome, Scheie syndrome)	252800	–	AFC + AFS +	CVS +	–	FBS +	FKSB (+)E	Kleijer et al. (1983), Rodeck et al. (1983b)
Mucopolysaccharidosis type II (Hunter syndrome)	309900	–	AFC + AFS +	CVS +	ILP (–) ELP (–)	MP (–)	FBS (+)E	Pannone et al. (1986), Lissens et al. (1988)
Mucopolysaccharidosis type IIIA (Sanfilippo A disease)	252900	–	AFC + AFS +	CVS +	–	–	Kleijer et al. (1986)
Mucopolysaccharidosis type IIIB (Sanfilippo B disease)	252920	–	AFC + AFS +	CVS +	–	–	Minelli et al. (1988)
Mucopolysaccharidosis type IIIC (Sanfilippo C disease)	252930	–	AFC (–) AFS +	CVS +	–	–	Di Natale et al. (1987)
Mucopolysaccharidosis type IIID (Sanfilippo D disease)	252940	–	AFC (–)	CVS (–)	–	MP (–)	Nowakowski et al. (1989)
Mucopolysaccharidosis type IVA (Morquio disease type A)	253000	–	AFC + AFS +	CVS +	–	–	Von Figura et al. (1982), Yuen and Fensom (1985), Zhao et al. (1990)
Mucopolysaccharidosis type IVB (Morquio disease type B)	253010	–	AFC (–)	CVS (–)	–	–	Guigliani et al. (1987)
Mucopolysaccharidosis type V	252800	–	–	–	–	–	See mucopolysaccharidosis type 1H, 1S

Disorder	MIM	US	AFC/AFS	CVS	ELP		MP		Reference
Mucopolysaccharidosis type VI (Maroteaux–Lamy disease)	253200	–	AFC + / AFS +	CVS +	–	–	–	–	Van Dyke et al. (1981), Rogoyski (1985)
Mucopolysaccharidosis type VII (Sly syndrome)	253220	–	AFC (+)E	CVS (+)E	–	–	MP (−)	–	Maire et al. (1979), Poenaru (1982)
Multiple carboxylase deficiency (late-onset variant, biotinidase deficiency)	253260	–	AFC (+)E / AFS (+)E	–	–	–	–	–	Secor McVoy et al. (1984)
Multiple carboxylase deficiency (neonatal form, holocarboxylase synthase deficiency)	253270	–	AFC (+)E / AFS (+)E	CVS (−)	–	–	–	–	Packman et al. (1982)
Multiple contracture syndrome, Finnish type	253310	US (+)E	–	–	–	–	–	–	Herva et al. (1985), Kirkinen et al. (1987)
Multiple endocrine neoplasia type I	131100	–	–	–	ELP (−)	–	–	–	Bale et al. (1989)
Multiple endocrine neoplasia type IIA	171400	–	–	–	ELP (−)	–	–	–	Mathew et al. (1987)
Multiple endocrine neoplasia type IIB	162300	–	–	–	ELP (−)	–	–	–	Jackson et al. (1988)
Multiple gestation	–	US +	–	–	–	–	–	–	Neilson et al. (1989), Winn et al. (1989), Filly et al. (1990)
Multiple pterygium syndrome	253290	US (+)E	–	–	–	–	–	–	Lockwood et al. (1988), Zeitune et al. (1988)
Multiple pterygium syndrome with concentric bone fusion	–	US (+)E	–	–	–	–	–	–	van Regemorter et al. (1984)
Multiple pterygium syndrome with spinal fusion	252390	US (+)E	–	–	–	–	–	–	Chen et al. (1984), Zeitune et al. (1988)
Multiple pterygium syndrome, X-linked variant	312150	US (+)E	–	–	–	–	–	–	Tolmie et al. (1987d)
Multiple sulphatase deficiency (mucosulphatidosis)	272200	–	AFC (−)	CVS +	–	–	–	–	Patrick et al. (1988)
Myasthenia gravis with fetal arthrogryposis	254200	US (+)E	–	–	–	–	–	–	Stoll et al. (1991)
Myotonic dystrophy	160900	–	–	–	ELP (+)E	–	MP +	–	Norman et al. (1989), Speer et al. (1990)
Myotubular myopathy, X-linked	310400	–	–	–	ELP (+)E	–	–	–	Bartley and Gies (1990)
Nager acrofacial dysostosis	154400	US (+)E	–	–	–	–	–	–	Benson et al. (1988)
Nephroblastomatosis	267000	US (+)E	–	–	–	–	–	–	Ambrosino et al. (1990)
Nephrogenic diabetes insipidus	304800	–	–	–	ELP (−)	–	–	–	Knoers et al. (1988)
Nephrotic syndrome, congenital (Finnish nephrosis)	256300	–	AFS +	–	–	–	–	–	Morin (1984)
Neu–Laxova syndrome	256520	US (+)E	–	–	–	–	–	–	Tolmie et al. (1987c), Mennuti et al. (1990)
Neuroblastoma, adrenal	256700	US (+)E	–	–	–	–	–	–	Ferraro et al. (1988)
Neuroblastoma, thoracic	–	US (+)E	–	–	–	–	–	–	De Filippi et al. (1986)
Neurofibromatosis type I	162200	–	–	–	ILP (+)E / ELP (−)	–	MP (−)	–	Viskochil et al. (1990), Lazard et al. (1992)
Neurofibromatosis type II	101000	–	–	–	ELP (−)	–	–	–	Rouleau et al. (1987)

Table 77.1 continued

Disease	MIM	Imaging	Biochemistry	DNA	Other	References
Neuronal ceroid lipofuscinosis (infantile type)	256730	–	CVS +	ELP (+)E	–	Rapola et al. (1990), Jarvela et al. (1991)
Neuronal ceroid lipofuscinosis (juvenile type, late-onset Batten's disease)	204200	–	CVS (+)E	ELP (–)	–	Conradi et al. (1989), Gardiner et al. (1990)
Neuronal ceroid lipofuscinosis (late infantile type, early-onset Batten's disease)	204500	–	–	ELP (–)	–	Jarvela et al. (1991)
Niemann–Pick, types A,B	257200	–	AFC + / AFS – / CVS +	–	–	Donnai et al. (1981), Vanier et al. (1985)
Niemann–Pick, type C	257220	–	AFC + / CVS +	–	–	Harzer et al. (1978), Vanier et al. (1989)
Nijmegen breakage syndrome	251260	–	–	–	CHR (+)E	Jaspers et al. (1990)
Noonan syndrome	163950	US (+)E	–	–	–	Benacerraf et al. (1989b)
Norrie disease	310600	–	–	ELP (+)E	–	Gal et al. (1988), Curtis et al. (1989)
Nucleoside phosphorylase deficiency	164050	–	AFC (+)E / AFS (+)E / CVS (+)E	ILP (–) / ELP (–) / MP (–)	FBS (–)	Linch et al. (1982), Kleijer (1989)
Obstructive uropathy	–	US +	–	–	–	Hobbins et al. (1984), Stiller (1989)
Occipital hair	–	US (+)E	–	–	–	Petrikovsky et al. (1989)
OEIS complex (omphalocoele, exstrophy of the bladder, imperforate anus and spinal defects)	–	US (+)	–	–	–	Kutzner et al. (1988)
Oesophageal atresia	189960	US (+)R	–	–	–	Pretorius et al. (1987)
Ohdo syndrome	–	US (+)E	–	–	–	Ohdo et al. (1987)
Oligodactyly	–	US (+)E	–	–	–	Russell (1973)
Opitz G syndrome (Opitz BBB syndrome)	145410	US (+)E	–	–	–	Patton et al. (1986), Hogdall et al. (1989)
Oral–facial–digital syndrome type I	311200	US (+)E	AFC (–)	–	–	Iaccarino et al. (1985)
Ornithinaemia, with gyrate atrophy	258870	–	–	MP (–)	–	O'Donnell (1981)
Ornithine transcarbamoylase deficiency	311250	–	–	–	–	See Hyperammonaemia I
Oromandibular limb hypogenesis syndrome	–	US (+)E	–	–	–	Shechter et al. (1990)
Orotic aciduria type I	258900	–	–	MP (–)	FBS (–)	Suttle et al. (1988)
Osteogenesis imperfecta type I (milder autosomal dominant variant)	166200	US (+)E	–	ILP (+)P / MP (+)P	–	Tsipouras et al. (1987), Pope et al. (1989)
Osteogenesis imperfecta type II (severe congenital form)	166210	US +	CVS (+)E	MP (+)P	–	Pope et al. (1989), Grange et al. (1990), Munoz et al. (1990), Constantine et al. (1991)
Osteogenesis imperfecta, other types	259400	US (+)E	–	MP (+)P	–	Carpenter et al. (1986), Robinson et al. (1987), Pope et al. (1989)

Disorder	MIM No.							References
Osteopetrosis (milder autosomal dominant variant)	166600	Other (+)E	–	–	–	–	–	Jenkinson et al. (1943), Camera et al. (1989)
Osteopetrosis (severe autosomal recessive variant)	259700	US (+)E	–	–	–	–	–	El Khazen et al. (1986), Camera et al. (1989)
Osteopoikilosis	166700	Other (+)E	–	–	–	–	–	Martincic (1952)
Otocephaly (synotia)	–	US (+)E	–	–	–	–	–	Cayea et al. (1985)
Ovarian cyst in fetus	–	US (+)E	–	–	–	–	–	Rizzo et al. (1989)
Parenti–Fraccaro syndrome	200600	–	–	–	–	–	–	See Achondrogenesis type IA
Patent urachus	–	US (+)E	–	–	–	–	–	Persutte et al. (1988b)
Pelizaeus–Merzbacher disease (myelin proteolipid protein deficiency)	312080	–	–	–	ILP (+)E ELP (+)E	MP (–)	–	Maenpaa et al. (1990), Bridge et al. (1991)
Pelvic kidney	–	US (+)E	–	–	–	–	–	Hill and Peterson (1987), Colley and Hooker (1989)
Pelvic-ureteric obstruction	–	US (+)	–	–	–	–	–	Grignon et al. (1986b), Kleiner et al. (1987)
Pena–Shokeir syndrome type I	208150	US (+)E	–	–	–	–	–	Ohlsson et al. (1988), Persutte et al. (1988a), Genkins et al. (1989)
Pena–Shokeir syndrome type II	214150	US (+)E	–	–	–	–	–	Preus et al. (1977)
Pentalogy of Cantrell	–	US (+)E	–	–	–	–	–	Abu-Yousef et al. (1987), Ghidini et al. (1988)
Pericardial effusion	–	US (+)E	–	–	–	–	–	Shenker et al. (1989)
Pericardial tumour	–	US (+)E	–	–	–	–	–	Cyr et al. (1988)
Peroxisomal 3-oxo-acyl-CoA thiolase deficiency (pseudo-Zellweger syndrome)	261510	–	AFC (+)E AFS (+)E	CVS (+)E	–	–	–	Schutgens et al. (1989)
Persistent cloaca	–	US (+)E	–	–	–	–	–	Holzgreve (1985)
Phenylketonuria type I (phenylalanine hydroxylase deficiency)	261600	–	–	–	ILP +	MP (+)P	FLB (–)	Woo et al. (1974), Daiger et al. (1986), Speer et al. (1986), Huang et al. (1990)
Phenylketonuria type II (dihydropteridine reductase deficiency)	261630	–	AFC (+)E	–	ILP (+)E	MP (–)	–	Dahl et al. (1988)
Phenylketonuria type III (dihydrobiopterin synthetase deficiency)	261640	–	AFS (+)E	–	–	–	FBS (+)E	Firgaira et al. (1983), Niederwieser (1986)
Phenylketonuria with neopterin deficiency	233910	–	–	–	–	–	–	See GTP cyclohydrolase I deficiency
Phocomelia	223340	US (+)E	–	–	–	–	–	Campbell and Pearce (1983)
Phosphoglycerate kinase deficiency	311800	–	–	–	–	–	–	Michelson et al. (1985)
Pierre Robin sequence	261800	US (+)E	–	–	–	MP (–)	–	Pilu et al. (1986b), Malinger et al. (1987)
Pituitary dysgenesis	262600	–	AFS +	–	–	–	–	Stoll et al. (1978)
Placenta, succenturiate lobe	–	US +	–	–	–	–	–	Spirt et al. (1987)
Placenta praevia	–	US (+)E	–	–	–	–	–	Gottesfeld (1978)
Placental haemangioma	–	US (+)E	–	–	–	–	–	Mann et al. (1983)
Placental tumour	–	US (+)E	–	–	–	–	–	Kapoor et al. (1989)
Placentomegaly	–	US +	–	–	–	–	–	Quagliariello et al. (1978)

1218

Table 77.1 *continued*

Disease	MIM	Imaging	Biochemistry	DNA	Other	References
Pleural effusion	–	US (+)E	–	–	–	Bruno et al. (1988), Lien et al. (1990)
Polycystic kidney disease	173900	–	–	–	–	See Infantile polycystic disease and Adult polycystic kidney disease
Polysplenia syndrome	208530	US (+)E	–	–	–	Chitayat et al. (1988a)
Pompe disease	232300	–	–	–	–	See Glycogen storage disease II
Porencephaly	175780	US (+)E	–	–	–	Vintzileos et al. (1987) (see also Schizencephaly)
Porphyria, acute intermittent	176000	–	AFC (+)E	ILP (–)	MP (–)	Sassa et al. (1975) Llewellyn et al. (1987)
Porphyria, congenital erythropoietic	263700	–	–	–	–	Nitowsky et al. (1978), Kaiser (1980)
Prolidase deficiency (peptidase D deficiency)	170100	–	AFS (+)E / AFC (–)	–	CVS (–)	Endo et al. (1990)
Properdin deficiency	312060	–	–	ELP (–)	–	Goonewardena et al. (1988)
Propionic acidaemia (ketotic hyperglycinaemia)	232000	–	AFC + / AFS +	–	CVS +	FBS +	Perez-Cerda et al. (1989), Rolland et al. (1990)
Protein C deficiency	176860	US +	–	–	–	FBS +	Mibashan et al. (1985)
Prune-belly syndrome	100100	–	–	–	–	Meizner et al. (1985)
Pseudo-Hurler syndrome	252600	–	–	–	–	See Mucolipidosis type III
Pulmonary atresia	178370	US (+)E	–	–	–	Allan et al. (1986)
Pulmonary cyst	–	US (+)E	–	–	–	Lebrun et al. (1985) (see also Bronchogenic cyst)
Pulmonary lymphangiectasia	265300	US (+)E	–	–	–	Wilson et al. (1985)
Pulmonary sequestration	–	US (+)E	–	–	–	Davies et al. (1989)
Pulmonary vein atresia	121000	US (+)E	–	–	–	Samuel et al. (1988)
Pyloric stenosis, congenital hypertrophic	179010	US (+)E	–	–	–	Katz et al. (1988)
Pyroglutamic aciduria	266130	–	AFC (–)	–	CVS (–)	Wellner et al. (1974)
Pyropoikilocytosis type II	266140	–	–	–	–	Morris et al. (1986)
Pyruvate carboxylase deficiency	266150	–	AFC +	–	–	FBS (+)E	Tsuchiyama et al. (1983), Robinson et al. (1985)
Pyruvate dehydrogenase deficiency	208800	US +	AFC (–)	–	CVS (–)	Blass (1980)
Radial aplasia	–	US +	–	–	–	Brons et al. (1990) (see also Holt–Oram syndrome and Thrombocytopenia–absent radius syndrome)
RAG syndrome	–	US (+)E	–	–	–	Saal (1986)
Refsum disease, adult form	266500	–	AFC (–)	–	CVS (–)	Billimoria et al. (1982)
Refsum disease, infantile form	266510	–	AFS +	–	CVS +	Poll-The et al. (1985), Schutgens et al. (1989)
Renal agenesis (bilateral)	191830	US +	–	–	–	Romero et al. (1985), Morse et al. (1987a)
Renal agenesis (unilateral)	–	US +	–	–	–	Jeanty et al. (1990b)
Renal duplication	–	US +	–	–	–	Sherer et al. (1989)
Renal multicystic dysplasia	–	US (+)E	–	–	–	Rizzo et al. (1987), Stiller et al. (1988)

Disorder	No.	US	AFC/AFS	CVS	ELP/ILP	MP	FBS	CHR	References
Renal vein thrombosis	–	US (+)E	–	–	–	–	–	–	
Retinitis pigmentosa, X-linked types	312600 / 312610	–	–	–	–	–	–	–	Wright et al. (1987)
Retinoblastoma	180200	–	–	–	ELP (+)E / ILP (–)	MP (–)	–	–	Horsthemke et al. (1987), Mitchell et al. (1988)
Retinoschisis	312700	–	–	–	ELP (–)	–	–	–	Gellert et al. (1988), Sieving et al. (1990)
Rhesus isoimmunization	–	–	AFS +	–	ELP (–)	–	FBS +	–	
Roberts syndrome	268300	US (+)E	–	–	–	–	–	CHR (+)R	Romke et al. (1987), Tomkins (1989)
Robin anomalad	261800	–	–	–	–	–	–	–	See Pierre Robin sequence
Robinow syndrome	180700	US (+)E	–	–	–	–	–	–	Loverro et al. (1990)
Sacral agenesis	182940	US (+)E	–	–	–	–	–	–	Fellous et al. (1982), Sonek et al. (1990)
Sacrococcygeal teratoma	–	US +	–	–	–	–	–	–	Chervenak et al. (1985), Holzgreve et al. (1985), Gross et al. (1987)
Saldino–Noonan syndrome	263530	–	–	–	–	–	–	–	See Short rib–polydactyly syndrome type I
Salla disease	268740		AFC + / AFS (+)E	CVS (+)E	–	–	–	–	Renlund and Aula (1987)
Sandhoff disease	268800		–	–	–	–	–	–	See Gangliosidosis, G_{M2} type II
Scheie syndrome	252800		–	–	–	–	–	–	See Mucopolysaccharidosis type IS
Schilder disease	300100	–	–	–	–	–	–	–	See Adrenoleucodystrophy
Schindler disease	104170	–	–	–	–	–	–	–	See Acetylgalactosaminidase deficiency
Schizencephaly	269250	US (+)E / Other (+)E	–	–	–	–	–	–	Lituania et al. (1989), Komarniski et al. (1990)
Schneckenbecken dysplasia	269250	US (+)E	–	–	–	–	–	–	Laxova et al. (1973), Borochowitz et al. (1986)
Schwartz–Jampel syndrome	255800	US (+)E	–	–	–	–	–	–	Hunziker et al. (1989)
Scoliosis	181800	US (+)E	–	–	–	–	–	–	Henry and Norton (1987) (see also Jarcho–Levin syndrome)
Seckel syndrome	210600	US (+)E	–	–	–	–	–	–	De Elejalde and Elejalde (1984)
Seizures	–	US (+)E	–	–	–	–	–	–	Landy et al. (1989) (see also Convulsions, benign familial neonatal)
Short chain acyl-CoA dehydrogenase deficiency	201470	–	AFC (–)	CVS (–)	–	MP (–)	–	–	Naito et al. (1989)
Short rib syndrome, Beemer type	269860	US (+)E	–	–	–	–	–	–	Balci et al. (1991)
Short rib-polydactyly syndrome type I (Saldino–Noonan syndrome)	263530	US (+)E / Other (+)E	–	–	–	–	–	–	Toftager-Larsen and Benzie (1984), Meizner and Bar-Ziv (1989)
Short-rib-polydactyly syndrome type II (Majewski syndrome)	263520	US (+)E / Other (+)E	–	–	–	–	–	–	Toftager-Larsen and Benzie (1984), Gembruch et al. (1985), Meizner and Bar-Ziv (1985)
Short rib-polydactyly syndrome type III (Spranger–Verma)	263510	US (+)E	–	–	–	–	–	–	Verma et al. (1975)
Short rib-polydactyly syndrome type IV (Piepkorn)	–	US (+)E	–	–	–	–	–	–	Piepkorn et al. (1977)

Table 77.1 continued

Disease	MIM	Imaging	Biochemistry	DNA	Other	References
Sialic acid storage disease	269920	–	AFC + AFS +	CVS +	–	Lake et al. (1989), Vamos et al. (1986)
Sialidosis	252400	–	–	–	–	See Mucolipidosis type I
Sickle-cell disease	142300	–	–	–	–	See Haemoglobin S
Simian crease	–	US (+)E	–	–	–	Jeanty et al. (1990) (see also Trisomy 21)
Single umbilical artery	–	US +	–	–	–	Spirt et al. (1987), Jauniaux et al. (1989)
Single ventricle	121000	–	–	–	–	See Univentricular heart
Sirenomelia	–	US (+)E	–	–	–	Fitzmorris-Glass (1989), Sirtori et al. (1989)
Situs inversus	270100	US (+)E	–	–	–	Stoker et al. (1983)
Sjögren–Larsen syndrome	270200	–	AFC (–)	CVS (–)	FKSB (+)E	Kouseff et al. (1982), Trepeta et al. (1984)
Skull deformation	–	US (+)E	–	–	–	Romero et al. (1981)
Skull fracture	–	Other (+)E	–	–	–	Alexander and Davis (1969), McRae et al. (1982)
Sly syndrome	253220	–	–	–	–	See Mucopolysaccharidosis VII
Smith–Lemli–Opitz syndrome	270400	US (+)E	–	–	–	Curry et al. (1987)
Spherocytosis	182900	–	–	MP (–)	–	Lux et al. (1990)
Spina bifida	182940	US +	AFS (+)R	–	–	Nicolaides et al. (1986), Chambers et al. (1989), Van den Hof et al. (1990)
Spinal and bulbar muscular atrophy (Kennedy disease)	313200	–		ELP (–)	MP (–)	Fischbeck et al. (1986)
Spinal muscular atrophy type I (Werdnig–Hoffmann disease)	253300	–		ELP (+)E		Gilliam et al. (1990)
Spinal muscular atrophy type II	253550	–		ELP (–)		Gilliam et al. (1990)
Spinal muscular atrophy type III (Kugelberg–Welander disease)	253400	–		ELP (–)		Gilliam et al. (1990)
Splenic cyst	–	US (+)E	–	–	–	Lichman and Miller (1988)
Spondyloepiphyseal dysplasia congenita	183900	US (+)E	–	–	–	Donnenfeld and Mennuti (1987), Kirk and Comstock (1990)
Spondylothoracic dysplasia	277300	US (+)E	–	–	–	Marks et al. (1989) (see also Jarcho–Levin syndrome)
Steroid sulphatase deficiency	308100	–	–	–	–	See Ichthyosis, X-linked
Stomach duplication	–	US (+)E	–	–	–	Bidwell and Nelson (1986)
Subdural haematoma	–	–	–	–	–	See Intracranial haemorrhage
Subdural hygroma	–	US (+)E	–	–	–	Ghidini (1988)
Supraventricular tachycardia	–	US (+)E Other +	–	–	–	Wiggins et al. (1986), Buissliem et al. (1987)
Takahara disease	115500	–	–	–	–	See Acatalasia
Talipes	119800	US (+)E	–	–	–	Bronshtein and Zimmer (1989)
Tangier disease (familial high density lipoprotein deficiency)	205400	–	AFC (–)	–	–	Gebhardt (1979)
Tay–Sachs disease	272800	–	–	–	–	See Gangliosidosis G_{M2} type I

Condition	No.	US	AFC/AFS	CVS	Other	MP	FBS	CHR	References
Tay–Sachs variant	272750	-	-	-	-	-	-	-	See Gangliosidosis
Testicular feminization	313700	-	-	-	-	-	-	-	See Androgen insensitivity syndrome
Testicular torsion	-	US (+)E	-	-	-	-	-	-	Hubbard et al. (1984)
Tetralogy of Fallot	185700	US (+)E	-	-	-	-	-	-	Allan et al. (1985)
Thalassaemia, alpha	141800	-	-	-	ILP + ELP +	MP (+)P	FBS +	-	Zeng and Huang (1985), Wang et al. (1986), Kazazian (1990)
Thalassaemia, beta	141900	-	-	-	ILP + ELP +	MP (+)P	FBS +	-	Cao et al. (1986), Camaschella et al. (1988), Ristaldi et al. (1989), Old et al. (1990), Kazazian (1990)
Thalidomide embryopathy	-	US (+)E	-	-	-	-	-	-	Gollop et al. (1987)
Thanatophoric dysplasia	187600	US (+)E	-	-	-	-	-	-	Pretorius (1986)
Thanatophoric dysplasia with cloverleaf skull	273670	US (+)E	-	-	-	-	-	-	Mahony et al. (1985b), Weiner et al. (1986)
Thoracic dysplasia–hydrocephalus syndrome	273730	US (+)E	-	-	-	-	-	-	Winter et al. (1987)
Thoracic gastroenteric cyst	-	US (+)E	-	-	-	-	-	-	Newnham et al. (1984), Albright et al. (1988)
Thoracoabdominal eventration	-	US (+)E	-	-	Other (+)E	-	-	-	Seeds et al. (1984)
Thrombocytopenia, neonatal alloimmune	-	-	-	-	-	-	FBS +	-	McFarland et al. (1991)
Thrombocytopenia–absent radius syndrome (TAR syndrome)	274000	US (+)E Other (+)E	-	-	-	-	FBS (+)E	-	Luthy et al. (1981), Filkins et al. (1984), Donnenfeld et al. (1990)
Thyrotoxicosis (hyperthyroidism)	275000	-	AFS (+)E	-	-	-	-	-	Pekonen et al. (1984) (see also Goitre)
Tracheo-oesophageal fistula	189960	-	-	-	-	-	-	-	See Oseophageal atresia
Transcobalamin II deficiency	275350	-	AFC (−)	-	-	-	-	-	Mayes et al. (1987), Rosenblatt (1987)
Treacher Collins syndrome	154500	-	-	-	-	-	-	-	See Mandibulofacial dysostosis
Tricuspid atresia	121000	US (+)E	-	-	-	-	-	-	De Vore et al. (1987)
Tricuspid incompetence	121000	US (+)E	AFC +	CVS +	-	-	FBS (+)E	-	Brown et al. (1986)
Triose phosphate isomerase deficiency	190450	-	-	-	-	-	-	-	Rosa et al. (1986), Dallapiccola et al. (1987), Bellingham et al. (1989)
Triploidy	-	US (+)R	-	-	-	-	-	CHR +	Pircon et al. (1989)
Trisomy 13	-	US (+)R	-	-	-	-	-	CHR +	Benacerraf et al. (1986b)
Trisomy 18	-	US (+)R	-	-	-	-	-	CHR +	Benacerraf et al. (1986b), Bundy et al. (1986)
Trisomy 21	-	US (+)R	-	-	-	-	-	CHR +	Benacerraf and Frigoletto (1987), Toi et al. (1987), Nyberg et al. (1990)
Truncus arteriosus	121000	US (+)E	-	-	ELP (+)P	-	-	-	Allan et al. (1985)
Tuberous sclerosis	191100	US (+)E	-	-	-	MP (−)P	-	-	Connor et al. (1987), Chitayat et al. (1988b)
Twin embolization syndrome	-	US (+)E	-	-	-	-	-	-	Patten et al. (1989)
Twin–twin transfusion syndrome	-	-	-	-	-	-	-	-	See Fetofetal transfusion syndrome
Twins, zygosity	-	-	-	-	-	-	-	-	See Multiple pregnancy
Tyrosinaemia, type I	276700	-	AFC + AFS +	CVS +	-	-	-	-	Gagne et al. (1982), Kvittingen et al. (1986), Jakobs et al. (1990)

Table 77.1 *concluded*

Disease	MIM	Imaging	Biochemistry	DNA	Other	References
Uhl anomaly	10790	US (+)E	—	—	—	Wager et al. (1988)
Umbilical cord, vesicoallantoic defect	—	US (+)E	—	—	—	Donnenfeld et al. (1989)
Umbilical cord angiomyxoma	—	US (+)E	—	—	—	Jauniaux et al. (1989)
Umbilical cord cyst	—	US (+)E	—	—	—	Rempen (1989)
Umbilical cord haemangioma	—	US (+)E	—	—	—	Ghidini et al. (1990)
Umbilical cord haematoma	—	US (+)E	—	—	—	Sutro et al. (1984)
Umbilical cord thrombosis	—	US (+)E	—	—	—	Abrams et al. (1985)
Umbilical vein ectasia	—	US (+)E	—	—	—	Vesce et al. (1987)
Univentricular heart	121000	US +	—	—	—	Allan et al. (1985)
Urachal cysts	—	US (+)E	—	—	—	Hill et al. (1990)
Ureterocele	191650	US (+)E	—	—	—	Fitzsimons et al. (1986)
Ureteropelvic junction obstruction	143400	US +	—	—	—	Hobbins et al. (1984), Corteville et al. (1991)
Urethral atresia	—	US +	—	—	—	Hill et al. (1985), Hayden et al. (1988)
Urethral valves	—	US (+)R	—	—	—	Hill et al. (1985), Hayden et al. (1988)
Uterovesical junction obstruction	—	US (+)E	—	—	—	Hobbins et al. (1984)
VATER syndrome	192350	(+)E	—	—	—	Claiborne et al. (1986), McGahan et al. (1988)
Ventricular arrhythmia	—	US (+)E Other +	—	—	—	Lingman et al. (1986)
Ventricular septal defect	121000	US (+)E	—	—	—	Allan et al. (1985)
Vesicoallantoic abdominal wall defect	—	—	—	—	—	See Umbilical cord, vesicoallantoic defect
Vitamin D-dependent rickets type II	277420	—	AFC (+)E	—	—	Weisman et al. (1990)
von Gierke disease	232200	—	—	—	—	See Glycogen storage disease IA
von Hippel–Lindau disease	193300	—	—	ELP (−)	—	Seizinger et al. (1988)
von Willebrand disease	193400	—	—	ILP (+)E ELP (−)	MP (−)	Shelton-Inloes et al. (1987), Bignell et al. (1990)
Walker–Warburg syndrome	236670	US (+)E	—	—	FBS +	Crow et al. (1986), Farrell et al. (1987)
Weyers syndrome	193530	US (+)E	—	—	—	Elejalde et al. (1983)
Wiskott–Aldrich syndrome	301000	—	—	ELP (+)E	FBS +	Holmberg et al. (1983), Schwartz et al. (1989), Lorenz et al. (1991)
Wolffian duct cyst	194200	US (+)E	—	—	—	Kapoor et al. (1989)
Wolff–Parkinson–White syndrome	—	Other +	—	—	—	Wiggins et al. (1986)
Wolman disease	278000	—	—	—	—	See Cholesterol ester storage disease
Xanthine oxidase deficiency (xanthinuria)	278300	—	AFC +	—	—	Desjacques et al. (1985)
Xeroderma pigmentosum	278700	—	AFC +	—	FBS (−) CHR (+)E	Halley et al. (1979), Arase et al. (1985), Savary et al. (1991)
Zellweger syndrome	214100	—	—	—	—	See Cerebrohepatorenal syndrome
Zellweger-like syndrome	214110	—	AFC (−)	—	—	Schutgens et al. (1989)

For explanation see text.

References

Abbitt, P.L. and McIhenny, J. (1990) Prenatal detection of gallstones. *JCU*, **18**, 202–204.

Abrams, S.L., Callen, P.W. and Filly, R.A. (1985) Umbilical vein thrombosis: sonographic detection *in utero*. *Journal of Ultrasound in Medicine*, **4**, 283–85.

Abrams, S.L. and Filly, R.A. (1985) Congenital vertebral malformations: prenatal diagnosis using ultrasonography. *Radiology*, **155**, 762.

Abu-Yousef, M.M., Wray, A.B., Williamson, R.A. and Bonsib, S.M. (1987) Antenatal ultrasound diagnosis of variant of pentalogy of Cantrell. *Journal of Ultrasound in Medicine*, **6**, 535–38.

Achiron, R., Malinger, G., Zaidel, L. and Zakut, H. (1988) Prenatal sonographic diagnosis of endocardial fibroelastosis secondary to aortic stenosis. *Prenatal Diagnosis*, **8**, 73–77.

Adam, A.H., Robinson, H.P., Pont, M. et al. (1979) Prenatal diagnosis of fetal lymphatic system abnormalities by ultrasound. *JCU*, **7**, 361–64.

Albright, E.B., Crane, J.P. and Shackelford, G.D. (1988) Prenatal diagnosis of a bronchogenic cyst. *Journal of Ultrasound in Medicine*, **7**, 91–95.

Alexander Jr, E. and Davis, C.H. (1969) Intrauterine fracture of the infant's skull. *Journal of Neurosurgery*, **30**, 446–54.

Allan, L.D. (1987) Prenatal diagnosis of congenital heart disease. *Hospital Update*, **13**, 553–60.

Allan, L.D., Crawford, D.C., Handerson, R. and Tynan, M. (1985) Spectrum of congenital heart disease detected echocardiographically in prenatal life. *British Heart Journal*, **54**, 523–26.

Allan, L.D., Crawford, D.C. and Tynan, M.J. (1986) Pulmonary atresia in prenatal life. *Journal of the American College of Cardiology*, **8**, 1131–36.

Allan, L.D., Desai, G. and Tynan, M.J. (1982). Prenatal echocardiographic screening for Ebstein's anomaly for mothers on lithium therapy. *Lancet*, **ii**, 875–76.

Almeida, M.R., Alves, I.L., Sakaki, Y. et al. (1990) Prenatal diagnosis of familial amyloidotic polyneuropathy: evidence for an early expression of the associated transthyretin methionine 30. *Human Genetics*, **85**, 623–26.

Alter, B.P. (1984) Advances in the prenatal diagnosis of hematologic diseases. *Blood*, **64**, 329–40.

Ambrosino, M.M., Hernanz-Schulman, M., Horii, S.C. et al. (1990) Prenatal diagnosis of nephroblastomatosis in two siblings. *Journal of Ultrasound in Medicine*, **9**, 49–51.

Ampola, M.G., Mahoney, M.J., Nakamura, E. and Tanaka, K. (1975). Prenatal therapy of a patient with vitamin B_{12} responsive methylmalonic acidemia. *New England Journal of Medicine*, **293**, 313–17.

Andersen, Jr, P.E., Hauge, M. and Bang, J. (1988) Dyssegmental dysplasia in siblings: prenatal ultrasonic diagnosis. *Skeletal Radiology*, **17**, 29–31.

Anneren, G., Andersson, T., Lindgren, P.G. and Kjartansson, S. (1991) Ectodactyly–ectodermal dysplasia–clefting syndrome (EEC), the clinical variation and prenatal diagnosis. *Clinical Genetics*, **40**, 257–62.

Anton-Lamprecht, I. (1981) Prenatal diagnosis of genetic disorders of the skin by means of electron microscopy. *Human Genetics*, **59**, 392–405.

Anton-Lamprecht, I., Rauskolb, R., Jovanovic, V. et al. (1981) Prenatal diagnosis of epidermolysis bullosa dystrophica Hallopeau–Siemens with electron microscopy of fetal skin. *Lancet*, **ii**, 1077–79.

Anyane-Yeboa, K., Kasznila, J., Malin, J. and Maidman, J. (1987) Herrmann–Opitz syndrome: report of an affected fetus. *American Journal of Medical Genetics*, **27**, 467–70.

Apuzzio, J.J., Diamond, N., Ganesh, V. and Desposito, F. (1987) Difficulties in the prenatal diagnosis of Jarcho–Levin syndrome. *American Journal of Obstetrics and Gynecology*, **156**, 916–18.

Apuzzio, J.J., Ganesh, V.V., Chervenak, J. and Sama, J.C. (1988) Prenatal diagnosis of dicephalous conjoined twins in a triplet pregnancy. *American Journal of Obstetrics and Gynecology*, **159**, 1214–15.

Apuzzio, J.J., Unwin, W., Adhate, A. and Nichols, R. (1986) Prenatal diagnosis of fetal renal mesoblastic nephroma. *American Journal of Obstetrics and Gynecology*, **154**, 636–37.

Arase, S., Bohnert, E., Fischer, E. and Jung, E.G. (1985) Prenatal exclusion of xeroderma pigmentosum (XP-D) by amniotic cell analysis. *Photodermatology*, **2**, 181–83.

Argubright, K.F. and Wicks, J.D. (1987) Third trimester ultrasonic presentation of infantile polycystic kidney disease. *American Journal of Perinatology*, **4**, 1–4.

Arizawa, M., Imai, S., Suehara, N. and Nakayama, M. (1989) Prenatal diagnosis of laryngeal atresia. *Nippon Sanka Fujinka Gakkai Zasshi*, **41**, 907–910.

Arnold, M.-L., Rauskolb, R., Anton-Lamprecht, I. et al. (1984) Prenatal diagnosis of anhidrotic ectodermal dysplasia. *Prenatal Diagnosis*, **4**, 85–98.

Auerbach, A.D., Min, Z., Ghosh, R. et al. (1986) Clastogen-induced chromosomal breakage as a marker for first trimester prenatal diagnosis of Fanconi anaemia. *Human Genetics*, **73**, 86–88.

Aula, P., Mattila, K., Piiroinen, O. et al. (1989) First-trimester prenatal diagnosis of aspartylglucosaminuria. *Prenatal Diagnosis*, **9**, 617–20.

Bachmann, C., Krahenbuhl, S., Colombo, J.P. et al. (1981) N-Acetylglutamate synthetase deficiency: a disorder of ammonia detoxification. *New England Journal of Medicine*, **304**, 543.

Bailey, W., Freidenberg, G.R., James, H.E. et al. (1990) Prenatal diagnosis of a craniopharyngioma using ultrasonography and magnetic resonance imaging. *Prenatal Diagnosis*, **10**, 623–29.

Bair, J.H., Russ, P.D., Pretorius, D.H. et al. (1986) Fetal omphalocele and gastroschisis: a review of 24 cases. *AJR*, **147**, 1047–1051.

Bakharev, V.A., Aivazyan, A.A., Karetnikova, N.A. et al. (1990) Fetal skin biopsy in prenatal diagnosis of some genodermatoses. *Prenatal Diagnosis*, **10**, 1–12.

Bakker, E., Bonten, E.J., Veenema, H. et al. (1989) Prenatal diagnosis of Duchenne muscular dystrophy: a three-year experience in a rapidly evolving field. *Journal of Inherited Metabolic Disease*, **12** (suppl. 1), 174–90.

Balci, S., Ercal, M.D., Onol, B. et al. (1991) Familial short rib syndrome, type Beemer, with pyloric stenosis and short intestine, one case diagnosed prenatally. *Clinical Genetics*, **39**, 298–303.

Bale, S.J., Bale, A.E., Stewart, K. et al. (1989) Linkage analysis of multiple endocrine neoplasia type I with INT2 and other markers on chromosome 11. *Genomics*, **4**, 320–322.

Ballabio, A., Carroxxo, R., Parenti, G. et al. (1989) Molecular heterogeneity of steroid sulfatase deficiency: a multicentre study on 57 unrelated patients at DNA and protein levels. *Genomics*, **4**, 36–40.

Barker, D.F., Hostikka, S.L., Zhou, J. et al. (1990) Identification of mutations in the COL4A5 collagen gene in Alport syndrome. *Science*, **248**, 1224–27.

Barr, Jr, M., Heidelberger, K.P. and Dorovini-Zis, K. (1986) Scalp neoplasm associated with cranium bifidum in a 24-week human fetus. *Teratology*, **33**, 153–57.

Barss, V.A., Benacerraf, B.R. and Frigoletto, F.D. (1985) Antenatal sonographic diagnosis of fetal gastrointestinal malformations. *Pediatrics*, **76**, 445–449.

Barth, R.A., Filly, R.A. and Sondheimer, F.K. (1990) Prenatal sonographic findings in bladder exstrophy. *Journal of Ultrasound in Medicine*, **9**, 359–61.

Bartley, J.A. and Gies, C.M. (1990) Prenatal diagnosis in X-linked myotubular myopathy (MTM1) with linkage to DXS52. *American Journal of Human Genetics*, **47**, A268.

Bass, H.N., Oliver, J.B., Srinivasan, M. et al. (1986) Persistently elevated AFP and AChE in amniotic fluid from a normal fetus following demise of its twin. *Prenatal Diagnosis*, **6**, 33–35.

Baty, B.J., Cubberley, D., Morris, C. and Carey, J. (1988) Prenatal diagnosis of distal arthrogryposis. *American Journal of Medical Genetics*, **29**, 501–10.

Baxi, L., Warren, W., Collins, M.H. and Timor-Tritsch, I.E. (1990) Early detection of caudal regression syndrome with transvaginal scanning. *Obstetrics and Gynecology*, **75**, 486–89.

Bellingham, A.J., Lestas, A.N., Williams, L.H.P. and Nicolaides, K.H. (1989) Prenatal diagnosis of a red cell enzymopathy: triose phosphate isomerase deficiency. *Lancet*, **ii**, 419–21.

Benacerraf, B.R. and Adzick, N.S. (1987) Fetal diaphragmatic hernia: ultrasound diagnosis and clinical outcome in 19 cases. *American Journal of Obstetrics and Gynecology*, **156**, 573–76.

Benacerraf, B.R. and Birnholz, J.C. (1987) The diagnosis of fetal hydrocephalus prior to 22 weeks. *JCU*, **15**, 531–36.

Benacerraf, B.R. and Frigoletto, F.D. (1987) Soft tissue nuchal fold in the second-trimester fetus: standards for normal measurements compared with those in Down syndrome. *American Journal of Obstetrics and Gynecology*, **157**, 1146–49.

Benacerraf, B.R. and Frigoletto, F.D. (1988) Prenatal ultrasonographic recognition of Goldenhar's syndrome. *American Journal of Obstetrics and Gynecology*, **159**, 950–52.

Benacerraf, B.R., Frigoletto, F.D. and Greene, M.F. (1986b) Abnormal facial features and extremities in human trisomy syndromes: prenatal UK appearance. *Radiology*, **159**, 243–46.

Benacerraf, B.R., Greene, M.F. and Barss, V.A. (1986a) Prenatal sonographic diagnosis of congenital hemivertebra. *Journal of Ultrasound in Medicine*, **5**, 257–59.

Benacerraf, B.R., Green, M.F. and Holmes, L.B. (1989b) The prenatal sonographic features of Noonan's syndrome. *Journal of Ultrasound in Medicine*, **8**, 59–63.

Benacerraf, B.R., Osathanondh, R. and Bieber, F.R. (1984) Achondrogenesis type I: ultrasound diagnosis *in utero*. *JCU*, **12**, 357–59.

Benacerraf, B.R., Saltzman, D.H. and Sanders, S.P. (1989a) Sonographic sign suggesting the prenatal diagnosis of coarctation of the aorta. *Journal of Ultrasound in Medicine*, **8**, 65–69.

Ben-Ami, A., Shalev, E., Romano, S. and Zuckerman, H. (1986) Mid-trimester diagnosis of endocardial fibroelastosis and atrial septal defect: a case report. *American Journal of Obstetrics and Gynecology*, **155**, 662–63.

Bennett, M.J., Allison, F., Lowther, G.W. et al. (1987) Prenatal diagnosis of medium-chain acyl coenzyme A dehydrogenase deficiency. *Prenatal Diagnosis*, **7**, 135–41.

Benson, C.B., Pober, B.R., Hirsh, M.P. and Doubilet, P.M. (1988) Sonography of Nager acrofacial dysostosis syndrome *in utero*. *Journal of Ultrasound in Medicine*, **7**, 163–67.

Benson, P.F. and Fensom, A.H. (1985) *Genetic Biochemical Disorders*, Oxford University Press, Oxford, p. 351.

Ben-Yoseph, Y., Mitchell, D.A. and Nadler, H.L. (1988) First trimester prenatal evaluation for I-cell disease by N-acetyl-glucosamine 1-phospho-transferase assay. *Clinical Genetics*, 33, 38–43.

Berkvens, T.M., Gerritsen, E.J.A., Oldenburg, M. *et al.* (1987) Severe combined immune deficiency due to a homozygous 3.2 kb deletion spanning the promoter and first axon of the adenosine deaminase gene. *Nucleic Acids Research*, 15, 9365–78.

Besley, G.T.N., Ferguson-Smith, M.E., Frew, C. *et al.* (1988) First trimester diagnosis of Gaucher disease in a fetus with trisomy 21. *Prenatal Diagnosis*, 8, 471–74.

Bick, D.P., Balkite, E.A., Baumgarten, A. *et al.* (1987) The association of congenital skin disorders with acetylcholinesterase in amniotic fluid. *Prenatal Diagnosis*, 7, 543–49.

Bidwell, J.K. and Nelson, A. (1986) Prenatal ultrasonic diagnosis of congenital duplication of the stomach. *Journal of Ultrasound in Medicine*, 5, 589–91.

Bignell, P., Standen, G.R., Bowen, D.J. *et al.* (1990) Rapid neonatal diagnosis of von Willebrand's disease by use of the polymerase chain reaction. *Lancet*, ii, 638–39.

Billimoria, J.D., Clemens, M.E., Gibberd, F.B. and Whitelaw, M.N. (1982) Metabolism of phytanic acid in Refsum's disease. *Lancet*, i, 194–96.

Blaakaer, J. (1986) Ultrasonic diagnosis of fetal ascites and toxoplasmosis. *Acta Obstetricia et Gynecologica Scandinavica*, 65, 633–38.

Blagowidow, N., Mennuti, M.T., Huff, D.S. *et al.* (1986) A possible X-linked lethal disorder characterised by brain, eye and urogenital malformations. *American Journal of Human Genetics*, 39, A53.

Blanchet-Bardon, C. and Dumez, Y. (1984) Prenatal diagnosis of harlequin fetus. *Journal of Dermatology*, 3, 225–28.

Blass, J.P. (1980) Pyruvate dehydrogenase deficiencies. In *Inherited Disorders of Carbohydrate Metabolism*, (eds D. Burman *et al.*) MTP Press, Lancaster, p. 293.

Bock, S.C. and Prochownik, E.V. (1987) Molecular genetic survey of 16 kindreds with hereditary antithrombin III deficiency. *Blood*, 70, 1273–78.

Bodmer, W.F., Bailey, C.J., Bodmer, J. *et al.* (1987) Localisation of the gene for familial adenomatous polyposis on chromosome 5. *Nature*, 328, 614–16.

Boomsa, J.H., Weemhoff, R.A. and Polman, H.A. (1982) Songraphic appearance of annular pancreas *in utero*: a case report. *Diagnostic Imaging*, 51, 288–290.

Borochowitz, Z., Jones, K.L., Silbey, R. *et al.* (1986) A distinct lethal neonatal chondrodysplasia with snail-like pelvis: Schneckenbecken dysplasia. *American Journal of Medical Genetics*, 25, 47–59.

Borresen, A.L., Hellerud, C., Moller, P. *et al.* (1987) Prenatal diagnosis of a glycerol kinase deficiency associated with a DNA deletion of the short arm of the X-chromosome. *Clinical Genetics*, 32, 254–59.

Boucher, M. and Yonekura, M.L. (1986) Perinatal listeriosis (early-onset): correlation of antenatal investigations and neonatal outcome. *Obstetrics and Gynecology*, 68, 593–97.

Boue, J., Oberle, I., Heilig, R. *et al.* (1985) First trimester prenatal diagnosis of adrenoleucodystrophy by determination of very long chain fatty acid levels and by linkage to a DNA probe. *Human Genetics*, 69, 253–54.

Bovicelli, L., Rizzo N., Orsini, L.F. and Calderoni, P. (1981) Ultrasonographic real-time diagnosis of fetal hydrothorax and lung hypoplasia. *JCU*, 9, 253–54.

Braunstein, G.D., Ziel, F.H., Allen, A. *et al.* (1976) Prenatal diagnosis of placental steroid sulfatase deficiency. *American Journal of Obstetrics and Gynecology*, 126, 716–19.

Brennan, J.N., Diwan, R.J., Rosen, M.G. and Bellon, E.M. (1982) Fetofetal tranfusion syndrome: a prenatal ultrasonographic diagnosis. *Radiology*, 143, 535–36.

Bridge, P.J., MacLeod, P.M. and Lillicrap, D.P. (1991) Carrier detection and prenatal diagnosis of Pelizaeus–Merzbacher disease using a combination of anonymous DNA polymorphisms and the proteolipid protein (PLP) gene cDNA. *American Journal of Medical Genetics*, 38, 616–21.

Brock, D.J.H. and Barron, L. (1991) First-trimester prenatal diagnosis of hypophosphatasia: experience with 16 cases. *Prenatal Diagnosis*, 11, 387–92.

Brock, D.J.H., Clarke, H.A.K. and Barron, L. (1988) Prenatal diagnosis of cystic fibrosis by microvillar enzyme assay on a sequence of 258 pregnancies. *Human Genetics*, 78, 271–75.

Brocker-Vriends, A.H.J.T., Briet, E., Kanhai, H.H.H. *et al.* (1988) First trimester prenatal diagnosis of haemophilia A: two years' experience. *Prenatal Diagnosis*, 8, 411–21.

Brons, J.T.J., Van der Harten, H.J., Van Geijn, H.P. *et al.* (1990) Prenatal ultrasonographic diagnosis of radial-ray reduction malformations. *Prenatal Diagnosis*, 10, 279–88.

Brons, J.T.J., van Geijn, H.P., Wladimiroff, J.W. *et al.* (1988a) Prenatal ultrasound diagnosis of the Holt–Oram syndrome. *Prenatal Diagnosis*, 8, 175–82.

Bronshtein, M. and Zimmer, E.Z. (1989) Transvaginal ultrasound diagnosis of fetal club feet at 13 weeks menstrual age. *JCU* 17, 518–20.

Brown, B.I. and Brown, D.H. (1989) Branching enzyme activity of cultured amniocytes and chorionic villi: prenatal testing for type IV glycogen storage disease. *American Journal of Human Genetics*, 44, 378–81.

Brown, D.L., Emerson, D.S., Shulman, L.P. and Carson, S.A. (1989) Sonographic diagnosis of omphalocele during 10th week of gestation. 153, 825–26.

Brown, J., Gunn, T.R., Mora, J.D. and Mok, P.M. (1986) The prenatal diagnosis of cardiomegaly due to tricuspid incompetence. *Pediatric Radiology*, 16, 440.

Brown, T.R., Lubahn, D.B., Wilson, E.M. *et al.* (1988) Deletion of the steroid-binding domain of the human androgen receptor gene in one family with complete androgen insensitivity syndrome: evidence for further genetic heterogeneity in this syndrome. *Proceedings of the National Academy of Sciences of the USA*, 85, 8151–55.

Bruinse, H.W., Sijmons, E.A. and Reuwer, P.J.H.M. (1989) Clinical value of screening for fetal growth retardation by Doopler ultrasound. *Journal of Ultrasound in Medicine*, 8, 207–209.

Bruno, M., Iskra, L., Dolfin, G. and Farina, D. (1988) Congenital pleural effusion: prenatal ultrasonic diagnosis and therapeutic management. *Prenatal Diagnosis*, 8, 157–59.

Buehler, B.A., Delimont, D., Van Waes, M. and Finnell, R.H. (1990) Prenatal prediction of risk of the fetal hydantoin syndrome. *New England Journal of Medicine*, 322, 1567–71.

Bui, T.H., Marsk, L., Eklof, D. and Theorell, K. (1984) Prenatal diagnosis of chondroectodermal dysplasia with fetoscopy. *Prenatal Diagnosis*, 4, 155–59.

Buiss-Liem, T.N., Ottenkamp, J., Meerman, R.H. and Verwey, R. (1987) The concurrence of fetal supraventricular tachycardia and obstruction of the foramen ovale. *Prenatal Diagnosis*, 7, 425–431.

Bundy, A.L., Saltzman, D.H., Pober, B. *et al.* (1986) Antenatal sonographic findings in trisomy 18. *Journal of Ultrasound in Medicine*, 5, 361–64.

Byrne, J.L.B., Ward, K., Kochenour, N.K. and Dolcourt, J.L. (1990) Prenatal sonographic diagnosis of fetal varicella syndrome. *American Journal of Human Genetics*, 47, A270.

Cacchio, M., Conti, M. and Plicchi, G. (1983) Anatomo-functional considerations and prenatal ultrasonic diagnosis of fetal cryptorchidism and hydrocele. *Minerva Ginecologica*, 35, 483–88.

Camaschella, C., Serra, A., Saglio, G. *et al.* (1988) Meiotic recombination in the beta globin gene cluster causing an error in prenatal diagnosis of beta thalassaemia. *Journal of Medical Genetics*, 25, 307–310.

Camera, G., Centa, A., Zucchinetti, P. *et al.* (1989) Osteopetrosis: description of 2 cases, non-familial of the fatal infantile form and of a case of the mild adult form. Impossibility of performing early prenatal diagnosis. *Pathologica*, 81, 617–25.

Campbell, S. and Pearce, J.M. (1983) The prenatal diagnosis of fetal structural anomalies by ultrasound. *Clinical Obstetrics and Gynecology*, 10, 475–506.

Campbell, S., Tsannatos, C. and Pearce, J.M. (1984) The prenatal diagnosis of Joubert's syndrome of familial agenesis of the cerebellar vermis. *Prenatal Diagnosis*, 4, 391–95.

Cao, A., Falchi, A.M., Tuveri, T. *et al.* (1986) Prenatal diagnosis of thalassaemia major by fetal blood analysis: experience with 1000 cases. *Prenatal Diagnosis*, 6, 159–67.

Carpenter, M.W., Abuelo, D. and Neave, C. (1986) Mid-trimester diagnosis of severe deforming osteogenesis imperfecta with autosomal dominant inheritance. *American Journal of Perinatology*, 3, 80–83.

Caspi, B., Gorbacz, S., Appelman, Z. and Elchalal, U. (1990) Antenatal diagnosis of diastematomyelia. *Journal of Clinical Ultrasound*, 18, 721–25.

Cayea, P.D., Bieber, F.R., Ross, M.J. *et al.* (1985) Sonographic findings in otocephaly (synotia). *Journal of Ultrasound in Medicine*, 4, 377–79.

Ceccherini, I., Lituania, M., Cordone, M.S. *et al.* (1989) Autosomal dominant polycystic kidney disease: prenatal diagnosis by DNA analysis and sonography at 14 weeks. *Prenatal Diagnosis*, 9, 751–58.

Chadefaux, B., Bonnefont, J.P., Rabier, D. *et al.* (1989) Potential for the prenatal diagnosis of hyperornithemia, hyperammonemia and homocitrulli-nuria syndrome. *American Journal of Medical Genetics*, 32, 264.

Chadefaux, B., Ceballos, I., Rabier, D. *et al.* (1990) Prenatal diagnosis of arginosuccinic aciduria by assay of arginosuccinate in amniotic fluid at the 12th week of gestation. *American Journal of Medical Genetics*, 35, 59.

Chalmers, R.A., Tracey, B.M., Mistry, J. *et al.* (1989) Prenatal diagnosis of 3-hydroxy-3-methylglutaric aciduria by GC–MS and enzymology on cultured amniocytes and chorionic villi. *Journal of Inherited Metabolic Disease*, 12, 283–85.

Chambers, J.E., Muir, B.B. and Bell, J.E. (1989) 'Bullet'-shaped head in fetuses with spina bifida: a pointer to the spinal lesion. 16, 25–28.

Chambers, S.E., Johnstone, F.D. and Laing, I.A. (1988) Ultrasound *in utero* diagnosis of choroid plexus haemorrhage. *British Journal of Obstetrics and Gynaecology*, 95, 1317–20.

Chatterjee, M.S., Bondoc, B. and Adhate, A. (1985) Prenatal diagnosis of occipital encephalocele. *American Journal of Obstetrics and Gynecology*, 153, 646–47.

Chen, H., Immken, L. and Lachman, R. (1984) Syndrome of multiple pterygia, camptodactyly, facial anomalies, hypoplastic lungs and heart, cystic hygroma and skeletal anomalies: delineation of a new entity and review of lethal forms of multiple pterygium syndrome. *American Journal of Medical Genetics*, 17, 809–26.

Chervenak, F.A., Berkowitz, R.L., Romero, R. *et al.* (1983) The diagnosis of fetal hydrocephalus. *American Journal of Obstetrics and Gynecology*, 147, 703–16.

Chervenak, F.A., Isaacson, G., Rosenberg, J.C. and Kardon, N.B. (1986) Antenatal diagnosis of frontal cephalocele in a fetus with atelosteogenesis. *Journal of Ultrasound in Medicine*, 5, 111–13.

Chervenak, F.A., Isaacson, G., Touloukian, R. *et al.* (1985) Diagnosis and management of fetal teratomas. *Obstetrics and Gynecology*, 66, 666–71.

Chervenak, F.A., Jeanty, P., Cantraine, F. *et al.* (1984a) The diagnosis of fetal microcephaly. *American Journal of Obstetrics and Gynecology*, 149, 512–17.

Chervenak, F.A., Tortora, M., Mayden, K. *et al.* (1984b) Antenatal diagnosis of median cleft face syndrome: sonographic demonstration of cleft lip and hypertelorism. *American Journal of Obstetrics and Gynecology*, 149, 94–97.

Chitayat, D., Hahm, S.Y.E., Marion, R.W. *et al.* (1987) Further delineation of the McKusick–Kaufman hydrometrocolpos–polydactyly syndrome. *American Journal of Diseases of Childhood*, 141, 1133–36.

Chitayat, D., Lao, A., Wilson, D. *et al.* (1988a) Prenatal diagnosis of asplenia/polysplenia syndrome. *American Journal of Obstetrics and Gynecology*, 158, 1085–87.

Chitayat, D., McGillivray, B.C., Diamant, S. *et al.* (1988b) Role of prenatal detection of cardiac tumours in the diagnosis of tuberous sclerosis – report of two cases. *Prenatal Diagnosis*, 8, 577–84.

Christensen, E. and Brandt, N.J. (1985) Prenatal diagnosis of 5,10-methylenetetrahydrofolate reductase deficiency. *New England Journal of Medicine*, 313, 50–51.

Chung, W.M. (1986) Antenatal detection of hepatic cyst. *JCU*, 14, 217–19.

Cicardi, M., Igarashi, T., Rosen, F.S. and Davis, A.E. (1987) Molecular basis for the deficiency of complement 1 in type I hereditary angioneurotic edema. *Journal of Clinical Investigation*, 79, 698–702.

Cidivalli, G., Yarkoni, S., Dar, H. and Kohn, G. (1983) Can infantile hereditary agranulocytosis be diagnosed prenatally? *Prenatal Diagnosis*, 3, 157–59.

Claiborne, A.K., Blocker, S.H., Martin, C.M. and McAllister, W.H. (1986) Prenatal and postnatal sonographic delineation of gastro-intestinal abnormalities in a case of the VATER syndrome. *Journal of Ultrasound in Medicine*, 5, 45–47.

Cobellis, G., Iannoto, P., Stabile, M. *et al.* (1988) Prenatal ultrasound diagnosis of macroglossia in the Wiedemann–Beckwith syndrome. *Prenatal Diagnosis*, 8, 79–81.

Colley, N. and Hooker, J.G. (1989) Prenatal diagnosis of pelvic kidney. *Prenatal Diagnosis*, 9, 361–63.

Collinge, J., Harding, A.E., Owen, F. *et al.* (1989) Diagnosis of Gerstmann–Straussler syndrome in familial dementia with prion protein gene analysis. *Lancet*, ii, 15–17.

Comstock, C.M. (1986) The antenatal diagnosis of diaphragmatic anomalies. *Journal of Ultrasound in Medicine*, 5, 391–96.

Connor, J.M., Connor, R.A.C., Sweet, E.M. *et al.* (1985) Lethal neonatal chondrodysplasias in the west of Scotland 1970–1983 with a description of a thanatophoric-like autosomal recessive disorder, Glasgow variant. *American Journal of Medical Genetics*, 22, 243–53.

Connor, J.M., Gatherer, D., Gray, F.C. *et al.* (1986) Assignment of the gene for dyskeratosis congenita to Xq28. *Human Genetics*, 72, 348–51.

Connor, J.M., Loughlin, S.A.R. and Whittle, M.J. (1987) First trimester prenatal exclusion of tuberous sclerosis. *Lancet*, i, 269.

Conradi, N.G., Uvebrandt, P., Hokegard, K.H. *et al.* (1989) First trimester diagnosis of juvenile neuronal ceroid lipofuscinosis by demonstration of finger-print inclusions in chorionic villi. *Prenatal Diagnosis*, 9, 283–87.

Constantine, G., McCormack, J., McHugo, J. and Fowlie, A. (1991) Prenatal diagnosis of severe osteogenesis imperfecta. *Prenatal Diagnosis*, 11, 103–10.

Cooper, C., Mahony, B.S., Bowie, J.D. and Pope II (1985) Prenatal ultrasound diagnosis of ambiguous genitalia. *Journal of Ultrasound in Medicine*, 4, 433–36.

Cordone, M., Lituania, M., Zampatti, C. *et al.* (1989) In utero ultrasonographic features of campomelic dysplasia. *Prenatal Diagnosis*, 9, 745–50.

Corney, G., Whitehouse, D.B., Hopkinson, D.A. *et al.* (1987) Prenatal diagnosis of alpha-1-antitrypsin deficiency by fetal blood sampling. *Prenatal Diagnosis*, 7, 101–108.

Corson, V.L., Sanders, R.C., Johnson Jr, T.R. and Winn, K.J. (1983) Mid-trimester fetal ultraasound: diagnostic dilemmas. *Prenatal Diagnosis*, 3, 47–51.

Corteville, J.E., Gray, D.L. and Crane, J.P. (1991) Congenital hydronephrosis: correlation of fetal ultrasonographic findings with infant outcome. *American Journal of Obstetrics and Gynecology*, 165, 384–88.

Crane, J.P. and Beaver, H.A. (1986) Mid-trimester sonographic diagnosis of mandibulofacial dysostosis. *American Journal of Medical Genetics*, 25, 251–55.

Cremers, F.P.M., Brunsmann, F., Van De Pol, T.J.R. *et al.* (1987) Deletion of the DXS16S locus in patients with classical choroideremia. *Clinical Genetics*, 32, 421–23.

Cremers, F.P.M., Van de Pol, D.J.R., Van Kerkhoff, P.M. *et al.* (1990) Cloning of a gene that is rearranged in patients with choroideremia. *Nature*, 347, 674–77.

Crowe, C., Jassani, M. and Dickerman, L. (1986) The prenatal diagnosis of the Walker–Warburg syndrome. *Prenatal Diagnosis*, 6, 177–85.

Cullen, M.T., Athanassiadis, A.P. and Romero, R. (1990) Prenatal diagnosis of anterior parietal encephalocele with transvaginal sonography. *Obstetrics and Gynecology*, 75, 489–91.

Curry, C.J.R., Carey, J.C., Holland, J.S. *et al.* (1987) Smith–Lemli–Opitz syndrome type II. Multiple congenital anomalies with male pseudohermaphroditism and frequent early lethality. *American Journal of Medical Genetics*, 26, 45–57.

Curtis, D., Blank, C.E., Parsons, M.A. and Hughes, H.N. (1989) Carrier detection and prenatal diagnosis in Norrie disease. *Prenatal Diagnosis*, 9, 735–40.

Cuthbertson, G., Weiner, C.P., Giller, R.H. and Grose, C. (1987) Prenatal diagnosis of second trimester congenital varicella syndrome by virus-specific immunoglobulin M. *Journal of Pediatrics*, 111, 592–95.

Cyr, D.R., Gunteroth, W.G., Nyberg, D.A. *et al.* (1988) Prenatal diagnosis of an intrapericardial teratoma. A cause for non-immune hydrops. *Journal of Ultrasound in Medicine*, 7, 87–90.

Daffos, F., Forestier, F., Capella-Pavlovsky, M. *et al.* (1988) Prenatal management of 746 pregnancies at risk for congenital toxoplasmosis. *New England Journal of Medicine*, 318, 271–75.

Daffos, F., Forestier, F., Mandelbrot, L. *et al.* (1989) Prenatal diagnosis of HIV infection: two attempts using fetal blood sampling. *Journal of Acquired Immune Deficiency Syndromes*, 2, 205–207.

Dahl, D.L., Warren, C.D., Rathke, E.J.S. and Jones, M.Z. (1986) Beta-mannosidosis: prenatal detection of caprine allantoic fluid oligosaccharides with thin layer, gel permeation and HPLC. *Journal of Inherited Metabolic Disease*, 9, 93–98.

Dahl, H.-H.M., Wake, S., Cotton, R.G.H. and Danks, D.M. (1988) The use of restriction fragment length polymorphisms in prenatal diagnosis of dihydropteridine reductase deficiency. *Journal of Medical Genetics*, 25, 25–28.

Daiger, S.P., Lidsky, A.S., Chakraborty, R. *et al.* (1986) Polymorphic DNA haplotypes at the phenylalanine hydroxylase locus in prenatal diagnosis of phenylketonuria. *Lancet*, i, 229–32.

Dallapiccola, B., Carbone, L.D.L., Ferranti, G. *et al.* (1985) Monitoring pregnancies at risk for Fanconi's anaemia by chorionic villi sampling. *Acta Haematologica (Basel)*, 73, 157–58.

Dallapiccola, B., Novelli, G., Cuoco, C. and Porro, E. (1987) First trimester studies of a fetus at risk for triose phosphate isomerase deficiency. *Prenatal Diagnosis*, 7, 289–94.

Dallapiccola, B., Novelli, G., Ferranti, G. *et al.* (1986) First trimester monitoring of a pregnancy at risk for glucose phosphate isomerase deficiency. *Prenatal Diagnosis*, 6, 101–107.

Danpure, C.J., Cooper, P.J., Jennings, P.R. *et al.* (1989) Enzymatic prenatal diagnosis of primary hyperoxaluria type I; potential and limitations. *Journal of Inherited Metabolic Disease*, 12 (suppl. 2), 286–88.

Danpure, C.J., Jennings, P.R. and Watts, R.W.E. (1987) Enzymological diagnosis of primary hyperoxaluria type I by measurement of hepatic alanine: glyoxylate aminotransferase activity. *Lancet*, i, 289–291.

Davies, R.P., Ford, W.D.A., Lequesne, G.W. and Orell, S.R. (1989) Ultrasonic detection of subdiaphragmatic pulmonary sequestration in utero and post-natal diagnosis by fine needle aspiration biopsy. *Journal of Ultrasound in Medicine*, 8, 47–49.

Davis, W.K., Mahony, B.S., Carroll, B.A. and Bowie, J.D. (1987) Antenatal sonographic detection of benign dacrocystoceles (lacrimal duct cysts). *Journal of Ultrasound in Medicine*, 6, 461–65.

De Elejalde, M.M. and Elejalde, B.R. (1984) Visualisation of the fetal face by ultrasound. *Journal of Craniofacial Genetics and Developmental Biology*, 4, 251–57.

De Filippi, G., Canestri, G. Bosio, U. *et al.* (1986) Thoracic neuroblastoma: antenatal detection in a case with unusual postnatal radiographic findings. *British Journal of Radiology*, 59, 704–706.

De Lange, M. and Rouse, G.A. (1990) Prenatal diagnosis of hypophosphatasia. *Journal of Ultrasound in Medicine*, 9, 115–17.

Dembure, P.P., Priest, J.H., Snoddy, S.C. and Elsas, L.J. (1984) Genotyping and prenatal assessment of collagen lysyl hydroxylase deficiency in a family with Ehlers–Danlos syndrome type VI. *American Journal of Human Genetics*, 36, 783–790.

Denholm, T.A., Crow, H.C., Edwards, W.H. *et al.* (1984) Prenatal sonographic appearance of meconium ileus in twins. *AJR*, 143, 371–372.

Derosa, R., Lenke, R.R., Kurczynski, T.W. *et al.* In utero diagnosis of benign fetal macrocephaly. *American Journal of Obstetrics and Gynecology*, 161, 690–92.

Desjacques, P., Mousson, B., Vianey-Ziaud, C. *et al.* (1985) Combined deficiency of xanthine oxidase and sulphite oxidase: a diagnosis of a new case followed by an antenatal diagnosis. *Journal of Inherited Metabolic Disease*, 8 (suppl.2), 117–18.

Deter, R.L., Rossavik, I.K. and Carpenter, R.J. (1989) Development of individual growth standards for estimated fetal weight: II. Weight prediction during the third trimester and at birth. *JCU*, 17, 83–88.

De Vita, G., Alcalay, M., Sampietro, M. *et al.* (1989) Two point mutations are responsible for G6PD polymorphism in Sardinia. *American Journal of Human Genetics*, 44, 233–40.

De Vore, G.R. and Hobbins, J.C. (1979) Diagnosis of structural abnormalities in the fetus. *Clinical Perinatology*, 6, 293–319.

De Vore, G.R., Siassi, B. and Platt, L.D. (1987) Fetal echocardiography: the prenatal diagnosis of tricuspid atresia (type 1c) during the second trimester of pregnancy. *JCU*, 15, 317–24.

Dhermy, D., Feo, C., Garbarz, M. *et al.* (1987) Prenatal diagnosis of hereditary elliptocytosis with molecular defect of spectrum. *Prenatal Diagnosis*, 7, 471–83.

Dhonot, J.L., Tilmont, P., Ringel, J. and Farriaux, J.P. (1990) Pterins analysis in amniotic fluid for the prenatal diagnosis of GTP cyclohydrolase deficiency. *Journal of Inherited Metabolic Disease*, 13, 879–82.

Dietz, H.C., Cutting, G.R., Pyeritz, R.E. *et al.* (1991) Marfan syndrome caused by a recurrent *de novo* missense mutation in the fibrillin gene. *Nature*, 352, 337–39.

Di Ferrante, N., Leachman, R.D., Angelini, P. *et al.* (1975) Lysyl oxidase deficiency in Ehlers–Danlos syndrome type V. *Connective Tissue Research*, 3, 49–53.

Di Natale, P., Pannone, N., D'Argenio, G. *et al.* (1987) First trimester prenatal diagnosis of Sanfilippo C disease. *Prenatal Diagnosis*, 7, 603–605.

Donnai, P., Donnai, D., Harris, R. *et al.* (1981) Antenatal diagnosis of Niemann–Pick disease in a twin pregnancy. *Journal of Medical Genetics*, 18, 359–61.

Donnenfeld, A.E., Gussman, D., Mennuti, M.T. and Zackai, E.H. (1986) Evaluation of an unknown fetal skeletal dysplasia: prenatal findings in hypochondrogenesis. *American Journal of Human Genetics*, 39, A252.

Donnenfeld, A.E. and Mennuti, M.I. (1987) Second trimester diagnosis of fetal skeletal dysplasias. *Obstetrics and Gynecology Survey*, 42, 199–217.

Donnenfeld, A.E., Mennuti, M.T., Templeton, J.M. and Gabbe, G.G. (1989) Prenatal diagnosis of a vesico-allantoic abdominal wall defect. *Journal of Ultrasound in Medicine*, 8, 43–45.

Donnenfeld, A.E., Wiseman, B., Lavi, E. and Weiner, S. (1990) Prenatal diagnosis of thrombocytopenia–absent radius syndrome by ultrasound and cordocentesis. *Prenatal Diagnosis*, 10, 29–35.

Dooley, T., Fairbanks, L.D., Simmonds, H.A. *et al.* (1987) First trimester diagnosis of adenosine deaminase deficiency. *Prenatal Diagnosis*, 7, 561–65.

Dreazen, E., Tessler, F., Sarti, D. and Crandall, B.F. (1989) Spontaneous resolution of fetal hydrocephalus. *Journal of Ultrasound in Medicine*, 8, 155–57.

Driscoll, D.A., Budarf, M.L. and Emanuel, B.S. (1991) Antenatal diagnosis of DiGeorge syndrome. *Lancet*, 338, 1390–91.

Duff, P., Harlass, F.E. and Milligan, D.A. (1990) Prenatal diagnosis of chondrodysplasia punctata by sonography. *Obstetrics and Gynecology*, 76, 497–500.

Dunn, V. and Glasier, C.M. (1985) Ultrasonographic antenatal demonstration of primary megaureters. *Journal of Ultrasound in Medicine*, 4, 101–103.

Duran, M., Schutgens, R.B.H., Ketel, A. *et al.* (1979) 3-Hydroxy-3-methylglutaryl coenzyme A lyase deficiency: postnatal management following prenatal diagnosis by analysis of maternal urine. *Journal of Pediatrics*, 95, 1004–1007.

Durandy, A., Cerf-Bensussan, N., Dumez, Y. and Griscelli, C. (1987) Prenatal diagnosis of severe combined immunodeficiency with defective synthesis of HLA molecules. *Prenatal Diagnosis*, 7, 27–34.

Durandy, A., Griscelli, G., Dumez, Y. *et al.* (1982a) Antenatal diagnosis of severe combined immunodeficiency from fetal cord blood. *Lancet*, 7, 852–53.

Durandy, A., Dury, C., Griscelli, C. *et al.* (1982b) Prenatal testing for inherited immune deficiencies by fetal blood sampling. *Prenatal Diagnosis*, 2, 109–13.

Eady, R.A.J., Gunner, D.B., Carbone, L.D.L. *et al.* (1986) Prenatal diagnosis of bullous ichthyosiform erythroderma: detection of tonofilament clumps in fetal epidermal and amniotic fluid cells. *Journal of Medical Genetics*, 23, 46–51.

Eady, R.A.J., Gunner, D.B., Garner, A. and Rodeck, C.H. (1983) Prenatal diagnosis of oculocutaneous albinism by electron microscopy of fetal skin. *Journal of Investigative Dermatology*, 80, 210–12.

Eady, R.A.J., Schofield, O.M.V., Nicolaides, K.H. and Rodeck, C.H. (1989) Prenatal diagnosis of junctional epidermolysis bullosa. *Lancet*, ii, 1453.

Elder, G.H., Evans, J.O., Thomas, N. *et al.* (1976) The primary enzyme defect in hereditary coproporphyria. *Lancet*, ii, 1217–19.

Elejalde, B.R., De Elejalde, M.M., Booth, C. *et al.* (1983) Prenatal diagnosis of Weyers syndrome (deficient ulnar and fibular rays with bilateral hydronephrosis). *American Journal of Medical Genetics*, 21, 439–44.

Elejalde, B.R., De Elejalde, M.M. and Pansch, D. (1985) Prenatal diagnosis of Jeune syndrome. *American Journal of Medical Genetics*, 21, 433–38.

El Khazen, N., Faverley, D., Vamos, E. *et al.* (1986) Lethal osteopetrosis with multiple fractures *in utero*. *American Journal of Medical Genetics*, 23, 811–19.

Elrad, H., Mayden, K.L., Ahart, S. *et al.* (1985) Prenatal diagnosis of choledochal cyst. *Journal of Ultrasound in Medicine*, 4, 553–55.

Endo, F., Tanoue, A., Kitano, A. *et al.* (1990) Biochemical basis of prolidase deficiency: polypeptide acid RNA phenotypes and relation to clinical phenotypes. *Journal of Clinical Investigation*, 85, 162–69.

Evans, M.I., Greb, A., Kunkel, L.M. *et al.* (1991) *In utero* fetal muscle biopsy for the diagnosis of Duchenne muscular dystrophy. *American Journal of Obstetrics and Gynecology*, 165, 728–32.

Evans, M.I., Zador, I.E., Qureshi, F. *et al.* (1988) Ultrasonographic prenatal diagnosis and fetal pathology of Langer mesomelic dwarfism. *American Journal of Medical Genetics*, 31, 915–20.

Farrell, S.A., Toi, A., Leadman, M.L. *et al.* (1987) Prenatal diagnosis of retinal detachment in Walker–Warburg syndrome. *American Journal of Medical Genetics*, 28, 619–24.

Feldman, E., Shalev, E., Weiner, E. *et al.* (1985) Microphthalmia – prenatal ultrasonic diagnosis: a case report. *Prenatal Diagnosis*, 5, 205–207.

Feldman, G.L., Lewiston, N., Fernbach, S.D. *et al.* (1989) Prenatal diagnosis of cystic fibrosis by any linked DNA markers in 138 pregnancies at 1 in 4 risk. *American Journal of Medical Genetics*, 32, 238–41.

Fellous, M., Boue, J., Malbrunot, C. *et al.* (1982) A five-generation family with sacral agenesis and spina bifida: possible similarities with the mouse T-locus. *American Journal of Medical Genetics*, 12, 465–87.

Fensom, A.H., Benson, P.F. and Baker, J.E. (1978) A rapid method for assay of branched-chain ketoacid decarboxylation in cultured cells and its application to prenatal diagnosis of maple syrup urine disease. *Clinica Chimica Acta*, 87, 169–74.

Fensom, A.H., Benson, P.F., Crees, M.J. *et al.* (1983) Prenatal exclusion of homocystinuria (cystathionine beta-synthase deficiency) by assay of phytohaemagglutinin-stimulated fetal lymphocytes. *Prenatal Diagnosis*, 3, 127–30.

Fensom, A.H., Benson, P.F., Neville, B.R.G. *et al.* (1979) Prenatal diagnosis of Farber's disease. *Lancet*, ii, 990–92.

Ferraro, E.M., Fakhry, J., Aruny, J.E. and Bracero, L.A. (1988) Prenatal adrenal neuroblastoma. Case report with review of the literature. *Journal of Ultrasound in Medicine*, 7, 275–78.

Filkins, K., Russo, J., Bilinki, I. *et al.* (1984) Prenatal diagnosis of thrombocytopenia–absent radius syndrome using ultrasound and fetoscopy. *Prenatal Diagnosis*, 4, 139–42.

Filly, R.A., Goldstein, R.B. and Callen, P.W. (1990) Monochorionic twinning: sonographic assessment. *AJR*, 154, 459–69.

Fine, J.D., Eady, R.A.J., Levy, M.L. *et al.* (1988) Prenatal diagnosis of dominant and recessive dystrophic epidermolysis bullosa: application and limitations in the use of KF-1 and LH 7:2 monoclonal antibodies and immunofluorescence techniques. *Journal of Investigative Dermatology*, 91, 465–471.

Fine, J.D., Holbrook, K.A., Elias, S. *et al.* (1990) Applicability of 19-DEJ-1 monoclonal antibody for the prenatal diagnosis or exclusion of junctional epidermolysis bullosa. *Prenatal Diagnosis*, 10, 219–29.

Fink, I.J. and Filly, R.A. (1983) Omphalocele associated with umbilical cord allantoic cyst: sonographic evaluation *in utero*. *Radiology*, 149, 473–76.

Firgaira, F.A., Cotton, R.G.H., Danks, D.M. *et al.* (1983) Prenatal determination of dihydropteridine reductase in a normal fetus at risk for malignant hyperphenylalanemia. *Prenatal Diagnosis*, 3, 7–11.

Fischbeck, K.H., Ionasecu, V., Ritter, A.W. *et al.* (1986) Localisation of the gene for X-linked spinal muscular atrophy. *Neurology*, 36, 1595–98.

Fisk, N.M., Dhillon, H.K., Ellis, C.E. *et al.* (1990) Antenatal diagnosis of megalourethra in a fetus with the prune belly syndrome. *JCU*, 18, 124–28.

Fitzgerald, E.J. and Toi, A. (1986) Antenatal ultrasound diagnosis of cystic adenomatoid malformation of the lung. *Journal of the Canadian Association of Radiology*, 37, 48–49.

Fitzmorris-Glass, R., Mattrey, R.F. and Cantrell, C.J. (1989) Magnetic resonance imaging as an adjunct to ultrasound in odigohydramnios. Detection of sirenomelia. *Journal of Ultrasound in Medicine*, 8, 159–62.

Fitzsimons, P.J., Frost, R.A., Millward, S. *et al.* (1986) Prenatal and immediate postnatal ultrasonographic diagnosis of ureterocele. *Journal of the Canadian Association of Radiology*, 337, 189–191.

Fleisher, L.D., Rassin, D.K., Desnick, R.J. *et al.* (1979) Argininosuccinicaciduria: prenatal studies in a family at risk. *American Journal of Human Genetics*, 31, 439–45.

Fletman, D., McQuown, D., Kanchanapoom, V. and Gyepes, M.T. (1980) 'Apple peel' atresia of the small bowel: prenatal diagnosis of the obstruction by ultrasound. *Pediatric Radiology*, 9, 118–19.

Foderaro, A.E., Abu-Yousef, M.M., Benda, J.A. *et al.* (1987) Antenatal ultrasound diagnosis of iniencephaly. *JCU*, 15, 550–54.

Fogarty, K., Cohen, H.L. and Haller, J.O. (1989) Sonography of fetal intracranial hemorrhage: unusual causes and a review of the literature. *JCU*, 17, 366–70.

Forestier, F., Daffos, F., Sole, Y. and Rainaut, M. (1986) Prenatal diagnosis of haemophilia by fetal blood sampling under ultrasound guidance. *Haemostasis*, 16, 346–51.

Foucar, E., Williamson, R.A., Yiu-Chiu, V. *et al.* (1983) Mesenchymal hamartoma of the liver identified by fetal sonography. *AJR*, 140, 970–72.

Foulon, W., Naessens, A., Mahler, T. *et al.* (1990) Prenatal diagnosis of congenital toxoplasmosis. *Obstetrics and Gynecology*, 76, 769–72.

Fowler, B., Borresen, A.L. and Boman, N. (1982) Prenatal diagnosis of homocystinuria. *Lancet*, ii, 875.

Fowler, B., Giles, L., Sardharwalla, I.B. *et al.* (1988) First trimester diagnosis of methylmalonic aciduria. *Prenatal Diagnosis*, 8, 207–13.

Fraser, W.D., Nimrod, C., Nicholson, S. and Harder, J. (1989) Antenatal diagnosis of restriction of the foremen ovale. *Journal of Ultrasound in Medicine*, 8, 281–83.

Friedman, J.M. and Santos-Ramos, R. (1984) Natural history of X-linked aqueductal stenosis in the second and third trimesters of pregnancy. *American Journal of Obstetrics and Gynecology*, 150, 104–106.

Fukuda, M.N., Dell, A. and Scartezzini, P. (1987) Primary defect of congenital dyserythropoietic anaemia type II: failure of glycosylation of erythrocyte lactosaminoglycan proteins caused by lowered N-acetylglucosaminyl transferase II. *Journal of Biological Chemistry*, **262**, 7195–206.

Gabrielli, S., Reece, E.A., Pilu, G. *et al.* (1989) The clinical significance of prenatally diagnosed choroid plexus cysts. *American Journal of Obstetrics and Gynecology*, **160**, 1207–10.

Gagne, R., Lescault, A., Grenier, A. *et al.* (1982) Prenatal diagnosis of hereditary tyrosinaemia: measurement of succinylacetone in amniotic fluid. *Prenatal Diagnosis*, **2**, 185–88.

Gal, A., Uhlhass, S., Glaser, D. and Grimm, T. (1988) Prenatal exclusion of Norrie disease with flanking DNA markers. *American Journal of Medical Genetics*, **31**, 449–53.

Gamble, C.N., Hershey, D.W. and Schaeffer, C.J. (1990) Femoral–facial syndrome detected in prenatal ultrasound. *American Journal of Human Genetics*, **47**, 274.

Garber, A., Shohat, M. and Sarti, D. (1990) Megacystis–microcolon–intestinal hypoperistalsis syndrome in two male siblings. *Prenatal Diagnosis*, **10**, 377–88.

Garcia-Munoz, M.J., Belloque, J., Merinero, B. *et al.* (1989) Non-ketotic hyperglycinaemia: glycine/serine ratio in amniotic fluid – an unreliable method for prenatal diagnosis. *Prenatal Diagnosis*, **9**, 473–76.

Gardiner, R.M., Sandford, A., Deadman, M. *et al.* (1990) Batten disease (Spielmeyer–Vogt; juvenile onset neuronal ceroid lipofuscinosis) maps to human chromosome 16. *Genomics*, **8**, 387–90.

Gatti, R.A., Berkel, I., Boder, E. *et al.* (1988) Localisation of an ataxia-telangiectasia gene to chromosome 11q22–23. *Nature*, **336**, 577–580.

Gatti, R., Lombardo, C., Filocamo, M. *et al.* (1985) Comparative study of 15 lysosomal enzymes in chorionic villi and cultured amniotic fluid cells. Early PND in seven pregnancies at risk for lysosomal storage diseases. *Prenatal Diagnosis*, **5**, 329–36.

Gazit, E., Brand, N., Harel, Y. *et al.* (1990) Prenatal diagnosis of Lowe's syndrome: a case report with evidence of *de novo* mutation. *Prenatal Diagnosis*, **10**, 257–60.

Gebhardt, D.O. (1979) Prenatal detection of Tangier disease. *Lancet*, **ii**, 754–55.

Gellert, G., Petersen, J., Krawczak, M. and Zoll, B. (1988) Linkage relationship between retinoschisis and four marker loci. *Human Genetics*, **79**, 382–84.

Gembruch, U., Chatterjee, M., Bald, R. *et al.* (1990b) Prenatal diagnosis of aortic atresia by colour Doppler flow mapping. *Prenatal Diagnosis*, **10**, 211–18.

Gembruch, U., Hansmann, M. and Fodisch, H.J. (1985) Early prenatal diagnosis of short rib–polydactyly (SRP) syndrome type II (Majewski) by ultrasound in a case at risk. *Prenatal Diagnosis*, **5**, 357–62.

Gembruch, U., Knople, G., Chatterjee, M. *et al.* (1990a) First-trimester diagnosis of fetal congenital heart disease by transvaginal two-dimensional and Doppler echocardiography. *Obstetrics and Gynecology*, **75**, 496–98.

Gembruch, U., Niesen, M., Kehrberg, G. and Hansmann, M. (1988) Diastrophic dysplasia: a specific prenatal diagnosis by ultrasound. *Prenatal Diagnosis*, **8**, 539–46.

Gembruch, U., Steil, E. Redel, D.A. and Hansmann, M. (1990c) Prenatal diagnosis of a left ventricular aneurysm. *Prenatal Diagnosis*, **10**, 203–209.

Gembruch, U., Steil, E. Redel, D.A. and Hansmann, M. (1990c) Prenatal diagnosis of a left ventricular aneurysm. *Prenatal Diagnosis*, **10**, 203–209.

Genkins, S.M., Hertzberg, B.S., Bowie, J.D. and Blow, O. (1989) Pena–Shokeir type I syndrome: *in utero* sonographic appearance. **17**, 56–61.

Geraghty, A.V., Knott, P.O. and Hanna, H.M. (1989) Prenatal diagnosis of fetal glioblastoma multiforme. *Prenatal Diagnosis*, **9**, 613–16.

Ghidini, A., Romero, R., Eisen, R.N. *et al.* (1990) Umbilical cord haemangioma. Prenatal identification and review of the literature. *Journal of Ultrasound in Medicine*, **9**, 297–300.

Ghidini, A., Sirtori, M., Romero, R. and Hobbins, J.C. (1988) Prenatal diagnosis of pentalogy of Cantrell. *Journal of Ultrasound in Medicine*, **7**, 567–72.

Ghidini, A., Sirtori, M., Vergani, P. *et al.* (1989) Fetal intracranial calcification. *American Journal of Obstetrics and Gynecology*, **160**, 86–87.

Ghidini, A., Vergani, P., Sirtori, M. *et al.* (1988) Prenatal diagnosis of subdural hygroma. *Journal of Ultrasound in Medicine*, **7**, 463–65.

Gibbs, D.A., Headhouse-Benson, C.M. and Watts, R.W.E. (1986) Family studies of the Lesch–Nyhan syndrome: the use of a restriction fragment length polymorphism (RFLP) closely linked to the disease gene for carrier state and prenatal diagnosis. *Journal of Inherited Metabolic Disease*, **9**, 45–57.

Giles, L., Cooper, A., Fowler, B. *et al.* (1987) Krabbe's disease: first trimester diagnosis confirmed on cultured amniotic fluid cells and fetal tissues. *Prenatal Diagnosis*, **7**, 329–32.

Giles, L., Cooper, A., Fowler, B. *et al.* (1988) First trimester prenatal diagnosis of Sandhoff's disease. *Prenatal Diagnosis*, **8**, 199–205.

Gillett, M.G., Holton, J.B. and MacFaul, R. (1983) Prenatal determination of uridine diphosphate galactose-4-epimerase activity. *Prenatal Diagnosis*, **3**, 57–59.

Gilliam, T.C., Brzustowicz, L.M., Castilla, L.H. *et al.* (1990) Genetic homogeneity between acute and chronic forms of spinal muscular atrophy. *Nature*, **345**, 823–25.

Glenn, L.W. and Teng, S.S.K. (1985) *In utero* sonographic diagnosis of achondrogenesis. *JCU*, **13**, 195–98.

Glick, P.L., Harrison, M.R. and Filly, R.A. (1983) Antepartum diagnosis of meconium peritonitis. *New England Journal of Medicine*, **309**, 1392.

Godfrey, M., Menashe, V., Weleber, R.G. *et al.* (1990) Cosegregation of elastin-associated microfibrillar abnormalities with the Marfan phenotype in families. *American Journal of Human Genetics*, **46**, 652–60.

Golbus, M.J., Sagebiel, R.W., Filly, R.A. *et al.* (1980) Prenatal diagnosis of congenital bullous ichthyosiform erythroderma (epidermolytic hyperkeratosis) by fetal skin biopsy. *New England Journal of Medicine*, **302**, 93–95.

Golbus, M.S., Simpson, T.J., Koresawa, M. *et al.* (1988) The prenatal determination of glucose-6-phosphatase activity by fetal liver biopsy. *Prenatal Diagnosis*, **8**, 401–404.

Goldstein, R.B., Filly, R.A. and Callen, P.W. (1989) Sonography of anencephaly: pitfalls in early diagnosis. *JCU*, **17**, 397–402.

Gollop, T.R., Eigier, A. and Neto, J.G. (1987) Prenatal diagnosis of thalidomide syndrome. *Prenatal Diagnosis*, **7**, 295–98.

Goodship, J., Levinsky, R. and Malcolm, S. (1989) Linkage of PGK1 to X-linked severe combined immunodeficiency (IMD4) allows predictive testing in families with no surviving male. *Human Genetics*, **84**, 11–14.

Goonewardena, P., Sjoholm, A.G., Nilsson, L.A. and Pettersson, V. (1988) Linkage analysis of the properdin deficiency gene: suggestion of a locus in the proximal part of the short arm of the X chromosome. *Genomics*, **2**, 115–18.

Gorczyca, D.P., McGahan, J.P., Lindfors, K.K. *et al.* (1989) Arthrogryposis multiplex congenita: prenatal ultrasonographic diagnosis. *JCU*, **17**, 40–44.

Gotoh, T., Adachi, Y., Nounaka, O. *et al.* (1989) Adrenal hemorrhage in the newborn with evidence of bleeding *in utero*. *Journal of Urology*, **141**, 1145–47.

Gottesfeld, K.R. (1978) Ultrasound in obstetrics. *Clinical Obstetrics and Gynecology*, **21**, 311–27.

Graham M. (1985) Congenital short femur: prenatal sonographic diagnosis. *Journal of Ultrasound in Medicine*, **4**, 361–63.

Grange, D.K., Lewis, M.B. and Marini, J.C. (1990) Analysis of cultured chorionic villi in a case of osteogenesis imperfecta type II: implications for prenatal diagnosis. *American Journal of Medical Genetics*, **36**, 258–64.

Gray, D.L., Martin, C.M. and Crane, J.P. (1989) Differential diagnosis of first trimester ventral wall defect. *Journal of Ultrasound in Medicine*, **8**, 255–58.

Gray, R.G.F., Green, A., Basu, S.N. *et al.* (1990) Antenatal diagnosis of molybdenum cofactor deficiency. *American Journal of Obstetrics and Gynecology*, **163**, 1203–204.

Grebner, E.E. and Jackson, L.G. (1979) Prenatal diagnosis of Tay–Sachs disease: reliability of amniotic fluid. *American Journal of Obstetrics and Gynecology*, **134**, 547–50.

Grebner, E.E. and Jackson, L.G. (1985) Prenatal diagnosis for Tay–Sachs disease using chorionic villus sampling. *Prenatal Diagnosis*, **5**, 313–20.

Greenberg, C.R., Hevenen, C.L. and Evans, J.A. (1988) The BOR syndrome and renal agenesis – prenatal diagnosis and further clinical delineation. *Prenatal Diagnosis*, **8**, 103–108.

Greenblatt, A.M., Beretsky, I., Lankin, D.H. and Phelan, L. (1985) *In utero* diagnosis of crossed renal ectopia using high-resolution real-time ultrasound. *Journal of Ultrasound in Medicine*, **4**, 105–107.

Grignon, A., Filiatrault, D., and Homsy, Y. *et al.* (1986b) Ureteropelvic junction stenosis: antenatal ultrasonographic diagnosis, postnatal investigation and follow-up. *Radiology*, **160**, 649–51.

Grignon, A., Filion, R., Filiatrault, D. *et al.* (1986a) Urinary tract dilatation *in utero*: classification and clinical applications. *Radiology*, **160**, 645–47.

Gross, S.J., Benzie, R.J., Sermer, M. *et al.* (1987) Sacrococcygeal teratoma: prenatal diagnosis and management. *American Journal of Obstetrics and Gynecology*, **156**, 393–96.

Gruel, Y., Boizard, B., Daffos, F. *et al.* (1986) Determination of platelet antigens and glycoprotein in the human fetus. *Blood*, **68**, 488–92.

Grundy, H., Glasmann, A., Burlbaw, J. *et al.* (1985) Hemangioma presenting as a cystic mass in the fetal neck. *Journal of Ultrasound in Medicine*, **4**, 147–50.

Guigliani, R., Jackson, M., Skinner, S.J. *et al.* (1987) Progressive mental retardation in siblings with Morquio disease type B (mucopolysaccharidosis IVB). *Clinical Genetics*, **32**, 313–25.

Guzman, E.R. (1990) Early prenatal diagnosis of gastroschisis with transvaginal sonography. *American Journal of Obstetrics and Gynecology*, **162**, 1253–54.

Hadi, H.A., Mashini, I.S., Devoe, L.D. *et al.* (1986) Ultrasonographic prenatal diagnosis of hydranencephaly. A case report. *Journal of Reproductive Medicine*, **31**, 254–56.

Haeusler, M.C.H., Hofmann, H.M.H., Hoenigl, W. *et al.* (1990) Congenital generalised cystic lymphangiomatosis diagnosed by prenatal ultrasound. *Prenatal Diagnosis*, **10**, 617–21.

Hahnel R., Hahnel, E., Wysocki, S.J. *et al.* (1982) Prenatal diagnosis of X-linked ichthyosis. *Clinica Chimica Acta*, **120**, 143–52.

Halley, D.J.J., Kleijler, W., Jaspers, N.G.J. *et al.* (1979) Prenatal diagnosis of xeroderma pigmentosum (group C) using assays of unscheduled DNA synthesis and post replication repair. *Clinical Genetics*, 16, 137–46

Hanauer, A., Alembik, Y., Gilgenkrantz, S. *et al.* (1988) Probable localisation of the Coffin–Lowry locus in Xp22.2–p22.1 by multipoint linkage analysis. *American Journal of Medical Genetics*, 30, 523–30.

Harper, A.K., Clark, J.A. and Koontz, W.L. and Holmes, M. (1989) Sonegraphic appearance of fetal extracranial hematoma. *Journal of Ultrasound in Medicine*, 8, 693–95.

Hartikainen-Sorri, A.L., Kirkinen, P. and Herva, R. (1983) Prenatal detection of hydrolethalus syndrome. *Prenatal Diagnosis*, 3, 219–24.

Harzer, K., Hager, H.-D. and Tariverdian, G. (1987) Prenatal enzymatic diagnosis and exclusion of Krabbe's disease (globoid cell leucodystrophy) using chorionic villi in five risk pregnancies. *Human Genetics*, 77, 342–44.

Harzer, K., Schlote, W., Peiffer, J. *et al.* (1978) Neurovisceral lipidosis compatible with Niemann–pick disease type C: morphological and biochemical studies of a later infantile case and enzyme and lipid assays in a prenatal case of the same family. *Acta Neuropathologica*, 43, 97–104.

Hastbacka, J., Kaitila, I., Sistonen, P. and de la Chapelle, A. (1990) Diastrophic dysplasia gene maps to the distal long arm of chromosome 5. *Proceedings of the National Academy of Sciences*, 87, 8056–59

Hatjis, C.G., Philip, A.G., Anderson, G.G. and Mann, L.I. (1981) The *in utero* ultrasonographic appearance of Klippel–Trenaunay–Weber syndrome. *American Journal of Obstetrics and Gynecology*, 139, 972–74.

Hayasaka, K., Tada, K., Fueki, N. and Aikawa, J. (1990) Prenatal diagnosis of nonketotic hyperglycinemia. Enzymatic analysis of the glycine cleavage system in chorionic villi. *Journal of Pediatrics*, 116, 444–45.

Hayden, M.R., Hewitt, J, Kastelein, J.J.P. *et al.* (1987) First-trimester prenatal diagnosis for Huntington's disease with DNA probes. *Lancet*, i, 1284–85.

Hayden, S.A., Russ, P.D., Pretorius, D.H. *et al.* (1988) Posterior urethral obstruction. Prenatal sonographic findings and clinical outcome in fourteen cases. *Journal of Ultrasound in Medicine*, 7, 371–75.

Hayes, M.E. and Robertson, E. (1981) Can oculocutaneous albinism be diagnosed prenatally? *Prenatal Diagnosis*, 1, 85–89.

Heagerty, A.H.M., Kennedy, A.R., Gunner, D.B. and Eady, R.A.J. (1986) Rapid prenatal diagnosis and exclusion of epidermolysis bullosa using novel antibody probes. *Journal of Investigative Dermatology*, 86, 603–605.

Heijne, L. *et al.* (1985) The development of fetal gallstones demonstrated by ultrasound. *Radiography*, 51, 155–56.

Hejtmancik, J.F., Holcomb, J.D., Howard, J. and Vanderford, M. (1989) *In vitro* amplification of the alpha-1-antitrypsin gene: application to prenatal diagnosis. *Prenatal Diagnosis*, 9, 177–86.

Hendricks, S.K., Cyr, D.R., Nyberg, D.A. *et al.* (1988) Exencephaly – clinical and ultrasonic correlation to anencephaly. *Obstetrics and Gynecology*, 72, 898–901.

Henrion, R., Oury, J.F., Aubry, J.P. and Aubry, M.C. (1980) Prenatal diagnosis of ectrodactyly. *Lancet*, ii, 319.

Henry, R.J.W. and Norton, S. (1987) Prenatal ultrasound diagnosis of fetal scoliosis with termination of the pregnancy: case report. *Prenatal Diagnosis*, 7, 663–66.

Hensleigh, P.A., Moore, W.V., Wilson, K. and Tulchinsky, D. (1978) Congenital X-linked adrenal hypoplasia. *Obstetrics and Gynecology*, 52, 228–32.

Herbert, W.N., Seeds, J.W., Cefalo, R.C. and Bowes, W.A. (1985) Prenatal detection of intraamniotic bands: implications and management. *Obstetrics and Gynecology*, 65, 36S–38S.

Herva, R., Leisti, J., Kirkinen, P. and Sappanen, U. (1985) A lethal autosmal recessive syndrome of multiple congenital contractures. *American Journal of Medical Genetics*, 20, 431–39.

Hill, L.M., Breckle, R. and Gehrking, W.C. (1985) Prenatal detection of congenital malformations by ultrasonography: Mayo Clinic experience. *American Journal of Obstetrics and Gynecology*, 152, 44–50.

Hill, L.M., Kislak, S. and Belfar, H.L. (1990) The sonographic diagnosis of urachal cysts *in utero*. *CU*, 18, 434–37.

Hill, L.M., Kislak, S. and Jones, N. (1988) Prenatal ultrasound diagnosis of a forearm constriction band, *Journal of Ultrasound in Medicine*, 7, 293–95.

Hill, L.M. and Peterson, C.S. (1987) Antenatal diagnosis of fetal pelvic kidneys. *Journal of Ultrasound in Medicine*, 6, 393–96.

Hill, L.M., Thomas, M.L. and Peterson, C.S. (1987) The ultrasonic detection of Apert syndrome. *Journal of Ultrasound in Medicine*, 6, 601–604.

Hill, S.J. and Hirsch, J.H. (1985) Sonographic detection of fetal hydrometrocolpos. *Journal of Ultrasound in Medicine*, 4, 323–25.

Hilpert, P.L. and Kurtz, A.B. (1990) Prenatal diagnosis of agenesis of the corpus callosum using transvaginal ultrasound. *Journal of Ultrasound in Medicine*, 9, 363–65.

Hine, D.G., Hack, A.M., Goodman, S.I. and Tanaka, K. (1986) Stable isotope dilution analysis of isovalerylglycine in amniotic fluid and urine and its application for the prenatal diagnosis of isovaleric acidemia. *Pediatric Research*, 20, 222–26.

Hirose, K., Koyanagi, T., Hara, K. *et al.* (1989) Antenatal ultrasound diagnosis of the femur–fibula–ulna syndrome. *JCU*, 16, 199–203.

Hirsch, M., Josefsberg, Z., Schoenfeld, A. *et al.* (1990) Congenital hereditary hypothyroidism: prenatal diagnosis and treatment. *Prenatal Diagnosis*, 10, 491–96.

Hiyama, K., Sakura, N., Matsumoto, T. and Kuhara, T. (1986) Deficient beta-

ketothiolase activity in a patient with 2-methylacetoacetic aciduria. *Clinica Chimica Acta*, 155, 189–94.

Hobbins, J.C., Romero, R., Grannum, P. *et al.* (1984) Antenatal diagnosis of renal anomalies with ultrasound. I. Obstructive uropathy. *AJR*, 148, 868–77.

Hoffmann, G., Gibson, K.M., Brandt, I.K. *et al.* (1986) Mevalonic aciduria – an inborn error of cholesterol and nonsterol isoprene biosynthesis. *New England Journal of Medicine*, 314, 1610–14.

Hogdall, C., Siegl-Bartelt, J., Toi, A. and Ritchie, S. (1989) Prenatal diagnosis of Opitz (BBB) syndrome in the second trimester by ultrasound detection of hypospadias and hypertelorism. *Prenatal Diagnosis*, 9, 783–93.

Hohlfeld, P., Vial, Y., Maillard-Brignon, C. *et al.* (1991) Cytomegalovirus fetal infection. Prenatal diagnosis. *Obstetrics and Gynaecology*, 78, 615–18.

Holbrook, K.A., Dale, B.A., Williams, M.L. *et al.* (1988) The expression of congenital ichthyosiform erythroderma in second trimester fetuses of the same family: morphologic and biochemical studies. *Journal of Investigative Dermatology*, 91, 521–31.

Holmberg, L., Gustavi, B. and Johnson, A. (1983) A prenatal study of fetal platelet count and size with application to fetus at risk for Wiskott–Aldrich syndrome. *Journal of Pediatrics*, 102, 773–76.

Holme, E., Kyllerman, M. and Lindstedt, S. (1989) Early prenatal diagnosis in two pregnancies at risk for glutaryl-CoA-dehydrogenase deficiency. *Journal of Inherited Metabolic Disease*, 12 (suppl.2), 280–82.

Holmes, R.D., Wilson, G.N. and Hajra, A.K. (1987) Peroxisomal enzyme deficiency in the Conradi–Hunerman form of chondrodysplasia punctata. *New England Journal of Medicine*, 316, 1608.

Holton, J.B., Allen, J.T. and Gillett, M.G. (1989) Prenatal diagnosis of disorders of galactose metabolism. *Journal of Inherited Metabolic Disease*, 12 (suppl.1), 202–206.

Holzgreve, W. (1985) Prenatal diagnosis of persistent common cloaca with prune belly and anencephaly in the second trimester. *American Journal of Medical Genetics*, 20, 729–32.

Holzgreve, W., Mahony, B.S., Glick, P.L. *et al.* (1985) Sonographic demonstration of fetal sacrococcygeal teratoma. *Prenatal Diagnosis*, 5, 245–57.

Honour, J.W., Goolamali, S.K. and Taylor, N.F. (1985) Prenatal diagnosis and variable presentation of recessive X-linked icthyosis. *British Journal of Dermatology*, 112, 423–30.

Horsthemke, B., Barnet, H.J., Greger, V. *et al.* (1987) Early diagnosis in hereditary retinoblastoma by detection of molecular deletions at gene locus. *Lancet*, i, 511–12.

Hsu, L.Y.F. (1986) Prenatal diagnosis of chromosome abnormalities, in *Genetic Disorders and the Fetus* 2nd edn (ed. A. Milunsky), Plenum Press, NY, pp. 115–83.

Huang, S.Z., Zhou, X.D., Ren, Z.R. *et al.* (1990) Prenatal detection of an Arg-Ter mutation at codon 111 of the PAH gene using DNA amplification. *Prenatal Diagnosis*, 10, 289–94.

Hubbard, A.E., Ayers, A.B., MacDonald, L.M. and James, C.E. (1984) *In utero* torsion of the testis: antenatal and postnatal ultrasonic appearances. *British Journal of Radiology*, 57, 644–46.

Hughes, I.A., Dyas, J. Riad-Fahmy, D. and Laurence, K.L. (1987) Prenatal diagnosis of congenital adrenal hyperplasia: reliability of amniotic fluid steroid analysis. *Journal of Medical Genetics*, 24, 344–47.

Hunziker, U.A., Savoldelli, G., Bolthauser, E. *et al.* (1989) Prenatal diagnosis of Schwartz–Jampel syndrome with early manifestation. *Prenatal Diagnosis*, 9, 127–31.

Huu, T.P., Dumez, Y., Marquetty, C., Durandy, A. *et al.* (1987) Prenatal diagnosis of chronic granulomatous disease (CGD) in four high risk male fetuses. *Prenatal Diagnosis*, 7, 253–60.

Iaccarino, M., Baldi, F., Persico, D. and Palagiano, A. (1986) Ultrasonographic and pathologic study of mucoid degeneration of umbilical cord. *JCU*, 14, 127–29.

Iaccarino, M., Lonardo, F., Guigliano, M. and Brunna, M.D. (1985) Prenatal diagnosis of Mohr syndrome by ultrasography. *Prenatal Diagnosis*, 5, 415–18.

Iavarone, A., Dolfin, G., Bracco, G. *et al.* (1989) First trimester prenatal diagnosis of Wolman disease. *Journal of Inherited Metabolic Disease*, 12 (suppl.2), 299–300.

Ives, E.J. and Houston, C.S. (1980) Autosomal recessive microcephaly and micromelia in Cree Indians. *American Journal of Medical Genetics*, 7, 351–60.

Izquierdo, L.A., Kushnir, O., Aase, J. *et al.* (1990) Antenatal ultrasonic diagnosis of dyssegmental dysplasia: a case report. *Prenatal Diagnosis*, 10, 587–92.

Jackson, C.A., Norum, R.A. and O'Neal, J.P. (1988) Linkage between MEN2B and chromosome 10 markers linked to MEN2A. *American Journal of Human Genetics*, 43, A147.

Jaffe, R., Schoenfeld, A. and Ovadia, J. (1990) Sonographic findings in the prenatal diagnosis of bladder exstrophy. *American Journal of Obstetrics and Gynecology*, 162, 675–78

Jakobs, C., Stellaard, F., Kvittingen, E.A. *et al.* (1990) First trimester prenatal diagnosis of tyrosinaemia type I by amniotic fluid succinylacetone determination. *Prenatal Diagnosis*, 10, 133–39.

Jakobs, C., Stellaard, F., Smit, L.M. *et al.* The first prenatal diagnosis of dihydropyrimidine dehydrogenase deficiency. *European Journal of Pediatrics*, 150, 291.

Jakobs, C., Sweetman, L., Wadman, S.K. *et al.* (1984) Prenatal diagnosis of glutaric aciduria type II by direct chemical analysis of dicarboxylic acids in amniotic fluid. *European Journal of Paediatrics*, 141, 153–57.

Jarvela, I., Rapola, J., Peltonen, L. *et al.* (1991) DNA-based prenatal diagnosis of the infantile form of neuronal ceroid lipofuscinosis (INCL, CLN1). *Prenatal Diagnosis*, 11, 323–28

Jaspers, N.G.J., Van der Kraan, M., Linssen, P.C.M.L. *et al.* (1990) First-trimester prenatal diagnosis of the Nijmegen breakage syndrome and ataxia telangiectasia using an assay of radioresistant DNA synthesis. *Prenatal Diagnosis*, 10, 667–74.

Jauniaux, E., Campbell, S. and Vyas, S. (1989) The use of color Doppler imaging for prenatal diagnosis of umbilical cord anomalies: report of three cases. *American Journal of Obstetrics and Gynecology*, 161, 1195–97.

Jauniaux, E., Vyas, S., Finlayson, C. *et al.* (1990) Early sonographic diagnosis of body stalk anomaly. *Prenatal Diagnosis*, 10, 127–32

Jeanty, P. (1990) Prental detection of simian crease. *Journal of Ultrasound in Medicine*, 9, 131–36.

Jeanty, P., Kepple, D., Roussis, P. and Shah, D. (1990a) *In utero* detection of cardiac failure from an aneurysm of the vein of Galen. *American Journal of Obstetrics and Gynecology*, 163, 50–51.

Jeanty, P. and Kleinman, G. (1989) Proximal femoral focal deficiency. *Journal of Ultrasound in Medicine*, 8, 639–42.

Jeanty, P., Romero, R., Kepple, D. *et al.* (1990b) Prenatal diagnosis in unilateral empty renal fossa. *Journal of Ultrasound in Medicine*, 9, 651–54.

Jenkinson, E.L., Pfisterer, W.H., Latteier, K.K. and Martin, H. (1943) A prenatal diagnosis of osteopetrosis. *AJR*, 49, 455–62.

Johnson, M.L., Dunne, M.G., Mack, L.A. and Rashbaum, C.L. (1980) Evaluation of fetal intracranial anatomy by static and real-time ultrasound. *JCU*, 8, 311–312.

Jones, M.Z., Rathke, E.J.S., Cavanagh, K. and Hancock, L.W. (1984) Beta-mannosidosis: prenatal biochemical and morphological characteristics. *Journal of Inherited Metabolic Disorders*, 7, 80–85.

Jones, S.M., Robinson, L.K. and Sperrazza, R. (1990) Prenatal diagnosis of a skeletal dysplasia identified postnatally as hypochondroplasia. *American Journal of Medical Genetics*, 36, 404–407.

Journel, H., Guyot, C., Barc, R.M. *et al.* (1989) Unexpected ultrasonographic prenatal diagnosis of autosomal dominant polycystic kidney disease. *Prenatal Diagnosis*, 9, 663–71.

Junien, C., Leroux, A., Lostanlen, D. *et al.* (1981) Prenatal diagnosis of congenital enzymopenic methemoglobinaemia with mental retardation due to generalized cytochrome B_5 reductase deficiency: first report of two cases. *Prenatal Diagnosis*, 1, 17–24.

Juul, S., Ledbetter, D., Wight, T.N. and Woodrum, D. (1990) New insights into idiopathic infantile arterial calcinosis. *American Journal of Diseases of Children*, 144, 229–33.

Kainulainen, K., Pulkkinen, L., Savolainen, A. *et al.* (1990) Location on chromosome 15 of the gene defect causing Marfan syndrome. *New England Journal of Medicine*, 323, 935–39.

Kaiser, I.H. (1980) Brown amniotic fluid in congenital erythropoietic porphyria. *Obstetrics and Gynecology*, 56, 383.

Kalugdan, R.G., Satoh, S., Koyanagi, T. *et al.* (1989) Antenatal diagnosis of pulmonary arteriovenous fistula using real-time ultrasound and color Doppler flow imaging. *JCU*, 17, 607–14.

Kaplan, C., Patereau, C., Reznikoff-Etievant, M.F. *et al.* (1985) Antenatal PL Al typing and detection of GP IIb–IIIa complex. *British Journal of Haematology*, 60, 586–88.

Kapoor, R., Gupta, A.K., Sing, S. *et al.* (1989) Antenatal sonographic diagnosis of chorioangioma of placenta. *Australasian Radiology*, 33, 288–89.

Kapoor, R., Saha, M.M. and Mandal, A.K. (1989) Antenatal sonographic detection of Wolffian duct cyst. *JCU*, 17, 515–17.

Kapur, S. and Van Vloten, A. (1986) Isolated congenital bowed long bones. *Clinical Genetics*, 29, 165–67.

Katz, S., Basel, D. and Branski, D. (1988) Prenatal gastric dilatation and infantile hypertrophic pyloric stenosis. *Journal of Pediatric Surgery*, 23, 1021–22.

Kazazian, Jr, H.H. (1990) The thalassemia syndromes: molecular basis and prenatal diagnosis in 1990. *Seminars in Hematology*, 27, 209–28.

Kazazian, Jr, H.H., Boehm, C.D. and Dowling, C.E. (1985) Prenatal diagnosis of hemoglobinopathies by DNA analysis. *Annals of the New York Academy of Sciences*, 445, 337–48.

Kazazian, Jr, H.H., Dover, G.L., Lightbody, K.L. and Park, I.J. (1978) Prenatal diagnosis in a fetus at risk for haemoblobin S–O Arab disease. *Journal of Pediatrics*, 93, 502–504.

Kazazian, Jr, H.H., Phillips, D.G., Dowling, C.E. and Boehm, C.D. (1988) Prenatal diagnosis of sickle cell anaemia. *Annals of the New York Academy of Sciences*, 565, 44–47.

Keller, E., Andreas, A., Scholz, S. *et al.* (1991) Prenatal diagnosis of 21-hydroxylase deficiency by RFLP analysis of the 21-hydroxylase, complement C4 and HLA class II genes. *Prenatal Diagnosis*, 11, 827–40.

Kennedy, K.A., Flick, K.J. and Thurmond, A.S. (1990) First trimester diagnosis of exencephaly. *American Journal of Obsterics and Gynecology*, 162, 461–63.

Khouzam, M.N. and Hooker, J.G. (1989) The significance of prenatal diagnosis of choroid plexus cysts. *Prenatal Diagnosis*, 9, 213–16.

Kirk, J.S. and Comstock, C.H. (1990) Antenatal sonographic appearance of spondyloepiphyseal dysplasia congenita. *Journal of Ultrasound in Medicine*, 9, 173–75.

Kirkinen, P., Herva, R. and Leisti, J. (1987) Prenatal diagnosis of a lethal syndrome of multiple congenital contractures. *Prenatal Diagnosis*, 7, 189–96.

Kirkinen, P. and Jouppila, P. (1986) Intrauterine membranous cyst: a report of antenatal diagnosis and obstetric aspects in two cases. *Obstetrics and Gynecology*, 67, 265–305.

Kishi, F., Matsuura, S., Murano, I. *et al.* (1991) Prenatal diagnosis of infantile hypophosphatasia. *Prenatal Diagnosis*, 11, 305–309.

Kishimoto, T.K., O'Connor, K. and Springer, T.A. (1989) Leucocyte adhesion deficiency. Aberrant splicing of a conserved integrin sequence causes a moderate deficiency phenotype. *Journal of Biological Chemistry*, 264, 3588–95.

Kitchiner, D., Leung, M.P. and Arnold, R. (1990) Isolated congenital left ventricular diverticulum: echocardiographic features in a fetus. *American Heart Journal*, 119, 1435–37.

Kjoller, M., Holm-Nielsen, G., Meiland, H. *et al.* (1985) Prenatal obstruction of the ileum diagnosed by ultrasound. *Prenatal Diagnosis*, 5, 427–30.

Kleijer, W.J., Hoogeveen, A., Verheijen, F.W. *et al.* (1979) Prenatal diagnosis of sialidosis with combined neuraminidase and beta-galactosidase deficiency. *Clinical Genetics*, 16, 60–61.

Kleijer, W.J., Hussarts-Odijk, L.M., Los, F.J. *et al.* (1989) Prenatal diagnosis of purine nucleoside phosphorylase deficiency in the first and second trimesters of pregnancy. *Prenatal Diagnosis*, 9, 401–407.

Kleijer, W.J., Hussarts-Odijk, L.M., Sachs, E.S. *et al.* (1987) Prenatal diagnosis of Fabry's disease by direct analysis of chorionic villi. *Prenatal Diagnosis*, 7, 283–87.

Kleijer, W.J., Janse, H.C., Vosters, R.P.L. *et al.* (1986) First trimester diagnosis of mucopolysaccharidosis IIIA (Sanfilippo A disease). *New England Journal of Medicine*, 314, 185–86.

Kleijer, W.J., Thompson, E.J. and Niermeijer, M.F. (1983) Prenatal diagnosis of the Hurler syndrome; report on 40 pregnancies at risk. *Prenatal Diagnosis*, 3, 179–86.

Kleiner, B., Callen, P.W. and Filly, R.A. (1987) Sonographic analysis of the fetus with ureteropelvic junction obstruction. *AJR*, 148, 359–63.

Kleinman, C.S., Donnerstein, R.L., Devore, G.V. *et al.* (1982) Fetal echocardiography for evaluation of *in utero* congestive heart failure. *New England Journal of Medicine*, 306, 568–75.

Kleinman, C.S., Donnerstein, R.L., Jaffe, C.C. *et al.* (1983) Fetal echocardiography. A tool for evaluation of *in utero* cardiac arrythmias and monitoring of *in utero* therapy: analysis of 71 patients. *American Journal of Cardiology*, 51, 237–43.

Klingensmith, W.C., Cioffi-Ragan, D.T. and Harvey, D.E. (1988) Diagnosis of ectopia cordis in the second trimester. *JCU*, 16, 204–206.

Knoers, N., Van der Heyden, H., Van Oost, B.A. *et al.* (1988) Nephrogenic diabetes insipidus-close linkage with markers from the distal long arm of the human X chromosome. *Human Genetics*, 80, 31–38.

Koga, Y., Mizumot, M., Matsumoto, M.D. *et al.* (1990) Prenatal diagnosis of fetal intracranial calcifications. *American Journal of Obstetrics and Gynecology*, 163, 1543–45.

Kohler, R., Sousa, P. and Jorge, O.S. (1989) Prenatal diagnosis of the ectodactyly, ectodermal dysplasia, cleft palate (EEC) syndrome. *Journal of Ultrasound in Medicine*, 8, 337–39.

Komrower, G.M. (1974) The philosophy and practice of screening for inherited diseases. *Pediatrics*, 53, 182–88.

Kormarniski, C.A., Cyr, D.R., Mack, L.A. and Weinberger, E. (1990) Prenatal diagnosis of schizencephaly. *Journal of Ultrasound in Medicine*, 9, 305–307.

Kourides, L.A., Berkowitz, R.L., Pang, S. *et al.* (1984) Antepartum diagnosis of goitrous hypothyroidism by fetal ultrasonography and amniotic fluid thyrotrophin concentration. *Journal of Clinical Endocrinology and Metabolism*, 59, 1016–18.

Kousseff, B.G., Matsuoka, L.Y., Stenn, K.S. *et al.* (1982) Prenatal diagnosis of Sjögren–Larsen syndrome. *Journal of Pediatrics*, 101, 998–1001.

Kurjak, A. and Latin, V. (1979) Ultrasound diagnosis of fetal abnormalities in multiple pregnancy. *Acta Obstetricia et Gynecologica Scandinavica*, 58, 153–61.

Kurtz, A.B., Filly, R.A., Wapner, R.J. *et al.* (1986) *In utero* analysis of heterozygous achondroplasia: variable time of onset as detected by femur length measurements. *Journal of Ultrasound in Medicine*, 5, 137–40.

Kushnir, O., Izquierdo, L., Vigil, D. and Curet, L.B. (1990) Early transvaginal sonographic diagnosis of gastroschisis. *JCU*, 18, 194–97.

Kutzner, D.K., Wilson, W.G. and Hogge, W.A. (1988) DETS complex (cloacal exstrophy): prenatal diagnosis in the second trimester. *Prenatal Diagnosis*, 8, 247–53.

Kvittingen, E.A., Guibaud, P.P., Divry, P. *et al.* (1986) Prenatal diagnosis of hereditary tyrosinaemia type I by determination of fumarylacetoacetase in chrorionic villus material. *European Journal of Pediatrics*, **144**, 597–98.

Lake, B.D., Young, E.P. and Nicolaides, K. (1989) Prenatal diagnosis of infantile sialic acid storage disease in a twin pregnancy. *Journal of Inherited Metabolic Disease*, **12**, 152–56.

Lamy, M.E., Mulongo, K.N., Gadisseux, J.F. *et al.* (1992) Prenatal diagnosis of fetal cytomegalovirus infection. *American Journal of Obstetrics and Gynecology*, **166**, 91–94.

Landy, H.J., Khoury, A.N. and Heyl, P.S. (1989) Antenatal ultrasonographic diagnosis of fetal seizure activity. *American Journal of Obstetrics and Gynecology*, **161**, 308.

Langer, R. and Kaufmann, H.J. (1986) Case report 363. Infantile cortical hyperostosis (Caffey disease ICH) of iliac bones, femora, tibiae and left fibula. *Skeletal Radiology*, **15**, 377–82.

Lau, Y.L., Levinsky, R.J., Malcolm, S. *et al.* (1988) Genetic prediction in X-linked agammaglobulinemia. *American Journal of Medical Genetics*, **31**, 437–48.

Laxova, R., O'Hara, P.T., Ridler, M.A.C and Timothy, J.A.D. (1973) Family with probable achondrogenesis and lipid inclusions in fibroblasts. *Archives of Disease in Childhood*, **48**, 212–16.

Lazaro, C., Ravella, A., Casals, T. *et al.* (1992) Prenatal diagnosis of sporadic neurofibromatosis 1. *Lancet*, **339**, 119–20.

Lebrun, D., Avni, E.F., Goolaerts, J.P. *et al.* (1985) Prenatal diagnosis of a pulmonary cyst by ultrasonography. *European Journal of Pediatrics*, **144**, 399–402.

Lehmann, A.R., Francis, A.J. and Gianelli, F. (1985) Prenatal diagnosis of Cockayne's syndrome. *Lancet*, **i**, 486–88.

Leithiser, Jr, R.E., Fyfe, D., Weatherby, E. *et al.* (1986) Prenatal sonographic diagnosis of atrial hemangioma. *AJR*, **147**, 1207–208.

Lemna, W.K., Reldman, G.L., Kerem, B.-S. *et al.* (1990) Mutation analysis for heterozygote detection and the prenatal diagnosis of cystic fibrosis. *New England Journal of Medicine*, **322**, 291–96.

Leppert, M., Anderson, V.E., Quattlebaum, T. *et al.* (1989) Benign familial neonatal convulsions linked to genetic markers on chromosome 20. *Nature*, **337**, 647–48.

Levinsky, R., Harvey, B., Nicolaides, K. and Rodeck, C. (1986) Antenatal diagnosis of chronic granulomatous disease. *Lancet*, **i**, 504.

Lewis, B.D., Doubilet, P.M., Heller, V.L. *et al.* (1986) Cutaneous and visceral hemangiomata in the Klippel–Trenaunay–Weber syndrome: antenatal sonographic detection. *AJR*, **147**, 598–600.

Lichman, J.P. and Miller, E.I. (1988) Prenatal ultrasonic diagnosis of a splenic cyst. *Journal of Ultrasound in Medicine*, **7**, 637–38.

Lien, J.M., Colmorgen, G.H.C., Gehret, J.F. and Evantash, A.B. (1990). Spontaneous resolution of fetal pleural effusion diagnosed during the second trimester. *JCU*, **18**, 54–56.

Linch, D.C., Beverley, P.C.L., Levinsky, R.J. and Rodeck, C.H. (1982) Phenotypic analysis of fetal blood leucocytes: potential for prenatal diagnosis of immunodeficiency disorders. *Prenatal Diagnosis*, **2**, 211–18.

Linch, D.C., Levinsky, R.J., Rodeck, C.H. *et al.* (1984) Prenatal diagnosis of three cases of severe combined immunodeficiency disease: severe T cell deficiency during the first half of gestation in fetuses with ADA deficiency *Clinical and Experimental Immunology*, **56**, 223–32.

Lindfors, K.K., McGahan, J.P. and Walter, J.P. (1986) Fetal omphalocele and gastroschisis: pitfalls in sonographic diagnosis. *AJR*, **147**, 797–800.

Lindlof, M., Kere, J., Ristola, M. *et al.* (1987) Prenatal diagnosis of X-linked chronic granulomatous disease using restriction fragment length polymorphism analysis. *Genomics*, **1**, 87–92.

Liner, R.I. (1990) Intrauterine listeria infection: prenatal diagnosis by biophysical assessment and amniocentesis. *American Journal of Obstetrics and Gynecology*, **163**, 1596–97.

Lingman, G., Lundstrom, N.R., Marsal, K. and Ohrlander, S. (1986) Fetal cardiac arrhythmia. Clinical outcome in 113 cases. *Acta Obstetricia et Gynecologica Scandinavia*, **65**, 263–67.

Liskowska-Grospierre, B., Bohler, M.-C., Fisher, A. *et al.* (1986) Defective membrane expression of the LFA-1 complex may be secondary to the absence of the beta chain in a child with recurrent bacterial infection. *European Journal of Immunology*, **16**, 205–208.

Lissens, W., Bril, T., Vercammen, M. *et al.* (1987) First trimester prenatal diagnosis of lysosomal storage disease. Study of alpha-L-fucosidase isoenzyme patterns in fetal and maternal tissue. *Annales de Biologie Clinique*, **45**, 464–68.

Lissens, W., Van Lierde, M., Decaluwe, J., *et al.* (1988) Prenatal diagnosis of Hunter syndrome using fetal plasma. *Prenatal Diagnosis*, **8**, 59–62.

Lituania, M., Cordone, M., Zampatti, C. *et al.* (1988) Prenatal diagnosis of a rare heteropagus. *Prenatal Diagnosis*, **8**, 547–51.

Lituania, M., Passamonti, U., Cordone, M.S. *et al.* (1989) Schizencephaly: prenatal diagnosis by computed tomography and magnetic resonance imaging. *Prenatal Diagnosis*, **9**, 649–55.

Llewellyn, D.H., Elder, G.H., Kalsheker, N.A. *et al.* (1987) DNA polymorphism of human porphobilinogen deaminase gene in acute intermittent porphyria. *Lancet*, **ii**, 706–708.

Lockwood, C., Irons, M., Troiani, J. *et al.* (1988) The prenatal sonographic diagnosis of lethal multiple pterygium syndrome: a heritable cause of

recurrent abortion. *American Journal of Obstetrics and Gynecology*, **159**, 474–76.

Loewy, J.A., Richards, D.G. and Toi, A. (1987). *In-utero* diagnosis of the caudal regression syndrome: report of three cases. *JCU*, **15**, 469–74.

Lonenz, P., Bollmann, R., Hinkel, G.K. *et al.* (1991) False-negative prenatal exclusion of Wiskott–Aldrich syndrome by measurement of fetal platelet count and size. *Prenatal Diagnosis*, **11**, 819–25.

Loverro, G., Guanti, G., Carso, G. and Selvaggi, L. (1990) Robinow's syndrome: prenatal diagnosis. *Prenatal Diagnosis*, **10**, 121–26.

Lowden, J.A., Cutz, E., Conen, P.E. *et al.* (1973) Prenatal diagnosis of GML-gangliosidosis. *New England Journal of Medicine*, **288**, 225–28.

Luthy, D.A., Mack, I., Hirsch, J. *et al.* (1981) Prenatal ultrasound diagnosis of thrombocytopenia with absent radii. *American Journal of Obstetrics and Gynecology*, **141**, 3350–51.

Lux, S.E., Tse, W.T., Menninger, J.C. *et al.* (1990) Hereditary spherocytosis associated with deletion of human erythrocyte ankyrin gene on chromosome 8. *Nature*, **345**, 736–39.

Lynch, L., Bussel, J., Goldberg, J.D. *et al.* (1988) The *in utero* diagnosis and management of autoimmune thrombocytopenia. *Prenatal Diagnosis*, **8**, 329–31.

Lynch, L., Daffos, F., Emanuel, D. *et al.* (1991) Prenatal diagnosis of fetal cytomegalovirus infection. *American Journal of Obstetrics and Gynecology*, **165**, 714–18.

Maasen, J.A., Lindhout, D., Reuss, A. and Kleijer, W.J. (1990) Prenatal analysis of insulin receptor autophosphorylation in a family with leprechaunism. *Prenatal Diagnosis*, **10**, 13–16.

McAlister, W.H., Wright, Jr, J.R., and Crane, J.P. (1987) Main-stem bronchial atresia: intrauterine sonographic diagnosis. *AJR*, **148**, 364–66.

McCabe, E., Sadava, P., Bullen, W. *et al.* (1982) Human glycerol kinase deficiency: enzyme kinetics and fibroblast hybridisation. *Journal of Inherited Metabolic Disease*, **5**, 177–82.

MacDermot, K.D., Morgan, S.H., Cheshire, J.K. and Wilson, T.M. (1987) Anderson–Fabry disease, a close linkage with highly polymorphic DNA markers DXS17, DXS87 and DXS88. *Human Genetics*, **77**, 263–66.

McFarland, J.G., Aster, R.H., Bussel, J.B. *et al.* (1991) Prenatal diagnosis of neonatal alloimmune thrombocytopenia using allele-specific oligonucleotide probes. *Blood*, **78**, 2276–82.

McFarland, S.L. (1929) Congenital dislocation of the knee. *Journal of Bone and Joint Surgery*, **11**, 281.

McGahan, J.P., Ellis, W., Lindfors, K.K. *et al.* Prenatal sonographic diagnosis of VATER association. *JCU*, **16**, 588–91.

McGahan, J.P., Haesslein, H.C., Meyers, M. and Ford, K.B. (1984) Sonographic recognition of *in utero* intraventricular hemorrhage. *AJR*, **142**, 171–73.

McGahan, J.P. and Hanson, J. (1983) Meconium peritonitis with accompanying pseudocyst: prenatal sonographic diagnosis. *Radiology*, **128**, 125–26.

McGahan, J.P., Nyberg, D.A. and Mack, L.A. (1990) Sonography of facial features of alobar and semilobar holoprosencephaly. *AJR*, **154**, 143–48.

McGahan, J.P. and Schneider, J.M. (1986) Fetal neck hemangiondothelioma with secondary hydrops fetalis: sonographic diagnosis. *JCU*, **14**, 384–88.

Mack, L., Gottesfeld, K. and Johnson, M.L. (1978) Antenatal detection of ectopic fetal liver by ultrasound. *JCU*, **6**, 226–27.

Macken, M.B., Grantmyre, E.B. and Vincer, M.L. (1989) Regression of nuchal cystic hygroma in utero. *Journal of Ultrasound in Medicine*, **8**, 101–103.

McKusick, V.A. (1990) *Mendelian Inheritance in Man. Catalogs of Autosomal Dominant, Autosomal Recessive and X-linked Traits*, 9th edn, Johns Hopkins University Press, Baltimore.

McRae, S.M., Speed, R.A. and Sommerville, A.J. (1982) Intrauterine skull fracture diagnosed by ultrasound. *Australian and New Zealand Journal of Obstetrics and Gynaecology*, **22**, 159–60.

Maenpaa, J., Lindahl, E., Aula, P. and Savontaus, M.-L. (1990) Prenatal diagnosis in Pelizaeus–Merzbacher disease using RFLP analysis. *Clinical Genetics*, **37**, 141–46.

Mahoney, M.J. and Hobbins, J.C. (1977) Prenatal diagnosis of chondroectodermal dysplasia (Ellis–Van Creveld syndrome) with fetoscopy and ultrasound. *New England Journal of Medicine*, **297**, 258–60.

Mahony, B.S., Filly, R.A., Callen, P.W. and Golbus, M.S. (1985a) The amniotic band syndrome: antenatal sonographic diagnosis and potential pitfalls. *American Journal of Obstetrics and Gynecology*, **152**, 63–68.

Mahony, B.S., Filly, R.A., Callen, P.W. and Golbus, M.S. (1985b) Thanatophoric dwarfism with the cloverleaf skull: a specific antenatal sonographic diagnosis. *Journal of Ultrasound in Medicine*, **4**, 151–54.

Mahony, B.S., Filly, R.A., Callen, P.W. *et al.* (1984b) Severe nonimmune hydrops fetalis: sonographic evaluation. *Radiology*, **151**, 757–61.

Mahony, B.S., Filly, R.A. and Cooperberg, P.L. (1984a) Antenatal sonographic diagnosis of achondrogenesis. *Journal of Ultrasound in Medicine*, **3**, 333–35.

Maire, I., Mandon, G. and Mathieu, M. (1989) First trimester prenatal diagnosis of glycogen storage disease type III. *Journal of Inherited Metabolic Disease*, **12** (suppl.2), 292–94.

Maire, I., Mandon, G., Zabot, M.T. *et al.* (1979) Beta-glucuronidase deficiency: enzyme studies in an affected family and prenatal diagnosis. *Journal of Inherited Metabolic Disease*, **2**, 29–34.

Majoor-Krakauer, D.F., Waldimiroff, J.W., Stewart, P.A. *et al.* (1987)

Microcephaly, micrognathia, and bird-headed dwarfism: prenatal diagnosis of a Seckel-like syndrome. *American Journal of Medical Genetics*, 27, 183–88.

Malinger, G., Rosen, N., Achiron, R. and Zakut, H. (1987) Pierre Robin sequence associated with amniotic band syndrome. Ultrasonographic diagnonsis and pathogenesis. *Prenatal Diagnosis*, 7, 455–59.

Mann, L., Alroomi, L., McNay, M. and Ferguson-Smith, M.A. (1983) Placental haemangioma: case report. *British Journal of Obstetrics and Gynaecology*, 90, 983–86.

Mao, K., and Adams, J. (1983) Antenatal diagnosis of intracranial arteriovenous fistula by ultrasonography. Case report. *British Journal of Obstetrics and Gynaecology*, 90, 872–73.

Marino, J., Martinez-Urrutia, M.J., Hawkins, F. and Gonzalez, A. (1990) Encysted adrenal haemorrhage. Prenatal diagnosis. *Acta Paediatrica Scandinavica*, 79, 230–31.

Mariona, F., McAlpin, G., Zador, I. et al. (1986) Sonographic detection of fetal extrathoracic pulmonary sequestration. *Journal of Ultrasound in Medicine*, 5, 283–85.

Marks, F., Hernanz-Schulman, M., Horri, S. et al. (1989) Spondylthoracic dysplasia. Clinical and sonographic diagnosis. *Journal of Ultrasound in Medicine*, 8, 1–5.

Marks, F., Thomas, P., Lustig, I. et al. (1990) *In utero* sonographic description of a fetal liver adenoma. *Journal of Ultrasound in Medicine*, 9, 119–22.

Martincic, N. (1952) Case reports: osteopoikilosis (spotted bones) *British Journal of Radiology*, 25, 612–14.

Martini, G., Toniolo, D., Vulliamy, T et al. (1986) Structural analysis of the X-linked gene encoding human glucose-6-phosphate dehydrogenase. *European Molecular Biology Organisation Journal*, 5, 1849–55.

Matalon, R., Michals, K., Gashkoff, P. and Kaul, R. (1992). Prenatal diagnosis of Canavan's disease. *Journal of Inherited Metabolic Disease*, 15, 392–94.

Mathew, C.G.P., Chin, K.S., Easton, D.F. et al. (1987) A linked genetic marker for multiple endocrine neoplasia type 2a on chromosome 10. *Nature*, 328, 528–30.

Mayes, J.S., Say, B. and Marcus, D.L. (1987) Prenatal studies in a family with transcobalamin II deficiency. *American Journal of Human Gentics*, 41, 686–87.

Meizner, I., Barki, Y. and Hertzanu, Y (1987) Prenatal sonographic diagnosis of agenesis of corpus callosum. *JCU*, 15, 262–64.

Meizner, I. and Bar-Ziv, J. (1987) Prenatal ultrasonic diagnosis of short-rib polydactyly syndrome (SRPS) type III: a case report and a proposed approach to the diagnosis of SRPS and related conditions. *JCU*, 13, 284–87.

Meizner, I. and Bar-Ziv, J. (1989) Prenatal ultrasonic detection of short rib polydactyly syndrome type I. A case report. *Journal of Reproductive Medicine*, 34, 668–72.

Meizner, I. and Bar-Ziv, J. (1987) Prenatal ultrasonic diagonisis of a rare case of iniencephaly apertus. *JCU*, 15, 200–203.

Meizner, I., Bar-Ziv, J., Barki, and Abeliovich D. (1986a) Prenatal ultrasonic diagnosis of radial-ray apiasa and renal anomalies (acrorenal syndrome). *Prenatal Diagnosis*, 6, 223–25.

Meizner, I., Bar-Ziv, J. and Katz, M. (1985) Prenatal ultrasonic diagnosis of the extreme form of prune belly syndrome. *JCU*, 13, 581–83.

Meizner, I., Carmi, R. and Bar-Ziv, J. (1986b) Congenital chylothorax: prenatal ultrasonic diagnosis and successful post partum management. *Prenatal Diagnosis*, 6, 217–21.

Menashe, Y., Baruch, G.B., Rabinovitch, O. et al. (1989) Exophthalmos: prenatal ultrasonic features for diagnosis of Crouzon syndrome. *Prenatal Diagnosis*, 9, 805–808.

Mennuti, M.T., Zackai, E.H., Curtis, M.T. et al. (1990) Early ultrasound diagnosis of Neu–Laxova syndrome. *American Journal of Human Genetics*, 47, A281.

Mensink, E.J.B.M., Thompson, A., Sandkuyl, L.A. et al. (1987) X-linked immunodeficiency with hyperimmunoglobulinaemia M appears to be linked to DXS42 restriction fragment length polymorphism locus. *Human Genetics*, 76, 96–99.

Merlob, P., Schonfeld, A., Grunebaum, M. et al. (1987) Autosomal dominant cerebro-costo-mandibular syndrome: ultrasonographic and clinical findings. *American Journal of Medical Genetics*, 26, 195–202.

Mibashan, R.S., Millar, D.S., Rodeck, C.H. et al. (1985) Prenatal diagnosis of hereditary protein C deficiency. *New England Journal of Medicine*, 313, 1607.

Mibashan, R.S. and Rodeck, C.H. (1984) Haemophilia and other genetic defects of haemostasis, in *Prenatal Diagnosis*, Proceedings of the 11th RCOG Study Group (eds C.H. Rodeck and K.H. Nicolaides), Wiley, Chichester.

Mibashan, R.S., Rodeck, C.H., Thumpston, J.K. et al. (1979) Plasma assay of fetal factors VIIIC and IX for prenatal diagnosis of haemophilia. *Lancet*, i, 1309–11.

Michelson, A.M., Blake, C.C.F., Evans, S.T. and Orkin, S.H. (1985) Structure of the human phosphoglycerate kinase gene and the intron-mediated evolution and dispersal of the nucleotide binding domain. *Proceedings of the National Academy of Sciences of the USA*, 82, 6965–69.

Middleton-Price, H.R., Harding, A.E., Monteiro, C. et al. (1990) Linkage of hereditary motor and sensory neuropathy type I to the pericentromeric region of chromosome 17. *American Journal of Human Genetics*, 46, 92–94.

Minelli, A., Danesino, C., Curto, F.L. et al. (1988) First trimester prenatal diagnosis of Sanfilippo disease (MPS III) type B. *Prenatal Diagnosis*, 8, 47–52.

Mintz, M.C., Arger, P.H. and Coleman, B.G. (1985) *In utero* sonographic diagnosis of intracerebral haemorrhage. *Journal of Ultrasound in Medicine*, 4, 375–76.

Miro, J. and Bard, H. (1988) Congenital atresia and stenosis of the duodenum: the impact of a prenatal diagnosis. *American Journal of Obstetrics and Gynecology*, 158, 555–59.

Mitchell, C., Nicolaides, K., Kingston, J. et al. (1988) Prenatal exclusion of hereditary retinoblastoma. *Lancet*, i, 826.

Mitchell, G.A., Brody, L.C., Sipila, I. et al. (1989) At least two mutant alleles of ornithine delta-aminotransfease cause gyrate atrophy of the chorioid and retina in Finns. *Proceedings of the National Academy of Sciences of the USA*, 86, 197–201.

Mitchell, G., Saudubray, J.M., Benoit, Y. et al. (1983) Antenatal diagnosis of glutaric aciduria type II. *Lancet*, i, 1099.

Moodley, T.R., Vaughan, J.E., Chuntapursat, I. et al. (1986) Congenital heart block detected *in utero*. A case report. *South African Medical Journal*, 70, 433–34.

Morgan-Capner, P., Rodeck, C.H., Nicolaides, K.H. and Cradock-Watson, J.E. (1985) Prenatal detection of rubella-specific IgM in fetal sera. *Prenatal Diagnosis*, 5, 21–26.

Morin, P.R. (1981) Prenatal detection of the autosomal recessive type of polycystic kidney disease by trehalase assay in amniotic fluid. *Prenatal Diagnosis*, 1, 5–9.

Morin, P.R. (1984) Prenatal detection of the congenital nephrotic syndrome (Finnish type) by trehalase assay in amniotic fluid. *Prenatal Diagnosis*, 4, 257–60.

Morris, M., Nichols, W. and Benson, M. (1991) Prenatal diagnosis of hereditary amyloidosis in a Portugese family. *American Journal of Medical Genetics*, 39, 123–24.

Morris, S.A., Ohanian V., Lewis, M.L. et al. (1986) Prenatal diagnosis of hereditary red cell membrane defect. *British Journal of Haematology*, 62, 763–72.

Morse, R.P., Rawnsley, E., Crowe, H.C. et al. (1987a) Bilateral renal agenesis in three consecutive siblings. *Prenatal Diagnosis*, 7, 573–79.

Morse, R.P., Rawnsley, E., Sargent, S.K. and Graham J.M. (1987b) Prenatal diagnosis of a new syndrome: holoprosencephaly with hypokinesia. *Prenatal Diagnosis*, 7, 631–38.

Mostello, D., Hoechstetter, L., Bendon, R.W. et al. (1991) Prenatal diagnosis of recurrent Larsen syndrome: further definition of a lethal variant. *Prenatal Diagnosis*, 11, 215–25.

Mulligan, G. and Meier, P. (1989) Lipoma and agenesis of the corpus callosum with associated choroid plexus lipomas. *In utero* diagnosis. *Journal of Ultrasound in Medicine*, 8, 583–88.

Munoz, C., Filly, R.A. and Golbus, M.S. (1990) Osteogenesis imperfecta type II: prenatal sonographic diagnosis. *Radiology*, 174, 181–85.

Nadler, H.L. and Egan, T.J. (1970) Deficiency of lysosomal acid phosphatase. A new familial metabolic disorder. *New England Journal of Medicine*, 282, 302–307.

Naides, S.J. and Weiner, C.P. (1989) Antenatal diagnosis and palliative treatment of non-immune hydrops fetalis secondary to fetal parvovirus B19 infection. *Prenatal Diagnosis*, 9, 105–114.

Naito, E., Ozasa, H., Ikeda, Y. and Tanaka, K. (1989) Molecular cloning and nucleotide sequence of complementary DNAs encoding human short chain acyl coenzyme A dehydrogenase and the study of the molecular basis of human short chain acyl-coenzyme A dehydrogenase deficiency. *Journal of Clinical Investigation*, 83, 1605–13.

Nakamoto, S.K., Dreilinger, A., Dattel, B. et al. (1983) The sonographic appearance of hepatic hemangioma *in utero*. *Journal of Ultrasound in Medicine*, 2, 239–41.

Nakamura, M., Imajoh-Ohmi, S., Kanegasaki, S. et al. (1990) Prenatal diagnosis of cytochrome-deficient chronic granulomatous disease. *Lancet*, 336, 118–19.

Nancarrow, P.A., Mattrey, R.F., Edwards, D.K. and Skram, C. (1985) Fibroadhesive meconium peritonitis: *in utero* sonographic diagnosis. *Journal of Ultrasound in Medicine*, 4, 213–15.

Narayan, H. and Scott IV (1991) Prenatal ultrasound diagnosis of Apert's syndrome. *Prenatal Diagnosis*, 10, 187–92.

Narisawa, K., Gibson, K.M., Sweetman, L. et al. (1986) Deficiency of 3-methylglutaconyl-coenzyme A hydratase in two siblings with 3-methylglutaconic aciduria. *Journal of Clinical Investigation*, 77, 1148–52.

Navon, R., Sandbank, U., Frisch, A. et al. (1986) Adult-onset GM_2 gangliosidosis diagnosed in a fetus. *Prenatal Diagnosis*, 6, 169–76.

Nazzaro, V., Nicolini, U., Deluca, L. et al. (1990) Prenatal diagnosis of junctional epidermolysis bullosa associated with pyloric atresia. *Journal of Medical Genetics*, 27, 244–48.

Neilson, J.P., Danskin, F. and Hastie, S.J. (1989) Monozygotic twin pregnancy: diagnostic and Doppler ultrasound studies. *British Journal of Obstetrics and Gynaecology*, 96, 1413–18.

Newgard, C.B., Fletterick, R.J., Anderson, L.A. and Lebo, R.V. (1987) The polymorphic locus for glycogen storage disease VI (liver glycogen phosphory-lase) maps to chromosome 14. *American Journal of Human Genetics*, 40, 351–64.

Newnham, J.P., Crues, J.V. III, Vinstein, A.L. and Medearis, A.L. (1984) Sonographic diagnosis of thoracic gastroenteric cyst *in utero*. *Prenatal Diagnosis*, 4, 467–71.

Mguyen, D.L. and Leonard, J.C. (1986) Ischemic hepatic necrosis: a cause of fetal liver calcification. *AJR*, 147, 596–97.

Nichols, W.C. and Benson, M.D. (1990) Hereditary amyloidosis: detection of variant prealbumin genes by restriction enzyme analysis of amplified genomic DNA sequences. *Clinical Genetics*, 37, 44–53.

Nichols, W.C., Padilla, L.-M. and Benson, M.D. (1989) Prenatal detection of a gene for hereditary amyloidosis. *American Journal of Medical Genetics*, 34, 520–24.

Nicolaides, K.H., Campbell, S., Gabbe, S.G. and Guidetti, R. (1986) Ultra-sound screening for spina bifida: cranial and cerebellar signs. *Lancet*, ii, 72–74.

Nicolaides, K.H., Johansson, D., Donnai, D. and Rodeck, C.H. (1984) Prenatal diagnosis of mandibulofacial dysostosis. *Prenatal Diagnosis*, 4, 201–205.

Niederwieser, A. (1986) Prenatal diagnosis of dihydrobiopterin synthetase deficiency: a variant form of phenylketonuria. *European Journal of Pedia-trics*, 145, 176–78.

Nitowsky, H.M., Sassa, S., Nakagawa, M. and Jagani, B. (1978) Prenatal diagnosis of congenital erythropoietic porphyria. *Pediatric Research*, 12, 455.

Norman, A.M., Floyd, J.L., Meredith, A.L. and Harper, P.S. (1989) Presymptomatic detection and prenatal diagnosis for myotonic dystrophy by means of linked DNA markers. *Journal of Medical Genetics*, 26, 750–54.

Northrup, H., Beaudet, A.L. and O'Brien, E.W. (1990) Prenatal diagnosis of citrullinaemia: review of a 10-year experience including recent use of DNA analysis. *Prenatal Diagnosis*, 10, 771–79.

Novelli, G., Frontali, M., Baldini, D. *et al.* (1989) Prenatal diagnosis of adult polycystic kidney disease with DNA markers on chromosome 16 and the genetic heterogeneity problem. *Prenatal Diagnosis*, 9, 759–67.

Nowakowski, R.W., Thompson, J.N. and Taylor, K.B. (1989) Sanfilippo syndrome, type D: a spectrophotometric assay with prenatal diagnostic potential. *Pediatric Research*, 26, 462–66.

Nyberg, D.A., Hallesy, D., Mahony, B.S. *et al.* (1990) Meckel–Gruber syndrome. Importance of prenatal diagnosis. *Journal of Ultrasound in Medicine*, 9, 691–96.

Nyberg, D.A., Hastrup, W., Watts, H. and Mack, L.A. (1987) Dilated fetal bowel. A sonographic sign of cystic fibrosis. *Journal of Ultrasound in Medicine*, 6, 257–60.

Nyberg, D.A., Resta, R.G., Luthy, D.A. *et al.* (1990) Prenatal sonographic findings of Down syndrome: review of 94 cases. *Obstetrics and Gynecology*, 76, 370–77.

O'Donnell, J. (1981) Gyrate atrophy of the retina and choroid. *International Ophthalmology*, 4, 33–36.

Ogier, H., Wadman, S.K., Johnson, J.L. *et al.* (1983) Antenatal diagnosis of combined xanthine and sulphite oxidase deficiencies. *Lancet*, ii, 1363–64.

Ohdo, S., Madokoro, H., Sonoda, T. *et al.* (1987) Association of tetra-amelia, octodermal dysplasia, hypoplastic lacrimal ducts and sacs opening towards the exterior, peculiar face and developmental retardation. *Journal of Medical Genetics*, 24, 609–12.

Ohlsson, A., Fong, K.W., Rose, T.H. and Moore, D.C. (1988) Prenatal sonographic diagnosis of Pena–Shokeir syndrome type I, or fetal akinesia deformation sequence. *American Journal of Medical Genetics*, 29, 59–65.

Old, J.M., Fitches, A., Heath, C. *et al.* (1986) First trimester fetal diagnosis for haemoglobinopathies: report on 200 cases. *Lancet*, ii, 763–67.

Old, J.M., Varawalla, N.Y. and Weatherall, D.J. (1990) Rapid detection and prenatal diagnosis of beta-thalassaemia in Indian and Cypriot populations in the UK. *Lancet*, ii, 834–37.

Ordorica, S.A., Marks, F., Frieden, F.J. *et al.* (1990) Aneurysm of the vein of Galen: a new cause for Ballantyne syndrome. *American Journal of Obstetrics and Gynecology*, 162, 1166–67.

Orney, A., Arnon, J., Grebner, E. *et al.* (1987) Early prenatal diagnosis of mucolipidosis IV. *American Journal of Medical Genetics*, 27, 983–85.

Pachi, A., Giancotti, A., Torci, F. *et al.* (1989) Meckel–Gruber syndrome. *Prenatal Diagnosis*, 9, 187–90.

Packman, S., Cowan, M.J., Golbus, M.S. *et al.* (1982) Prenatal treatment of biotin-responsive multiple carboxylase deficiency. *Lancet*, i, 1435–39.

Pagliano, M., Mossetti, M. and Ragno, P. (1990) Echographic diagnoses of omphalocele in the first trimester of pregancy. *JCU*, 18, 658–60.

Pannone, N., Gatti, R., Lombardo, C. *et al.* (1986) Prenatal diagnosis of Hunter syndrome. *Prenatal Diagnosis*, 6, 107–10.

Parvy, P., Rabier, D., Boue, J. *et al.* (1990) Glycine/serine ratio and prenatal diagnosis of non-ketotic hyperglycaemia. *Prenatal Diagnosis*, 10, 303–305.

Patel, P., Kolawole, T., Ba'Agueel, H. *et al.* (1989) Antenatal sonographic findings in congenital chloride diarrhea. *JCU*, 17, 115–18.

Patrick, A., Young, E., Ellis, C. *et al.* (1988) Multiple sulphatase deficiency. *Prenatal Diagnosis*, 8, 303–306.

Patrick, A., Young, R., Mossman, J. *et al.* (1987) First trimester diagnosis of cystinosis. *Prenatal Diagnosis*, 7, 71–74.

Patten, R.M., Mack, L.A. Nyberg, D.A. and Filly, R.A. (1989) Twin

embolisation syndrome: prenatal sonographic detection and significance. *Radiology*, 173, 685–89.

Patton, M., Baraister, M., Nicolaides, K. *et al.* (1986) Prenatal treatment of hydrops (Opitz-G syndrome). *Prenatal Diagnosis*, 6, 109–15.

Pekonen, F. Teramo, K., Makinen, T. *et al.* (1984) Prenatal diagnosis and treatment of fetal thyrotoxicosis. *American Journal of Obstetrics and Gynecology*, 150, 893–94.

Peleg, D., Golichowski A.M. and Ragan W.D. (1985) Fetal hydrothorax and bilateral pulmonary hypoplasia. Ultrasonic diagnosis. *Acta Obstetricia and Gynecologica Scandinavica*, 64, 451–53.

Pennel, R.G. and Baltarowich, O.H. (1986) Prenatal sonographic diagnosis of a fetal facial haemangioma. *Journal of Ultrasound in Medicine*, 5, 525–23.

Perelman, A.H., Johnson, R.H. Clemons, R.D. *et al.* (1990) Intrauterine diagnosis and treatment of fetal goitrous hypothyroidism. *Journal of Clinical Endocrinology and Metabolism*, 71, 618–21.

Perez-Cerda, C., Merinero, B, Sanz, P. *et al.* (1989) Successful first trimester diagnosis in a pregnancy at risk for propionic acidemia. *Journal of Inherited Metabolic Disease*, 12, (suppl. 2), 274–76.

Perry, T.B., Holbrook, K.A. Hoff, M.S. *et al.* (1987) Prenatal diagnosis of congenital non-bullous ichthyosiform erythroderma (lamellar ichthyosis). *Prenatal Diagnosis*, 7, 145–55.

Persutte, W.W., Lenke, R.R. and Derosa, R.T. (1990) Prenatal ultrasono-graphic appearance of the agnathia malformation complex. *Journal of Ultrasound in Medicine*, 9, 725–28.

Persutte, W.W., Lenke, R.R., Kropp, K. and Ghareeb, C. (1988b) Antenatal diagnosis of fetal patent uracus. *Journal of Ultrasaound in Medicine*, 7, 399–403.

Persutte, W.H., Lenke, R.R., Kruczynski, T.W. and Brinker, R.A. (1988a) Antenatal diagnosis of Pena–Skokeir syndrome (type I) with ultrasonography and magnetic resonance imaging. *Obstetrics and Gynecology*, 72, 472–75.

Peters, M.T. and Nicolaides, K.H. (1990) Cordocentesis for the diagnosis and treatment of human fetal parvovirus infection. *Obstetrics and Gynecology*, 75, 501–504.

Petres, R.E., Redwine, F.O. and Cruikshank, D.P. (1982) Congenital bilateral chylothorax. Antepartum diagnosis and successful intrauterine surgical management. *JAMA* 248, 1360–61.

Petrikovsky, B.M., Vintzileos, A.M. and Rodis, J.F. (1989) Sonographic appearance of occipital fetal hair. *JCU*, 17, 425–27.

Petrikovsky, B.M., Walzak, M.P., and D'Addario, P.F. (1988) Fetal cloacal anomalies: prenatal sonographic findings and differential diagnosis. *Obstetrics and Gynecology*, 72, 464–69.

Petrova-Benedict, R., Robinson, B.H., Stacey, T.E. *et al.* (1987) Deficient fumarase activity in an infant with fumaricacidemia and its distribution between different forms of the enzyme seen on isoelectric focussing. *American Journal of Human Genetics*, 40, 257–266.

Phillips, J.A., Hjelle, B.L., Seeburg, P.H. and Zachmann, M. (1981) Molecular basis for familial isolated growth hormone deficiency. *Proceedings of the National Academy of Sciences of the USA*, 78, 6372–75.

Piepkorn, M., Karp, L.E., Hickok, D. *et al.* (1977) A lethal neonatal dwarfing condition with short ribs, polysyndactyly, cranial synostosis, cleft palate, cardiovascular and urogenital anomalies and severe ossification defect. *Teratology*, 16, 345–50.

Pilu, G., Reece, A., Romero, R. *et al.* (1986a) Prenatal diagnosis of craniofacial malformations with ultrasonography. *American Journal of Obstetrics and Gynecology*, 155, 45–50.

Pilu, G., Romero, R., Reece, A. *et al.* (1986b) The prenatal diagnosis of Robin anomalad. *American Journal of Obstetrics and Gynecology*, 154, 630–32.

Pircon, R.A., Porto, M., Towers, C.V. *et al.* (1989) Ultrasound findings in pregnancies complicated by fetal triploidy. *Journal of Ultrasound in Medicine*, 8, 507–11.

Poenaru, L (1982) Prenatal diagnosis of a heterozygote for mucopolysacchari-dosis type VII (beta-glucuronidase deficiency). *Prenatal Diagnosis*, 2, 251–56.

Poenaru, L (1987) First trimester prenatal diagnosis of metabolic diseases: a survey in countries from the European community. *Prenatal Diagnosis*, 7, 333–41.

Poenaru, L., Castelnau, L., Besancon, A.-M. *et al.* (1988) First trimester prenatal diagnosis of metachromatic leucodystrophy on chorionic villi by 'immunoprecipitation electrophoresis'. *Journal of Inherited Metabolic Dis-ease*, 11, 123–30.

Poenaru, L., Girard, S., Thepot, F. *et al.* (1979) Antenatal diagnosis in three pregnancies at risk for mannosidosis. *Clinical Genetics*, 16, 428–32.

Poenaru, L., Mezard, C., Akli, S. *et al.* (1990) Prenatal diagnosis of mucolipidosis type II on first-trimester amniotic fluid. *Prenatal Diagnosis*, 10, 231–35.

Pollitt, R.J. (1989) Disorders of mitochondrial beta-oxidation: prenatal and early postnatal diagnosis and their relevance to Reye's syndrome and sudden infant death. *Journal of Inherited Metabolic Disease*, 12 (suppl. 1), 215–30.

Poll-The, B.T., Poulos, A., Sharp, P. *et al.* (1985) Antenatal diagnosis of infantile Refsum's disease. *Clinical Genetics*, 27, 524–26.

Pope, F.M., Daw, S.C.M., Narcisi, P. *et al.* (1989) Prenatal diagnosis and prevention of inherited disorders of collagen. *Journal of Inherited Metabolic Disease*, 12 (suppl.), 135–73.

Pretorius, D.H., Drose, J.A., Dennis, M.A. et al. (1987) Tracheoesophageal fistula in utero: twenty-two cases. Journal of Ultrasound in Medicine, 6, 509–13.

Pretorius, D., Manchester, D., Barkin, S. et al. (1988) Doppler ultrasound of twin transfusion syndrome. Journal of Ultrasound in Medicine, 7, 117–24.

Pretorius, D.H., Rumack, C.M., Manco-Johnson, M.L. et al. (1986) Specific skeletal dysplasia in utero: sonographic diagnosis. Radiology, 159, 237–42.

Preus, M., Kaplan, P. and Kirkham, T.H. (1977) Renal anomalies and oligohydramnios in the cerebro-oculofacio-skeletal syndrome. American Journal of Diseases of Children, 131, 62–64.

Puck, J.M., Kraus, C.M., Puck, S.M. et al. (1990) Prenatal test for X-linked severe combined immunodeficiency by analysis of maternal X-chromosome inactivation and linkage analysis. New England Journal of Medicine, 322, 1063–66.

Quagliarello, J.R., Passalaqua, A.M., Greco, M.A. et al. (1978) Ballantyne's triple edema syndrome: prenatal diagnosis with ultrasound and maternal renal biopsy findings. American Journal of Obstetrics and Gynecology, 132, 580–81.

Quan, F., Korneluk, R.G., Tropak, M.B. and Gravel, R.A. (1986) Isolation and characterisation of the human catalase gene. Nucleic Acids Research, 14, 5321–35.

Quarrell, O.W.J., Meredith, A.L., Tyler, A. et al. (1987) Exclusion testing for Huntington's disease in pregnancy with a closely linked DNA marker. Lancet, i, 1281–83.

Quigg, M.H., Evans, M.I., Zador, I. et al. (1985) Ultrasonographic prenatal diagnosis of Langer-type mesomelic dwarfism. American Journal of Human Genetics, 37, A225.

Quinlan, R.W., Cruz, A.C. and Huddleston, J.F. (1986) Sonographic detection of fetal urinary tract anomalies. Obstetrics and Gynecology, 67, 558–65.

Ramsing, M., Rehd, H., Holzgreve, W. et al. (1990) Fraser syndrome (cryptophthalmos with syndactyly) in the fetus and newborn. Clinical Genetics, 37, 84–96.

Rapola, J., Salonen, R., Ammala, P. and Santavuori, P. (1990) Prenatal diagnosis of the infantile type of neuronal ceroid lipofuscinosis by electron microscopic investigation of human chorionic villi. Prenatal Diagnosis, 10, 553–59.

Rasore-Quartino, A., Vignola, G. and Camera, G. (1985) Hereditary enlarged parietal foramina (foramina parietalia permagna). Prenatal diagnosis, evolution and family study. Pathologica, 77, 449–55.

Reiter, A.A., Hunta, J.C., Carpenter, R.J. et al. (1986) Prenatal diagnosis of arteriovenous malformation of the vein of Galen. JCU, 14, 623–28.

Rempen, A. (1989) Sonographic first-trimester diagnosis of umbilical cord cyst. JCU, 17, 53–55.

Rempen, A., Feige, A. and Wunsch, P. (1987) Prenatal diagnosis of bilateral cystic adenomatoid malformation of the lung. JCU, 15, 3–8.

Renlund, M. and Aula, P. (1987) Prenatal detection of Salla disease based upon increased free sialic acid in amniocytes. American Journal of Medical Genetics, 28, 377–84.

Reuss, A., Den Hollander, J.C., Niermeijer, M.F. et al. (1989) Prenatal diagnosis of cystic renal disease with ventriculomegaly: a report of six cases in two related sibships. American Journal of Medical Genetics, 33, 385–89.

Reuss, A., Waldimiroff, J.W. and Stewart, P.A. (1990) Prenatal diagnosis by ultrasound in pregnancies at risk for autosomal recessive polycystic kidney disease. Ultrasound in Medicine and Biology, 16, 355–59

Richards, R.I., Holman, K., Kozman, H. et al. (1991) Fragile X syndrome: genetic localisation by linkage mapping of two microsatellite repeats FRAXAC1 and FRAXAC2 which immediately flank the fragile site. Journal of Medical Genetics, 28, 818–23.

Ristaldi, M.S., Piratsu, M., Rosatelli, C. et al. (1989) Prenatal diagnosis of beta-thalassaemia in Mediterranean populations by dot-blot analysis with DNA amplification and allele specific oligonucleotide probes. Prenatal Diagnosis, 9, 629–38.

Ritchie, G., Jequier, S. and Lussier-Lazaroff, J. (1988) Prenatal renal ultrasound of Laurence–Moon–Biedl syndrome. Pediatric Radiology, 19, 65–66.

Rizzo, G., Arduini, D., Pennestri, F. et al. (1987) Fetal behaviour in growth retardation: its relationship to fetal blood flow. Prenatal Diagnosis, 7, 229.

Rizzo, N., Gabrielli, S., Perolo, A. et al. (1989) Prenatal diagnosis and management of fetal ovarian cysts. Prenatal Diagnosis, 9, 97–104.

Rizzo, N., Gabrielli S., Pilu, G. et al. (1987) Prenatal diagnosis and obstetrical management of multicystic dysplastic kidney disease. Prenatal Diagnosis, 7, 109–18.

Roberson, D.A. and Silverman, N.H. (1989) Ebstein's anomaly: echocardiographic and clinical features in the fetus and neonate. Journal of the American College of Cardiology, 14, 1300–307.

Robinson, B.H., Toone, J.R., Benedict, R.P. et al. (1985) Prenatal diagnosis of pyruvate carboxylase deficiency. Prenatal Diagnosis, 5, 67–71.

Robinson, L.P., Worthen, N.J., Lachman, R.S. et al. (1987) Prenatal diagnosis of osteogenesis imperfecta type III. Prenatal Diagnosis, 7, 7–15.

Rodeck, C.H., Patrick, A.D., Pembrey, P.F. et al. (1982) Fetal liver biopsy for prenatal diagnosis of ornithine carbamyl transferase deficiency. Lancet, ii, 297–300.

Rodeck, C.H., Tansley, L.R., Benson, P.F. et al. (1983b) Prenatal exclusion of Hurler's disease by leucocyte alpha-L-iduronidase assay. Prenatal Diagnosis, 3, 61–63.

Rogoyski, A. (1985) Postnatal and prenatal diagnosis of Maroteaux–Lamy syndrome. Acta Anthropogenetica, 9, 109–16.

Rolland, M.O., Divry, P., Mandon, G. et al. (1990) Early prenatal diagnosis of propionic acidaemia with simultaneous sampling of chorionic villus and amniotic fluid. Journal of Inherited Metabolic Disease, 13, 345–48.

Rolland, M., Sarramon, M.F., and Bloom, M.C. (1991) Astomia-agnathia-holoprosencephaly association. Prenatal diagnosis of a new case. Prenatal Diagnosis, 11, 199–203.

Romero, R., Chevenak, F.A., Devore, G. et al. (1981) Fetal head deformation and congenital torticollis associated with a uterine tumour. American Journal of Obstetrics and Gynecology, 141, 839–40.

Romero, R., Cullen. M., Grannum, P. et al. (1985) Antenatal diagnosis of renal anomalies with ultrasound. III. Bilateral renal agenesis. American Journal of Obstetrics and Gynecology, 151, 38–43.

Romero, R., Cullen, M., Jeanty, P. et al. (1984) The diagnosis of congenital renal anomalies with ultrasound. II. Infantile polycystic kidney disease. American Journal of Obstetrics and Gynecology, 150, 259–62.

Romero, R., Ghindi, A., Eswara, M.S. et al. (1988) Prenatal findings in a case of spondylocostal dysplasia type I (Jarcho–Levin syndrome). Obstetrics and Gynecology, 71, 988–91.

Romke, C., Froster-Iskenius, U., Heyne, K. et al. (1987) Roberts syndrome and SC phocomelia: a single genetic entity. Clinical Genetics, 31, 170–77.

Rosa, R., Prehu, M,O., Calvin, M.C. et al. (1986) Possibility of prenatal diagnosis of hereditary triose phosphate isomerase deficiency. Prenatal Diagnosis, 6, 231–34.

Rosenblatt, D.S., (1987) Expression of transcobalamin II by amniocytes. Prenatal Diagnosis, 7, 35–39.

Rosenblatt, D.S., Cooper, B.A., Schmutz, S.M. et al. (1985) Prenatal vitamin B_{12} therapy of a fetus with methylcobalamin deficiency (cobalamin E disease) Lancet, i, 1127–29.

Rosler, A., Lieberman, E., Rosenmann, A. et al. (1979) Prenatal diagnosis of 11beta-hydroxylase deficiency congenital adrenal hyperplasia. Journal of Clinical Endocrinology and Metabolism, 49, 546–51.

Rotmensch, S., Grannum, P.A., Nores, J.A. et al. (1991) In utero diagnosis and management of fetal subdural haematoma. American Journal of Obstetrics and Gynecology, 164, 1246–48.

Rouleau, G.A., Wertelecki, W., Haines, J.L. et al. (1987) Genetic linkage of bilateral acoustic neurofibromatosis to a DNA marker on chromosome 22. Nature, 329, 246–48.

Rowley, K.A. (1955) Coronal cleft vertebra. Journal of the Faculty of Radiologists, 6, 267.

Rozear, M.P., Pericak-Vance, M.A., Fischbeck, K. et al. (1987) Hereditary motor and sensory neuropathy, X-linked: a half century follow-up. Neurology, 37, 1460–65.

Rudiger, H.W., Bartram, C.R., Harder, W. and Passarge, E. (1980) Rate of sister chromatid exchanges in Bloom syndrome fibroblasts reduced by co-cultivation with normal fibroblasts. American Journal of Human Genetics, 32, 150–57.

Ruitenbeek, W., Sengers, R., Albani, M. et al. (1988) Prenatal diagnosis of cytochrome C oxidase deficiency by biopsy of chorionic villi. New England Journal of Medicine, 319, 1095.

Ruitenbeek, W., Sengers, R.C.A., Trijbels, J.M.F. et al. (1992). The use of chorionic villi in prenatal diagnosis of mitochondropathies. Journal of Inherited Metabolic Disease, 15, 303–306.

Russ, P.D., Pretorius, P.M. and Johnson, M.J. (1989) Dandy–Walker syndrome: a review of fifteen cases evaluated by prenatal sonography. American Journal of Obstetrics and Gynecology, 161, 401–406.

Russell, J.G.B. (1973) Radiology in Obstetrics and Antenatal Paediatrics, Butterworth, London, pp. 79–80.

Saal, H.M., Deutsch, L., Herson V. et al. (1986) The RAG syndrome: a new autosomal recessive syndrome with Robin sequence, ancreolia and profound growth and developmental delays. American Journal of Human Genetics, 39, A78.

Sabbagha, R.E., Tamura, R.K., Compo, S.D. et al. (1980) Fetal cranial and craniocervical masses: ultrasound characteristics and differential diagnosis. American Journal of Obstetrics and Gynecology, 138, 511–17.

Sada, I., Shiratori, H. and Nakamura, Y. (1986) Antenatal diagnosis of fetus in fetu. Asia–Oceania Journal of Obstetrics and Gynaecology, 12, 353–56.

Sahn, D.J., Shenker, L., Reed, K.L. et al. (1982) Prenatal ultrasound diagnosis of hypoplastic left heart syndrome in utero associated with hydrops fetalis. American Heart Journal, 104, 1368–72.

Sakuma, T., Sugiyama, N., Ichiki, T. et al. (1991) Analysis of acylcarnitines in maternal urine for prenatal diagnosis of glutaric aciduria type 2. Prenatal Diagnosis, 11, 77–82.

Saltzman, D.H., Benacerraf, B.R. and Frigoletto, F.D. (1986) Diagnosis and management of fetal facial clefts. American Journal of Obstetrics and Gynecology, 155, 377–79.

Saltzman, D.H., Krauss, C.M., Goldman, J.M. and Benacerraf, B.R. (1991) Prenatal diagnosis of lissencephaly. Prenatal Diagnosis, 11, 139–43

Salvo, A.F. (1981) *In utero* diagnosis of Kleeblattschadel (cloverleaf skull) *Prenatal Diagnosis*, 1, 141–45.

Samuel, N., Dicker, D., Landman, J. *et al.* (1986) Early diagnosis and intrauterine therapy of meconium plug syndrome in the fetus: risks and benefits. *Journal of Ultrasound in Medicine*, 5, 425–28.

Samuel, N., Sirotta, L., Bar-Ziv, J. *et al.* (1988) The ultrasonic appearance of common pulmonary vein atresia *in utero*. *Journal of Ultrasound in Medicine*, 7, 25–28.

Samueloff, A., Navot, D., Bickenfeld, A. and Schenker, J.G. (1987) Fryns syndrome: a predictable, lethal pattern of multiple congenital anomalies. *American Journal of Obstetrics and Gynecology*, 156, 86–88.

Sassa, S., Solish, G., Levere, R.D. and Kappas, A. (1975) Studies in porphyria IV. Expression of the gene defect of acute intermittent porphyria in cultured human skin fibroblasts and amniotic fluid cells: PND of the porphyric trait. *Journal of Experimental Medicine*, 142, 722–31.

Savary, J.B., Vasseur, F. and Deminatti, M.M. (1991) Routine autoradiographic analysis of DNA excision-repair. Report of prenatal and postnatal diagnosis in eleven families. *Annales de Génétique*, 34, 76–81.

Savary, J.B., Vasseur, F., Vinatier, D. *et al.* (1991) Prenatal diagnosis of PIBIDS. *Prenatal Diagnosis*, 11, 859–66.

Savodelli, G. and Schinzel, A. (1983) Prenatal ultrasound detection of humeroradial synostosis in a case of Antley–Bixler syndrome. *Prenatal Diagnosis*, 2, 219–33.

Schaffer, R.M., Cabbad, M., Minkoff, H. *et al.* (1986) Sonographic diagnosis of fetal cardiac rhabdomyoma. *Journal of Ultrasound in Medicine*, 5, 531–33.

Schauer, G.M., Dunn, L.K., Godmilow, L. *et al.* (1990) Prenatal diagnosis of Fraser syndrome at 18.5 weeks gestation with autopsy findings at 19 weeks. *American Journal of Medical Genetics*, 37, 583–91.

Schechter, A.G., Fakhry, J., Shapiro, L.R. and Gewitz, M.H. (1987) *In utero* thickening of the chordae tendinae: a cause of intracardiac echogenic foci. *Journal of Ultrasound in Medicine*, 6, 691–695.

Schindler, D., Bishop, D.F., Wolfe, D.E. *et al.* (1989) Neuroaxonal dystrophy due to lysosomal α-*N*-acetylgalactosaminidase deficiency. *New England Journal of Medicine*, 320, 1735–40.

Schinzel, A., Savodelli, G., Briner, J. and Schubiger, G. (1985) Prenatal sonographic diagnosis of Jeune syndrome. *Radiology*, 154, 777–78.

Schinzel, A., Savoldelli, G., Briner, J. *et al.* (1983) Antley–Bixler syndrome in sisters: a term newborn and a prenatally diagnosed fetus. *American Journal of Medical Genetics*, 14, 139–47.

Schmidt, K.G., Birk, E., Silverman, N.H. and Scagnelli, S.A. (1989) Echocardiographic evaluation of dilated cardiomyopathy in the human fetus. *American Journal of Cardiology*, 63, 599–605.

Schmidt, W., Harms, E. and Wolf, D. (1985) Successful prenatal treatment of non-immune hydrops fetalis due to congenital chylothorax. Case report. *British Journal of Obstetrics and Gynaecology*, 92, 685–87.

Schneider, J.A., Verroust, F.M., Kroll, W.A. *et al.* (1974) Prenatal diagnosis of cystinosis. *New England Journal of Medicine*, 290, 878–82.

Schroeder, D., Smith, L. and Prain, H.C. (1989) Antenatal diagnosis of choledochal cyst at 15 weeks' gestation: etiologic implications and management. *Journal of Pediatric Surgery*, 24, 936–38.

Schumert, Z., Rosenmann, A., Landau, H. and Rosler, A. (1980) 11-Deoxycortisol in amniotic fluid: prenatal diagnosis of congenital adrenal hyperplasia due to 11 beta-hydroxylase deficiency. *Clinical Endocrinology*, 12, 257–60.

Schutgens, R.B.H., Schrakamp, G., Wanders, R.J.A. *et al.* (1989) Prenatal and perinatal diagnosis of peroxisomal disorders. *Journal of Inherited Metabolic Disease*, 12 (suppl. 1), 118–34.

Schuurman, H.J., Huber, J., Zegers, B.J.M. and Roord, J.J. (1985) Placental diagnosis of bare lymphocyte syndrome. *New England Journal of Medicine*, 313, 757.

Schwartz, M., Mibashan, R. and Nicolaides, K.H. (1989) First-trimester diagnosis of Wiskott–Aldrich syndrome by DNA markers. *Lancet*, ii, 1405.

Schwartz, S., Flannery, D.B. and Cohen, M.M. (1985) Tests appropriate for prenatal diagnosis of ataxia telangiectasia. *Prenatal Diagnosis*, 5, 9–14.

Secor McVoy, J.R., Heard, G.S. and Wolf, B. (1984) Potential for prenatal diagnosis of biotinidase deficiency. *Prenatal Diagnosis*, 4, 317–18.

Seeds, J.W., Cefalo, R.C., Lies, S.C. and Koontz, W.L. (1984) Early prenatal sonographic appearance of rare thoracoabdominal eventration. *Prenatal Diagnosis*, 4, 437–41.

Seeds, J.W. and Powers, S.K. (1988) Early prenatal diagnosis of familial lipomyelomeningocele. *Obstetrics and Gynecology*, 72, 469–71.

Seizinger, B.R., Rouleau, G.A., Ozelius, L.J. *et al.* (1988) Von Hippel–Lindau disease maps to the region of chromosome 3 associated with renal cell carcinoma. *Nature*, 332, 268–69.

Seligsohn, V., Mibashan, R.S., Rodeck, C.H. (1985) Prenatal diagnosis of Glanzmann's thrombasthenia. *Lancet*, ii, 1419.

Serini, L.P., Bachmann, C., Pfister, U. *et al.* (1988) Prenatal diagnosis of carbamoyl-phosphate synthetase deficiency by fetal liver biopsy. *Prenatal Diagnosis*, 8, 307–309.

Sewell, A.C. and Pontz, B.F. (1988) Prenatal diagnosis of galactosialidosis. *Prenatal Diagnosis*, 8, 151–55.

Shah, Y.G. and Metlay, L. (1990) Prenatal ultrasound diagnosis of Beckwith–Wiedemann syndrome. *JCU*, 18, 597–600.

Shalev, E. (1983) Prenatal ultrasound diagnosis of intestinal calcification with imperforate anus. *Acta Obstetricia et Gynecologica Scandinavica*, 62, 95–96.

Shalev, E., Romano, S., Nseit, T. and Zuckerman, H. (1988) Klippel–Trenaunay syndrome: ultrasonic prenatal diagnosis. *JCU*, 16, 268–70.

Shalev, J., Frankel, Y., Avigad, I. and Mashiach, S. (1982) Spontaneous intestinal perforation *in utero*: ultrasonic diagnostic criteria. *American Journal of Obstetrics and Gynecology*, 144, 855–57.

Shapiro, L.R., Wilmot, P.L., Murphy, P.O. and Breg, W.R. (1988) Experience with multiple approaches to the prenatal diagnosis of the fragile X syndrome: amniotic fluid, chorionic villi, fetal blood and molecular methods. *American Journal of Medical Genetics*, 30, 347–54.

Shechter, S.A., Sherer, D.M., Geilfuss, C.J. *et al.* (1990) Prenatal sonographic appearance and subsequent management of a fetus with oromandibular limb hypogenesis syndrome associated with pulmonary hypoplasia. *JCU*, 18, 661–65.

Shelton-Inloes, B.B., Chehab, F.F., Mannucci, P.M. *et al.* (1987) Gene deletions correlate with the development of alloantibodies in von Willebrand disease. *Journal of Clinical Investigation*, 79, 1459–65.

Shenker, L., Reed, K.L., Anderson, C.F. and Kern, W. (1989) Fetal pericardial effusion. *American Journal of Obstetrics and Gynecology*, 160, 1505–508.

Sherer, D.M., Cullen, J.B.H., Thompson, H.O. *et al.* (1990) Prenatal sonographic findings associated with a fetal horseshoe kidney. *Journal of Ultrasound in Medicine*, 9, 477–79.

Sherer, D.M., Menashe, M., Lebensart, P. *et al.* (1989) Sonographic diagnosis of unilateral fetal renal duplication with associated ectopic ureterocele. *JCU*, 17, 371–73.

Shin, Y.S., Rieth, M., Tausenfreund, J. and Endres, W. (1989) First trimester diagnosis of glycogen storage disease type II and type III. *Journal of Inherited Metabolic Disease*, 12 (suppl. 2), 289–91.

Siebert, J.R., Warkany, J. and Lemire, R.J. (1986) Atelencephalic microcephaly in a 21-week human fetus. *Teratology*, 34, 9–19.

Sieck, U.V. and Ohlsson, A. (1984) Fetal polyuria and hydramnios associated with Bartter's syndrome. *Obstetrics and Gynecology*, 63, 226–245.

Sieving, P.A., Bingham, E.L., Roth, M.S. *et al.* (1990) Linkage relationships of X-linked juvenile retinoschisis with Xp22.1–p22.3 probes. *American Journal of Human Genetics*, 47, 616–21.

Siffring, P.A., Forrest, T.S. and Frick, M.P. (1991) Sonographic detection of hydrolethalus syndrome. *JCU*, 19, 43–47.

Silver, D.N., Lewis, R.A. and Nussbaum, R.L. (1987) Mapping the Lowe oculocerebro-renal syndrome to Xq24–q26 by use of restriction fragment length polymorphisms. *Journal of Clinical Investigation*, 79, 282–85.

Silverman, N.H., Enderlein, M.A. and Golbus, M.S. (1984) Ultrasonic recognition of aortic valve atresia *in utero*, *American Journal of Cardiology*, 53, 391–92.

Sirtori, M., Ghidini, A., Romero, R. and Robbins, J.C. (1989) Prenatal diagnosis of sirenomelia. *Journal of Ultrasound in Medicine*, 8, 83–88.

Skare, J.C., Milunsky, A., Byron, K.S. and Sullivan, J.L. (1987) Mapping the X-linked lymphoproliferative syndrome. *Proceedings of the National Academy of Sciences of the USA*, 84, 2015–18.

Skrede, S., Bjorkhem, I., Kvittingen, E.A. *et al.* (1986) Demonstrations of 26-hydroxylation of C-27 steroids in human skin fibroblasts and a deficiency of this activity in cerebrotendinous xanthomatosis. *Journal of Clinical Investigation*, 78, 729–735.

Smith, H.J., Hanken, H. and Brundelet, P.J. (1981) Ultrasound diagnosis of interstitial pregnancy. *Acta Obstetricia et Gynecologica Scandinavia*, 60, 413–16.

Snyder, J.R., Lustig-Gillman, I., Milio, L. *et al.* (1986) Antenatal ultrasound diagnosis of an intracranial neoplasm (craniopharyngioma). *JCU*, 14, 304–306.

Socol, M.L., Sabbagha, R.E., Elias, S. *et al.* (1985) Prenatal diagnosis of congenital muscular dystrophy producing arthrogryposis. *New England Journal of Medicine*, 313, 1230.

Sonek, J.D., Gabbe, S.G., Landon, M.B. (1990) Antenatal diagnosis of sacral agenesis syndrome in a pregnancy complicated by diabetes mellitus. *American Journal of Obstetrics and Gynecology*, 162, 806–808.

Spear, R., Mack, L.A., Benedetti, T.J. and Cole, R.E. (1990) Idiopathic infantile arterial calcification: *in utero* diagnosis. *Journal of Ultrasound in Medicine*, 9, 473–76.

Spector, E.B., Kiernan, M., Bernard, B. and Cederbaum, S.D. (1980) Properties of fetal and adult red blood cell arginase deficiency. *American Journal of Human Genetics*, 32, 79–97.

Speer, A., Bollman, R., Michel, A. *et al.* (1986) Prenatal diagnosis of classical phenylketonuria by linked restriction fragment length polymorphism analysis. *Prenatal Diagnosis*, 6, 447–50.

Speer, M.C., Pericak-Vance, M.A., Yamacka, L. *et al.* (1990) Presymptomatic and prenatal diagnosis in myotonic dystrophy by genetic linkage studies. *Neurology*, 40, 671–76

Speiser, P.W., Laforgia, N., Kato, K. *et al.* (1990) First trimester prenatal treatment and molecular genetic diagnosis of congenital adrenal hyperplasia (21-hydroxylase deficiency). *Journal of Clinical Endocrinology and Metabolism*, 70, 838–48.

Spence, J.E., Maddalena, A., O'Brien, W.E. *et al.* (1989) Prenatal diagnosis and heterozygote detection by DNA analysis in ornithine transcarbamylase deficiency. *Journal of Pediatrics*, 114, 582–88.

Spirt, B.A., Gordon, L.P. and Oliphant, M. (1987) *Prenatal Ultrasound: A Colour Atlas with Anatomic and Pathologic Correlation*, Churchill Livingstone, Edinburgh.

Spritz, R.A., Strunk, K.M., Giebel, L.B. and King, R.A. (1990) Detection of mutations in the tyrosinase gene in a patient with type IA oculocutaneous albinism. *New England Journal of Medicine*, 322, 1724–28.

Stamm, E., King, G. and Thickman, D. (1991) Megacystic–microcolon–intestinal hypoperistalsis syndrome: prenatal identification in siblings and review of the literature. *Journal of Ultrasound in Medicine*, 10, 599–602.

Stamm, E.R., Pretorius, D.H., Rumack, C.M. and Manco-Johnson, M.L. (1987) Kleeblattschadel anomaly. In utero sonographic appearance. *Journal of Ultrasound in Medicine*, 6, 319–24.

Stanford, W., Abu-Yousef, M. and Smith, W. (1987) Intracardiac tumour (rhabdomyoma) diagnosed by in utero ultrasound: a case report. *JCU*, 15, 337–41.

Steinfeld, L., Rappaport, H.L., Rossbach, H.C. and Martinez, E. (1986) Diagnosis of fetal arrhythmias using echocardiographic and Doppler techniques. *Journal of the American College of Cardiology*, 9, 1425–33.

Steinherz, R. (1985) Prenatal diagnosis of cystinosis upon exposure of amniotic cells to cystine dimethyl ester. *Israeli Journal of Medical Science*, 21, 537–39.

Steinman, L., Tharp, B.R., Dorfman, L.J. et al. (1980) Peripheral neuropathy in the cherry-red spot myoclonus syndrome (sialidosis type I). *Annals of Neurology*, 7, 450–56.

Stellaard, F., Langelaar, S.A., Kok, R.M. et al. (1988) Prenatal diagnosis of Zellweger syndrome by determination of trihydroxycoprostanic acid in amniotic fluid. *European Journal of Pediatrics*, 148, 175–76.

Stephens, J.D. (1984) Prenatal diagnosis of testicular feminisation. *Lancet*, ii, 1038.

Stewart, P.A., Buis-Liem, T., Verwey, R.A. and Wladimiroff, J.W. (1986) Prenatal ultrasonic diagnosis of familial asymmetric septal hypertrophy. *Prenatal Diagnosis*, 6, 249–56.

Stewart, P.A., Wladimiroff, J.W. and Becker, A.E. (1985) Early prenatal detection of double outlet right ventricle by echocardiography. *British Heart Journal*, 54, 340–42.

Stiller, R.J. (1989) Early ultrasonic appearance of fetal bladder outlet obstruction. *American Journal of Obstetrics and Gynecology*, 160, 584–85.

Stiller, R.J., Pinto, M., Heller, C. and Hobbins, J.C. (1988) Oligohydramnios associated with bilateral multicystic dysplastic kidneys: prenatal diagnosis at 15 weeks gestation. *JCU*, 16, 436–39.

Stoker, A.F., Jonnes, S.V. and Spence, J. (1983) Ultrasound diagnosis of situs inversus in utero. A case report. *South African Medical Journal*, 64, 832–34.

Stoll, C., Ehret-Mentre, M.-C., Treisser, A. and Tranchant, C. (1991) Prenatal diagnosis of congenital myasthenia with arthrogryposis in a myasthenic mother. *Prenatal Diagnosis*, 11, 17–22.

Stoll, C., Willard, D., Czernichow, P. and Boue, J. (1978) Prenatal diagnosis of primary pituitary dysgenesis. *Lancet*, i, 932.

Stoll, C., Willard, D., Czernichow, P. and Boue, J. (1985) Prenatal diagnosis of hypochondroplasia. *Prenatal Diagnosis*, 5, 423–26.

Sugita, T., Ikenaga, M., Suchara, N. et al. (1982) Prenatal diagnosis of Cockayne syndrome using assay of colony-forming ability in ultraviolet light irradiated cells. *Clinical Genetics*, 22, 137–42.

Sutro, W.H., Tuck, S.M., Loesevitz, A. et al. (1984) Prenatal observation of umbilical cord hematoma. *AJR*, 142, 801–802.

Suttle, D.P., Bugg, B.Y., Winkler, J.K. and Kanalas, J.J. (1988) Molecular cloning and nucleotide sequence for the complete coding region of human UMP synthase. *Proceedings of the National Academy of Sciences of the USA*, 85, 1754–58.

Suzumori, K. and Kanzaki, T. (1991) Prenatal diagnosis of harlequin ichthyosis by total skin biopsy, report of two cases. *Prenatal Diagnosis*, 11, 451–57.

Taylor, P., Jeenah, M., Seed, M. and Humphries, S. (1988) Four DNA polymorphisms in the LDL receptor gene: their genetic relationship and use in the study of variation at LDL receptor locus. *Journal of Medical Genetics*, 25, 653–59.

Teichler-Zallen, D. and Doherty, R.A. (1983) Fetal ABO blood group typing using amniotic fluid. *Clinical Genetics*, 23, 120–24.

Terry, G.M., Ho-Terry, L., Warren, R.C. et al. (1986) First trimester prenatal diagnosis of congenital rubella: a laboratory investigation. *BMJ*, 292, 930–33.

Thiagarajah, S., Abbitt, P.L., Hogge, W.A. and Leason, S.H. (1990) Prenatal diagnosis of eventration of the diaphragm. *JCU*, 18, 46–49.

Thomas, C.S., Leopold, G.R., Hilton, S. et al. (1986) Fetal hydrops associated with extralobar pulmonary sequestration. *Journal of Ultrasound in Medicine*, 5, 668–71.

Toftager-Larsen, K. and Benzie, R.J. (1984) Fetoscopy in prenatal diagnosis of the Majewski and the Saldino–Noonan types of the short rib–polydactyly syndromes. *Clinical Genetics*, 26, 56–60.

Toi, A., Simpson, G.F. and Filly, R.A. (1987) Ultrasonically evident fetal nuchal skin thickening: is it specific for Down syndrome? *American Journal of Obstetrics and Gynecology*, 156, 150–53.

Tolmie, J.L., McNay, M.B. and Connor, J.M. (1987a) Prenatal diagnosis of severe autosomal recessive spondylothoracic dysplasia (Jarcho–Levin type). *Prenatal Diagnosis*, 7, 129–34.

Tolmie, J.L., McNay, M.B., Stephenson, J.B.P. et al. (1987b) Microcephaly:

genetic counselling and antenatal diagnosis. *American Journal of Medical Genetics*, 27, 583–94.

Tolmie, J.L., Mortimer, G., Doyle, D. et al. (1987c) The Neu–Laxova syndrome in female sibs: clinical and pathological features with prenatal diagnosis in the second sib. *American Journal of Medical Genetics*, 27, 175–82.

Tolmie, J.L., Patrick, A. and Yates, J.R.W. (1987d) A lethal multiple pterygium syndrome with apparent X-linked recessive inheritance. *American Journal of Medical Genetics*, 27, 913–19.

Toma, P., Costa, A., Magnano, G.M. et al. (1990) Holoprosencephaly: prenatal diagnosis by sonography and magnetic resonance imaging. *Prenatal Diagnosis*, 10, 429–36.

Toma, P., Dell'Acqua, A., Cordone, M. et al. (1991) Prenatal diagnosis of hydrosyringomyelia by high-resolution ultrasonography. *JCU*, 19, 51–54.

Tomkins, D.J. (1989) Premature centromere separation and the prenatal diagnosis of Roberts syndrome. *Prenatal Diagnosis*, 9, 450–51.

Tonnensen, T. and Horn, N. (1989) Prenatal and postnatal diagnosis of Menkes disease, an inherited disorder of copper metabolism. *Journal of Inherited Metabolic Disease*, 12 (suppl. 1), 207–14.

Trecet, J.C., Claramunt, V., Larraz, J. et al. (1984) Prenatal ultrasound diagnosis of fetal teratoma of the neck. *JCU*, 12, 509–11.

Trepeta, R., Stenn, K.S. and Mahoney, M.J. (1984) Prenatal diagnosis of Sjögren–Larsson syndrome. *Seminars in Dermatology*, 3, 221–24.

Triggs-Raine, B.L., Archibald, A., Gravel, R.A. and Clarke, J.T.R. (1990) Prenatal exclusion of Tay–Sachs disease by DNA analysis. *Lancet*, i, 1164.

Tsipouras, P., Schwartz, R.C., Goldberg, J.D. et al. (1987) Prenatal prediction of osteogenesis imperfecta (OI type IV): exclusion of inheritance using a collagen gene probe. *Journal of Medical Genetics*, 24, 406–409.

Tsuchiyama, A., Oyanagi, K., Hirano, S. et al. (1983) A case of pyruvate carboxylase deficiency with later prenatal diagnosis of an unaffected sibling. *Journal of Inherited Metabolic Disease*, 6, 85–88.

Tuck, S.M., Slack, J. and Buckland, G. (1990) Prenatal diagnosis of Conradi's syndrome. Case report. *Prenatal Diagnosis*, 10, 195–98.

Vamos, E., Libert, J., Elkhazen, N. et al. (1986) Prenatal diagnosis and confirmation of infantile sialic acid storage disease. *Prenatal Diagnosis*, 6, 437–46.

Van Dam, L.J., de Groot, C.J., Hazebroek, F.W. and Waldimiroff, J.W. (1984) Case report. Intrauterine demonstration of bowel duplication by ultrasound. *European Journal of Obstetrics, Gynecology and Reproductive Biology*, 18, 229–32.

Van den Hof, M.C., Nicolaides, K.H., Campbell, J. and Campbell S. (1990) Evaluation of the lemon and banana signs in one hundred and thirty fetuses with open spina bifida. *American Journal of Obstetrics and Gynecology*, 162, 322–27.

Van Dyke, D.L., Fluharty, A.L., Schafer, I.A. et al. (1981) Prenatal diagnosis of Maroteaux–Lamy syndrome. *American Journal of Medical Genetics*, 8, 235–42.

Van Egmond-Linden, A., Waldimiroff, J., Jahoda, M. et al. (1983) Prenatal diagnosis of X-linked hydrocephaly. *Prenatal Diagnosis*, 13, 245–48.

Vanier, M.T., Boue, J. and Dumez, Y. (1985) Niemann–Pick diseases type 8. First trimester prenatal diagnosis on chorionic villi. *Clinical Genetics*, 28, 348–50.

Vanier, M.T., Rousson, R.M., Mandon, G. et al. (1989) Diagnosis of Niemann–Pick disease type C on chorionic villus cells. *Lancet*, i, 1014–15.

Van Regemorter, H., Wilkin, P., Englert, Y. et al. (1984) Lethal multiple pterygium syndrome. *American Journal of Medical Genetics*, 17, 827–34.

Verkerk, A.J.M.H., Pieretti, M., Sutcliffe, J.S. et al. (1991) Identification of a gene (*FMR-1*) containing a CGG repeat coincident with a breakpoint cluster region exhibiting length variation in the fragile X syndrome. *Cell*, 65, 905–14.

Verma, I.C., Bhargava, S. and Agarwal, S. (1975) An autosomal recessive form of lethal chondrodystrophy with severe thoracic narrowing, rhizoacromelic type of micromelia, polydactyly, and genital anomalies. *Birth Defects*, 11, 167–74.

Vermesh, M., Mayden, K.L., Confino, E. et al. (1986) Prenatal sonographic diagnosis of Hirschsprung's disease. *Journal of Ultrasound in Medicine*, 5, 37–39.

Vesce, F., Guerrini, P., Perri, G. et al. (1987) Ultrasonographic diagnosis of ectasia of the umbilical vein. *JCU*, 15, 346–49.

Vimal, C.M., Fensom, A.H., Heaton D. et al. (1984) Prenatal diagnosis of argininosuccinic aciduria by analysis of cultured chorionic villi. *Lancet*, ii, 521–22.

Vintners, H.V., Murphy, J., Wittman, B. and Norman, M.G. (1982) Intracranial teratoma: antenatal diagnosis at 31 weeks' gestation by ultrasound. *Acta Neuropathologica*, 58, 233–36.

Vintzileos, A.M. Hovick, T.J., Escoto, D.T. et al. (1987) Congenital midline porencephaly: prenatal sonographic findings and review of the literature. *American Journal of Perinatology*, 4, 125–28.

Viskochil, D., Buchberg, A.M., Xu, G. et al. (1990) Deletions and a translocation interrupt a cloned gene at the neurofibromatosis type I locus. *Cell*, **62**, 187–92.

Visser, G.H.A., Desmedt, M.C.H. and Meijboom, E.J. (1988) Altered fetal cardiac flow patterns in pure red cell anaemia (the Blackfan–Diamond syndrome). *Prenatal Diagnosis*, **8**, 525–29.

Von Figura, K., Van de Kamp, J.J. and Niermeijer, M.F. (1982) Prenatal diagnosis of Morquio's disease type A (*N*-acetyl-galactosamine 6-sulphate sulphatase deficiency). *Prenatal Diagnosis*, **2**, 67–69.

Vora, S., Dimauro, S., Spear, D. *et al.* (1987) Characterisation of the enzymatic defect in late onset muscle phosphofructokinase deficiency: a new subtype of glycogen storage disease type VII. *Journal of Clinical Investigation*, **80**, 1479–85.

Wager, G.P., Couser, R.J., Edwards, O.P. *et al.* (1988) Antenal ultrasound findings in a case of Uhl's anomaly. *American Journal of Perinatology*, **5**, 164–67.

Wallis, J., Shaw, J., Wilkes, D. *et al.* (1989) Prenatal diagnosis of Friedreich ataxia. *American Journal of Medical Genetics*, **34**, 458–61.

Wanders, P.J.A and Ijlst, L. (1992) Long chain 3-hydroxyacyl-CoA dehydrogenase in leucocytes and chorionic villus fibroblasts: potential for pre- and postnatal diagnosis. *Journal of Inherited Metabolic Disease*, **15**, 356–58.

Wanders, R.J.A., Schelen, A., Feller, N. *et al.* (1990) First prenatal diagnosis of acyl-CoA oxidase deficiency. *Journal of Inherited Metabolic Disease*, **13**, 371–74.

Wang, L.M., Zhang, J., Wu, G. *et al.* (1986) First trimester prenatal diagnosis of severe alpha thalassaemia. *Prenatal Diagnosis*, **6**, 89–95.

Ward, P.A., Hejmancik, J.F., Witkowski, J.A. *et al.* (1989) PND of Duchenne muscular dystrophy: prospective linkage analysis and retrospective dystrophin cDNA analysis. *American Journal of Human Genetics*, **44**, 270–81.

Warner, T.G., Robertson, A.D., Mock, A.K. *et al.* (1983) Prenatal diagnosis of G_{M1} gangliosidosis by detection of galactosyl-oligosaccharides in amniotic fluid with high performance liquid chromatography. *American Journal of Human Genetics*, **35**, 1034–45.

Weatherall, D.J., Old, J.M., Thein, S.L. *et al.* (1985) Prenatal diagnosis of the common haemoglobin disorders. *Journal of Medical Genetics*, **22**, 422–30.

Webb, T.P., Bundey, S. and McKinley, M. (1989) Missed prenatal diagnosis of fragile X syndrome. *Prenatal Diagnosis*, **9**, 777–81.

Weaning, R.S., Bredius, R.G.M., Wolf, H. and van der Schoot, C.E. (1991) Prenatal diagnosis procedure for leucocyte adhesion deficiency. *Prenatal Diagnosis*, **11**, 193–97.

Weiner, C.P., Williamson, R.A. and Bonsib, S.M. (1986) Sonographic diagnosis of cloverleaf skull and thanatophoric dysplasia in the second trimester. *JCU*, **14**, 463–65.

Weisman, Y., Jaccard, N., Legum, C. *et al.* (1990) Prenatal diagnosis of vitamin D-dependent rickets, type II: response to 1,25-dihydroxyvitamin D in amniotic fluid cells and fetal tissues. *Journal of Clinical Endocrinology and Metabolism*, **71**, 937–43.

Wellner, V.P., Sekura, R., Meister, A. and Larsson, A. (1974) Glutathione synthetase deficiency, an inborn error of metabolism involving the gamma-glutamyl cycle in patients with 5-oxoprolinuria (pyroglutamic aciduria). *Proceedings of the National Academy of Sciences of the USA*, **71**, 2505–509.

Wendel, U. and Claussen, U. (1979) Antenatal diagnosis of maple syrup urine disease. *Lancet*, i, 161–62.

Wendel, U., Claussen, U. and Diekmann, E. (1983) Prenatal diagnosis for methylene tetrahydrofolate reductase deficiency. *Journal of Pediatrics*, **102**, 938–40.

Wenstrom, K.D., Williamson, R.A., Hoover, W.W. and Grant, S.S. (1989) Achondrogenesis type II (Langer–Saldino) in association with jugular lymphatic obstruction sequence. *Prenatal Diagnosis*, **9**, 527–32.

Wenstrom, K.D., Williamson, R.A., Weiner, C.P. *et al.* (1991) Magnetic resonance imaging of fetuses with intracranial defects. *Obstetrics and Gynecology*, **77**, 529–32.

Westergaard, J.G., Chemnitz, J., Teisner, B. *et al.* (1983) Pregnancy associated plasma protein A: possible marker in the classification and prenatal diagnosis of Cornelia de Lange syndrome. *Prenatal Diagnosis*, **3**, 225–32.

Wexler S., Baruch A., Ekshtein N. *et al.* (1985) An acardiac acephalic anomaly detected on sonography. *Acta Obstetricia et Gynecologica Scandinavica*, **64**, 93–94.

Whitley, C.B., Burke, B.A., Granroth, G. and Gorlin, R.J. (1986) de la Chapelle dysplasia. *American Journal of Medical Genetics*, **25**, 29–39.

Wieacker, P., Griffin, J.E., Wienker, T. *et al.* (1987) Linkage analysis with RFLPs in families with androgen resistance syndromes: evidence for close linkage between the androgen receptor locus and the DXS1 segment. *Human Genetics*, **76**, 248–252.

Wiggins, J.W., Bowes, W., Clewell, W. *et al.* (1986) Echocardiographic diagnosis and intravenous digoxin management of fetal tachyarrhythmias and congestive heart failure. *American Journal of Diseases of Children*, **140**, 202–204.

Wijmenga C., Frants R.R., Brouwer O.F. *et al.* (1990) Location of facioscapulohumeral muscular dystrophy gene on chromosome 4. *Lancet*, **336**, 651–53.

Wilson, R.H.J.K., Duncan, A., Hume, R. and Bain, A.D. (1985) Prenatal pleural effusion associated with congenital pulmonary lymphangiectasia. *Prenatal Diagnosis*, **5**, 73–76.

Winn, H.N., Gabrielli, S., Reece, F.A. *et al.* (1989) Ultrasonographic criteria for the prenatal diagnosis of placental chorionicity in twin gestations. *American Journal of Obstetrics and Gynecology*, **161**, 1540–42.

Winter, R.K., McKnight, L., Byrne, R.A. and Wright, C.H. (1989) Diastematomyelia: prenatal ultrasonic appearances. *Clinical Radiology*, **40**, 291–94.

Winter, R.M., Campbell, S., Wigglesworth, J.S. and Nevrkla, E.J. (1987) A previously undescribed syndrome of thoracic dysplasia and communicating hydrocephalus in two sibs, one diagnosed prenatally by ultrasound. *Journal of Medical Genetics*, **24**, 204–206.

Witter, F.R. and Molteni, R.A. (1986) Intrauterine intestinal volvulus with hemoperitoneum presenting as fetal distress at 34 weeks' gestation. *American Journal of Obstetrics and Gynecology*, **155**, 1080–81.

Woo, S.L.C., Gillam, S.S. and Woolf, L.I. (1974) The isolation and properties of phenylalanine hydroxylases from human liver. *Biochemical Journal*, **139**, 741–49.

Wood, S., Shukin, R.J., Yong, S.L. *et al.* (1987) Prenatal diagnosis in Becker muscular dystrophy. *Clinical Genetics*, **31**, 45–47.

Wright, A.F., Bhattacharya, S.S., Clayton, J.F. *et al.* (1987) Linkage relationships between X-linked retinitis pigmentosa and nine short arm markers: exclusion of the disease locus from Xp21 and localisation between DXS7 and DXS14. *American Journal of Human Genetics*, **41**, 644–53.

Yagel, S., Mandelberg, A., Hurwitz, A. and Jlaser, Y. (1986) Prenatal diagnosis of hypoplastic left ventricle. *American Journal of Perinatology*, **3**, 6–8.

Yang, B.-Z., Ding, J.-H., Brown, B.I. and Chen, Y.-T. (1990) Definitive prenatal diagnosis of type III glycogen storage disease. *American Journal of Human Genetics*, **47**, 735–39.

Yates, J.R.W., Affara, N.A., Jamieson, D.M. *et al.* (1986) Emery–Dreifus muscular dystrophy: localisation to Xq27.3-qter confirmed by linkage to factor VIII gene. *Journal of Medical Genetics*, **23**, 587–90.

Yates, J.R.W., Gillard, E.F., Cooke, A. *et al.* (1987) A deletion of Xp21 maps congenital adrenal hypoplasia distal to glycerol kinase deficiency. *Journal of Medical Genetics*, **24**, 241.

Yokota, I., Tanaka, K., Coates, P.M. and Ugarte, M. (1990) Mutations in medium chain acyl-CoA dehydrogenase deficiency. *Lancet*, **336**, 748.

Young, I.D., McKeever, P.A., Brown, L.A. and Lang, G.D. (1989) Prenatal diagnosis of the megacystis–microcolon–intestinal hypoperistalsis syndrome. *Journal of Medical Genetics*, **26**, 403–406.

Yuen, M. and Fensom, A.H. (1985) Diagnosis of classical Morquio's disease: *N*-acetyl-galactosamine 6-sulphate sulphatase activity in cultured fibroblasis, leucocytes, amniotic fluid cells and chorionic villi. *Journal of Inherited Metabolic Disease*, **8**, 80.

Zanke, S. (1986) Prenatal ultrasound diagnosis of acardius. *Ultraschall in der Medizin*, **7**, 172–75.

Zeitune, M., Fejgin, M.D., Abramowicz, J. *et al.* (1988) Prenatal diagnosis of the pterygium syndrome. *Prenatal Diagnosis*, **8**, 145–49.

Zeng, Y.T. and Huang, S.Z. (1985) Alpha-globin gene organisation and prenatal diagnosis of alpha-thalassaemia in Chinese. *Lancet*, i, 304–307.

Zeng, Y.T., Zhang, M.-L., Ren, Z.-R. *et al.* (1987) Prenatal diagnosis of haemophilia B in the first trimester. *Journal of Medical Genetics*, **24**, 632.

Zerfowski, J. and Sandhoff, K. (1974) Juvenile GM_2 Gangliosidose mit veranderter Sub-stratspezifitat der Hexosaminidase A. *Acta Neuropathologica (Berlin)*, **27**, 225–32.

Zerres, K., Hansmann, M., Mallmann, R. and Gembruch, U. (1988) Autosomal recessive polycystic kidney disease. Problems of prenatal diagnosis. *Prenatal Diagnosis*, **8**, 215–29.

Zerres, K., Schwanitz, G., Niesen, M. *et al.* (1990) Prenatal diagnosis of acute non-lymphoblastic leukaemia in Down syndrome. *Lancet*, i, 117.

Zhao, H., Van Diggelen, D.P., Thoomes, R. *et al.* (1990) Prenatal diagnosis of Morquio disease type A using a simple fluorometric enzyme assay. *Prenatal Diagnosis*, **10**, 85–92.

Zimmerman, H.B. (1978) Prenatal demonstration of gastric and duodenal obstruction by ultrasound. *Journal of the Canadian Association of Radiologists*, **29**, 138–41.

Zlotogora, J., Chakraborty, S., Knowlton, R.G. and Wenger, D.A. (1990) Krabbe disease locus mapped to chromosome 14 by genetic linkage. *American Journal of Human Genetics*, **47**, 37–44.

Zonana, J., Schinzel, A., Upadhyaya, M. *et al.* (1990) Prenatal diagnosis of X-linked hypohidrotic ectodermal dysplasia by linkage analysis. *American Journal of Medical Genetics*, **35**, 132–35.

Zoref-Shani, E., Bromberg, Y., Goldman, B. *et al.* (1989) Prenatal diagnosis of Lesch–Nyhan syndrome: experience with three fetuses at risk. *Prenatal Diagnosis*, **9**, 657–661.

PART SIX

MANAGEMENT OF THE AT RISK FETUS AND NEWBORN

Edited by F. Cockburn, J.P. Neilson and D. Stevenson

78 INTRODUCTION TO MANAGEMENT OF THE HIGH-RISK FETUS AND NEWBORN

G.B. Reed

78.1 Introduction

The text concerning management and care of the 'high-risk' fetus and newborn is divided into five subsections:

- investigation of fetal conditions (Chapters 79–83);
- treatment of certain fetal conditions (Chapters 84–88);
- preparation for delivery (Chapters 89–91);
- birth resuscitation and care (Chapters 92–94);
- newborn medical and surgical conditions (Chapters 95–101 and 103–106); neonatal support systems (Chapters 98–102); perinatal laboratory support (Chapters 107–108); the neonatal intensive care unit (Chapters 90–95).

A flow chart (Figure 78.1) outlines 'high-risk' situations which are reviewed in Table 78.1. The definition of 'high-risk' is related to the anticipated as well as the unexpected findings and/or events involving the fetus or newborn. In general this involves those infants who have anomalies, are of low birth weight or are products of premature birth [1–10].

There is intentionally a moderate amount of overlap of the subject matter in the subsections, e.g. fetal and neonatal sepsis and fetal and neonatal lung disorders.

Certain procedures or interventions described are still under investigation; often few cases have been reported. In such instances these 'procedures' are briefly mentioned. As editors, we have tried to be conservative. In our view the mother is the primary patient and the fetus is the other patient. The reader should note that certain areas of management are discussed in Part Four (Chapters 53–55) and Part Five (Chapters 59, 60 and 63).

Different approaches to *in utero* intervention exist, based on the questions: Who is the primary patient? When should a (singleton) pregnancy be terminated? When should multifetal pregnancies be reduced? When should delivery be made early? When should a neonate

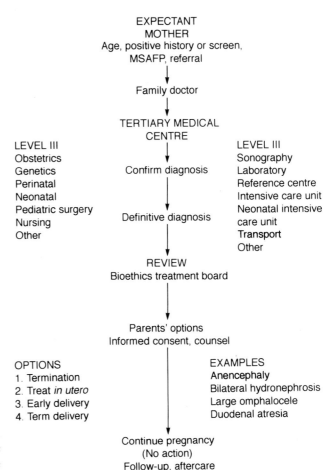

Figure 78.1 Management of the 'high-risk' pregnant population. MSAFP = maternal serum α-fetoprotein.

be treated, not treated or have treatment withdrawn? Many of these difficult decisions are made by physicians daily, with parental consent.

Several themes recur in all these subsections. First, the concept of 'a team approach'. The team should be composed of: (1) the family physician; (2) the obstetri-

Diseases of the Fetus and Newborn, 2nd edn, Edited by G.B. Reed, A.E. Claireaux and F. Cockburn. Published in 1995 by Chapman & Hall, London. ISBN 0 412 39160 0

Table 78.1 'High-risk' groups

Mother	Age; recurrent abortion; a previous large abnormal fetus, stillbirth, pregnancy complication (hydramnios, premature rupture of membranes, rhesus RhD, phenylketonuria, diabetes, elevated blood pressure – >90 mmHg diastolic, >140 mmHg systolic); consanguineous union; exposure (TORCH – toxoplasmosis, other, rubella, cytomegalovirus, syphilis); substance abuse; alcohol, balanced translocation; hemoglobinopathy; ethnic group; positive screen (inborn errors of metabolism, sexually transmitted diseases)
Fetus	Positive sonogram, presentation, viability, intrauterine growth retardation, major anomaly, fetal number; positive screen, decreased fetal movement, abnormal fundal height; X-linked male, question of dating, diethylstilbestrol exposure, medications; fetal Apgar, biophysical profile, amniotic fluid index; long–short cord; placental situs; pelvic mass; preterm premature rupture of membranes; premature rupture of membranes >72 hours
Newborn	Depressed Apgar score at birth, clinical risk index for babies (CRIB) score or score for neonatal acute physiology (SNAP) at 12–24 hours; preterm premature rupture of membranes, premature rupture of membranes, breech; nuchal cord, heavy meconium; major or large anomalies, birth weight/gestational age, <2000 g/<32 weeks; diseases of immaturity (respiratory distress syndrome, necrotizing enterocolitis, cerebral palsy, retinopathy of prematurity, bronchopulmonary dysplasia); very low birth weight (<1500 g) or extremely low birth weight (<1000 g); perinatal insults; asphyxia; group B streptococci/herpesvirus/ hepatitis B virus (serum)/human immunodeficiency virus (AIDS)/*Neisseria gonorrheae*/chlamydiae; acidosis, sepsis, severe anemia, polycythemia, jaundice, shock, seizures; acute small molecule inborn errors of metabolism; infants of diabetic mother; macrosomia; postmature; intrauterine growth retardation; infant birth weight ↑ or ↓ 2 standard deviations

cian, (3) the peri- or neonatologist; (4) appropriate subspecialist(s), e.g. ultrasonographer, geneticists; (5) nursing staff; and (6) others. Second is continuity of care, which should include long-term clinical follow-up of the infant, and counsel and aftercare for the family and parents when indicated. Third is the application of common sense, humanitarianism and the restrained hand of wisdom when intervention is considered, taking into account the long-term effects, whether biological, medical, social, economic or familial. A list of references concerning 'at-risk' (maternal, fetal or neonatal) criteria is given [1–10] and some current 'interventions' are cited [11–18].

78.2 Synopsis

Medical management is ideally a continuum and is a multidisciplinary effort in the care of the conceptus *in utero* or *ex utero*. The leader of the team may change as the fetus progresses toward birth. The leader's cap may pass from perinatal obstetrician to neonatologist or on to a subspecialist. Informed written consent, understood by both parents, is essential. Ethical concerns in obstetrics, perinatology and neonatology practice are discussed (Table 78.2).

A brief review of the present state of fetal and neonatal medicine and surgery is given. The diagnosis of many malformations can be made sonographically. When to treat? How to treat? A 'high-risk' fetus is now being defined. Which conditions should be treated remain contentious. Management guidelines have been proposed for antenatally diagnosed disorders and for subsequent medical or surgical care after birth.

Table 78.2 Overview of genetics, pathology and medical care

Preconceptual, prenatal screening, diagnosis
Indirect or invasive methods, maternal markers
Fetal blood, amniotic fluid or chorionic villous samples
Infections, teratogens and environmental hazards
Reproductive pathology, embryopathology, teratology
Obstetric and placental pathology
Fetal pathology, dysmorphology
Neonatal pathology, hematology, oncology, immunology
Medical genetics, counseling and aftercare
Molecular, biochemical, cytogenetic and developmental genetics
Disease of immaturity and sequelae
Results of medical, surgical and genetic therapy (*in utero* or *ex utero*), iatrogenic and forensic medicine
Ultrasonography and other imaging techniques confirmed by pathology and laboratory tests

Laboratory services for obstetrics, fetal medicine and surgery, and neonatology
Virology, serology, immunology
Microbiology
Chemistry – blood gases, electrolytes, osmolality; bedside – neonatal intensive care unit
Blood and tissue banks
Tissue culture and long-term storage
Molecular diagnostic pathology (DNA banks)
Endocrinology – metabolism
Genetic medicine – diagnosis and treatment, pharmacogenetics
Transplantation (HLA, tissue typing) – diagnosis and treatment
Nuclear medicine, spectroscopy

These sections begin with a discussion which assumes that a young fetus *in utero* can be a patient. The critical investigations which are needed before *in utero* treatment are discussed. The exchange and communication of information between specialists concerned in the care of the patient are always assumed to take place.

78.2.1 FETAL INVESTIGATIONS

These include significant conditions associated with oligohydramnios and polyhydramnios, fetal hydrops (immune and non-immune), fetal hemodynamics, fetal metabolism, fetal nutritional and growth disturbances, fetal and neonatal coagulopathies, *in utero* viral infections and fetal alloimmunization. The management of fetal cardiac disorders is discussed in Chapter 54.

78.2.2 FETAL TREATMENT

Treatment includes indirect and direct fetal therapy, closed and open fetal surgery and *in utero* transplacental hematopoietic cell transplantation.

78.2.3 PREPARATION FOR DELIVERY

This covers the use of prenatal maternal steroids to accelerate fetal lung maturation, intrapartum management of the anomalous fetus and the monitoring of the fetus during labor.

78.2.4 AT BIRTH

Neonatal asphyxia and delivery room resuscitation are reviewed, as is neonatal intensive care of the preterm and very low birth weight infant; support by the nursery staff of families of a dying infant is described.

78.2.5 NEONATAL AND POSTNATAL CONDITIONS

A number of conditions and treatments are described. These are: neonatal apnea and pulmonary hypoplasia, respiratory distress syndrome and postnatal respiratory support, neonatal cerebrovascular monitoring, metabolism, total parenteral nutrition, extracorporeal membrane oxygenation, congenital heart disease and therapeutic options including transplantation, medical and surgical care of necrotizing enterocolitis and surgical care of severe gastrointestinal malformations and congenital diaphragmatic hernia. Basic criteria for a perinatal laboratory are outlined (Table 78.2).

78.2.6 SUMMARY

There were several subjects which were to be, but have not been, reviewed. Time and Murphy's laws can intervene. 'Fetal breathing and hypoplastic lungs' are touched on in Chapters 32 and 79. Similarly 'fetal cardiac adaptations' to hypoxia and 'fetal metabolic responses' to nutritional deprivation are mentioned in

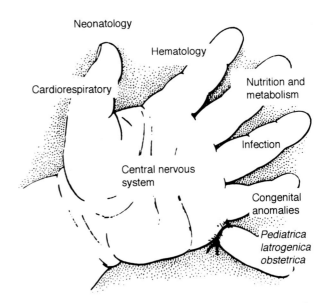

Figure 78.2 A good mnemonic: a 'six-finger' exercise for fetology and neonatology. (Adapted with permission from Andrews [16] and the American Medical Association.)

Chapters 20, 54 and 81. Finally, the treatment of the fetus *in utero* (or its compartments) by way of the mother's 'systems' has not been reviewed. All these subjects are essentially obstetrics and can be found in current obstetrical textbooks or in the expanding medical literature of fetal medicine and/or perinatology [5]; see also Figure 78.2.

It is worth recapitulating two points raised earlier in this book. First, primary prevention is at present available for certain birth defects and disorders of prematurity, and includes dietary folates, immunization and steroids antenatally and surfactant postnatally. Using these methods preconceptually, antenatally or postnatally a number of conditions – which are discussed in Part Six – could be avoided, or at least the incidence reduced significantly. Second, this approach has been vindicated by programs involving β-thalassemia in Sardinia, RhD immunization and improved care of maternal diabetics. Antenatal care and hygiene were proposed in 1900 in Scotland by John Ballantyne. Now, a century later, we are just beginning to approach these goals.

References

'HIGH-RISK' CRITERIA AND ASSESSMENT

1. Fanaroff, A., Martin, R. and Miller, M. (1989) Identification and management of high risk problems in the neonate, in *Maternal–Fetal Medicine* 2nd edn (eds R. Resnick and R. Creasy), W.B. Saunders, Philadelphia, pp. 1150–93 [neonate].
2. Pernoll, M., Benda, G. and Babson, S. (eds) (1986) *Diagnosis and Management of the Fetus and Neonate At Risk*, 5th edn, C.V. Mosby, St.

Louis, pp. 1, 16–20, 103–107, 329–33 ['High', 'middle' and 'low' risk, at-risk perinate?]

3. Klaus, M. and Fanaroff A. (eds) (1993) *Care of the High-Risk Neonate*, 4th edn, W.B. Saunders, Philadelphia, pp. 1–37 [neonate].

4. Mattison, D. and Jelovsek, F. (1992) Environmental and occupational exposures, in *Reproductive Risks and Prenatal Diagnoses* (ed. M. Evans), Appleton and Lange, Norwalk, CT, pp. 91–94. [Maternal, fetal toxicity].

5. Reece, E., Hobbins, J. Mahoney, M. and Petrie, R. (1992) *Medicine of the Fetus and Mother*, Lippincott, Philadelphia [fetus].

6. Knuppel, R. and Drukker, J. (eds) (1993) *High Risk Pregnancy*, 2nd edn, W.B. Saunders, Philadelphia [fetus].

7. Daffos, F. (1989) Access to the other patient. *Semin. Perinatol.*, **13**, 252–59 [fetus].

8. Harrison, M., Golbus, M. and Filly, R. (eds) (1991) *The Unborn Patient*, 2nd ed, W.B. Saunders, Philadelphia [fetus].

9. Brock, D., Rodeck, C. and Ferguson-Smith, M. (eds) (1992) *Prenatal Diagnosis and Screening*, Churchill Livingstone, Edinburgh [fetus].

10. Goldberg, J. (ed.) (1993) Fetal medicine. *West. J. Med.*, **159** [whole issue: fetus].

INTERVENTIONS

11. Bennett, P. (1993) Ethics and late termination of pregnancy (letter). *Lancet*, **342**, 929.

12. Keirse, M. (1993) Frequent prenatal ultrasound: time to think again. *Lancet*, **342**, 878–79.

13. Hedrich, M., Jennings, R., MacGillivray, T. *et al.* (1993) Chronic fetal vascular access. *Lancet*, **342**, 1086–87.

14. Harrison, M. and Adzick, S. (1994) Fetal surgical therapy. *Lancet*, **343**, 897–902.

15. Schulman, J. (1990) Treatment of the embryo and fetus. *Am. J. Med. Genet.*, **35**, 197–200.

16. Andrews, B. (1994) Neonatology. *Arch. Pediatr. Adolesc. Med.*, **148**, 132.

17. Hustin, J. and Jauniaux, E. (1993) Curing the human embryo – curing the placenta. *Hum. Reprod. Update*, **8**, 1966–82.

18. Marwick, C. (1993) Coming to terms with indications for fetal surgery. *JAMA*, **270**, 2025–29.

79 OLIGOHYDRAMNIOS AND POLYHYDRAMNIOS

N.M. Fisk and A.C. Moessinger

79.1 Introduction

Amniotic fluid surrounds the fetus in intrauterine life, providing both protection against external trauma, and a low resistance space within which the fetus moves. It arises from secondary partitioning of water within the fetoplacental extracellular space, and reflects fetal fluid balance. Although amniotic fluid is normally controlled within a wide range of volumes, oligohydramnios and polyhydramnios are both associated with increases in perinatal morbidity and mortality, in relation to the degree of aberrant amniotic fluid volume [1,2].

79.1.1 DETERMINANTS OF AMNIOTIC FLUID VOLUME

(a) Source and control

The factors determining amniotic fluid volume regulation remain poorly understood. In early pregnancy, amniotic fluid is considered firstly a maternal dialysate, and then a fetal transudate, since its composition resembles that of maternal and then fetal serum [3]. After 20–25 weeks with progressive impermeability of fetal skin [4], amniotic fluid becomes increasingly hypotonic with greater concentrations of urea and creatinine, implicating fetal urine as the major contributor [5,6]. Certainly, failure of fetal urination results in oligohydramnios in clinical [7,8] and experimental studies [9,10]. Radiosotope studies in both human and ovine near-term fetuses suggest that 550–650 ml/day of urine enters the amniotic cavity [11,12]. Ultrasonic studies reporting human fetal urine production rates of up to 50 ml/hour [13] suggest an even higher figure.

Fetal swallowing is a major route of clearance. Radio-opaque contrast medium is observed in the fetal intestines within 20 minutes of intra-amniotic injection [14]. Human fetuses with lesions preventing swallowing often develop polyhydramnios [15,16], as do sheep after oesophageal occlusion [17]. Radiotracer studies indicate that near-term human fetuses swallow 234–326 ml less per day than they void [18,19],

suggesting additional pathways of clearance. The respiratory tract is not a site of net resorption of significant amounts of amniotic fluid [19]; indeed there is a net outflow of lung liquid from the fetal trachea, calculated as 200–345 ml/24 hours in late gestation sheep [20,21], although swallowing may prevent much of this reaching the amniotic cavity [22,23].

The other major route of clearance is bulk flow across permeable membranes between maternal, fetal and amniotic compartments [24,25] in response to osmotic and hydrostatic gradients [26–30]. Consistent with this is the correlation between maternal plasma and amniotic fluid volumes in human pregnancies with both normal and abnormal quantities of amniotic fluid [31]. In experimental ovine studies, bulk flows across the membranes account for most of the clearance of intra-amniotically infused fluids [11,32,33], almost all by the intramembranous route (from amniotic cavity via vascularized membranes into the fetal circulation), rather than the transmembranous pathway (from amniotic cavity to the maternal circulation). This suggests that alterations in amniotic fluid volume in response to changes in maternal fluid balance [34,35] occur via their effect on fetal fluid balance. The fetus is known to be able to decrease its urine production by releasing vasopressin in response to fetal hypovolaemia [36], maternal hypertonicity [37], and maternal water deprivation [34,35] and increase it in response to hypervolaemia [38].

The relative constancy of amniotic fluid volume at any stage during pregnancy, in the presence of a high turnover rate and a large number of potential pathways of exchange, indicates remarkable co-ordination in its control. The literature suggests that such control is chiefly determined by the state of fetal hydration.

(b) Measurement

Amniotic fluid volume has been measured in normal human pregnancy by direct collection [39], or by

Diseases of the Fetus and Newborn, 2nd edn, Edited by G.B. Reed, A.E. Claireaux and F. Cockburn. Published in 1995 by Chapman & Hall, London. ISBN 0 412 39160 0

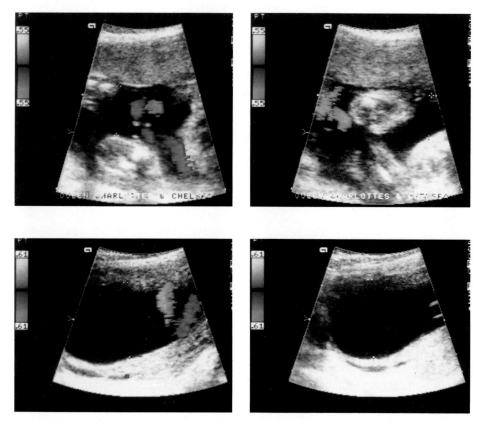

Figure 79.1 Ultrasound views of four quadrants, with colour flow mapping used to highlight the presence of umbilical cord loops. The amniotic fluid index is the sum of the deepest vertical pool devoid of cord or limbs in each quadrant.

indicator-dye dilution techniques [40]. The best estimate comes from data pooled from 12 publications [41], showing that mean amniotic fluid volume increases rapidly to 630 ml at 22 weeks, and then more slowly to a peak of 817 ml at 33 weeks, declining thereafter to 715 ml at 40 weeks. The 95% reference range is wide, encompassing values within 1/2.57 to 2.57 times the mean at any given gestational age (for example 318–2100 ml at 30 weeks).

Quantitation of amniotic fluid volume is not performed in clinical practice, since it necessitates two amniocenteses with attendant risks [40,42], and relies on the dubious supposition that complete mixing of the indicator-dye occurs within a 15–30-minute interval [43]. Accordingly, definitions of increased and decreased amniotic fluid volume are based on non-invasive criteria. Clinical assessment is considered inaccurate, while calculation of total intrauterine volume is cumbersome, poorly reproducible, and requires an outmoded static scanner [44]. Using real-time ultrasound, subjective assessment of amniotic fluid volume as normal, increased or decreased has been used widely. Next the depth (in centimetres) of the deepest vertical pool devoid of cord or limbs [45,46] became popular, but a weakness was that it made no reference to gestational age.

Polyhydramnios has been arbitrarily defined as a deepest pool ≥ 8 cm [2,47], while oligohydramnios has been variously defined as a deepest pool ≤ 3, 2 or 1 cm [1,45,46], the more stringent indicating moderate to severe oligohydramnios. The amniotic fluid index (AFI), the sum of the deepest pool in each of four quadrants (Figure 79.1), was initially developed for use in late pregnancy to increase the sensitivity of detection of oligohydramnios [48], but a recent modification allows it to be used throughout pregnancy with good reproducibility [49]. The regression curve between AFI and gestational age is similar in shape to that between amniotic fluid volume and gestational age [41], and has been used to derive a reference range for AFI from 16 to 42 weeks [49] (Figure 79.2). The AFI appears superior to the deepest pool in diagnosis and classification of severity of both oligohydramnios and polyhydramnios [50,51].

79.2 Oligohydramnios

79.2.1 BACKGROUND

Oligohydramnios is found in 3–5% of pregnancies in the third trimester [1,52,53] but only 0.2% in the

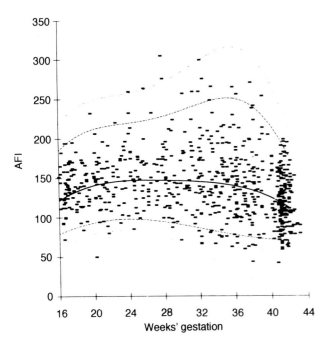

Figure 79.2 Normal range for amniotic fluid index (AFI) between 16 and 44 weeks. (Reproduced with permission from Moore and Cayle [49]).

midtrimester [54]. Severe oligohydramnios is less frequent than are milder degrees [53,55,56].

(a) Aetiology

Oligohydramnios may be due to urinary obstruction, absence of renal function, rupture of the membranes or intrauterine growth retardation (IUGR), their relative frequency depending on the gestation and severity of oligohydramnios. In late pregnancy, IUGR and ruptured membranes predominate [1,52,55], whereas urinary tract anomalies leading to oligohydramnios are usually detected on routine ultrasound in the midtrimester. The aetiology in the remainder is idiopathic, oligohydramnios being significantly less severe than in the other aetiological groups [57].

Preterm premature rupture of the membranes (PPROM) complicates 3–17% of pregnancies [58,59], and is responsible for a quarter of cases of oligohydramnios [52]. The earlier the gestation, the lower is the incidence of PPROM [60]. The mechanism seems to be the obvious physical one of leakage through the membranous defect, as fetal urine output is unaltered [61]. Nevertheless, only 5–44% of patients with PPROM have ultrasonic evidence of oligohydramnios [62–64]. Oligohydramnios from PPROM is usually short-lived, as the latent period to onset of labour exceeds a week in only 2–5% of those with term [65,66], and 20–40% with PPROM [60,67,68].

IUGR leads to oligohydramnios [1,46,53,69], the deepest pool measurement being significantly lower in

small for gestational age (SGA) compared with appropriate for gestational age fetuses [70]. Furthermore, 80–85% of SGA births are preceded by oligohydramnios [46,53]. Oligohydramnios in IUGR seems secondary to fetal oliguria, with human ultrasonic studies showing reduced fetal urine output in 70–100% of SGA fetuses [71,72]. Fetal oliguria in IUGR probably reflects a renovascular response to hypoxia, with reflex redistribution of blood flow away from kidneys and viscera towards the brain [73,74]. Renal hypoperfusion as the mechanism is supported by human studies showing correlations between increased resistance in the renal artery and reduced amniotic fluid volume [75] and between reduced urine production and fetal hypoxaemia [76]. Hypoxia-induced vasopressin release [77] may also contribute.

Major congenital abnormalities are found in 4–7% of pregnancies with oligohydramnios [1,52], this figure rising to 26–35% in the midtrimester [57,78]. The frequency of anomalies is also greater if oligohydramnios is severe (52 versus 14% if mild/moderate) [57]. Between 33 and 57% will be urinary tract anomalies [52,78,79], either bilateral fetal renal pathologies such as agenesis and multicystic/polycystic disease, or lower urinary tract obstruction. Experimental animal studies [9,10] and observation in humans of restoration of amniotic fluid volume after vesicoamniotic shunting [80,81] indicate that lack of the urinary contribution to amniotic fluid volume is the mechanism for oligohydramnios in fetuses with urinary tract anomalies.

(b) Perinatal mortality

Perinatal mortality is significantly increased in oligohydramnios, as a result of the underlying aetiology such as congenital malformations and IUGR, of preterm delivery, and of oligohydramnios sequelae such as pulmonary hypoplasia. Among a series of 7562 high risk pregnancies with 52 perinatal deaths, mortality was higher in those with, compared to without, oligohydramnios (18.8 and 0.5% respectively), even after correction for congenital anomalies (10.9 and 0.2%) [1]. Perinatal mortality is infrequent in mild oligohydramnios in the third trimester [53,56]. In contrast, 43 and 88% of perinates succumbed in two series of midtrimester oligohydramnios [57,78]. The prognosis is worse when maternal serum α-fetoprotein is raised [82,83]. The severity of oligohydramnios also influences prognosis, with a mortality rate of 88% in severe compared with 11% in mild/moderate midtrimester oligohydramnios [57].

Poor outcome in PPROM is largely confined to pregnancies with rupture prior to 29 weeks, in which mortality rates of 37–76% have been reported [60,68,84-86]. Gestational age at delivery is the most important variable, with little survival before 24–25 weeks [68,84,86]. Perinatal death in PPROM is more common in association with oligohydramnios than with normal amniotic fluid volume [63]. Early gestational age at rupture is also associated with poor outcome [68,84].

(c) Perinatal morbidity

Some of the fetal complications may be attributed to reduced amniotic fluid volume, such as pulmonary hypoplasia and soft tissue deformites, while others result from the underlying condition such as IUGR renal anomalies or PPROM. Series of midtrimester PPROM are characterized by neonatal complications of prematurity, including respiratory distress in 45–70%, intraventricular haemorrhage in 29–50%, and long-term sequelae in 32–71% [68,84,86]. Proven neonatal sepsis occurs in only 17–29%, confirming that prematurity rather than infection is the greater cause of perinatal morbidity and mortality in PPROM [68,86]. PPROM with oligohydramnios leads to a higher frequency of neonatal sepsis than PPROM with normal amniotic fluid volume (1 of 54 versus 7 of 36 respectively) [63]. This difference may partly be a gestational age effect [62], as marked reduction in bacteriostatic amniotic fluid is less likely after 32 weeks when fetal urine output increases and the frequency of chorioamnionitis declines [87]. Another explanation is that amniotic fluid volume distinguishes those with definite PPROM and oligohydramnios from 'high leaks' with preserved liquor volume, which have a lower risk of infection due to more minor disruption in membrane integrity [88].

Oligohydramnios is also associated with an increased risk of fetal distress and birth asphyxia [46,52,56]. These may reflect the underlying condition, as both IUGR and postmaturity predispose to fetal compromise. In the group of fetuses with early onset of oligohydramnios, such as in the midtrimester, the high incidence of breech presentation may also complicate delivery. Nevertheless, the high frequency of fetal heart rate decelerations in labouring patients with ruptured membranes [63,89] suggests that oligohydramnios *per se* may adversely affect fetal well-being. Animal experiments indicate that variable decelerations in oligohydramnios are the result of umbilical cord compression [90]. In human pregnancy, controlled trials demonstrate that intrapartum amnioinfusion to restore amniotic fluid volume reduces the frequency of variable fetal heart rate decelerations [91–93]. On the other hand, oligohydramnios in the absence of labour does not appear to affect fetal well-being, as in oligohydramnios fetal Doppler waveforms are normal in the absence of IUGR [94–96], and are unaltered by restoration of amniotic fluid volume [97].

The relationship between oligohydramnios and pulmonary hypoplasia was recognized 50 years ago by Edith Potter [98], but the identification of the causality in the association (i.e. that lack of amniotic fluid leads to pulmonary hypoplasia) is more recent. The recognition of this causal link has been made by extrapolation from 'experiments of nature' by Douglas Bain [99,100], to whom this book is dedicated, and by William Blanc [101]. This causal link was later confirmed by a number of animal studies (reviewed in Fisk [102]). In the human fetus, the association is strong when there are urological anomalies such as renal agenesis, polycystic kidneys or posterior urethral valves. Fortunately, when oligohydramnios results from PPROM alone, or in the twin-to-twin syndrome, the association is less constant and is determined by the gestational age at the onset of oligohydramnios and the latent period until delivery. The earlier the onset and the longer the duration of oligohydramnios, the more marked will be the inhibition of fetal lung growth [103,104]. However, it is important to realize that, even with early onset of PPROM and a prolonged latent period, neonatal outcome is not consistently bad [104].

Given this last observation, i.e. lack of consistency in the association following PPROM, it would be of considerable benefit to develop diagnostic modalities to identify in time which fetuses will develop pulmonary hypoplasia and which fetuses will not be affected. It is only fair to say that despite an abundant literature on both the physiopathology of oligohydramnios-induced pulmonary hypoplasia and *in utero* ultrasound diagnosis (reviewed in Fisk [102], this issue is unresolved and leaves the obstetrician faced with a major clinical dilemma. The earlier hopes that the evaluation of fetal breathing movements would allow the identification of affected fetuses have not been supported by the recent literature. Likewise, the assessment of fetal lung size by ultrasound using various anatomical predictive ratios is exceedingly difficult in the presence of oligohydramnios in the midtrimester, when it would be of clinical relevance.

Pulmonary hypoplasia is discussed in Chapter 32. Other oligohydramnios sequelae are the soft tissue and skeletal deformities, comprising flattened facies, flexion contractures and talipes [8,105]. Their relationship to oligohydramnios seems different from that of pulmonary hypoplasia, in that the severity and duration are more important than gestation at onset [106]. Because amniotic pressure is low in oligohydramnios [107,108], they are more likely to result from immobilization of fetal extremities [109–111] than fetal compression.

79.2.2 DIAGNOSTIC APPROACH

The aim is to determine the underlying aetiology, the presence of associated anomalies and the severity of oligohydramnios. History and physical examination reveal most cases of amniorrhexis, except for a few very early in gestation in whom the small quantities of fluid lost vaginally go unnoticed [112]. High resolution ultrasound is performed next; however, just when detailed examination of fetal anatomy is crucial, the ultrasonic view is impaired by lack of an acoustic window and the degree of fetal flexion.

(a)   Ultrasound

In the absence of amniotic fluid, renal agenesis is a notoriously difficult diagnosis which rests on demonstration of vacant renal fossae [113]. If the fetal abdomen is within the lower half of the uterus, transvaginal ultrasound may facilitate views of the fetal renal fossae [114,115]. Maternal administration of frusemide (furosemide) has been used in an attempt to provoke fetal diuresis in the presence of a structurally normal renal tract [72,116]. However, numerous false-negative diagnoses have been reported [113,117,118], and it is now known that maternally administered frusemide, at least in sheep, neither produces a fetal diuresis nor indeed crosses the placenta [119]. In contrast, lower urinary tract obstruction is a relatively easy diagnosis, with a large cystic structure found in the fetal abdomen. Nevertheless, visualization of other urinary structures of prognostic value (i.e. renal cortex, upper urethra; see Chapter 52) and of extra renal anatomy for associated anomalies, remains suboptimal.

The severity of oligohydramnios is also assessed, not only for clues to aetiology, but also for prognosis. Colour flow mapping improves the differentiation of residual pockets of amniotic fluid from umbilical cord loops (Figure 79.1). This facilitates both the assessment of severity and the performance of invasive procedures.

(b)   Karyotyping

Since it may be impossible to inspect minor structures such as the face, limbs, etc. for features of aneuploidy, rapid karyotyping is recommended in midtrimester oligohydramnios. Chromosomal abnormalities will be found in 5–10% [94,120].

(c)   Amnioinfusion

Thus, the underlying aetiology often remains elusive when conventional modalities are used. Diagnostic amnioinfusion, in which amniotic volume is restored by transabdominal infusion [112,120], overcomes these constraints.

A needle is guided under ultrasound control into the amniotic cavity; in the absence of an identifiable pool of fluid, the needle is instead guided towards a potential amniotic space in the vicinity of fetal limbs or neck, and

correct intra-amniotic positioning confirmed by visualization of dispersal of injected saline within the amniotic space. Next, a warmed physiological solution is administered, care being taken to avoid bubbles. As the optimal volume of infusate has yet to be determined, it seems prudent to administer only the minimum required to improve the ultrasound view. This requires <200 ml for most midtrimester pregnancies [112,120]. A dye may be added to the fluid, so that its subsequent identification in the lower genital tract indicates ruptured membranes [121]. Indigo carmine is used, in view of the association of neonatal intestinal obstruction with *in utero* exposure to methylene blue [122].

The resolution of the ultrasound examination after infusion is superior to that beforehand, providing that vaginal leakage does not prevent retention of infused fluid. Most fetal abnormalities suspected before amnioinfusion are then confirmed. Such confirmation is nevertheless important, especially if termination of pregnancy is to be offered. An example is bilateral renal agenesis, with amnioinfusion in one series being considered necessary for definitive diagnosis in five of 16 cases [123]. Not all, however, will have suspected anomalies confirmed: in one report, bilateral renal agenesis was suspected in three fetuses on the preinfusion scan, but kidneys were clearly demonstrated after infusion [112]. Alternatively, fetal intraperitoneal infusion has been used to facilitate diagnoses of renal agenesis (Figure 79.3) [124].

In addition, amnioinfusion improves ultrasonic demonstration of other fetal structures, revealing unsuspected anomalies in 9–18% [112,120] and thus

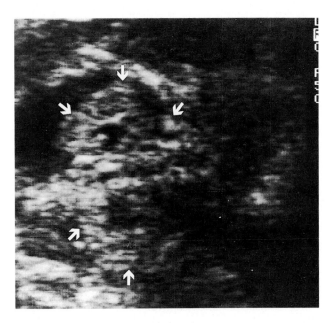

Figure 79.3 The fetal kidneys are clearly seen in this case of anhydramnios, outlined (arrows) by the fluid within the fetal abdomen surrounding the renal capsule.

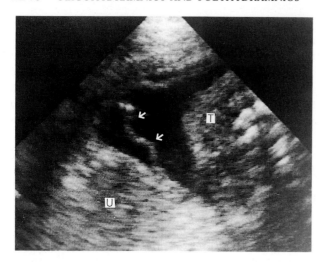

Figure 79.4 Ultrasound scan after amnioinfusion revealing membranous detachment (arrows). U = uterine wall; T = fetal trunk [112].

facilitating prognostication. A further advantage of amnioinfusion is that it facilitates diagnosis of ruptured membranes, both by demonstrating liquor leakage, and by revealing membranous detachment on ultrasound (Figure 79.4) [112]. In one series of diagnostically unclear oligohydramnios, the most likely diagnosis was revised in 13% as a result of information yielded by amnioinfusion [112].

79.2.3 THERAPIES

The aim of therapies in oligohydramnios is chiefly to restore amniotic fluid volume to allow continued lung development during the canalicular phase (Chapter 32). In animal models, the experimental basis for restitution of amniotic volume preventing lung pulmonary hypoplasia has been well established [80,125]. In human oligohydramnios, several approaches have been tried, but no controlled data yet exist to confirm any benefit.

(a) Vesicoamniotic shunting

In fetuses with lower obstructive uropathy, urinary decompression [126,127] aims not only to relieve obstruction to prevent renal dysplasia (Chapter 86) but also to restore amniotic fluid volume to facilitate lung development. However pulmonary hypoplasia was the cause of death in almost all of the 59% of shunted fetuses that died in the International Registry [127]. There is considerable scepticism about this procedure [128,129], in particular as to whether it can restore amniotic fluid volume in fetuses with severe oligohydramnios.

(b) Cervical occlusion

In patients with PPROM, attempts have been made to restore amniotic fluid volume by plugging the leak. Occluding the cervix with a fibrin gel does not appear to prevent continued amniotic fluid drainage [130], nor does fixation of a double balloon catheter [131] within the cervical canal. However, physiological saline can be infused intra-amniotically via the catheter to maintain the deepest pool $\geq$ 5 cm [132]. This device has been mainly used to prevent infective complications of PPROM in late pregnancy [133], rather than in the midtrimester to prevent pulmonary hypoplasia.

(c) Serial amnioinfusions

Another option is repeated therapeutic amnioinfusions [112,120]. In a pilot study in nine women with appropriately-grown fetuses with severe midtrimester oligohydramnios, 40 infusions were performed to restore amniotic volume at weekly intervals until the end of the canalicular phase of lung development [112]. Lung hypoplasia was found in only two of nine pregnancies (22%) with severe oligohydramnios diagnosed at $\leq$22 weeks, which compared favourably with 60% reported in severe oligohydramnos diagnosed at $\leq$28 weeks [57].

If serial amnioinfusion is confirmed by other studies as beneficial, only a small proportion of patients seem eligible for this strategy, since idiopathic oligohydramnios is rare, while the rate and degree of leakage render this approach impractical in many with ruptured membranes.

79.3 Polyhydramnios

79.3.1 BACKGROUND

The prevalence varies depending on the criteria used. Older studies used the subjective finding of $\geq$ 2 litres at delivery [15,134] to report prevalences of 0.25–0.7% [134–137], whereas ultrasound studies seem more sensitive, finding prevalences of 1.0–3.2% using the 8-cm pool definition [2,47]. Polyhydramnios complicates 9–13% of twin pregnancies assessed on ultrasound [138,139].

(a) Aetiology

The more severe the polyhydramnios, the more likely it is that an underlying cause will be found. Whereas 83% of mild polyhydramnios were idiopathic in a series of 102 cases, only 8% of severe polyhydramnios remained unexplained [47].

Congenital anomalies were found in 20–27% in older studies [15,134,136,137] and 9–13% in more recent ultrasonic series [47,140]. The largest category is central nervous system defects, mostly anencephaly, followed by gastrointestinal and musculoskeletal abnormalities [134,137,141]. Impairment of fetal swallowing, which causes polyhydramnios in animal experiments [17], seems the predominant mechanism [15] and explains the high frequency of polyhydramnios in fetuses with upper gastrointestinal obstruction [142], with intrathoracic space-occupying lesions such as diaphragmatic hernia [143] and pleural effusions [144], with skeletal dystrophies affecting the thorax, and with neurological deficits such as myotonic dystrophy [145,146]. Nevertheless, only 65% of anencephalic fetuses develop polyhydramnios [147], although almost all do not swallow [19], suggesting alternative mechanisms may contribute, such as meningeal transudation or vasopressin deficiency producing fetal polyuria [148].

Maternal diabetes as a cause for polyhydramnios has recently declined in frequency to 5–13% [47,141] from 22–26% in older series [134,136,137]. This seems to be due to tighter control, since polyhydramnios is least common in diabetics with the lowest mean glucose levels [149]. Although fetal polyuria secondary to an osmotic diuresis might seem an obvious mechanism, Van Otterlo, Waldimiroff and Wallenburg [150] found normal fetal urine production rates in 12 of 13 diabetic pregnancies with mild polyhydramnios. Their measurement technique is now known to underestimate fetal urine output considerably [13], but nevertheless has been used to demonstrate polyuria in a fetus with diabetes insipidus and polyhydramnios [151]. Polyuria is presumably also the cause of polyhydramnios in fetuses with Bartter syndrome [152] or nephrogenic diabetes insipidus secondary to maternal lithium therapy [153,154]. Similarly, recipient fetuses in fetofetal transfusion syndrome have been shown to be polyuric [151] *in vivo*, and histologically have enlarged glomeruli and dilated distal collecting tubules [151,155]. The suggested mechanism is increased cardiac output, which might also explain polyhydramnios in some cases of hydrops and in Rh alloimmunized fetuses. Work in sheep suggests this may be an oversimplification, as raised fetal lactate, such as found in Rh disease [156], causes an osmotic diuresis to produce polyhydramnios [157]. Further, fetal infusions of angiotensin I cause polydramnios by an unknown mechanism [158].

The term 'acute polyhydramnios' indicates the rapid increase in amniotic fluid volume, associated with uterine distension and severe maternal symptoms [134,159], which occurs approximately once in 4000 pregnancies [159,160]. Although there is argument about this definition and its application to singleton pregnancies [134,161], most cases occur before 24–26 weeks in one sac of monochorial multiple pregnancies as a manifestation of fetofetal transfusion syndrome (FFTS) [134,159].

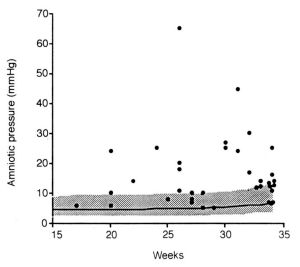

Figure 79.5 Amniotic pressure in 36 pregnancies complicated by polyhydramnios shown against the reference range (continuous line = mean; shaded area = upper/lower limits) [163].

(b) Maternal complications

Polydramnios may produce abdominal discomfort, respiratory embarrassment and uterine irritability [145]. The preterm delivery rate is increased [47,138,162], although the high incidence of anomalies and multiple pregnancy makes derivation of an exact risk for spontaneous preterm labour difficult. A rate corrected for congenital anomalies of 22% has been reported [47]. In many cases, PPROM precedes the onset of preterm labour [145,162]. Amniotic pressure is raised in polyhydramnios [108] (Figure 79.5), and thus the above complications have been attributed to uterine distension. The incidence of caesarean section is also increased [137,140], due largely to unstable fetal lie. A further risk is abruption, associated with rapid decompression of the uterus at amniotomy [164]. These risks are largely confined to those with severe polyhydramnios, i.e. an AFI >24 cm or a deepest pool ≥ 15 cm [51,108], and thus are almost universal in acute polyhydramnios [159].

(c) Fetal complications

Perinatal mortality rates are high at 13–29% [15, 47,51,134], reflecting the increased incidence of congenital malformations, preterm labour and asphyxial complications such as abruption, cord prolapse and placental insufficiency. Three main variables influence perinatal survival in polyhydramnios: the presence of congenital anomalies, gestational age at delivery, and severity of polyhydramnios. In a series of 537 singletons with polyhydramnios, perinatal mortality was 61% in the presence of fetal or placental malforma-

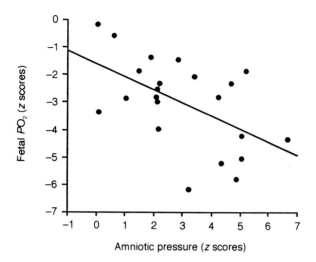

Figure 79.6 The relationship between the degree of fetal hypoxaemia in polyhydramnios and the degree of elevation in amniotic pressure, expressed in z scores (= standard deviations from reference mean) [173].

tions, and 10% in the presence of maternal diabetes, compared with only 2.4% in their absence [141]. Perinatal mortality more than doubles in the presence of anomalies [47,134]. Similarly, it is much higher in singletons with acute as opposed to chronic polyhydramnios [161].

Perinatal mortality exceeds 50% in FFTS [165,166], when polyhydramnios is present and the diagnosis made *in utero* [167]. When detected prior to 28 weeks, mortality rates of 80–100% have been reported [159,168,169]. Acute polyhydramnios complicating FFTS accounts for 17% of overall perinatal mortality in twins [160]. Approximately one-third are intrauterine deaths [160], and in this regard fetal hypoxaemia/acidaemia have recently been demonstrated in four of six affected pregnancies investigated by fetal blood sampling [170].

Although this excess perinatal morbidity and mortality has been attributed to preterm delivery and congenital malformations [47,134], these associations do not entirely account for the adverse outcome attributed to polyhydramnios. In large series, 6–14% of perinatal deaths occurred antepartum in normally formed singletons [51,171]. It has been suggested that raised amniotic pressure in polyhydramnios impairs uteroplacental perfusion [172], based on observations during iatrogenic polyhydramnios from intrapartum amnioinfusion. Indeed, in a study of fetuses with polyhydramnios investigated by blood sampling, fetal pH and Po_2 were inversely correlated with amniotic pressure [173] (Figure 79.6), and thus severity [108]. In a sheep model, however, fetal blood gas status did not change when amniotic pressure was raised by amnioinfusion [174].

79.3.2 DIAGNOSTIC APPROACH

The aim is to determine the underlying aetiology, the presence of associated anomalies and the severity of the polyhydramnios.

(a) Ultrasound

A detailed scan is performed for structural malformations, with particular emphasis on the upper gastro-intestinal tract and its surrounds. Fetal neurological function is assessed by observing the presence of fetal movements. As discussed earlier, repeated sonographic measurements of bladder size (every 2–5 minutes for up to an hour) [13] may be used to calculate the hourly fetal urine production rate, in order to distinguish polyhydramnios due to fetal polyuria from that due to other causes [151]. In our experience this is unnecessary in polyhydramnios because frequent and incomplete emptying give the polyuric bladder the appearance of being chronically full, which can be simply determined from three to four observations during the course of the scan.

Severity of polyhydramnios should also be assessed, both as a baseline and for prognosis.

(b) Karyotyping

In view of a 5% chance of chromosomal abnormality, rapid karyotyping warrants consideration, especially in moderate/severe polyhydramnios associated with a structural anomaly [51].

(c) Others

Maternal diabetes should be excluded by carbohydrate tolerance testing. In twin pregnancies, chorionicity should be determined if not previously done. In the 15–17% with a single placental mass concordant for fetal sex, the dividing membrane is measured, with values <2.0 mm predicting monochorial placentation with sensitivities and specificities of 80–90% [175]. One group has reported even greater accuracy by counting the number of layers in the septum on ultrasound [176], but in our experience this technique is poorly reproducible. In FFTS, visualization of any membrane around the 'stuck' twin can be exceptionally difficult [167]. In unclear cases, zygosity determination by DNA techniques can help by indicating dichorial placentation if dizygotic, but provides no additional information if monozygotic [177].

79.3.3 THERAPIES

Treatment of polyhydramnios has two aims: (1) relief of maternal symptoms; and (2) prolongation of gestation. As many with polyhydramnios are not at risk of either complication, treatment is only warranted in severe or acute polyhydramnios in the midtrimester or early third trimester. Polyhydramnios secondary to FFTS is the most frequent indication.

(a) Indomethacin

Following recognition of decreased urinary flow in neonates given indomethacin [178], maternally administered indomethacin has been shown to reduce hourly fetal urine production [179] and amniotic fluid volume [42]. It crosses the placenta freely [180], and acts by either a renovascular mechanism [181] or by reduced prostaglandin E inhibition of antidiuretic hormone [182]. The amniotic cavity and fetal bladder are monitored daily on ultrasound so that the dose (75–200 mg/day) can be adjusted to ensure sufficient response without causing oligohydramnios. In eight singleton pregnancies with symptomatic polyhydramnios between 21 and 34 weeks, Cabrol et al. [183] found that indomethacin reduced fundal height, umbilical perimeter and qualitative amniotic fluid volume, all of which increased after cessation of therapy. Similarly, a significant fall in qualitative amniotic fluid volume has been reported following treatment in both singleton [184] and twin pregnancies [185].

Indomethacin appears a promising drug for treatment of polyhydramnios, although there remains concern regarding potential fetal side-effects of oligohydramnios [186], premature closure of the ductus [187] and cerebral vasoconstriction [188]. Monitoring ductal patency by Doppler has been recommended [186], although the risks of neonatal complications from premature closure of the ductus in utero seem remote, providing therapy is discontinued by 32 weeks. A further disadvantage is that amelioration in amniotic volume is not rapid, one study reporting a median time to achieve normal volume of 12.5 days. Accordingly, one group advocates initial amnioreduction followed by maternal indomethacin [42]. Indomethacin is not used in FFTS because of concern about further jeopardizing renal function in the already oliguric donor [189].

Sulindac, another prostaglandin synthetase inhibitor used in obstetric practice, has a much weaker effect on fetal urine output [190], and therefore is not used to treat polyhydramnios.

(b) Amnioreduction

Since the first description of therapeutic drainage of amniotic fluid [191], known as amnioreduction or therapeutic or decompression amniocentesis, numerous case reports have been published attributing relief of maternal symptoms and prolongation of gestation to this procedure in both singleton [134] and twin pregnancies [192–197]. On the other hand, others have found that rapid reaccumulation of fluid renders this procedure of little benefit [198,199]. Chronic drainage catheters, although theoretically attractive, are complicated by a high incidence of infection and blockage [200], and therefore are not used.

Recent series of polyhydramnios secondary to FFTS suggest that serial amnioreduction is beneficial in prolonging gestation. The median diagnosis-to-delivery interval of 43 days in one series of nine repeatedly drained pregnancies [139] was greater than the 10-day interval reported in 18 cases not subjected to drainage. Another group noted better perinatal survival in eight pregnancies managed by serial amnioreduction compared with those managed conservatively (69 versus 20%), despite similar mean gestational ages at diagnosis [201]. Combining their figures with those in the literature, these authors confirmed a significant difference in survival between 29 pregnancies managed with, and 48 without, serial amnioreduction (69 versus 16%). The small number of such patients seen in any one centre renders it unlikely that the efficacy of this procedure can be evaluated without a randomized multicentre trial.

There is some controversy over the amount of fluid which should be removed. Most authors have been conservative in selecting volumes in view of concerns regarding precipitation of abruption or preterm labour [197,202]. Indeed, raised amniotic pressure in severe polyhydramnios is restored to normal by removal of relatively small volumes [108]. On the other hand, Urig, Clewell and Elliott [169], who drained a mean of 1826 ml (range 900–5000 ml) in 29 procedures, consider restitution of normal amniotic fluid volume the more important goal. This group's promising results in terms of reversal of hydrops in the recipient and oligohydramnios in the donor support their claim [203]. They speculated that raised pressure in the recipient's sac secondary to polyhydramnios impairs placental perfusion in the donor twin, and that this results in further hypovolaemia and oliguria [169,203]. Using 'aggressive therapeutic amniocentesis', survival rates of 69–79% have recently been reported [162, 201,203], leading one group to suggest that decompression 'effectively reverses the physiology of twin–twin transfusion syndrome' [203].

Patients having contractions at the time of amnioreduction are known to have a greater risk of preterm delivery following the procedure [204], and therefore amnioreduction should be performed before the onset of preterm labour [169].

(c) Others

In selected pathologies, correction of the underlying aetiology is preferable to empirical treatment of polyhydramnios. Medical causes of hydrops, as discussed in Chapter 80, may respond to transfusion or drug therapy. In fetuses with bilateral hydrothoraces, chronic *in utero* drainge by pleuroamniotic shunting corrects polyhydramnios, providing lung hypoplasia does not prevent lung re-expansion [144] (Chapter 86). Open fetal surgical correction of intrathoracic lesions, such as diaphragmatic hernia [205] or cystic adenomatoid lung malformation [206], is theoretically also beneficial in restoring transit of amniotic fluid through the upper gastrointestinal tract, but at this stage remains experimental.

A number of techniques have been tried in FFTS with variable results, including selective fetocide of the donor [198,207] and fetoscopic laser ablation of vascular anastomoses [208]. These drastic procedures were performed primarily for prolongation of pregnancies threatened by gross polyhydramnios, in which case the simpler therapies discussed deserve consideration first.

79.4 Conclusions

Aberrant amniotic fluid volume complicates up to 7% of pregnancies, although, in many, the derangement will be mild, idiopathic, occur in the third trimester and not produce sequelae. In contrast, severe oligohydramnios and polyhydramnios in the midtrimester are associated with substantial perinatal morbidity and mortality, reflecting both the underlying aetiology and the complications of disordered amniotic volume.

Severe oligohydramnios, which may be due to ruptured membranes, growth retardation, absent fetal renal function or fetal urinary tract obstruction, poses a diagnostic challenge because it impairs ultrasound resolution. Transabdominal amnio-infusion facilitates visualization of fetal anatomy and determines membranous integrity. Karyotyping and transvaginal ultrasound may also be indicated. In order to prevent pulmonary hypoplasia, vesicoamniotic shunting and serial amnio-infusion have been used to maintain amniotic volume in selected euploid fetuses with functioning renal tissue. Despite their sound experimental basis, no controlled data exist to indicate benefit of these procedures in human pregnancies.

Polyhydramnios may be due to fetal polyuria or impairment of fetal deglutition. The investigation of polyhydramnios involves detection of anomalies by ultrasound, karyotyping and exclusion of carbohydrate intolerance. Transplacental indomethacin reduces fetal urine output and has been used in severe polyhydramnios to prolong gestation. It is inappropriate in twin–twin transfusion, the most common aetiology of severe polyhydramnios, because it further impairs the donor's renal function. Serial amnioreduction is associated with perinatal survival rates of 69–79% in midtrimester twin–twin transfusion with gross polyhydramnios, a considerable improvement on the uniformly poor prognosis associated with conservative management.

References

1. Chamberlain, P.F., Manning, F.A., Morrison, I. *et al.* (1984) Ultrasound evaluation of amniotic fluid volume. I. The relationship of marginal and decreased amniotic fluid volumes to perinatal outcome. *Am. J. Obstet. Gynecol.*, **150**, 245–49.
2. Chamberlain, P.F., Manning, F.A., Morrison, I. *et al.* (1984) Ultrasound evaluation of amniotic fluid volume. II. The relationship of increased amniotic fluid volume to perinatal outcome. *Am. J. Obstet. Gynecol.*, **150**, 250–54.
3. Lind T., Kendall, A. and Hytten, F.E. (1972) The role of the fetus in the formation of amniotic fluid. *J. Obstet. Gynaecol. Br. Commonw.*, **79**, 289–98.
4. Parmley, T.H. and Seeds, A.E. (1970) Fetal skin permeability to isotopic water (THO) in early pregnancy. *Am. J. Obstet. Gynecol.*, **108**, 128–31.
5. Lind, T., Billewicz, W.Z. and Cheyne, G.A. (1971) Composition of amniotic fluid and maternal blood throughout pregnancy. *J. Obstet. Gynecol. Br. Commonw.*, **78**, 505–12.
6. Benzie, R., Doran, T.A., Harkins, J.L. *et al.* (1974) Composition of the amniotic fluid and maternal serum in pregnancy. *Am. J. Obstet. Gynecol.*, **119**, 798–810.
7. Perlman, M. and Levin, M. (1974) Fetal pulmonary hypoplasia, anuria and oligohydramnios: clinicopathologic observations and review of the literature. *Am. J. Obstet. Gynecol.*, **118**, 1119–23.
8. Thomas, I.T. and Smith, D.W. (1974) Oligohydramnios, cause of the non-renal features of Potter's syndrome, including pulmonary hypoplasia. *J. Pediatr.*, **84**, 811–4.
9. Minei, L.J. and Suzuki, K. (1976) Role of fetal deglutition and micturition in the production and turnover of amniotic fluid in the monkey. *Obstet. Gynecol.*, **48**, 177–81.
10. Harrison, M.R., Ross, N.A., Noall, R. and de Lorimier, A.A. (1983) Correction of congenital hydronephrosis *in utero*. I: The model: fetal urethral obstruction produces hydronephrosis and pulmonary hypoplasia in fetal lambs. *J. Pediatr. Surg.*, **18**, 247–56.
11. Tomoda, S., Brace, R.A. and Longo, L. (1987) Amniotic fluid volume regulation, basal volumes and responses to fluid infusion or withdrawal in sheep. *Am. J. Physiol.*, **252**, R380–87.
12. Abramovich, D.R., Garden, A., Jandial, L. and Page, K.R. (1978) Fetal swallowing and voiding in relation to hydramnios. *Obstet. Gynecol.*, **54**, 15–20.
13. Rabinowitz, R., Peters, M.T., Vyas, S. *et al.* (1989) Measurement of fetal urine production in normal pregnancy by real-time ultrasonography. *Am. J. Obstet. Gynecol.*, **161**, 1264–66.
14. McLain, C.R. (1963) Amniography studies of the gastrointestinal motility of the human fetus. *Am. J. Obstet. Gynecol.*, **86**, 1079–87.
15. Moya, F., Apgar, V., James, L.S. and Berrien, C. (1960) Hydramnios and congenital anomalies. *JAMA*, **173**, 1552–56.
16. Pritchard J.A. (1966) Fetal swallowing and amniotic fluid volume. *Obstet. Gynecol.*, **28**, 606–10.
17. Fujino, Y., Agnew, C.L., Schreyer, P.G. *et al.* (1991) Amniotic fluid volume response to esophageal occlusion in fetal sheep. *Am. J. Obstet. Gynecol.*, **165**, 1620–26.
18. Gitlin, D., Kumate, J., Morales, C. *et al.* (1972) The turnover of amniotic fluid protein in the human conceptus. *Am. J. Obstet. Gynecol.*, **113**, 632–45.
19. Abramovich, D.R. (1970) Fetal factors influencing the volume and composition of liquor amnii. *J. Obstet. Gynaecol. Br. Commonw.*, **77**, 865–77.
20. Harding, R., Sigger, J.N., Wickham, P.J.D. and Bocking, A.D. (1984) The regulation of flow of pulmonary fluid in fetal sheep. *Respir. Physiol.*, **57**, 47–59.
21. Harding, R., Bocking, A.D. and Sigger, J.N. (1986) Influence of upper respiratory tract on liquid flow to and from fetal lungs. *J. Appl. Physiol.*, **61**, 68–74.
22. Adams, F.H., Desilets, D.T. and Towers, B. (1967) Control of flow of fetal lung fluid at the laryngeal outlet. *Resp. Physiol.*, **2**, 302–309.
23. Harding, R., Bocking, A.D., Sigger, J.N. and Wickham, P.J.D. (1984) Composition and volume of fluid swallowed by fetal sheep. *Q. J. Exp. Physiol.*, **69**, 487–95.
24. Hutchinson, D.L., Gray, M.J., Plentl, A.A. *et al.* (1959) The role of the fetus in the water exchange of the amniotic fluid of normal and hydramniotic patients. *J. Clin. Invest.*, **38**, 971–80.
25. Seeds, A.E. (1980) Current concepts of amniotic fluid dynamics. *Am. J. Obstet. Gynecol.*, **138**, 575–86.

26. Battaglia, F., Prystowsky, H., Smisson, C. *et al.* (1960) Fetal blood studies. XIII. The effect of the administration of fluids intravenously to mothers upon the concentrations of water and electrolytes in plasma of human fetuses. *Pediatrics*, 25, 2–10.

27. Schruefer, J.J., Seeds, A.E., Behrman, R.E. *et al.* (1972) Changes in amniotic fluid volume and total solute concentration in the rhesus monkey following replacement with distilled water. *Am. J. Obstet. Gynecol.*, 112, 807–15.

28. Kerenyi, T.D. and Muzsnai, D. (1975) Volume and sodium concentration studies in 300 saline-induced abortions. *Am. J. Obstet. Gynecol.*, 121, 590–96.

29. Basso, A., Fernandez, A., Aldabe, O. *et al.* (1977) Passage of mannitol from mother to amniotic fluid and fetus. *Obstet. Gynecol.*, 49, 628–31.

30. Ross, M.G., Ervin, M.G., Oakes, G. *et al.* (1983) Bulk flow of amniotic fluid water in response to maternal osmotic challenge. *Am. J. Obstet. Gynecol.*, 147, 697–701.

31. Goodlin, R.C., Anderson, J.C. and Gallagher, T.F. (1983) Relationship between amniotic fluid volume and maternal volume expansion. *Am. J. Obstet. Gynecol.*, 146, 505–11.

32. Gilbert, W.M. and Brace R.A. (1989) The missing link in amniotic fluid volume regulation: intramembranous absorption. *Obstet. Gynecol.*, 74, 748–54.

33. Ross, M.G., Sherman, D.J., Schreyer, P. *et al.* (1991) Fetal rehydration via intra-amniotic fluid: contribution of fetal swallowing. *Pediatr. Res.*, 29, 214–17.

34. Bell, R.J., Congiu, M., Hardy, K.J. and Wintour, E.M. (1984) Gestation-dependent aspects of the response of the ovine fetus to the osmotic stress induced by maternal water deprivation. *Q. J. Exp. Physiol.*, 69, 187–95.

35. Stevens, A.D. and Lumbers, E.R. (1985) The effect of maternal fluid intake on the volume and composition of fetal urine. *J. Dev. Physiol.*, 7, 161–6.

36. Schroder, H., Gilbert, R.D. and Power, G.G. (1984) Urinary and hemodynamic responses to blood volume changes in fetal sheep. *J. Dev. Physiol.*, 6, 131–41.

37. Lumbers, E.R. and Stevens, A.D. (1983) Changes in fetal renal function in response to infusions of a hyperosmotic solution of mannitol to the ewe. *J. Physiol.*, 343, 439–46.

38. Brace, R.A. (1989) Fetal blood volume, urine flow, swallowing, and amniotic fluid volume responses to long term intravascular infusions of saline. *Am. J. Obstet. Gynecol.*, 161, 1049–54.

39. Abramovich, D.R. (1968) The volume of amniotic fluid in early pregnancy. *J. Obstet. Gynecol. Br. Commonw.*, 75, 728–31.

40. Queenan, J.T., Thompson, W., Whitfield, C.R. and Shah, S.I. (1972) Amniotic fluid volumes in normal pregnancies. *Am. J. Obstet. Gynecol.*, 114, 34–38.

41. Brace, R.A. and Wolf, E.J. (1989) Normal amniotic fluid volume changes throughout pregnancy. *Am. J. Obstet. Gynecol.*, 161, 382–88.

42. Kirshon, B., Mari, G. and Moise, K.J. (1990) Indomethacin therapy in the treatment of symptomatic polyhydramnios. *Obstet. Gynecol.*, 75, 202–205.

43. Brans, Y., Andrew, D.S., Dutton, E.R. *et al.* (1989) Dilution of chemicals used for estimation of water content of body compartments in perinatal medicine. *Pediatr. Res.*, 25, 377–82.

44. Gohari, P., Berkowitz, R.L. and Hobbins, J. (1977) Prediction of intrauterine growth retardation by determination of total intrauterine volume. *Am. J. Obstet. Gynecol.*, 127, 255–60.

45. Crowley, P. (1980) Non-quantitative measurement of amniotic fluid volume in prolonged pregnancy. *J. Perinat. Med.*, 8, 249–51.

46. Manning, F.A., Hill, L.M. and Platt, L.D. (1981) Qualitative amniotic fluid volume determination by ultrasound: antepartum detection of intrauterine growth retardation. *Am. J. Obstet. Gynecol.*, 139, 254–58.

47. Hill, L.M., Breckle, R., Thomas M.L. and Fries, J.K. (1987) Polyhydramnios: ultrasonically detected prevalence and neonatal outcome. *Obstet. Gynecol.*, 69, 21–25.

48. Phelan, J.P., Smith, C.V., Broussard, P. and Small, M. (1987) Amniotic fluid volume assessment with the four-quadrant technique at 36–42 weeks gestation. *J. Reprod. Med.*, 32, 540–2.

49. Moore, T.R. and Cayle, J.E. (1990) The amniotic fluid index in normal human pregnancy. *Am. J. Obstet. Gynecol.*, 162, 1168–73.

50. Moore, T.R. (1990) Superiority of the four-quadrant sum over the single-deepest-pocket technique in ultrasonic identification of abnormal amniotic fluid volumes. *Am. J. Obstet. Gynecol.*, 163, 762–67.

51. Carlson, D.E., Platt, L.D., Medearis, A.L. and Horenstein, J. (1990) Quantifiable polyhydramnios: diagnosis and management. *Obstet. Gynecol.*, 75, 989–93.

52. Mercer, L.J., Brown, L.G., Petres, R.E. and Messer R.H. (1984) A survey of pregnancies complicated by decreased amniotic fluid. *Am. J. Obstet. Gynecol.*, 149, 355–61.

53. Philipson, E.H., Sokol, R.J. and Williams, T. (1983) Oligohydramnios: clinical associations and predictive value for intrauterine growth retardation. *Am. J. Obstet. Gynecol.*, 146, 271–8.

54. Barss, V., Benacceraf, B. and Frigoletto, F. (1984) Second trimester oligohydramnios: a predictor of poor fetal outcome. *Obstet. Gynecol.*, 64, 608–10.

55. Hill, L.M. Breckle, R., Wolfgram, K.R. and O'Brien, P.C. (1983) Oligohydramnios: ultrasonically detected incidence and subsequent fetal outcome. *Am. J. Obstet. Gynecol.*, 147, 407–10.

56. Crowley, P., O'Herlihy, C. and Boylan, P. (1984) The value of ultrasound measurement of amniotic fluid volume in the management of prolonged pregnancies. *Br. J. Obstet. Gynaecol.*, 91, 444–48.

57. Moore, T.R., Longo, J., and Leopold, G.R. *et al.* (1989) The reliability and predictive value of an amniotic fluid scoring system in severe second trimester oligohydramnios. *Obstet. Gynec.*, 73, 739–42.

58. Gunn, G.C., Mishell, D. and Morton, D.G. (1970) Premature rupture of the fetal membranes. *Am. J. Obstet. Gynecol.*, 106, 469–83.

59. Grant, J. and Keirse, M.J. (1989) Prelabour rupture of the membranes at term, in *Effective Care in Pregnancy and Childbirth*, vol. 2 (eds I. Chalmers, M. Enkin and M.J. Keirse), Oxford University Press, Oxford, pp. 1112–17.

60. Taylor, J. and Garite, T.J. (1984) Premature rupture of membranes before fetal viability. *Obstet. Gynecol.*, 64, 615–20.

61. Watson, W.J., Latz, V.L. and Seeds, J.W. (1991) Fetal urine output does not influence residual amniotic fluid volume after premature rupture of membranes. *Am. J. Obstet. Gynecol.*, 164, 64–65.

62. Gonik, B., Bottoms, S.F. and Cotton, D.B. (1985) Amniotic fluid volume as a risk factor in preterm premature rupture of the membranes. *Obstet. Gynecol.*, 65, 456–59.

63. Vintzileos, A.M., Campbell, W.A., Nochimson, D.J. and Weinbaum, P.J. (1985) Degree of oligohydramnios and pregnancy outcome in patients with premature rupture of the membranes. *Obstet. Gynecol.*, 66, 162–67.

64. Robson, M.S., Turner, M.J., Strong, J.M. and O'Herlihy, C.O. (1990) Is amniotic fluid quantitation of value in the diagnosis and conservative management of prelabour membrane rupture at term? *Br. J. Obstet. Gynaecol.*, 97, 324–278.

65. Kappy, K.A., Cetrulo, C.L., Knuppel, R.A. *et al.* (1979) Premature rupture of the membranes; a conservative approach. *Am. J. Obstet. Gynecol.*, 134, 655–61.

66. Kappy, K.A., Cetrulo, C.L., Knuppel, R.A. *et al.* (1982) Premature rupture of the membranes at term: a comparison of induced and spontaneous labours. *J. Reprod. Med.*, 27, 29–33.

67. Johnson, J.W.C., Daikoku, N.H., Niebyl, J.R. *et al.* (1981) Premature rupture of the membranes and prolonged latency. *Obstet. Gynecol.*, 57, 547–56.

68. Moretti, M. and Sibai, B.M. (1988) Maternal and perinatal outcome of expectant management of premature rupture of membranes in the midtrimester. *Am. J. Obstet. Gynecol.*, 159, 390–96.

69. Paterson, R.M., Prihoda, T.J. and Pouliot, M.R. (1987) Sonographic amniotic fluid measurement and fetal growth retardation: a reappraisal. *Am. J. Obstet. Gynecol.*, 157, 1406–10.

70. Bottoms, S.F., Welch, R.A., Zador, I.E. and Sokol, R.J. (1986) Limitations of using maximal vertical pocket and other sonographic evaluations of amniotic fluid volume to predict fetal growth: technical or physiologic? *Am. J. Obstet. Gynecol.*, 155, 154–58.

71. Wladimiroff, J.W. and Campbell S. (1974) Fetal urine-production rates in normal and complicated pregnancy. *Lancet*, i, 151–54.

72. Kurjak, A., Kirkinen, P., Latin, V. and Ivankovic, D. (1981) Ultrasonic assessment of fetal kidney function in normal and complicated pregnancies. *Am. J. Obstet. Gynecol.*, 141, 266–70.

73. Cohn, H.E., Sacks, E., Heyman, M.A. and Rudolph, A.M. (1974) Cardiovascular responses to hypoxemia and acidemia in fetal lambs. *Am. J. Obstet. Gynecol.*, 120, 817–24.

74. Peeters, L.L.H., Sheldon, R.E., Jones, M.D. *et al.* (1979) Blood flow to fetal organs as a function of arterial oxygen content. *Am. J. Obstet. Gynecol.*, 135, 637–46.

75. Ardiuni, D. and Rizzo, G. (1991) Fetal renal artery velocity waveforms and amniotic fluid volume in growth-retarded and post-term fetuses. *Obstet. Gynecol.*, 77, 370–73.

76. Nicolaides, K.H., Peters, M.T., Vyas, S. *et al.* (1990) Relation of rate of urine production to oxygen tension in small-for-gestational-age fetuses. *Am. J. Obstet. Gynecol.*, 162, 387–91.

77. Robillard, J.E., Weitzman, R.E., Burmeister, L. and Smith, F.G. (1981) Development aspects of the renal response to hypoxemia in the fetal lamb *in utero*. *Circ. Res.*, 48, 128–38.

78. Mercer, L.J. and Brown, L.G. (1986) Fetal outcome with oligohydramnios in second trimester. *Obstet. Gynecol.*, 67, 840–42.

79. Rosendahl, H. and Kivinen, S. (1989) Antenatal detection of congenital malformations by routine ultrasonography. *Obstet. Gynecol.*, 73, 947–51.

80. Harrison, M.R., Nakayama, D.K., Noall, R. and de Lorimier, A.A. (1982) Correction of congenital hydronephrosis *in utero* II: Decompression reverses the effects of obstruction on the fetal lung and urinary tract. *J. Pediatr. Surg.*, 17, 965–74.

81. Nicolini, U., Rodeck, C.H. and Fisk, N.M. (1987) Shunt treatment for fetal obstructive uropathy, *Lancet*, ii, 1338–39.

82. Dyer, S.N., Burton, B.K. and Nelson, L.H. (1987) Elevated maternal serum α-fetoprotein levels and oligohydramnios: poor prognosis for pregnancy outcome. *Am. J. Obstet. Gynecol.*, 157, 336–39.

83. Richards, D.S., Seeds, J.W., Katz, V.L. *et al.* (1988) Elevated maternal serum alpha-fetoprotein with oligohydramnios, ultrasound evaluation and outcome, *Obstet. Gynecol.*, 72, 337–41.

84. Beydoun, S.N. and Yasin, S.Y. (1986) Premature rupture of the membranes before 28 weeks: conservative management. *Am. J. Obstet. Gynecol.*, 155, 471–79.

85. Bengtson, J.M., Van Marter, L.J., Barss, V.A. *et al.* (1989) Pregnancy outcome after premature rupture of the membranes at or before 26 weeks gestation. *Obstet. Gynecol.*, 73, 921–26.

86. Major, C.A. and Kitzmiller, J.L. (1990) Perinatal survival with expectant management of midtrimester rupture of the membranes. *Am. J. Obstet. Gynecol.*, 163, 838–44.

87. Russell, P. (1979) Inflammatory lesions of the human placenta. I. Clinical significance of acute chorioamnioinitis. *Am. J. Diagn. Obstet. Gynecol.*, 1, 127–37.

88. Fisk, N.M. (1988) Modifications to selective conservative management in preterm premature rupture of the membranes. *Obstet. Gynecol. Surv.*, 43, 328–34.

89. Moberg, L.J., Garite, T.J. and Freeman, R.K. (1984) Fetal heart rate patterns and fetal distress in patients with preterm premature rupture of membranes. *Obstet. Gynecol.*, 64, 60–64.

90. Gabbe, S.G., Ettinger, B.B., Freeman, R.K. and Martin, C.B. (1976) Umbilical cord compression associated with amniotomy; laboratory observations. *Am. J. Obstet. Gynecol.*, 126, 353–55.

91. Miyazaki, F.S. and Nevarez, F. (1985) Saline amnioinfusion for relief of repetitive variable decelerations: a prospective randomised study. *Am. J. Obstet. Gynecol.*, 153, 301–306.

92. Nageotte, M.P., Freeman, R.K., Garite, T.J. and Dorchester, W. (1985). Prophylactic intrapartum amnioinfusion in patients with preterm premature rupture of membranes. *Am. J. Obstet. Gynecol.*, 153, 557–62.

93. Strong, T.H., Hetzler, G., Sarno, A.P. and Paul, R.H. (1990) Prophylactic intrapatum amnioinfusion: a randomised clinical trial. *Am. J. Obstet. Gynecol.*, 162, 1370–75.

94. Hackett, G.A., Nicolaides, K.H. and Campbell, S. (1987) Doppler ultrasound assessment of fetal and uteroplacental circulations in severe second trimester oligohydramnios. *Br. J. Obstet. Gynecol.*, 159, 1074–77.

95. Cruz, A.C., Frentzen, B.H., Gomez, K.J. *et al.* (1988) Continous-wave Doppler ultrasound and decreased amniotic fluid volume in pregnant women with intact and ruptured membranes. *Am. J. Obstet. Gynecol.*, 159, 708–14.

96. Lombardi, S., Rosemund, R., Ball, R. *et al.* (1989) Umbilical artery velocimetry as a predictor of adverse outcome in pregnancies complicated by oligohydramnios. *Obstet. Gynecol.*, 74, 338–41.

97. Fisk, N.M., Welch, C.R., Ronderos-Dumit, D. *et al.* (1992) Relief of presumed compression in oligohydramnios: amnioinfusion does not affect umbilical Doppler waveforms. *Fetal Diagn. Ther.*, 7, 180–85.

98. Potter, E.L. (1946) Bilateral renal agenesis. *J. Pediatr.*, 29, 68–76.

99. Bain, A.D. and Scott, J.S. (1960) Renal agenesis and severe urinary tract dysplasia. A review of 50 cases with particular reference to the associated anomalies. *BMJ*, 1, 841–46.

100. Bain, A.O., Smith, J.J. and Gauld, I.K. (1964) Newborn after prolonged leakage of liquor amni. *BMJ*, 2, 598–99.

101. Blanc, W.A., Apperson, J.W. and McNally, J. (1962) Pathology of the newborn and of the placenta in oligohydramnios. *Bull. Sloane Hosp. Women*, 8, 51–64.

102. Fisk, N.M. (1991) Oligohydramnios-related pulmonary hypoplasia. *Contemp. Rev. Obstet. Gynaecol.*, 4, 191–201.

103. Moessinger, A.C., Collins, M.H., Blanc, W.A., Rey, H.R. and James, L.S. (1986) Oligohydramnios-induced lung hypoplasia: the influence of timing and duration in gestation. *Pediatr. Res.*, 20, 951–54.

104. Nimrod, C., Varela-Gittings, F., Machin, G., Campbell, D. and Wesenberg, R. (1984) The effect of very prolonged membrane rupture on fetal development. *Am. J. Obstet. Gynecol.*, 148, 540–43.

105. Potter, E.L. (1946) Facial characteristics of infants with bilateral renal agenesis. *Am. J. Obstet. Gynecol.*, 51, 885–88.

106. Rotschild, A., Ling, E.W., Puterman, M.L. and Farquharson, D. (1990) Neonatal outcome after prolonged preterm rupture of the membranes. *Am. J. Obstet. Gynecol.*, 162, 46–52.

107. Nicolini, U., Fisk, N.M., Rodeck, C.H. *et al.* (1989) Low amniotic pressure in oligohydramnios: is this the cause of pulmonary hypoplasia? *Am. J. Obstet. Gynecol.*, 161, 1098–101.

108. Fisk, N.M., Tannirandorn, Y., Nicolini, U. *et al.* (1990) Amniotic pressure in disorders of amniotic fluid volume. *Obstet. Gynecol.*, 76, 210–14.

109. DeMyer, W. and Baird, I. (1969) Mortality and skeletal malformations from amniocentesis and oligohydramnios in rats: cleft palate, club foot, microstomia, and adalactyly. *Teratology*, 2, 33–38.

110. Thibault, D.W., Beatty, E.C., Hall, R.T. *et al.* (1985) Neonatal pulmonary hypoplasia with premature rupture of fetal membranes and oligohydramnios. *J. Pediatr.*, 107, 273–77.

111. Pringle, K.C. (1986) Human fetal lung development and related animal models. *Clin. Obstet. Gynecol.*, 29, 502–13.

112. Fisk, N.M., Ronderos-Dumit, D., SoIaini, A. *et al.* (1991) Diagnostic and therapeutic transabdominal amnioinfusion in oligohydramnios. *Obstet. Gynecol.*, 78, 270–78.

113. Romero, R., Cullen, M., Grannum, P. *et al.* (1985) Antenatal diagnosis of renal anomalies with ultrasound. III. Bilateral renal agenesis. *Am. J. Obstet. Gynecol.*, 151, 38–43.

114. Fisk, N.M., and Rodeck, C.H. (1990) Detection of congenital abnormalities of the renal and urinary tract by ultrasound, in *Modern Antenatal Care of the Fetus* (ed. G. Chamberlain), Blackwell Scientific, Oxford, pp. 359–88.

115. Benacerraf, B.R. (1990) Examination of the severe second trimester fetus with severe oligohydramnios using transvaginal scanning. *Obstet. Gynecol.*, 75, 491–93.

116. Wladimiroff, J.W. (1975) Effect of frusemide on fetal urine production. *Br. J. Obstet. Gynecol.*, 82, 221–24.

117. Goldenberg R.L., Davis, R.O. and Brumfield, C.G. (1984) Transient fetal anuria of unknown etiology: a case report. *Am. J. Obstet. Gynecol.*, 149, 87.

118. Harman, C.R. (1984) Maternal furosemide may not provoke urine production in the compromised fetus. *Am. J. Obstet. Gynecol.*, 150, 322–23.

119. Chamberlain, P.F., Cumming, M., Torchia, M.G. *et al.* (1985) Ovine fetal urine production following maternal intravenous furosemide administration. *Am. J. Obstet. Gynecol.*, 151, 815–19.

120. Germbruch, U. and Hansmann, M. (1988) Artificial instillation of amniotic fluid as a new technique for the diagnostic evaluation of cases of oligohydramnios. *Prenat. Diagn.*, 8, 33–45.

121. Atlay, R.D. Sutherst, J.R. (1970) Premature rupture of the fetal membranes confirmed by intra-amniotic injection of dye (Evans blue T-1824). *Am. J. Obstet. Gynecol.*, 108, 993–94.

122. Nicolini, U. and Monni, G. (1990) Intestinal obstruction in babies exposed *in utero* to methylene blue. *Lancet*, ii, 1258–59.

123. Reuss, A., Wladimiroff J.W., Wijngard, J.A. *et al.* (1987) Fetal renal anomalies, a diagnostic dilemma in the presence of intrauterine growth retardation and oligohydramnios. *Ultrasound Med. Biol.*, 10, 619–24.

124. Nicolini, U., Santolaya, J., Hubinont, C. *et al.* (1989) Visualization of fetal intra-abdominal organs in second trimester severe oligohydramnios by intraperitoneal infusion. *Prenat. Diagn.*, 9, 191–94.

125. Nakayama, D.K., Glick, P.L., Harrison, M.R. *et al.* (1983) Experimental pulmonary hypoplasia due to oligohydramnios and its reversal by relieving thoracic compression. *J. Pediatr. Surg.*, 18, 347–53.

126. Harrison, M.R., Golbus, M.S., Filly, R.A. *et al.* (1982) Fetal surgery for congenital hydronephrosis. *N. Engl. J. Med.*, 306, 591–3.

127. Manning, F.A., Harrison, M.R., Rodeck, C.H. and members of the International Fetal Medicine and Surgery Society (1986) Catheter shunts for fetal hydronephrosis and hydrocephalus. *N. Engl. J. Med.*, 315, 336–40.

128. Elder, J.S., Duckett, J.W. and Snyder, H.M. (1987) Intervention for fetal obstructive uropathy: has it been effective? *Lancet*, ii, 1007–10.

129. Reuss, A., Wladimiroff J.W., Stewart, P.A. and Scholtmeijer, R.J. (1988) Non-invasive management of fetal obstructive uropathy. *Lancet*, ii, 949–51.

130. Baumgarten, K. and Moser, S. (1986) The technique of fibrin adhesion for premature rupture of the membranes during pregnancy. *J. Perinat. Med.*, 14, 43–49.

131. Ogita, S., Imanaka, M., Matsumoto, M. and Hatanaka, K. (1984) Premature rupture of the membranes managed with a new cervical catheter. *Lancet*, i, 1330–31.

132. Imanaka, M., Ogita, S. and Sugawa, T. (1989) Saline solution amnioinfusion for oligohydramnios after premature rupture of the membranes. *Am. J. Obstet. Gynecol.*, 161, 102–106.

133. Ogita, S., Mizuno, M., Takeda, Y. *et al.* (1988) Clinical effectiveness of a new cervical indwelling catheter in the management of premature rupture of the membranes: a Japanese collaborative study. *Am. J. Obstet. Gynecol.*, 159, 336–41.

134. Queenan, J.T. and Gadow E.C. (1970) Polyhydramnios, chronic versus acute. *Am. J. Obstet. Gynecol.*, 108, 349–55.

135. Barry, A.P. (1958) Hydramnios. *Obstet. Gynecol.*, 11, 667–75.

136. Murray, S.R. (1964) Hydramnios – a study of 864 cases. *Am. J. Obstet. Gynecol.*, 88, 65–67.

137. Jacoby, H.E. and Charles, D. (1966) Clinical conditions associated with hydramnios. *Am. J. Obstet. Gynecol.*, 94, 910–19.

138. Hashimoto, B., Callen, P.W., Filly, R.A. and Laros, R.K. (1984) Ultrasound evaluation of polyhydramnios and twin pregnancy. *Am. J. Obstet. Gynecol.*, 154, 1069–72.

139. Schneider, K.T.M., Vetter, K., Huch, R. and Huch, A. (1985) Acute polyhydramnios complicating twin pregnancies. *Acta Genet. Med. Gemellol.*, 34, 179–84.

140. Zamah, N.M., Gillieson, M.S., Walters, J.H. and Hall, P.F. (1982) Sonographic detection of polyhydramnios, a five-year experience. *Am. J. Obstet. Gynecol.*, 143, 523–27.

141. Desmedt, E.J., Henry, O.A. and Beischer N.A. (1990) Polyhydramnios and associated maternal and fetal complications in singleton pregnancies. *Br. J. Obstet. Gynecol.*, 97, 1115–22.

142. Lloyd, J.R. and Clatworthy, H.W. (1958) Hydramnios as an aid to the early diagnosis of congenital obstruction of the alimentary tract: a study of the maternal and fetal factors. *Pediatrics*, **21**, 903–909.

143. Adzick, N.S., Harrison, M.R., Glick, P.L. *et al.* (1985) Diaphragmatic hernia in the fetus: prenatal diagnosis and outcome in 94 cases. *J. Pediatr. Surg.*, **20**, 357–61.

144. Rodeck, C.H., Fisk, N.M., Fraser, D.I. and Nicolini, U. (1988) Long-term *in utero* drainage of fetal hydrothorax. *N. Engl J. Med.*, **319**, 1135–38.

145. Cardwell, M.S. (1987) Polyhydramnios: a review. *Obstet. Gynecol. Surv.*, **42**, 612–17.

146. Phelan, J.P. and Martin, G.I. (1989) Polyhydramnios: fetal and neonatal implications. *Clin. Perinatol.*, **16**, 987–94.

147. Nichols, J. and Schrepfer, R. (1966) Polyhydramnios in anencephaly. *JAMA*, **197**, 549–51.

148. Naeye, R.L., Milic, A.M.B. and Blanc, W. (1970) Fetal endocrine and renal disorders: clues to the origin of hydramnios. *Am. J. Obstet. Gynecol.*, **108**, 1251–56.

149. Kitzmiller, J.L., Cloherty, J.P., Younger, M.D. *et al.* (1978). Diabetic pregnancy and perinatal morbidity. *Am. J. Obstet. Gynecol.*, **131**, 560–80.

150. Van Otterlo, L.C. Wladimiroff, J.W. and Wallenburg, H.C.S. (1977) Relationship between fetal urine production and amniotic fluid volume in normal pregnancy and pregnancy complicated by diabetes. *Br. J. Obstet. Gynaecol.*, **84**, 205–209.

151. Kirshon, B. (1989) Fetal urine output in hydramnios. *Obstet. Gynecol.*, **73**, 240–42.

152. Sieck, U.V. and Ohlsson, A. (1984). Fetal polyuria and hydramnios associated with Bartter's syndrome. *Obstet. Gynecol.*, **63**, 22S–24S.

153. Krause, S., Ebbeson, F. and Lange, A.P. (1990) Polyhydramnios with maternal lithium treatment. *Obstet. Gynecol.*, **75**, 504–506.

154. Ang, M.S., Thorp, J.A. and Parisi, V.M. (1990) Maternal lithium therapy and polyhydramnios. *Obstet. Gynecol.*, **76**, 517–19.

155. Achiron, R., Rosen, N. and Zakut, H. (1987) Pathophysiologic mechanism of hydramnios development in twin transfusion syndrome. *J. Reprod. Med.*, **32**, 305–308.

156. Soothill, P.W., Nicolaides, K.H., Rodeck, C.H. *et al.* (1987) Relationship of fetal hemoglobin and oxygen content to lactate concentration in Rh iso-immunized pregnancies. *Obstet. Gynecol.*, **69**, 268–70.

157. Powell, T.L. and Brace, R.A. (1991) Elevated fetal plasma lactate produces polyhydramnios in the sheep. *Am. J. Obstet. Gynecol.*, **165**, 1595–607.

158. Anderson, D.F. and Faber, J.J. (1989) Animal model for polyhydramnios. *Am. J. Obstet. Gynecol.*, **160**, 389–90.

159. Weir, P.E., Ratten, G.J. and Beischer, N.A. (1979) Acute polyhydramnios: a complication of monozygous twin pregnancy. *Br. J. Obstet. Gynaecol.*, **86**, 849–53.

160. Steinberg, L.H., Hurley, V.A., Desmedt, E. and Beischer, N.A. (1990). Acute polyhydramnios in twin pregnancies. *Aust. N. Z. J. Obstet. Gynaecol.*, **30**, 196–200.

161. Desmedt, E.J., Henry, O.A., Steinberg, L.H. and Beischer, N.A. (1990) Acute and subacute polyhydramnios in singleton pregnancies. *Aust. N. Z. J. Obstet. Gynecol.*, **30**, 191–95.

162. Barry, A.P. (1953) Hydramnios: a survey of 100 cases. *Irish J. Med. Sci.*, **331**, 257–64.

163. Fisk, N.M. (1992) Amniotic pressure in disorders of amniotic fluid volume. University of London Ph.D thesis.

164. Pritchard, J.A., Mason, R., Corley, M. and Pritchard, S. (1970) Genesis of severe placental abruption. *Am. J. Obstet. Gynecol.*, **108**, 22–25.

165. Pretorius, D.H., Manchester, D., Barkin, S. *et al.* (1988) Doppler ultrasound of twin–twin transfusion syndrome. *J. Ultrasound. Med.*, **7**, 117–24.

166. Bebbington, M.W. and Wittman, B.K. (1989) Fetal transfusion syndrome: antenatal factors predicting outcome. *Am. J. Obstet. Gynecol.*, **160**, 913–15.

167. Brown, D.G., Benson, C.B., Driscoll, S.G. and Doubilet, P.M. (1989) Twin–twin transfusion syndrome: sonographic findings. *Radiology*, **170**, 61–63.

168. Gonsoulin, W., Moise, K.J., Kirshon, B. *et al.* (1990) Outcome of twin–twin transfusion syndrome diagnosed before 28 weeks of gestation. *Obstet. Gynecol.*, **75**, 214–16.

169. Urig, M.A., Clewell, W.H. and Elliott, J.P. (1990) Twin–twin transfusion syndrome. *Am. J. Obstet. Gynecol.*, **163**, 1522–26.

170. Fisk, N.M., Borrell, A., Hubinont, C. *et al.* (1990) Fetofetal transfusion syndrome: do the neonatal criteria apply *in utero*? *Arch. Dis. Child.*, **65**, 657–61.

171. Barkin, S.Z., Pretorius, D.H., Beckett, M.K. *et al.* (1987) Severe polyhydramnios; incidence of anomalies. *AJR*, **148**, 155–59.

172. Tabor, B.L. and Maier, J.A. (1987) Polyhydramnios and elevated intrauterine pressure during amnioinfusion. *Am. J. Obstet. Gynecol.*, **156**, 130–31.

173. Fisk, N.M., Vaughan J. and Talbert D. (1994) Impaired fetal blood gas status in polyhydramnios and its relation to raised amniotic pressure. *Fetal. Diagn. Ther.*, **9**, 7–13.

174. Fisk, N.M., Giussani, D.A., Parkes, M.J. *et al.* (1991) Amnioinfusion increases amniotic pressure in pregnant sheep but does not alter fetal acid base status. *Am. J. Obstet. Gynecol.*, **165**, 1459–63.

175. Winn, N.W., Gabrielli, S., Reece, E.A. *et al.* (1989) Ultrasonographic criteria for the prenatal diagnosis of placental chorionicity in twin gestations. *Am. J. Obstet. Gynecol.*, **161**, 1540–42.

176. D'Alton, M.E. and Dudley, D.K. (1989). The ultra-sonographic prediction of chorionicity in twin gestation. *Am. J. Obstet. Gynecol.*, **160**, 557–61.

177. Bennett, P., Henderson, D., Stanier, P. *et al.* (1992) Determination of twin zygosity by DNA hybridisation to wild type bacteriophage M13. *Br. J. Obstet. Gynaecol.*, **99**, 85–88.

178. Cifuentes, R.F., Olley, P.M., Balfe, J.W. *et al.* (1979) Indomethacin and renal function in premature infants with persistent patent ductus arteriosus. *J. Pediatr.*, **95**, 583–87.

179. Kirshon, B., Moise, K.J., Wasserstrum, N. *et al.* (1988) Influence of short-term indomethacin therapy on fetal urine output. *Obstet. Gynecol.*, **72**, 51–53.

180. Moise, K.J., Ou, C.N., Kirshon, B. *et al.* (1990) Placental transfer of indomethacin in the human pregnancy. *Am. J. Obstet. Gynecol.*, **162**, 549–54.

181. Millard, R.W., Baig, H. and Vatner, S.F. (1979) Prostaglandin control of the renal circulation in response to hypoxemia in the fetal lamb *in utero*. *Circ. Res.*, **45**, 172–79.

182. Seyberth, H., Rascher, W. Hackenthal, R. and Wille, L. (1983) Effect of prolonged indomethacin therapy on renal function and selected vasoactive hormones in very low birth weight infants with symptomatic patent ductus arteriosus. *J. Pediatr.*, **103**, 979–84.

183. Cabrol, D., Landesman, R., Muller, J. *et al.* (1987) Treatment of polyhydramnios with prostaglandin synthetase inhibitor (indomethacin). *Am. J. Obstet. Gynecol.*, **157**, 422–26.

184. Mamopoulos, M., Assimakopoulos, E., Reece, E.A. *et al.* (1990) Maternal indomethacin therapy in the treatment of polyhydramnios. *Am. J. Obstet. Gynecol.*, **162**, 1225–29.

185. Lange, I.R., Harman, C.R., Ash, K.M. *et al.* (1989) Twins with hydramnios: treating premature labor at source. *Am. J. Obstet. Gynecol.*, **160**, 552–57.

186. Hendricks, S.D., Smith, J.R. Moore, D.E. and Brown, Z.A. (1990) Oligohydramnios associated with prostaglandin synthetase inhibitors in preterm labour. *Br. J. Obstet. Gynaecol.*, **97**, 312–16.

187. Moise, K.J., Huhta, J.C., Sharif, D.S. *et al.* (1988) Indomethacin in the treatment of premature labor. Effects on fetal ductus arteriosus. *N. Engl J. Med.*, **319**, 327–31.

188. Cowan, F. (1986) Indomethacin, patent ductus arteriosus, and cerebral blood flow. *J. Pediatr.*, **109**, 341–44.

189. Buderus, S., Thomas B., Fahnenstich H. and Kowalewski, S. (1992) Renal failure in two preterm infants: toxic effect of prenatal maternal indomethacin treatment? *Br. J. Obstet. Gynaecol.*, **100**, 97–98.

190. Carlan, S.J., O'Brien, W.F., O'Leary, T.D. and Mastrogiannis, D. (1992) Randomized comparative trial of indomethacin and sulindac for the treatment of refractory preterm labor. *Obstet. Gynecol.*, **79**, 223–28.

191. Rivett, L.C. (1933). Hydramnios. *J. Obstet. Gynaecol. Br. Empire*, **40**, 522–25.

192. Erskine, J.P. (1944) A case of acute hydramnios successfully treated by abdominal paracentesis. *J. Obstet. Gynaecol. Br. Empire*, **51**, 549–51.

193. Danziger, R.W. (1948) Twin pregnancy with acute hydramnios treated by paracentesis uteri. *BMJ*, **ii**, 205–206.

194. Brown, G.R. (1958) Acute hydramnios treated by abdominal paracentesis. *J. Obstet. Gynaecol. Br. Empire*, **65**, 61–63.

195. Brandt, A.J. and Bates, J.S. (1961) Transabdominal amniocentesis in hydramnios. *Obstet. Gynecol.*, **17**, 392–94.

196. Brown, G.R. and Macaskill, S. (1961) Acute hydramnios, with twins, successfully treated by abdominal paracentesis. *BMJ*, **i**, 1739.

197. Feingold, M., Cetrulo, C.L., Newton, E. *et al.* (1986) Serial amniocenteses in the treatment of twin of twin transfusion complicated with acute polyhydramnios. *Acta Genet. Med. Gemellol.*, **35**, 107–13.

198. Weiner, C.P. (1987) Diagnosis and treatment of twin to twin transfusion in the mid-second trimester of pregnancy. *Fetal Ther.*, **2**, 71–74.

199. Chescheir, N.C. and Seeds, J.W. (1988) Polyhydramnios and oligohydramnios in twin gestations. *Obstet. Gynecol.*, **71**, 882–84.

200. Pearce, M.J., Fisk, N.M. and Rodeck, C.R. (1992) The operative management of abnormalities of amniotic fluid volume, in *Textbook of Ultrasound in Obstetrics and Gynecology* (eds. F. Chervenak, G. Isaacson and S. Campbell), Little, Brown, Boston, pp. 1357–60.

201. Mahoney, B.S., Petty, C.N., Nyberg, D.A. *et al.* (1990) The 'stuck twin' phenomenon: ultrasonographic findings, pregnancy outcome, and management with serial amniocenteses. *Am. J. Obstet. Gynecol.*, **163**, 1513–22.

202. Cabrera-Ramirez, L. and Harris, R.E. (1976) Controlled removal of amniotic fluid in hydramnios, *South. Med. J.*, **69**, 239–40.

203 Elliott, J.P., Urig, M.A. and Clewell, W.H. (1991) Aggressive therapeutic amniocentesis for treatment of twin–twin transfusion syndrome. *Obstet. Gynecol.*, 77, 537–40.

204. Caldeyro-Barcia, R., Pose, S.V. and Alvarez, H. (1957) Uterine contractility in polyhydramnios and the effects of withdrawal of the excess of amniotic fluid. *Am. J. Obstet. Gynecol.*, 73, 1238–54.

205. Harrison, M.R., Adzick, N.S., Longaker, M.T. *et al.* (1990) Successful repair *in utero* of a fetal diaphragmatic hernia after removal of herniated viscera from the left thorax. *N. Engl. J. Med.*, 322, 1582–84.

206. Harrison, M.R., Adzick, N.S., Jennings, R.W. *et al.* (1990) Antenatal intervention for congenital cystic adenomatoid malformation. *Lancet,* 336, 965–67.

207. Wittman, B.K., Farquharson, D.F., Thomas, W.D. *et al.* (1986) The role of feticide in the management of severe twin transfusion syndrone. *Am. J. Obstet. Gynecol.*, 155, 1023–26.

208. de Lia, J.E., Cruickshank, D.P. and Keye, W.R. (1990) Fetoscopic neodymium:YAG laser occlusion of placental vessels in severe twin–twin transfusion syndrome. *Obstet. Gynecol.*, 75, 1046–53.

80 IMMUNE AND NON-IMMUNE FETAL HYDROPS

G. Ryan and M.J. Whittle

80.1 Definition and history

Hydrops is defined as an abnormal accumulation of serous fluid in body cavities or tissues. If a maternal circulating antibody against red blood cells is identified, the hydrops is 'immune' in origin, otherwise it is 'non-immune'. Before the widespread introduction of rhesus (Rh) immunoglobulin prophylaxis [1,2], most cases of hydrops were immune [3] whereas today most are non-immune. Non-immune hydrops (NIH) was unknowingly described in 1892 in a series of hydropic cases [4] and was only reported separately in 1943 in a 'fetus unassociated with erythroblastosis' [5]. Recent reviews document the changing face of hydrops over later years [6–9].

80.2 Immune hydrops

80.2.1 PATHOGENESIS

Immune hydrops is due primarily to the haemolysis which occurs when circulating anti-red blood cell IgG antibodies cross the placenta and attack antigen-positive fetal red cells. The majority of cases still occur in the presence of Rh antibodies but other systems, such as Kell, can produce devastating disease. The result is anaemia, extramedullary erythropoiesis, hepatosplenomegaly, hypoalbuminaemia, and an outpouring of immature nucleated red blood cells (erythroblastosis fetalis). Ultimately, tissue hypoxia, fetal hydrops, cardiac failure and death occur. Hydrops develops when the fetal haemoglobin (Hb) deficit is ≥ 7 g/dl [10], probably because of reduced oncotic pressure secondary to hypoalbuminaemia. Eventually there is fetal decompensation, with metabolic and lactic acidosis [10–12].

80.2.2 TREATMENT

This type of alloimmune disease is discussed in Chapter 84, and we shall restrict ourselves to the hydropic fetus.

Immune hydrops is an absolute indication for fetal blood sampling and transfusion *in utero*. This procedure was intially performed fetoscopically [13], a technique superseded by needling under ultrasound guidance [14].

Intravascular fetal transfusion has proved life saving in the hydropic and/or moribund fetus, in whom intraperitoneal transfusion is often unsuccessful because of poor absorption of blood from the peritoneal cavity, possibly due to reduced fetal breathing movements [15]. With intravascular fetal transfusion, 70–85% of hydropic and 85–95% of non-hydropic fetuses can survive [16–19].

80.3 Non-immune hydrops

80.3.1 INTRODUCTION

Non-immune hydrops (NIH) occurs in between 1 of 1500 and 1 of 4000 pregnancies [20]. It can occur at any gestation, and is a common pathological finding in first and second trimester spontaneous abortions. The aetiology varies worldwide. In North America and Europe, the most common causes are cardiovascular, infectious and chromosomal [8,9].

80.3.2 PATHOGENESIS

NIH usually represents the terminal stage for many conditions (Table 80.1), and several different pathogenic mechanisms may act simultaneously. These include anaemia, hepatitis, hypoproteinaemia, arrhythmia, heart failure, infection and obstructed venous or lymphatic return. NIH is the end-result of a redistribution of body fluids among the intravascular, intracellular and interstitial compartments, secondary to an imbalance in capillary hydrostatic pressure, plasma oncotic pressure and/or capillary permeability [21]. Capillary damage is often hypoxic in origin, resulting in plasma protein loss.

Diseases of the Fetus and Newborn, 2nd edn, Edited by G.B. Reed, A.E. Claireaux and F. Cockburn. Published in 1995 by Chapman & Hall, London. ISBN 0 412 39160 0

Table 80.1   Causes of hydrops fetalis

A. Immune		
	Anaemia	*Rhesus alloimmunization*
		Other red cell antigen alloimmunization
B. Non-immune		
1. Fetal		
(a) Cardiovascular		
	(i) Malformation	Left or right heart hypoplasia
		Atrioventricular canal
		Single ventricle
		Transposition
		Tetralogy of Fallot
		Closure of foramen ovale or ductus arteriosus
		Any absent/atretic valves
		Endocardial fibroelastosis
		Ebstein's anomaly
		Major septal defects
		Cardiac tumours
		Myocarditis
	(ii) *Tachyarrhythmia*	*Supraventricular tachycardia*
		Paroxysmal atrial tachycardia
		Atrial flutter
		Wolff–Parkinson–White syndrome
	(iii) *Bradyarrhythmia*	*Complete heart block*
		Unspecified bradycardia
	(iv) High output failure	Placental chorioangioma
		Other large fetal angiomas
		Sacrococcygeal teratoma
		Vein of Galen aneurysm
		Twin–twin transfusion (recipient usually)
		Acardiac twin (donor)
(b) Neck/thoracic anomalies		Cystic hygroma
		Chylothorax–hydrothorax
		Congenital cystic adenomatoid malformation
		Diaphragmatic hernia
		Pulmonary sequestration
		Thoracic tumours
(c) Gastrointestinal anomalies		Hepatic: cirrhosis; hepatitis; tumour
		Atresias
		Volvulus
		Meconium peritonitis
(d) Urinary tract anomalies		Congenital nephrotic syndrome
		Lower urinary tract obstruction
		Upper urinary tract obstruction
		Prune-belly syndrome
		Polycystic kidneys
(e) Chromosomal		45,X
		Trisomy 21
		Trisomy 18
		Triploidy
		Trisomy 13
(f) Anaemia		α-Thalassaemia (homozygous)
		Human parvovirus (HPV) B19 infection
		Glucose-6-phosphate dehydrogenase deficiency
		Fetomaternal haemorrhage
		Twin–twin transfusion (donor)
(g) Infection		Cytomegalovirus
		Parvovirus (HPVB19)
		Toxoplasmosis
		Syphilis
		Coxsackie
		Rubella
		Listeriosis

Table 80.1 *continued*

(h) Genetic		
	(i) Metabolic disorders	Gaucher's disease
		G_{M1} gangliosidosis
		Sialidosis
		Mucopolysaccharidosis
		Hurler's syndrome
	(ii) Skeletal dysplasias	Achondroplasia
		Achondrogenesis
		Osteogenesis
		Thanatophoric dysplasia
		Asphyxiating thoracic dystrophy
		Short rib–polydactyly syndromes
	(iii) Fetal hypokinesis	Arthrogryposis
		Neu–Laxova syndrome
		Pena–Shokeir syndrome
		Multiple pterygia
(i) Idiopathic (approx. 15–20%)		
2. Maternal		Severe diabetes
		Severe anaemia
		Severe hypoproteinaemia
3. Placental		Chorioangioma
		Venous thrombosis
		Cord torsion, knot or tumour

Conditions where prenatal therapy has been successful are shown in italics.

80.3.3 CLASSIFICATION

Causes of NIH may be maternal, placental or most commonly fetal. **Maternal** causes are rare and should be differentiated from maternal complications which are secondary to fetal hydrops (e.g. pre-eclampsia). **Placental** causes usually represent high output failure states.

A classification scheme for **fetal** causes is suggested in Table 80.1. There is some overlap in the groupings which may only represent associations and not causations. Many reports are from specialized units [22], so certain conditions tend to be over-represented. Machin [8] has extensively reviewed cases from the last decade, and has taken into account both general and specialized series.

(a) Cardiovascular

The most common causes in most series are cardiovascular [7–9,23–26]. These can be subdivided into malformations, conduction disorders, valvular disorders, tumours, premature closure of communicating structures, and high output failure states. Most result in congestive cardiac failure *in utero* with associated increased hydrostatic pressure. Some also have rhythm disturbances. Maternal SS-A (Ro) or SS-B (La) antibodies are present in 30–50% of cases of fetal complete heart block. Complete heart block is associated with a high incidence of cardiac malformation, and a fetal echo is always warranted [9,22]. Umbilical vein pulsa-

tions have been reported as a poor prognostic sign suggesting cardiac failure.

(b) Neck/thoracic anomalies

Hydrops results from obstruction of venous or lymphatic return due to maldevelopment, compression or kinking, or from cardiac tamponade. Diaphragmatic hernias may also cause NIH by similar mechanisms.

(c) Gastrointestinal anomalies

These rare causes of NIH may be related to other primary pathology (e.g. infection). Abdominal masses presumably act by compression of venous return, although hypoproteinaemia or arteriovenous shunting may also play a role.

(d) Urinary tract anomalies

These are rare causes of NIH, probably related to hypoproteinaemia. It is unclear why hydrops occurs in lower urinary tract obstruction, although the ascites may, in fact, be urine following bladder rupture.

(e) Chromosome anomalies

These comprise the second most common group [8,9,24,27]. Turner's syndrome is classically associated with cystic hygromas. Many of these disorders result in early spontaneous abortion. Trisomies 21, 18 and 13 and triploidy have all been associated with NIH, although it is often unclear why hydrops occurs.

(f) Anaemia

Anaemia is due to decreased production, increased haemolysis or haemorrhage. If the process is gradual, the fetus mounts a compensatory erythropoietic response and NIH only develops when the anaemia exceeds its ability to keep pace. Hydrops seems to result from a combination of hypoxic capillary damage, causing protein leakage, and high output cardiac failure.

In α-thalassaemia, homozygotes cannot manufacture α-globin chains, either in utero, to form haemoglobin F (HbF), or after birth to form haemoglobin A (HbA) [28]. In utero, haemoglobin Bart's is formed, which has such a high oxygen affinity that tissue hypoxia results, leading to capillary damage, protein leakage, cardiac failure and hydrops. Other causes of decreased production include a generalized marrow aplasia, as found in parvovirus infection [29], or fetal leukaemia [26]. Glucose-6-phosphate dihydrogenase deficiency is a rare cause of NIH, resulting from increased haemolysis.

Haemorrhage may occur either into another fetus (twin–twin transfusion) [30], into the fetus itself (e.g. intracranial), into a tumour (e.g. sacrococcygeal), or transplacentally [8]. In twin–twin transfusion syndrome the donor is usually growth restricted, anaemic and may have severe oligohydramnios ('stuck twin'), whereas the recipient is usually larger, polycythaemic, and has a persistently large bladder and associated hydramnios. Usually the recipient becomes hydropic because of volume overload, although this can also happen in the donor as a result of anaemia and tissue hypoxia [3]. Twin–twin transfusion only occurs in monochorionic placentae, because of their vascular communications.

(g) Infection

Intrauterine infections may cause NIH as a result of either multiple organ damage, hepatitis causing decreased protein production, or capillary damage causing protein leakage. Parvovirus and cytomegalovirus have a predilection for erythroid precursors, and cause a generalized marrow aplasia [23,29]. The marrow may be particularly sensitive to infection from 17 to 22 weeks' gestation. In contrast to most other congenital infections, parvovirus has not been associated with any adverse long-term sequelae, although follow-up is only 1 year so far [31]. Toxoplasmosis may also cause calcifications and can pose a difficult diagnostic challenge [32]. Rubella and syphilis are still encountered as causes of NIH in developing countries.

(h) Genetic anomalies

A host of non-chromosomal genetic conditions may cause NIH [27]; some are listed in Table 80.1. The mechanism is poorly understood and is probably multifactorial. In storage diseases the most likely mechanism is hepatic infiltration.

(i) Idiopathic

The number of 'idiopathic' cases of NIH for which we can still find no obvious cause has decreased in recent series [8,9,24] and will continue to do so as our investigative abilities improve.

80.3.4 INVESTIGATION

A thorough systematic prenatal evaluation can establish a cause in 80–85% of cases, which is important for the management of the index pregnancy and also for future genetic counselling [9,23,25]. Table 80.2 outlines a suggested protocol, in which some investigations are recommended universally unless a cause is immediately obvious, whereas others are done selectively.

A detailed history may provide the first clues to aetiology, and may help prioritize subsequent investigations. Homozygous α-thalassaemia is particularly prevalent in south-east Asians; a maternal history of systemic lupus erythematosus or diabetes may be relevant; previous losses may be related to one of the inborn errors of metabolism, and the family history may suggest other genetic conditions.

A comprehensive sonographic evaluation should be the initial step. Hydramnios is commonly associated and often prompts the ultrasound examination which first identifies the problem. The collections of fluid in the body cavities and tissues are unmistakeable (Figure 80.1), and their relative distribution may give a clue to the aetiology [25]. A detailed anatomical scan may identify the responsible structural anomaly (e.g. sacrococcygeal teratoma), or ultrasound 'markers' may suggest a chromosomal cause [33]. The degree of hydramnios should be assessed as this may pose an imminent threat of premature rupture of the membranes or labour. If appropriate, fetal well-being should be simultaneously assessed [34]. Fetal Doppler evaluation may give some indication of anaemia [12], cardiac failure [35] and well-being. Fetal echocardiography should be performed whenever conventional ultrasound does not provide an answer.

The initial maternal blood work should establish blood type and the presence of red blood cell antibodies to exclude immune hydrops. Other baseline tests are a complete blood count and indices, Kleihauer–Betke, glucose and viral serology. Further selective investigations are suggested in Table 80.2.

Table 80.2 Investigation of non-immune hydrops

HISTORY

Age, racial background:	
Occupation:	e.g. ?schoolteacher
Medical history:	e.g. diabetes mellitus, systemic lupus erythematosus, haemoglobinopathy
Obstetric history:	e.g. stillbirth, neonatal deaths
Family history:	e.g. stillbirths, congenital anomalies, inherited conditions
Are parents related?	
Complications during index pregnancy:	e.g. vaginal bleeding, viral illness

INVESTIGATIONS	**In all cases**	**In selected cases only**
Mother	Indirect Coombs' test	Karyotype
	Blood group	Maternal serum α-fetoprotein
	Complete blood count and indices	Hb electrophoresis
	Kleihauer–Betke	SS-A, SS-B antibodies
	Glucose screen	Glucose tolerance test
	TORCH/HPVB19, IgM, IgG	G6PD pyruvate kinase
	VDRL	Uric acid, liver function tests
		HLA typing
Father	–	Hb electrophoresis
		Karyotype
Fetus	Ultrasound:	Fetal echocardiogram:
	Detailed anatomy	Structure (two-dimensions)
	Amniotic fluid volume	M-mode
	Doppler	Doppler
	Biophysical profile	Colour flow
	Non-stress test	
Fetal blood	Complete blood count, platelets	Hb electrophoresis
	Direct Coombs' test	Blood gas
	Blood group	
	Karyotype	Liver function tests
	WBC differential	Specific enzyme assays
	TORCH/HPVB19 IgM	TORCH/HPVB19 DNA
	Protein/albumin	Electron microscopy
Placenta	Karyotype (CVS)	Specific metabolic tests
Amniotic fluid	Karyotype	Viral DNA
	Cytomegalovirus culture	Lecithin/sphingomyelin ratio
	Other viral culture and sensitivity	Restriction endonucleases
	Bacterial culture and sensitivity	Amniotic fluid α-fetoprotein
Fetal effusions	Lymphocyte count (pleural)	Karyotype
	Protein/albumin	Viral culture and sensitivity and/or DNA
Post mortem	Placental pathology	
	Full autopsy	–
	Skeletal survey	
	Clinical genetics consult	
Neonate	Similar work-up to above as considered appropriate	

CVS = chorionic villus sampling; G6PD = glucose-6-phosphate dehydrogenase; VDRL = Venereal Disease Research Laboratory.

Fetal karyotype should be determined from fetal blood, chorionic villi, amniotic fluid or one of the fetal body cavities, as appropriate, depending on gestation, accessibility and the urgency of the need for results [36]. Basic fetal blood work should include a direct Coombs' test, complete blood count and indices, karyotype, protein, albumin and viral-specific IgM. Other tests are done selectively (Table 80.2) [37], and some samples can be kept in storage for subsequent

evaluation. With this approach, one can find an answer in the majority of cases within 48 hours.

Blood sampling yields most information. The risks of fetal loss due to this procedure are approximately 1% [14,38], although in the fetus with NIH loss rates of up to 7% may be more realistic [39,40]. Blood is usually sampled from the fixed cord root [14], although alternatives are a free loop, the intrahepatic vein [41], or the heart [42]. If it is anticipated that the fetus may

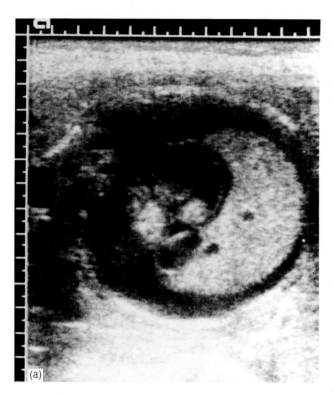

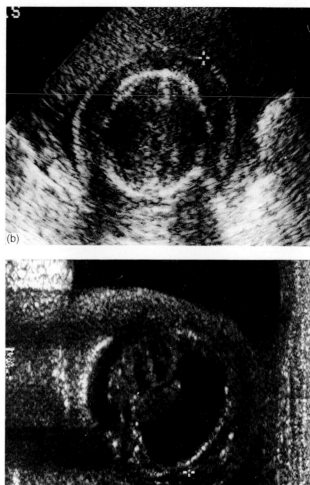

Figure 80.1 (a) Ascites (NIH due to parvovirus infection, Hb = 3 g/dl). (b) Severe skull oedema (NIH associated with trisomy 21). (c) Massive pleural effusions and chest wall oedema (NIH due to congenital chylothorax, associated with trisomy 21).

require transfusion (e.g. parvovirus infection), it is prudent to have some cross-matched blood ready, to avoid the risks of a second procedure. It is usually a simple matter simultaneously to advance the needle into the fetal chest, abdomen or amniotic fluid, as this can be both diagnostic (e.g. chylothorax) and occasionally therapeutic (e.g. hydramnios), and does not increase the overall procedure risk. Amniotic fluid is preferable for cytomegalovirus or bacterial culture, and, later on, can give an indication of lung maturity. Chorionic villous sampling is an alternative at any gestation for obtaining a rapid karyotype or DNA results.

After birth, the placenta should be sent for pathology and a skeletal survey and clinical genetics opinion considered. If the baby is dead, permission for a postmortem examination should be obtained. Further investigations may be prompted by additional physical findings. A comprehensive evaluation of each case greatly aids subsequent genetic counselling.

80.3.5 PROGNOSIS

The overall mortality in NIH as a whole is still approximately 80% [9,23]. Some of this improvement over earlier reports [3,7] is attributable to the growing number of causes which are amenable to *in utero* therapy. The majority of cases still represent a terminal process which may be irreversible, hence the grim outlook for many fetuses. Attempts have been made to identify predictors of outcome in NIH, with limited success [35,43]. The key to further improvement in prognosis lies in early comprehensive evaluation, accurate diagnosis and refinements of prenatal therapy. Pregnancies should no longer be automatically referred for termination, as prenatal treatment may be possible in carefully selected cases.

80.3.6 PRENATAL THERAPY

In Table 80.1 the conditions shown in italics denote those in which some form of prenatal therapy has been successful, as determined by the birth of a healthy child.

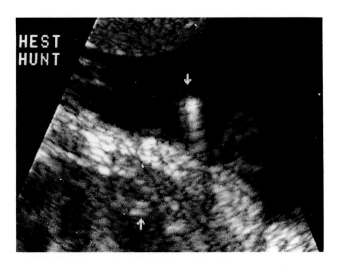

Figure 80.2 Pleuroamniotic shunt *in situ* after successful drainage of congenital chylothorax and subsequent resolution of NIH.

Many of the tachyarrhythmias are amenable to antiarrhythmic therapy, almost always transplacentally. Rarely, direct fetal administration may be required [44]. Digoxin, verapamil, flecainide and amiodarone at standard paediatric dosages (mg/kg) have been used. Digoxin has also been given when intrauterine congestive failure due to other causes is suspected, and has even been empirically combined with frusemide (furosemide), albumin and blood [9]. Cardiac pacing *in utero* may be an option in severe cases [45].

Twin–twin transfusion syndrome still has a very high mortality [30] and various interventions have been attempted. Aggressive amniocentesis has some merit [46]; selective transfusion/phlebotomy has been uniformly disappointing; and recently dramatic success with embryoscopic laser ablation of communicating vessels has been reported [47]; selective feticide is contraindicated because of the risks to the other twin. Cord occlusion has been attempted in an acardiac twin to prevent cardiac failure in the donor [9].

Thoracic causes of NIH such as chylothorax, lung sequestration and congenital cystic adenomatoid malformation type 1 have been successfully treated by chest shunt insertion *in utero* [48,49] (Figures 80.1b and 80.2). The main rationale for invasive therapy in these cases is to prevent pulmonary hypoplasia, and prevent or even reverse hydrops and hydramnios. Cases must be carefully selected, as some effusions resolve spontaneously whereas others proceed to develop NIH, hydramnios and die [50,51]. We drain all isolated large effusions initially, as this usually suggests a diagnosis (e.g. high lymphocyte count), gives a karyotype, and may even be therapeutic. Effusions which re-collect rapidly may benefit from chronic drainage. Therapeutic drainage immediately prior to delivery may facilitate neonatal resuscitation. Urinary tract obstructions are

rarely associated with NIH, and, using a similar rationale, vesicoamniotic drainage may have a role. All prenatal drainage procedures have yet to be subjected to scrutiny by randomized trials.

NIH related to a diaphragmatic hernia has been successfully treated by thoracocenteses [52]. Several cases of diaphragmatic herniae [53] and congenital cystic adenometoid malformation [54] have been definitively repaired antenatally.

The most significant application of fetal therapy is in fetal anaemia. Initially, fetal transfusion was confined to Rh disease [55], but the same principles and expertise have been applied to non-immune causes of anaemia, such as parvovirus infection [56], and severe fetomaternal haemorrhage [57]. Theoretically, there might be a role in glucose-6-phosphate dehydrogenase deficiency, unlike α-thalassaemia which is fatal regardless. Stem cell transfusion is an exciting potential future option for some genetic causes of NIH [58].

Maternal or fetal antibiotic therapy is possible in various fetal infections leading to NIH [14], however, in most, apart from parvovirus, there are adverse long-term sequelae which pre-empt such treatment. By the time hydrops occurs, the damage has usually been done. Some sequelae may be prevented by early diagnosis and antibiotic therapy.

80.3.7 MATERNAL COMPLICATIONS, OBSTETRIC AND NEONATAL MANAGEMENT

Maternal complications may occur with NIH. Hypoproteinaemia, oedema, hypertension and laboratory findings consistent with a diagnosis of pre-eclampsia may develop [59]. This association was noted previously with severe Rh disease. We have seen a dramatic resolution of this condition once the fetal problem has resolved. The maternal condition may occasionally be severe enough to warrant delivery.

Ongoing viable pregnancies should be closely monitored for fetal well-being, until delivery, by biophysical profile scoring, including non-stress test [34] and Doppler analysis of fetal haemodynamics.

Mode of delivery should be decided on usual obstetric grounds, taking into account the underlying prognosis. Uterine overdistension secondary to hydramnios carries the dangers of abruptio placentae or cord prolapse when the membranes rupture and thus a controlled amniotomy in labour may be safer. Because of the risk of postpartum haemorrhage due to uterine atony, all such mothers should receive a prophylactic oxytocic post partum. Prematurity secondary to hydramnios is a major contributing factor to the poor outcome of some neonates, and indomethacin may be worth considering to decrease the amniotic fluid volume [60].

Where appropriate, all viable pregnancies should be

delivered in a tertiary care centre with neonatal and paediatric surgical facilities. Immediate measures such as pericardiocentesis or thoracocentesis may be necessary to allow ventilation, and blood product replacement via an umbilical catheter may be crucial. Neonatal investigations should follow on from those outlined above, and a multidisciplinary approach is recommended [61].

80.4 Conclusions

Hydrops represents a terminal stage for may conditions, most of which are fetal in origin, and its onset usually signifies fetal decompensation. Immune causes can be successfully treated *in utero*, and we have dwelt on the non-immune causes as these pose the major diagnostic and therapeutic challenge today. Parents can be counselled that the mortality is no longer close to 100%, and a steadily growing number of carefully selected cases may be amenable to some form of prenatal therapy, with expectation of a good outcome. A comprehensive approach must be taken in the investigation of hydrops, both for the management of the index case and for future counselling. Early referral to a tertiary care centre is encouraged for complete evaluation of each case.

References

1. Freda, V.J., Gorman, J.G. and Pollack, W. (1966) Rh factor: prevention of immunization and clinical trial on mothers. *Science*, **151**, 828–30.
2. Bowman, J.M. (1978) The management of Rh-isoimmunization. *Obstet. Gynecol.*, **52**, 19–78.
3. Macafee, C.A.J., Fortune, D.W. and Beischer, N.A. (1970) Non-immunological hydrops fetalis. *Br. J. Obstet. Gynaecol.*, **77**, 226–37.
4. Ballantyne, J.W. (1892) *The Diseases and Deformities of the Fetus*, Oliver & Boyd, Edinburgh.
5. Potter, E.L. (1943) Universal edema of the fetus associated with erythroblastosis. *Am. J. Obstet. Gynecol.*, **43**, 130–34.
6. Andersen, H.M., Drew, J.H., Beischer, N.A. *et al.* (1983) Non-immune hydrops fetalis: changing contribution to perinatal mortality. *Br. J. Obstet. Gynaecol.*, **90**, 636–39.
7. Machin, G.A. (1981) Differential diagnosis of hydrops fetalis. *Am. J. Med. Genet.*, **9**, 341–50.
8. Machin, G.A. (1989) Hydrops revisited: literature review of 1414 cases published in the 1980s. *Am. J. Med. Genet.*, **34**, 366–90.
9. Hansmann, M., Gembruch, U. and Bald, R. (1989) New therapeutic measures in non immune hydrops fetalis based on 402 prenatally diagnosed cases. *Fetal Ther.*, **4**, 29–36.
10. Nicolaides, K.H., Warenski, J.C. and Rodeck, C.H. (1985) The relationship of fetal plasma protein concentration and hemoglobin level to the development of hydrops in rhesus isoimmunization. *Am. J. Obstet. Gynecol.*, **152**, 341–34.
11. Soothill, P.W., Nicolaides, K.H. and Rodeck, C.G. (1987) Effect of anaemia on fetal acid–base status. *Br. J. Obstet. Gynaecol.*, **94**, 880–83.
12. Nicolaides, K.H. (1989) Studies on fetal physiology and pathophysiology in Rhesus disease. *Semin Perinatol.*, **13**, 328–37.
13. Rodeck, C.H., Kemp, J.R., Holman, C.A. *et al.* (1981) Direct intravascular fetal blood transfusion in severe rhesus isoimmunization. *Lancet*, **i**, 625–27.
14. Daffos, F. Capella-Povolsky, M. and Forestier, F. (1985) Fetal blood sampling during pregnancy with use of a needle guided by ultrasound. A study of 606 consecutive cases. *Am. J. Obstet. Gynecol.*, **153**, 655–60.
15. Menticoglou, S.M., Harman, C.R., Bowman, J.M. and Manning, F.A. (1987) Intraperitoneal blood transfusion: paralysis inhibits red cell absorption. *Fetal Ther.*, **2**, 154–57.
16. Bowman, J.M. (1994) Haemolytic disease, in *Maternal Fetal Medicine – Principles and Practice*, 3rd edn (eds R.K. Creasy and R. Resnik), W.B. Saunders, Philadelphia.
17. Harman, C.R., Bowman, J.M., Manning, F.A. and Menticoglou, S.M. (1990) Intrauterine transfusion – intraperitoneal versus intravascular approach: a case-control comparison. *Am. J. Obstet. Gynecol.*, **162**, 1053–59.
18. Nicolaides, K.H., Soothill, P.W., Rodeck, C.H. *et al.* (1986) Rh disease: intravascular fetal blood transfusion by cordocentesis. *Fetal Ther.*, **1**, 185–92.
19. Tannirandorn, Y. and Rodeck, C.H. (1991) Management of immune haemolytic disease in the fetus. *Blood Rev.*, **5**, 1–14.
20. Romero, R. (1987) Non immune hydrops fetalis, in *Prenatal Diagnosis of Congenital Anomalies*, Appleton & Lange, Norwalk, CT, pp. 414–26.
21. Fadnes, H.O. and Oian, P. (1989) Transcapillary fluid balance and plasma volume regulation: a review. *Obstet. Gynecol. Surv.*, **44**, 769–73.
22. Allan, L.D., Crawford, D.C., Sheridan, R. *et al.* (1986) Aetiology of nonimmune hydrops: the value of echocardiography. *Br. J. Obstet. Gynaecol.*, **93**, 223.
23. Holzgreve, W., Curry, C.J.R., Golbus, M.S. *et al.* (1984) Investigation of nonimmune hydrops fetalis. *Am. J. Obstet. Gynecol.*, **150**, 805–12.
24. Poeschmann, R.P., Verheijen, R.H.M. and Van Dongen, P.W.J. (1991) Differential diagnosis and causes of nonimmunological hydrops fetalis: a review. *Obstet. Gynecol. Surv.*, **46**, 223–31.
25. Salzman, D.H., Frigoletto, F.D., Harlow, B.L. *et al.* (1989) Sonographic evaluation of hydrops fetalis. *Obstet. Gynecol.*, **74**, 106–11.
26. Watson, J. and Campbell, S. (1986) Antenatal evaluation and management in nonimmune hydrops fetalis. *Obstet. Gynecol.*, **67**, 589–92.
27. Jauniaux, E., Van Maldergem, L., De Munter, C. *et al.* (1990) Nonimmune hydrops fetalis associated with genetic abnormalities. *Obstet. Gynecol.*, **75**, 568–72.
28. Tan, S.L., Tseng, A.M. and Thong, P.W. (1989) Bart's hydrops fetalis – clinical presentation and management: an analysis of 25 cases. *Aust. N.Z. J. Obstet. Gynaecol.*, **29**, 233–37.
29. Anand, A., Gray, E.S., Brown, T. *et al.* (1987) Human parvovirus infection in pregnancy and hydrops fetalis. *N. Engl J. Med.*, **316**, 183–86.
30. Blickstein, I. (1990) The twin–twin transfusion syndrome. *Obstet. Gynecol.*, **76**, 714–22.
31. PHLS Working Party on Fifth Disease (1990) Prospective study of human parvovirus (B19) infection in pregnancy. *BMJ*, **300**, 1166–70.
32. Daffos, F., Forestier, F., Capella-Povolsky, M. *et al.* (1988) Prenatal management of 746 pregnancies at risk for congenital toxoplasmosis. *N. Engl. J. Med.*, **318**, 271–75.
33. Benacerraf, B. (1991) Prenatal sonography of autosomal trisomies. *Ultrasound Obstet. Gynecol.*, **1**, 66–75.
34. Manning, F.A. (1985) Assessment of fetal condition and risk: analysis of single and combined biophysical variable monitoring. *Semin. Perinatol.*, **9**, 168.
35. Gudmundsson, I., Huhta, J.C., Wood, D.C. *et al.* (1991) Venous Doppler ultrasonography in the fetus with nonimmune hydrops. *Am. J. Obstet. Gynecol.*, **164**, 33–37.
36. Nicolaidés, K.H., Snijders, R.J.M., Cheng, H.H. and Gosden, C. (1992) Fetal gastro-intestinal and abdominal wall defects: associated malformations and chromosomal abnormalities. *Fetal Diagn. Ther.*, **7**, 102–15.
37. Galjaard, H. (1987) Fetal diagnosis of inborn errors of metabolism. *Baillière's Clin. Obstet. Gynecol.*, **1**, 547–67.
38. Ghidini, A., Sepulveda, W., Lockwood, C.J. and Romero, R. (1993) Complications of fetal blood sampling. *Am. J. Obstet. Gynecol.*, **168**, 1339–44.
39. Maxwell, D.J., Johnson, P., Hurley, P. *et al.* (1991) Fetal blood sampling and pregnancy loss in relation to indication. *Br. J. Obstet. Gynaecol.*, **98**, 892–97.
40. Weiner, C.P., Wenstrom, K.D., Sipes, S.L. and Williamson, R.A. (1991) Risk factors for cordocentesis and fetal intravascular transfusion. *Am. J. Obstet. Gynecol.*, **165**, 1020–25.
41. Nicolini, U., Nicolaidis, P., Fisk, N.M. *et al.* (1990) Fetal blood sampling from the intrahepatic vein: analysis of safety and clinical experience with 214 procedures. *Obstet. Gynecol.*, **76**, 47–53.
42. Westgren, M., Selbing, A. and Stangenberg, M. (1988) Fetal intracardiac transfusions in patients with severe rhesus isoimmunisation. *BMJ*, **296**, 885–86.
43. Carlson, D.E., Platt, L.D., Medearis, A.L. and Horenstein, J. (1990) Prognostic indicators of the resolution of nonimmune hydrops fetalis and survival of the fetus. *Am. J. Obstet. Gynecol.*, **163**, 1785–87.
44. Hansmann, M., Gembruch, U., Bald, R. *et al.* (1991) Fetal tachyarrhythmias: transplacental and direct treatment of the fetus – a report of 60 cases. *Ultrasound Obstet. Gynecol.*, **1**, 162–70.
45. Carpenter, R.J. (1976) Fetal ventricular pacing for hydrops secondary to complete atrioventricular block. *J. Am. Coll. Cardiol.*, **8**, 1434.
46. Elliott, J.P., Urig, M.A. and Clewell, W.H. (1991) Aggressive therapeutic amniocentesis for the treatment of twin–twin transfusion syndrome. *Obstet. Gynecol.*, **77**, 537–40.

47. Ville, Y., Hecher, K., Ogg, D. *et al.* (1992) Successful outcome after Nd: YAG laser separation of chorioangiopagus-twins under sonoendoscopic control. *Ultrasound Obstet. Gynecol.*, 2, 429–31.

48. Rodeck, C.H., Fisk, N.M., Fraser, D.I. and Nicolini, U. (1988) Long-term *in utero* drainage of fetal hydrothorax. *N. Engl. J. Med.*, 319, 1135–38.

49. Weiner, C.P., Varner, M., Pringle, K. *et al.* (1986) Antenatal diagnosis and palliative treatment of nonimmune hydrops fetalis secondary to pulmonary extralobar sequestration. *Obstet. Gynecol.*, 68, 275–80.

50. Weber, A.M. and Philipson, E.H. (1992) Fetal pleural effusion: a review and meta-analysis for prognostic indicators. *Obstet. Gynecol.*, 79, 281–86.

51. Hagay, Z, Reece, A.E., Roberts, A. and Hobbins, J.C. (1993) Isolated fetal pleural effusion: a prenatal management dilemma. *Obstet. Gynecol.*, 81, 147–52.

52. Benacerraf, B. and Frigoletto, F. (1986) *In utero* treatment of a fetus with diaphragmatic hernia complicated by hydrops. *Am. J. Obstet. Gynecol.*, 155, 817–18.

53. Harrison, M.R., Adzick, N.S., Longaker, M.T. *et al.* (1990) Successful repair *in utero* of a fetal diaphragmatic hernia after removal of herniated viscera from the left thorax. *N. Engl. J. Med.*, 322, 1582–84.

54. Harrison, M.R., Adzick, N.S., Jennings, R.W. *et al.* (1990) Antenatal intervention for congenital cystic adenomatoid malformation. *Lancet*, 336, 965–67.

55. Whittle, M.J. (1992) Rhesus haemolytic disease. *Arch. Dis. Child.*, 67, 65–68.

56. Peters, M. and Nicolaides, K.H. (1990) Cordocentesis for the diagnosis and treatment of human fetal parvovirus infection. *Obstet. Gynecol.*, 75, 501–504.

57. Cardwell, M.S. (1988) Successful treatment of hydrops fetalis caused by fetomaternal hemorrhage: a case report. *Am. J. Obstet. Gynecol.*, 158, 131.

58. Johnson, J. and Elias, S. (1988) Prenatal treatment: medical and gene therapy in the fetus. *Clin. Obstet. Gynecol.*, 31, 390–406.

59. Van Selm, M., Kanhai, H.H.H. and Bennebroek Gravenhorst, J. (1991) Maternal hydrops syndrome: a review. *Obstet. Gynecol. Surv.*, 46, 785–788.

60. Kirshon, B., Mari, G. and Moise, K.J. (1990) Indomethacin therapy in the treatment of symptomatic polyhydramnios. *Obstet. Gynecol.*, 75, 202–205.

61. Carlton, D.P., McGillivray, B.C. and Schreiber, M.D. (1989) Nonimmune hyrops fetalis: a multidisciplinary approach. *Clin. Perinatol.*, 16, 839–51.

81 FETAL METABOLISM

F. Cockburn

81.1 Introduction

Genetic material contained in the fertilized ovum controls cell division and tissue development, and when the environment surrounding the embryo and fetus, provided by the mother, is satisfactory a normal, well-grown, well-formed infant should result. Fetal growth takes place within the uterus and uterine size is a major determinant of fetal growth which can override genetic factors [1,2]. Extrauterine pregnancies generally result in light-for-date infants when the pregnancy reaches viability. This small size could result from many factors but effective placental blood supply is likely to be a major determinant of fetal growth. Maternal diet, maternal metabolic disorder and exposure to environmental toxins can clearly affect fetal metabolic activities. Disorders of placental structure and function can also influence fetal metabolic activities, as can inherited defects within the developing embryo and fetus.

81.2 Maternal influences

81.2.1 NUTRIENT AVAILABILITY

There is still considerable controversy about the extra energy requirements of pregnancy and lactation. These requirements can be calculated on a theoretical basis with considerable accuracy but well-controlled longitudinal studies which confirm these theoretical requirements are scarce.

(a) Energy requirements in pregnancy

Additional energy is required to:

1. increase uterine mass;
2. form the fetal placental unit;
3. increase effective breast tissue;
4. enlarge maternal fat stores to create an energy reserve for lactation;
5. expand blood volume.

These factors have been described as the 'capital gains' associated with pregnancy [3]. There are also the

Table 81.1 Mean energy cost of pregnancy: 'capital' costs

Subject or tissue	Energy cost	
	kcal	MJ
Fetus (3.5 kg)		
Fat 490 g	5 390	23
Protein 420 g	2 940	12
Placenta (0.64 kg)		
Fat 4 g	40	0.2
Protein 98 g	690	3
Maternal fat 2.4 kg	26 400	110
Uterus, blood volume, amniotic fluid, extracellular fluid, breasts (total 5.8 kg)		
Fat 41 g	450	2
Protein 435 g	3 040	13
Total	38 950	163

additional 'running costs' required to meet the increased energy requirements of these enlarging organs and tissue. The larger body mass of the pregnant woman requires her to expend a relatively greater amount of energy for normal daily activities such as walking and working at home than she would in the non-pregnant state. There are energy savings and there are reports of remarkable adaptations in basal metabolic rates in women on a marginal energy intake [4]. Table 81.1 shows the mean energy cost of pregnancy (capital costs) for an average pregnancy, together with the energy required to deposit fat and protein in various tissues. The average fat gain in European women between the beginning and end of pregnancy is between 2.0 and 2.4 kg [5,6]. In order to lay down this amount of energy reserve for lactation and late pregnancy there is an energy cost of between 20 000 and 30 000 kcal (84–126 MJ). This represents about one-third of the total theoretical energy cost of pregnancy. Women who do not breast feed their infants or do so for only a limited time may find themselves having to diet if they wish to remove this fat reserve. Although the fat reserve

Diseases of the Fetus and Newborn, 2nd edn, Edited by G.B. Reed, A.E. Claireaux and F. Cockburn. Published in 1995 by Chapman & Hall, London. ISBN 0 412 39160 0

Table 81.2 Energy cost of pregnancy: Scotland and the Netherlands [5,6]

Subject or tissue	Energy cost (kcal) Scotland	The Netherlands
Fetus	8 330	8 230
Placenta	730	740
Uterus Breasts Blood volume Amniotic fluid Extracellular fluid	3 490	2 950
Maternal fat	26 400	22 000
Basal metabolic rate	30 100	34 700
Total	69 050 (or 290 MJ)	68 620 (or 288 MJ)

laid down during late pregnancy is important in terms of energy, it is probably just as important to ensure that the quality of that fat is appropriate to the fetal needs, particularly in terms of long chain polyunsaturated fatty acids supplying the developing brain *in utero* [7]. The total energy cost of pregnancy found in Scotland and the Netherlands is shown in Table 81.2 [8]. The total extra energy need for pregnancy in these healthy women was 69 000 kcal (290 MJ). Current recommendations, that pregnant women should increase their food intake to supply an extra 300 kcal (1.3 MJ) per day made by the US National Research Council [9], 240 kcal (1.0 MJ) per day made by the UK Department of Health and Social Security [10] or 285 kcal (1.2 MJ) per day made by FAO/WHO/UNU [11] are unrealistic for a population of healthy women living in a developed society without the need for constant strenuous activity throughout pregnancy. An extra 100 kcal (0.4 MJ) per day during the second and third trimester would appear to be adequate.

(b) Variations in individual nutrient intake

Increased carbohydrate consumption during pregnancy can increase prenatal and postnatal growth and might account for some of the increased fetal and infant growth rates observed over the past two generations [12]. A randomized controlled trial of the effect of fish oil supplementation from week 30 of pregnancy in healthy Danish women showed that pregnancies in the fish oil group were on average 4 days longer than the control olive oil group and the infants weighed 100 grams more [13]. Whether the increased weight of the infants was due to the increased energy supplied, to long chain ω-3 fatty acid effects or to fat-soluble

vitamins in the fish oil is unknown, and whether the supplements enhanced or damaged the longer-term health prospects of the infants is also unknown. In many reports from developing countries nutrional supplements have been shown to improve the reproductive ability of women and to increase the birth weight of their infants [14,15]. Aspects of the environment of disadvantaged women known to affect pregnancy outcome include poverty, bad climatic conditions, inadequate housing, increased smoking, increased alcohol and other drugs intake, poor education, poor availability or uptake of medical provision as well as inadequate nutrition. That dietary supplements can improve pregnancy outcome without any change in the other negative factors indicates that poor nutrition is a significant correctable factor.

Apart from low birth weight and preterm onset of labour, other potential indices of poor maternal nutrition are higher rates of congenital malformations. Congenital malformations have been associated with folate deficiency, zinc deficiency and alcohol ingestion. There are several possible mechanisms whereby nutrient deficiencies and excesses can inhibit embryonic and fetal organ development. There is evidence that folate and zinc deficiency, together with alcohol excess, influence the closure of the neural tube in the early weeks of pregnancy [16–18]. A recent UK Medical Research Council study [19] has shown that folic acid suplementation will significantly reduce the risk of neural tube defect. There are a number of nutrients which have a role in gene expression, either directly on nucleoprotein enzyme systems where zinc is a major cofactor or through the antioxidant effects of vitamin C. Dietary fatty acids, vitamin E, selenium and copper can also alter antioxidant activities in tissues. Abnormalities in embryos can be caused by maternal ingestion of excessive quantities of vitamins A, D and K. The molecular structure and function of cell receptors and nucleotide regulatory proteins (e.g. G (guanosine) protein) are also likely to be disordered by nutritional factors. Cellular dysfunction induced by nutrient deficiencies and excesses might result in a reduction of final organ size and structure (e.g. small hypoplastic kidney, reduced brain size, abnormal liver or brain structure or even frank malformation such as congenital heart disease). The effects of nutritional stress depend on the stage of development of the individual organ or tissue at the time of stress. The brain has two peak periods of growth. The first, in early pregnancy, peaks at around 15 weeks' gestation and is almost entirely due to neuroblast division to form the neurons which migrate to the cerebral cortex. From about 30 weeks of gestational age through to 100 weeks of postnatal age there is further cell division but this is mainly in glial cells. The peak of the second phase of cellular proliferation is in the first month after birth.

Malnutrition and undernutrition may predispose the developing embryo to insults from teratogens and infections. The association of vitamin B deficiency and alcohol-induced abnormalities is a possible example. Contamination of food with agrochemicals, insecticides and possibly from aflatoxins produced from fungal food damage during storage might also induce embryonic maldevelopments.

Evolutionary processes have produced a robust system for ensuring species survival in the human so that a wide range of maternal nutrition can allow birth and survival of the human infant, who may grow to maturity and in turn achieve reproduction. However, this may be at the cost of increased morbidity and decreased life span for the growth-retarded and preterm low-birth-weight infant. David Barker and his colleagues in the MRC Environmental Epidemiology Unit [20–24] have shown that infants of low birth weight and poor infant growth have a greater risk of ischaemic heart disease, chronic bronchitis, hypertension, stroke and non-insulin-dependent diabetes.

81.2.2 MATERNAL METABOLIC DISORDER

Major cardiac abnormalities, hepatic failure, severe gastrointestinal disease, renal failure and respiratory failure may all have adverse effects on the developing embryo and fetus. Cardiac lesions that produce right-to-left shunts are the most dangerous for fetus and mother. Because systemic pressure drops during pregnancy and fluctuates widely during labour and delivery, the risk of increased shunting is high. Increasing numbers of women born with congenital heart disease are reaching childbearing age. Many of these conditions have been corrected in childhood and carry an increased risk of maternal morbidity and mortality during pregnancy. Some cardiac anomalies, such as idiopathic hypertrophic subaortic stenosis are transmitted as an autosomal dominant trait and the infant has a 50% chance of developing the same abnormality [25]. Eclampsia and pre-eclampsia are important causes of fetal and neonatal morbidity and mortality. The intrauterine growth retardation which occurs in the moderate to severe cases of pre-eclampsia appear related to chronic hypoxia, blood hyperviscosity and hypoglycaemia associated with decreased glycogen stores and an inability to mobilize glucose.

(a) Endocrine disorders

The deleterious effects of maternal diabetes mellitus on the outcome for the fetus have long been recognized. The general insulin resistance of pregnancy makes hyperglycaemia in women with true diabetes mellitus difficult to control, particularly after the first trimester.

Ketoacidosis may develop more rapidly and occur at relatively low blood glucose values. Severe maternal ketoacidosis can have disastrous effects on the fetus, with a mortality rate of around 50%. Fetal overgrowth due to maternal hyperglycaemia–fetal hyperglycaemia and secondary fetal hyperinsulinaemia is the consequence of the metabolic effects of the fetal insulin. Insulin is the major growth-promoting hormone of the fetus; it is responsible for increased protein synthesis, growth, and the deposition of glycogen and fat [26]. Although macrosomia is most marked in infants born to women with poor diabetic control, some infants have exposure to excess insulin due to the transplacental passage of insulin–anti insulin antibody complex [27,28]. Macrosomic infants have organomegaly, particularly involving the liver, adrenal glands and heart, although brain growth is not excessive. Infants with marked cardiomegaly may have hypertrophic cardiomyopathy with congestive heart failure. Cardiomegaly related to macrosomia of the infant of the diabetic mother usually resolves by the age of 6 weeks. The major metabolic problem of the infant is hypoglycaemia between 1 and 5 hours after birth. The infants do not appear to produce sufficient catecholamine and glucagon to compensate for the hypoglycaemia. Early infant feeding is usually sufficient to maintain plasma glucose concentrations, although occasionally infusions of 10% dextrose may be required. There would appear to be a delay in fetal lung maturation but with good medical and obstetric management more pregnancies are continuing to term and the incidence of respiratory distress syndrome is now much less than in earlier times. Many infants of diabetic mothers have transient difficulties in clearing pulmonary fluid (wet lung). Congenital abnormalities of the heart and vertebrae (caudal regression syndrome) as well as central nervous system defects, such as holoprosencephaly, anencephaly and meningomyelocele, can occur. The Atlanta birth defects case control study found the relative risks for major malformations among infants of insulin-dependent diabetic mothers to be 7.9%, with a relative risk for major central nervous system and cardiovascular system defects of 15.5 and 18% respectively. There is increasing evidence that the incidence of anomalies is reduced when maternal diabetes is well controlled before conception [29]. The classic description of infants of diabetic mothers was given by Farquhar in Edinburgh [30]. 'These infants are remarkable not only because like fetal versions of Shadrach, Meshach and Abednego they emerged at least alive from within the fiery metabolic furnace of diabetes mellitus, but because they resemble one another so closely that they might be related. They are plump, sleek, liberally covered with vernix caseosa, full-faced and plethoric. The umbilical cord and placenta share in the gigantism.' In addition to the problems of hypoglycaemia the infants may have hypocalcaemia and hypomagnesaemia, and polycythaemia is frequently associated with dehydration.

Hyperthyroidism, which occurs in approximately 0.2% of pregnancies, is most commonly due to Graves' disease but acute thyroiditis, Hashimoto's disease, hydatidiform mole, choriocarcinoma, toxic nodular goitre or toxic adenoma may be the cause. Approximately 1% of infants born to mothers with some degree of thyrotoxicosis will themselves have thyrotoxicosis. The transfer of abnormal thyroid-stimulating immunoglobulins (IgG) across the placenta can result in stillbirth or preterm delivery. Some affected infants have widespread evidence of autoimmune disease, including thrombocytopenic purpura and generalized hypertrophy of lymphatic tissues. Hyperthyroidism can occur shortly after birth and may last from 1 to 5 months.

Maternal hypothyroidism is usually due to chronic lymphocytic thyroiditis and previous treatment for Graves' disease. Pregnancies complicated by untreated hypothyroidism may be associated with increased fetal loss or prolongation of gestation. Treatment of the mother with replacement of thyroid hormone is usually well tolerated and there is some evidence that there is movement of thyroid hormone from the fetus to the mother, decreasing the severity of her disease during pregnancy.

Graves' disease in pregnancy carries risks and the choice lies between antithyroid drugs, with or without thyroid hormone replacement, and subtotal thyroidectomy. Surgery is rarely indicated when medical treatment has failed because too large doses have to be used, the patient is unwilling or unable to comply or toxic reaction to antithyroid drugs occurs. Carbimazole, which acts by blocking thyroid hormone synthesis, together with propranolol for a short time to control the peripheral effects of the disease is the most commonly used combination. Propylthiouracil is an alternative drug to carbimazole. Small doses of thyroxine (0.1–0.2 mg daily) may be used to keep the mother euthyroid. Both drugs can be reduced and usually stopped before delivery as hyperthyroidism generally becomes milder towards the end of pregnancy. The smallest dose necessary to maintain normal maternal concentrations of free thyroxine and thyroid-stimulating hormone is used. Antithyroid drugs cross the placenta and may cause abortion, hypothyroidism and goitre in the fetus. If the euthyroid state has been maintained throughout pregnancy the infant may be expected to be normal. All infants should be examined for hyperthyroidism which, if present, usually remits within 4–6 weeks when maternal immunoglobulins are eliminated. In the presence of severe tachycardia propranolol will control the infant heart rate and prevent heart failure.

(b) Adrenal gland disorder

During pregnancy the two major adrenal cortical steroids, cortisol and aldosterone, are produced in increased quantities by the enlarged maternal adrenal gland from cholesterol, progesterone and 17α-hydroxy progesterone. Aldosterone concentration increases markedly after week 16 of pregnancy, partly in response to an increased plasma renin concentration. Catecholamine production and metabolism remain remarkably unchanged during pregnancy. Disorders of the adrenal cortex in pregnancy are rare and include adrenal failure (Addison's disease) and excessive secretion (Cushing's syndrome). Disorders of the adrenal medulla include excessive catecholamine secretion from a phaeochromocytoma. Cushing's syndrome resulting from adenoma or carcinoma of the adrenal cortex or bilateral adrenal hyperplasia with an adrenocorticotrophin-secreting pituitary tumour is rarely compatible with pregnancy. Successful management with metyrapone, a drug inhibiting adrenal cortisol production, has been achieved in a pregnancy associated with an active adrenal adenoma [31]. Children successfully treated for congenital virilizing adrenal hyperplasia are surviving in increasing numbers and those with 21-hydroxylase and 11-hydroxylase deficiencies have been reported to have given birth to normal infants. Mothers with congenital adrenal hypoplasia have a one in four risk of passing the condition on to the fetus but prenatal diagnosis through measurement of 17-hydroxyprogesterone in amniotic fluid allows prenatal diagnosis and early infant treatment. Pregnancy is rare in the untreated Addison's disease state. Most treated cases are due to autoimmune disease and pregnancy does not carry a significant risk to mother or fetus as long as replacement therapy with hydrocortisone and fludrocortisone is maintained. Phaeochromocytoma may develop or become active during pregnancy, when it carries a high risk for both mother and fetus [32]. Treatment of prolonged episodes of hypertension requires initial alpha blockade with phentolamine followed by beta blockade and surgical removal, which can be performed safely during pregnancy.

Functioning and non-functioning adenomas and deficiency of one or more pituitary trophic hormones may rarely be encountered during pregnancy. The prolactin-secreting adenomas, particularly microadenomas, have been successfully treated with bromocriptine with no obvious problems with pregnancy or with congenital abnormality [33].

(c) Enzyme abnormalities

It has been postulated that deficient alcohol dehydrogenase activity may predispose some women to develop fetal alcohol syndrome and fetal alcohol effects at relatively low alcohol intakes [34].

Phenylketonuria is one of the more common inherited metabolic diseases which, if not effectively managed during pregnancy, can result in severe fetal problems. Dr Charles E. Dent in 1956 reported the chance observation made by a Dr Richards that a mentally handicapped phenylketonuric mother had three children whose fathers were presumed to be different. All three children had gross mental handicap from birth and Dr Dent felt that the mental handicap in the children might well have been the result of the toxicity of the mother's high blood phenylalanine concentrations on the developing brain *in utero* [35]. Since that time there have been many reports of fetal abnormalities associated with uncontrolled or poorly controlled maternal phenylketonuria (PKU) [36–40]. Abnormalities reported in children with mothers whose intrapartum plasma phenylalanine concentration exceeded 1.2 mmol/l (PKU phenotype) include mental handicap (92%), microcephaly (72%), intrauterine growth delay (40%) and congenital heart malformation (12%). Thankfully there is now sufficient evidence to show that the incidence of such abnormalities can be reduced, given that the mother has appropriate dietary management to ensure 'safe' maternal plasma phenylalanine and tyrosine concentrations from before the time of conception and throughout pregnancy [39–45]. Good longitudinal data on plasma amino acid concentrations in ovulating women and in pregnant women are not available. Thomson and his colleagues [46] quote 'a therapeutic control range for phenylalanine of between 50 and 150 μmol/l and for tyrosine 60 and 90 μmol/l'. There is some evidence which suggests that fetal liver phenylalanine hydroxylase activity is sufficiently developed by 20 weeks to begin to influence the rate of utilization of phenylalanine by the fetus. The mother's phenylalanine requirements increase from about 20 weeks' gestation to meet the increasing demands of the fetus and additional tyrosine may require to be supplied in order to meet the maternal and fetal demand, particularly during the first trimester. Phenylalanine and tyrosine cross the placenta by an active transport process which results in higher plasma water concentrations of phenylalanine in the embryo and fetus than in the mother. The ratio of fetal to maternal plasma water amino acid concentrations vary throughout pregnancy, with a tendency to higher ratios in the earlier months [47]. The observed ratio of fetal to maternal plasma phenylalanine is 1.48, with a range of 1.13–2.19 and for plasma tyrosine 1.93 with a range of 1.32–2.53 [47–49]. Deficiencies and excesses of maternal dietary phenylalanine and tyrosine are very promptly manifest in placental tissue and fetal plasma phenylalanine and tyrosine concentrations. These concentrations of phenylalanine and tyrosine in fetal plasma are reflected in cerebrospinal fluid (CSF) and presumably in brain tissue. For example, when the plasma phenylalanine in a 16-week fetus was 1150 μmol/l the CSF values were 425 μmol/l. Control 16-week fetal values were 102 μmol/l in the plasma and 23 μmol/l in the CSF. Values of 278 μmol/l for plasma tyrosine were reflected in the CSF at 106 μmol/l. In a control 16-week fetus the CSF tyrosine concentration was 19 μmol/l when the plasma tyrosine concentration was 95 μmol/l [48]. In untreated maternal phenylketonuria there is a very high phenylalanine to tyrosine ratio. This disturbed ratio could affect neurological development and neurotransmitter synthesis, which in turn could adversely affect developing embryonic organs, including the heart. There is competition across the placental and blood–brain barrier for amino acid transport systems, and disturbances of phenylalanine and tyrosine could inhibit or enhance uptake of other amino acids or other essential nutrients [49]. There is some evidence that tyrosine deficiency may not cause maternal phenylketonuria syndrome in the rat [50]. There are undoubtedly detrimental effects of the hyperphenylalaninaemia, and possibly hypotyrosinaemia, on embryogenesis and fetal development [51]. The embryopathy affects predominantly the face and heart, producing a range of defects, and in brain there are neuronal loss, immature cortical pyramidal cell bodies and dendritic spines [52]. In addition to the dangers to the embryo and fetus there are, in the uncontrolled women, problems of relative infertility, an increased rate of spontaneous abortion and a high incidence of pregnancy termination. For those mothers who conceive while plasma phenylalanine concentrations are 900 μmol/l or above, pregnancy termination should be offered because of the high risk of malformations. Even below this concentration hyperphenylalaninaemia poses some risk to brain growth and intellectual development so that the offer of detailed fetal ultrasound assessment and possible termination should extend to patients with phenylalanine concentrations of 700 μmol or more. Phenylalanine concentrations in pregnancy need to be very strictly controlled. Biochemical monitoring should be undertaken at least twice a week, both in the period before conception and during pregnancy, aiming at values of 60–250 μmol/l. Effective contraception should be continued until control has been achieved. Pregnancies require careful monitoring, using ultrasound to assess fetal growth and anatomy so that any fetal abnormalities can be identified as early as possible [53].

(d) Other inherited metabolic disorders

Disorders in which pregnancy outcome has been reported include cystic fibrosis, histidinaemia, Hartnup's disorder, homocystinuria, lysinuric protein intolerance, isovaleric acidaemia, galactosaemia and phenyl-ketonuria.

In cystic fibrosis there are problems of infertility in both females and males but no evidence of embryopathy or fetal disorder, given an adequate maternal nutritional status during pregnancy [54].

Maternal histidinaemia is probably benign to the fetus. At least 53 children from 21 histidinaemic mothers, most of whom were normal, have been reported [55].

At least 14 children of women with Hartnup's disease are known and all are normal [56].

Homocystinuria comprises a group of autosomal recessive disorders in which there are increased concentrations of homocystine and methionine in blood and urine, with physical features including mental handicap, epilepsy, ectopia lentis, osteoporosis, skeletal anomalies, fatty liver and thrombotic vascular disease. There may be deficiency of the enzyme cystathionine synthetase and in some instances this disorder is pyridoxine responsive [57]. Pregnancies with normal outcome have been reported in both pyridoxine responsive and non-responsive mothers [58–60]. In the pyridoxine non-responsive mother strict dietary control is maintained to reduce the risk of maternal vascular complications associated with platelet abnormalities and thrombosis.

Lysinuric protein intolerance is a rare condition and seven pregnancies have been reported in four women [61]. Treatment instituted before conception involves protein restriction and L-citrulline supplements of between 3 and 5 g/day.

Maternal isovaleric acidaemia has been reported, with little difficulty during the pregnancy and no ill effect on the offspring [62]. Treatment is with protein restriction with additional glycine and carnitine to reduce the risk of attacks of metabolic acidosis during the pregnancy.

One pregnancy in a mother with non-ketotic hyperglycinaemia has been managed by the author, with a normal outcome. Treatment of the mother throughout pregnancy with oral sodium benzoate kept the glycine concentrations at a reasonable level during the pregnancy. It was easier to maintain a low glycine level during the pregnancy than in the prepregnancy phase.

The long-term outcome for patients with galactosaemia is recognized to be unsatisfactory [63,64]. Ovarian dysfunction is an almost universal consequence of the disorder, even in the best controlled women [65]. Part of the explanation for the poor outcome may relate to the endogenous synthesis of galactose by the tissues of the galactosaemic child and part may be due to the fact that even though the heterozygous mother of the affected homozygous infant is given a lactose-free diet, the homozygous galactosaemic fetal tissues will still accumulate galactose and galactitol in utero [66]. There is no apparent advantage in restricting the lactose intake of the heterozygous carrier mother. There are very few reports on the outcome of pregnancy in homozygous galactosaemic mothers [63,67–69]. Reports so far indicate that the outcome for the obligate heterozygote infant is good but that mothers should be discouraged from breastfeeding because of the risk of autointoxication with galactose-1-phosphate and galactitol produced in her breast tissue as a by-product of lactose biosynthesis [70].

81.2.3 MATERNAL TOXINS (Chapters 6, 23 and 24)

Since the first edition of this book was published there has been a dramatic increase in the number of women of childbearing age who use legal and illegal substances that have adverse affects on fetal metabolism and development. In New York City the proportion of women in the known addicted population rose from 14% in 1968 to 25% in 1973 and is now estimated to be 40% [71]. In the USA women make up approximately 30% of the drug treatment admissions and 25% of the alcohol treatment admissions. In addition to the side-effects produced by alcohol, nicotine and prescription drugs (Table 81.3), there are major problems now arising from the abuse of amphetamine, heroin and cocaine. A survey conducted by the National Association for Perinatal Addiction Research and Education found a consistent 11% incidence of documented illicit drug use during pregnancy in 36 urban, suburban and rural hospitals examined [72]. With the emergence of cocaine, especially in its 'crack' or smoked form, amounting to a new cocaine epidemic, there has been an alarming increase in the incidence of fetal exposure to this drug. Studies in the USA indicate that 10–15% of major urban area newborn births are affected by cocaine use [73–74]. The same pattern of maternal cocaine use is spreading throughout major cities in northern Europe. A majority of women who use cocaine during pregnancy are 'polydrug' users and take alcohol, marijuana and heroin in addition to the cocaine [75]. Cocaine's low molecular weight and high water and lipid solubility allow it to cross placental and fetal blood–brain membrane barriers readily to enter the fetal central nervous system. It acts by inhibiting active reuptake of catecholamine and serotonin, produces vasoconstriction and tachycardia as well as blocking nerve conduction. Animal studies show that a pattern of congenital defects can be regularly produced and are similar to those found among infants born to mothers using cocaine during pregnancy [76]. The types of defects which have been found in animals and in humans may well result from vascular effects, with limb defects and genitourinary malformations [77–79]. In practice it is always difficult to differentiate malformations due to cocaine and the other drugs, particularly alcohol, which these women regularly ingest.

Table 81.3   Effects of drugs taken by the mother on the embryo and fetus *in utero*

Drug/agent	Organs affected
Alcohol	Eyes, cranium, face, skeleton, brain; stunted
Aminopterin	Cranium, face, skin, ears; death
Amphetamines	Heart, lip, skeleton, urogenital
Anaesthetics	Skeletal and face suggested – very rare: affects theatre staff
Androgens and synthetic progestogens	Masculinized females
Antiemetics	All probably harmless save diphenhydramine
Antithyroid drugs	Thyroid, brain
Atropine	Tachycardia
Aspirin	Probably nil
Beta-blockers	Diminished adaptive response to asphyxia
Busulphan	Eyes, palate; stunted
Chlorambucil	Urogenital
Chloroquine	Deafness and choriodoretinitis possible
Cigarette smoking	Reduced birth weight
Corticosteroids	Probably nil
Cyclophosphamide	Palate
Diazepam	Cleft lip and palate possible + respiratory depression
Diethylstilboestrol	In first trimester predisposes to vaginal carcinoma and adenosis (after 15 years)
Diuretics	Reduced birth weight
Folic acid deficiency	Brain, neural tube
Hydralazine	Hypotension
Iodine excess or deficiency	Goitre, hypothyroidism, brain
Lithium	Heart, great vessels
Methotrexate	Skeletal
Paramethadione	Heart, palate, face, brain
Phenytoin and barbiturates	Lips, skull, skeleton, ear, heart
Progestogens	Virilization
Quinine	Hypoplasia of optic nerve; deafness in high doses
Radiation	Neural tube, skeleton; microcephaly
Ritodrine	Hypoglycaemia
Streptomycin	Deafness
Tetracycline	Teeth discoloured and enamel hypoplasia
Thalidomide	Skeleton, heart, ears, eyes
Troxidone (trimethadione)	Heart, palate, face, brain
Vitamin A deficiency	Brain, eyes, palate, skeleton
Vitamin D excess	Infantile hypercalcaemia possible
Valproate	Face and neural tube
Warfarin	Nose, skeleton, eyes, brain; nasal hypoplasia, chondrodysplasia punctata in first trimester, optic atrophy, microcephaly, mental handicap in second and third trimester

It seems that cocaine is a relatively weak teratogen but there is evidence that there is impaired body growth with decreased head circumference and subsequent learning difficulties. In the immediate postnatal period the infants show many of the same behavioural differences observed in alcohol and marijuana exposed infants. These features include an inability to co-ordinate feeding reflexes and the infants therefore feed poorly and develop coarse features. There have been many published studies investigating the neuro-behavioural sequelae of cocaine-exposed infants during the first month of life but it is difficult to draw specific conclusions from these neonatal studies. In one study, with a sample adequate to control for other drug use, neonatal complications and observer variations, cocaine was found to have independent effects on infant motor behaviour, state regulation and abnormal reflexes at 28 days [80]. There are may variables involved in infants born to drug-abusing mothers, including premature delivery, intrauterine growth re-tardation and exposure to many drugs. However, it seems likely that just as most children exposed to alcohol during gestation do not develop fetal alcohol syndrome but develop educational difficulties and short

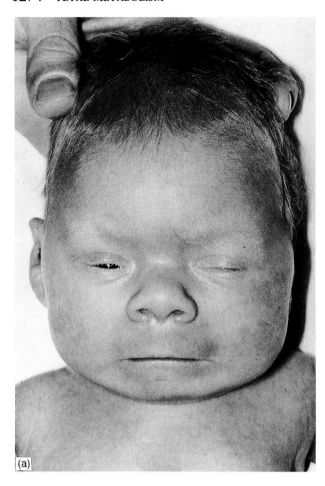

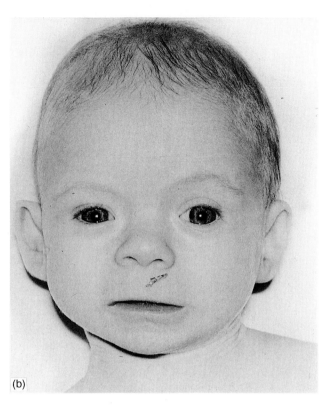

Figure 81.1 (a,b) The appearance of an infant affected by the fetal alcohol syndrome.

attention span. There seems to be a similar relationship between fetal cocaine exposure and long-term behavioural problems. Some cocaine-exposed infants under certain conditions, such as prenatal maternal drug treatment and intensive infant intervention, function within normal developmental limits within the first 3 years of life [81]. Figure 81.1 shows the appearance of an infant affected by the fetal alcohol syndrome. Similar facial features may appear in infants born to mothers with phenylketonuria and with a history of multiple substance abuse.

Amphetamines, like cocaine, are psychomotor stimulants, previously used primarily by those involved in sports and entertainment to enhance performance. They also potentiate the action of noradrenaline, dopamine and serotonin but unlike cocaine they appear to exert their central nervous system effects primarily by enhancing the release of neurotransmitters from presynaptic neurons. They may also stimulate postsynaptic catecholamine receptors. Cardiovascular malformations have been described [82]. The children can subsequently exhibit disturbed behaviour, including hyperactivity, aggressiveness and sleep disturbances [83].

Narcotic derivatives of opium, including morphine, meperidine, heroin, methadone and codeine, have been used as analgesics for centuries. During this last decade specific opiate receptors have been identified in the brain for associated opiate-like substances: the endorphins and enkephalins [84,85]. Heroin is the most extensively used derivative during pregnancy and it can have potentially devastating effects on the outcome of pregnancy. These are associated mainly with the intravenous injection of heroin, although it can be ingested by smoking or by the intranasal route. Intravenous use may result in septicaemia, thrombophlebitis, hepatitis, AIDS and endocarditis. The high rate of preterm and low-birth-weight delivery is likely to be multifactorial, related to the malnutrition, anaemia and other results of the heroin addiction in the mother. Once diagnosed in pregnancy most women are treated with methadone maintenance until the end of the pregnancy. This can improve the fetal outcome. However, methadone-dependent mothers who have inadequate prenatal care have many of the same problems seen in heroin addicted mothers [86]. Head circumference and growth of infants born to heroin and methadone-dependent women are smaller than those infants born to socioeconomically comparable drug-free women. Long-term follow-up studies of narcotic-exposed infants show significant developmental and learning deficits in both methadone and heroin-exposed children [87].

The effects on the fetus of maternal ingestion of alcohol were first described in Europe by Lemoine *et al.* in 1968 [88]. Many studies throughout the world have now revealed a consistent picture of prenatal and postnatal growth deficiency with microcephaly, mental handicap and characteristic facies. The microcephaly is secondary to the disordered brain development resulting from alcohol exposure. The typical facial features consist of short palpable fissures, flat nasal bridge, micrognathia, hypoplastic maxilla and thin upper lip [89]. Speech, language and behavioural problems, including severe hyperactivity and attention deficit disorders, contribute to the learning disabilities characteristically found in these children. Fetal alcohol syndrome is estimated to occur in 30–40% of pregnant women consuming 3 oz (85 ml) of absolute alcohol per day. Lesser degrees of alcohol consumption are associated with intrauterine growth retardation and learning difficulties. During the neonatal period the infant may show jitteriness and poor feeding similar to those features found with misuse of other substances. The term 'alcohol-related birth defects' is now used to reflect the range of anomalies associated with alcohol consumption during pregnancy.

In North America and the UK it is estimated that about 25% of pregnant women smoke cigarettes during pregnancy. The effect of cigarette smoking on fetal growth has revealed that intrauterine growth retardation is correlated with the number of cigarettes smoked. One pack (20 cigarettes) per day correlates with a 280-g weight loss in a term newborn.

Many women who misuse drugs and other substances have high-risk behaviour which puts the fetus at risk of intrauterine infection and premature delivery. As well as the high incidence of disorders related to intrauterine growth retardation and infection the infants are at high risk for subsequent physical abuse and neglect.

81.3 Fetoplacental influences

81.3.1 PLACENTAL STRUCTURE AND FUNCTION

The haemochorial placenta and fetus abstract from the mother the necessary materials required for the cellular growth of the fetoplacental unit. Throughout pregnancy there is an ever-increasing demand of this unit for fuel and this demand is met through increased maternal caloric intake, hyperinsulinaemia, insulin resistance and maternal pancreatic islet cell hypertrophy. In young mothers not yet fully grown there is competition between the growth requirements of maternal tissues and those of the fetoplacental unit. It

appears from animal studies that the needs of the developing young woman probably take precedence over the needs of her developing embryo and fetus. The production of pregnancy-related hormones begins with the implantation of trophoblast and these hormones immediately alter the metabolism of nutrients, in particular glucose, to shift the priority of metabolic products towards the growing fetus, given that the mother is fully developed. Maternal glucose homoeostasis through these maternal hormones is designed to increased maternal fat storage, decrease energy expenditure and delay glucose clearance. Fetal hormones from the conceptus can affect metabolic processes, uteroplacental blood flow and cellular differentiations. Glucose crosses the placenta by carrier-mediated facilitated diffusion and the uterus and placenta use a considerable amount of glucose. In contrast, amino acids are actively transported to the fetus [91]. Free fatty acids cross the placenta in small amounts by gradient-dependent diffusion and are esterified to triglyceride by fetal adipocytes. There is little evidence for selective transfer of different fatty acids and net transfer from mother to fetus is predominantly determined by the free fatty acid concentrations in maternal plasma [92]. The growing fetus accumulates inorganic ions such as potassium, calcium, sodium and chloride in large amounts but neither the route nor the mechanisms of ion transport across the placental trophoblast are fully understood. It is not clear how far the net transport of ions can be accounted for by aqueous diffusion via an extracellular route in response to electrochemical driving forces [93] or how much the transcellular route involving ion transporters and channels is involved [94,95].

The changes in carbohydrate metabolism of the mother and fetus are brought about by the diabetogenic hormones: oestrogen, prolactin, human chorionic somatomammotrophin, cortisol and progesterone.

Although glucose is the primary source of energy for the fetus, protein accretion is an essential component for fetal growth and the synthesis of new fetal and placental tissue. Direct and indirect chemical analysis of fetal and maternal tissue in the human suggests that the total protein cost of pregnancy is approximately 925 g, or 128 g nitrogen [96]. Nitrogen balance studies have shown that nitrogen retention is in excess of the theoretical protein cost [97]. Maternal plasma water amino acid concentrations are low in early pregnancy compared with the non-pregnant state [98,99]. This early gestation hypoaminoacidaemia is not simply due to maternal volume expansion but is possibly related to progesterone and placental lactogen effects [100,101]. Light-for-date infants born to mothers with preeclampsia and heavy-for-date infants born to mothers with diabetes mellitus have alterations in the gradients of amino acids between the maternal plasma water and fetal plasma water [102]. Maternal plasma amino acid concentrations in the pre-eclamptic mothers tend to go towards non-pregnant values, whilst in diabetic pregnancies the effect of fetal hyperinsulinaemia may 'drive' amino acids from placental tissue into fetal cells. These studies suggest that the homoeostatic changes in maternal amino acids may have important influences on both maternal metabolism and on fetal growth and body weight.

In late gestation, studies in human pregnancy suggest a maternal adaptive response to conserve nitrogen, as evidenced by a decrease in urea excretion. The available data also suggest that there is decreased ureagenesis, possibly as a result of decreased hepatic uptake of amino acids. Whole body protein turnover studies during pregnancy are difficult to conduct and the results difficult to interpret [103,104].

There are no direct quantitive measurements of fetal protein turnover in man. Data for the preterm and term human infant, however, do indicate a higher rate of protein turnover in the fetus than in the adult [105,106].

In 1847, Virchow reported lipaemia during pregnancy [107]. The maternal fats store and circulating fat is derived from exogenous or dietary sources as well as endogenous synthesis. The two essential fatty acids (linoleic acid ($C_{18:2}$,ω-6) and α-linolenic acid ($C_{18:3}$,ω-3)) must be provided from the diet or mobilized from the triglyceride stores or phospholipid membrane. The ω-6 series can be converted in the adult to arachidonic acid (AA – $C_{20:4}$,ω-6) and the α-linolenic acid to docosahexaenoic acid (DHA – $C_{22:6}$,ω-3). There is some uncertainty about the ability of placental trophoblast to elongate and desaturate the essential fatty acids into the long chain polyunsaturated fatty acids AA and DHA. Even the term human newborn infant seems unable to synthesize DHA from the essential fatty acid precursor α-linolenic acid. The ω-6 series fatty acids become precursors for prostaglandin and leukotriene metabolism, whereas the ω-3 series are converted to prostaglandins which may have competitive or alternative effects as well as being essential constituents of the phospholipids in neuronal synaptosomes and photoreceptors. The mother is capable of synthesizing all other fats, including cholesterol and fatty acids of varied lengths and saturations, that are required for normal physiological functions by the placenta and fetus. A recycling system exists in the body for delivering cholesterol and fatty acids, the two main fats of the body, to sites where they are required for new cell synthesis, energy provision and a host of metabolic signalling processes involving phospholipids, prostaglandins and their metabolites. This system is mediated by lipoproteins. Little is known about the kinetics of lipoprotein metabolism in pregnancy. There are increased very-low-density lipoprotein (VLDL) triglyceride concentrations in mid and late gestation and it

may be that low-density lipoprotein (LDL) cholesterol clearance is enhanced in pregnancy, but this is still a matter of debate. Plasma triglyceride concentration is significantly positively associated with plasma oestriol concentrations and VLDL triglyceride correlates positively with insulin. LDL cholesterol is negatively associated with progesterone concentration and high-density lipoprotein (HDL) cholesterol is positively associated with both oestradiol and progesterone concentrations [108]. The fetus probably does not use fatty acids for oxidation but does use them for new tissue growth and for storage in subcutaneous adipocyte triglyceride. Phospholipids do not cross the placenta but they can be hydrolysed into their constituent parts and transferred to the fetus for reassembly [109].

When lipid disorders occur during pregnancy they may result in severe hypertriglyceridaemia and this can cause severe haemorrhagic pancreatitis in the pregnant woman. The disorder is usually associated with a deficiency of LDL [110]. Low-fat diet for the mother, together with enriched fatty acids (fish oil), can reduce plasma triglyceride concentrations in this condition [111]. Hypercholesterolaemia in the mother has no known deleterious effect on the fetus but it would be reasonable to implement dietary management in the mother without the introduction of lipid-lowering drugs as these could potentially inhibit fetal growth and development. At term newborn subcutaneous fat triglyceride contains virtually no essential fatty acid. There are small quantities of DHA and AA available for new tissue synthesis but this supply would be quickly depleted unless replaced in the diet. Unfortunately many currently available infant formulae contain inadequate amounts of precursor essential fatty acid (linolenic acid) and little or no DHA. The effect of this is a reduction in DHA in the synaptosomes of the cerebral cortex of artificially fed infants, with an excess of the ω-6 series of fatty acids, particularly docosapentaenoic (reference 112 and J. Farquharson et al., unpublished data). There is some evidence that in the preterm, low-birth-weight infant there are differences in umbilical vascular endothelium in relation to maternal dietary intake of essential fatty acids [7,113].

Fetal concentrations of fat-soluble vitamins A (retinol), D (cholecalciferol), E (tocopherol) and K (phylloquinone and menaquinone) are not as great as in the mother. Water-soluble vitamins B and C transfer readily from mother to fetus so that at term fetal tissue concentrations of these vitamins exceed maternal concentrations.

During this past decade the fetus has been revealed in more and more detail and studies of metabolic processes in vivo are beginning to be derived. Many new fetal and placental growth factors, such as epidermal, neuronal and insulin-like growth factors, together with their carrier proteins and cell surface receptors, have been identified and their functions studied [114]. The foundation for the 'new' science of fetal medicine is now being rapidly developed, and improved understanding of fetal metabolic processes should allow us to understand the pathogenesis of adult diseases better, and hopefully prevent them.

81.3.2 FETAL ENZYME DEFECTS

Prenatal diagnosis of enzyme defects by chorionic villus sampling, early amniocentesis and improved DNA analysis and diagnosis of genetic errors in preimplantation embryos has increased enormously in recent years. It is now possible to investigate the molecular basis of over 250 different genetic diseases using recombinant DNA techniques, as well as providing a reliable prenatal diagnosis for the first time in some cases. However, DNA methods have confirmed the enormous heterogeneity of diseases such as phenylketonuria and cystic fibrosis. About 20 lysosomal enzymes have now been cloned and molecular genetic cell analysis has similarly revealed tremendous heterogeneity in the different lysosomal storage diseases. Therefore it seems that each family or subpopulation will require specific DNA tests for a single or small number of mutations before prenatal fetal diagnosis can be assured. Fetal cells can be isolated from the maternal circulation and presently the technique can be used to determine the presence of a Y chromosome in X-linked fetal disorders. Similarly, *in vitro* sexing of preimplantation embryos has reduced the risks to couples of X-linked disorders such as adrenoleucodystrophy by transferring only female embryos. For a small number of enzyme defects treatment *in utero* is an alternative to prenatal diagnosis and pregnancy termination [115]. This treatment may take the form of vitamin supplementation for disorders responsive to co-factors, e.g. cobalamin E disease, or the use of glucocorticoid to suppress adrenal production of androgenic steroids in adrenal hyperplasia due to a deficiency of steroid 21-hydroxylase. First trimester DNA analysis permits initiation of this treatment at about 9–10 weeks before masculinization of genitalia begins [116]. Considerable progress has also been made in clarifying the defects in peroxisomal disorders and in developing methods for prenatal diagnosis in the first trimester [117]. Mitochondrial defects in the fetus can result in severe disturbance of central nervous function and the presence of congenital malformations, including absent corpus callosum and congenital cysts in the fetal brain [118].

Inherited metabolic diseases affecting the fetus and the newborn have become much more important causes of neonatal pathology as advances in obstetric, prenatal and perinatal management have reduced the classical causes of neonatal damage and distress. The incidence of inherited defects is still underestimated as in many instances accurate diagnosis of the underlying defect is not considered and made. Accurate pathological diagnosis is, however, essential if appropriate genetic counselling and prenatal diagnosis of subsequent pregnancies, especially in those conditions where there is a good response to early therapy, are to be made.

References

1. Walter, A. and Hammond, J. (1938) The maternal effects on growth and information in Shire horse–Shetland pony crosses. *Proc. R. Soc. Lond. [Biol.]*, 125, 311–35.
2. Penrose, L.S. (1952) Data on the genetics of birthweight. *Ann. Eugen.*, 16, 378–80.
3. Hytten, F.E. and Pointin, D.B. (1963) Increase in plasma volume during normal pregnancy. *J. Obstet. Gynaecol. Br. Commonw.*, 70, 402–407.
4. Lawrence, M., Lawrence, F., Coward, W.A. *et al.* (1987) Energy requirements of pregnancy in the Gambia. *Lancet.*, ii, 1072–76.
5. Van Raay, J.M.A., Vermatt -Miedema, S.H., Schonk, C.M. *et al.* (1987) Energy requirements of pregnancy in the Netherlands, *Lancet*, ii, 953–55.
6. Durnin, J.V.G.A., McKillop, F.M., Grant, S. *et al.* (1987). Energy requirements of pregnancy in Scotland. *Lancet*, ii, 897–900.
7. Crawford, M.A., Doyle, W., Drury, P. *et al.* (1989) N-6 and n-3 fatty acids during early human development. *J. Intern. Med.*, 225 (suppl. 1), 159–69.
8. Durnin, V.G.A. (1991) Energy metabolism in pregnancy, in *Principles of Perinatal–Neonatal Metabolism* (ed. R.M. Cowett), Springer, New York, pp. 228–36.
9. National Research Council, Food and Nutrition Board (1989), *Recommended Dietary Allowances*, National Academy Press, Washington, DC.
10. Department of Health and Social Security (1979) Recommended daily amounts of food energy and nutrients for groups of people in the United Kingdom. *Report on Health and Social Subjects, Subject No. 15*, HMSO, London.
11. FAO/WHO/UNU (1985) Energy and protein requirements: report of a joint FAO/WHO/UNU Expert Consultation. *WHO Tech. Rep. Ser. 724*, 84–87.
12. Schaefer, O. (1970) Pre- and post-natal growth acceleration and increased sugar consumption in Canadian Eskimos. *Can. Med. Assoc. J.*, 103, 1059–68.
13. Olsen, S., Sorensen, J.D., Secher, N.J. *et al.* (1992) Randomised controlled trial of effect of fish-oil supplementation on pregnancy duration. *Lancet*, 339, 1003–1007.
14. Prentice, A.M., Whitehead, R.G. and Watkinson, M. *et al.* (1983) Prenatal dietary supplementation of African women and birthweight. *Lancet*, i, 489–92.
15. Prentice, A.M., Cole, T.J., Lamb, W.H. and Whitehead, R.J. (1987) Effect of prenatal supplementation on birthweight and subsequent growth of infants. *Am. J. Clin. Nutr.*, 46, 912–25.
16. Smithells, R.W., Shepherd, S. and Schorah, C.J. (1976) Vitamin deficiency and neural tube defects. *Arch. Dis. Child.*, 51, 944–50.
17. Cavdar, O.A., Arcasoy, A., Boycu, T. and Himmetoglu, O. (1980) Zinc deficiency and anencephaly in Turkey. *Teratology*, 22, 141.
18. Jameson, S. (1976) Variations in maternal zinc during pregnancy and correlations with congenital malformations, dysmaturity and abnormal parturition. *Acta Paediatr. Scand. Suppl.*, 593, 21–37.
19. MRC Vitamin Study Research Group (1991) Prevention of neural tube defects: result of the Medical Research Council Vitamin Study. *Lancet*, ii, 131–36.
20. Barker, D.J.P., Winder, P.D., Osmond, C. *et al.* (1989) Weight in infancy and death from ischaemic heart disease. *Lancet*, ii, 577–80.
21. Barker, D.J.P., Bull, A.R., Osmond, C. and Simmonds, S.J. (1990) Fetal and placental size and risk of hypertension in adult life. *BMJ*, 301, 259–62.
22. Barker, D.J.P., Osmond, C., Golding, J. *et al.* (1989) Growth *in utero*, blood pressure in childhood and adult life and mortality from cardiovascular disease. *BMJ*, 298, 564–67.
23. Hales, C.N., Barker, D.J.P., Clark, P.M.S. *et al.* (1991) Fetal and infant growth and impaired glucose tolerance at age 64. *BMJ*, 303, 1019–22.
24. Barker, D.J.P. and Martyn, C.N. (1992) The maternal and fetal origins of cardiovascular disease. *J. Epidemiol. Community Health*, 46, 8–11.
25. Burrow, G.N. and Ferris, T.F. (1988) *Medical Complications During Pregnancy*, 3rd edn, W.B. Saunders, Philadelphia.
26. Pedersen, J. (1954) Weight and length at birth of infants of diabetic mothers. *Acta Endocrinol.*, 16, 330–42.
27. Menon, R.K., Cohen, R.M., Sperling, M.A. *et al.* (1990) Transplacental passage of insulin in pregnant women with insulin-dependent diabetes mellitus. *N. Engl. J. Med.*, 323, 309–10.

28. Schwartz, R. (1990) Hyperinsulinemia and macrosomia. *N. Engl. J. Med.*, 323, 340–42.
29. Kitzmiller, J.L., Gavin, L.A., Gin, D.G. *et al.* (1988) Managing diabetes and pregnancy. *Curr. Probl. Obstet. Gynecol. Fertil.*, 12, 107–17.
30. Farquhar, J.W. (1959) The child of the diabetic woman. *Arch. Dis. Child.*, 34, 76–96.
31. Gormley, M.J., Hadden, D.R., Kennedy, T.L. *et al.* (1982) Cushing's syndrome in pregnancy – treatment with metyrapone. *Clin. Endocrinol.*, 16, 283–93.
32. Shenker, J.G. and Chowers, I. (1971) Pheochromocytoma and pregnancy: review of 89 cases. *Obstet. Gynecol. Surv.*, 26, 739–47.
33. McGregor, A.M. and Ginsberg, J. (1981) Dilemmas in the management of functioning pituitary tumours. *Br. J. Hosp. Med.*, 25, 344–47.
34. Véghelyi, P.V. (1983) Fetal abnormality and maternal alcohol metabolism. *Lancet*, 11, 53–54.
35. Dent, C.E. (1957) *Report of the 23rd Ross Conference*, Ross Laboratories, Columbus, Ohio, pp. 32–33.
36. Lenke, R.R. and Levy, H.L. (1980) Maternal phenylketonuria and hyperphenylalaninemia. An international survey of untreated and treated pregnancies. *N. Engl. J. Med.*, 303, 1202–208.
37. Koch, R., Friedman, E.G., Wenz, E. *et al.* (1986) Maternal phenylketonuria. *J. Inherited Metab. Dis.*, 9 (suppl. 2), 159–68.
38. Platt, L.D., Koch, R., Azen, C. *et al.* (1992) Maternal phenylketonuria collaborative study, obstetric aspects and outcome; the first 6 years. *Am. J. Obstet. Gynecol.*, 166, 1150–62.
39. Drogari, E., Beasley, M., Smith, I. and Lloyd, J.K. (1987) Timing of strict diet in relation to fetal damage in maternal phenylketonuria, *Lancet*, ii, 927–30.
40. Smith, I., Glossop, J. and Beasley, M. (1990) Fetal damage due to maternal phenylketonuria: effects of dietary treatment and maternal phenylalanine concentrations around the time of conception (an interim report from the UK phenylketonuria register). *J. Inherited Metab. Dis.*, 13, 651–57.
41. Nielson, K.B., Wamberg, G. and Weber, J. (1979) Successful outcome of pregnancy in a phenylketonuric woman after low phenylalanine diet introduced before conception. *Lancet*, i, 1245.
42. Tenbrinck, M.S. and Stroud, H.W. (1982) Normal infant born to a mother with phenylketonuria. *JAMA*, 247, 2139–40.
43. Bush, R.T. and Dukes, P.C. (1985) Women with phenylketonuria: successful management of pregnancy and implications. *N. Z. Med. J.*, 98, 181–83.
44. Lynch, B.C., Pitt, D.B., Meddison, T.G. *et al.* (1988) Maternal phenylketonuria: successful outcome in four pregnancies treated prior to conception. *Eur. J. Pediatr.*, 148, 72–75.
45. Clark, B.J. and Cockburn, F. (1991) Management of inborn errors of metabolism during pregnancy. *Acta Paediatr. Scand. Suppl.*, 373, 43–45.
46. Thompson, G.N., Francis, D.E.M., Kirby, D.M. and Compton, R. (1991) Pregnancy in phenylketonuria: dietary treatment aimed at normalising maternal plasma phenylalanine concentration. *Arch. Dis. Child.*, 66, 1346–49.
47. Cockburn, F., Farquhar, J.W., Forfar, J.O. *et al.* (1972) Maternal hyperphenylalaninaemia in the normal and phenylketonuric mother and its influence on maternal plasma and fetal fluid amino acid concentrations. *J. Obstet. Gynaecol. Br. Commonw.*, 79, 698–707.
48. Cockburn, F., Giles, M., Robins, F.P. and Forfar, J.O. (1973) Free amino acid composition of human amniotic fluid at term, *J. Obstet. Gynaecol. Br. Commonw.*, 50, 10–18.
49. Kudo, Y. and Boyd, C.A.R. (1990) Transport of amino acids across the blood–brain barrier: implications for treatment of maternal phenylketonuria. *J. Inherited Metab. Dis.*, 13, 617–26.
50. Lewis, S.A., Lyon, I.C. and Elliott, R.B. (1985) Outcome of pregnancy in the rat with mild hyperphenylalaninaemia: implications for the management of 'human maternal PKU'. *J. Inherited Metab. Dis.*, 8, 113–17.
51. Fisch, R.O., Burke, B., Bass, J. *et al.* (1986) Maternal phenylketonuria – chronology of the detrimental effects in embryogenesis and fetal development: pathological report, survey, clinical application. *Pediatr. Pathol.*, 5, 449–61.
52. Lacey, D.J. and Terplan, K. (1987) Abnormal cerebral cortical neurones in a child with maternal PKU syndrome. *J. Child. Neurol.*, 2, 201.
53. Cockburn, F., Clark, B.J., Byrne, A. *et al.* (1992) Maternal phenylketonuria: diet, dangers and dilemmas. *Int. Pediatr.*, 7, 67–74.
54. Cohen, L.F., di Sant'Agnese, P.A. and Friedlander, J. (1980) Cystic fibrosis and pregnancy. A national study. *Lancet*, ii, 824–44.
55. Levy, H.L. (1989) Disorders of histidine metabolism, in *The Metabolic Basis of Inherited Disease*, 6th edn. (eds C.R. Scriver, A.L. Beaudet, W.S. Sly and D. Valle), McGraw-Hill, New York, pp. 563–76.
56. Levy, H.L. (1989) Hartnup disorder, in *The Metabolic Basis of Inherited Disease*, 6th edn (eds C.R. Scriver, A.L. Beaudet, W.S. Sly and D. Valle), McGraw-Hill, New York, pp. 2515–27.
57. Gaull, G.E., Rassin, D.K. and Struman, J.A. (1968) Pyridoxine dependency in homocystinria (letter). *Lancet*, ii, 1302.
58. Bittle, A.H. and Carson, N.A.J. (1973) Tissue culture techniques as an aid to prenatal diagnosis and genetic counselling in homocystinuria. *J. Med. Genet.*, 10, 120–21.
59. Kurczynski, T.W., Muir, W.A., Fleisher, L.D. *et al.* (1980) Maternal homocystinuria: studies of an untreated mother and fetus. *Arch. Dis. Child.*, 55, 721–23.
60. Rassin, D.K., Fleisher, L.D., Muir, A. *et al.* (1979) Fetal tissue amino acid concentrations in argininosuccinic aciduria and in maternal homocystinuria. *Clin. Chim. Acta.*, 94, 101–108.
61. Simell, O. (1989) Lysinuric protein intolerance, *The Metabolic Basis of Inherited Disease*, 6th edn (eds C.R. Scriver, A.L. Beaudet, W.S. Sly and D. Valle), McGraw-Hill, New York, p. 2500.
62. Shih, V.E., Aubrey, R.H., De Grande, G. *et al.* (1984) Maternal isovaleric acidemia. *J. Pediatr.*, 105, 77–78.
63. Komrower, G.M. (1982) Galactosaemia – thirty years on. The experience of a generation. *J. Inherited Metab. Dis.*, 5 (suppl. 2), 96–104.
64. Waggoner, D.D., Buist, N.R.M. and Donnell, G.N. (1990) Long term prognosis in galactosaemia: results of a survey of 350 cases. *J. Inherited Metab. Dis.*, 13, 802–18.
65. Kaufman, F.R., Kogut, M.D., Donnell, G.N. *et al.* (1981) Hypergonadotrophic hypogonadism in female patients with galactosemia. *N. Engl. J. Med.*, 304, 994–98.
66. Jakobs, C., Kleijer, W.J., Bakker, H.D. *et al.* (1988) Dietary restriction of maternal lactose intake does not prevent accumulation of galactitol in the amniotic fluid of fetuses affected with galactosemia. *Prenat. Diagn.*, 8, 641–45.
67. Roe, T., Hallatt, J., Donnell, G. and Ng, W. (1971) Child bearing by galactosemic women. *J. Pediatr.*, 78, 1026.
68. Tedesco, T.A., Marro, G. and Mellman, W.J. (1972) Normal pregnancy and childbirth in a galactosemic woman. *J. Pediatr.*, 81, 1158.
69. Sardharwalla, I.B., Komrower, G.M. and Schwarz, V. (1980) Pregnancy in classical galactosaemia, in *Inherited Disorders of Carbohydrate Metabolism* (eds D. Burman, J.B. Holton and C.A. Pennock), MTP Press, Lancaster, pp. 125–32.
70. Brivet, M., Raymond, J.P., Konopka, P. *et al.* (1989) Effect of lactation in a mother with galactosemia, *J. Pediatr.*, 115, 280–82.
71. Kestner, E., Frank, B., Marel, R. and Schneldeler, J. (1986) Substance use among females in New York State catching-up with males. *Adv. Alcohol Subst. Abuse*, 5, 29–35.
72. Chasnoff, I.J. (1989) Drug use and women: establishing a standard of care. *Ann. N.Y. Acad. Sci.*, 562, 208–10.
73. Chasnoff, I.J., Landress, H. and Barrett, M. (1990) The prevalence of illicit drug or alcohol use during pregnancy and discrepancies in mandatory reporting in Pinellas County, Florida. *N. Engl. J. Med.*, 322, 1202–206.
74. Gillogley, K., Evans, A., Hansen, R. *et al.* (1990) The perinatal impact of cocaine, amphetamine and opiate use detected by universal intrapartum screening. *Am. J. Obstet. Gynecol.*, 163, 1535–42.
75. Streissguth, A.P., Grant, T.M., Barr, H.M. *et al.* (1991) Cocaine and the use of alcohol and other drugs during pregnancy. *Am. J. Obstet. Gynecol.*, 164, 1239–43.
76. Simmerman, E.F. (1991) Substance abuse in pregnancy: teratogenesis. *Pediatr. Ann.*, 20, 541–47.
77. Bingol, N., Fuchs, M., Diaz, V. *et al.* (1987) Teratogenicity of cocaine in humans. *J. Pediatr.*, 110, 93–96.
78. Chasnoff, I.J., Chisum, G.M. and Kaplan, E.W. (1988) Maternal cocaine use and genitourinary tract malformations. *Perinatology*, 37, 201–204.
79. Little, B.B., Snell, L.M., Klein, B.R. *et al.* (1989) Cocaine abuse during pregnancy: maternal and fetal implications. *Obstet. Gynecol.*, 73, 157–60.
80. Coles, C.D., Platzman, K.A., Smith, I. *et al.* (1991) Effects of cocaine, alcohol and other drugs used in pregnancy on neonatal growth and neuro behavioral status. *Neurotoxicol. Teratol.*, 13, 229–33.
81. Mayes, L.C., Granger, R.H., Bornstein, M.H. *et al.* (1992) The problems of prenatal cocaine exposure. *JAMA*, 267, 406–408.
82. Fein, A.F., Shviro, Y., Manoach, M. and Nebel, L. (1987) Teratogenic effect of D-amphetamine sulfate: histo differentiation and electrocardiogram pattern of mouse embryonic heart. *Teratology*, 35, 27–30.
83. Billings, L., Eriksson, M., Steneroth, G. and Zetterstrom, R. (1985) Preschool children of amphetamine-addicted mothers. 1: Somatic and psychomotor development. *Acta Pediatr. Scand.*, 74, 179–84.
84. Platt, J.J. (1986) *Heroin Addiction: Theory, Research and Treatment*, Robert E, Kriegier, Malabar, FL.
85. Snyder, S.H. (1984) Drug and neurotransmitter receptors in the brain. *Science*, 224, 22–31.
86. Lee, M.I., Stryker, J.C, and Sokol, R.J. (1985) Perinatal care for narcotic-dependent gravidas. *Perinatology/Neonatology*, Nov/Dec., 35.
87. Wilson, G.S., McCreary, R., Kean, J. and Baster, J.C. (1979) The development of pre-school children of heroin-addicted mothers: a controlled study. *Pediatrics*, 63, 135–41.
88. Lemoine, P., Harrousseau, H., Bortequ, J.P. and Menuet, J.C. (1968) Les enfants de parents alcooliques; anomalies observés à propos de 127 cas. *Quest. Med.*, 21, 476–82.
89. Abel, E.A., Jacobson, S. and Sherman, B.T. (1983) *In utero* alcohol exposure; functional and structural brain damage. *Neurobehav. Toxicol. Teratol.*, 5, 363–66.

90. Stern, Z.A. and Susser, M. (1984) Intrauterine growth retardation: epidemiological issues and public health significance. *Semin. Perinatol.*, **8**, 5–14.

91. Battaglia, F.C. (1979) Principal substrates of fetal metabolism: fuel and growth requirements of the ovine fetus. *Ciba Found. Symp.*, **63**, 57–74.

92. Hull, D. and Elphick, M.G. (1979) Evidence for fatty acid transfer across the human placenta. *Ciba Found. Symp.*, **63**, 77–91.

93. Stulc, J. (1989) Extracellular transport pathways in the haemochorial placenta. *Placenta*, **10**, 113–9.

94. Shennan, D.B. and Boyd, C.A.R. (1987) Ion transport by the placenta: a review of membrane transport systems. *Biochim. Biophys. Acta*, **906**, 437–57.

95. Greenwood, S.L. Boyde, R.D. and Sibley, C.P. (1993) Transtrophoblast and microvillus membrane potential difference in mature intermediate human placental villi. *Am. J. Physiol.*, **265**, C460–66.

96. Hytten, F.E. and Leitch, I. (1971) The gross composition of the component of weight gain, in *The Physiology of Human Pregnancy*, 2nd edn, Blackwell Scientific, London, pp. 371–387.

97. King, J.C. (1975) Protein metabolism during pregnancy. *Clin. Perinatol.*, **2**, 243–54.

98. Cockburn, F., Robins, S.P. and Forfar, J.O. (1970) Free amino acid concentrations in fetal fluids. *BMJ*, **iii**, 747–50.

99. Cockburn, F., Giles, M., Robins, S.P. and Forfar, J.O. (1973) Free amino acid composition of human amniotic fluid at term. *J. Obstet. Gynaecol., Br. Commonw.*, **80**, 10–18.

100. Landau, R.L. and Lugibihl, K. (1967) The effect of progesterone on the concentration of plasma amino acids in man. *Metabolism*, **16**, 1114–22.

101. Handwerger, S., Fellows, R.E., Crenshaw, M.C. *et al.* (1976) Ovine placental lactogen; acute effects on intermediary metabolism in pregnant and non pregnant sheep. *J. Endocrinol.*, **69**, 133–37.

102. Cockburn, F., Blagden, A., Michie, E.A. and Forfar, J.O. (1971) The influence of pre-eclampsia and diabetes mellitus on plasma free amino acids in maternal umbilical vein and infant blood. *J. Obstet. Gynaecol. Br. Commonw.*, **78**, 215–31.

103. DeBenoist, B., Jackson, A.A., Hall, J. St. E. *et al.* (1985) Whole body protein turnover in Jamaican women during pregnancy. *Hum. Nutr. Clin. Nutr.*, **39C**, 167–79.

104. Fitch, L. and King, J.C. (1987) Protein turnover and 3 methylhistidine excretion in non pregnant, pregnant and gestational diabetic women. *Hum. Nutr. Clin. Nutr.*, **41C**, 327–39.

105. Meier, P.R., Peterson, R.G., Bonds, D.R. *et al.* (1981) Rates of protein synthesis and turnover in fetal life. *Am. J. Physiol.*, **240**, E320–24.

106. Pencharz, P.B. (1988) The 1987 Borden Award Lecturer: Protein metabolism in premature human infants. *Can. J. Physiol. Pharmacol.*, **66**, 1247–52.

107. Virchow, R. (1847) Zur Entwicklungsgeschichte des Krebses: Bemerkungen ubër Fettbildung im thierischen Körper und pathologische Resorption. *Virchows Arch* [A], 1, 94.

108. Knopp, R.H., Warth, M.R., Charles, D. *et al.* (1986) Lipoprotein metabolism in pregnancy, fat transport to the fetus and the effects of diabetes. *Biol. Neonate*, 31, 913–21.

109. Biezenski, J.J., Carrozza, J. and Li, J. (1971) Role of placenta in fetal lipid metabolism III. Formation of rabbit plasma phospholipids. *Biochim. Biophys. Acta*, **239**, 92–97.

110. Knopp, R.H. (1984) Physiological and clinical significance of hyperlipidemia in pregnancy. *Perspect. Lipid Disord.*, 2, 12–16.

111. Knopp, R.H. (1988) What's new in the nutritional management of hyperlipidemia? in *Programme of the American Dietetic Association Annual Meeting*, San Francisco, p. 14.

112. Farquharson, J., Cockburn, F., Patrick, W.A. *et al.* (1992) Infant cerebral cortex phospholipid fatty acid composition and diet. *Lancet*, **340**, 810–13.

113. Leaf, A.A., Leighfield, M.J., Costeloe, K. and Crawford, M.A. (1992) Factors affecting long chain fatty acid composition of plasma choline phosphoglycerides in preterm infants. *J. Pediatr. Gastroenterol. Nutr.*, **14**, 300–308.

114. Wang, H.S. and Chard, T. (1992) The role of insulin-like growth factor-I and insulin-like growth factor-binding protein-1 in the control of human fetal growth. *J. Endocrinol.*, **132**, 11–19.

115. Schulman, J.D. (1990) Treatment of the embryo and the fetus in the first trimester. *Am. J. Med. Genet.*, **35**, 197–200.

116. Pang, S., Pollack, M.S., Marshall, R.N. and Immken, L. (1990) Prenatal treatment of congenital adrenal hyperplasia due to 21-hydroxylase deficiency. *N. Engl. J. Med.*, **322**, 111–15.

117. Schutgens, R.B.H., Schrakamp, G., Wanders, R.G.A. *et al.* (1990) Prenatal and perinatal diagnosis of peroxisomal disorders. *J. Inherited Metab. Dis.*, **12** (suppl.), 118–34.

118. Brown, G.K., Hann, E.A., Kirby, D.M. *et al.* (1988) Cerebral lactic acidosis: defects in pyruvic metabolism with profound brain damage and minimal systemic acidosis. *Eur. J. Pediatr.*, **147**, 10–14.

82 FETAL AND NEONATAL COAGULATION

B.E.S. Gibson

82.1 Development of haemostasis in the newborn

Coagulation factors do not cross the placental barrier to any significant degree but are synthesized by the fetus from 10 weeks of gestational age onwards. Concentrations of many of the procoagulants, anticoagulants and proteins involved in fibrinolysis are gestation dependent and gradually increase towards term, with adult values for most parameters being reached by 6 months of age [1]. The physiological immaturity of the newborn's haemostatic system causes no clinical problem for the healthy newborn but may contribute to morbidity in the sick and preterm infant (Chapter 39).

82.1.1 PROCOAGULANTS

Factors I, V, VIII:C and von Willebrand factor (vWF) are within the normal adult range from the beginning of the third trimester onwards. All other procoagulants are reduced at birth to variable levels and are dependent on gestational age (Table 82.1). A fibrinogen level of 1.5 g/l at birth represents the lower limit of normal in both the term and preterm infant. The factor VIII:C level of a term infant is above, and of a preterm infant within, the normal adult range. Both term and preterm infants have raised von Willebrand factor antigen (vWF:Ag) values with disproportionately elevated levels of high molecular weight (HMW) vWF multimers, in addition to unusually large vWF multimers not present in normal adult plasma [2]. Levels of the vitamin K-dependent factors (II, VII, IX, X) and the contact factors (XI, XII, prekallikrein (PK) and high-molecular-weight kininogen (HMWK)) are gestation dependent with values approximately 50% and 30–50% respectively of normal adult levels at term. Factor XIII levels are about 70% of adult values in the term infant. Only small quantities are required for clot stabilization and this minor decrease in activity has no clinical significance.

Table 82.1 Mean values for the procoagulants in the fetus and newborn infant

Age	Cofactors				VitaminK-dependent factors				Contact factors				
	I (g/l)	*V* (iu/dl)	*VIII:C* (iu/dl)	*vWF:Ag* (iu/dl)	*II* (iu/dl)	*VII* (iu/dl)	*IX* (iu/dl)	*X* (iu/dl)	*XI* (iu/dl)	*XII* (iu/dl)	*PK* (iu/dl)	*HMWK* (iu/dl)	*XIII* (u/dl)
Adult	3.4	100	100	100	100	100	100	100	100	100	100	100	100
Term newborn (37–41 weeks)	2.4	100	150	160	52	57	35	45	42	44	35	64	61
Preterm newborn (33–36 weeks)	3.0	82	93	166	45	59	41	44	–	25	33	–	–
Preterm newborn (25–32 weeks)	2.5	80	75	150	32	37	22	38	20	22	26	28	11–40
Fetus (≃20 weeks)	0.96	70	50	65	16	21	10	19	–	–	–	–	≃30

All values are venous and for the first 24 hours of life.
All subjects received vitamin K at birth.
Adapted from Hathaway, W.E. and Bonnar, J. (1987) *Hemostatic Disorders of the Pregnant Woman and Newborn Infant*, Elsevier, Amsterdam, pp. 58–59, with permission of the publishers.

Diseases of the Fetus and Newborn, 2nd edn, Edited by G.B. Reed, A.E. Claireaux and F. Cockburn. Published in 1995 by Chapman & Hall, London. ISBN 0 412 39160 0

Table 82.2 Mean values for the anticoagulants in the fetus and newborn infant

	AT III (iu/dl)	α_2-Antiplasmin (iu/dl)	C_1-esterase inhibitor (u/dl)	α_2-Macro-globulin (u/dl)	Plasminogen (u/dl)	Protein C:Ag (iu/dl)	Protein S:Ag (u/dl)
Adult	100	100	100	100	100	100	100
Term newborn (37–41 weeks)	56	83	100	180	49	50[a]	24[a]
Preterm newborn (33–36 weeks)	40	73	–	129	38	38	–
Preterm newborn (25–32 weeks)	35	74	–	158	35	29	–
Fetus ($\approx$20 weeks)	23	–	–	–	–	10	–

[a] Cord, all other values are venous and for the first 24 hours of life.
All subjects received vitamin K at birth.
Adapted from McDonald, M.M. and Hathaway, W.E. (1983) Perinatal hematology/oncology. *Seminars in Perinatology*, 7, 213–25, with permission of the publishers.

82.1.2 ANTICOAGULANTS

Antithrombin III (AT III), heparin co-factor II (HC II), protein C and protein S are all reduced at birth (Table 82.2). AT III levels in the term and preterm infant parallel the reduction in its substrates, factors II and X. In contrast, protein C and its co-factor, protein S, are reduced to levels similar to those of the other vitamin K-dependent factors in the term and preterm infant, whilst their substrates, factors Va and VIII:C, are in the adult range at birth. Newborns have very low levels of C4b-binding protein, which results in most, if not all, protein S existing in the free and active form. Only protein C levels remain low at 6 months of age. α_2-Macroglobulin, C_1-esterase inhibitor and α_1-antitrypsin are near or above adult values at birth. α_2-Macroglobulin inhibits significantly more thrombin and AT III less thrombin in the newborn, compared with the adult.

Plasminogen concentrations are gestation dependent and about 50% of adult values at term. Tissue-plasminogen activator and plasminogen activator inhibitor are both high at term, whilst the major inhibitor of plasmin, α_2-antiplasmin, is within the normal adult range.

The result of the physiological changes in the newborn's coagulation system is that thrombin generation is both decreased and delayed, thrombin inhibition slower and plasmin generation decreased compared with that of adult plasma [3]. Reference ranges for postnatal development are available for the procoagulants, anticoagulants and proteins involved in fibrinoly-sis [1,4]. Normal values for very premature infants are difficult to define because these infants often have disease processes which activate the coagulation system.

82.1.3 PLATELETS

The neonate's platelet count is in the adult range ($>150 \times 10^9$/l) from the second trimester onwards and the bleeding time (performed with a device designed for newborns) similar to or shorter than that of the adult [5]. The presence of platelet membrane receptors (GPIb and GPIIb/IIIa) in adult amounts from early fetal life, coupled with normal levels of vWF and fibrinogen, should secure adequate platelet adhesion and aggregation. Despite this, formal platelet aggregation studies are variably impaired, except for the response to ristocetin, which is enhanced, reflecting increased levels of HMW multimers of vWF. This, in addition to enhanced vWF function, high haematocrit and large size of red cells, explains the neonates short bleeding time.

82.2 Investigation and diagnosis of disorders of haemostasis

The cause of bleeding and/or thrombosis in the newborn is usually obvious and acquired secondary to infection or indwelling catheters. However, this is also the age at which inherited disorders present. The assessment of a bleeding neonate begins with a detailed history, examination, laboratory investigations, interpretation and diagnosis.

82.2.1 HISTORY

This should include that of the family (i.e. inherited bleeding disorders), the sex of the child, the obstetric history (e.g. of maternal idiopathic thrombocytopenic purpura, intrauterine infection or drug ingestion), the route of vitamin K administration and the presence or not of an intravenous catheter.

82.2.2 EXAMINATION

The most important factor is whether the neonate is well or unwell. Bleeding in an otherwise healthy neonate suggests immune-mediated or inherited thrombocytopenia, a hereditary bleeding disorder or vitamin K deficiency. Bleeding in a sick neonate is usually associated with infection and disseminated intravascular coagulation (DIC). Dysmorphic features, jaundice and hepatosplenomegaly suggest congenital infection, and organomegaly with petechiae and bruising may indicate an underlying haematological disorder. Acquired disorders, e.g. DIC, tend to present with generalized bleeding, whilst inherited coagulation deficiencies are characterized by localized bleeding. Purpura fulminans can be precipitated by acute infection but is also characteristic of homozygous protein C deficiency.

82.2.3 LABORATORY INVESTIGATION

This section is intended only as a brief overview of laboratory coagulation tests. Investigation of a bleeding neonate starts with screening tests which are designed to detect the presence of an abnormality, but fall short of specific identification. They include a full blood count with platelet number, blood film, prothrombin time (PT), activated partial thromboplastin time (APTT) and a thrombin clotting time (TCT). The PT principally tests the extrinsic coagulation pathway (factors I, II, V, VII and X) and the APTT assesses the intrinsic pathway (factors I, II, V, VIII, IX, X, XI, XII, PK, HMWK). The TCT measures the conversion of fibrinogen to fibrin and is prolonged in hypofibrinogenaemia, dysfibrinogenaemia or by inhibitors of thrombin e.g. heparin or fibrin degradation products. Other routine tests include measurement of the fibrinogen level and a simple test to detect fibrinolysis, e.g. fibrin degradation products (generated by the lysis of fibrinogen and non-cross-linked fibrin) or D-dimers (generated by the lysis of cross-linked fibrin by plasmin). Specific coagulation factor assays employ a variation of the PT or APTT. Factor XIII deficiency is screened for with 5 mol/l urea or 1% monochloracetic acid and clots from deficient plasma dissolve more rapidly than normal. AT III, protein C, protein S and HC II can all be measured by functional or immunological methods or both. The bleeding time can be measured by a modified template method. Monoclonal antibodies detecting the presence or absence of glycoprotein membrane receptors facilitate the diagnosis of the more common inherited platelet disorders, Bernard–Soulier syndrome (GP1b) and Glanzmann's thrombasthenia (GPIIb/IIIa).

Interpretation of coagulation results in the newborn is complicated, not only because of the differing 'normal' range in the preterm and term neonate but also because of problems with small samples (relying on the use of microtechniques), heparin contamination from the lines (usually detected by prolongation of the TCT), and the necessity for anticoagulant ratios to be based on plasma rather than whole blood volume. Abnormal results which are not in keeping with the clinical picture should be repeated in the first instance. Values for the PT, APTT and TCT are very reagent and technique dependent. Values in Tables 82.3 and 82.4 are based on a 6-month longitudinal study of healthy full term and preterm infants [1,4] and employed venous samples from infants who had received 1 mg of vitamin K at birth.

82.3 Inherited haemostatic deficiencies

The diagnosis of inherited haemostatic defects in the newborn period is complicated by the low physiological levels of many of the coagulation parameters. Inherited coagulation disorders which have been successfully diagnosed antenatally include haemophilia A and B, severe type III von Willebrand's disease and homozygous protein C deficiency. Only severe disorders which would warrant termination of pregnancy are appropriate for antenatal diagnosis, which can be based

Table 82.3 Reference values for screening tests in the healthy fullterm infant during the first 6 months of life [After Ref. 1, with permission of the publishers]

Tests	Day 1	Day 5	Day 30	Day 90	Day 180	Adult
PT (s)	13.0±1.43	12.4±1.46	11.8±1.25	11.9±1.15	12.3±0.79	12.4±0.78
APTT (s)	42.9±5.80	42.6±8.62	40.4±7.42	37.1±6.52	35.5±3.71	33.5±3.44
TCT (s)	23.5±2.38	23.1±3.07	24.3±2.44	25.1±2.32	25.5±2.86	25.0±2.66

All values are expressed as mean ± 1 SD.

Table 82.4 Reference values for screening tests in healthy premature infants (30–36 weeks' gestation) during the first 6 months of life [After Ref. 4, with permission of the publishers]

Tests	Day 1 M	Day 1 B	Day 5 M	Day 5 B	Day 30 M	Day 30 B	Day 90 M	Day 90 B	Day 180 M	Day 180 B	Adult M	Adult B
PT (s)	13.0	(10.6–16.2)	12.5	(10.0–15.3)	11.8	(10.0–13.6)	12.3	(10.0–14.6)	12.5	(10.0–15.0)	12.4	(10.8–13.9)
APTT (s)	53.6	(27.5–79.4)	50.5	(26.9–74.1)	44.7	(26.9–62.5)	37.5	(28.3–50.7)	37.5	(21.7–53.3)	33.5	(26.6–40.3)
TCT (s)	24.8	(19.2–30.4)	24.1	(18.8–29.4)	24.4	(18.8–29.9)	25.1	(19.4–30.8)	25.2	(18.9–31.5)	25.0	(19.7–30.3)

M = mean; B = lower and upper boundary encompassing 95% of the population.

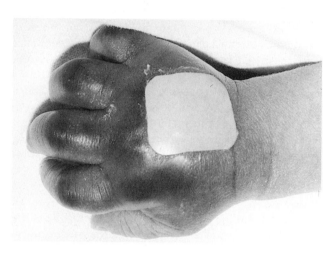

Figure 82.1 Haematoma at the site of a venepuncture performed on the second day of life to check the bilirubin level in an undiagnosed severe haemophiliac with a factor VIII:C level of <1 iu/dl.

on DNA analysis or immunological assays of coagulation proteins on fetal samples.

82.3.1 INHERITED BLEEDING DISORDERS

(a) Haemophilia A and B

Haemophilia A (incidence of 1 in 10 000) and B (incidence of 1 in 50 000) and von Willebrand's disease account for more than 90% of inherited clotting factor deficiencies. The haemophilias are the most common bleeding disorders to present in the newborn period, but less than 10% do so and these infants will be severely affected. The majority will have no problems until they begin crawling and bumping into objects or attempt standing and fall. Oozing after heel prick screening for phenylketonuria or haematoma formation at the site of a venepuncture (Figure 82.1) or following intramuscular vitamin K may draw attention to an underlying coagulopathy. Bleeding may occur from the cord or from a circumcision site, if this has been performed on an undiagnosed haemophiliac. Spontaneous bleeding occurs and, although intracranial bleeding is rare [6,7], cephalohaematoma is seen. Splenic and adrenal haemorrhage have also been described [8,9].

Two-thirds of infant boys with haemophilia will have a family history and present for diagnosis in the immediate newborn period, as even families who have decided to risk a haemophiliac child are anxious to have their worst fears erased or confirmed. Severe (factor VIII:C <2 iu/dl), moderate (factor VIII:C 2–10 iu/dl) and mild (factor VIII:C >10–40 iu/dl) haemophilia A can be diagnosed confidently in the newborn period because factor VIII:C levels in the term and preterm infant are within the normal adult range at birth: factor VIII:C >50–150 iu/dl. The diagnosis of haemophilia B, which is clinically indistinguishable from haemophilia A, is more complicated because factor IX is a vitamin K-dependent factor and gestationally reduced at birth. Factor IX:C levels in mild haemophilia B (factor IX:C >10–40 iu/dl) overlap with the lower end of the physiological normal range, necessitating retesting of such infants in later infancy. Severely affected infants (factor IX:C <2 iu/dl) should be easily identified [4], although the accuracy of the diagnosis of moderate haemophilia B is questionable. Infants severely affected with haemophilia A or B and requiring treatment should receive high purity, viricidally treated factor concentrates and should be protected with hepatitis B vaccine.

(b) Von Willebrand's disease

Von Willebrand's disease (vWF) is an acute phase reactant and the elevated levels at birth and in early infancy mask the presence of the more common types of von Willebrand's disease at this time. Bleeding requiring treatment rarely occurs, but severe type III von Willebrand's disease (with concomitant factor VIII:C deficiency) and type IIb von Willebrand's disease (with associated thrombocytopenia) can be, and have been, diagnosed in infancy [10]. These infants should be treated with viricidally treated factor VIII concentrate rich in HMW multimers or a specific vWF concentrate.

(c) Rarer coagulation deficiencies

Infants homozygous for deficiencies of factors II, V, VII, X and XI may present in the newborn period, when they can be identified by their low level of the deficient factor (<10 iu/dl), which is below the normal physiological range. In contrast, values of the deficient factor in heterozygotes may overlap with the lower end of the physiological range and confident identification is not possible. Infants homozygous for deficiencies of factors II, V, VII, X and XI who require treatment should receive fresh frozen plasma (FFP) 10–15 ml/kg, which will raise the deficient factor by 10–20 iu/dl or specific concentrate, where available.

(d) Disorders of fibrinogen and factor XIII deficiency

Cryoprecipitate or a specific viricidally treated concentrate are the best replacement products for abnormalities of fibrinogen (hypofibrinogenaemia, afibrinogenaemia, dysfibrinogenaemia), which should be easily identified in the newborn who has a fibrinogen level in the adult range. Levels of factor XIII are very low in homozygotes for factor XIII deficiency (<1 u/dl), who often experience bleeding from the umbilical cord and are at significant risk of spontaneous intracranial haemorrhage. Only tiny quantities of factor XIII (2–3 u/dl) are required for fibrin stabilization; factor XIII has a long half-life of 6 days and FFP (10 ml/kg), cryoprecipitate (10 ml/kg) or specific factor XIII concentrate are suitable vehicles for replacement.

82.3.2 INHERITED THROMBOTIC DISORDERS

The physiological anticoagulants are autosomally inherited and heterozygous deficiency rarely produces problems in infancy unless a second prethrombotic factor coexists. The homozygous states for AT III, protein S and HC II deficiency should be identifiable in the newborn period, although this has not been confirmed clinically. Homozygous protein C deficiency presents at this time with extensive life-threatening thrombosis characterized by purpura fulminans, DIC, central nervous system thrombi, blindness and venous thrombosis. Physiological levels may be very low, therefore caution should be exercised with diagnosis, which should include a typical clinical presentation, confirmation of the heterozygous state in the parents and a protein C level below the reference range. Although levels in heterozygotes probably lie outside the physiological range, this has to be established and diagnosis is best deferred until later in infancy.

82.4 Acquired haemostatic defects

82.4.1 THROMBOCYTOPENIA

A unique set of conditions surrounds the newborn, producing unusual susceptibility to thrombocytopenia, for example maternal antibodies, congenitally acquired infections and hypoxia. These combine to make thrombocytopenia (platelet count <150 × 10^9/l) probably the most common haemostatic abnormality in newborns, with approximately 22% of neonates admitted to one tertiary care intensive therapy unit developing the problem, of which over half of affected infants had platelet counts <100 × 10^9/l [11]. This cohort followed a remarkably consistent pattern with thrombocytopenia developing on day 2 of life, reaching a nadir on day 4 and resolving by day 10. Increased platelet consumption appeared to be the underlying mechanism in most cases.

Thrombocytopenia may result from increased platelet destruction, decreased platelet production, splenic sequestration, or be of combined pathogenesis (Table 82.5). Increased platelet consumption associated with infection is the most common cause, with regenerative thrombocytopenia accounting for less than 5% of cases.

(a) Autoimmune thrombocytopenia

Maternal chronic idiopathic thrombocytopenic purpura and systemic lupus erythematosus may result in neonatal thrombocytopenia due to placental transfer of maternal IgG antiplatelet autoantibodies and account for 80% of all cases of immune-mediated neonatal thrombocytopenia; alloimmune thrombocytopenia is responsible for the remaining 20%. Antenatally, autoimmune thrombocytopenia differs in two major aspects from neonatal alloimmune thrombocytopenia: the mother herself has a low platelet count and intracranial haemorrhage in utero is exceedingly rare. There is no reliable non-invasive means of predicting which infants will be severely affected. Neither the maternal platelet count, platelet-associated IgG nor free antiplatelet antibodies are predictive. Direct measurement of the fetal platelet count is becoming common practice, but cordocentesis may be associated with as high a risk to the fetus as the thrombocytopenia, and fetal scalp sampling has fallen into disfavour because of falsely low counts due to platelet clumping and the haemorrhagic risk to the fetus, if the count is low [12].

The period of greatest risk for an affected infant is generally thought to be the time of delivery, and many obstetricians would elect to deliver infants with a platelet count of <50 × 10^9/l by caesarean section. The clinical problems of an affected infant may be confined

Table 82.5 Causes of neonatal thrombocytopenia

Immune-mediated
Neonatal alloimmune thrombocytopenia
Autoimmune maternal idiopathic thrombocytopenic
   purpura, systemic lupus erythematosus, drugs, etc.

Non-immune DIC
Infection – bacterial, viral, protozoal
Asphyxia
Necrotizing enterocolitis
Haemangioma
Respiratory distress syndrome
Polycythaemia

Bone marrow infiltration
Congenital leukaemia
Neuroblastoma
Osteopetrosis
Histiocytosis
Familial erythrophagocytic lymphohistiocytosis

Bone marrow aplasia
Thrombocytopenia with absent radii
Fanconi's anaemia
Trisomy syndrome (13,18)
Congenital megakaryocyte hypoplasia

Hereditary thrombocytopenia
Wiskott–Aldrich syndrome
Bernard–Soulier syndrome
May–Hegglin anomaly

Miscellaneous
Hyperbilirubinaemia
Phototherapy
Assisted ventilation
Rhesus haemolytic disease
Post-exchange transfusion
Inborn errors of metabolism – hyperglycinaemia,
   methylmalonic acidaemia, isovaleric acidaemia
Congenital thrombotic thrombocytopenic purpura
Intralipid
Type IIB von Willebrand's disease
Maternal hyperthyroidism

to bruising or may be more serious; intracranial haemorrhage is the most serious complication. These infants should be monitored closely as the platelet count may fall in the first few days of life. However, the disorder is self-limiting and the platelet count usually starts to rise by the third week, reaching normal values before the second or third postnatal month. Once safely delivered, many infants, particularly those mildly affected, will require no treatment. Postnatal therapeutic options include steroid therapy (2 mg/kg per day) and high-dose intravenous immunoglobulin (i.v. IgG 400 mg/kg × 5 days; i.v. IgG 1 g/kg × 2 days) and are indicated for a platelet count of $<50 \times 10^9/l$. The latter will raise the platelet count faster than steroids. In the event of significant haemorrhage, random donor platelets should be transfused, but these may be rapidly destroyed. Alloimmune neonatal thrombocytopenia is dealt with elsewhere in the text (Chapters 39 and 84).

(b) Management of platelet problems and specific considerations for platelet transfusions

Bleeding is less likely to occur when thrombocytopenia is due to increased consumption rather than decreased production, and the risk is greatest when there is an associated platelet function defect. Any level accepted as an indication for platelet transfusion is to some extent arbitrary. Specific management depends upon the underlying cause, but serious beleeding is a risk, even in healthy full term infants, when the platelet count falls below $30 \times 10^9/l$. Although a platelet level in this range is often adopted for replacement, some would argue that this value is too low and that a platelet count of $50 \times 10^9/l$ is more appropriate, especially for premature, sick or unstable infants. In the presence of active bleeding, the platelet count should be kept above $50 \times 10^9/l$.

A trial of platelet concentrate should be transfused in the face of active bleeding or significant thrombocytopenia. A single platelet concentrate (10–15 ml/kg) will raise the platelet count into a safe range unless the thrombocytopenia is specifically immune mediated and secondary to antibody directed platelet destruction, when transfused platelets will be consumed. If the aetiology of the thrombocytopenia is unclear, it is prudent to document the increment postplatelet transfusion. Transfused platelets should be ABO homologous and rhesus compatible, wherever possible. They carry the risk of transmitting cytomegalovirus and causing graft-versus-host disease when transfused to the fetus and specific groups of infants. Infants considered candidates for cytomegalovirus screened and/or irradiated red cells should receive cytomegalovirus-negative and/or irradiated platelet concentrates.

82.4.2 HAEMORRHAGIC DISEASE OF THE NEWBORN

The vitamin K-dependent procoagulant factors (factors II, VII, IX and X) are physiologically low in the neonate and commonly fall further in the first 3 days of life. This can be prevented by the prophylactic administration of vitamin K at birth and is therefore, at least in part, due to deficiency of this vitamin [13].

Haemorrhagic disease of the newborn (HDN) has three recognized patterns dependent on the time of presentation.

- Early HDN. Severe and sometimes fatal bleeding presenting in the first 24 hours of life, typically, but not exclusively, in infants whose mothers are taking drugs which cross the placenta and affect vitamin K metabolism, e.g. anticonvulsants, warfarin, rifampicin and isoniazid.

- Classic HDN. Bruising or bleeding from the gastrointestinal tract during the 2–5 days of life, usually in breast-fed, fullterm, otherwise healthy infants. Breast feeding is a significant risk factor as not only are vitamin K levels low in breast milk [14], but breast-fed babies tend to have a smaller intake of milk in the first days of life than do formula-fed infants and the volume may be as important as the vitamin K concentration.

- Late HDN. Presentation may be delayed until after the first month of life and it is this pattern of disease which is presently the subject of much controversy. Haemorrhage is delayed when an infant (usually breast fed) has not received any or adequate vitamin K prophylaxis or when an infant has an underlying condition predisposing to impaired vitamin K absorption. Breast-fed babies are particularly vulnerable and intracranial haemorrhage is a common complication. Dietary deficiency alone may not explain late onset HDN in the breast-fed infant, but mild malabsorption or cholestasis related to infection may play a role [15]. Vitamin K deficiency may be secondary to chronic diarrhoea, diarrhoea in the breast-fed infant, or antibiotic therapy, and HDN may be the initial manifestation of cystic fibrosis, biliary atresia, α_1-antitrypsin deficiency, hepatitis, coeliac disease and abetalipoproteinaemia.

(a) Diagnosis

Differentiating between vitamin K deficiency and another acquired or inherited coagulation disorder may be difficult. In vitamin K deficiency haemorrhage is usually generalized and the infant otherwise healthy with a normal platelet count and fibrinogen level, but a prolonged PT and APTT. Functional factor assays (II, VII, IX and X) are lower than would be expected for the gestational age. A shortening of screening tests values or a rise in factor levels following the administration of vitamin K suggests a previous vitamin deficiency. More precise diagnosis requires measurement of circulating non-carboxylated vitamin K-dependent factors, e.g. PIVKA:II (protein induced in vitamin K's absence: prothrombin) or demonstration of a discrepancy between coagulant activity and immunological concentrations of the vitamin K-dependent factors. Vitamin K levels can be measured directly.

(b) Prophylaxis

Both the necessity for and the safety of vitamin K prophylaxis have recently been questioned. Newborn stores of vitamin K are known to be low from studies of vitamin K levels in cord blood and livers of aborted fetuses. Marginal vitamin K stores at birth combined with physiologically reduced levels of vitamin K factors may overchallenge the newborn's ability to maintain acceptable haemostasis, and the infant who develops vitamin K deficiency may be at particular risk of

haemorrhage. Daily vitamin K requirements for newborns are approximately 1–5 μg/kg and this is generally given as 0.5–1.0 mg intramuscularly or 2–4 mg orally at birth. Additional prophylaxis is indicated for high-risk infants, and some might include exclusively breast-fed infants in this category.

The incidence of HDN in the absence of vitamin K prophylaxis is largely dependent upon the frequencies of breast versus formula feeding in the population. A 2-year prospective study (1988–1990) in the UK identified an incidence of classic or late HDN of 1.62 per 100 000 live births [16]. No infant in receipt of intramuscular vitamin K developed HDN. The relative risk ratios for no or oral vitamin K when compared with intramuscular vitamin K prophylaxis were 81.1 and 13.1 respectively. Twenty-four of the 27 affected infants were solely breast-fed, and although the study was not designed to assess the role of breast-feeding, it carried an estimated relative risk ratio of 12.0. Ten infants with HDN suffered an intracranial haemorrhage. Intramuscular vitamin K affords the best protection. Oral vitamin K appears to prevent classic HDN but the efficacy of a single dose against late-onset HDN in exclusively breast-fed infants must be questioned. Concerns about administering vitamin K orally relate to doubts about optimal absorption and possible regurgitation. Intestinal malabsorption or mild cholestasis may play a role and breast-fed infants who develop diarrhoea or infants who receive antibiotic therapy are at particular risk of vitamin K deficiency.

Recently concerns have surfaced about the safety of intramuscular vitamin K, which may influence future practice. An association with intramuscular vitamin K and childhood cancer (odds ratio of 1.97), particularly leukaemia, has been reported in a birth cohort [17]. Very much higher plasma concentrations of vitamin K are achieved after parenteral administration compared with oral administration, and high concentrations of vitamin K have been reported to increase sister chromatid exchanges in sheep fetal lymphocytes *in vivo* [18], but no evidence of genetic toxicity has been found following the intramuscular administration of 1 mg vitamin K to newborn infants [19]. Other alternative pathogeneses suggested include the role of phenol present in the preparation and that of possible protection afforded by the deficiency state.

(c) Management of HDN

It is clear that all infants should receive vitamin K prophylaxis, although the optimal regimen may not be established. High-risk groups require additional prophylaxis. If vitamin K deficiency is suspected, 1 mg vitamin K by slow intravenous (to avoid anaphylaxis) or subcutaneous injection should be given, while laboratory confirmation is awaited. Intramuscular administration may lead to haematoma formation. After parenteral administration correction will occur within a few hours. In the presence of non-serious bleeding, vitamin K-dependent factors can be raised immediately by FFP, 10–15 ml/kg. Intracranial haemorrhage or other life-threatening bleeding may require treatment with factor IX complex concentrate to increase vitamin K-dependent factors to haemostatic levels immediately, although the risk of DIC and hepatitis must be taken into consideration. Several recent reviews on this topic are recommended [13,20–22].

82.4.3 DISSEMINATED INTRAVASCULAR COAGULATION

DIC is always associated with an underlying disorder (Table 82.6) which triggers the coagulation system by stimulating either the intrinsic clotting cascade via endothelial injury or the extrinsic cascade via tissue factor. Poor tissue perfusion, hypoxia and acidosis, common in neonates, further aggravate consumption from any other cause. The pathophysiology of DIC results from excessive thrombin generation; platelets and coagulation factors (I, V, VIII:C) are consumed and natural inhibitors (AT III, HC II and protein C) overwhelmed. The result is haemorrhage, organ ischaemia and microangiopathic haemolytic anaemia. The consumptive coagulopathy in neonates is generally acute and uncompensated. Bleeding is the main clinical problem and although thrombosis, particularly of the small vessels, occurs, this is usually clinically insignificant, but falling AT III levels may predispose to thrombosis in the presence of indwelling catheters.

Table 82.6 Causes of DIC in the neonate

Fetal disorders
Hypoxia–acidosis: birth asphyxia; respiratory distress syndrome; polycythaemia
Infection: bacterial, viral, protozoal, parasitic, mycotic
Meconium aspiration
Hypothermia
Erythroblastosis fetalis
Necrotizing enterocolitis
Giant haemangioma (Kasabach–Merritt syndrome)
Purpura fulminans (homozygous protein C deficiency)
Brain injury
Neoplasms and leukaemia

Maternal/obstetric disorders
Abruptio placentae
Dead twin fetus
Amniotic fluid embolism
Small-for-gestation
Maternal hypertensive syndromes (eclampsia)

(a) Diagnosis

Laboratory abnormalities include a prolonged PT, APTT, TCT, reduced fibrinogen, thrombocytopenia, elevated fibrin degradation products or D-dimers and possible evidence of red cell fragmentation on the blood film. Both term and preterm infants may have D-dimer plasma concentrations above the accepted adult range [23].

(b) Management of DIC

Treatment of the underlying disorder, thereby removing the stimulus to further consumption, is the most important aspect of management. This includes correction of hypotension, hypoxia and acidosis. Treating the coagulopathy is purely supportive. The mainstay of treatment is with FFP (10–15 ml/kg) which provides consumed procoagulants (particularly I, V, VIII:C) and anticoagulants (AT III and protein C). Cryoprecipitate (10 ml/kg) provides fibrinogen and factor VIII:C in a higher concentration per unit volume. Red cell and platelet concentrates (10–15 ml/kg) may also be required. Exchange transfusion may be necessary to avoid overload, but is not without risk in a sick neonate. Although treatment should be based on clinical rather than laboratory indicators, laboratory monitoring is often necessary to guide replacement therapy and it is reasonable to aim for a platelet count $>50 \times 10^9$/l, a fibrinogen level of >1.0 g/l and a PT normal for the gestational age. The newborn compensates poorly for factor consumption because of hepatic immaturity. AT III concentrates are of unproven value. The use of heparin in the treatment of DIC remains controversial [24], although its role is better established in some situations than others, such as in purpura fulminans [25]. However, the possible benefits of heparin must be carefully weighed against the risk of inducing further bleeding.

82.4.4 INTRACRANIAL HAEMORRHAGE

Intracranial haemorrhage is the most common manifestation of late-onset haemorrhagic disease of the newborn. These infants are almost exclusively breast fed and have either received none or oral vitamin K. Any infant with intracranial haemorrhage should be carefully evaluated for an underlying coagulopathy, either acquired or inherited.

82.4.5 INTRAVENTRICULAR HAEMORRHAGE

Intraventricular haemorrhage remains a major cause of morbidity and mortality in term and low-birth-weight infants, with an incidence variably reported between 30 and 40% [26–29]. Intraventricular haemorrhage is associated with prematurity, perinatal asphyxia, acidosis, chronic hypoxia, assisted ventilation and hypercapnia. The use of low-dose heparin has been causally linked with intraventricular haemorrhage [30], but it must be appreciated that it is the preterm infant at the highest risk of intraventricular haemorrhage who is most likely to require an indwelling catheter for venous access and monitoring.

Intraventricular haemorrhage is characterized by bleeding from the fragile microvasculature of the subependymal germinal matrix and can extend into the lateral ventricles or into the brain parenchyma. The pathogenesis is poorly understood and probably multi-factorial. Immaturity and fragility of the subependymal or germinal matrix vessels, decreased perfusion of brain tissue secondary to abnormal regulation of cerebral blood flow, oxidative damage to the endothelium and haemostatic defects may contribute. A significant co-agulopathy or thrombocytopenia is associated with intraventricular haemorrhage, but the role of the physiological immaturity of the preterm infant's coagu-lation system remains controversial. Attempts have been made to evaluate this by correcting abnormal coagulation parameters. In a few studies FFP appeared to reduce the incidence of intraventricular haemor-rhage, although not significantly, and did not have a noticeable effect on mortality. Improvement in the coagulation parameters were short lived [31,32]. It is unclear whether FFP extended its positive effect by improving haemostasis or by an alternative route such as stabilization of the blood pressure and cerebral blood flow.

A number of drugs with possible protective roles against intraventricular haemorrhage have been studied, with no constant positive benefit, and include vitamin E [33–35] and ethamsylate [36]. Further controlled studies are required to assess the different therapies available.

82.4.6 LIVER DISEASE

Liver disease in neonates can occur secondary to a number of disorders including viral heptatitis, inherited inborn errors of metabolism, fetal hydrops, cirrhosis due to α_1-antitrypsin deficiency and hypoxic liver damage. The coagulopathy is complex and due to both failure of synthesis of procoagulants and anticoagulants and to consumption of clotting factors and platelets secondary to activation of the coagulation and fibrino-lytic systems, and possibly to hypersplenism.

Treatment is supportive and consists of replacement therapy with platelets, FFP and cryoprecipitate until improvement or recovery of normal function occurs.

82.4.7 CONGENITAL HEART DISEASE AND CARDIAC SURGERY (Chapter 103)

A variety of haemostatic defects are recognized in cyanotic and acyanotic heart disease, including mild to moderate thrombocytopenia, platelet dysfunction, hyperfibrinolysis and an acquired abnormality of the vWF. Cardiac surgical procedures employing cardio-pulmonary bypass are often complicated by both intraoperative and postoperative haemorrhage. Haem-orrhage is more likely to complicate lengthy pump procedures and surgery for cyanotic heart disease. Bleeding may result from:

- thrombocytopenia and/or platelet dysfunction;
- primary fibrinolysis;
- incomplete neutralization of heparin by protamine sulphate;
- DIC;
- reduced clotting factors secondary to dilution;
- surgical techniques.

Platelet abnormalities and hyperfibrin(ogen) lysis are the most common sources of problems. Hyperfibrino-lysis complicating cardiopulmonary bypass is short lived. Treatment is directed at correcting precipitating factors, e.g. hypoxia, sepsis, heparin reversal with prot-amine sulphate and supportive treatment with appro-priate blood products.

82.4.8 THROMBOSIS

The peak incidence of thrombosis in the paediatric age group is in the neonatal period [37], when events are most frequently associated with indwelling catheters, but not exclusively so. Thrombosis in the absence of a catheter usually occurs in sick, and often preterm infants, with underlying sepsis, asphyxia, respiratory distress syndrome, dehydration or shock. The triad of factors, first proposed by Virchow, which predispose to thrombosis may be present in the neonate.

(a) Factors predisposing to thrombosis

Abnormalities of the vessel wall

All intra-arterial and intravenous catheters carry a risk of thrombosis and all vessels accessed have been affected, although umbilical catheters are associated with the majority of catheter-related thrombosis because of their popularity. Catheters may act as a nidus for thrombus formation, may damage the endothelium of the vessel wall and may produce mechanical occlusion, vasospasm and alterations in blood flow.

Although symptomatic thrombosis with vessel obstruction is relatively unusual (approximately 1%

after catheterization of the umbilical artery) [38], clinically silent thrombi encasing the catheter are much more common, with reported incidences, dependent on the criteria employed for diagnosis, as high as 59% by autopsy [39] and 20–95% by angiography [40,41]. The use of low-dose heparin prolongs catheter patency but does not appear to reduce the incidence of catheter-related thrombosis [42].

Disturbances of blood flow

In newborns, as in adults, there is a strong correlation between blood viscosity and haematocrit. True polycythaemia and dehydration both result in an elevated haematocrit and hyperviscosity. The larger diameter of neonatal red cells is associated with significantly increased platelet adhesion [43].

Changes in blood coagulability

There is no real evidence that the physiological reduction of natural anticoagulants in the neonate contributes to thrombosis in the well infant. Damage to the vessel wall and disturbances of blood flow are more important. Hereditary protein C, protein S, and AT III deficiencies have already been discussed. Heterozygotes probably have levels below the physiological normal ranges and these individuals may be at increased risk in the presence of a second insult.

(b) Treatment of thrombosis in the neonate

In the absence of an obvious identifiable cause for thrombosis, a congenital deficiency of one of the natural anticoagulants should be considered. The thrombus should be demonstrated by appropriate investigation. Optimal treatment in the neonatal period is still very controversial. Heparin therapy, thrombolytic drugs and surgery have all been employed therapeutically for clinically obvious thrombi.

Heparin acts by enhancing AT III which is physiologically low in the neonate, perhaps indicating the need for greater amounts of heparin for the same therapeutic effect. Low levels of thrombin and AT III compromise the assay systems used for monitoring [44].

Thrombolytic therapy may have a role to play in the treatment of major thrombosis associated with impaired blood flow. Urokinase, streptokinase and tissue-plasminogen activator have all been used both systemically and locally. Thrombolytic agents are not without risk in preterm infants with an immature coagulation system and an increased risk of intracranial/intraventricular haemorrhage, and their therapeutic effect may be modified by reduced levels of their substrate, plasminogen.

Oral anticoagulation with drugs such as warfarin has little place in the treatment of neonatal thrombotic disease, with the possible exception of the long-term management of homozygous protein C deficiency, which is initially treated with protein C concentrate or FFP and heparin. Surgery has been used for the management of major arterial thrombosis, but the small calibre of the neonate's vessels reduces the chance of a successful outcome; advances in microsurgery may improve this.

References

1. Andrew, M., Paes, B., Milner, R. et al. (1987) Development of the human coagulation system in the full-term infant. Blood, 70, 165–72.
2. Weinstein, M.J., Blanchard, R., Moake, J.L. et al. (1989) Fetal and neonatal von Willebrand factor (vWF) is unusually large and similar to the vWF in patients with thrombotic thrombocytopenic purpura. British Journal of Haematology, 72, 68–72.
3. Schmidt, B., Ofosu, F.A., Mitchell, L. et al. (1989) Anticoagulant effects of heparin in neonatal plasma. Pediatric Research, 25, 405–408.
4. Andrew, M., Paes, B., Milner, R. et al. (1988) Development of the human coagulation system in the healthy premature infant. Blood, 72, 1651–57.
5. Andrew, M., Paes, B., Bowker, J. et al. (1990) Evaluation of automated bleeding time device in the newborn. American Journal of Hematology, 35, 275–77.
6. Olsen, T.A., Alving, B.M., Cheshire, J.L. et al. (1985) Intracerebral and subdural haemorrhage in a neonate with hemophilia A. American Journal of Pediatric Hematology/Oncology, 7, 384–87.
7. Yonker, P.G., Graham-Pole, J. and Mehta, P. (1985) Presentation of haemophilia A in the newborn period. Journal of the Florida Medical Association, 72, 99–101.
8. Jannoccone, G. and Pasquino, A.M. (1981) Calcifying splenic haematoma in a haemophiliac newborn. Pediatric Radiology, 10, 183–85.
9. Schmidt, B. and Ziprusky, A. (1986) Disseminated intravascular coagulation masking neonatal hemophilia. Journal of Pediatrics, 109, 886–88.
10. Donnér, M., Holmberg, L. and Nilsson, I.M. (1987) Type IIB von Willebrand's disease with probable autosomal recessive inheritance and presenting as thrombocytopenia in infancy. British Journal of Haematology, 66, 349–54.
11. Castle, V., Andrew, M., Kelton, J. et al. (1986) Frequency and mechanism of neonatal thrombocytopenia. Journal of Pediatrics, 108, 749–55.
12. Scott, J.R., Cruickshank, D.P., Kochenouri, N.K. et al. (1980) Fetal platelet counts in the obstetric managment of immunologic purpura. American Journal of Obsetrics and Gynecology, 136, 495–99.
13. Lane, P.A. and Hathaway, W.E. (1985) Vitamin K in infancy. Journal of Pediatrics, 106, 351–59.
14. Harron, Y., Shearer, M.J., Rahim, S. et al. (1982) The content of phylloquinine (vitamin K) in human milk, cow's milk and infant formula foods determined by high-performance liquid chromatography. Journal of Nutrition, 112, 1105–17.
15. von Kries, R., Reifenhauser, A., Gobel, U. et al. (1985) Late onset haemorrhagic disease of newborn with temporary malabsorption of vitamin K₁. Lancet, i, 1035.
16. McNinch, A. and Tripp, J. (1991) Haemorrhagic disease of the newborn in the British Isles: two year prospective study. BMJ, 303, 1105–109.
17. Golding, J., Greenwood, R. Birmingham, K. and Mott M. (1992) Childhood cancer, intramuscular vitamin K and pethidine during labour. BMJ, 305, 341–46.
18. Israels, L.G., Friesen, E., Jansen, A.H. et al. (1987) Vitamin K₁ increases sister chromatoid exchange in vitro in human leukocytes and in vivo in fetal sheep cells: a possible role for 'vitamin K deficiency' in the fetus. Pediatric Research, 22, 405–408.
19. Cornelissen, M., Smeets, D., Merkx, G. et al. (1991) Analysis of chromosome aberrations and sister chromatid exchanges in peripheral blood lymphocytes of newborns after vitamin K prophylaxis at birth. Pediatric Research, 30, 550–53.
20. Von Kries, R. and Gobel, U. (1988) Vitamin K prophylaxis: oral or parenteral? American Journal of Diseases of Children, 142, 14–15.
21. Hathaway, W.E. (1987) New insights on vitamin K. Hematology/Oncology Clinics of North America, 1, 367–79.
22. Shearer, M.J. (1990) Vitamin K and vitamin K-dependent proteins. British Journal of Haematology, 75, 156–62.

23. Hudson, I.R.B., Gibson, B.E.S., Brownlie, J. *et al.* (1990) Increased concentrations of D-dimers in newborn infants. *Archives of Disease in Childhood*, **65**, 383–89.
24. Yamada, K., Shirahata, A., Inagaki, M. *et al.* (1983) Therapy for DIC in newborn infants. *Bibliotheca Haematologica*, **49**, 329–41.
25. Chenaille, P.J. and Horowitz M.E. (1989) Purpura fulminans. *Clinical Pediatrics*, **28**, 95–98.
26. Volpe, J.J. (1981) Neonatal intraventricular haemorrhage. *New England Journal of Medicine*, **304**, 886–91.
27. Tarby, T.J. and Volpe, J.J. (1982) Intraventricular haemorrhage in the premature infant. *Pediatric Clinics of North America*, **19**, 1077–104.
28. Beverley, D.W., Chance, G.W. and Coates, C.F. (1984) Intraventricular haemorrhage – timing of occurrence and relationship to perinatal events. *British Journal of Obstetrics and Gynaecology*, **91**, 1007–13.
29. McDonald, M.M., Koops, B.L., Johnson, M.L. *et al.* (1984) Timing and antecedents of intracranial haemorrhage in the newborn. *Pediatrics*, **74**, 32–36.
30. Lesko, S.M., Mitchell, A.A., Epstein, M.F. *et al.* (1986) Heparin use as a risk factor for intraventricular hemorrhage in low-birth-weight infants. *New England Journal of Medicine*, **314**, 1156–60.
31. Beverley, D.W., Pitts-Tucker, T.J., Congdon, P.J. *et al.* (1985) Prevention of intraventricular haemorrhage by fresh frozen plasma. *Archives of Disease in Childhood*, **60**, 710–13.
32. Turner, T.L., Prowse, C.V., Prescott, R.J. and Cash, J.D. (1981) A clinical trial on the early detection and correction of haemostatic defects in selected high-risk neonates. *British Journal of Haematology*, **47**, 65–75.
33. Sinha, S., Davies, J., Toner, N. *et al.* (1987) Vitamin E supplementation reduces frequency of periventricular haemorrhage in very preterm babies. *Lancet*, **i**, 466–71.
34. Spear, M.E., Blifeld, C., Rudolph, A.J. *et al.* (1984) Intraventricular haemorrhage and vitamin E in the very low birth weight infant: evidence for efficacy of early intramuscular vitamin E administration. *Pediatrics*, **74**, 1107–12.
35. Phelps, D.L. (1984) Vitamin E and CNS haemorrhage (editorial). *Pediatrics*, **74**, 113–114.
36. Benson, J.W., Drayton, M.R., Hayward, C. *et al.* (1986) Multicentre trial of ethamsylate for prevention of periventricular haemorrhage in very low birthweight infants. *Lancet*, **ii**, 1297–1300.
37. Schmidt, B. and Zipursky, A. (1984) Thrombotic disease in newborn infants. *Clinics in Perinatology*, **11**, 461–88.
38. O'Neill, J.A., Neblett III, W.W. and Born, M.L. (1981) Management of major thromboembolic complications of umbilical arterial catheters. *Journal of Pediatric Surgery*, **16**, 972–78.
39. Tyson, J.E., deSa, D.J. and Moore, S. (1976) Thromboatheromatous complications of umbilical arterial catheterisation in the newborn period: clinicopathological study. *Archives of Disease in Childhood*, **51**, 744–54.
40. Neal, W.A., Reynolds, J.W., Jarvis, C.W. and Williams, H.J. (1972) Umbilical artery catheterization: demonstration of arterial thrombosis by aortography. *Pediatrics*, **50**, 6–13.
41. Goetzman, B.W., Stadalnik, R.C., Bogren, H.G. *et al.* (1975) Thrombotic complications of umbilical artery catheters: a clinical and radiographic study. *Pediatrics*, **56**, 374–79.
42. Horgan, M.J., Bartoletti, A. and Polansky, S. (1987) Effect of heparin infusates in umbilical arterial catheters on frequency of thrombotic complications. *Journal of Pediatrics*, **111**, 774–78.
43. Piet, A.A.M.M., Piet, B.A., Kjell, S.S. *et al.* (1983) Red cell size is important for adherence of blood platelets to artery subendothelium. *Blood*, **62**, 214–17.
44. Andrew, M. and Schmidt, B. (1988) Use of heparin in newborn infants. *Seminars in Thrombosis and Hemostasis*, **14**, 28–32.

83 VIRAL INFECTION DURING PREGNANCY

A.B. MacLean

83.1 History

John Hunter in 1780 noted that pregnant women suffering with smallpox often miscarried. This risk appeared as high as 50% when viraemia occurred during early pregnancy. Further it was recognized that vaccination against smallpox during the first trimester was associated with transplacental spread, the development of generalized vaccinia of the fetus and subsequent abortion or fetal death.

The fetal damage that may follow viral infection during pregnancy was recognized in 1941 when Gregg [1] reported the association between congenital cataract and maternal rubella occurring in early pregnancy during an epidemic the previous summer.

The work of Semmelweis, Pasteur and Lister recognized the importance of bacterial infection during pregnancy and the puerperium, and the availability of antimicrobials (antibiotics) has meant that bacteria now seem less pathogenic than viruses. However, it must not be forgotten that elsewhere in the world syphilis, malaria, and tuberculosis pose major threats to the fetus or neonate whereas *Listeria* sp., *Toxoplasma* spp. and group B streptococci remain just as prevalent or fetotoxic as many of the viruses.

83.2 Virology

The clinician previously regarded virology as an area of medical science with little application to real-life problems. The positive identifications of viruses came too late to change management and the lack of antiviral agents meant such a diagnosis was academic anyway.

Much development of laboratory sophistication follows funding and incentives subsequent to the appearance of human immunodeficiency virus, to improve sensitivity, specificity and speed to obtain a result. Other viruses which have appeared or been identified during the last 10 years as being clinically important include human parvovirus B19 and the non-A, non-B hepatitis viruses.

Virological diagnosis still relies heavily on serological screening of the mother, but techniques are now enhanced by enzyme-linked or fluorescein-labelled immunological techniques for IgG or IgM antibody or viral antigen detection. Identification in fetal blood or tissue of viral DNA/RNA by Southern/Northern blot hybridization or protein products by Western blotting allows confirmation. Use of polymerase chain reaction techniques gives high sensitivity but has been handicapped by false-positive results arising from contamination from DNA within the laboratory.

Prevention of viral transmission to the fetus or modification of replication by antiviral agents is already available for some viruses.

83.3 Effects of viral infection on the mother

The mother is not immunocompromised during pregnancy; she will still show seroconversion, e.g. with rubella. However, there is evidence to suggest that cell-mediated immunity is altered by reduction in T-helper lymphocytes [2] and natural killer cells [3]; the latter appear important in the response to the herpes group of viruses, including cytomegalovirus and varicella-zoster virus.

Some viral infections appear to be more serious if the woman is pregnant. Varicella-zoster infection during pregnancy may be associated with severe pneumonia, sometimes with fatal consequences. In a series of 43 women who developed varicella [4], four cases were complicated by pneumonia and there was one maternal death. In a recent series from Glasgow (J.C.P. Kingdom, personal communication), of 31 pregnant women with varicella, cough and tachypnoea were often associated with the rash; ten had evidence of lung involvement, three required ventilation and there was one death. The severity of respiratory problems correlated

Diseases of the Fetus and Newborn, 2nd edn, Edited by G.B. Reed, A.E. Claireaux and F. Cockburn. Published in 1995 by Chapman & Hall, London. ISBN 0 412 39160 0

with smoking habits, and with the delay between the patient being seen with her rash and being referred for treatment with acyclovir. Currently, acyclovir is not licensed for use in pregnancy but should be considered when the benefits against life-threatening infection outweigh what appears to be minimal fetal risk.

The clinical courses of hepatitis A and B are not usually affected by pregnancy unless the acute illness occurs in the last trimester, when there is a small risk of massive hepatic necrosis. However, non-A, non-B hepatitis appears to be more life threatening if infection occurs during pregnancy. During an epidemic of non-A, non-B hepatitis in Bombay [5] the incidence of hepatitis was increased in pregnant compared with non-pregnant women, or men, and the increase was highest in late pregnancy. Infection during pregnancy was more likely to be associated with progression to hepatic failure, and again this risk was greatest with infection in late pregnancy.

Human papilloma virus produces genital condyloma acuminata which frequently increase in size during pregnancy and undergo regression in the puerperium. Similar changes may occur while a woman is on the oral contraceptive pill and may relate to hormonal as well as immunological changes.

It now seems unlikely that human immunodeficiency virus (HIV) is influenced by pregnancy. Several of the earliest North American reports commented on rapid progression with development of acquired immune deficiency syndrome (AIDS) soon after pregnancy. These women had been identified retrospectively after their infants had developed AIDS; vertical transmission from an HIV-positive woman appears more likely as CD4 counts fall and viral antigen levels rise due to advancing disease rather than the pregnancy. More recently data from Edinburgh [6] showed that women who had pregnancies after seroconversion had better CD4 (T4 lymphocyte) counts than those women who did not have pregnancies, perhaps reflecting differences in continuing drug abuse rather than any beneficial effect of the pregnancy. Even when drug use continues during the pregnancy, as reported in a New York City study [7], pregnancy does not accelerate HIV disease status.

Maternal response to the presence of virus, e.g. the development of pyrexia or production of prostaglandins or cytokines, may lead to fetal damage or loss [8].

83.4 Effects of viral infection on the fetus

Virus usually reaches the fetus transplacentally, or is transmitted to the emerging neonate during delivery. It is likely that some sexually transmitted viruses reach the fetus by ascending through the uterine cervix, with or without intact membranes (e.g. cytomegalovirus).

Transmission may occur during fetal investigation, either from the mother, e.g. enterovirus reaching the fetus as the needle traverses peritoneum and enters uterus and fetus, or from the staff performing the procedure.

The effect of the virus on the fetus may be nothing, i.e. the majority of episodes of viral infection in pregnancy do not have consequences. In the minority, early pregnancy loss, congenital abnormality, growth retardation, late pregnancy fetal death, preterm labour or vertical transmission to cause congenital or neonatal infection can result. The effect will depend on the gestation at which exposure occurs, the affinity of some viruses for certain tissues (tropism), alterations in placental function due to vasculitis, and concurrent but coincidental factors.

83.5 Individual viruses

83.5.1 RUBELLA

Gregg [1], an Australian ophthalmologist, reported the association between cataracts, usually, bilateral, diagnosed in young children who often appeared smaller than expected, and a history of rubella illness of the mother occurring during the pregnancy. Subsequent associations were made between maternal rubella infection and congenital cardiac defects and deafness. The pattern of congenital abnormalities depends on when viraemia occurs in relation to the timing of specific organogenesis. The risks of damage appear greatest (up to 50%) early in the pregnancy and damage is uncommon following infection after 16 weeks, although mental handicap, microcephaly and expanded rubella syndrome (hepatosplenomegaly, thrombocytopenic purpura and defective bone formation) are described.

Rubella embryopathy occurs in women who have not been infected during childhood or have not been immunized as schoolgirls. However, examples of fetal damage following reinfection during pregnancy are recorded [9,10].

(a) Diagnosis and management

The woman usually presents after noticing an illness with malaise, slight pyrexia, upper respiratory tract symptoms and a rash. This appears first on the face and thence spreads to body and limbs, is pink with discrete macules initially before becoming confluent on the second day and disappearing by the third day. Lymph nodes, especially occipital, will enlarge and persist after the rash has gone. Sometimes the symptoms will be minimal, but will follow exposure to a known contact 2–3 weeks earlier. Unfortunately, asymptomatic or subclinical infection can be just as damaging to the fetus as symptomatic infection [10].

Confirmation of diagnosis is based on serological testing. Most laboratories have replaced haemagglutination inhibition titres with single radial haemolysis. If a pregnant woman presents soon after exposure or development of a rash, she should be tested for rubella antibody status. She can be reassured if she is immune, with rubella-specific IgG antibodies greater than 15 iu/ml. If she has no antibodies, or they exist at a level less than 15 iu/ml, she should have repeat testing 7 days later; if seroconversion has occurred, specific IgG titres have risen fourfold, or if specific IgM is detected she should be counselled about the risk of fetal damage. If there is a delay before the woman presents, the presence of IgG may not represent old immunity but recent infection; then IgM should be measured using IgM capture radioimmunoassay (MACRIA) or enzyme-linked immunosorbent assay (ELISA) [11]. The concern of fetal damage following reinfection seems greatest if the woman develops a rash; it appears that asymptomatic infection is rarely followed by fetal damage.

83.5.2 CYTOMEGALOVIRUS

It is likely that cytomegalovirus (CMV) is now the most common infectious cause of fetal damage, with a risk of 1 in 30 after primary maternal infection, or 3–4 infants with congenital CMV per 1000 livebirths [12]. Fetal damage can occur in any trimester, usually with the virus crossing the placenta, but sometimes ascending from the cervix. The infected mother is usually asymptomatic, but may occasionally experience an influenza like illness.

Some women may carry the virus in a chronic state, or may become reinfected; the presence of antibodies does not protect against reinfection. Although fetal infection will occur in about half of the fetuses where the mother is seronegative, maternal immunoglobulins seem to protect the fetus and only 2% will be infected when the mother is reinfected [13]. When the fetus is infected, about 10% will suffer damage, usually to the central nervous system but also to other organs. The affected infant may present later with microcephaly, choroidoretinitis, optic atrophy, sensorineural deafness, mental handicap or delayed neurodevelopment.

(a) Diagnosis and management

The diagnosis of CMV infection during pregnancy is usually made retrospectively after the infant shows clinical features and CMV particles are found in the urine (where they may be found for several months after birth). CMV-specific IgM may be found on serological testing. Characteristic intracranial calcification can be seen on the skull radiograph of older children. Most maternal infections are asymptomatic but if the patient presents after a non-specific or

influenza-like illness CMV-specific IgM will confirm a diagnosis. However, screening of asymptomatic women for seroconversion is not recommended in clinical practice [14,15], particularly as the presence of maternal antibodies will not protect the fetus. Fetal blood sampling may allow detection of those fetuses who become infected [16] but will not determine which ones have become damaged. Continuing to test for seroconversion in susceptible individuals seems impractical after 24 weeks, and yet the fetus still runs the risk of infection up to and during delivery. An alternative approach would be to treat the mother with a non-fetotoxic antiviral agent; ganciclovir produces profound neutropenia and is unsuitable in these circumstances. Suitable antiviral agents have still to be found.

The question of whether termination of pregnancy should be offered after intrauterine infection has been diagnosed is a vexing one as only 10% of infected fetuses will have serious handicap, i.e. if half of the fetuses are infected after maternal seroconversion, only 5% will be damaged, and 95% of aborted fetuses will be normal. Until methods are found to differentiate damaged from undamaged infected fetuses, termination of pregnancy is thought to be unjustified [17].

83.5.3 PARVOVIRUS B19

This virus is one of the causes of erythematous rash in children; it is known variously as erythema infectiosum, fifth disease or slapped-cheek syndrome. It is also a cause of aplastic crises in patients with sickle-cell disease. Although parvovirus in various animals (unrelated to B19) is a known cause of congenital abnormality, stillbirth and neonatal death, it is only in the last 10 years that it has been recognized as a cause of abortion and fetal death, usually occurring in the second trimester and sometimes associated with non-immune hydrops. Cases tend to occur in clusters coinciding with outbreaks of erythema infectiosum. Most mothers will have a rash, similar to rubella, and will be asymptomatic; otherwise when symptoms do occur they are usually transient arthralgia.

Cumulative evidence from the literature of reported cases in the UK [11] suggests that the relative risk of an adverse fetal outcome due to B19 infection is around 6%. The virus attacks fetal erythroid precursors and although subsequent fetal death or hydrops is associated with anaemia, normal bilirubin levels are found, suggesting that haemolysis is not the cause. A possible mechanism for the development of hydrops is the myocardial damage described by Morey and colleagues [18]. There is no evidence that the virus is teratogenic.

(a) Diagnosis and management

If the mother presents with a maculopapular rash she should be tested for serological markers for rubella or parvovirus B19 infections, i.e. specific IgM which may persist for up to 18 weeks. The presence of elevated maternal serum α-fetoprotein has been described as an early marker for predicting fetal involvement [10] and may represent leakage across a damaged placenta.

Fetal blood sampling for B19-specific IgM is not always useful if infection occurs before 22 weeks or if there is an interval of more than 12 weeks between infection and development of, for example, hydrops. Newer techniques for detecting B19 DNA in fetal blood may be more conclusive.

The histological features of fetal damage have been described [18] and include erythroid precursors with characteristic eosinophilic intranuclear inclusions and marginated chromatin found in sites of extramedullary erythropoiesis and especially in liver. Vasculitis of the placenta, with a perivascular inflammatory infiltrate around villous capillaries, and myocardial round cell infiltrate with focal subendocardial fibroelastosis are described.

Management of an infected mother, following rash and/or symptoms and confirmatory serology, may be helped by determining maternal α-fetoprotein levels and giving serial intrauterine transfusions to treat fetal anaemia, although spontaneous resolution of hydropic changes is also recognized.

83.5.4 VARICELLA-ZOSTER VIRUS

Reference has been made to the serious maternal sequelae of infection with varicella-zoster virus (VZV) during pregnancy. McGregor et al. [19] estimate that approximately 10% of pregnant women will not have antibodies. However, primary chicken-pox infections in adults are uncommon, while episodes of zoster are seen more frequently but are less complicated.

Congenital varicella syndrome is described, usually following exposure of the fetus during the first 20 weeks and consisting of microphthalmia, cataracts, microcephaly, rudimentary fingers, hypoplastic limbs, muscle atrophy, cutaneous scarring and contractures. Balducci et al. [20] found no evidence of these features in 36 infants after exposure to varicella in the first trimester, while Preblud, Cochi and Orenstein [21] reviewed the literature and found abnormalities in 2–3% of infants exposed in the first trimester and 0.6% (3 of 461) for the whole of pregnancy.

Other sequelae of VZV infection during pregnancy include preterm delivery and the development of neonatal varicella with mild to severe pneumonitis, as well as skin lesions following exposure in late pregnancy (especially within 4 days of labour and delivery).

(a) Diagnosis and management

Diagnosis of varicella and zoster in the mother are usually made on clinical grounds. Confirmation can be by electron microscopy, virus culture or by labelled monoclonal antibodies.

If the mother is exposed, especially in late pregnancy, she should have her serological status assessed by VZV-specific IgG and IgM. If she is immune she can be reassured. If she is susceptible and exposure has been less than 96 hours earlier, she should be given human varicella-zoster immunoglobulin. If the mother develops VZV after exposure, immunoglobulin has no role. Acyclovir has been used to treat pregnant women with severe varicella pneumonitis, and should be used if infection is diagnosed in late pregnancy or during labour, continuing its administration to the neonate.

There is little support for termination of the pregnancy if VZV infection occurs in the first 20 weeks of gestation.

83.5.5 HERPES SIMPLEX VIRUS

Herpes simplex virus (HSV) is second to human papilloma virus as the most frequent sexually transmitted virus. Epidemics of infection (herpes progenitalis) have been recorded since the last century, and there was a large increase in cases in the UK a decade or more ago. Despite well-documented consequences of HSV infection during pregnancy, such cases are seen infrequently.

Congenital abnormality may follow viraemia, with meningoencephalitis, hydrocephaly, microcephaly, chorioretinitis, cataracts, conjunctivitis, pneumonitis and hepatitis. Infection in early pregnancy may produce abortion/or intrauterine death. Although the antiviral agent used for HSV, acyclovir, interferes with thymidine metabolism, there is no evidence from retrospective and prospective studies [2] that its use in pregnancy is associated with any increase in birth defects.

HSV (type 2 but occasionally type 1) can cause neonatal encephalitis or hepatitis when the fetus is exposed to active lesions during delivery. The greatest risk is when delivery coincides with a primary genital lesion in the mother, with transmission rates greater than 50% [23]; the risk of transmission with a recurrent or secondary lesion appears to be less than 5% [24] because maternal neutralizing antibodies crossing the placenta provide protective benefit for the neonate [25].

(a) Diagnosis and management

HSV grows on certain cell lines and produces a cytopathic effect visible within 2–4 days. New faster methods of diagnosis are available, based on centrifugation enhanced culture, DNA probes, or antigen detection by immunofluorescence, enzyme immunoassay and latex agglutination [26]. HSV can also be identified from vesicular fluid by electron microscopy, but obtaining the fluid may be very painful and the virus cannot be distinguished from, for example, VZV.

Previous recommendations involved identifying pregnancies at risk from maternal history and taking vulval, vaginal and cervical swabs at weekly intervals from between 30–34 weeks and delivery. If the mother went into labour, was seen within 4 hours of membrane rupture and had a positive HSV result from the previous week, she was delivered by caesarean section [27]. There was debate as to whether ascending infection occured quickly after rupture of the membranes, and after what duration of membrane rupture caesarean section ceased to be of benefit.

Such policy is now questioned [15,25]: it now appears that screening for shedding of virus has limited diagnostic merit, as events last week (and last week's swab result) have little relationship to reactivation of virus during events at the onset of labour. It is estimated that such a policy of screening will have only 25% correlation with results on swabs taken during labour [24]. In addition, the risks of transmission of virus to the neonate, certainly in the UK, seem less than earlier estimates. Binkin, Koplan and Cates [24] have calculated that the former policy, as practised in USA, would save only 31 babies from neonatal herpes each year, would cost $1.8 million for each baby saved and that the additional caesarean sections would be responsible for up to four additional maternal deaths.

Current recommendations [28] are that women who develop primary herpetic lesions in late pregnancy should be treated with acyclovir and be followed for disappearance of virus; if labour threatens during a primary attack and viral presence, caesarean section is suggested. If a recurrent episode is noted during labour, section is recommended; alternatively, vaginal delivery followed by close surveillance of the neonate, with antiviral therapy if virus is detected, seems appropriate [15].

83.5.6 HUMAN PAPILLOMA VIRUS

Some infants will develop laryngeal or cutaneous (genital) condylomata due to human papilloma virus (HPV) which are thought to be caused by perinatal exposure. There is no evidence that this virus causes congenital abnormality, abortion or stillbirth and is probably not associated with preterm labour. The risk of laryngeal lesions developing in infants born to women with condylomas has been calculated to be between 1 in 80 and 1 in 1500 after a survey of North American otolaryngologists and estimating that condylomas are present in 2–5% of pregnant women [29]. However, polymerase chain reaction techniques to detect HPV would suggest that the virus is present in 20% or more of sexually active women. Review of laryngeal biopsy material in Glasgow found only two

new cases per year from an area with more than 25 000 deliveries per year. Thus the risks of perinatal transmission would seem small and certainly do not justify trying to eradicate HPV or even condylomas from the genital tract during pregnancy.

83.5.7 HEPATITIS VIRUSES

The recognition of carriage of hepatitis B during pregnancy enables the risk of vertical transmission to be reduced by the neonatal administration of immunoglobulin and subsequent immunization. The fetus does not appear to be at risk during the pregnancy; it is unlikely that either hepatitis A or C cause risk for the fetus unless maternal illness is severe enough to cause abortion or preterm labour.

83.5.8 HUMAN IMMUNODEFICIENCY VIRUS

This virus has made a major impact on several areas of pregnancy care. In some areas of the world, e.g. central Africa, at least one in five pregnant women will be HIV positive; elsewhere, estimated rates among antenatal patients are 20 per 1000 in New York and 0.24 per 1000 in London [30]. The virus can be transmitted to the fetus at the time of delivery but there is evidence of transplacental transmission, occurring as early as 15 weeks and with either viral antigen detected or virus isolated in fetal tissues.

Marion and colleagues [31] have suggested that HIV may cause embryopathy, describing 20 infants or children with craniofacial abnormalities including box-like appearance of forehead, hypertelorism, flattening of the nasal bridge, obliquity of the eyes, long palpebral fissures with blue sclera, short nose with flattened columella and well-formed triangular philtrum, as well as microcephaly and delayed growth.

The risk of vertical transmission to the fetus, as mentioned earlier, appears to correlate with maternal symptoms, viral load and CD4 count. Earlier estimates of transmission rates of up to 50% [6] have been reviewed after the European Collaborative Study [32] reported a rate of only 12.9% for 372 children with at least 18 months of follow-up. A recent study of twin pregnancies [33] suggests that exposure to virus following rupture of the membranes places the first twin at greater risk than the second, and that delivery by caesarean section might reduce, though not prevent, the risk of vertical transmission (Chapters 7 and 18).

(a) Diagnosis and management

The diagnosis of HIV infection is based on an initial serological (ELISA) screening for specific antibody, usually against core (p24) or envelope (gp44) antigens. Positive results are usually confirmed by a Western blot assay for core and/or envelope proteins. An increasing number of commercially produced kits has become available, using recombinant or partially purified viral antigens attached to polystyrene beads or microtitre wells, with conventional or competitive binding assays to detect anti-HIV IgG or IgM antibodies. These kits have high sensitivity and specificity [26]. Other recent advances include techniques for rapid screening, and detection of virus before antibodies appear (during the 'window phase') or are eliminated (e.g. clearing of maternal IgG in the infant), such as with polymerase chain reaction. Whether screening of antenatal patients for HIV should be selective, elective or compulsory is still being debated.

The management of HIV infection during pregnancy currently may include the use of azidothymidine (AZT) and antimicrobials to prevent *Pneumocystis carinii* pneumonia. Although AZT might interfere with nucleic acid synthesis if taken at the time of conception or during embryogenesis, there has been no evidence of teratogenicity [34]. There is a theoretical risk that AZT taken in later pregnancy could induce fetal marrow suppression and cause hydrops fetalis. To date there is no evidence of any adverse effects on the neonate [35]. Although the use of AZT at the end of pregnancy might help protect the fetus from vertical transmission during labour, its efficacy is not proven; studies to evaluate this and its safety are underway [36]. An alternative would be to use a topical antiviral agent, e.g. as a douche, in late pregnancy to reduce the risks to the fetus.

The prophylactic use of pentamidine aerosol to prevent *P. carinii* pneumonia appears safe because there is little absorption. Co-trimoxazole (sulphamethoxazole + trimethoprim) appears safe in early pregnancy (despite the antifolate action of trimethoprim) but as the sulphamethoxazole will cross the placenta and displace the bilirubin binding with protein, it is better avoided during the last month of pregnancy.

83.5.9 OTHER VIRUSES

Viral infections of the respiratory or gastrointestinal tracts are common and therefore occur during pregnancy; apart from a report from a Dublin study of increased neural tube defects after an influenza epidemic [36], these viruses do not appear to be teratogenic. Influenza, mumps and measles viruses are associated with increased early pregnancy loss and preterm labour. Infection in late pregnancy, and also with polio, echovirus type II and coxsackie B viruses, has been associated with perinatal transmission (transplacental for some if not all these viruses) and development of neonatal infection with sequelae [11] (Chapters 7 and 99).

References

1. Gregg, N.M. (1941) Congenital cataract following German measles in the mother. *Transactions of the Ophthalmological Society of Australia*, 3, 35–45.
2. Sridama, V., Pacini, F., Yang, S.-L. et al. (1982) Decreased levels of helper T cells – a possible cause of immunodeficiency in pregnancy. *New England Journal of Medicine*, 397, 352–56.
3. Kurashige, T., Morita, H., Ogura, H. et al. (1986) Natural killer cell activity in pregnancy and the effect of pregnant women's sera. *Asia-Oceania Journal of Obstetrics and Gynaecology*, 12, 305–19.
4. Paryani, S.G. and Arvin, A.M. (1986) Intrauterine infection with varicella-zoster virus after maternal varicella. *New England Journal of Medicine*, 314, 1542–46.
5. Khuroo, M.S., Teli, M.R., Skidmore, S. et al. (1981) Incidence and severity of viral hepatitis in pregnancy. *American Journal of Medicine*, 70, 252–55.
6. Johnstone, F.D. and Mok, J. (1990) HIV infection in obstetrics, in *Clinical Infection in Obstetrics and Gynaecology* (ed. A.B. MacLean), Blackwell Scientific, Oxford, pp. 72–94.
7. Selwyn, P.A., Schoenbaum, E.E., Davenny, K. et al. (1989) Prospective study of human immunodeficiency virus infection and pregnancy outcomes in intravenous drug users. *JAMA*, 261, 1289–94.
8. Pleet, H., Graham, J.M. and Smith, D.W. (1981) Central nervous system and facial defects associated with maternal hyperthermia at four to fourteen weeks' gestation. *Paediatrics*, 67, 785–89.
9. Smithells, R., Sheppard, S., Holzel, H. and Jones, G. (1991) Congenital rubella in Great Britain 1971–1988. *Health Bulletin*, 49, 266–72.
10. Carrington, D. (1991) Rubella and parvovirus in pregnancy. *Current Obstetrics and Gynaecology*, 1, 72–77.
11. Carrington, D. (1990) Viral infections during pregnancy, in *Clinical Infection in Obstetrics and Gynaecology* (ed. A.B. MacLean), Blackwell Scientific, Oxford, pp. 39–71.
12. Editorial (1989) Screening for congenital CMV. *Lancet*, ii, 599–600.
13. Stagno, S., Pass, R.F., Dworsky, M.E. et al. (1982) Congenital cytomegalovirus infection. The relative importance of primary and recurrent maternal infection. *New England Journal of Medicine*, 306, 945–49.
14. Jeffries, D.J. (1984) Cytomegalovirus infection in pregnancy. *British Journal of Obstetrics and Gynaecology*, 91, 305–306.
15. Rudd, P. and Peckham, C. (1988) Infection of the fetus and the newborn: prevention, treatment and related handicap. *Clinical Obstetrics and Gynecology*, 2, 55–71.
16. Lange, I., Rodeck, C.H., Morgan-Capner, P. et al. (1982) Prenatal serological diagnosis of intrauterine cytomegalovirus infection. *BMJ*, 284, 1673–74.
17. Griffiths, P.D. and Baboonian, C. (1984) A prospective study of primary cytomegalovirus infection during pregnancy: final report. *British Journal of Obstetrics and Gynaecology*, 91, 307–15.
18. Morey, A.L., Keeling, J.W., Porter, H.J. and Fleming, K.A. (1992) Clinical and histopathological features of parvovirus B19 infection in the human fetus. *British Journal of Obstetrics and Gynaecology*, 99, 566–74.
19. McGregor, J.A., Mark, S., Crawford, G.P. and Levin, M.J. (1987) Varicella zoster antibody testing in the care of pregnant women exposed to varicella. *American Journal of Obstetrics and Gynecology*, 157, 281–84.
20. Balducci, J., Rodis, J.F., Rosengren, S. et al. (1992) Pregnancy outcome following first trimester varicella infection. *Obstetrics and Gynecology*, 79, 5–6.
21. Preblud, S.R., Cochi, S.L. and Orenstein, W.A. (1986) Varicella zoster infection in pregnancy (letter). *New England Journal of Medicine*, 315, 1416–17.
22. Andrews, E.B., Yankaskas, B.C., Cordero, J.F. and The Acyclovir in Pregnancy Registry Advisory Committee (1992) Acyclovir in pregnancy registry: six years' experience. *Obstetrics and Gynecology*, 79, 7–13.
23. Nahmias, A.J., Keyserling, H.H. and Kerrick, G. (1983) Herpes simplex, in *Infectious Diseases of the Fetus and Newborn Infant*, 2nd edn (eds J.S. Remington and J.O. Klein), W.B. Saunders, Philadelphia, pp. 156–90.
24. Binkin, N.J., Koplan, J.P. and Cates, W. (1984) Preventing neonatal herpes: the value of weekly viral cultures in pregnant women with recurrent genital herpes. *JAMA*, 251, 2816–21.
25. Prober, C.G., Sullender, W.M., Yasukawa, L.L. et al. (1987) Low risk of herpes simplex virus infections in neonates exposed to the virus at the time of vaginal delivery to mothers with recurrent genital herpes simplex virus infection. *New England Journal of Medicine*, 316, 240–44.
26. Lee, P.C. and Hallsworth, P. (1990) Rapid viral diagnosis in perspective, *BMJ*, 300, 1413–18.
27. Grossman, J.H., Wallen, W.C. and Sever, J.L. (1981) Management of genital herpes simplex virus infection during pregnancy. *Obstetrics and Gynecology*, 58, 1–4.
28. Editorial (1988) Virological screening for herpes simplex virus during pregnancy, *Lancet*, ii, 722–23.
29. Shah, K., Kashima, H., Polk, B.F. et al. (1986) Rarity of cesarean delivery in cases of juvenile-onset respiratory papillomatosis. *Obstetrics and Gynecology*, 68, 795–99.

30. Johnstone, F. (1991) HIV infection in pregnancy. *Current Obstetrics and Gynaecology*, **1**, 78–83.

31. Marion, R.W., Wiznia, A.A., Hutcheon, R.G. and Rubinstein, A. (1986) Human T-cell lymphotropic virus type III (HTLV-III) embryopathy. *American Journal of Diseases of Children*, **140**, 638–40.

32. European Collaborative Study (1991) Children born to women with HIV-1 infection: natural history and risk of transmission, *Lancet*, **337**, 253–60.

33. Goedert, J.J., Duliege, A.M., Amos, C.I. and the International Registry of HIV Exposed Twins (1991) High risk of HIV-1 infection for first-born twins. *Lancet*, **338**, 1471–75.

34. Sperling, R.S., Stratton, P. and the members of the Obstetrics – Gynecologic Working Group of the AIDS Clinical Trials Group of the National Institute of Allergy and Infectious Diseases (1992) Treatment options for human immunodeficiency virus infected pregnant women, *Obstetrics and Gynecology*, **79**, 443–8.

35. Watts, D.H., Brown, Z.A., Tartaglione, T. *et al.* (1991) Pharmacokinetic disposition of zidovudine during pregnancy. *Journal of Infectious Diseases*, **163**, 226–32.

36. Coffey, A.P. and Jessop, W.J.E. (1963) Maternal influenza and congenital deformities: a follow up study, *Lancet*, **i**, 748–51.

84 RHESUS ALLOIMMUNIZATION

K.J. Moise Jr and G.G. Ashmead

84.1 Introduction

4.1.1 ETIOLOGY

When fetomaternal hemorrhage causes foreign red cell antigens to enter the maternal circulation, the production of antibodies is initiated. This process has been classically described as **red cell isoimmunization**. In recent times, red cell alloimmunization has been adapted as the new terminology to describe this disease. Although the rhesus antigen (D antigen) is the most common cause of **red cell alloimmunization**, more than 43 other red cell antigens have been implicated in hemolytic disease of the newborn [1]. The antigens that produce severe fetal disease necessitating intrauterine transfusion are however limited in number. Often the D antibody is found in conjunction with other rhesus antibodies (c, C, E, e) of weaker titer. An indirect Coombs' test, positive only for c or Kell antibody, has been associated with severe *in utero* disease. Duffy (FyA) and Kidd (JkA, JkB) on rare occasions will cause fetal anemia that requires intrauterine transfusion.

84.1.2 INCIDENCE

Before the use of rhesus immunoglobulin (RhIg) 0.5–1.0% of all pregnant women were Rh-alloimmunized [2]. In 1968, RhIg was approved by the Food and Drug Administration for use in the USA. Thereafter, Rh-negative patients delivering Rh-positive infants were administered 300 μg of RhIg intramuscularly within 72 hours of delivery. A rapid fall in the incidence of rhesus sensitization was noted as a result of this practice. In 1978, Bowman *et al.* [3] reported that the incidence of rhesus alloimmunization could be reduced 5–10-fold if RhIg was administered at 28 and 34 weeks of gestation. In 1984, the American College of Obstetricians and Gynecologists [4] recommended routine antenatal prophylaxis at 28 weeks of pregnancy. Despite these measures, patients continue to become sensitized due to subclinical fetomaternal hemorrhage in early gestation or failures to appropriately administer RhIg. Recent data published from the Centers for Disease Control noted that the incidence of rhesus hemolytic disease of the newborn in the USA in 1984 was 10.6 cases per 10 000 total births [5]. Red cell alloimmunization to irregular antibodies continues to be a problem since prophylactic immune globulin is not available to prevent these cases. In a series of 131 898 Rh-positive pregnant patients, the incidence of a positive indirect Coombs' test was 1 in 330 patients [6]. Thirty of the infants in the series required exchange transfusions for hemolytic disease of the newborn.

84.2 Physiologic adaptions in the anemic fetus

In 1983, Daffos, Capella-Pavlovsky and Forestier [7] described the use of ultrasound to guide a 20-gauge needle into an umbilical cord vessel to obtain fetal blood. This advancement opened the field of fetal hematology. Normal reference ranges for hematocrit increase with gestational age while the fetal reticulocyte and erythroblast counts decrease [8,9].

Fetal anemia is defined as a value less than 2 standard deviations below the mean for gestational age, although most authorities will begin intrauterine transfusions when the hematocrit falls below 30%. Nicolaides *et al.* [10] found that hydrops fetalis is usually not seen until the fetal hemoglobin concentration falls more than 7 g/dl below the mean value for gestational age. Mild anemia appears to be well tolerated by the fetus. An increase in circulating reticulocytes is noted when the hemoglobin deficit exceeds 2 g/dl [10]. An increase in both serum erythropoietin and circulating erythroblasts is not seen until the hemoglobin deficit is greater than 7 g/dl [10,11]. Despite the decreased oxygen-carrying capacity that occurs with significant anemia, tissue hypoxia does not usually occur in the fetus until the anemia becomes severe. It is not until the fetal hemoglobin declines to less than 50% of the mean

Diseases of the Fetus and Newborn, 2nd edn, Edited by G.B. Reed, A.E. Claireaux and F. Cockburn. Published in 1995 by Chapman & Hall, London. ISBN 0 412 39160 0

value for gestational age that a fall in pH can be detected [12]. Serum lactate becomes elevated only after the fetal hemoglobin is less than 30% of norm. The exact mechanisms by which the fetus is able to adapt to severe anemia are poorly understood. Doppler studies have demonstrated increased cardiac output in association with anemia [13]. In addition, the 2,3-diphosphoglycerate (2,3-DPG) concentration of the red cells increases with the severity of fetal anemia, thereby enhancing oxygen release at the tissue level [14]. The relative hyperthyroid status of the anemic fetus that has been recently reported may be the explanation for enhanced myocardial contractility and elevated 2,3-DPG levels [15].

The etiology of hydrops fetalis as a result of anemia has yet to be elucidated. Theories that have been proposed include myocardial failure, depressed protein synthesis by the liver secondary to extramedullary hematopoiesis, enhanced capillary permeability secondary to tissue hypoxia and portal hypertension [16,17]. We studied the serum colloid osmotic pressure (COP) and umbilical venous pressure (UVP) prior to intravascular transfusion [18]. Fifteen hydropic fetuses were matched for gestational age to 15 anemic fetuses without evidence of hydrops by ultrasound. Both COP and UVP were noted to be elevated in the hydropic fetuses although the difference in the UVP between affected infants and controls did not achieve statistical significance. We did not feel that the minimal derangements in Starling forces found were of sufficient magnitude to establish clearly an etiology for fetal hydrops. Studies in the fetal lamb indicate that for every 1-mm increase in venous pressure, a 13% reduction in lymphatic flow occurs [19]. As the UVP values in our study were above the norms found by Weiner *et al.* [20], it may be that this slight increase in central venous pressure may be sufficient to compromise lymphatic return to the heart. A slow accumulation of extracellular fluid with subsequent hydrops would then be the end-result. A recent study in fetal lambs made anemic by euvolemic exchanges of plasma has noted an increase in central venous pressure with the onset of hydrops [21]. Further investigation, particularly in the animal model, is necessary to confirm this theory.

84.3 Diagnosis

Diagnostic modalities used in the assessment of fetal disease can be divided into non-invasive and invasive techniques. Non-invasive methods include real-time and Doppler ultrasound and maternal serum testing for antibody titer. Invasive tests include percutaneous umbilical blood sampling and amniocentesis.

Ultrasound has played a key role in the improved survival of the fetus affected by maternal red cell alloimmunization. It is used to establish the correct gestational age since such parameters as the normal fetal hematocrit and the zones of the Liley curve are based on gestational age. Unfortunately, its use in the diagnosis of fetal anemia is relatively limited until overt fetal hydrops is present. Although some investigators have advocated the use of serial ultrasound examinations to detect signs of impending hydrops, Nicolaides and co-workers [22] were unable to correlate fetal hematocrit with such parameters as increased placental thickness or increased umbilical vein diameter. Two studies [23,24] have proposed that an increase in fetal hepatic dimensions is a good predictor of anemia since this organ increases in size as a source of extramedullary hematopoiesis. The use of Doppler ultrasound to measure blood velocities in various fetal vessels in an attempt to predict the fetal hematocrit has not proven reliable [25,26].

Maternal antibody titers can be used to assess the degree of risk for fetal disease. Although titers performed with saline or albumin techniques were once routinely used, most centers now employ human antiglobulin (indirect Coombs') testing. A critical titer is defined as the titer at which there is a significant risk of fetal hydrops. Although the actual titer will vary with institution, methodology and incidence of hydrops, most centers will use a titer value between 8 and 32 (dilution: 1:8 and 1:32) as their definition of a critical value. Once a patient is found to have this titer, further invasive fetal testing is indicated.

Since its introduction by Daffos, Capella-Pavlovsky and Forestier in 1983 [7], percutaneous umbilical blood sampling (also known as PUBS, cordocentesis and fetal blood sampling (FBS)) has come to play a major role in the treatment of hemolytic disease of the fetus. Complications of the procedure include cord hematoma and fetal bradycardia [27,28]. In our experience, the bradycardia is usually transient and can be observed. Vasospasm is felt to play a major role in the etiology of the decline in the fetal heart rate. In addition, a fetal loss rate of 1.2% has been attributed to PUBS undertaken for diagnostic purposes [29]. Fetuses with severe anemia do not appear to tolerate puncture of the umbilical vessels as well as fetuses with normal hematocrits and therefore a higher fetal mortality can be expected in these cases. Paternal genotype testing for the particular red cell antigen involved in maternal alloimmunization is available in most blood banks. PUBS can be used in cases of a heterozygous paternal genotype to determine the fetal blood type. In half of such cases, the specific antigen will be absent from the fetal red cells and the fetus will be unaffected. Care should be taken to avoid the placenta as a disruption of chorionic villi with leakage of fetal cells into the maternal circulation may result in a rise in the maternal

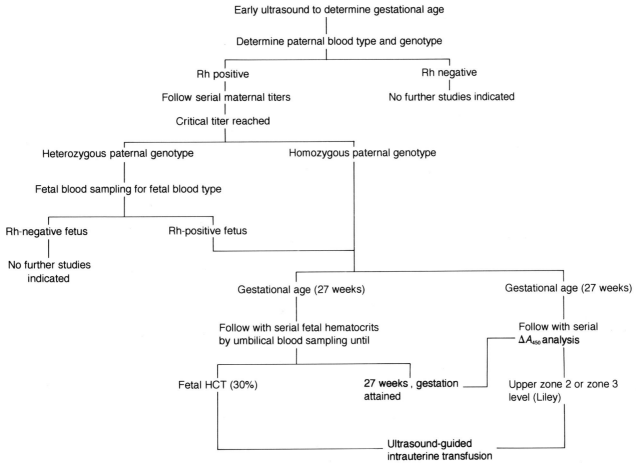

Figure 84.1   Management scheme for red cell alloimmunization. HCT = hematocrit. (Modified from Moise, Carpenter and Milam [35].)

antibody level and subsequent worsening of fetal disease [30,31].

Until the advent of PUBS, measurement of amniotic fluid bilirubin was the primary means for determining the severity of fetal anemia in hemolytic disease. Bevis [32] was the first to note a relationship between bile pigments in the amniotic fluid and the severity of erythroblastosis fetalis. In 1961, Liley [33] spectrophotometrically analyzed amniotic fluid for bilirubin at an absorbance (optical density) of 450 nm (A_{450}) and proposed three prognostic zones for the value ΔA_{450}. For the next 25 years, the Liley curve became the cornerstone of management for the pregnant patient with red cell alloimmunization. As neonatal survival at early gestational ages improved, 'modified' Liley curves were created by extrapolating the Liley zones backward to assess change in absorbance at 450 nm before 27 weeks of gestation. The usefulness of the Liley curve came into question when Nicolaides and coworkers [34] correlated fetal hematocrits obtained by PUBS in alloimmu-

nized pregnancies between 18 and 25 weeks with ΔA_{450} values from a 'modified' Liley curve. These authors found that 70% of anemic fetuses had values in zone 2 of the Liley curve and would therefore have been misdiagnosed. Subsequent to this investigation, many centers abandoned amniocentesis as a useful tool for predicting fetal disease. At the authors' center, both amniocentesis and PUBS are used in the treatment algorithm (Figure 84.1). Patients are followed with monthly titers until a critical titer of 16 is reached. If a heterozygous paternal genotype for the involved antigen is noted, PUBS is offered to determine the fetal blood type. In cases of a homozygous paternal genotype or a fetus found to be positive for the red cell antigen at the initial PUBS, serial umbilical blood samplings to determine the fetal hematocrit or serial amniocentesis to determine ΔA_{450} values can be undertaken, depending upon gestational age. Invasive testing is repeated at 2-week intervals until a fetal hematocrit of less than 30% or a A_{450} value at the 80th percentile of zone 2 of the Liley curve is noted. Intrauterine transfusion is then undertaken.

84.4 Treatment and outcome

84.4.1 TREATMENT

A variety of unsuccessful treatments have been attempted to reduce the maternal antibody level in patients with red cell alloimmunization. These include plasmapheresis and the oral administration of promethazine and Rh-positive red cell fragments [36–38]. The maternal administration of large doses of pooled intravenous immunoglobulin has achieved some success in one report [39].

The only truly effective treatment for hemolytic disease of the fetus has been the intrauterine transfusion. In 1963, Liley [40] introduced the technique of intraperitoneal transfusion (IPT). This remained the only method of transfusion until 1982. In that year, Bang, Bock and Trolle described the use of umbilical cord puncture under ultrasound guidance to perform the first intravascular transfusion (IVT). Since that time, both simple and exchange intravascular methods have been proposed as the optimal technique for fetal transfusion. Although most centers use the umbilical vein as the source of access to the fetal circulation, such diverse sites as the fetal left ventricle and the intrahepatic portion of the umbilical vein have been described. After the introduction of the IVT, the IPT was virtually abandoned. The new intravascular approach appeared to be a major technical advancement. An actual measure of fetal disease could be determined, the hematocrit. In addition, red blood cells could be administered directly into the fetal circulation. In a comparative study between fetuses treated with IVT and matched historical controls treated with IPT, Harman et al. [42] demonstrated a marked improvement in the survival of the hydropic fetus treated with IVT. Survival in the non-hydropic fetus was not clearly improved by IVT.

Despite its advantages, complications such as umbilical cord hematoma, fetal bradycardia and porencephalic cysts not previously described in fetuses treated with IPT have been reported after IVT [27,28,43]. In addition, analysis of serial hematocrits from fetuses transfused with IVT techniques reveal wide swings between transfusions. We evaluated a combined IPT/IVT transfusion method and found it to result in a more stable hematocrit between procedures than either the exchange or direct IVT [44]. In addition, a combined transfusion technique allows for longer intervals between transfusions. Our transfusion technique involves administering enough packed red cells to achieve a final fetal hematocrit of 35–40%. An IPT is

then performed (volume of blood to be transfused (ml) = (gestational age in weeks − 20) × 10). An intravenous dose of vecuronium (0.1 mg/kg of ultrasound estimated fetal weight) is given at the start of the IVT, producing immediate cessation of fetal movement that lasts 1–2 hours. This eliminates troublesome fetal movement during the procedure that may result in fetal injury. Transfusions are undertaken at 2-week intervals for the first two transfusions: the interval is lengthened to 3–4 weeks thereafter.

The end-point of intrauterine transfusion is subject to debate among therapists. Most centers use a target hematocrit to decide when to complete a transfusion. Advocates of direct IVT will usually transfuse to a final fetal hematocrit of 50–65%, whereas advocates of the combined transfusion technique will use 35–40% as a final value. The hydropic or severely anemic fetus that presents early in the second trimester does not appear to tolerate an IVT as well as an older or less severely affected fetus. A post-transfusion increase in fetal hematocrit by more than four-fold or an increase in umbilical venous pressure of greater than 10 mmHg have both been associated with a marked increased in mortality in this subgroup of fetuses [45,46]. For this reason, we transfuse these fetuses to a final fetal hematocrit of 20–25% at the first IVT. A second transfusion is then performed 48 hours later to achieve a final hematocrit of 35%.

When to deliver the fetus undergoing intrauterine transfusions is also a source of continued debate. When IPTs were used as the sole means of in utero therapy, fetuses were routinely delivered at 32 weeks' gestation. Hyaline membrane disease and the need for neonatal exchange transfusions for the treatment of hyperbilirubinemia were common. As experience with IVT became widespread, pregnancies were delivered at later gestational ages. Most authorities will now perform the final transfusion at 35 weeks' gestation with delivery anticipated at 37–38 weeks.

In the past, O-negative, cytomegalovirus (CMV)-negative, heterologous red blood cells were used as the primary source of blood for intrauterine transfusion. Patient concern regarding the transmission of the human immunodeficiency virus has led several centers to use maternal blood for intrauterine transfusion. Advantages include the availability of fresh blood and the decreased chance for sensitization to new red cell antigens if some of the transfused blood escapes back into the maternal circulation. With folate and iron supplementation, these young patients are easily able to maintain an adequate hemoglobin level [47]. Routine donor screening for the various infectious agents should be employed. The red cells are washed to remove the offending antibody and tightly packed to achieve a final hematocrit of 75–85%. The unit is then filtered through a leukocyte-poor filter and irradiated with

25 Gy of external beam radiation to prevent graft-versus-host reaction. If the mother is positive for CMV antibody, the blood may still be used as the dormant CMV virus resides in the white blood cells that have been removed by the filtering process. On some occasions an ABO incompatibility may be detected between the mother and her fetus after the initial cordocentesis. In these cases, maternal blood should not be used secondary to the risk of sensitization of the fetus.

84.4.2   OUTCOME

A survival rate after IVT of up to 96% has been reported by at least one center [48]. A more realistic statistic can be gleaned from a survey of 1087 intravascular transfusions (389 fetuses) performed at 16 centers in the USA and Canada [29]. The survival rate for non-hydropic fetuses was 90%, while survival of hydropic fetuses was 82%.

Immediate follow-up studies of infants treated with IVTs in utero have revealed a need for 'top up' transfusions in the early weeks of life in as many as 50% of cases [49]. The exact mechanism for this depressed hematopoiesis has yet to be determined. Since these infants do not require exchange transfusions in the immediate neonatal period, the passively acquired maternal antibody remains elevated in the neonatal circulation for at least 6 weeks. One of the predominant theories conjectures that high levels of anti-D cause lysis of reticulocytes in the bone marrow. Because of this phenomenon, weekly hematocrit and reticulocyte determinations are recommended for the first 1–2 months of life in these infants [50]. One proposed criterion for transfusion includes a hemoglobin of less than 5–6 g/dl in the symptom-free infant [50]. In addition, any infant with symptoms related to anemia, such as poor weight gain, lethargy or feeding difficulties, should be transfused [50].

Although previous studies regarding the developmental outcome of infants who had undergone IPTs for severe anemia have shown no major deficits, long-term follow-up studies of infants after IVT have not been reported to date [51].

84.5   Future therapy

It is doubtful that fetal survival can be improved much beyond that now achieved with ultrasound-guided IVT. Future therapy for red cell alloimmunization will probably involve selective suppression of the maternal B-lymphocyte cell line that produces the offending red cell antibody. Such therapy would make invasive therapy unnecessary except in the moribund fetus.

Another option for the sensitized patient with a heterozygous paternal genotype may involve the use of in vitro fertilization. The cloning of the Rh gene on the first chromosome will allow for blastocyst biopsy to be employed to determine the blood type of the developing embryo [52]. Only Rh-negative embryos would then be transferred back into the uterus, guaranteeing an unaffected infant.

Such therapies will prove useful since it is unlikely that red cell alloimmunization in pregnancy will ever be totally eliminated despite the widespread use of prophylactic immunoglobulin.

References

1. American College of Obstetricians and Gynecologists (1986) Management of Isoimmunization in Pregnancy (ACOG Technical Bulletin 90), ACOG, Washington, DC.
2. Bowman, J. (1989) Maternal blood group immunization, in Maternal-Fetal Medicine: Principles and Practice, 2nd edn (eds R.K. Creasy and R. Resnik), W.B. Saunders, Philadelphia, pp. 613–49.
3. Bowman, J., Chown, B., Lewis, M. and Pollock, J. (1978) Rh isoimmunization during pregnancy: antenatal prophylaxis. Can. Med. Assoc. J., 118, 623–27.
4. American College of Obstetricians and Gynecologists (1984) Prevention of Rho (D) Isoimmunization (ACOG Technical Bulletin 79), ACOG, Washington, DC.
5. Chavéz, G., Mulinare, J. and Edmonds, L. (1991) Epidemiology of Rh hemolytic disease of the newborn in the United States. JAMA, 265, 3270–74.
6. Solola, A., Sibai, B. and Mason, J. (1983) Irregular antibodies: an assessment of routine prenatal screening. Obstet. Gynecol., 61, 25–30.
7. Daffos, F., Capella-Pavlovsky, M. and Forestier, F. (1983) A new procedure for fetal blood sampling in utero: preliminary results of fifty-three cases. Am. J. Obstet. Gynecol., 146, 985–87.
8. Leduc, L., Moise, K., Carpenter, J. and Cano, L. (1990) Fetoplacental blood volume estimation in pregnancies with Rh alloimmunization. Fetal Diagn. Ther., 5, 138–46.
9. Nicolaides, K., Thilaganathan, B. and Mibashan, R. (1989) Cordocentesis in the investigation of fetal erythropoiesis. Am. J. Obstet. Gynecol., 161, 1197–2000.
10. Nicolaides, K., Thilaganathan, B., Rodeck, C. and Mibashan, R. (1988) Erythroblastosis and reticulocytosis in anemic fetuses. Am. J. Obstet. Gynecol., 159, 1063–65.
11. Thilaganathan, B., Salvesen, D., Abbas, A. et al. (1992) Fetal plasma erythropoietin concentration in red cell-isoimmunized pregnancies. Am. J. Obstet. Gynecol., 167, 1292–97.
12. Westergen, M., Selbing, A., Stangenberg, M. and Phillips, R. (1989) Acid–base status in fetal heart blood in erythroblastic fetuses: a study with special reference to the effect of transfusions with adult blood. Am. J. Obstet. Gynecol., 160, 1134–38.
13. Copel, J., Grannum, P., Green, J. et al. (1989) Fetal cardiac output in the isoimmunized pregnancy: a pulsed Doppler-echocardiographic study of patients undergoing intravascular intrauterine transfusion. Am. J. Obstet., Gynecol. 161, 361–65.
14. Soothill, P., Lestas, A., Nicolaides, K. et al. (1988) 2,3-Disphosphoglycerate in normal, anemic and transfused human fetuses. Clin. Sci., 74, 527–30.
15. Thorpe-Beeston, J., Nicolaides, K., Snijders, R. and Felton, C. (1990) Thyroid function in anemic fetuses. Fetal Diagn. Ther., 5, 109–13.
16. Diamond, L., Blackfan, K. and Baty, J. (1932) Erythroblastosis fetalis and its association with universal edema of the fetus, icterus gravis neonatorum and anemia of the newborn. J. Pediatr., 1, 269–309.
17. Bowman, J. (1978) The management of Rh-isoimmunization. Obstet. Gynecol., 52, 1–16.
18. Moise, K., Carpenter, R. and Hesketh, D. (1992) Do abnormal Starling forces cause fetal hydrops in red cell alloimmunization? Am. J. Obstet. Gynecol., 167, 907–12.
19. Brace, R. (1989) Effects of outflow pressure on fetal lymph flow. Am. J. Obstet. Gynecol., 160, 494–97.
20. Weiner, C., Heilskov, J., Pelzer, G. et al. (1989) Normal values for human umbilical venous and amniotic fluid pressures and their alteration by fetal disease. Am. J. Obstet. Gynecol., 161, 714–17.
21. Blair, D., Vander Straten, M. and Gest, A. (1992) Edema occurs in anemic

fetal sheep when central venous pressure is increased. *Pediatr. Res.*, **31**, 193A.

22. Nicolaides, K., Fontanarosa, M., Gabbe, S. and Rodeck, C. (1988) Failure of ultrasonographic parameters to predict the severity of fetal anemia in rhesus isoimmunization. *Am. J. Obstet. Gynecol.*, **158**, 920–26.

23. Vintzileos, A., Campbell, W., Storlazzi, E. *et al.* (1986) Fetal liver ultrasound measurements in isoimmunized pregnancies. *Obstet. Gynecol.*, **68**, 162–67.

24. Roberts, A., Mitchell, J. and Pattison, N. (1989) Fetal liver length in normal and isoimmunized pregnancies. *Am. J. Obstet. Gynecol.*, **161**, 42–46.

25. Rightmire, D., Nicolaides, K., Rodeck, C. and Campbell, S. (1986) Fetal blood velocities in Rh isoimmunization: relationship to gestational age and to fetal hematocrit. *Obstet. Gynecol.*, **68**, 233–36.

26. Copel, J., Grannum, P., Belanger, K. *et al.* (1988) Pulsed Doppler flow–velocity waveforms before and after intrauterine intravascular transfusion for severe erythroblastosis fetalis. *Am. J. Obstet. Gynecol.*, **158**, 768–74.

27. Moise, K., Carpenter, R., Huhta, J. and Deter, R. (1987) Umbilical cord hematoma secondary to *in utero* intravascular transfusion for Rh isoimmunization. *Fetal Ther.*, **2**, 65–70.

28. Benacerraf, B., Barss, V., Saltzman, D. *et al.* (1987) Acute fetal distress associated with percutaneous umbilical blood sampling. *Am. J. Obstet. Gynecol.*, **156**, 1218–20.

29. Proceedings of the Fourth International Conference on Percutaneous Fetal Umbilical Blood Sampling, October, 1989, Philadelphia, PA.

30. Nicolini, U., Kochenour, N., Greco, P. *et al.* (1988) Consequences of fetomaternal haemorrhage after intrauterine transfusion. *BMJ*, **297**, 1379–81.

31. MacGregor, S., Silver, R. and Sholl, J. (1991) Enhanced sensitization after cordocentesis in a rhesus-isoimmunized pregnancy. *Am. J. Obstet. Gynecol.*, **165**, 382–3.

32. Bevis, D. (1956) Blood pigments in haemolytic disease of the newborn. *J. Obstet. Gynaecol. Br. Commonw.*, **63**, 68–75.

33. Liley, A. (1961) Liquor amnii analysis in the management of the pregnancy complicated by rhesus sensitization. *Am. J. Obstet. Gynecol.*, **82**, 1359–70.

34. Nicolaides, K., Rodeck, C., Mibashan, R. and Kemp, J. (1986) Have Liley charts outlived their usefulness? *Am. J. Obstet. Gynecol.*, **155**, 90–94.

35. Moise, K.J., Carpenter, R.J. and Milam, J.D. (1987) Changing trends in the diagnosis and treatment of Rh alloimmunization. *Tex. Med.*, **83**, 27–32.

36. Graham-Pole, J., Barr, W. and Wiloughby, M. (1977) Continuous-flow plasmapheresis in management of severe rhesus disease. *BMJ*, **i**, 1185–88.

37. Gudson, J. and Witherow, C. (1973) Possible ameliorating effects of erythroblastosis by promethazine hydrochloride. *Am. J. Obstet. Gynecol.*, **117**, 1101–108.

38. Gold, W., Queenan, J., Woody, J. and Sacher, R. (1983) Oral desensitization in Rh disease. *Am. J. Obstet. Gynecol.*, **146**, 980–81.

39. Margulies, M., Voto, L., Mathet, E. and Margulies, M. (1991) High-dose intravenous IgG for the treatment of severe rhesus alloimmunization. *Vox Sang.*, **61**, 181–89.

40. Liley, A. (1963) Intrauterine transfusion of foetus in haemolytic disease. *BMJ*, **2**, 1107–109.

41. Bang, J., Bock, J. and Trolle, D. (1982) Ultrasound-guided fetal intravenous transfusion for severe rhesus haemolytic disease. *BMJ*, **284**, 373–74.

42. Harman, C., Bowman, J., Manning, F. and Menticoglou, S. (1990) Intrauterine transfusion – intraperitoneal versus intravascular approach: a case-control comparison. *Am. J. Obstet. Gynecol.*, **162**, 1053–59.

43. Didly, G., Smith, L., Moise, K. *et al.* (1991) Porencephalic cyst: a complication of fetal intravascular transfusion. *Am. J. Obstet. Gynecol.*, **165**, 76–78.

44. Moise, K., Carpenter, R., Kirshon, B. *et al.* (1989) Comparison of four types of intrauterine transfusion: effect on fetal hematocrit. *Fetal Ther.*, **4**, 126–37.

45. Radunovic, N., Lockwood, C., Alvarez, M. *et al.* (1992) The severely anemic and hydropic isoimmune fetus: changes in fetal hematocrit associated with intrauterine death. *Obstet. Gynecol.*, **79**, 390–93.

46. Hallak, M., Moise, K., Hesketh, D. *et al.* (1992) Intravascular transfusion of fetuses with rhesus incompatibility: prediction of fetal outcome by changes in umbilical venous pressure. *Obstet. Gynecol.*, **8**, 1–5.

47. Gonsulin, W., Moise, K., Milam, J. *et al.* (1990) Serial maternal blood donations for intrauterine transfusion. *Obstet. Gynecol.*, **75**, 158–62.

48. Weiner, C., Williamson, R., Wenstrom, K. *et al.* (1991) Management of fetal hemolytic disease by cordocentesis II. Outcome of treatment. *Am. J. Obstet. Gynecol.*, **165**, 1302–307.

49. Saade, G., Moise, K., Belfort, M. *et al.* (1993) Fetal and neonatal hematologic parameters in red cell alloimmunization: predicting the need for late neonatal transfusions. *Fetal Diagn. Ther.*, **8**, 161–64.

50. Millard, D., Gidding, S., Socol, M. *et al.* (1990) Effects of intravascular, intrauterine transfusion on prenatal and postnatal hemolysis and erythropoiesis in severe fetal isoimmunization. *J. Pediatr.*, **117**, 447–54.

51. White, C., Goplerud, C., Kisker, C. *et al.* (1978) Intrauterine fetal transfusion, 1965–1976, with an assessment of the surviving children. *Am. J. Obstet. Gynecol.*, **130**, 933–42.

52. Kim, C., Mouro, I., Chérif-Zahar, B. *et al.* (1992) Molecular cloning and primary structure of the human blood group RhD polypeptide. *Proc. Natl Acad. Sci. USA*, **89**, 10925–29.

85 DIRECT FETAL THERAPY

D. Maxwell and P. Johnson

85.1 Introduction

Developments in fetal therapy over the past 10 years have been technology led and consequent upon advances in prenatal diagnosis. The expanded range of conditions amenable to diagnosis has sometimes created an artificial pressure to attempt prenatal therapy. The ideal sequel of treatment following diagnosis has led to therapeutic attempts which have sometimes been opportunistic and unstructured. Therapy has not always predated knowledge of the underlying pathophysiology and natural history.

In addition, therapeutic attempts centralized in referral centres have been hampered by the difficulties that patients face in travel or accessing appropriate facilities. The appropriate medical care for pregnant women who carry a fetus with malformation is undeniable, but therapy for the fetus is frequently regarded as an academic or research activity. The issue has been further clouded by the inability of health care systems to accept therapies that are innovative or unproven, but are not research techniques.

85.1.1 AIMS

The aims of fetal therapy can be considered under the following headings.

- To provide supportive therapy for an ongoing process which is capable of being ameliorated *in utero*, until the fetus is mature enough to be delivered and the condition definitively treated.
- To provide therapy which is specific for an *in utero* condition and where the *in utero* therapy mimics the *ex utero* treatment.
- To provide therapy which is aimed at the treatment of a primary condition in order to prevent, reverse or minimize its secondary deleterious effects.
- To provide *in utero* therapy where expectant management would make *ex utero* treatment poor or impossible due to advanced disease.
- To avoid/minimize the need for postnatal therapy.

These concepts are arbitrary, overlap, are not exhaustive for all fetal conditions, and are meant as an attempt to understand what prenatal therapy has tried to achieve.

85.2 Therapeutic methods

In order to fulfil the perceived clinical need, the repertoire of fetal therapy has widened considerably since the pioneering work of Liley in 1963. Methods can be described under three broad technical approaches.

1. Maternal transplacental therapy
2. Open uterus surgery
3. Closed uterus procedures:
   (a) ultrasound-guided techniques:
       (i) simple aspiration
       (ii) fetal shunting
       (iii) fetal injection
       (iv) prenatal infusion
       (v) fetal balloon valvoplasty;
   (b) direct vision techniques.

Maternal transplacental therapy and open uterus surgery are considered elsewhere in the text and will not be considered in this section.

85.2.1 CLOSED UTERUS TECHNIQUES

Imaging by ultrasound or endoscopy is the foundation of therapy in this area and both techniques have been successfully applied across a wide spectrum of fetal conditions. Maternal morbidity is minimal and the risks of premature labour are less by comparison with open uterus surgery. Closed uterus techniques will form the focus for the remainder of this chapter. A definitive exploration of all management options will not be attempted: attention will be focused on how the techniques have been utilized and current favoured options.

Diseases of the Fetus and Newborn, 2nd edn, Edited by G.B. Reed, A.E. Claireaux and F. Cockburn. Published in 1995 by Chapman & Hall, London. ISBN 0 412 39160 0

85.3 Ultrasound-guided therapies

Using high-resolution ultrasound, it is possible to place a needle or cannula with precision at, in or on almost any anatomical point within the uterine cavity. The method most frequently adopted is a free-hand ultrasound-guided approach [1]. The ultrasound transducer is held in one hand, and the needle in the other. With due care to avoid sepsis and after local anaesthesia if desired, the needle is advanced under continuous vision through the maternal skin and uterine wall and on to the chosen site. Alternatively, a needle-guided approach can be used [2]. The methodology described by Daffos, Capella-Pavlovsky and Forestier [1] fostered the very rapid application of an ultrasound-guided approach to therapeutic attempts and is recognized as the contribution which provided the turning point away from fetoscopic techniques.

Once in position, the needle becomes a simple conduit able to be utilized for numerous diagnostic and therapeutic purposes. In general, the access gained can be used for aspiration or as a delivery system for therapeutic agents, including blood, drugs or mechanical devices.

85.3.1 ASPIRATION

The most straightforward application of an aspiration technique is that of amniocentesis. Performed at any gestation, it is the gold standard test for karyotyping. Further standard applications include the assessment from 18 weeks of the severity of haemolytic disorder *in utero* and estimation of fetal lung maturity in late pregnancy.

When the needle is positioned in the intravascular compartment, pure fetal blood can be aspirated. Normal ranges exist for a wide variety of fetal haematological [3,4] and biochemical [5,6] parameters, allowing the fetal status to be explored in almost the same detail as the newborn. The fetal karyotype can be determined from circulating lymphocytes within 48–72 hours, forming an integral part of most assessments. Knowledge of the fetal chromosomal status is frequently essential to allow accurate counselling prior to determining the applicability of therapy. Intravascular sites amenable to sampling include the placental and fetal insertion of the umbilical cord, free loops, the intrahepatic vein and the fetal heart. Choice of site and attendant complications are dealt with elsewhere in this text. Diagnostic purposes normally require only 0.5–2 ml of blood, depending on gestational age and the range of investigations required.

This inherently simple technique can also be used to aspirate fluid-filled spaces or cystic areas in the fetus for specific therapeutic purposes. These applications can be considered for each organ system.

(a) Central nervous system

The fetal central nervous system was amongst the first thought amenable to *in utero* treatment. Initial attempts at *in utero* decompression of fetal hydrocephalus were by serial drainage [7,8]. The limitations of this approach led to the implantation of valved ventriculoamniotic shunts to provide continuing drainage [8,9]. Earlier attempts did not adhere to uniform selection criteria and the results, though difficult to assess, were apparently disappointing. Neither procedure is presently performed as therapy, although considerable research has been performed in the interim [10].

(b) Respiratory system

Cyst aspiration has been used in the management of congenital cystic adenomatoid malformation of the lung (CCAML). In a suspected case of multilocular CCAML with associated mediastinal shift and ascites, aspiration was performed at 27 weeks [11]. The mediastinal structures returned to the midline and the ascites lessened. By 30 weeks the cyst had resumed its original size, polyhydramnios had developed and the ascites increased. Further aspiration was performed and although the cyst did reaccumulate, the ascites and polyhydramnios resolved. The fetus was delivered at 35 weeks, but died at day 20 after surgery. Unsuspected microscopic CCAML was later discovered in the other lung. Other successful attempts at aspiration have been performed on unilocular cysts [12,13]; however, both of these did have transthoracic shunts inserted subsequently. In one case, a single aspiration at 28 weeks resulted in minimal reaccumulation with no further need for therapy *in utero* [14].

The precise role of this type of intervention in the prenatal treatment of CCAML remains undefined. Single or even repeated aspirations do not seem to prevent fluid reaccumulation. They may, however, reduce mediastinal shift, avoiding the need for more invasive therapy or premature delivery. Careful consideration of treatment aims in individual cases is essential.

Fetal pleural effusions have also been treated with drainage by thoracocentesis. It is notable that resolution has occurred spontaneously without treatment, or following single and repeated drainage procedures [15]. In most cases, the fluid reaccumulates within 24 hours and, on balance, evidence would favour pleuroamniotic shunting as the definitive treatment of choice [16–18]. It seems clear that outcomes are most dependent on the variables such as gestational age at delivery, presence or absence of hydrops and antenatal therapy. Management should take these factors into account. An initial assessment of these cases requires karyotyping. As part of this initial assessment, simple aspiration may avoid further therapy in a limited number of cases.

(c) Genitourinary system

The insertion of vesicoamniotic shunts in the fetus can provide definitive relief in the management of lower urinary tract obstruction [19]. The selection of cases appropriate for an *in utero* procedure involves exclusion of accompanying abnormality, karyotyping and knowledge of renal function. The assessment of renal function by inference from liquor volume and the ultrasound appearance of the kidneys is unreliable [20] and has been augmented by aspiration of bladder urine [21,22]. Examination of fetal urine biochemistry has been used to exclude cases in which renal function is thought non-salvageable and to predict those cases where vesicoamniotic shunts might prevent renal deterioration if the fetus is not mature. There is still no universal agreement on the criteria to be met prior to intervention [23,24].

Considerable attention has focused on the best use of the technique of ultrasound-guided bladder tapping. In some cases a single aspiration has proved successful in relieving the underlying cause. 'Poor function' and 'good function' groups have been established [21,22,25] dependent upon the absolute levels of sodium, chloride, osmolality and more recently β_2-microglobulin [26], although it may be important to remember that fetal urine electrolytes vary with gestational age [27]. In addition, rather than rely on a single spot urine sample, serial aspirations may prove superior in establishing prognosis [28]. Biochemistry, which was considered suboptimal on the first tap, improved after decompression, indicating an unsuspected functional reserve. Further evaluation of this approach is awaited with interest.

The criticisms of early cephalocentesis can also be applied to drainage of lower urinary tract obstruction [23,24]. However, with robust evaluation of the biochemical parameters mentioned, greater rigour can be applied to case selection and a consensus would now favour intervention for lower tract obstruction. A similar consensus has not been reached in cases of upper tract obstruction [29].

Central reporting, pooling of data and the ability to be able to evaluate results internationally are fundamental to structured advance in this area.

(d) Intra-abdominal cysts

It is technically possible prenatally to aspirate intra-abdominal cysts diagnosed in fetal life. However, caution should be exercised and the procedure must have a clearly stated therapeutic aim. A fetal intrarenal cyst has been drained with subsequent resolution of associated polyhydramnios and threatened premature labour [30]. In addition, ovarian cysts have been drained *in utero* in a number of cases. In one, developing cardiac failure resolved following drainage and, in an innovative step, sclerosant was introduced into the cyst cavity to prevent recurrence [31]. The necessity for such procedures seems infrequent, the indications generally being deleterious secondary effects on other organ systems.

The dangers of ill-considered intervention have been documented by Purkiss, Brereton and Wright [32], highlighting the need for a multidisciplinary team evaluation before *in utero* treatment.

(e) Fetal tumours

The correct method of delivery in the presence of structural malformation is often controversial. *In utero* intervention in selected cases has allowed an expansion of the available management options. A cystic sacrococcygeal teratoma has been decompressed at 38 weeks' gestation to allow vaginal delivery [33]. A total of 2.75 litres were withdrawn on two consecutive days with substantial reduction in the size of the lesion. Labour was then induced with subsequent normal delivery of a liveborn child with good Apgar scores. Difficulty can also be anticipated at caesarean section in such cases, which may be lessened by drainage prior to operation. Management must be tailored to the needs of individual cases.

Simple aspiration has also been applied in the acute management of an intrapericardial teratoma at 34 weeks' gestation [34]. The associated pericardial effusion had rapidly increased in size over the course of 1 week, threatening cardiac tamponade. Pericardiocentesis was performed with reversion of cardiac function to normal. The effusion did not reaccumulate to the same degree and the fetus was delivered by caesarean section at 37 weeks' gestation. Good neonatal outcome after surgery was obtained.

(f) Amniotic fluid

Drainage of amniotic fluid in pregnancies complicated by polyhydramnios has the clinical purpose of reducing maternal discomfort and potentially reducing the change of preterm labour. At Guy's Hospital, we have recorded the intra-amniotic pressure in 14 such cases (P. Johnson and D.J. Maxwell, unpublished data). The measurements were made at the time of fetal blood sampling and the methods previously described [35]. Four cases had pressures above the 95th centile for gestation and the other ten were within our reference range. The existence of high and normal pressure groups in pregnancies complicated by polyhydramnios confirms the findings of earliers workers [36]. The diagnosis to delivery intervals appeared greater in the normal pressure group. In seven cases in our series, drainage of liquor was performed to alleviate maternal discomfort. In all cases, intra-amniotic pressure was lessened, regardless of the volume aspirated. In one case in the high pressure and one in the normal pressure group, the polyhydramnios resolved. A further case with pressure in the normal range resolved spontaneously. Unfortunately, the small number of cases and variation in underlying fetal disorder precluded any statement of clinical relevance. It is open to speculation that the finding of a raised pressure may help to predict those cases most at risk of premature labour [37].

85.3.2 FETAL SHUNTING

These procedures are discussed in detail elsewhere in this text and will not be considered further in this section (Chapter 86).

85.3.3 INJECTION

A veritable pharmacopoeia has become established for the purpose of fetal treatment. Intramuscular or intravascular injection of agents are used to immobilize the fetus during therapy [38,39], or to resuscitate it if cardiorespiratory arrest has occurred during an invasive procedure. These agents include pancuronium, diazepam, adrenaline, atropine, isoprenaline and calcium infusion [40,41].

The most usual method of prenatal treatment of fetal atrial tachycardia is by maternal transplacental drug therapy [42,43]. In addition, direct fetal administration of a variety of injectables has been utilized in cases refractory to maternal treatment. Drugs administered include digoxin, verapamil, amiodarone, propafenone and flecainide [42,43]. All choices of route have been utilized; intravascular, intramuscular and intraperitoneal. We have most recently administered adenosine via the placental cord insertion and directly into the right ventricle, achieving conversion in a case of fetal supraventricular tachycardia with accompanying hydrops (Chapter 54).

The intra-amniotic route has been employed in the treatment of fetal thyroid goitre. Following ultrasound diagnosis, thyroid function was assessed by amniocentesis at 23 weeks' gestation and then by fetal blood sampling at 27 weeks. Intra-amniotic L-thyroxine [44] administration was performed at 35 weeks to reduce goitre size and avoid dystocia at delivery and possible neonatal respiratory distress. Hormone supplementation following delivery allowed normal development to the age of 2 years at follow-up. Repeated intra-amniotic administration of thyroxine [45], resulting in successful treatment of fetal hypothyroidism, has also been reported.

85.3.4 INFUSION

A wide variety of infusion mediums have been utilized.

(a) Blood transfusion

Treatment of fetal haemolytic disease secondary to maternal alloimmunization provides the best illustration of successful intrauterine therapy. Following Liley's [46] introduction of the intraperitoneal infusion of rhesus-negative donor blood, the technique remained largely unchanged until 1974 when the fetoscope was utilized [47,48]. This new approach provided direct access to the fetal circulation and allowed detailed assessment of fetal haematology. Free-hand ultrasound-guided needling of the umbilical cord provided the next stimulus to development [1,49]. There are numerous excellent accounts of the application of this technique for intravascular and intraperitoneal infusion [50–54]. The transfusion methodology has been simplified and procedure times drastically reduced, with excellent neonatal outcomes. For intravascular transfusion, the placental insertion of the umbilical cord is most frequently utilized, although the intraheptic vein has its advocates [55]. Direct intracardiac transfusion has also been performed [56] (Chapter 84).

At Guy's Hospital, all patients referred for the investigation and management of a pregnancy complicated by red cell antibodies are managed in the affiliated Rhesus Unit at Lewisham Hospital. The Fetal Medicine Unit at Guy's and the Rhesus Unit at Lewisham are under the same management with the same staff. Management protocols in both are identical. In addition, the clinics are attended by a neonatologist and a haematologist. Consistently between 90 and 100 new tertiary referrals are seen per annum. From July 1988, ultrasound guided intravascular transfusion has largely replaced the intraperitoneal technique as the mainstay of treatment. In the 4 years to 1 August 1992, a total of 134 transfusions were performed on 48 patients. One hundred and five were intravascular, 19 were intraperitoneal and combined intravascular and intraperitoneal transfusions were performed in a further 10 cases. Of the 48 patients, 34 have had successful pregnancies resulting in a living child.

In utero transfusion has also been utilized in the treatment of hydrops fetalis secondary to fetomaternal haemorrhage [57] and fetal anaemia following parvovirus B19 infection [58].

(b) Platelet infusion

The underlying principle of treatment based on direct fetal evaluation has been applied to the management of congenital thrombocytopenia [59]. In alloimmune disease, therapy aims to identify those fetuses most at risk of antenatal and perinatal intracranial haemorrhage. Cordocentesis provides an exact measure of fetal platelet count, allowing prelabour decision-making with regard to the most appropriate method of delivery. Unnecessary operative measures can be avoided. In addition, platelet transfusion prior to delivery may allow a safer attempt at vaginal delivery.

Earlier in pregnancy, fetal thrombocytopenia may prompt consideration of the need for a weekly series of platelet transfusions as prophylaxis against cerebral haemorrhage [60]. Alternatively, a maternal treatment programme of intravenous immunoglobulin with or without steroids can be implemented [61]. This can be backed up by cordocentesis later in pregnancy to confirm a satisfactory fetal platelet response. The correct choice of management remains unclear [62–64]. The intensive nature and risk of serial platelet transfusions cannot be overstated, outlining the difficulty of management choice. In considering therapy, the fetal platelet count, severity of disease in previously affected neonates and gestational age at referral are important variables.

(c) **Electrolyte infusion**

Amnioinfusion involves the instillation of warmed electrolyte solution into the amniotic cavity in an attempt to replenish liquor volume in cases of oligohydramnios or anhydramnios [65]. In these circumstances, the underlying aetiology may be unclear from history and examination and optimal ultrasound viewing can be difficult or impossible. The infusion of even relatively small volumes of fluid (40–100 ml) will generally create a more favourable environment in which to image fetal structure. Furthermore, the addition of a sweetening agent to the infusion has been claimed to promote fetal swallowing, allowing the stomach and bladder to be visualized when they are present. The authors have found amnioinfusion to be particularly useful in the investigation of suspected fetal renal disease. Optimal viewing conditions are best obtained a few hours after the instillation, when microbubbles have had time to dissipate. A dye added to the infusion is helpful in the diagnosis of unsuspected midtrimester rupture of membranes.

Therapeutically, creation of an artificial liquor environment has been claimed to minimize lung hypoplasia related to the reduced amniotic fluid [66]. This requires repeated infusions on a regular basis for many weeks. Hitherto limited accounts of the success of this technique do not constitute a firm foundation for its clinical value [67,68].

Amnioinfusion has been used antepartum in cases of preterm prelabour rupture of membranes [69] and also intrapartum to relieve cord compression [70–72] or achieve a dilutional effect in cases of meconium-stained liquor [73–75]. Such instances of therapy are considered beyond the scope of this chapter but have been well reviewed [76].

In a further application, the instillation of saline directly into the fetal peritoneal cavity has proved beneficial in enhancing visualization of intra-abdominal organs where other measures had failed [77].

85.3.5 BALLOON VALVOPLASTY

Critical aortic stenosis (CAS) in infants carries a high mortality irrespective of treatment modality. When the condition has been diagnosed in fetal life, the outlook is hopeless. In a series of 12 cases diagnosed prenatally, there were no survivors despite technically successful postnatal valvoplasty in some [78]. The left ventricle had become so hypoplastic that neonatal therapy was not possible, or progressive severe fibroelastosis had occurred which did not allow the ventricle to support circulation after relief of valvular obstruction.

We have combined the technique of ultrasound guided cannula placement with paediatric balloon valvoplasty in the management of fetal CAS. The method used has been previously described [40]. In summary, an 18-gauge needle was passed through the maternal abdominal wall and into the amniotic cavity and then into the left ventricle at its apex in line with the aortic root. After removal of the stylette, a steerable wire was passed through the needle and advanced across the aortic valve. A custom-made Numed balloon catheter was passed over the wire into the left ventricle to lie within the valve ring. The balloon was inflated to 5 mm within the valvular ring and then withdrawn.

Of two cases of fetal CAS treated by this method, technical success was achieved in both. In the first case, the child survived for 1 month [40] and the second is now well at age 2 years (L.D. Allan and D.J. Maxwell, unpublished data).

Technical difficulties have been considerable. In both cases, portions of the catheter became detached on withdrawal of the assembly. In neither case did this cause fetal or neonatal problems. Bradycardia occurring after inflation of the balloon required treatment with isoprenaline. The correct line of entry is crucial, which can be appreciated when one considers the distance of needle travel, the number of tissue interfaces to be traversed and the tiny size of the aortic ring. A suitable entry path to the cardiac apex can only be obtained when the fetus is thorax uppermost, therefore the procedure is completely dependent on fetal position. Furthermore, the disordered architecture characteristic of CAS makes access to the aortic ring from within the left ventricle more difficult and substantially interferes with ultrasound viewing during the course of the procedure. As with all forms of fetal therapy, robust selection of cases is paramount.

Allied to the development of the fetal balloon valvoplasty has been research directed towards extending knowledge of fetal intravascular and intracardiac pressures. The authors have been able to establish reference ranges for pressures in the umbilical vein and artery, and all four cardiac chambers [35] (P. Johnson and D.J. Maxwell, unpublished data). An elevated end-diastolic pressure in the left ventricle associated with severe endocardial fibroelastosis would suggest unsuitability for *in utero* valvoplasty. This type of therapy underscores the potential of multidisciplinary collaboration.

A further benefit of the pressure manometry technique has been the validation of the cardiothoracic ratio as a non-invasive index of cardiac failure [79].

85.4   Direct vision

Direct endoscopic viewing of the fetus is conceptually attractive. Earliest attempts using an operating fetoscope in the second trimester allowed only a limited visual field with a short focal range. The technique, a significant advance at the time [80], was limited in its utility, difficult to learn and accompanied by a high pregnancy loss rate. Its use in middle pregnancy has now been supplanted by high resolution ultrasound to view the fetus. Fetal blood sampling and fetal tissue sampling can most easily be performed by the ultrasound-guided techniques previously outlined. However, even more recent developments suggest that fetal endoscopy may be about to undergo a resurgence.

Embryoscopy is a procedure which allows viewing of the embryo through an operating hysteroscope passed transcervically under ultrasound control [81,82]. It can then pierce the chorion and allow direct viewing through the amnion. The procedure can be performed from 5 weeks of menstrual age and reliable views can be obtained in more than 90% of cases. We have been able to confirm the excellent views obtained by this technique in a smaller series of cases. Embryonic blood sampling, embryonic tissue biopsy, a detailed study of the yolk sac and perhaps realistic attempts at gene therapy can be contemplated. Indeed, some of these procedures have already been performed and publication of results is awaited (Chapter 66).

The extraordinary advances in miniaturization of instrumentation coupled with refinements in laparoscopic cameras and monitors have led to the emergence of minimally invasive surgery. These techniques have begun to be applied to the fetus. Fetoscopic laser ablation of aberrant placental vasculature in the human [83] and fetoscopic excimer laser surgery in animals [84] have been performed. A multiportal laparoscopic approach to fetal surgery seems an inevitable next step.

85.5   Therapeutic applications

Offering a prognosis in the presence of fetal malformation requires an accurate knowledge of the nature and severity of the condition, its underlying pathophysiology and the natural history *in utero* and following delivery. This will frequently mean referral to a specialized centre, which is to be encouraged. A diligent search for accompanying abnormalities is essential. Karyotyping or other invasive investigative procedures may be necessary in the initial stages and the purpose and risks of these should be explained fully to the parents. Chromosomal status, in particular, may have relevance when discussing future pregnancies. Further vital determinants in considering available options are an accurate knowledge of gestational age plus consideration of potential obstetric problems in later pregnancy.

At the most fundamental level, pregnant women and their partners, when faced with the knowledge of a congenital malformation in a desired pregnancy ask straightforward questions that are remarkably similar irrespective of personal and clinical circumstance.

- What is wrong?
- Is there anything else wrong?
- Why did it happen?
- Will it happen again?
- Can anything be done?

To these questions can be added a further consideration directed at both the patient and her advisers: 'Should anything be done?' The parents have a right to expect honest, simple and, as far as possible, accurate answers to these questions. They expect to reach an informed choice of management, in conjunction with their advisers and in keeping with their own wishes. If therapy is to be considered, a clear outline of the purpose and likely benefit of the procedure is essential. This should be given against the background of previous experience. This explanation must also contain an active consideration of the possible untoward consequences of intervention.

The issues to be considered are frequently complex and mandate the involvement of a multidisciplinary team. At Guy's Hospital, fortnightly meetings are held in the Fetal Medicine Unit at which geneticists, radiologists and the paediatric subspecialities attend. All of the cases are discussed, whether intervention is planned or not. In addition, colleagues from other disciplines regularly demonstrate their commitment to this team approach by coming to the Fetal Medicine Unit to discuss individual cases to counsel parents as soon as the diagnosis has been made. This team approach has not resulted in sharp divisions of opinion between obstetrician and paediatrician, but has rather strengthened the links between the two disciplines. The authors believe that this is the only way in which a fetal diagnostic and treatment programme can function to the full benefit of the fetus and parents.

There is no dedicated medical ethicist on the staff, but the team approach does allow rational discussion of any religious and moral issues. Liberal use of the Hospital Ethical Committee has been made in developing new techniques and, on the few occasions where clinical urgency did not allow this, a 'three wise men' approach has been adopted.

Parents are often not in a frame of mind that is receptive to the assimilation of complicated information. The facts may need to be repeated a number of times, in different ways and on separate occasions. It is prudent to offer a sympathetic contact person who is available to be telephoned for advice and for further follow-up sessions.

The counselling method that is adopted by the authors' team is non-directive and non-judgemental. Frequently, however, the authors are asked to recommend an option or are asked what they would do in similar circumstances. These questions are some of the most difficult to answer. They are generally best dealt with by careful and patient repetition of the essential information. Although never actually recommending a particular option, it is sometimes possible to indicate that the evidence may favour one or other course of action.

85.6 Conclusion

Fetal therapy has much to offer. The options available following the diagnosis of fetal malformation have expanded enormously in recent years. At the core of management is information: information with regard to the condition itself, its associations, the natural history and prognosis if untreated and a clear appraisal of the benefits and risks of intervention. Information needs to be pooled and shared between centres practising in this field. Counselling of the parents should contain neither excessive zeal for unproven therapies nor undue pessimism. Information given to the parents needs to be couched in clear and unambiguous terms so that they can reach what they feel is an informed decision.

Practitioners in this field cannot work in isolation. There are few other fields in medicine where multidisciplinary collaboration has such exciting potential. The dangers in not entering into it are already becoming manifest.

References

1. Daffos, F., Capella-Pavlovsky, M. and Forestier, F. (1983) Fetal blood sampling via the umbilical cord using a needle guided by ultrasound. *Prenat. Diag.*, 3, 271–77.
2. Bovicelli, L., Orsini, L.F., Grannum, P.A.T. *et al.* (1989) A new funipuncture technique: two-needle ultrasound and needle biopsy-guided procedure. *Obstet. Gynecol.*, 73, 428–31.
3. Ludomirsky, A., Weiner, S., Ashmead, G.G. *et al.* (1988) Percutaneous fetal umbilical blood sampling: procedure, safety and normal fetal hematological indices. *Am. J. Perinatol.*, 5, 264–66.
4. Nicolaides, K.H., Thilaganathan, B. and Mibashan, R.S. (1989) Cordocentesis in the investigation of fetal erythropoiesis. *Am. J. Obstet. Gynecol.*, 161, 1197–200.
5. Khoury, A.D., Moretti, M.L., Barton J.R. *et al.* (1991) Fetal blood sampling in patients undergoing elective caesarean section: a correlation with cord blood gas values obtained at delivery. *Am. J. Obstet. Gynecol.*, 165, 1026–29.
6. Thorpe-Beeston, J.G., Nicolaides, K.H., Felton, C.V. *et al.* (1991) Maturation of the secretion of thyroid hormone and thyroid stimulating hormone in the fetus. *N. Engl. J. Med.*, 324, 532–36.
7. Birnholz, J.C. and Frigoletto, F.D. (1981) Antenatal treatment of hydrocephalus. *N. Engl. J. Med.*, 303, 1021–23.
8. Chervenak, F.A., Berkowitz, R.L., Tortora, M. and Hobbins, J.C. (1985) The management of fetal hydrocephalus. *Am. J. Obstet. Gynecol.*, 151, 933–42.
9. Clewell, W.H., Johnson, M.C., Meier, P.R. *et al.* (1982) A surgical approach to fetal hydrocephalus. *N. Engl. J. Med.*, 306, 1320–25.
10. Michejda, M. (1989) Antenatal treatment of central nervous system defects: current and future developments in experimental therapies. *Fetal Ther.*, suppl. 1, 108–31.
11. Chao, A. and Monoson, R.F. (1990) Neonatal death despite fetal therapy for cystic adenomatoid malformation. *J. Reprod. Med.*, 35, 655–57.
12. Clark, S.L., Vitale, D.J., Minton, S.D. *et al.* (1987) Successful fetal therapy for cystic adenomatoid malformation associated with second trimester hydrops. *Am. J. Obstet. Gynecol.*, 157, 294–95.
13. Nicolaides, K.H., Blott, M. and Greenough, A. (1987) Chronic drainage of fetal pulmonary cyst. *Lancet*, i 618.
14. Nugent, C.E., Hayashi, R.H. and Rubin, J. (1989) Prenatal treatment of type I congenital cystic adenomatoid malformation by intrauterine fetal thoracentesis. *J. Clin. Ultrasound*, 17, 675–7.
15. Longaker, M.T., Blaberge, J.M., Danserean, J. *et al.* (1989) Primary fetal hydrothorax: natural history and management. *J. Pediatr. Surg.*, 24, 573–76.
16. Rodeck, C.H., Fisk, N.M., Fraser, D.I. and Nicolini, U. (1988) Longterm in-utero drainage of fetal hydrothorax. *N. Engl. J. Med.*, 319, 1135–38.
17. Nicolaides, K.H. and Azar, G.B. (1990) Thoraco-amniotic shunting. *Fetal Diagn. Ther.*, 5, 153–64.
18. Weber, A.M. and Philipson, E.H. (1992) Fetal pleural effusion: a review and meta-analysis for prognostic indicators. *Obstet. Gynecol.*, 79, 281–86
19. Manning, F.A., Harman, C.R., Lange, I.R. *et al.* (1993) Antepartum chronic fetal vesicoamniotic shunts for obstructive uropathy. *Am. J. Obstet. Gynecol.*, 145, 819–22.
20. Mahoney B.S., Filley, R.A., Callen, P. *et al.* (1984) Sonographic evaluation of fetal renal dysplasia. *Radiology*, 144, 563–68.
21. Glick, P.L., Harrison, M.R., Golbus, M.S. *et al.* (1985) Management of the fetus with congential hydronephrosis. II: Prognostic criteria and selection for treatment. *J. Pediatr. Surg.*, 20, 376–87.
22. Grannum, P.A., Ghidini, A., Scioscia, A. *et al.* (1989) Assessment of fetal renal reserve in low level obstructive uropathy *Lancet*, i, 281–82.
23. Elder, J.S., Duckett, J.W. and Snyder, H.M. (1987) Intervention for fetal obstructive uropathy: has it been effective? *Lancet*, ii, 1007–10.
24. White, R.H.R. (1989) Fetal uropathy. *BMJ*, 298, 1408–9.
25. Crombleholme, T.M., Harrison, M.R., Golbus, M.S. *et al.* (1990) Fetal intervention in obstructive uropathy: prognostic indicators and efficacy of intervention. *Am. J. Obstet. Gynecol.*, 162, 1239–44.
26. Nolte, S., Mueller, B. and Pringshein, W. (1991) Serum alpha-microglobulin and beta-microglobulin for the estimation of fetal glomerular renal function. *Pediatr. Nephrol.*, 5, 573–77.
27. Nicolini, U., Fisk, N.M. and Rodeck, C.H. (1992) Fetal urine biochemistry: an index of renal maturation and dysfunction. *Br. J. Obstet. Gynecol.*, 99, 46–50.
28. Evans, M.I., Sacks A.J., Johnson, M.P. *et al.* (1991) Sequential invasive assessment of fetal renal function and the intrauterine treatment of fetal obstructive uropathies. *Obstet. Gynecol.*, 77, 545–50.
29. Arthur, R.J., Irving, H.C., Thomas, D.F.M. and Watters, J.K. (1989) Bilatering fetal uropathy: what is the outlook? *BMJ*, 298, 1419–20.
30. Broecker, B.H., Redwine, F.O. and Petres, R.E. (1988) Reversal of acute polyhydramnios after fetal renal decompression. *Urology* 31, 60–62.
31. Giorlandino, C., Rivosecchi, M., Bilancioni, E. *et al.* (1990) Successful intrauterine therapy of a large fetal ovarian cyst. *Prenat. Diagn.*, 10, 473–75.
32. Purkiss, S., Brereton, R.J. and Writh, V.M. (1988) Surgical emergencies after prenatal treatment for intra-abdominal abnormality. *Lancet*, i, 289–90.

33. Weston, M.J. and Andrews, H. (1990) Case report: *in utero* aspiration of sacococcygeal cyst. *Clin. Radiol.*, **44**, 119–20.

34. Benatar, A., Vaughan, J., Nicolini, U. *et al.* (1992) Prenatal pericardiocentesis: its role in the management of intrapericardial teratoma. *Obstet. Gynecol.*, **79**, 857–59.

35. Johnson, P. and Maxwell, D.J. (1990) Intrauterine measurement of fetal cardiac pressures. *Contemp. Rev. Obstet. Gynecol.*, **2**, 141–44

36. Caldeyro-Barcia, R., Pose, S.V. and Alvarez, H. (1957) Uterine contractility in polyhydramnios and the effects of withdrawal of the excess amniotic fluid. *Am. J. Obstet. Gynecol.*, **73**, 1238–54.

37. Fisk, N.M., Tannisandorn, Y., Nicolini, V. *et al.* (1990) Amniotic pressure in disorders of amniotic fluid volume. *Obstet. Gynecol.*, **76**, 210–14.

38. De Crespigny, L.C., Robinson, H.P., Quinn, M. *et al.* (1985) Ultrasound guided fetal blood transfusion for severe rhesus isoimmunisation. *Obstet. Gynecol.*, **66**, 529–32.

39. Seeds, J.W., Corke, C. and Spielman, F.J. (1986) Prevention of fetal movement during invasive procedures with pancuronium bromide. *Am. J. Obstet. Gynecol.*, **155**, 818–19.

40. Maxwell, D.J., Allan, L.D. and Tynan, M. (1991) Balloon aortic valvoplasty in the fetus: a report of two cases. *Br. Heart J.* **65**, 256–58.

41. Soothill, P., Kypros, H., Nicolaides, H.K. and Rodeck, C.H. (1987) Invasive techniques for prenatal diagnosis and therapy. *J. Perinat. Med.*, **15**, 117–27.

42. Maxwell, D.J., Crawford, D.C., Curry, P.N. *et al.* (1988) Obstetric importance, diagnosis and management of fetal tachycardias. *BMJ*, **297**, 107–10.

43. Hansmann, M., Gembruck, U., Bald, R. *et al.* (1991) Fetal tachyarrhythmias: transplacental and direct treatment of the fetus – a report of 60 cases. *Ultrasound Obstet. Gynecol.*, **1**, 162–70.

44. Sagot, P., David, A., Yvinec, M. *et al.* (1991) Intrauterine treatment of thyroid goiters. *Fetal Diagn. Ther.*, **6**, 28–33.

45. Davidson, K.M., Richards, D.S., Schatz, D.A. and Fisher, D.A. (1991) Successful *in utero* treatment of fetal goiter and hypothyroidism. *N. Engl. J. Med.*, **324**, 543–46.

46. Liley, A.W. (1963) Intrauterine transfusion of foetus in haemolytic disease. *BMJ*, **ii**, 1107–109.

47. Hobbins, J.C., Mahoney, M.J. and Goldstein, M.A. (1974) New method of intrauterine evaluation by the combined use of fetoscopy and ultrasound. *Am. J. Obstet. Gynecol.*, **118**, 1069–72.

48. Rodeck, C.H., Nicolaides, K.H. and Warsof, S. (1984) The management of severe rhesus isoimmunisation by fetoscopic intravascular transfusions. *Am. J. Obstet. Gynecol.*, **150**, 769–74.

49. Bang, J., Bock, J.E. and Trolle, D. (1982) Ultrasound-guided fetal intravenous transfusion for severe hemolytic disease. *BMJ*, **284**, 373–74.

50. Berkowitz, R.L., Chitkara, U., Goldberg, J.D. *et al.* (1986) Intrauterine intravascular transfusion for severe red blood cell isoimmunisation, ultrasound-guided approach. *Am. J. Obstet. Gynecol.*, **155**, 574–81.

51. Grannum, P.A., Capel, J.A., Plaxe, S.C. *et al.* (1986) *In utero* exchange transfusion by direct intravascular injection in severe erythroblastosis fetalis. *N. Engl. J. Med.*, **314**, 1431–34.

52. Grannum, P.A., Copel, J.A., Moya, F.R. *et al.* (1988) The reversal of hydrops fetalis by intravascular intrauterine transfusion in severe isoimmune fetal anemia. *Am. J. Obstet. Gynecol.*, **158**, 914–19.

53. Westgren, M., Jabbar, F., Larsen, J.F. *et al.* (1988) Introduction of a programme for intravascular transfusions at severe rhesus isoimmunisation. *J. Perinat. Med.*, **16**, 417–22.

54. Pattison, N.S., Roberts, A.B. and Mantell, N. (1992) Intrauterine fetal transfusion 1963–90. *Ultrasound Obstet. Gynecol.*, **2**, 329–32.

55. Nicolini, U., Santolaya, J., Ojo, O.E. *et al.* (1988) The fetal intrahepatic umbilical vein as an alternative to cord needling for prenatal diagnosis and therapy. *Prenat. Diagn.*, **8**, 665–71.

56. Westgren, M., Selbing, M. and Stangenberg, M. (1988) Fetal intracardiac transfusions in patients with severe rhesus isoimmunisation. *BMJ*, **296**, 885–86.

57. Cardwell, M.S. (1988) Successful treatment of hydrops fetalis caused by fetomaternal hemorrhage: a case report. *Am. J. Obstet. Gynecol.*, **158**, 131–32.

58. Peters, M.T. and Nicolaides, K.H. (1990) Cordocentesis for the diagnosis and treatment of human fetal parvovirus infection. *Obstet. Gynecol.*, **75**, 501–504.

59. Kaplan, C., Daffos, F., Forestier, F. *et al.* (1988) Management of alloimmune thrombocytopenia: antenatal diagnosis and *in utero* transfusion of maternal platelets. *Blood*, **72**, 340–43.

60. Nicolini, U., Rodeck, C.H., Kochenour, N.K. *et al.* (1988) *In utero* platelet transfusion for alloimmune thrombocytopenia. *Lancet*, **ii**, 506.

61. Poulain, P., Kaplan, C., Leberre, C. *et al.* (1992) Alloimmune thrombocytopenia: *in utero* treatment by high doses of intravenous gamma globulins. *Fetal Diagn. Ther.*, **7**, 144–46.

62. Mueller-Eckhardt, C., Kiefel, V., Jovanovic, V. *et al.* (1988) Prenatal treatment of fetal alloimmune thrombocytopenia. *Lancet*, **ii**, 910.

63. Bussel, J., Berkowitz, R., McFarland, J. *et al.* (1988) *In utero* platelet transfusion for alloimmune thrombocytopenia. *Lancet*, **ii**, 1307–308.

64. Editorial (1989) Management of alloimmune neonatal thrombocytopenia. *Lancet*, **i**, 137–38.

65. Gembruch, U. and Hansmann, M. (1988) Artificial instillation of amniotic fluid as a new technique for the diagnostic evaluation of cases of oligohydramnios. *Prenat. Diagn.*, **8**, 33–45.

66. Nicolini, U., Fisk, N.M., Rodeck, C.H. *et al.* (1989) Low amniotic pressure in oligohydramnios – is this the cause of pulmonary hypoplasia? *Am. J. Obstet. Gynecol.*, **161**, 1098–101.

67. Stringer, M., Librizzi, R. and Weiner, S. (1990) Management of midtrimester oligohydramnios: a case for amnioinfusion. *J. Perinatol.*, **10**, 143–45.

68. Fisk, N.M., Ronderos-Dumit, D., Soliani, A. *et al.* (1991) Diagnostic and therapeutic transabdominal amnioinfusion in oligohydramnios. *Obstet. Gynecol.*, **78**, 270–78.

69. Imanaka, M., Ogita, S. and Sugawa, T. (1989) Saline solution amnioinfusion for oligohydramnios after premature rupture of the membranes. A preliminary report. *Am. J. Obstet. Gynecol.*, **161**, 102–106.

70. Miyazaki, F.S. and Nevarez, F. (1985) Saline amnioinfusion for relief of repetitive variable decelerations: a prospective randomised study. *Am. J. Obstet. Gynecol.*, **153**, 301–306.

71. Owen, J., Henson, B.V. and Hauth, J.C. (1990) A prospective randomised study of saline solution amnioinfusion. *Am. J. Obstet. Gynecol.*, **162**, 1146–49.

72. Strong, T.H., Hetzler, G., Sarno, A.P. and Paul, R.H. (1990) Prophylactic intrapartum amnioinfusion: a randomised clinical trial. *Am. J. Obstet. Gynecol.*, **162**, 1370–75.

73. Sadovsky, Y., Amon, E., Bade, M.E. and Petrie, R.H. (1989) Prophylactic amnioinfusion during labor complicated by meconium: a preliminary report. *Am. J. Obstet. Gynecol.*, **161**, 613–17.

74. Adam, K., Cano, L. and Moise, K.J. (1989) The effect of intrapartum amnioinfusion on the outcome of the fetus with heavy meconium stained amniotic fluid. *Ninth Annual Meeting, Society of Perinatal Obstetricians*, February 1–4, New Orleans.

75. Macri, C.J., Schrimmer, D.B., Leung, A. *et al.* (1991) Amnioinfusion improves outcome in labour complicated by meconium and oligohydramnios. *Am. J. Obstet. Gynecol.*, **164**, 252.

76. Hofmeyer, G.J. (1992) Amnioinfusion: a question of benefits and risks. *Br. J. Obstet. Gynaecol.*, **99**, 449–51.

77. Nicolini, U., Santolaya, J., Hubinont, C. *et al.* (1989) Visualisation of fetal intra-abdominal organs in second-trimester severe oligohydramnios by intraperitoneal infusion. *Prenat. Diagn.*, **9**, 191–94.

78. Sharland, G.K., Chita, S.K., Fagg, N. *et al.* (1991) Left ventricular dysfunction in the fetus: relationship to aortic valve anomalies and endocardial fibroelastosis. *Br. Heart J.*, **66**, 219–24.

79. Johnson, P., Sharland, G., Allan, L.D. *et al.* (1992) Umbilical venous pressure in nonimmune hydrops fetalis: correlation with cardiac size. *Am. J. Obstet. Gynecol.*, **167**, 1309–13.

80. Rodeck, C.H. (1981) Fetoscopy, In *Progress in Obstetrics and Gynaecology*, vol. I (ed. J. Studd), Churchill Livingstone, Edinburgh, pp. 79–91.

81. Cullen, M.T., Reece, A., Whetham, J. and Hobbins, J.C. (1990) Embryoscopy: description and utility of a new technique. *Am. J. Obstet. Gynecol.*, **162**, 82–86.

82. Reece, E.A., Rotmensch, S., Whetham, J. *et al.* (1992) Embryoscopy: a closer look at first-trimester diagnosis and treatment. *Am. J. Obstet. Gynecol.*, **166**, 775–80.

83. De Lia, J.E., Cruikshank, D.P. and Keye, W.R. (1990) Fetoscopic neodymium:YAG laser occlusion of placental vessels in severe twin–twin transfusion syndrome. *Obstet. Gynecol.*, **75**, 1046–53.

84. Schmidt, S., Decleer, W., Wagner, U. *et al.* (1991) An approach to fetal surgery: endoscopic use of excimer laser. *Eur. J. Obstet. Gynaecol. Reprod. Biol.*, **42** (suppl.), 84–86.

86 SHUNTS IN CLOSED FETAL SURGERY

G.G. Ashmead and W.R. Burrows

86.1 Overview and history

The fetus in times past was perceived as an 'homunculus' – an imaginary creature curled within the head of a sperm [1]. There was little further advancement in knowledge of the fetus until Vesalius, the famous anatomist, made the first analytical observations on living mammalian specimens. These descriptive studies eventually led to experimental ablative surgical procedures performed on mammalian fetuses *in utero* early in the twentieth century [2].

Later in this century, the focus of experimentation was on chronic animal preparations. Congenital defects were replicated, providing information about their etiologies [3]. Within the last 40 years, ultrasound techniques have evolved to the point of accurate diagnosis of congenital anomalies [4]. Simultaneously, amniocentesis entered the modern era in 1952 [5]. In 1963, successful intrauterine transfusion via the fetal peritoneal cavity was reported [6]. Later reports involved the use of indwelling catheters for transfusion [7,8]. This chapter addresses a further advance of the 1980s: indwelling stents (or shunts) to drain fetal pathological fluid collections.

86.2 Ethical and medicolegal considerations

The ethical and medicolegal considerations in this field are controversial and involve four perspectives. The mother and fetus have common goals, as well as individual interests. The four points of view are those of the fetus (presumed), the mother, the clinician and society as a whole [9–11].

The fetal perspective requires that the anomaly considered for treatment be fatal or debilitating. The proposed surgery should correct or improve the situation with a lower risk than immediate delivery. The mother must also be aware of risks to herself, and of alternatives to the procedure [12]. The clinician must evaluate each individual for potential risks and benefits before proposing the procedure. The personal goals of the physician must not conflict with the ultimate goal of the mother and fetus.

The societal perspective has two functions. One is protecting the possibly conflicting goals of the persons involved. Local review boards to evaluate specific cases and assign a 'fetal advocate' have been proposed [13]. When individual interests conflict sufficiently, the medicolegal system is the review board of last resort. Other societal goals are often set by default. How does a clinician acquire adequate training for these techniques? How many clinicians are required for a given population? Much to their credit, the founders of the field of fetal surgery have addressed some of these broader questions. The International Fetal Medicine and Surgery Society has established guidelines and registries specifically for these purposes [14].

86.3 Obstructive urinary tract lesions

Obstructive fetal urinary tract lesions have the best prospects for successful *in utero* treatment by shunt procedures. Fetuses with bladder outlet obstruction severe enough to compromise renal and pulmonary development, but not severe enough to have irreversible renal and pulmonary damage, are appropriate candidates for *in utero* fetal surgical therapy. Severely affected fetuses in the third trimester are probably best treated by prompt early delivery and neonatal treatment.

Animal models provided the initial impetus for development of shunt procedures in human congenital obstructive uropathies. The fetal dog model showed that different lesions resulted from bladder neck ligation at different times in pregnancy [15]. Urethra ligation early in gestation produced a patent urachus; later ligation caused hydronephrosis and bladder trabeculation. The lamb model was subsequently developed for its applicability to the human situation, and demonstrated the value of decompression of the

Diseases of the Fetus and Newborn, 2nd edn, Edited by G.B. Reed, A.E. Claireaux and F. Cockburn. Published in 1995 by Chapman & Hall, London. ISBN 0 412 39160 0

obstruction [16,17]. This rapidly led to clinical applications [18–20]. Using ultrasound guidance, the shunt is placed to drain the distended bladder into the amniotic fluid cavity. Multiple attempts may be required for adequate placement.

An ideal fetal bladder shunt candidate should be of appropriate gestational age (20–32 weeks), have bilateral hydronephrosis, dilated bladder, oligohydramnios and no associated severe structural anomalies or chromosomal abnormalities [21–23]. Shunting an irreversible defect is not advantageous, so dysplasia should not be present, as determined by cortical cysts on ultrasound [24]. Adequate fetal renal function can be demonstrated on intrauterine fetal bladder aspiration. Fetal urinary sodium of less than 100 mmol/l, chloride of less than 90 mmol/l, osmolarity of less than 210 mosmol/l and urine output of more than 2 ml/hour may indicate adequate fetal renal function [25,26]. These parameters are used to differentiate a 'good' and a 'poor' prognostic group. Not all fetuses in the poor group have renal dysplasia [26,27] Elder et al. [27] reported five cases in which fetal urine electrolytes were not predictive of ultimate renal function. Others have recommended repeated evaluations after decompression of 'stale' urine, with improvement in subsequent biochemical analysis [28]. There are also advocates of β_2-microglobulin as an indicator of fetal renal status [28] (Chapter 101).

Technique

The shunt procedure is performed using sterile technique and under continual ultrasound guidance. A needle is inserted into the fetal bladder and a plastic catheter with memory (Rocket of London) (Figure 86.1) is placed in the fetal bladder. The lower coil of the catheter is positioned in the fetal bladder and the upper coil in the amniotic space. In cases of severe oligohydramnios, an *in utero* amnio-infusion can create an amniotic space to facilitate catheter placement.

Follow-up after bladder stent placement should consist of evaluation of amniotic fluid, initially biweekly for 2–3 weeks and then less frequently. If bladder dilatation and hydronephrosis recur then a repeat shunt procedure may be indicated. Complications include rupture of membranes, urinary ascites, displacement of the bladder stent, infection and premature labor.

The International Fetal Surgery Registry statistics from two reports indicate the success of these procedures [29,30]. Posterior urethral valves treated with stents have acceptable survival statistics. All other diagnoses either involve dismal survival or very few patients. Even for posterior urethral valves, there is controversy about these procedures. The mortality rate (approximately 5%), complication rate (44%) and rate of multiple

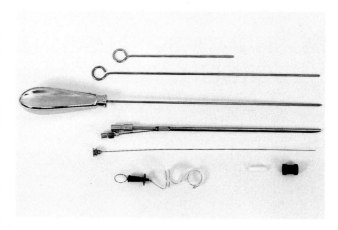

Figure 86.1 Parts for the KCH catheter (Rocket, USA) are, from top to bottom: first pusher rod, second pusher rod, trocar, cannula with irrigation channel, stilette for irrigation channel, catheter pusher with guide wire and seals for the cannula.

placement attempts to achieve success (92%) justify a re-evaluation of the technique [31]. As of 1992 there were 98 fetuses reported to the International Fetal Surgery Registry who were treated *in utero* for obstructive uropathy. Eight (8%) fetuses had multiple anomalies and eight (8%) had karyotypic anomalies. Thirty-four (35%) fetuses treated *in utero* died in the neonatal period from pulmonary hypoplasia. Of 79 fetuses reported to the International Fetal Surgery Registry with a diagnosis of bladder outlet obstruction who were followed with ultrasound but not treated, only five (6%) survived. Of the five survivors two had normal renal function and three had chronic renal failure and were awaiting kidney transplantation. A survival rate of 95% is reported for infants with obstructive uropathy due to posterior urethral valves who survive the neonatal period. It is difficult to make meaningful comparisons between the *in utero* treated group, the *in utero* untreated group, and the infants treated postnatally because of selection bias for each group (F.A. Manning, personal communication, 1992). It is time to compare these therapies with more conservative approaches in a prospective, randomized fashion.

86.4 Hydrocephalus

Fetal hydrocephalus is an obvious choice for *in utero* drainage. Unfortunately, *in utero* shunting for hydrocephalus shows no advantage to conservative therapy after birth.

Congenital hydrocephalus occurs in 0.3–0.8 per 1000 births [32]. The most common forms are aqueductal stenosis, communicating hydrocephalus and Dandy–Walker malformation, in decreasing order of frequency [33]. The neurological impairments from hydrocephalus are thought to be the result of excessive pressure on brain tissue with subsequent cerebral damage [34].

Fetal animal models produced simple ventriculomegaly by vascular occlusion [35]. Actual hydrocephalus can be produced with timed administration of synthetic corticosteroids to pregnant rhesus monkeys [36,37]. Another model involves kaolin injection into the cisterna magna [34]. This recreates some, but not all, histological changes seen in the human [38]. Both these techniques have been used to show the efficacy of *in utero* shunting in sheep and rhesus monkeys, with improved survival and/or neurological status [34,37,39–41].

A report of repetitive percutaneous cephalocentesis in a human fetus appeared in 1981 [42]. Neonatal outcome was poor, but there was an unsuspected Becker muscular dystrophy. A more favorable result was reported in June 1982 [43]. A November 1982 report involved shunt placement on the third attempt. The infant had severe neurological problems and died 5½ months after delivery at 28 weeks [44]. A more encouraging report appeared in 1983 [45].

While animal data were encouraging, Fetal Surgery Registry data on 39 cases treated with shunts were not [29]. Looking at neonatal data, early reports suffered a selection bias. Only neonates surviving to reach surgery were evaluated. When the diagnosis is established antenatally, perinatal death and associated anomalies (including some sought, but not recognized on ultrasound) are much more common [32,46,47]. Also, animal data were encouraging for survival, but not always for reversal of cerebral damage [41]. The problem may simply be in selecting the right candidates for shunting. Given the success of therapy after birth [48], until the pathophysiology of human hydrocephalus is better understood this procedure will not be generally applicable.

86.5 Pleuritic, ascitic and other fluid collections

The use of *in utero* fetal shunt procedures to treat pleuritic, ascitic and other fluid collections is experimental and controversial. Indications for *in utero* therapy are currently highly individualized.

Multiple reports of catheter placement for drainage of pulmonary congenital cystic adenomatoid malformation (CCAM) have appeared [49–51]. CCAM is subdivided into types I–III in decreasing order of cyst size [52]. Only type I is amenable to therapy. A case of neonatal death after repeated cyst aspirations *in utero*

was complicated by contralateral type III CCAM on postmortem examination [54]. While these results are favorable, so is the prognosis of type I CCAM without therapy [52,54].

A very promising area is shunting of fetal pleural effusions [55]. Unilateral hydrothorax without midline shift or non-immune hydrops, or with spontaneous resolution, has a favorable prognosis without treatment [55]. Hydrops, even secondary to chylothorax, has a more dismal prognosis. Antenatal stent procedures, however, have been effective even in the presence of non-immune hydrops.

Reports of *in utero* paracentesis for isolated ascites and drainage/sclerosis of large ovarian cysts have been described [58,59]. These can cause distension sufficient to produce heart failure. It is conceivable that chronic drainage might be required for such potentially lethal benign fluid collections pending pulmonary maturation. Shunting these fluid collections could prove efficacious in the future.

86.6 Conclusions and future directions

The fetus, originally depicted as an homunculus, has become a separate patient. Increasingly sophisticated ultrasound and amniocentesis adaptations have afforded access to the traditionally secluded intrauterine environment. This chapter briefly reviewed the recent development of fetal stent procedures derived from this technology.

Based on animal models, stent procedures have been developed for chronic drainage of pathological fluid collections. At this time, hydronephrosis from posterior urethral valves and chylothorax with development of non-immune hydrops appear to be the antenatal diagnoses which have benefited most from these procedures. Other attempts to utilize them have been less successful in humans, despite encouraging results in animal models. Perhaps this is because no reproducible animal model can faithfully recreate human congenital defects in all their myriad complexities. Expanded indications for stent procedures await further research. When shunting has seemed successful, it is imperative that it be compared with less invasive therapy in controlled, randomized, prospective trials. After a decade of experimentation, fetal shunts have passed through the homunculus stage of their development and require more sophisticated evaluation.

References

1. Harrison, M.R. (1982) Unborn: historical perspective of the fetus as a patient. *Pharos*, **45**, 19–24.
2. Pringle, K.C. (1986) *In utero* surgery. *Adv. Surg.*, **19**, 101–38.
3. Louw, J.H. and Barnard, C.N. (1955) Congenital intestinal atresia – observations on its origin. *Lancet*, ii, 1065–67.
4. Campbell, S., Johnstone, F.D., Holt, E.M. and May, P. (1972) Anencephaly: early ultrasonic diagnosis and active management. *Lancet*, ii: 1226–29.

5. Bevis, D.C.A. (1952) The antenatal prediction of haemolytic disease of the newborn. *Lancet,* i: 395–98.

6. Liley, A.W. (1963) Intrauterine transfusion of foetus in haemolytic disease. *BMJ,* ii, 1107–109.

7. Liggins, G.C. (1966) A self-retaining catheter for fetal peritoneal transfusion. *Obstet. Gynecol.,* 27, 323–26.

8. Asensio, S.H., Figueroa-Longo, J.G. and Pelegrina, I.A. (1968) Intrauterine exchange transfusion. A new technic. *Obstet. Gynecol.,* 32, 350–55.

9. Evans, M.I., Drugin, A., Manning, F.A. and Harrison, M.R. (1989) Fetal surgery in the 1990s. *Am. J. Dis. Child.,* 143, 1431–36.

10. Karp, L.E. (1982) Fetal surgery. *Am. J. Med. Genet.,* 13, 357–58.

11. Wilkinson, A.W. (1975) Fetal surgery. *Dev. Med. Child. Neurol.,* 17, 795–97.

12. Fost, N.C., Bartholome, W.G., Bell, W.R. *et al.* (Committee on Bioethics, American Academy of Pediatrics) (1988) Fetal therapy: ethical considerations. *Pediatrics,* 81, 898–99.

13. Porter, K.B., Wagner, P.C. and Cabaniss, M.L. (1988) Fetal board: a multidisciplinary approach to the management of the abnormal fetus. *Obstet. Gynecol.,* 72, 275–78.

14. Harrison, M.R., Filly, R.A. and Golbus, M.S. (1982) Fetal treatment 1982. *N. Engl. J. Med.,* 307, 1651–52.

15. Javadpour, N., Graziano, M.F. and Terrill, R. (1974) Experimental induction of patent allantoic duct by intrauterine bladder outlet obstruction. *J. Surg. Res.,* 17, 341–45.

16. Harrison, M.R., Ross, N.A., Noall, R.A. and deLorimier, A.A. (1983) Correction of congenital hydronephrosis *in-utero* I. The model: fetal urethral obstruction produces hydronephrosis and pulmonary hypoplasia in fetal lambs. *J. Pediatr. Surg.,* 18, 247–56.

17. Glick, P.L., Harrison, M.R., Adzick, N.S. *et al.* (1984). Correction of congenital hydronephrosis *in-utero* IV. *In-utero* decompression prevents renal dysplasia. *J. Pediatr. Surg.,* 19, 649–56.

18. Golbus, M.S., Harrison, M.R., Filly, R.A. *et al.* (1982) *In utero* treatment of urinary tract obstruction. *Am. J. Obstet. Gynecol.,* 142, 383–88.

19. Vallancien, G., Dumez, Y., Aubrey, M.C. *et al.* (1982) Percutaneous nephrostomy *in-utero. Urology,* 20, 647–49.

20. Manning, F.A., Harman, C.R., Lange, I.R. *et al.* (1983) Antepartum chronic fetal vesicoamniotic shunts for obstructive uropathy: a report of two cases. *Am. J. Obstet. Gynecol.,* 145, 819–22.

21. Romero, R., Pilu, G., Jeanty, P. *et al.* (1988) *Prenatal Diagnosis of Congenital Anomalies,* Appleton & Lange, Norwalk, CT, pp. 255–90.

22. Josephson, S. (1990) Suspected pyelo-ureteral junction obstruction in the fetus: when to do what? I. A clinical update. *Eur. Urol.,* 18, 267–75.

23. Brumfield, C.G., Davis, R.O., Joseph, D.B. and Cosper, P. (1991) Fetal obstructive uropathies. Importance of chromosomal abnormalities and associated anomalies to perinatal outcome. *J. Reprod. Med.,* 36, 662–66.

24. Crombleholme, T.M., Harrison, M.R., Golbus, M.S. *et al.* (1990) Fetal intervention in obstructive uropathy: prognostic indicators and efficacy of intervention. *Am. J. Obstet. Gynecol.,* 162, 1239–44.

25. Glick, P.L., Harrison, M.R., Golbus, M.S. *et al.* (1985) Management of the fetus with congenital hydronephrosis II: prognostic criteria and selection for treatment. *J. Pediatr. Surg.,* 20, 376–87.

26. Wilkins, I.A., Chitkara, U., Lynch, L. *et al.* (1987) The nonpredictive value of fetal urinary electrolytes: preliminary report of outcomes and correlations with pathologic diagnosis. *Am. J. Obstet. Gynecol.,* 157, 694–98.

27. Elder, J.S., O'Grady, J.P., Ashmead, G., *et al.* (1990) Evaluation of fetal renal function: unreliability of fetal urinary electrolytes. *J. Urol.,* 144, 574–78.

28. Evans, M.I., Sacks, A.J., Johnson, M.P. *et al.* (1991) Sequential invasive assessment of fetal renal function and the intrauterine treatment of fetal obstructive uropathies. *Obstet. Gynecol.,* 77, 545–50.

29. Manning, F.A., Harrison, M.R., Rodeck, C. *et al.* (1986) Catheter shunts for fetal hydronephrosis and hydrocephalus. *N. Engl. J. Med.,* 315, 336–40.

30. Manning, F.A. (1991) The fetus with obstructive uropathy: the fetal surgery registry, in *The Unborn Patient: Prenatal Diagnosis and Treatment,* 2nd edn (eds. M. Harrison, M. Golbus and R. Filly), W.B. Saunders, Philadelphia pp. 394–98.

31. Elder, J.S., Duckett, J.W. and Snyder, H.M. (1987) Intervention for fetal obstructive uropathy: has it been effective? *Lancet,* ii, 1007–10.

32. Williamson, R.A., Schauberger, C.W., Varner, M.W. and Aschenbrener, C.A. (1984) Heterogeneity of prenatal onset hydrocephalus: management and counseling implications. *Am. J. Med. Genet.,* 17, 497–508.

33. Romero, R., Pilu, G., Jeanty, P. *et al.* (eds) (1988) *Prenatal Diagnosis of Congenital Anomalies,* Appleton & Lange, Norwalk, C.T., pp. 21–34.

34. Nakayama, D.K., Harrison, M.R., Berger, M.S. *et al.* (1983) Correction of congenital hydrocephalus *in-utero* I. The model: intracisternal kaolin produces hydrocephalus in fetal lambs and rhesus monkeys. *J. Pediatr. Surg.,* 18, 331–38.

35. Myers, R.E. (1969) Brain pathology following fetal vascular occlusion: an experimental study. *Invest. Ophthalmol. Vis. Sci.,* 8, 41–50.

36. Hodgen, G.D. (1981) Antenatal diagnosis and treatment of fetal skeletal malformations. *JAMA,* 246, 1079–83.

37. Michejda, M. and Hodgen, G.D. (1981) *In-utero* diagnosis and treatment of non-human primate fetal skeletal anomalies I. Hydrocephalus. *JAMA,* 246, 1093–97.

38. Weller, R.O., Mitchell, J., Griffin, R.L. and Gardner, M.J. (1978) The effects of hydrocephalus upon the developing brain. *J. Neurol. Sci.,* 36, 383–402.

39. Michejda, M., Patronas, N., Chiro, G. and Hodgen, G.D. (1984) Fetal hydrocephalus II. Amelioration of fetal porencephaly by *in-utero* therapy in nonhuman primates. *JAMA,* 251, 2548–52.

40. Cambria, S., Gambardella, G., Cardia, E., and Cambria, M. (1984) Experimental endo-uterine hydrocephalus in foetal sheep and surgical treatment by ventriculo-amniotic shunt. *Acta Neurochir,* 72, 235–40.

41. Glick, P.L., Harrison, M.R., Halks-Miller, M. *et al.* (1984) Correction of congenital hydrocephalus *in-utero* II. Efficacy of *in-utero* shunting. *J. Pediatr. Surg.,* 19, 870–80.

42. Birnholz, J.C. and Frigoletto, F.D. (1981) Antenatal treatment of hydrocephalus. *N. Engl J. Med.* 304, 1021–23.

43. Clewell, W.H., Johnson, M.L., Meier, P.R. *et al.* (1982) A surgical approach to the treatment of fetal hydrocephalus. *N. Engl J. Med.* 306, 1320–25.

44. Frigoletto, F.D., Birnholz, J.C. and Greene, M.F. (1982) Antenatal treatment of hydrocephalus by ventriculoamniotic shunting. *JAMA,* 248, 2496–97.

45. Depp, R., Sabbagha, R.E., Brown, T. *et al.* (1983) Fetal surgery for hydrocephalus: successful *in-utero* ventriculoamniotic shunt for Dandy–Walker syndrome. *Obstet. Gynecol.,* 61, 710–14.

46. Chervenak, F.A., Ment, L.R., McClure, M. *et al.* (1984) Outcome of fetal ventriculomegaly. *Lancet,* ii, 179–81.

47. Glick, P.L., Harrison, M.R., Nakayama, D.K. *et al.* (1984) Management of ventriculomegaly in the fetus. *J. Pediatr.,* 105 97–105.

48. McCullough, D.C. and Balzer-Martin, L.A. (1982) Current prognosis in overt neonatal hydrocephalus. *J. Neurosurg.* 57, 378–83.

49. Bernashek, G., Deutinger, J., Gruber, W. and Helmer, F. (1989) Intrauterine treatment of a fetal pulmonary cyst by chorioamniotic shunt. *Arch. Gynecol. Obstet.,* 244, 129–32.

50. Clark, S.L., Vitale, D.J., Minton, S.D., *et al.* (1987) Successful fetal therapy for cystic adenomatoid malformation: prenatal diagnosis and natural history. *Am. J. Obstet. Gynecol.,* 157, 294–95.

51. Nicolaides, K.H., Blott, M. and Greenough, A. (1987) Chronic drainage of fetal pulmonary cyst. *Lancet,* i, 618.

52. Romero, R., Pilu, G., Jeanty, P. *et al.* (eds) (1988) *Prenatal Diagnosis of Congenital Anomalies,* Appleton & Lange, Norwalk, C.T., pp. 198–201.

53. Chao, A. and Monoson, R.F. (1990) Neonatal death despite fetal therapy for cystic adenomatoid malformation. *J. Reprod. Med.,* 35, 655–57.

54. Adzick, N.S., Harrison, M.R., Glick, P.K. *et al.* (1985) Fetal cystic adenomatoid malformation: prenatal diagnosis and natural history. *J. Pediatr. Surg.,* 20, 483–88.

55. Blott, M., Nicolaides, K.H. and Greenough, A. (1988) Pleuroamniotic shunting for decompression of fetal pleural effusions. *Obstet. Gynecol.,* 71, 798–800.

56. Longaker, M.T., Laberge, J. M., Dansereau, J. *et al.* (1989) Primary fetal hydrothorax: natural history and management. *J. Pediatr. Surg.,* 24, 573–76.

57. Rodeck, C.H., Fisk, N.M., Fraser, D.I. and Nicolini, U. (1988) Long-term *in-utero* drainage of fetal hydrothorax. *N. Engl. J. Med.,* 319, 1135–38.

58. Winn, H.N., Stiller, R., Grannum, P.A.T. *et al.* (1990) Isolated fetal ascites: prenatal diagnosis and management. *Am. J. Perinatol.,* 7, 370–73.

59. Giorlandino, C., Rivosecchi, M., Bilancioni, E. *et al.* (1990) Successful intrauterine therapy of a large fetal ovarian cyst. *Prenat. Diagn.,* 10, 473–75.

87 CONGENITAL DIAPHRAGMATIC HERNIA AND OPEN FETAL SURGERY

F. Bargy, E. Sapin, Y. Rouquet, S. Beaudoin, D. Hamza, C. Esteve, F. Toubas, F. Lewin and O. Gaudiche

87.1 Introduction

One of the most recent innovations in the perpetual quest to find new and better techniques of medical care for treating malformations in human babies is fetal surgery.

Progress in prenatal diagnosis has brought physicians into increasingly intimate contact with the fetus, encouraging them to consider it as a true patient. At the moment the fetal indications for such surgery are congenital malformations with a very poor prognosis, even if neonatal surgery and resuscitation and sophisticated techniques are used. Severe forms of congenital diaphragmatic hernia (CDH) thus represent a very good indication for the fetus and the main experiments on fetal surgery have been done for this malformation, which is why CDH and fetal surgery are described in the same chapter.

87.2 Congenital diaphragmatic hernia

CDH results from an embryological disorder during the formation of the diaphragm. The neonatal incidence is about 1 in 3000 to 1 in 5000. The most common anatomical form is a defect of the costal part of the diaphragm (Bochdalek's hernia) or a total aplasia of the dome. Between these two forms all sorts of intermediate conditions are encountered. The consequence of the diaphragmatic defect is the ascension and development of the abdominal viscera in the chest, compressing the lungs (Figure 87.1).

The other forms of diaphragmatic hernia, such as oesophageal hiatus hernia or retrosternal hernia, represent less than 5% of the total, and the clinical symptomatology is completely different. These forms are also congenital, but usually the term congenital diaphragmatic hernia refers only to the defective costal part of the diaphragmatic dome. Only CDH is described here.

Despite progress in neonatal surgery and resuscitation the prognosis for CDH is poor; the overall survival rate is about 50%. In the severe forms, with dome aplasia, the survival rate is less than 10%; in the more favourable forms, with a slight posterolateral defect, the survival rate is in excess of 70% [1,2].

87.2.1 EMBRYOLOGY OF CDH

CDH is the consequence of a maldevelopment of the septum transversum between 6 and 10 weeks of amenorrhoea. Several forms of the disease can be observed, depending on the time at which it occurs. As the defect appears very early in the pregnancy, associated anomalies are sometimes encountered [3–5] (Table 87.1). In cases of a large defect, the abdominal viscera, particularly the liver, will develop in the chest, and it is possible to observe a part of the dorsal mesogastrium in the mediastinum. If there is only a posterolateral defect (Bochdalek's hernia), the abdominal viscera grows initially in the abdomen and progressively herniates into the thorax. During the formation of the septum transversum, the intestinal tract elongates into the umbilical pouch and the dorsal mesenterium is in its initial position. That is the reason why the severe forms (earliest) combine diaphragmatic aplasia, mesenterium commune and intrathoracic liver.

The proliferation of the primitive hepatic cells around vitelline and umbilical vessels, beneath the heart, induces the growth of the septum transversum backward to the dorsal mesenterium. These events take place during the division of the foregut (6–8 weeks of

Diseases of the Fetus and Newborn, 2nd edn, Edited by G.B. Reed, A.E. Claireaux and F. Cockburn. Published in 1995 by Chapman & Hall, London. ISBN 0 412 39160 0

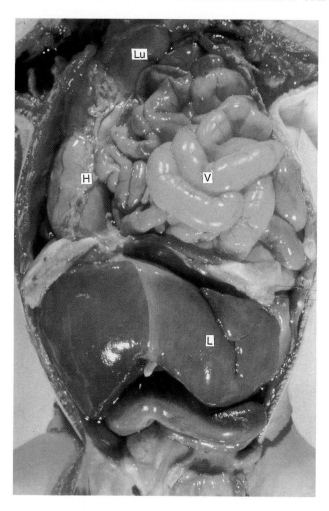

Figure 87.1 Bochdalek hernia with a partial defect: there is a ventral part of the diaphragm; the liver (L) is reduced from the thorax. The consequence of the diaphragmatic defect is the ascension of the abdominal viscera (V) into the chest and the compression of the lungs (Lu). The heart (H) is displaced.

Table 87.1 Anomalies associated with CDH (160 cases)

Anomaly	Number
Karyotype	7
Cardiac	5
Coelosomia	3
Multiple malformation	2
Total	17

amenorrhoea), before the formation of the tracheo-bronchial tree and the first stage of lung development (week 16) [6]. The formation of the diaphragm is completed at week 11 of amenorrhoea. The left side usually closes later than the right and 90% of cases of CDH are left-sided. Muscles fibres derived from cervical myotomes grow later [7,8] (Figure 87.2). If there

is a true membranous sac in CDH, the hernia results from failure of muscular elements to reinforce the diaphragm properly. The abdominal viscera compress the lungs and induce pulmonary hypoplasia [3,9,10]. Some authors, after teratologic studies, contend that CDH results from pre-existing pulmonary hypoplasia [4,11]. Regarding embryological chronology, this does not seem to be logical. Experimental studies of the genesis of pulmonary hypoplasia [3,9,10] have demonstrated compression of the lung by herniated viscera and showed the possible regression of the condition after decompression or surgical correction [12].

In humans, the growth of pulmonary alveoli begins at 28 weeks [6] so CDH should be repaired *in utero* before this time in order to obtain satisfactory lung growth. Regarding the anatomical and histological evolution (by Emery and Mithal's count of alveoli [13]) of the lungs during the pregnancy, it is possible to conclude that the lesions increase week after week [14,15] (Figure 87.3), not only on the herniated side but also in the opposite one.

87.2.2 CLINICAL CONDITIONS

After analysis of several large clinical series, differences between severe and relatively less severe forms appear to emerge [1,14,16]. In our experience of 180 cases seen between 1981 and 1991, 20% were of the severe form. More recently (1991–1992), out of 40 cases diagnosed prenatally, 28 were of the severe form, only 12 were 'good' in the sense of possible treatment and or survival. The clinical aspect of the disease changes as prenatal diagnosis progresses. Many severe cases are never seen in paediatric centres and constitute a 'hidden mortality' [17]. Nowadays the associated anomalies can be detected by careful prenatal sonographic examination. The progressive generalization of prenatal diagnosis in the medical management of pregnancies may decrease the hidden mortality; discussion on treatment and management of a baby with CDH requires consideration of prenatal data.

87.2.3 DIAGNOSIS

(a) Prenatal diagnosis

Before birth, the diagnosis of CDH can be made by sonography. The abdominal viscera appears in the pleural space (Figure 87.4); the heart and mediastinum are displaced towards the opposite side. The sonographic interface which represents the diaphragm is not seen, and this sign is sometimes very useful for differentiating CDH from cystic adenomatoid malformation. At this time, the problem for the physician is to estimate the prognosis for this unborn patient, and to identify anatomical criteria. It has been established that

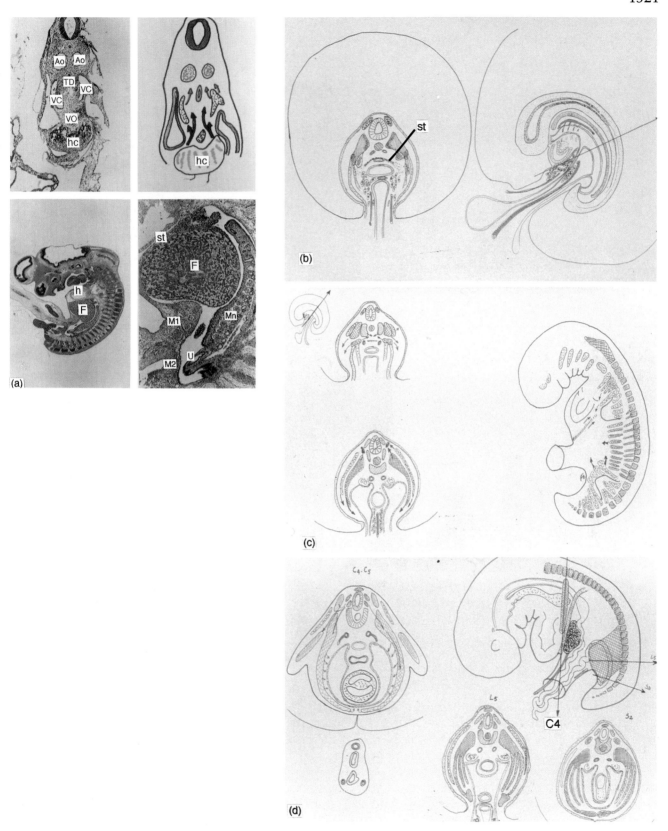

Figure 87.2 The formation of the septum transversum and diaphragm. (a,b) Embryo of 5 and 6 weeks of amenorrhoea: the septum transversum (st) appears between the heart (h) and the liver (F); the proliferation of the hepatocytes (hc) induces the formation of the septum transversum during the division of the foregut and before the formation of the tracheobronchial tree. MN = mesonephros; Ao = aorta; VC = cardinalis venae; U = ureter. (c,d) At 6 and 8 weeks of amenorrheoa: the muscle fibres derive from the cervical myotomes (C4). The phrenic nerve follows the migration of the muscular cells.

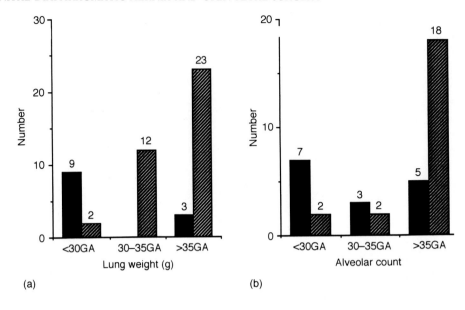

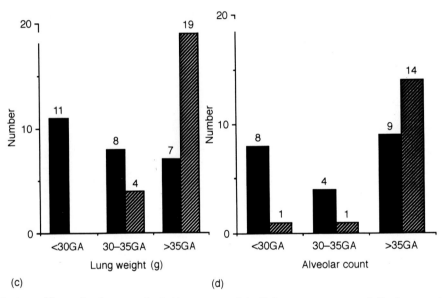

Figure 87.3 Evolution of lung development in (a,b) severe and (c,d) less severe cases of diaphragmatic hernia. (a,c) Lung weight and (b,d) alveolar count (taken from Emery [13]), on the side of the hernia (solid bar) and on the opposite side (cross-hatched), during pregnancy. GA = gestational age.

intrathoracic liver and abdominal diameter under 2 standard deviations mean a survival rate of less than 10% [14]. For some authors, intrathoracic stomach and polyhydramnios are associated with high mortality [1,18]. In the same way, functional hypotrophy of the left ventricle diagnosed by cardiac sonography appears to represent another factor for poor prognosis. With all these criteria it is possible to estimate the survival probability for the newborn (Table 87.2). This is only a clinical assessment, and these criteria are not really correlated with the histological aspect of the lungs. On the other hand, the sonographic pattern can change during the pregnancy and it is possible to observe the

liver in the abdomen at 20 weeks and to find it shifted into the thorax later in the same pregnancy. This indicates that repeated sonographic examinations are essential for the prenatal follow up of the fetus.

Associated anomalies can be detected by sonography; chromosomal abnormalities require amniocentesis or fetal blood sampling for chromosome analysis. An evaluation for cardiac abnormalities by fetal echocardiography is also necessary. Associated anomalies are present in almost 20% of cases [19–21] (Table 87.1). Patent ductus arteriosus must not be considered as an associated anomaly, but is related to a hypoplastic pulmonary vascular bed. A further step after diagnosis

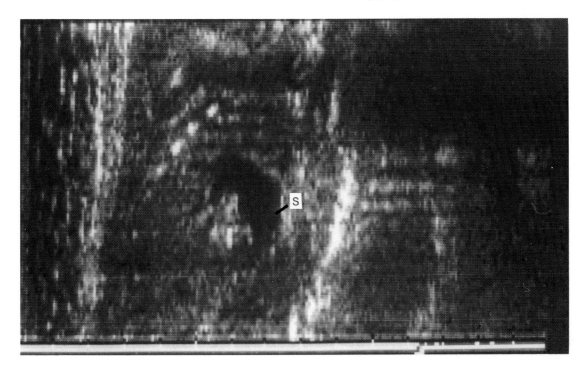

Figure 87.4 At sonography, the stomach (S) is visible in the pleural space.

Table 87.2 Survival probability (calculated)

Anomaly	P
Intrathoracic liver	<0.2
Small abdominal diameter	<0.15
Intrathoracic liver and small abdominal diameter	<0.1
Intrathoracic stomach	<0.4
Hydramnios	<0.4
Intrathoracic dilated stomach and polyhydramnios	<0.15
Functional hypoplasia of the left ventricle	<0.25

is the discussion about the best treatment before or after birth.

(b) Postnatal diagnosis

Sometimes there is no prenatal diagnosis if the ascension of the abdominal viscera into the chest occurs only after birth (which explains a previous normal sonographic examination), or if a pregnancy has not been surveyed ultrasonographically.

Signs and symptoms at birth vary in their gravity and appear immediately or a few hours later. Rarely a CDH can be diagnosed later in the life but it is obviously a different disease. Dyspnoea, cyanosis and respiratory distress are the main signs. At physical examination, the abdomen is scaphoid and heart sounds are displaced in the opposite direction. Radiology confirms

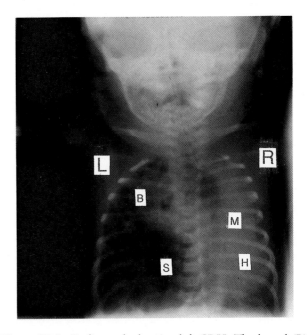

Figure 87.5 Radiograph showing left CDH. The bowel (B) and stomach (S) are in the chest. The heart (H) and mediastinum (M) are displaced towards the opposite side. L = left; R = right.

the diagnosis; gas, bowel and stomach are seen in the pleural space, with displacement of the mediastinum (Figure 87.5). Neonatal resuscitation has to be started immediately.

87.2.4 TREATMENT TECHNIQUES

Postnatal management

Several techniques can be proposed, alone or combined, for the treatment of CDH, before and after surgical repair [22]. The challenge is how to fight pulmonary hypoplasia and pulmonary hypertension which leads to persistent fetal circulation. Pulmonary hypertension is the consequence of anatomical and functional factors. Both must be overcome for recovery. Surgery creates the condition for lung growth by decompression, when the abdominal viscera return to the abdomen. But after surgery it takes time to obtain a *restitutio ad integrum* of the pulmonary vascular bed, and during this time the baby can die from pulmonary hypertension. In order to reduce the functional part of pulmonary hypertension, several techniques or medications are used. Prostaglandins or tolazoline induce vasodilatation in both pulmonary and systemic circulation, therefore the shunt increases and the persistent fetal circulation cannot really disappear. Nitric oxide used with artificial ventilation has a specific effect on the pulmonary vessels, so it could be more efficient. Extracorporeal membrane oxygenation (ECMO) can be used in severe forms [23,24], it requires an arteriovenous or a venovenous bypass. The results of ECMO in the treatment of respiratory failure in neonates is now well known, and it is an effective means of improving survival in selected patients. But in the treatment of CDH the results of ECMO are not as good as for other indications [25]. In many cases ECMO improves the oxygenation of the neonate during the procedure but cannot reverse the anatomical pulmonary hypoplasia. Theoretically, it needs a very long-term bypass before lung growth is effective.

The usual treatment is preoperative stabilization [22]. The aim of this management is to obtain the best haemodynamic conditions before surgery. In case of severe forms ECMO can be used before surgery. The surgical procedures for the repair of CDH use a transabdominal subcostal approach to the defective diaphragm, and a reduction of the herniated viscera. The diaphragm is repaired with simple interrupted stiches, if possible, and with a Silastic (or Gore-tex) prosthesis, if not. The abdominal wall is also closed with a patch if it is not possible to reintegrate all the viscera without tension, which leads to intestinal ischaemia.

Despite recent advances, the prognosis for patients with CDH, particularly in severe forms, is still poor. As prenatal diagnosis progresses, more and more severe forms are diagnosed before birth; then the mortality will not stay hidden.

Because pulmonary hypoplasia results from compression of the growing lungs during fetal life, repair *in utero* before 28 weeks seems to be a way of reversing pulmonary maldevelopment [18].

(b) Prenatal management

Prenatal surgery may be indicated in severe forms diagnosed prenatally. Both indications for the fetus and for the mother have to be considered. A decision to carry out fetal surgery can only be made after carefully considering how, when and why it can best be attempted, and by weighing the risks against expected results. Close communication between all those involved is an essential aspect of the whole process.

During the period 1991–1993 we encountered 40 cases of prenatally diagnosed CDH. Twelve cases were 'good' forms with an intra-abdominal liver at sonography; eight babies survived. Of the 28 cases with intra-thoracic liver and small abdominal diameter, five had associated anomalies (chromosomal, omphalocele, cardiac) and four were diagnosed after 29 weeks; 19 cases were carefully considered for fetal surgery on the basis of fetal indication. For the mother, the obstetric future was considered and only the women over 35 years old and/or those treated for infertility were considered as having good maternal indications. There were only six and, of these, three couples chose *in utero* surgery. Prenatal treatment requires a precise indication, and it can be considered as a therapeutic possibility among the range of techniques.

The procedure will be fully described further. In severe forms with dome aplasia and a very small abdominal cavity, the authors use a Silastic (or Gore-Tex) patch to repair the diaphragm and a second abdominal prosthesis to enlarge the abdominal cavity. The surgical technique has now been perfected and the main difficulty is to control tocolysis. Preterm labour occured in all cases. For the fetus, in *utero* surgery induces the risk of prematurity, coupled to that of the CDH. On the other hand, even if the fetus stays a short time in the maternal uterus after the operation, this creates the best condition for pulmonary circulation. The postoperative intensive care is done by the maternal placenta. During these few days or weeks, the lungs grow without compression, and this facilitates resuscitation after birth in respect of the anatomical part of the pulmonary hypertension. The use of artificial surfactant combats hyaline membrane disease. It is also possible to find a specific anomaly of the surfactant in CDH [26]. The use of exogenous surfactant before ventilation is possible at birth [27].

The remarkable stability of the operative conditions during fetal surgery leads us to consider the possibility of prenatal surgery at term.

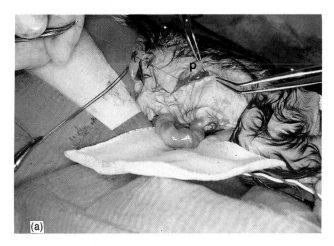
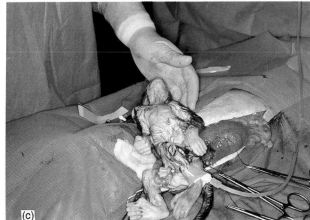
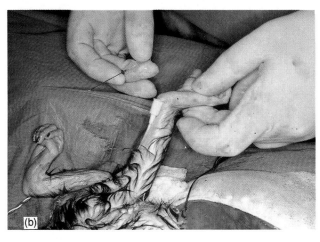
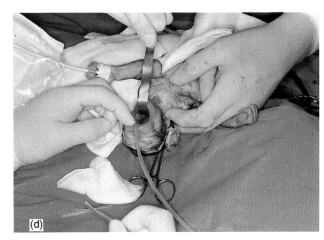

Figure 87.6   Prenatal surgery on monkeys. (a) The fetus is partially exteriorized and operated on. p = Parietal prosthesis. (b) A venous access is placed on the leg; (c) complete exteriorization; (d) a tracheal tube is placed.

(c)   Prenatal surgery at term (investigational)

Prenatal surgery at term could be considered in cases where prenatal surgery before 28 weeks is not possible or not indicated. The procedure begins as a classical caesarean section, but anaesthesia is performed with halothane or isoflurane to obtain uterine myorelaxation. Perfect haemostasis is obtained by a double running suture on the edges of the uterine incision. The fetus is partially exteriorized by the legs; fetal anaesthesia and analgesia are performed via the umbilical cord. The surgical repair starts and continues, while the placenta secures fetal oxygenation. After the surgery, a venous access is placed and the newborn is completely exteriorized. Tracheal intubation is then performed, and exogenous surfactant injected after manual ventilation. Artificial ventilation works in harmony with the placental blood flow. After a few minutes the umbilical flow is interrupted and the newborn is committed to the care of the neonatologist. Experimental studies on monkeys have been extremely encouraging (Figure 87.6) and such management is now possible in humans.

For the mother, the indication is easier to consider because there is only one caesarean section near term. For the fetus, as the procedure takes place at 35–36 weeks, it will be less effective than prenatal surgery in terms of pulmonary growth but more effective in terms of premature delivery.

87.2.5   INDICATIONS

If the prenatal diagnosis is made before 28 weeks and shows anatomical criteria of poor prognosis at sonography, such as intrathoracic liver, small abdominal diameter and functional hypotrophy of the left ventricle, fetal surgery is indicated on condition that there are no associated anomalies and the mother has good maternal indications. In the same conditions of prenatal diagnosis, without maternal indication for fetal surgery, a prenatal or postnatal procedure at term can be proposed. If there are no anatomical criteria for a bad prognosis, and if none appears further in the pregnancy, neonatal surgery with preoperative stabilization gives a survival rate of more than 70%; prenatal surgery at term is not yet evaluated but can be proposed in some cases. If bad criteria appear during a subsequent sonographic survey, prenatal surgery versus immediate ECMO prior to surgery can be discussed. If the prenatal diagnosis takes place after 28 weeks, only prenatal or postnatal management is adequate.

87.3 Open fetal surgery

As the fetus becomes a true patient fetal medicine and surgery appear as a new specialization of human medicine. The concept of fetal surgery is rather 'old' and began about 20 years ago with *in utero* transfusions for rhesus disease. Open fetal surgery became a reality with the work of Harrison and Golbus in the 1980s. The first operation on a baby would not have been attempted had it not been preceded by a stringent and extensive experimental programme on non-human primates to determine the safety and efficiency of the procedure. In the experience of the authors, experimental studies lasted more than 5 years, checking the technique and evaluating the results [28]. Michael Harrison was the first to perform a successful *in utero* procedure in 1982: a bilateral ureterostomy for bilateral hydronephrosis [29]. Subsequent growth of the fetus was normal, but after delivery at 35 weeks the newborn died of pulmonary hypoplasia. Despite this lack of success, this attempt did prove that it was possible to operate on a fetus partially outside the uterus and to keep uterine contractility under control so that pregnancy could continue.

The Harrison team (University of California, San Francisco; UCSF) [18] reported failure in six subsequent cases of CDH that underwent *in utero* surgery. Three cases with intrathoracic liver died during the removal of the liver into the abdomen. In the other cases the neonates died of other complications but the lung growth was satisfactory. These operations did, however, demonstrate the safety of the procedure from the mother's point of view. No maternal complications were reported and four of the mothers have since had another child.

A similar intervention was attempted in 1989 at Saint Vincent de Paul hospital in Paris. The mother was 42 years old and had been treated for infertility. The fetus presented a single left CDH with intrathoracic liver and a lower abdominal diameter under 2 standard deviations. The operation was successful in terms of obstetric and anaesthesic management, and although complete dome aplasia was repaired with a small prosthesis, the baby died 8 hours after the procedure because of a twist of the umbilical vein.

The first successful *in utero* operation to treat CDH was achieved in 1990 by the UCSF team. Performed on a 26-week-old fetus, it involved partial exteriorization of the left arm and repair of the diaphragm with a Gore-Tex patch. After tocolysis became unmanageable, the child was delivered by caesarean section and placed in intensive care. Birth weight was 1920 g and the Apgar score 7 at the first minute. There was no intrathoracic liver [30]. Three years later, the child is growing well. The UCSF team has now performed about 40 fetal operations for several indications without maternal complication. Only 4 of 20 cases of CDH have survived.

In our experience, only four patients have been operated on, all with a left-sided severe form of CDH; one baby survived. The two last unsuccessful attempts were in January and July 1992. In the first case, the surgery worked perfectly well, without technical problems and without fetal hypoxaemia. The difficulties occurred when the fetus had to be replaced into the uterine cavity. Uterine retraction and contraction compressed the umbilical cord and led to fetal hypoxaemia (Sao_2 <36%) for 10 minutes; the procedure was stopped because of the possible neurological risk. In the second case, everything went perfectly well during the procedure, and the tocolysis was well controlled after it. The fetus died 2 days later from renal failure caused by a toxic reaction to indomethacin, the tocolytic agent used. Research is underway to find an alternative so that this, albeit very rare, accident [5,31] can be prevented.

87.3.1 RISKS OF FETAL SURGERY

(a) Fetal risks

Indications for fetal surgery involve many factors. The most important of these is prenatal diagnosis, and so it is essential that this is accurate. There should be no more than one malformation, whatever that may be, and it should be one that jeopardizes the fetus. Such a diagnosis must be carefully checked before a decision as to whether or not to intervene is taken.

Next, the proposed techniques should be tested for their safety, efficiency and repeatability. This can be done in experimental studies on non-human primates whose physiology closely resembles that of humans [28].

The risks of the intervention itself can be divided into anaesthetic, surgical and resuscitative. The low weight of the fetus and its need for an excellent placental blood flow makes anaesthesia a very delicate business. Maternal blood pressure should not fall below 80% of maxima, so that placental exchange can be maintained. Halothane allows good uterine relaxation but induces maternal hypotension; the safety margin here is difficult to judge. Isoflurane is easier to use. It is also important to prevent any endogenous catecholamine release caused by pain, stress or hypoxia, since this leads to uterine vasoconstriction. Fetal bleeding or hypoxaemia, which lead to fetal acidosis, must be prevented. In cases of CDH, the risk of liver injury with subsequent haemorrhage is important. Peroperative management focuses on temperature and haemo-dynamic condition. Transcutaneous monitoring of fetal oxygenation is performed throughout the procedure.

(b) Maternal risks

As regards the mother, the operative risks may be immediate or delayed [3]. Placing the mother in slight left lateral decubitus position during the operation will prevent caval compression by the pregnant uterus. Gravid uterus section at this gestation is very prone to haemorrhage and perfect haemostasis is necessary when the uterus is opened. The running suture placed on the edges of the uterine incision for haemostasis can also prevent the risk of amniotic fluid embolism. The next major risk is uncontrolled tocolysis, resulting in pre-mature delivery. The success of fetal surgery depends entirely on efficient tocolysis. Beta mimetics and indo-methacin are used combined, but indomethacin can be toxic to the fetus [5,31]. Because of the risk of uterine rupture, sutures should be strong and tight, on two levels, with the help of biological glue. There have been no reported incidents of late uterine rupture to date. When tocolysis becomes unmanageable, delivery should be by caesarean section, making the incision away from the placenta and cervix area. Precautions should be taken against infection and thromboembol-ism, as for all pelvic surgery.

The delayed risks arise from hysterotomia. The uterus is opened twice and becomes cicatricial. This induces a theoretical risk of uterine rupture for the next pregnancy. Any new pregnancy must be kept under close surveillance and the baby delivered by caesarean section.

87.3.2 INDICATIONS

In the case of many malformations therapeutic proto-cols are not yet advanced enough to be applied on human fetuses. Neurological abnormalities that have been studied so far include spina bifida and exen-cephaly. Maria Michedja's work with monkeys has demonstrated the possibility of preventing paraplegia by closing the meningeal defect in utero, but it is difficult to achieve this success in humans. Some other malformations, such as gastroschisis or cleft palate, could be very well treated in utero, but the results of postnatal surgery are obviously good, and fetal surgery nowadays is only proposed if the expected results are better than those obtained by postnatal treatment.

Bilateral hydronephrosis caused by posterior urethral valves at first seemed to be an excellent indication. In

practice, experiments have failed to prove any signifi-cant improvement in renal prognosis. The potential pressure gradient between bladder and amniotic fluid could result in amniotic reflux into the urinary tract, in which case open fetal surgery versus diversion by bladder or kidney catheter may de discussed. Despite the use of precise biological criteria to evaluate the renal function in utero (β_2-microglobulin, calcium and sodium in fetal urine), it appears to be difficult to evaluate renal function early enough to have a chance of restoring renal units that are at risk. Collective studies and international registries produce new in-formation on this subject each year.

Cystic adenomatoid malformation of the lung is a very good indication in its severe forms with fetal hydrops. Harrison [32] reported six successes with open fetal surgery. Open fetal surgery appears to be indicated if the catheter diversion is unsuccessful after 24 hours.

Exceptional indications for fetal surgery are such rare malformations as sacrococcygeal teratoma, especially in the case of complication (internal haemorrhage affecting vital prognosis). It is possible to detect a complication at repeat sonography when the teratoma is growing faster than the fetus.

At the moment the most frequent indication for open fetal surgery is the severe forms of CDH. That is the reason why the procedure is described in detail.

87.3.3 THE PROCEDURE

To perform surgery on the fetus, the mother has to be operated on. Preoperative investigations are necessary (biological control, physical and cardiological examina-tion with cardiosonography) to check maternal health. If there is enough time it is possible to organize a protocol of autotransfusion but in the authors' experi-ence no blood transfusions were necessary.

The mother is positioned on the operating table slightly on the left side to prevent caval compression by the pregnant uterus. Anaesthetic induction is obtained with halothane or isoflurane [33,34] and completed with curarization and analgesia, supplied via a peri-dural catheter which is kept in place for several days. Laparotomy is performed through a large Pfannenstiel's incision, and the placental area is marked by sonogra-phy. The amniotic fluid is partially removed prior to section of the uterus and kept sterile at constant temperature. The uterus is then sectioned and haemo-stasis is achieved with a continuing running suture on the edges of the incision (Figure 87.7). The fetus is exteriorized by the legs and attached to monitoring equipment (Figure 47.8). This method is different from Harrison's technique in which the fetus is exteriorized by the left arm (in the case of left CDH), but provides a large upper abdominal operative area for reducing

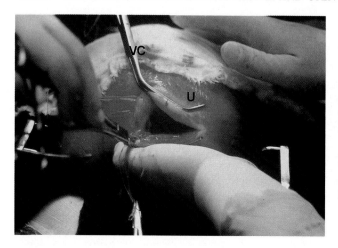

Figure 87.7 The haemostasis is performed on the edges of the uterine incision. U = uterus; VC = vascular clamp. (Copyright Philippe Plailly, Eurelios, 148 rue de Grenelle, 75007 Paris, France.)

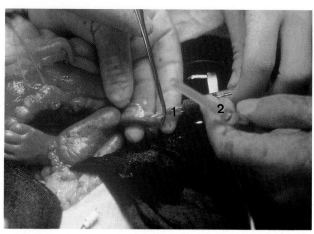

Figure 87.9 The umbilical cord is accessed for fetal blood analysis (1) and fetal anaesthesia (2). (Copyright Philippe Plailly, Eurelios.)

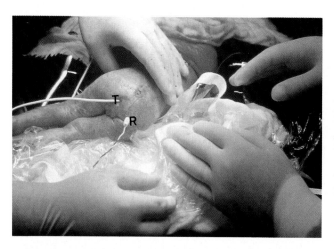

Figure 87.8 The fetus is attached to monitoring equipment (T = temperature; R = cardiac rhythm). (Copyright Philippe Plailly, Eurelios.)

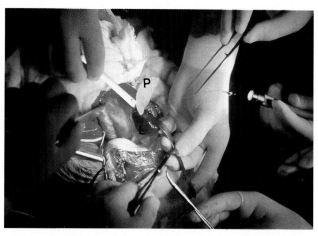

Figure 87.10 A Silastic prosthesis (P) is placed on the edge of the diaphragm. L = liver. (Copyright Philippe Plailly, Eurelios.)

an intrathoracic liver. The umbilical cord is accessed for administration of fetal anaesthesia and analgesia, and also for analysis of blood pH and blood gas tensions (Figure 87.9). Fetal laparotomy is performed through a left abdominal approach, preserving the umbilical vein. The herniated viscera are removed from the thorax so that the diaphragmatic edges can be identified. Removal and replacement of the visera mark a particularly critical phase of the operation, especially during the section of the left peritoneum of the liver, and the umbilical blood flow must be preserved. A Silastic (or Gore-Tex) prosthesis is placed on the edge of the diaphragm (Figure 87.10) and the pleural space is filled with Ringer's lactate solution. During the replacement

of the bowel, care must be taken to preserve the mesenterium commune, if it is a complete one. A second prosthesis is placed on the abdominal wall in order to enlarge the abdominal cavity and avoid any compression of the abdominal viscera (Figure 87.11). The skin is just sutured over the prosthesis. Reintegration of the fetus into the maternal uterus is also a critical stage, requiring perfect uterine relaxation without any compression of the umbilical cord. The uterus is closed carefully with two levels of interrupted stiches, and the amniotic fluid is reinfused into the uterine cavity (Figure 87.12). In the postoperative period, fetal vitality and efficiency of tocolysis are monitored by sonography and percutaneous Doppler signal.

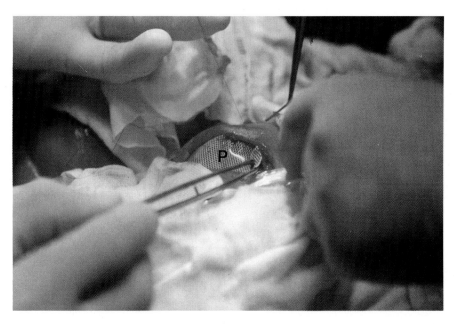

Figure 87.11   A second prosthesis (P) is placed on the abdominal wall. (Copyright Philippe Plailly, Eurelios.)

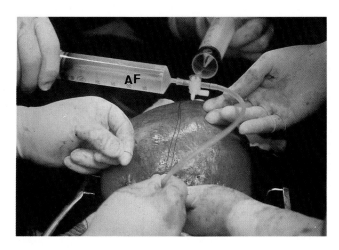

Figure 87.12   The amniotic fluid (AF) is reinfused into the uterine cavity. (Copyright Philippe Plailly, Eurelios.)

87.3.4   RESULTS

The results of fetal surgery must be compared with those of neonatal surgery for the same malformation. In cases of severe forms of CDH the survival rate is less than 10% and the success with fetal surgery is 25%. Statistically, it is not possible to reach a conclusion because of such small series (20 cases at UCSF and four cases in Paris). In specific cases, with a very precise indication for the fetus and for the mother, it is obviously better to propose *in utero* surgery. Similarly in cases of cystic adenomatoid malformation, with fetal hydrops, if catheter diversion is unsuccessful there is no chance for the fetus except fetal surgery.

Because of fetal anaesthesia and intraoperative haemodynamic stability, there is no risk of fetal hypoxia unless the umbilical cord is compressed during reinstatement of the fetus. This makes this method of malformation repair less aggressive for the fetus than the standard procedure, particularly in CDH repair. Fetal resuscitation is, in fact, facilitated by the placenta.

Most of the complications relate to tocolysis. The longest period sustained after fetal surgery for CDH is 34 weeks, reported by the UCSF team under Harrison. In our successful experiment, tocolysis escaped control on day 10. Research and animal experiments to find new tocolytic treatments should be a priority for the future.

87.4   Conclusions

The decision to operate has to be based on both fetal and maternal indications, in which ethical factors have to be considered. The mother's obstetric future needs to be taken into account. The procedure concerns mothers over 35 years of age, and/or those who have fertility difficulties, or those who explicitly ask for prenatal intervention. Psychologically, for parents, prenatal surgery could be an alternative to termination, and eliminates the sense of guilt due to the impression of doing nothing for their baby. During the pregnancy the feeling of waiting for the death of the baby in 90% of cases is absolutely overwhelming and prenatal surgery may be a way of settling the problem as soon as possible, with a slightly increased chance of saving the baby. Both parents must therefore be clearly and honestly informed, and ideally should initiate the request for fetal surgery, without prompting or persuasion. Both the benefits and risks of fetal surgery must be carefully considered and discussed, so that there is full agreement and cooperation between the parents and medical team (obstetrician, paediatric surgeon, anaesthesists, sonographer – all specialized in fetal therapy and trained on non-human primates). Fetal surgery has a fine future but good surgery proceeds from good indications. New techniques using endoscopy or radiotelemetry monitoring [35] will be developed in the future, and research is continuing. The main purpose of fetal surgery is to save the baby with the least aggressive technique for the mother.

References

1. Adzick, N.S., Harrison, M.R, Glick, P.L. et al. (1985) Diaphragmatic hernia in the fetus, prenatal diagnosis and outcome in 94 cases. J. Pediatr. Surg., 20, 357–61.
2. Kurzenne, J.Y., Sapin, E., Bargy, F. et al. (1988) Hernies diaphragmatiques congenitales: 120 cas neonataux, étude preliminaire. (Congenital diaphragmatic hernia: 120 neonatal cases, preliminary study.) Chir. Pediatr., 29, 11–17.
3. Rouquet, Y. and Bargy, F. (1990) La chirurgie foetal, in Mise à Jour en Gynécologie et Obstetrique (ed. M. Tournaire), Vigot, Paris, 177–95.
4. Tibboel, D., Tenbrinck, R., Bos, A.P. et al. (1990) An experimental model of congenital diaphragmatic hernia, in Defaut Congenitaux de la Paroi Abdominale (eds F. Beaufils, Y. Aigrain and Y. Nivoche), Arnette, Paris, 1 99–105.
5. Bavoux, F. (1992) Toxicité foetale des anti inflammatoires non steroidiens. (Non steroidal anti inflammatory drugs and fetal toxicity.) Presse Med., 11, 4–11.
6. Barbet, J.P., Houette, A., Barres, D. and Durigon, M. (1988) Histological assessment of gestational age in human embryo and fetuses. Am. J. Forensic Med. Pathol., 19, 40–44.
7. Hamilton, W.J., Boyd, J.D. and Mossmann, A.W. (1976) Human Embryology, Prenatal Development of Form and Function, 4th Edn, Macmillan, London.
8. Moore, K.L. (1988) The Developing Human, W.B. Saunders, Philadelphia.
9. Harrison, M.R., Jester, J.A. and Roos, N.A. (1980) Correction of congenital diaphragmatic hernia in utero I. Intrathoracic balloon produces fetal pulmonary hypoplasia. Surgery, 88, 174–82.
10. Pringle, K.C., Turner, J.W., Schofield, J.C. and Sopert, R.T. (1984) Creation and repair of diaphragmatic hernia in the fetal lamb. J. Pediatr. Surg., 19, 131–40.
11. Iritani, I. (1984) Experimental study on embryogenesis of congenital diaphragmatic hernia. Anat. Embryol, 169, 133–39.
12. Sopert, R.T., Pringle, K.C. and Schofield, J.C. (1984) Creation and repair of diaphragmatic hernia in fetal lamb. J. Pediatr. Surg., 19, 33–40.
13. Emery, J.L. and Mithal, A. (1960) The number of alveoli in the terminal respiratory unit of man during late intrauterine life and childhood. Arch. Dis. Child., 35, 544–47.
14. Bargy, F., Barbet, J.P., Houette, A. et al. (1989) Solutions a l'hypoplasie pulmonaire foetale dans la hernie diaphragmatique congenitale, in Les Malformations Congenitales: Diagnostic Ante-natal et Devenir (eds A. Couture, C. Veyrac and C. Baud), Sauramps, Montpellier, pp. 550–55.
15. Bargy, F., Sapin, E., Wakim, A. et al. (1992) La chirurgie à uterus ouvert pour la réparation des hernies diaphragmatiques. Med. Foetale, 11, 17–24.
16. Beals, D.A., Schloo, D.L., Vacanti, J.P. et al. (1992) Pulmonary growth and remodeling in infants with high risk congenital diaphragmatic hernia. J. Pediatr. Surg., 12, 997–102.
17. Harrison, M.R., Bjordac, R.I., Golbus, M.S. et al. (1979) Congenital diaphragmatic hernia: the hidden mortality. J. Pediatr. Surg., 13, 227–30.
18. Harrison, M.R., Langer, J.C., Adzick, N.S. et al. (1990) Correction of congenital diaphragmatic hernia in utero V. Initial clinical experience. J. Pediatr. Surg., 25, 47–57.
19. Aymé, S., Julian, C., Gambarelli, D. et al. (1989) Fryns syndrome: report of 8 cases. Clin. Genet., 35, 191–201.
20. Czeizel, A. and Kovars, M. (1985) A family study of congenital diaphragmatic hernia. Am. J. Med. Genet., 21, 105–115.
21. Puri, P. and Gorman, F. (1984) Lethal non pulmonary anomalies associated with congenital diaphragmatic hernia. J. Pediatr. Surg., 19, 29–32.
22. Nakayama, D.K., Motoyama, E.K. and Tagge, E.M. (1991) Effect of preoperative stabilization on respiratory system compliance, and outcome in newborn infants with congenital diphragmatic hernia. J. Pediatr., 118, 793–99.
23. Brands, W., Kachel, W., Wirth, H. et al. (1992) Indication for using extra corporeal membrane oxygenation in congenital diaphragmatic hernia. Eur. J. Pediatr. Surg., 12, 81–83.
24. O'Rourke, P., Lillehei, C.W., Crone, R.K. et al. (1991) The effect of extra corporeal membrane oxygenation on the survival of neonates with high risk congenital diaphragmatic hernia: 45 cases from a single institution. J. Pediatr. Surg., 126, 147–152.
25. Wilson, J.M., Lund, D.P., Lillehei, C.W. et al. (1992) Delayed repair and pre operative ECMO does not improve survival in high risk congenital diaphragmatic hernia. J. Pediatr. Surg., 27, 368–75.
26. Alfonso, L.F., Vilanova, J., Aldzabal, P. et al. (1993) Lung growth and maturation in the rat model of experimentally induced congenital diaphragmatic hernia. Eur. J. Pediatr. Surg., 13, 6–12.
27. Glick, P.L., Leach, C.L., Besner, G.E. et al. (1992) Physiopathology of congenital diaphragmatic hernia III. Exogenous surfactant therapy for the high risk neonate with CDH. J. Pediatr. Surg., 127, 866–69.
28. Bargy, F., Sapin, E., Wakim, A. et al. (1990) La chirurgie à uterus ouvert pour la réparation des hernies diaphragmatiques. (Open fetal surgery for repair of congenital diaphragmatic hernia.) Rech. Gynecol., 2, 4–6.
29. Harrison, M.R., Golbus, M.S. and Filley, R.A. (1982) Fetal surgery for hydronephrosis. N. Engl. J. Med., 306, 591.
30. Harrison, M.R., Adzick, S.N., Longacker, N.T. et al. (1990) Successful repair in utero of fetal diaphragmatic hernia after removal of the herniated viscera from the thorax. N. Engl. J. Med., 322, 1582–84.
31. Guignard, J.P. (1988) Influence of indomethacin (short term) on fetal urine output. Obstet. Gynecol., 72, 51–53.
32. Harrison, M.R., Adzick, N.S., Jennings, R.W. et al. (1990) Antenatal intervention for congenital cystic adenomatoid malformation. Lancet, 336, 1582–84.
33. Esteve, C., Toubas, F., Gaudiche, O. et al. (1992) Le bilan de 5 années de chirurgie expérimentale in utero pour la réparation des hernies diaphragmatiques. (Five years of experimental surgery for the repair of congenital diaphragmatic hernia in utero.) Ann. Fr. Anesth. Reanim., 11, 193–200.
34. Naftalin, N.J., McKay, D.H., Phear, W.P. et al. (1977) The effects of halothane on pregnant and non pregnant human myometrium. Anesthesiology, 118, 793–99.
35. Jennings, R.W., Adzick, S.N., Longaker, M.T. et al. (1992) New techniques in fetal surgery. J. Pediatr. Surg., 27, 1329–33.

88 *IN UTERO* HEMATOPOIETIC STEM CELL TRANSPLANTATION

A.W. Flake

88.1 Introduction

Prenatal therapy has evolved rapidly over the last few decades and now includes surgical and medical treatment of selected fetuses [1]. A potential method of fetal therapy which could treat far more patients than all other types of prenatal therapy combined is the prenatal transplantation of hematopoietic stem cells (HSCs) [2]. There are three obvious applications for this approach:

1. reconstitution of fetal hematopoietic disease;
2. prenatal tolerance induction for postnatal allogeneic or xenogeneic organ transplantation;
3. prenatal somatic gene therapy.

In this chapter, I will review the clinical and experimental progress with this unique approach to fetal therapy.

88.2 Reconstitution of fetal hematopoietic disease

Modern techniques of prenatal diagnosis have allowed the early gestational diagnosis of the majority of congenital diseases of hematopoietic origin. Table 88.1 is an incomplete list of hematopoietic diseases which are potentially curable by bone marrow transplantation after birth. Among these are some of the most common hereditary diseases in the world. With our ability to diagnose these conditions *in utero*, the obvious question is, would they be better treated *in utero*?

88.2.1 RATIONALE FOR *IN UTERO* HSC TRANSPLANTATION

All of these diseases could potentially be cured by conventional postnatal bone marrow transplantation (BMT). Unfortunately, application of conventional BMT has serious limitations [3,4]. Only 35% of candidates for BMT have an HLA-identical donor available for optimal transplantation. In addition,

Table 88.1 Congenital hematopoietic diseases potentially amenable to *in utero* HSC transplantation

Disorders of erythropoiesis
Thalassemia major
Sickle-cell anemia
Diamond–Blackfan syndrome
Fanconi's anemia

Disorders of lymphopoiesis
Severe combined immunodeficiency syndrome
Bare lymphocyte syndrome

Disorders of myelopoiesis
Chronic granulomatous disease
Chediak–Higashi syndrome
Wiskott–Aldrich syndrome
Infantile agranulocytosis (Kostman's syndrome)
Lazy leukocyte syndrome (neutrophil actin deficiency)
Neutrophil membrane GP-180 deficiency
Cartilage–hair syndrome

Metabolic errors of lysosomes of reticuloendothelial cells
Mucopolysaccharidoses
Hurler's disease (MPS-I) (α-iduronidase deficiency)
Hurler–Scheie syndrome
Hunter's disease (MPS-II) (iduronate sulfatase deficiency)
Sanfilippo (MPS-IIIB) (α-glycosaminidase deficiency)
Morquio's syndrome (MPS-IV) (hexosamine-6-sulfatase deficiency)
Maroteaux–Lamy syndrome (MPS-VI) (arylsulfatase B deficiency)
Mucolipidoses
Fabry's disease (α-galactosidase A deficiency)
Gaucher's disease (glucocerebrosidase deficiency)
Krabbe's disease (galactosylceramidase deficiency)
Metachromatic leukodystrophy (arylsulfatase A deficiency)
Niemann–Pick disease (sphingomyelinase deficiency)
Adrenal leukodystrophy

Disorder of osteoclast
Infantile osteopetrosis

myeloablation, with its associated immunosuppression and risk of lethal infection, is required. Even after successful engraftment, rejection and graft-versus-host disease (GVHD) are constant threats requiring further immunosuppressive therapy. By the time postnatal

Diseases of the Fetus and Newborn, 2nd edn, Edited by G.B. Reed, A.E. Claireaux and F. Cockburn. Published in 1995 by Chapman & Hall, London. ISBN 0 412 39160 0

transplants are performed, most recipients have been ravaged by their underlying disease. Finally, in many of the storage diseases, the neurologic damage begins early, perhaps *in utero*, and, is not reversed by BMT [5]. In these fetuses, *in utero* treatment is not only advantageous, but may be required to cure the disease [6].

The potential advantages of prenatal HSC transplantation arise from aspects of immunologic and hematologic ontogeny which are unique to fetal development [7,8]. During human fetal development hematopoiesis is first observed in the yolk sac blood islands. By 7 weeks' gestation, migration of HSCs has occurred to the fetal liver which remains the predominant hematopoietic organ through most of gestation. The fetal bone marrow contains only stromal elements until around 16 weeks' gestation when hematopoietic elements begin to appear. Migration of stem cells from the liver to the bone marrow is not largely complete until around 34 weeks' gestation. Thus, fetal hematopoietic ontogeny provides a 'window of opportunity' for engraftment of cells in a relatively empty fetal bone marrow.

The early gestational fetus is uniquely tolerant of foreign antigen. Recent evidence documents a pivotal role of the thymic microenvironment in establishment of tolerance [9,10]. T-cell progenitors first appear in the fetal thymus at 9–10 weeks' gestation, and mature CD4 or CD8+ lymphocytes are not found in the circulation until 14–16 weeks' gestation. Exposure of the 'pre-immune' fetus to foreign antigen results in processing of the antigen in the fetal thymus through a complex process of positive and negative selection of antigen reactive lymphocytes. The end-result is clonal deletion of T lymphocytes which recognize the foreign antigen in association with self-MHC (major histocompatibility complex) and specific tolerance of the foreign antigen as 'self'.

Thus early gestational transplantation of HSCs could theoretically avoid all of the complications of postnatal bone marrow transplantation. The recipient would be tolerant of the graft, no bone marrow ablation would be required and, with the use of early gestational fetal cells or enriched HSCs from adult donors, GVHD could be avoided. As pluripotent HSCs have the remarkable properties of multilineage differentiation as well as self-replication (immortality), permanent reconstitution of a wide variety of diseases could potentially be accomplished. Finally, prenatal reconstitution would avoid the clinical manifestations of the disease, preventing the associated human suffering and cost to society.

88.2.2 EXPERIMENTAL STUDIES

In 1945, Owen [11] observed that early gestational placental cross-circulation between bovine dizygotic twins resulted in permanent hematopoietic chimerism. In the 1950s and 1960s the classic experiments of Billingham, Brent and Medawar [12,13], as well as subsequent investigators, confirmed the phenomenon of acquired tolerance in a number of animal models by early gestational exposure to foreign antigen. More recently we performed early gestational fetal-to-fetal HSC transplantation in sheep [14] and monkey [15] and documented long-standing, multilineage hematopoietic chimerism without the need for immunosuppression or GVHD. More detailed analysis of the monkey chimeras confirms that the animals have normal immune response [16] and that their donor hematopoietic cells can respond normally to anemia-induced stress [17]. We have also investigated the use of T-cell-depleted and partially reconstituted adult marrow as a donor source in the sheep model and have found that the ability to engraft and the occurrence of GVHD are directly proportional to the number of mature T cells, analogous to postnatal BMT [18]. These and other studies in large animal models are summarized in Table 88.2.

Experimental work has been promising but leaves some doubt about the ability to achieve levels of engraftment necessary to ameliorate clinical disease. The level of engraftment required to cure the hemoglobinopathies is unknown and probably much higher than that required for immunodeficiencies. In addition, levels of engraftment achieved in a normal recipient probably do not reflect what could be achieved in an abnormal recipient and also probably do not reflect what could be achieved in a disease state in which there was a competitive advantage for normal cells. Although we are currently pursuing various methods of improving engraftment in our experimental models, some of these questions can only be answered clinically.

88.2.3 CLINICAL EXPERIENCE

Current techniques of prenatal diagnosis and fetal transfusion make prenatal HSC transplantation feasible in humans well within the immunologic and hematopoietic 'window of opportunity'. In spite of an absence of practical limitations, reported clinical experience has been limited. In the USA, because of the Government moratorium on funding for use of fetal tissue for therapeutic purposes [22], and the difficulty of obtaining intact fetal tissue, we are aware of only a few attempts at fetal reconstitution. The world's reported clinical experience is summarized in Table 88.3. In most cases no engraftment was achieved. In many instances the indication, timing, dose or source of donor cells has been suboptimal, providing an explanation for failure. Unequivocal cure of one patient with bare lymphocyte syndrome has been achieved by

Table 88.2 Summary of experimental data for successful large animal models of allogeneic *in utero* HSC transplantation[a] [19–21]

Animal model	Gestation (days)	Donor age (days)	Recipient age (days)	Cell type	Detection method[b]	BM (%)	PBL (%)	Hb (%)	GVHD
Sheep	145	35–50	55–62	FL	Karyotype Hb type	10–12	25	14–29	No
Sheep	145	Adult	100	BM	Hb type	–	–	22–36	Yes
	145	Adult	55–65	BM	Hb type	–	–	6–18	Yes
Sheep	145	Adult	55–65	TCD	Hb type	–	–	3–8	No
				TCD+TC 9.3%		–	–	14–22	Yes
				TCD+TC 4.4%		–	–	12–16	Yes
				TCD+TC 1.2%		–	–	8–12	No
Rhesus monkey	165	60–62	60–62	FL	Karyotype	5–15	3–8	–	No
Goat	145	43 Adult	60–79	FL BM	Karyotype	–	1–2 0	–	No
Baboon	180	Adult	80	BM	GPI	–	–	0.1–0.6 (%RBC)	?[c]

BM = bone marrow; PBL = peripheral blood leukocyte; FL = fetal liver; TCD = T-cell-depleted adult marrow; TCD + TC = T-cell-depleted adult marrow with reconstitution by autologous T cells (normal marrow = 9.3% T cells).
[a] In all cases donor cells were injected intraperitoneally. In sheep and goats the injections were given under direct visualization. Monkeys were injected under ultrasound guidance.
[b] Karyotype analyses were done on phytohemagglutinin-stimulated peripheral blood lymphocytes. Hb type was determined by carboxymethyl-cellulose chromatography of peripheral blood Hb. Baboon red cells were analyzed by glucose-phosphate isomerase (GPI).
[c] *In utero* deaths. GVHD not excluded.

Table 88.3 Summary of reported clinical experience with fetal stem cell transplantation[a]

Gestational age (weeks)	Donor cell source	Disease treated	No. cases	Postnatal outcome	Ref no.
17	T-cell depleted adult BM	Rh disease	1	Survived with no engraftment	23
28	Fetal liver and fetal thymus, 7 and 7.5 weeks	Bare lymphocyte syndrome	1	Clinically normal; lymphocytes have donor HLA expression	24–29
26	Fetal liver and fetal thymus, 7.5 weeks	SCIDS	1	Alive; remains immunodeficient in protective isolation; low level donor cell engraftment	24–29
12	Fetal liver, 9.5 weeks	Thalassemia major	1	Alive; remains anemic at less than 1 year; low level donor cell engraftment	24–29
34, 23, and 25	T-cell depleted adult BM	MCLD (2) Thalassemia (1)	3	No evidence of engraftment Clinical status consistent with primary disease	30
18	Maternal BM	α-Thalassemia	1	Terminated at 23 weeks; autopsy extramedullary maternal cells	31
19 and 26	Maternal BM	SCIDS and Chediak–Higashi	1	Terminated at 26 weeks; no engraftment	31
			1	No engraftment at birth	

BM = bone marrow; SCIDS = severe combined immunodeficiency syndrome; MCLD = metachromatic leukodystrophy.
[a] A total of ten cases have been reported by four different investigators. Engraftment was achieved postnatally in three fetuses given fetal donor cells. Attempts to engraft T-cell depleted adult marrow have been unsuccessful.

Touraine and colleagues [24–29], promising hope for the future (Chapter 106).

88.3   Prenatal tolerance induction

88.3.1   RATIONALE FOR PRENATAL TOLERANCE INDUCTION

Although now a routine procedure in older children and adults, organ transplantation remains a formidable challenge in the newborn [32,33]. Organ shortage is most critical for the newborn recipient. Technical considerations and size mismatch become limiting factors. The long-term ramifications of neonatal and lifelong immunosuppression are unknown and disturbing [34–36]. Nevertheless, a large number of fetuses continue to be born with hopelessly damaged or defective organs from congenital and developmental abnormalities. Examples include:

1. congenital diaphragmatic hernia with secondary severe pulmonary hypoplasia [37];
2. hypoplastic left heart and other severe inoperable cardiac defects [38];
3. obstructive uropathy with irreversible renal damage [39];
4. hepatic ornithine transcarbamoylase deficiency with neonatal hyperammonemia [40].

These diseases all have in common organ failure which is lethal, can be prenatally diagnosed, and could theoretically be cured by organ transplantation after birth. New and innovative approaches are desperately needed.

A potential solution would be the induction of specific transplantation tolerance by the *in utero* transplantation of allogeneic or xenogeneic hematopoietic stem cells. The specifically tolerant neonate could then be transplanted after birth with a size-matched xenogeneic or cut-down allogeneic organ. This approach could potentially solve the organ shortage problem for neonates, supply size-matched organs, and avoid, or reduce the need for immunosuppression.

88.3.2   EXPERIMENTAL STUDIES

Owen's [11] observation of hematopoietic chimerism in dizygotic cattle twins with shared placental circulation suggested the possibility of specific transplantation tolerance between chimeric siblings. This was confirmed in subsequent studies which revealed complete specific tolerance of skin and organ transplants [41–43]. This 'experiment of nature' has been reproduced by man in a number of animal models by exposure of immunologically 'immature' fetuses to protein or cellular antigen with subsequent demonstration of partial or complete, specific, immunologic tolerance [12,13,44,

45]. More recently xenogeneic hematopoietic chimerism has been achieved by the *in utero* HSC transplantation approach in a human into sheep model [46], a human into mouse model [47], and a pig into sheep model (A.W. Flake, unpublished data). These are the first successful models of hematopoietic chimerism in immunocompetent recipients between widely disparate species combinations. Further studies are required to determine whether these recipients are specifically tolerant for organ transplantation and are currently underway.

88.4   Gene therapy

Advances in molecular biology have made human gene therapy a clinical reality [48,49]. However, many obstacles remain prior to general application [50]. Gene therapy may be directed at either somatic cells or germ cells. Because of the ethical issues raised by germ cell therapy [51,52], most effort has been directed toward somatic cell targets. Experimentally the challenge is to develop methods to efficiently introduce genetic material into an appropriate target cell, with minimal toxicity, and in a manner in which expression of the gene product is normally regulated or, at least, within an appropriate range for therapeutic effect. The closest method to achieving this ideal is the use of retroviral vectors as gene delivery systems [53]. Because of its immortality, multilineage expression and ease of manipulation, and the frequency of hematopoietically based genetic disease, HSCs have been the most promising and frequently studied target cells.

88.4.1   RATIONALE FOR PRENATAL GENE THERAPY

Because most genetic disease is progressive, it could be argued that the earlier therapy is initiated, the better, particularly for storage diseases with devastating neurologic manifestations which may begin *in utero*. Although the non-CNS manifestations of these diseases can be reversed by postnatal BMT, the neurologic disease is, at best, arrested [5,6,54]. In addition to these clinical arguments, however, there are theoretical arguments and experimental data which support a physiologic advantage for prenatal gene therapy.

Postnatal studies of retroviral transfection of HSCs, particularly in large animals, using bone marrow, have generally been disappointing [55,56]. Although gene expression can be achieved, the level of expression has been low and frequently transient. This has primarily been due to inefficiency of transduction of the gene into cells rather than inefficient expression of the gene from transduced cells. Efficient transduction of retroviral vectors requires replicating cells. Normal hematopoiesis is felt to result from sequential activation of HSC clones rather than continuous cell cycling. Therefore at any given time the majority of HSC are quiescent [57,58]. Taken with the fact that less than 1% of postnatal bone marrow cells are pluripotential HSCs, transduction of a significant number of HSCs is unlikely.

It is established that fetal liver, bone marrow and peripheral blood contain a higher relative number of early progenitors than postnatal hematopoietic tissues. In addition, these cells may be less quiescent, with a higher proportion of cells cycling at any particular time. Therefore, fetal hematopoietic cells should be more efficiently transfected.

88.4.2 EXPERIMENTAL STUDIES

In collaborative studies, we have investigated *in utero* gene transfer in the sheep and monkey models [59,60] using an *ex vivo* infection technique. These studies can be summarized by stating that the efficiency of transduction is higher with fetal-derived HSCs than with postnatal HSCs and that persistence of durably transduced stem cells *in vivo* can be achieved; a result not achieved in any large animal postnatal model to date. In addition, *in vitro* studies of human cord blood and premature blood support improved efficiency of transduction of fetal derived HSC [61].

A promising approach to *in utero* gene therapy is the *in vivo* transfection of cells using either supernatant, containing raw vector, or injection of packaging cells that will release the retroviral vectors. Clapp *et al.* [62] have performed *in utero* injections in fetal mice with successful transfection of somatic target cells. The concern about this approach is the possibility of germ cell transfection and subsequent alteration of the gene pool.

Clinical application of prenatal gene therapy awaits further investigation. Obviously replacement therapy which requires unregulated expression of a deficient or defective enzyme, such as adenosine deaminase deficiency, will be far easier to achieve than corrective therapy for an abnormal protein, which will require site-specific recombination and normal regulation. If methods of safely transducing vector into a large number of fetal cells are developed, there will undoubtedly be wide application. Improved efficiency in such systems will require improvement of vectors, and potentially techniques to cycle HSCs so that maximal efficiency can be achieved.

88.5 Summary

Human *in utero* transplantation is now technically feasible for a variety of hematopoietic diseases. Experimental data are promising but efficacy remains unproven for most applications. Remaining obstacles for success include the current ethical debate over use of fetal tissue and gene therapy, the inability to engraft adult cells without GVHD, and, for some therapeutic applications, the low level of donor cell expression achieved thus far. If these can be overcome, *in utero* HSC transplantation may reduce the morbidity, mortality, and human and societal cost of prenatally diagnosed hematopoietic disease.

References

1. Harrison, M.R., Golbus, M.S. and Filly, R.A. (eds) (1990) *The Unborn Patient: Prenatal Diagnosis and Therapy*, 2nd edn, W.B. Saunders, Philadelphia.
2. Flake, A.W., Harrison, M.R. and Zanjani, E.D. (1991) In utero stem cell transplantation. *Exp. Hematol.*, 19, 1061–64.
3. Clark, J. (1990) The challenge of bone marrow transplantation. *Mayo Clin. Proc.*, 65, 111–14.
4. Sullivan, K. (1989) Current status of bone marrow transplantation. *Transplant. Proc.*, 21, 41–50.
5. Parkman, R. (1986) The application of bone marrow transplantation to the treatment of genetic diseases. *Science*, 232, 1373–78.
6. Krivit, W., Shapiro, E., Kennedy, W. *et al.* (1990) Treatment of late infantile metachromatic leukodystrophy by bone marrow transplantation. *N. Engl. J. Med.*, 322, 28–32.
7. Metcalf, D. and Moore, M.A.S. (1971) Embryonic aspects of hemopoiesis, in *Frontiers of Biology–Hematopoietic Cells* (eds A. Neuberger and E.L. Tatum), North Holland, Amsterdam, pp. 172–271.
8. Soloman, J. (1971) *Fetal and Neonatal Immunology*, North Holland, Company, Amsterdam, pp. 234–306.
9. Schwartz, R. (1989) Acquisition of immunologic self-tolerance. *Cell*, 57, 1073–80.
10. Marrack, P., Lo, D., Brinster, R. *et al.* (1988) The effect of the thymic microenvironment on T-cell development and tolerance. *Cell*, 53, 627–34.
11. Owen, R.D. (1945) Immunologic consequences of vascular anastomoses between bovine twins. *Science*, 102, 400–401.
12. Billingham, R., Brent, L. and Medawar, P.B. (1953) Actively acquired tolerance of foreign cells. *Nature*, 172, 603–606.
13. Billingham, R., Brent, L. and Medawar, P.B. (1956) Quantitative studies on tissue transplantation immunity. III. Actively acquired tolerance. *Philos. Trans. R. Soc. Lond. [Biol.]*, 239, 357–65.
14. Flake, A.W., Harrison, M.R., Adzick, N.S. and Zanjani, E.D. (1986) Transplantation of fetal hematopoietic stem cells *in utero*: the creation of hematopoietic chimeras. *Science*, 233, 776–78.
15. Harrison, M.R., Slotnick, R.N., Crombleholme, T.M. *et al.* (1989) In-utero transplantation of fetal liver haematopoietic stem cells in monkeys. *Lancet*, ii, 1425–27.
16. Duncan, B.W., Harrison, M.R., Flake, A.W. *et al.* (1991) Immune response in hematopoietic chimeric rhesus monkeys. *Surg. Forum*, 42, 373–75.
17. Duncan, B.W., Harrison, M.R., Crombleholme, T.M. *et al.* (1992) Effect of erythropoeitic stress on donor hematopoietic cell expression in chimeric rhesus monkeys transplanted *in utero*. *Exp. Hematol.*, 20, 350–53.
18. Crombleholme, T.M., Harrison, M.R. and Zanjani, E.D. (1990) In utero transplantation of hematopoietic stem cells in sheep: the role of T cells in engraftment and graft-versus-host disease. *J. Pediatr. Surg.*, 25, 885–92.
19. Zanjani, E.D., Mackintosh, F.R. and Harrison, M.R. (1991) Hematopoietic chimerism in sheep and non-human primates by *in utero* transplantation of fetal hematopoietic cells. *Blood Cells*, 17, 349–63.
20. Pearce, R.D., Kiehm, D., Armstrong, D.T. *et al.* (1989) Induction of hemopoietic chimerism in the caprine fetus by intraperitoneal injection of fetal liver cells. *Experientia*, 45, 307–10.
21. Roodman, G.D., Kuehl, T.J., Vandeberg, J.L. and Muirhead, D.Y. (1991) *In utero* bone marrow transplantation of fetal baboons with mismatched adult baboon marrow. *Blood Cells*, 17, 367–75.
22. Mason, J. and Ryan, K.J. (1990) Fetal tissue transplantation research. *Fetal Diagn. Ther.*, 5, 2–4.
23. Linch, D.C., Rodeck, C.H., Jones, H.M. and Brent, L. (1986) Attempted bone marrow transplantation in a 17-week fetus (letter). *Lancet*, ii, 1453.
24. Touraine, J.L., Raudrant, D., Royo, C. *et al.* (1989) In-utero transplantation of stem cells in bare lymphocyte syndrome (letter). *Lancet*, i, 1382.
25. Touraine, J.L. (1990) In utero transplantation of stem cells in humans. *Nouv. Rev. Fr. Hematol.*, 32, 441–44.
26. Touraine, J.L. (1991) Stem cell transplantation in primary immunodeficiency, with special reference to the first prenatal, *in utero*, transplants. *Allergol. Immunopathol. (Madr.)*, 19, 49–51.
27. Touraine, J.L. (1991) In utero transplantation of fetal liver stem cells in humans. *Blood Cells*, 17, 379–87.
28. Rebaud, A., Barbier, F., Roncarolo, M.G. *et al.* (1991) In utero transplantation of hemopoietic stem cells in humans. *Transplant. Proc.*, 23, 1706–708.

29. Touraine, J.L. (1992) *In utero* transplantation of fetal liver stem cells into human fetuses. *Hum. Reprod.*, 7, 44–48.

30. Slavin, S., Neparstek, E., Ziegler, M. *et al.* (1990) Intrauterine bone marrow transplantation for correction of genetic disorders in man [abstract]. *Exp. Hematol.*, 18, 658.

31. Golbus, M.S. (1991) *In utero* stem cell transplantation. *Am. J. Hum. Genet.*, 49, A155.

32. Mavroudis, C., Harrison, M.R., Klein, J.B. *et al.* (1988) Infant orthotopic cardiac transplantation. *J. Thorac. Cardiovasc. Surg.*, 96, 912–18.

33. Najarian, J., Frey, D.J., Matas, A.J. *et al.* (1990) Renal transplantation in infants. *Ann. Surg.*, 212, 353–60.

34. Fricker, F., Griffith, B.P., Hardesty, R.L. *et al.* (1987) Experience with heart transplantation in children. *Pediatrics*, 79, 138–43.

35. Krull, F., Hoyer, P.F., Offner, G. *et al.* (1988) Renal handling of magnesium in transplanted children under cyclosporin A treatment. *Eur. J. Pediatr.*, 148, 148–55.

36. Tagge, E., Campbell Jr, D.A., Dafoe, D.C. *et al.* (1987) Pediatric renal transplantation with an emphasis on the prognosis of patients with chronic renal insufficiency since infancy. *Surgery*, 102, 692–701.

37. Harrison, M.R., Adzick, N.S., Longaker, M.T. *et al.* (1990) Successful repair *in utero* of a fetal diaphragmatic hernia after removal of herniated viscera from the left thorax. *N. Engl. J. Med.*, 322, 1582–84.

38. Johston, J. and Sakala, E.P. (1990) Neonatal cardiac allotransplantation facilitated by *in utero* diagnosis of hypoplastic left-sided heart syndrome. The Loma Linda University Heart Transplant Group. *West. J. Med.*, 152, 70–72.

39. Harrison, M.R., Filly, R.A., Parer, J.R.T. *et al.* (1981) Management of the fetus with a urinary tract malformation. *JAMA*, 246, 635–39.

40. Grompe, M., Jones, S.N. and Caskey, C.T. (1990) Molecular detection and correction of ornithine transcarbamylase deficiency. *Trends Genet.*, 6, 335–39.

41. Cragle, R. and Stone, W.H. (1967) Preliminary results of kidney grafts between cattle chimeric twins. *Transplantation*, 5, 328–32.

42. Simonsen, M. (1955) The acquired immunity concept in kidney homotransplantation. *Ann. N.Y. Acad. Sci.*, 59, 448–52.

43. Anderson, D., Billingham, R.E., Lampkin, G.H. and Medawar, P.B. (1951) The use of skin grafting to distinguish between monozygotic and dizgotic twins in cattle. *Heredity*, 5, 379–92.

44. Binns, R. (1967) Bone marrow and lymphoid cell injection of the pig foetus resulting in transplantation tolerance or immunity, and immunoglobulin production. *Nature*, 214, 179–81.

45. Porter, K. (1960) Runt disease and tolerance in rabbits. *Nature*, 185, 789–90.

46. Zanjani, E.D., Pallavicini, M.G., Ascensao, J.L. *et al.* (1992) Engraftment and long-term expression of human fetal hemopoeitic stem cells in sheep following transplantation *in utero*. *J. Clin. Invest.*, 89, 1178–88.

47. Pallavicini, M.G., Flake, A.W., Madden, D. *et al.* (1992) Hemopoietic chimerism in rodents transplanted *in utero* with fetal human hemopoietic cells. *Transplant. Proc.*, 24, 542–43.

48. Culliton, B. (1990) Gene therapy begins, *Science*, 249, 1372.

49. Anderson, W. (1990) Clinical protocols: the N2-TIL human gene transfer clinical protocol. *Hum. Gene Ther.*, 1, 73–92.

50. Anderson, W.F. (1986) Prospects for human gene therapy in the born and unborn patient. *Clin. Obstet. Gynecol.* 29, 586–94.

51. Berger, E.M. and Gert, B.M. (1991) Genetic disorders and the ethical status of germ-line gene therapy. *J. Med. Philos.*, 16, 667–83.

52. Annas, G.J. and Elias, S. (1990) Legal and ethical implications of fetal diagnosis and gene therapy. *Am. J. Med. Genet.*, 35, 215–18.

53. Bernstein, A., Berger, S., Huszar, D. *et al.* (1985) Gene transfer with retrovirus vectors, in *Genetic Engineering: Principles and Methods*, vol. 7 (eds J. Setlow and A. Hollaender), Plenum Press, New York, pp. 235–67.

54. Muenzer, J. (1986) Mucopolysaccharidoses. *Adv. Pediatr.*, 33, 269–302.

55. Kohn, D.B., Kantoff, P.W., Eglitis, M.A. *et al.* (1987) Retroviral-mediated gene transfer into mammalian cells. *Blood Cells*, 13, 285–98.

56. Kantoff, P.W., Gillio, A., McLachlin, J. *et al.* (1987) Expression of human adenosine deaminase in non-human primates after retroviral mediated gene transfer. *J. Exp. Med.*, 166, 219–34.

57. Lemischka, I.R., Raulet, D.H. and Milligan, R.C. (1986) Developmental potential and dynamic behavior of hematopoietic stem cells. *Cell*, 45, 917–22.

58. Mintz, B., Anthony, D. and Litwin, S. (1984) Monoclonal derivation of mouse myeloid and lymphoid lineages from totipotent hematopoietic stem cells experimentally engrafted in fetal hosts. *Proc. Natl Acad. Sci. USA.*, 81, 7835–42.

59. Kantoff, P.W., Flake, A.W., Eglitis, M.A. *et al.* (1989) *In utero* gene transfer and expression: a sheep transplantation model. *Blood*, 73, 1066–73.

60. Kantoff, P.W., Gillio, A., McLachlin, J.R. *et al.* (1986) Retroviral-mediated gene transfer into hematopoietic cells. *Trans. Assoc. Am. Physicians.*, 99, 92–102.

61. Ekhterae, D., Crombleholme, T.M., Karson, E. *et al.* (1988) Comparison of the efficiency of Neo R transfer into fetal and adult hematopoietic progenitors *in vitro*. *Blood*, 72 (suppl. 5), 386a.

62. Clapp, D.W., Dumenco, L.L., Hatzoglou, M. and Gerson, S.L. (1991) Fetal liver hematopoietic stem cells as a target for *in utero* retroviral gene transfer. *Blood*, 78, 1132–39.

89 LUNG MATURATION IN PRENATAL PREPARATION OF THE FETUS

R.A. Ballard and P.L. Ballard

89.1 Pulmonary disease in the preterm infant

89.1.1 OCCURRENCE

Pulmonary disease remains the most common complication of preterm infants. The classical description of respiratory distress syndrome (RDS) as a surfactant deficiency disease has been modified as smaller and smaller preterm infants are resuscitated and survive to receive intensive care. Their respiratory distress results from a combination of surfactant deficiency, delayed clearance of lung water and immaturity of lung structure. Indeed, in the smallest infants (<1000 g) a weak chest wall also often contributes. These factors which lead to the requirement for oxygen therapy and mechanical ventilation are frequently the background upon which more prolonged respiratory distress develops in these infants as a result of antioxidant damage, edema, barotrauma, infection and inflammatory responses. It is clear that the group at greatest risk for morbidity and mortality from respiratory distress are the very-low-birth-weight infants (<1500 g). The Neonatal Network of the National Institute of Child Health and Human Development (NICHHD) in the USA has recently reported that in these very-low-birth-weight infants, the reported incidence of RDS was 43%, with an additional 27% with the diagnosis of 'respiratory insufficiency'. Thus a total of 70% of these infants had some significant pulmonary problem in the neonatal period [1].

89.1.2 ASSOCIATED PROBLEMS

During the past decade the number of infants actually dying of RDS has decreased due both to advances in perinatal–neonatal care and to prophylactic antenatal steroid therapy [2]. These infants therefore survive, often to suffer from a number of other diseases associated with prematurity. The NICHHD study [1] reported that in addition to being highly susceptible to septicemia and meningitis, approximately 25% of these infants had a significant patent ductus arteriosus, 45% had some degree of intracranial hemorrhage, 26% of the survivors were still on oxygen at 28 days of life and 60% of survivors under 1000 g were still on oxygen at 28 days of life. Any therapy which is being used in an effort to prevent pulmonary disease must therefore be evaluated for its effect on these other complications of prematurity.

89.2 Agents used to prevent respiratory distress in the preterm infant

A number of agents have been evaluated for their potential effect on lung development (Table 89.1). It is clear from laboratory studies that maturation of the lung is a complex process and that some agents stimulate, while others inhibit aspects of maturation by several different mechanisms. The only agent which has been extensively studied both in the laboratory and in

Table 89.1 Agents affecting lung development

Stimulators
Glucocorticoids
Thyroid hormones
cAMP
Epidermal growth factor
Interferon-γ

Inhibitors
Insulin
Transforming growth factor β
Testosterone
Phorbol esters

Questionable role
Prolactin
Estradiol
Ambroxol

Diseases of the Fetus and Newborn, 2nd edn, Edited by G.B. Reed, A.E. Claireaux and F. Cockburn. Published in 1995 by Chapman & Hall, London. ISBN 0 412 39160 0

controlled clinical trials is antenatal glucocorticoid therapy. The first clinical study was reported by Liggins and Howie [3], and Table 89.2 presents the results of this and 25 other studies reported in the literature [4–30]. Thirteen of these studies found decreased mortality in treated infants and 22 showed a decrease in RDS, while two additional studies reported a trend toward a decrease. Crowley [31] has recently reviewed studies that were randomized prospective trials (marked with an asterisk in Table 89.2) and performed a meta-analysis on 12 trials involving over 3000 women. She found a reduction in the overall incidence of RDS from 20% to 11% in the entire group (odds ratio of 0.48, 95% confidence limits 0.4–0.58); in the

'optimally treated' group (delivered > 24 hours but ≤ 7 days) the incidence increased from 21.6% to 8.9%.

89.3 Glucocorticoid issues affecting efficacy

89.3.1 GENDER

Although early reports [32,33] suggested that the male fetus was less responsive to antenatal glucocorticoid therapy, Crowley [31] found significant efficacy of corticosteroid therapy in both the male and the female. The incidence of RDS decreased in the male from 27.9% to 15.4% (odds ratio 0.43, 95% confidence limits 0.29–0.64) and in the female from 23.5% to

Table 89.2 Clinical studies of antenatal glucocorticoids

Investigators	Type of study	Less RDS	Less severe RDS	Less mortality	ROM effect	Other
Liggins and Howie [3]* } Howie and Liggins [4]* }	Prospective blind	Yes	Yes	Yes	No	No difference with double dose; no difference in infection
Fargier et al. [5]	Retrospective	Yes	NE	Yes	NE	
Bureau et al. [6]	Retrospective	Trend	NE	No	NE	
Kennedy [7]	Retrospective paired	Yes	NE	Trend	NE	No difference in infection; follow-up satisfactory after 3 years
Caspi et al. [8]	Retrospective	Yes	NE	Yes	No	Increased L/S ratio with therapy; no effect on infection
Dluholucky, Babic and Taufer [9]	Prospective 'random'	Yes	NE	Yes	No	No effect in 24 hours
Thornfeldt et al. [10]	Retrospective paired	Yes	NE	NE	NE	No difference with different dosages
Osler et al. [11]	Retrospective 'controls'	Yes	NE	Yes	NE	160 'controls' not concurrent
Block, Kling and Crosby [12]*	Prospective blind 'Beta'	Yes	NE	Trend	Yes	No effect of time of therapy to delivery
Morrison et al. [13]*	Prospective blind	Yes	Yes	Trend	NE	No effect on infection; trend to lower RDS at 18 h therapy
Ballard et al. [14]	Retrospective	Yes	Yes	Yes	No	No effect on infection
Papageorgiou [15]	Prospective blind	Yes	Yes	Yes	No	Less effect in male; hypoglycemia in treated patients; no effect on infection
Taeusch et al. [16]*	Prospective blind	Yes	Yes	Yes	No	Increased maternal infection with PROM; no effect admission to delivery time
Young et al. [17]	'Matched controls'	Yes	Yes	Yes	No	Increased infection in treated patients; PROM
Teramo, Hallman and Raivio [18]	Prospective	No	NE	No	NE	

cont.

Table 89.2 *continued*

Investigators	Type of study	Less RDS	Less severe RDS	Less mortality	ROM effect	Other
Doran et al. [19]*	Prospective blind	Yes	Yes	Yes	No	Less RDS in whole group; trend in 24–32 weeks
Caspi et al. [20]	Retrospective	Yes	NE	No	No	Increased RDS in any group with low Apgar score
Schutte et al. [21]*	Prospective blind	Yes	Yes	No	NE	Increased RDS in infants born <12 to >3 weeks after admission
Garite et al. [22]	'Random' with PROM	Trend 30 weeks	No	No	NE	Increased infection with Beta + PROM
Collaborative Group [23]*	Prospective blind	Yes	NE	No	Yes	No effect in twins; effect decreased in male; decreased hospital stay; no difference in infection
Kuhn et al. [24]	Prospective 'random'	Yes	NE	Yes	Yes	Increased infection with cerclage; increased infection in male 27–20 weeks
Schmidt et al. [25]*	Prospective blind	Yes	Yes	No	No	Increased maternal infection with hydrocortisone; no effect on neonatal infection
Doyle et al. [26]	Prospective non-random	Yes	Yes	Yes	NE	No difference in infection; improved growth at 2 years
Morales et al. [27]*	Prospective blind random	Yes	NE	No	All	Decreased intraventricular hemorrhage; decreased hospital costs
Papageorgiou, Doray and Ardilia [28]	Prospective non-random	Yes	Yes	Yes	NE	Decreased hospitalization; decreased patent ductus arteriosus
Gamsu et al. [29]*	Prospective randomized	Yes	NE	No	NE	No effect on infections; decreased jaundice

Beta = betamethasone; L/S = lecithin/phophatidylcholine/sphingomyelin; NE = not evaluated; PROM = premature rupture of membranes; ROM = (spontaneous) rupture of membranes.
* Study used by Crowley [31] in meta-analysis.

9.6% (odds ratio 0.36, 95% confidence limits 0.23–0.57).

89.3.2 MULTIPLE BIRTH

It is well known that the second of twins is more likely to suffer from RDS, an effect which is considered to be related to the increased likelihood of asphyxia in the second twin. Although a number of trials have attempted to examine this problem, it is currently impossible to determine whether the apparent lack of responsiveness to antenatal steroids for twins is due to the likelihood of asphyxia or whether glucocorticoids are less effective in multiple gestation infants for other reasons.

89.3.3 GESTATIONAL AGE

Although initial reports [3,23] did not report on glucocorticoid efficacy in early gestation infants, subsequent studies were examined by Crowley [31]. Results of seven randomized studies demonstrated efficacy of corticosteroids prior to 31 weeks with a reduction in incidence from 48.6% to 26.7% (odds ratio 0.38, 95% confidence limits 0.24–0.60).

89.3.4 PROLONGED RUPTURE OF MEMBRANES

The treatment of the woman who presents in preterm labor with prolonged rupture of membranes (PROM) remains a somewhat controversial area of management in the perinatal community. Initial reports [34–36] suggested that PROM alone was associated with a decrease in incidence of RDS, although other studies found that steroids provide an additional benefit to women with ruptured membranes [24]. Ohlsson [37] reviewed this literature and performed a meta-analysis of five studies and demonstrated a reduction of RDS in the treatment group. However, if one of the studies [27] is removed there is no significant reduction in RDS. In addition there has been concern that administration of steroids to women with ruptured membranes might result in increased maternal or neonatal infection. Although many institutions have developed a protocol for the use of antenatal betamethasone in the presence of ruptured membranes, other investigators feel that further randomized controlled trials are needed in order to demonstrate the safety of glucocorticoid treatment in the presence of preterm PROM.

89.3.5 SURFACTANT REPLACEMENT

In studies with premature animals the combination of antenatal steroid and postnatal surfactant replacement results in better outcome than with either therapy alone [38]. Data from the recent multicenter trials of surfactant treatment (Survanta and Exosurf) indicate that infants receiving prenatal corticosteroid had a better response to surfactant with regard to overall mortality, respiratory mortality, air leaks, patent ductus arteriosus and intraventricular hemorrhage [39] (A. Jobe, personal communication). In the Survanta study, for example, no infants receiving both surfactant and steroid died, compared with 6.5% for steroid alone, 7.3% for surfactant alone, and 19.6% for no treatment. These findings emphasize that surfactant replacement should not be considered as an alternative treatment to prenatal corticosteroids.

89.4   Other effects, risks and benefits of glucocorticoids

Antenatal steroid therapy has been subjected to a more careful examination of theoretical and demonstrated risks than virtually any other intervention used in perinatal medicine. Initial concerns about maternal and infant infection, growth, neurological development, immunologic competence, metabolic and hormonal disturbances as well as placental function have all been carefully addressed and no deleterious effects have been demonstrated. A particular area of concern, infant sepsis, was evaluated by Crowley [31] and in a meta-analysis of eight studies there was no evidence of increased risk either with or without PROM.

On the other hand, the established benefits of antenatal glucocorticoid include not just decreased mortality and RDS, but also decreased severity of respiratory distress, some evidence of decreased occurrence of bronchopulmonary dysplasia [40] and decreased incidence of patent ductus arteriosus, necrotizing enterocolitis, intraventricular hemorrhage, average length of hospital stay and cost of care (reviewed in ref. 30).

89.5   Recommendations for therapy

Administration of antenatal glucocorticoids is indicated in women with preterm labor between 24 and 34 weeks gestation, or after 34 weeks if studies show that the fetal lung is immature. Contraindications include signs of fetal distress, maternal distress, amnionitis, or severe maternal or fetal bleeding. We also recommend administration of antenatal glucocorticoids to women with PROM as long as there is no sign of maternal infection. The current method for administering glucocorticoids (betamethasone 12 mg in two doses every 24 hours) produces a physiologic stress level of steroids which is virtually the same as the endogenous steroid exposure of an untreated fetus who develops RDS and a steroid response after birth. It is of note that the dose of steroids commonly used [41] to treat postnatal chronic lung disease (the complication of severe RDS) in the preterm infant is tenfold higher (0.07 mg/kg for prenatal steroids versus 0.5-0.6 mg/kg for chronic lung disease) and administered for a much longer duration (antenatal steroids are cleared with 72 hours).

89.6   Long-term outcome after prenatal glucocorticoids

Multiple follow-up studies have been done on infants exposed to antenatal steroids, some through age 12 years of life [42–45]. No significant differences in growth or development or other complications have been found, in spite of improved survival of more very-low-birth-weight infants.

89.7   Other agents that have been evaluated

89.7.1 THYROID HORMONES

The acceleration of pulmonary development by thyroid hormone has been evaluated primarily in the laboratory and in experimental animals [46,47]. Some preliminary studies using intra-amniotic administration of thyroxine or triiodothyronine to women in premature labor have suggested the possibility of some benefit in the human [48,49]. One of the major problems with thyroxine administration in the human is the difficulty in getting the hormone to the fetus. For this reason recent studies have evaluated thyrotropin-releasing hormone (TRH), which crosses the placenta, in combination with antenatal glucocorticoids. In the first report of combined hormonal therapy, Morales *et al.* [50] found a decrease in RDS from 44% to 28% (not statistically significant) as well as a decrease in incidence of chronic lung disease from 24% to 8% (p ≤ 0.05). Three additional studies [51–53] in abstract form also suggest a decrease in severity of respiratory distress or requirement for mechanical ventilation.

Results from the first multi-center double-blind trial to examine the effect of TRH + betamethasone on infant outcome were recently published [54]. In this study women in preterm labor who were receiving betamethasone (12 mg two doses every 24 hours) were randomized to receive either four doses of TRH (400 μg in 50 ml of saline every 8 hours) or placebo. None of the infants received surfactant replacement. Although there was no decrease in incidence of respiratory distress, there was a trend toward less severe disease. Among the fully treated infants of less than 1500 g birth weight the incidence of chronic lung disease (requirement for oxygen at 28 days) was reduced from 43.9% in the betamethasone alone group to 17.6% in the TRH + betamethasone group (Figure 89.1). Additional trials are underway using prenatal TRH + glucocorticoid, combined with appropriate use of postnatal surfactant as needed, to evaluate further the effectiveness and possible risks of combined therapy.

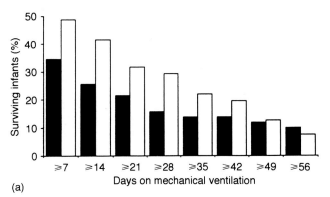

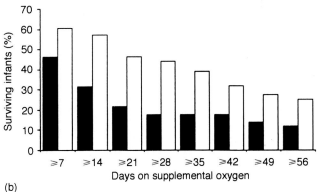

Figure 89.1 Percentage of surviving, fully treated infants in each treatment group requiring (a) assisted ventilation and (b) supplemental oxygen during the first 8 weeks of life. Results are for infants with birth weight ≤ 1500 g, whose mothers had four doses of TRH or placebo, and who were born less than 10 days after entry into the trial. At 8 weeks, there were 51 survivors of 55 infants in the TRH + S (steroid) group (■) and 40 survivors of 48 infants in the S-alone (□) group. For days on supplemental oxygen, Wilcoxon rank test P = 0.032, log rank test P = 0.042. Statistical analysis of mechanical ventilation was not possible since some infants needed further ventilation after initial withdrawal of ventilatory support.

89.7.2 AMBROXOL

Bromhexine metabolite VIII (ambroxol) is a drug with mucolytic action that has been investigated in Europe for efficacy in preventing RDS. Several studies in animals indicate that ambroxol stimulates synthesis and content of pulmonary phospholipids (reviewed in ref. 55). However, this effect of ambroxol requires therapy for 5–7 days. In the only double-blind trial of prenatal therapy, Wauer *et al* [56] were unable to demonstrate any benefit of ambroxol in infants of 30–34 weeks' gestation, and there is no evidence from other reports that this drug is effective in infants under 32 weeks' gestation. Thus, there is insufficient information to recommend treatment with ambroxol. In addition, a disadvantage of therapy is that there are significant side-effects including nausea, vomiting and headache in the women, increased fetal heart rate, and requirement for intravenous administration over at least 5 days.

89.7.3 CYCLIC ADENOSINE MONOPHOSPHATE MEDIATING AGENTS

There has been significant interest (reviewed in refs 30, 47 and 57) in the agents such as aminophylline and β-adrenergic agonists which would increase endogenous cyclic adenosine monophosphate (cAMP). There have been conflicting reports on decreased RDS associated with the use of β-adrenergic agents and currently these agents are not accepted modes of treatment for prevention of RDS.

89.8 Summary

Pulmonary disease as it affects the very-low-birthweight infant is a complex entity and antenatal therapeutic interventions must address other complications of prematurity such as patent ductus arteriosus, necrotizing enterocolitis and intraventricular hemorrhage, as well as long term pulmonary morbidity. The only currently well established agent for improving pulmonary as well as other outcomes for the preterm infant is antenatal glucocorticoid administration. The possibility of combining glucocorticoid with TRH antenatally, with appropriate administration of surfactant replacement after birth, is very promising.

References

1. Hack, M., Horbar, J.D., Malloy, M.H. et al. (1991) Very low birth weight outcomes of the National Institute of Health and Human Development neonatal network. Pediatrics, 87, 587–97.
2. Malloy M.H., Hartford, R.B. and Kleinman, J.C. (1987) Trends in mortality caused by respiratory distress in the United States, 1969–83. Am. J. Public Health, 77, 1511–14.
3. Liggins, G.C. and Howie, R.N. (1972) A controlled trial of antepartum glucocorticoid treatment for prevention of the respiratory distress syndrome in premature infants. Pediatrics, 50, 515–20.
4. Howie, R.N. and Liggins, G.C. (1982) The New Zealand study of antepartum glucocorticoid treatment in lung development, in Lung Development, vol. II Biological and Clinical Perspectives (ed., P.M. Farrell), Academic Press, New York, pp. 255–65.
5. Fargier, P., Salle, B., Baud Gagnaire, J.C. et al. (1974) Prévention du syndrome de détresse respiratoire chez le prématuré. Nouv. Presse Med., 3, 1595–97.
6. Bureau, M., Stocker, J., Deleon, A. et al. (1975) Utilization de la betamethasone dans la prévention du syndrome de déstresse respiratoire du nouveau prématuré. Union Med. Can., 104, 99–106.
7. Kennedy, J.L. (1976) Clinical experience with betamethasone for the prevention of respiratory distress syndrome, in Lung Maturation and the Prevention of Hyaline Membrane Disease, Proceedings of the Seventieth Ross Conference on Pediatric Research, Ross Laboratories, Columbus, Ohio, pp. 181–84.
8. Caspi, E., Schreyer, P., Weinraub, Z. et al. (1976) Prevention of the respiratory distress syndrome in premature infants by antepartum glucocorticoid therapy. Br. J. Obstet. Gynaecol., 83, 187–93.
9. Dluholucky, S., Babic, J. and Taufer, I. (1976) Reduction of incidence and mortality of respiratory distress syndrome by administration of hydrocortisone to mother. Arch. Dis. Child., 51, 420–23.
10. Thornfeldt, R.E., Franklin, R.W., Pickering, N.A. et al. (1978) The effect of glucocorticoids on the maturation of premature lung membranes, preventing the respiratory syndrome by glucocorticoids. Am. J. Obstet. Gynecol., 131, 143–47.
11. Osler, M., Faero, O., Friis-Hansen, B. and Trolle, D. (1978) Prevention of the respiratory syndrome (RDS) by antepartum glucocorticoid (betamethasone) therapy combined with phenobarbitone and ritodrine. Dan. Med. Bull., 25, 225–29.
12. Block, M., Kling, O. and Crosby, W. (1977) Antenatal glucocorticoid therapy for the prevention of respiratory distress syndrome in the premature infant. Obstet. Gynecol., 50, 186–90.
13. Morrison, J.C., Whybrew, W.D., Bucovaz, E.T. and Schneider, J.M. (1978) Injection of corticosteroids into mother to prevent neonatal respiratory distress syndrome. Am. J. Obstet. Gynecol., 131, 358–66.
14. Ballard, R.A., Ballard, P.L., Granberg, J.P. and Sniderman, S. (1979) Prenatal administration of betamethasone for prevention of respiratory distress syndrome. J. Pediatr., 94, 97–101.
15. Papageorgiou, A.N., Desgranges, M.F., Masson, M. et al. (1979) The antenatal use of betamethasone in the prevention of respiratory distress syndrome: a controlled double-blind study. Pediatrics, 63, 73–79.
16. Taeusch Jr, W.H., Frigoletto, F., Kitzmiller, J. et al. (1979) Risk of respiratory distress syndrome after prenatal dexamethasone treatment. Pediatrics, 63, 64–72.
17. Young, B.K., Klein, S.A., Katz, M. et al. (1980) Intravenous dexamethasone for prevention of neonatal respiratory distress: a prospective controlled study. Am. J. Obstet. Gynecol., 138, 203–209.
18. Teramo, K., Hallman, M. and Raivio, K.O. (1980) Maternal glucocorticoid in unplanned premature labor. Controlled study on the effects of betamethasone phosphate on the phospholipids of the gastric aspirate and on the adrenal cortical function of the newborn infant. Pediatr. Res., 14, 326–29.
19. Doran, T.A., Swyer, P., MacMurray, B. et al. (1980) Results of a double-blind controlled study on the use of betamethasone in the prevention of respiratory distress syndrome. Am. J. Obstet. Gynecol., 136, 313–20.
20. Caspi, E., Schreyer, P., Reif, R. and Goldberg, M. (1980) An analysis of

21. Schutte, M.F., Treffers, P.E., Koppe, J.G. and Breur, W. (1980) The influence of betamethasone and orciprenaline on the incidence of respiratory distress syndrome in the newborn after preterm labour. Br. J. Obstet. Gynaecol., 87, 127–31.
22. Garite, T.J., Freeman, R.K., Linzey, E.M. et al (1981) Prospective randomized study of corticosteroids in the managment of premature rupture of the membranes and the premature gestation. Am J. Obstet. Gynecol., 141, 508–15.
23. Collaborative Group on Antenatal Steroid Therapy (1981) Effect of antenatal dexamethasone administration on the prevention of respiratory distress syndrome. Am. J. Obstet. Gynecol., 141, 276–86.
24. Kuhn, R.J.P., Speirs, A.L., Pepperell, R.J. et al. (1982) Betamethasone, albuterol and threatened premature delivery: benefits and risks. Obstet. Gynecol., 60, 403–408.
25. Schmidt, P.L., Sims, M.E., Strassner, H.T. et al. (1984) Effect of antepartum glucocorticoid administration upon neonatal respiratory distress syndrome and perinatal infection. Am. J. Obstet. Gynecol., 148, 178–86.
26. Doyle, L.W., Kitchen, W.H. and Ford G.W. (1986) Effects of antenatal steroid therapy on mortality and morbidity in very low birth weight infants. J. Pediatr., 108, 287–92.
27. Morales, W.J., Diebel, D., Lazar, A.J. and Zadrozny, D. (1986) The effect of antenatal dexamethasone administration on the prevention of respiratory distress syndrome in preterm gestations with premature rupture of membranes. Am. J. Obstet. Gynecol., 154, 591–95.
28. Papageorgiou, A.N., Doray, J.L. and Ardilia, R. (1989) Reduction of mortality, morbidity and respiratory distress syndrome in infants weighing less than 1000 grams by treatment with betamethasone and ritodrine. Pediatrics, 83, 493–97.
29. Gamsu, H.R., Mullinger, B.M., Donnai, P. and Dash, C.H. (1989) Antenatal administration of betamethasone to prevent respiratory distress syndrome in preterm infants: report of a UK multicentre trial. Br. J. Obstet. Gynecol., 96, 401–10.
30. Ballard, R.A. and Ballard, P.L. (1992) Prevention of neonatal respiratory distress syndrome by pharmacological methods, in The Pulmonary Surfactant System (eds B. Robertson, L.M.G. Van Golde and J.J. Batenburg), Elsevier, Amsterdam, pp. 539–60.
31. Crowley, P. (1989) Promoting pulmonary maturity, in Effective Care in Pregnancy, vol. 1 (eds I.M. Chalmers and M.J.N.C. Keirse), Oxford University Press, Oxford, pp. 746–64.
32. Taeusch Jr, H.W. and Tulchinsky, D. (1979) Obstetric Factors Affect Risk of Respiratory Distress Syndrom. Perinatal Developmental Symposium on Premature Labor, Vail, Colorado. Mead Johnson, Evansville, IN, pp 48–55.
33. Ballard, P.L., Ballard, R.A., Granberg, J.P. et al. (1980) Fetal sex and prenatal betamethasone therapy. J. Pediatr., 97, 451–54.
34. Yoon, J.J. and Harper, R.G. (1973) Observations on the relationship between duration of rupture of the membranes and the development of idiopathic respiratory distress syndrome. Pediatrics, 52, 161–68.
35. Bauer C.R., Stein, L. and Colle, E. (1974) Prolonged rupture of membranes associated with a decreased incidence of respiratory distress syndrome. Pediatrics, 73, 7–12.
36. Berkowitz, R.L., Bonta, B.W. and Warshaw, J.E. (1976) The relationship between premature rupture of the membranes and the respiratory distress syndrome. Am. J. Obstet. Gynecol., 124, 7–12.
37. Ohlsson, A. (1989) Treatment of preterm premature rupture of the membranes: a meta-analysis. Am. J. Obstet Gynecol., 160, 890–906.
38. Ikegami, M., Jobe, A.H. and Pettenazo, A. et al. (1987) Effects of maternal treatment with corticosteroids, T3, TRH and their combinations on lung function of ventilated preterm rabbits with and without surfactant treatments. Am. Rev. Respir. Dis., 136, 892–98.
39. Andrews, E.B., White, A.D. and Weinberg, J.M. et al. (1992) Antenatal steroids and neonatal outcomes in infants receiving surfactants in the Exosurf® treatment IND (abstract). Pediatr. Res., 31, 241A.
40. Van Marter, L.J., Leviton, A. and Kuban, K.C.K. et al. (1990) Maternal glucocorticoid therapy and reduced risk of bronchopulmonary dysplasia. Pediatrics, 86, 331–36.
41. Cummings, J.J., D'Eugenio, D.B. and Gross, S.J. (1989) A controlled trial of dexamethasone in preterm infants at high risk for bronchopulmonary dysplasia. N. Engl. J. Med., 320, 1505–10.
42. MacArthur, B.A., Howie, R.N., Dezoete, J.A. and Elkins, J. (1982) School progress and cognitive development of 6-year-old children whose mothers were treated antenatally with betamethasone. Pediatrics, 70, 99–105.
43. Collaborative Group on Antenatal Steroid Therapy (1984) Effects of antenatal dexamethasone administration in the infant: long-term followup. J. Pediatr., 104, 259–67.
44. Schmand, B., Neuvel, J., Smolders-de Haas, H. et al. (1990) Psychological development of children who were treated antenatally with corticosteroids to prevent respiratory distress syndrome. Pediatrics, 86, 58–64.
45. Smolders-de Haas, H., Neuvel, J. and Schmand, B. et al. (1990) Physical development and medical history of children who were treated with

corticosteroids to prevent respiratory distress syndrome: a 10- to 12-year follow-up. *Pediatrics*, **86**, 65–70.

46. Wu, B., Kikkawa, Y. and Roazalesi, M.M. *et al.* (1973) The effect of thyroxine on the maturation of fetal rabbit lungs. *Biol. Neonate*, **22**, 161–68.

47. Ballard, P.L. (1986) Hormones and lung maturation. *Monogr. Endocrinol.*, **28**, 1–354.

48. Maschiah, S., Barkai, G., Sack, J. *et al.* (1978) Enhancement of fetal lung maturity by intra-amniotic administration of thyroid hormone. *Am. J. Obstet. Gynecol.*, **130**, 289–93.

49. Romaguera, J., Zorrilla, C., de la Vega, A. *et al.* (1990) Responsiveness of L-S ratio of the amniotic fluid to intra-amniotic administration of thyroxine. *Acta Obstet. Gynecol. Scand.*, **69**, 119–22.

50. Morales, W.J., O'Brien, W.F., Angel, J.F. *et al.* (1989) Fetal lung maturation: the combined use of corticosteroids and thyrotropin-releasing hormone. *Obstet. Gynecol.*, **73**, 111–16.

51. Knight, D., Liggins, G.C. and Wealthall, S.R. (1994) A randomized controlled trial of ante-partum thyrotropin releasing hormone in the prevention of respiratory disease in preterm infants. *Am. J. Obstet. Gynecol.* (in press).

52. Althabe, F., Fustinana, C., Althabe, O. and Ceriani Cernadas, J.M. (1991) Controlled trial of prenatal betamethasone plus TRH vs. betamethasone plus placebo for prevention of RDS in preterm infants (abstract). *Pediatr. Res.*, **29**, 200A.

53. Jikihara, H., Sawada, Y., Imai, S. *et al.* (1990) *Maternal Administration of Thyrotropin-releasing Hormone for Prevention of Neonatal Respiratory Distress Syndrome*. Proceedings of the 6th Congress of the Federation of Asia-Oceana Perinatal Societies, October, Perth, W. Australia, Abstract No. 87

54. Ballard, R.A., Ballard, P.L., Creasy, R.K., and the TRH Study Group (1992) Respiratory disease in very-low-birthweight infants after prenatal thyrotropin-releasing hormone and glucocorticoid. *Lancet*, **339**, 510–15.

55. Wauer, R.R., Schmalisch, G., Hammer, H. *et al.* (1989) Ambroxol for prevention and treatment of hyaline membrane disease. *Eur. Respir. J.*, **2** (suppl. 3), 57s–65s.

56. Wauer, R.R., Schmalisch, G., Menzel, K. *et al.* (1982) The antenatal use of ambroxol (bromhexine metabolite VIII) to prevent hyaline membrane disease: a controlled double-blind study. *Int. J. Biol. Res. Pregnancy*, **3**, 84–91.

57. Ballard, P.L. (1989) Hormonal regulation of pulmonary surfactant. *Endoc. Rev.*, **10**, 165–81.

90 INTRAPARTUM MANAGEMENT OF FETAL ANOMALIES

J. Manley and S. Weiner

90.1 Anomalies affecting the timing of delivery

Occasionally, continued gestation allows progression of an anomalous pathologic process resulting in a worsened prognosis. In general, the management of anomalous fetuse stresses the importance of the attainment of fetal lung maturity as determined by amniocentesis (lecithin : sphingomyelin ratio, presence of phosphatidyl glycerol). Neonatal stabilization may already be difficult without the addition of respiratory distress syndrome. However the rate of progression of the pathologic process may not afford time to delay delivery until the achievement of lung maturity. Congestive heart failure may develop in cases of vascular compression as in cystic adenomatoid malformation of the lung [1], tumor hemorrhage as in sacrococcygeal teratoma [2,3], arteriovenous anastomoses in hemangiomas [4] and cardiac dysrhythmias [5]. The ultrasonographic signs of intestinal obstruction and mural thickening correlate well with the extent of intestinal damage [6] and can be used to select those fetuses with gastroschisis who will benefit from early delivery. Fetal ovarian cysts may undergo torsion and hemorrhage, signs which may indicate early delivery [7].

It is thought that prolonged compression of the cerebral cortex in cases of ventriculomegaly adversely affects the neurologic outcome [8]. Results of *in utero* shunting have been disappointing. Reports of 44 fetuses by the Registry of the International Society of Fetal Medicine and Surgery revealed a loss rate of 10%, 35% were developing normally, and the remainder had mild or severe handicaps. For these reasons, many authors have recommended delivery as soon as lung maturity has been documented [9]. An exception may be in the case of rapidly enlarging ventricles [10].

Obstructive uropathy may result in varying degrees of renal dysplasia and pulmonary hypoplasia. The severity of dysplasia is related to the degree and timing in gestation of the obstruction. Decompression between 20 and 30 weeks' gestation during the most active period of nephrogenesis may allow normal development without further damage [11–15]. Unlike shunting *in utero* for ventriculomegaly, *in utero* vesicoamniotic shunting has shown some promise, particularly in 'good prognosis' patients, as determined by urinary electrolyte assessment of renal function [16–21]. However, shunt placement has been associated with chorioamnionitis and preterm labor [22–24], and early delivery may be preferable when oligohydramnios develops in the third trimester (Chapter 79).

In addition to progression of the pathologic process, the frequently associated intrauterine growth retardation or poor biophysical testing may be indications for early delivery (Chapters 85–87).

90.2 Anomalies affecting the mode of delivery

Cesarean section clearly carries higher maternal morbidity and mortality rates compared with vaginal delivery [25]. The risks of infection, blood loss and anesthesia complications are increased, in addition to prolonged hospital stays and long-term recovery. Use of cesarean section should be reserved for instances where benefits to the fetus have been proven and outweigh maternal risks.

Cesarean delivery is frequently used when vaginal delivery is unlikely to be successful due to anticipated dystocia. Causes of dystocia include macrocephaly resulting from hydrocephalus. Attempts at decompression of the fetal skull by cephalocentesis in order to allow vaginal delivery carry an unacceptably high perinatal mortality (about 90%) [26]. Thickness of the cortical mantle correlates poorly with outcome [27]. This procedure should be reserved for those cases associated with other anomalies or aneuploidies with

Diseases of the Fetus and Newborn, 2nd edn, Edited by G.B. Reed, A.E. Claireaux and F. Cockburn. Published in 1995 by Chapman & Hall, London. ISBN 0 412 39160 0

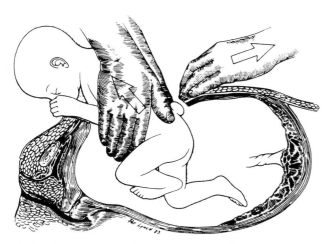

Figure 90.1 Fetus with meningomyelocele is delivered through a low transverse uterine incision. Both fetal flanks are grasped, and gentle traction is applied in an outward direction. The assistant retracts the edge of the uterine incision as the body is delivered.

poor outcomes. Vaginal delivery is recommended for those with normal head biometry (less than 2 standard deviations above the mean). Soft tissue dystocia can be caused by external masses, including large omphalocele or sacrococcygeal teratoma [28]. Dystocia has been reported with large intra-abdominal masses, including polycystic kidneys, ovarian cysts [29] and prune-belly syndrome [30]. Face presentation may result from hyperextension of the fetal head caused by anterior neck masses such as cervical teratoma, goiter, sarcoma and melanoma.

Abdominal delivery has been used for its presumed benefits of decreased trauma to the affected system and the preservation of sterility. This issue is particularly controversial in cases of neural tube defects and ventral wall defects. Cesarean section has been advocated to reduce the risk of infection and the traumatic forces of labor and delivery on the meningomyelocele sac [10,31]; Chervenak has described a technique for this purpose [32] (Figure 90.1). Bensen, Billard and Burton [32] reviewed retrospectively 32 infants born by cesarean section and 40 delivered vaginally and found no difference in neonatal mortality, meningitis, hospital stay or neurologic and developmental status at 1 year of age. Luthy *et al.* [33] reviewed 119 cases of meningomyelocele diagnosed at the time of birth and 81 diagnosed antenatally. They found that those infants exposed to labor (whether delivered abdominally or vaginally) were 2.2 times more likely to have severe paralysis and higher level paralysis. However, the study has the drawbacks of a retrospective study. Of those diagnosed antenatally, only one infant was delivered vaginally. Most reports fail to show any improvement in mortality when fetuses with gastroschisis or

omphalocele are delivered by cesarean section [34–37]. Chescheir *et al.* [38] found a decrease in the incidence of necrotizing enterocolitis in those fetuses delivered abdominally.

Cesarean section may be used in cases where timing is critical with regards to availability of the operating room staff and surgeon or specialists required for resuscitation. Abdominal delivery may be chosen for cases where fetal distress during labor is anticipated. Intrauterine growth retardation is frequently seen in the anomalous fetus and is associated with a 50% incidence of intrapartum asphyxia [39]. Similarly, the hydropic fetus may not be expected to tolerate labor. Conversely, some anomalies resulting in difficult neonatal courses have uncomplicated labors, as in isolated hypoplastic left heart syndrome [40].

Vaginal delivery may not be possible in cases where intrapartum surveillance cannot be achieved. Though frequent scalp pH determinations may permit continued labor, cesarean section is often performed in cases of congenital heart block because of difficulty in interpreting fetal heart rate monitoring [41]. Similar difficulty may be encountered in irregular fetal heart rates and tachydysrhythmias.

90.3 Anomalies affecting the location of delivery

The key to successful perinatal management of the anomalous fetus is the co-ordination of the multidisciplinary team that will care for the infant. This includes the obstetrician, anesthesiologist, neonatologist, obstetric and neonatal nurses, blood bank staff, pediatric surgeon, neurosurgeon and urologist. The nature of the anomaly dictates which aspects of neonatal management will present problems.

Difficult resuscitation may be anticipated from airway obstruction in cases of large goiter, cervical teratoma and epignathus. Fluid and electrolyte management may be complex in abdominal wall defects and in renal failure associated with urinary tract obstruction. Problems of acidosis and perfusion often complicate congenital heart disease. The prognosis associated with many defects is improved with very early neonatal surgery [42]. Success of surgery is strongly influenced by the preoperative stabilization of the neonate [43,44]. Maternal transport to, and delivery in a tertiary care center is mandatory for many antenatally diagnosed anomalies for the integration of all aspects of care. Transport to a perinatal center should be considered not only for anticipated problems, but for undiagnosed defects: as in anomalies with a high incidence of associated anomalies (omphalocele, aneuploidy) and where there are limitations on the diagnostic accuracy (oligohydramnios).

90.4 Intrapartum monitoring
(Chapters 21 and 91)

90.4.1 MONITORING TECHNIQUES

Oxygen deprivation in the fetus results in a shift in ATP production from the Kreb's cycle to the Embden–Meyerhof pathway, resulting in the production of pyruvate and subsequently lactate. Acidosis renders the cell membrane permeable to water, allowing the cell to swell and undergo lysis. This process is irreversible in brain cells and results in neurologic damage. The goal of intrapartum monitoring is to evaluate fetal oxygenation, which is potentially remediable, and to maintain normal acid–base status.

Intrapartum monitoring focuses primarily on the fetal heart rate (by external Doppler or internal fetal scalp electrode) in relation to uterine contractions (by external tocodynamometer or intrauterine pressure catheter). Specific periodic and non-periodic heart rate changes suggest the presence of hypoxia and/or acidosis and possible etiologies. Periodic decelerations are those recurring, bearing some relationship to the uterine contractions. Early decelerations begin at the onset of a contraction and reach a nadir at the peak of the contraction; they are thought to be benign, resulting from pressure on the head in the birth canal through meningeal stimulation and vagal output. Variable decelerations are characterized by their abrupt onset and recovery, variable shape and variable relationship to contractions [45]. They are thought to be vagally mediated, resulting from cord compression or head compression [46]. Cord compression results in increased peripheral resistance and P_{CO_2} and decreased P_{O_2}. Stimulation of baroreceptors and chemoreceptors results in vagal output. Late decelerations begin after the onset of the contraction and recover after the end of the contraction and are due to impaired intervillous blood flow resulting in fetal hypoxia. Non-periodic changes include accelerations which are indicative of an adequately oxygenated fetus. The heart rate variability is the variation in heart rate seen on a beat-to-beat basis and long-term (3–5 cycles per minute) basis. Though variability may be decreased by fetal sleep states and central nervous system depressants, its presence may be the most reliable indicator of intact cortical input and nomal acid–base status. If there is evidence of ongoing hypoxia, attempts should be made to alleviate this. If attempts at *in utero* resuscitation are unsuccessful or heart rate monitoring does not provide reassurance against the possibility of acidosis, scalp stimulation or acoustic stimulation may be employed. The presence of accelerations in response to these stimuli provides reasonable reassurance against acidosis [47,48]. Ultimately, a capillary blood pH determination via the scalp may be necessary to allow further labor or to mandate immediate delivery.

Continuous electronic monitoring has not been shown to be more effective than intermittent auscultation in reducing perinatal morbidity and mortality in large studies [49,50]. However, continuous electronic fetal monitoring with its high sensitivity is usually used in the high-risk fetus because of the reassurance normal monitoring gives, the labor-intensive effort required for intermittent auscultation and the significance of poor monitoring in warning of potentially correctable problems.

90.4.2 SPECIAL CONSIDERATIONS FOR THE ANOMALOUS FETUS

The management of labor often involves the appraisal of obstetrical interventions with regards to their risk to the mother and the benefits to the fetus. Chervenak and McCullough [51] dissected the management dilemma to produce an ethically justified, clinically comprehensive management strategy for third trimester pregnancies complicated by fetal anomalies. Essentially, the physician has obligations to the mother and to the fetus as a patient. The physician's responsibility to the

Table 90.1 Classification of fetal anomalies by degree of probability of antenatal diagnosis and degree of probability of outcome

Category	Probability of antenatal diagnosis	Probability of death or absence of cognitive developmental capacity	Example
A	Certainty	Certainty	Anencephaly
B	Certainty	Very high probability	Trisomy 18
B	Very high probability	Certainty	Renal agenesis
B	Very high probability	Very high probability	Thanatophoric dysplasia
C	Less than very high probability	Very high probability or certainty	Lissencephaly
C	Very high probability or certainty	Less than very high probability	Isolated hydrocephalus
C	Less than very high probability	Less than very high probability	Achondroplasia

mother is to respect her autonomy, allowing her to make decisions about the management of her pregnancy. This means providing her with the available alternatives: agressive management (intervention on behalf of the fetus), non-aggressive management (withholding intervention that increases risk for the mother), and termination of the pregnancy. Depending on the prognosis of the fetus, the physician may have beneficence-based obligations to the fetus. Both the certainty of prognosis associated with a particular diagnosis and the certainty of diagnosis must be factored into the management plan. If the lack of potential for cognitive development or survival is certain for a diagnosis, and the diagnosis is certain (Chervenak's group A), choices recommended to the patient include termination and non-aggressive management. This type of management does not use monitoring and would not include cesarean section for fetal distress. The access to third trimester pregnancy termination may be logistically limited and is affected by legal restrictions. If there is less certainty about the prognosis associated with the diagnosis and less certainty about the diagnosis (Chervenak's group B), either non-aggressive or aggressive management would be recommended (Table 90.1). Further along this continuum, the physician would recommend aggressive management because of beneficence-based obligations to the fetus (Chervenak's group C).

Once the management plan is established, it is critical that all involved members of the team (attending staff, resident staff and nurses) are aware of it. Ethical conflicts may limit a team member's participation. Complete co-operation of all members is necessary for optimal care for the mother and fetus.

References

1. Halloran, L.G., Silverberg, S.G. and Salzberg, A.M (1972) Congenital cystic adenomatoid malformation of the lung. *Arch. Surg.*, **104**, 715–719.
2. Alter, D.N., Reed, R.L. and Marx, G.R. *et al.* (1988) Prenatal diagnosis of congestive heart failure in a fetus with sacrococcygeal teratoma. *Obstet. Gynecol.*, **71**, 978–81.
3. Langer, J.C., Harrison, M.R. and Schmidt, K.G. *et al.* (1989) Fetal hydrops and demise from sacrococcygeal teratoma: rationale for fetal surgery. *Am. J. Obstet. Gynecol.*, **160**, 1145–50.
4. Seifer, D.B., Ferguson II, J.E., Behrens, C.M. *et al.* (1985) Nonimmune hydrops fetalis in association with hemangioma of the umbilical cord. *Obstet. Gynecol.*, **66**, 283–286.
5. Kleinman, C.S., Copel, J.A. and Weinstein, E.M. *et al.* (1985) *In utero* dianosis and treatment of fetal supraventricular tachycardia. *Semin. Perinatol.*, **9** 113–129.
6. Bond, S.J., Harrison, M.R., Filly, R.A. *et al.* (1988) Severity of intestinal damage in gastroschisis: correlation with prenatal sonographic findings. *J. Pediatr. Surg.*, **23**, 520–25.
7. Rizzo, N., Gabrielli, S. and Perolo, A. *et al.* (1989) Prenatal diagnosis and management of fetal ovarian cysts. *Prenat. Diagn.*, **9**, 97–104.
8. Michejda, M. and Hodgen, G.D. (1981) *In utero* diagnosis and treatment of non-human primate fetal skeletal anomalies. I. Hydrocephalus. *JAMA*, **246**, 1093–97.
9. Manning, F.A., Harrison, M.R., Rodeck, E. *et al.* (1986) Catheter shunts for fetal hydronephrosis and hydrocephalus. Reports of the International Fetal Registry. *N. Engl. J. Med.*, **315**, 336–40.
10. Chervenak, F.A., Duncan, C., Ment, L.R. *et al.* (1984) Perinatal management of meningomyelocoele. *Obstet. Gynecol.* **63**, 376–80.
11. Bernstein, J. (1971) Heritable cystic disorders of the kidney: the mythology of polycystic disease. *Pediatr. Clin North Am.*, **18**, 435–44.
12. Harrison, M.R., Ross, N.A., Noall, R.A. *et al.* (1988) Correction of congenital hydronephrosis *in utero*. I. The model: fetal urethral obstruction produces hydronephrosis and pulmonary hypoplasia in fetal lambs. *J. Pediatr. Surg.*, **18**, 247–56.
13. Harrison, M.R., Ross, N.A., Noall, R.A., *et al.* (1982) Correction of congenital hydronephrosis *in utero*. II: Decompression reverses the effects of obstruction on the fetal lung and urinary tract. *J. Pediatr. Surg.*, **17**, 965–74.
14. Harrison, M.R., Ross, N.A., Noall, R.A. *et al.* (1983) Correction of congenital hydronephrosis *in utero*. III: Early mid-trimester ureteral obstruction produces renal dysplasia. *J. Pediatr. Surg.*, **18**, 681–86.
15. Harrison, M.R., Ross, N.A., Noall, R.A. *et al.* (1984) Correction of congenital hydronephrosis *in utero*. IV: *In utero* decompression prevents renal dysplasia. *J. Pediatr. Surg.*, **19**, 649–56.
16. Golbus, M.S., Harrison, M.R., Filly, R.A. *et al.* (1982) *In utero* treatment of urinary tract obstruction. *Am. J. Obstet. Gynecol.*, **142**, 383–88.
17. Harrison, M.R., Golbus, M.S., Filly, R.A. *et al.* (1982) Management of the fetus with congenital hydronephrosis. *J. Pediatr. Surg.*, **17**, 728–42.
18. Golbus, M.S., Filly, R.A., Callen, P.W. *et al.* (1985) Fetal urinary tract obstruction: management and selection for treatment. *Semin. Perinatol.*, **9** 91–97.
19. Crombleholme, R.M., Harrison, M.R., Golbus, M.S. *et al.* (1990) Fetal intervention in obstructive uropathy: prognostic indicators and efficacy of intervention. *Am. J. Obstet. Gynecol.*, **162**, 1239–44.
20. Nicolaides, K.H., Cheng, H.H., Snijders, R.J.M. and Moniz, C.F. (1992) Fetal urine biochemistry in the assessment of obstructive uropathy. *Am. J. Obstet. Gynecol.*, **166**, 932–37.
21. Nicolini, U., Fisk, N.M. and Rodeck, C.H. (1992) Fetal urine biochemistry: an index of renal maturation and dysfunction. *Br. J. Obstet. Gynaecol.*, **99**, 46–50.
22. McFayden, I.R., Wigglesworth, J.S. and Dillon, M.J. (1983) Fetal urinary tract obstruction: is active intervention before delivery indicated? *Br. J. Obstet. Gynaecol.*, **90**, 342–49.
23. Shalev, E., Weiner, E., Feldman, E. *et al.* (1984) External bladder–amniotic fluid shunt for fetal urinary tract obstruction. *Obstet. Gynecol.*, **63**, 31S–34S.
24. Sholder, A.J., Maizels, M., Depp, R. *et al.* (1988) Caution in antenatal intervention. *J. Urol.*, **139**, 1026–29.
25. Cunningham, F.G., MacDonald, P.C. and Gant, N.F. (eds) (1989) *Williams Obstetrics*, 18th edn. Cesarean Section and Cesarean Hysterectomy, Appleton Lange, Norwalk, CT, p. 443–44.
26. Chervenak, F.A., Tortora, M. and Hobbins, J.C. (1985) The management of fetal hydrocephalus. *Am. J. Obstet. Gynecol.*, **151**, 933–42.
27. Lorber, J. (1967) The prognosis of occipital encephalocele. *Dev. Med. Child Neurol.*, **13** (suppl.), 75–86.
28. Gross, S.J., Benzie, R.J. and Sermer, M. (1987) Sacrococcygeal teratoma: prenatal diagnosis and management. *Am. J. Obstet. Gynecol.*, **156**, 393–96.
29. Carlson, D.H. and Griscom, N.T. (1972) Ovarian cysts in the newborn. *AJR*, **116**, 664–72.
30. Clark, S., Devore, G.R. and Platt, L.D. (1985) The role of ultrasound in the aggressive management of obstructed labor secondary to fetal malformations. *Am. J. Obstet. Gynecol.*, **152**, 1042–44.
31. Vintzileos, A.M., Campbell, W.A., Weinbaum, P.J. *et al.* (1987) Perinatal management of fetal ventriculomegaly. *Obstet. Gynecol.*, **69**, 5–11.
32. Bensen, J.T., Dillard, R.G. and Burton, B.K. (1988) Open spina bifida: does cesarean section delivery improve prognosis? *Obstet. Gynecol.*, **71**, 532–34.
33. Luthy, D.A., Wardinsky, T., Shurtleff, D.B. *et al.* (1991) Cesarean section before the onset of labor and subsequent motor function in infants with meningomyelocoele diagnosed antenatally. *N. Engl. J. Med.*, **324**, 662–66.
34. Carpenter, M., Curci, M., Dobbins, A. and Haddon, J. (1984) Perinatal management of ventral wall defects. *Obstet. Gynecol.*, **64**, 646–51.
35. Kirk, E. and Wah, R. (1983) Obstetric management of the fetus with omphalocoele or gastroschisis; a review of one hundred twelve cases. *Obstet. Gynecol.*, **146**, 512–18.
36. Sermer, M., Benzie, R.J., Pitson, L. *et al.* (1987) Prenatal diagnosis and management of congenital defects of the anterior abdominal wall. *Am. J. Obstet. Gynecol.*, **156**, 308–12.
37. Narayama, D.K., Harrison, M.R., Gross, B.H. *et al.* (1984) Management of the fetus with an abdominal wall defect. *J. Pediatr. Surg.*, **19**, 408–13.
38. Chescheir, N.C., Azizkan, R.G., Seeds, J.W. *et al.* (1991) Counseling and care for the pregnancy complicated by gastroschisis. *Am. J. Perinatol.*, **8**, 323–29.
39. Low, J.A., Boston, R.W. and Pancham, S.R. (1972) Fetal asphyxia during the intrapartum period in intrauterine growth-retarded infants. *Am. J. Obstet. Gynecol.*, **113**, 351–57.

40. Jackson, G.M., Ludmir, J., Castlebaum, A.J. *et al.* (1991) Intrapartum course of fetuses with isolated hypoplastic left heart syndrome. *Am. J. Obstet. Gynecol.*, **165**, 1068–72.
41. Freeman, R.K., Garite, T.J. and Nacelotte, M.P. (1991) *Fetal Heart Rate Monitoring*, 2nd edn, Williams & Wilkins, Baltimore, MD.
42. Ghory, M.J. and Sheldon, C.A. (1985) Newborn surgical emergencies of the gastrointestinal tract. *Surg. Clin. North Am.*, **65**, 1083.
43. Cartidge, P.H.T., Mann, N.P. and Kapila, L. (1986) Preoperative stabilization in congenital diaphragmatic hernia. *Arch. Dis. Child.* **61**, 1226.
44. Chang, A.C., Huhta, J.C., Norwood, W.I. and Mennutti, M.T. (1989) *In Utero Transport for Critical Left Ventricular Outflow Tract Obstruction.* Proceedings of the North-East Pediatric Cardiological Society, September 22–24, Newport, RI (abstract).
45. Hon, E.H. (1968) *An Atlas of Fetal Heart Rate Patterns*, Hartly Press, New Haven, CT.
46. Ball, R.H. and Parer, J.T. (1992) The physiologic mechanisms of variable decelerations. *Am. J. Obstet. Gynecol.*, **166**, 1683–89.
47. Clark, S., Gimovsky, M.L. and Miller, F.C (1982) Fetal heart rate response to scalp blood sampling. *Am. J. Obstet. Gynecol.*, **144**, 706–708.
48. Polzin, G.B., Blakemore, K.J., Petrie, R.H. and Amon, E. (1988) Fetal vibroacoustic stimulation: magnitude and duration of fetal heart rate accelerations as a marker of fetal health. *Obstet. Gynecol.*, **72**, 621–26.
49. Banta, H.D. and Thacker, S. (1979) Assessing the costs and benefits of electronic fetal monitoring. *Obstet. Gynecol. Surv.*, **34**, 627.
50. Macdonald, D., Grant, A., Sheridan-Pereira, M. *et al.* (1985) The Dublin randomized controlled trial of intrapartum fetal heart rate monitoring. *Am. J. Obstet. Gynecol.*, **152**, 524–39.
51. Chervenak, F.A. and McCullough, L.B. (1990) An ethically justified, clinically comprehensive management strategy for third-trimester pregnancies complicated by fetal anomalies. *Obstet. Gynecol.*, **75**, 311–16.

91 INTRAPARTUM FETAL MONITORING

N.C. Smith

91.1 The high-risk fetus

Identification of the high-risk fetus is useful: firstly, for the clinician who can then concentrate and utilize his or her skills appropriately to the management of such a pregnancy and, secondly, to the mother who will benefit from the expertise devoted to her care. The development of significant intrapartum asphyxia resulting in the birth of a compromised baby is a relatively rare event and to predict the exact degree of risk in an individual pregnancy is difficult. This results in the clinical dilemma of whether to monitor all fetuses during labour or to concentrate resources on those considered to be at greater risk of developing hypoxia (Table 91.1) (Chapter 21).

When all fetuses are monitored by continual fetal heart rate assessment alone, overtreatment results in inappropriate interventions which are detrimental to good care. The problem with continuous fetal heart rate monitoring is not the technique but the interpretation of the degree of abnormality [1]. The use of intrapartum fetal heart rate monitoring in association with fetal scalp blood pH measurement has been shown to reduce by 50% the risk of neonatal seizures [2], the

Table 91.1 Indications for continuous fetal heart rate monitoring

Abnormal antenatal cardiotocograph
Absent end-diastolic umbilical artery blood flow
Intrauterine growth retardation
Severe pre-eclampsia
Significant antepartum haemorrhage
Maternal medical problem
Prolonged pregnancy
Multiple pregnancy
Structural abnormality in a viable fetus
Malposition or malpresentation
Oligohydramnios or polyhydramnios
Meconium-stained amniotic fluid
Induced or augmented labour

occurrence of which has been shown to be the best prognostic index for long-term outcome [3], although the positive predictive value is poor.

Each fetus reacts differently to the stress of labour. During each contraction there is a degree of impairment to the uteroplacental blood flow which may cause hypoxia and subsequent acidosis over a period. Clinicians and scientists have been striving to understand these physiological mechanisms and to develop accurate methods of detection of events which may lead to irreversible or fatal pathological changes.

91.2 Pathophysiology of intrauterine hypoxia

Although Little [4] stated in 1861 that birth asphyxia could cause death or neurological impairment, it is only in the last 30 years that a clearer understanding of the pathophysiological mechanisms have evolved, and much remains uncertain.

The pathological consequences of acute fetal hypoxia are illustrated in Figure 91.1, which has been collated from work on monkeys [5,6] and from the autopsies of asphyxiated human infants [7]. If the hypoxia is sustained, myocardial infarction and cerebral haemorrhage and infarction will inevitably result. In the monkey experiments, severe hypoxia resulted in death from heart failure due to myocardial damage. When the hypoxia was less severe, the survivors were mostly normal, although a small number exhibited brain damage affecting the middle third of the paracentral area of the cerebral hemispheres and also frequently the basal ganglia. The pathological changes produced in the term monkeys resembled those seen in human babies who suffer birth asphyxia. Subsequent research on the effects of anoxia [8] and hypoxia [9] have suggested that it is the accumulation of lactic acid in the brain tissue which causes the development of oedema, the breakdown of the blood–brain barrier and widespread tissue necrosis. However, the animal studies

Diseases of the Fetus and Newborn, 2nd edn, Edited by G.B. Reed, A.E. Claireaux and F. Cockburn. Published in 1995 by Chapman & Hall, London. ISBN 0 412 39160 0

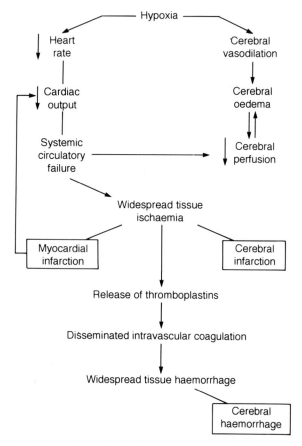

Figure 91.1 The pathological consequences of fetal hypoxia.

which implied acidaemia as the cause of brain damage have been criticized [10] because the effects of anaesthesia and the stress of surgery were not fully taken into account and the wide range of arterial pH values did not correlate closely with outcome.

All studies on the developmental follow-up of human infants who have suffered asphyxia at birth confirm the concept put forward in 1951 by Lilienfeld and Parkhurst [11] of a 'continuum of reproductive casualty'. They theorized that asphyxia may be severe and lethal causing intrapartum or neonatal death; it may be severe and sublethal causing cerebral palsy and/or mental handicap; or it may be less severe causing minimal brain damage.

In human parturition, severe acute hypoxia only occurs in cases of cord prolapse and abruptio placentae. The more common situation is longer-term hypoxia from cord compression or 'uteroplacental insufficiency', the latter being a non-specific term which masks our ignorance of the aetiology of intrapartum hypoxia. We have little knowledge of the degree and duration of hypoxia which the human fetus can tolerate in labour and each one has a different level of tolerance which makes assessment and development of guidelines for practice extremely difficult. The other confounding

variable is the antenatal course before the onset of labour which can be subject to an enormous array of obvious or occult complications during which time the fetus may sustain hypoxia and be neurologically damaged, but subsequently demonstrate normal biophysical parameters during labour. Such an infant may later reveal signs of neurological deficit similar to a baby born severely asphyxiated at birth.

The early work of James and co-workers [12] related abnormal cord blood pH, $P\text{CO}_2$ and buffer base to low Apgar scores. The association was not strong but, nevertheless, these findings were used to support the need to assess fetal blood acid–base status during labour. Of more concern is the lack of any associated neurological deficit in follow-up studies of infants who were born with low cord blood pH values [13,14]. It has even been suggested that the anaerobic metabolic response and development of acidosis is physiological and protective [10]. The onset of very early neonatal seizures has been shown to be the strongest predictor of death and disability in term babies, although up to 70% will survive without obvious disability [3].

There still exists uncertainty about the precise pathological and clinical sequelae of intrapartum hypoxia. It seems that of those babies who survive severe intrapartum hypoxia, most become normal children or die, but a small proportion live with substantial neurological handicap. Research into reliable methods of fetal surveillance must continue.

91.3 Current methods of intrapartum fetal surveillance

91.3.1 DETECTION OF MECONIUM-STAINED AMNIOTIC FLUID (MSAF)

Long before the introduction of continuous fetal heart rate monitoring, the presence of meconium in the liquor amnii was regarded as a sign of possible fetal distress. Active peristalsis of the gut has been shown to occur as a consequence of hypoxia [15], and this response in association with anal sphincter relaxation is thought to cause the passage of meconium [16]. However, increased vagal tone in a well-oxygenated fetus will cause a similar response [17] and therefore the correlation between MSAF and the birth of an asphyxiated baby is poor. There is undoubtedly an associated increased risk of perinatal death and morbidity associated with MSAF. This association was considered to be of such importance that patients with evidence of meconium staining were excluded from entry in the Dublin randomized trial of fetal heart rate monitoring [2]. All these labours had continuous fetal heart rate monitoring but, nevertheless, the perinatal mortality (corrected for lethal malformation) was 11.4

per 1000 compared with 2.1 in patients with clear or only lightly MSAF [18].

MSAF found at the onset of labour reflects a previous event which may or may not have been hypoxia and so the significance of such a finding is not clear. Routine amnioscopy, amniocentesis or artificial rupture of membranes to observe the colour of liquor have each been suggested and put into practice with varying degrees of enthusiasm. However, such screening methods have not been subjected to evaluation by prospective randomized controlled trials [1].

Exactly why some babies suffer varying degrees of the meconium aspiration syndrome and others do not is unclear but two important observations, strongly associated with bad outcome, require mention.

(a) Thick, viscid MSAF

Such a finding implies that there has been coexisting oligohydramnios, which in itself is associated with fetal compromise. It is rare to observe MSAF in preterm labours and the passage of meconium appears to be a sign associated with maturity. When MSAF occurs in the postmature fetus and oligohydramnios supervenes, an often fatal combination seems to coexist. The airways become inspissated with this tenuous material which cannot be easily cleared by the neonate and so any pre-existing hypoxia appears exaggerated.

Some suggest that the collection of amniotic fluid and observation in a test-tube is essential to ensure accurate grading of the degree of meconium [19]. Clinical observation of external pads may be misleading because absorption of fluid makes the staining appear more extreme. MSAF and oligohydramios is a particularly difficult clinical problem because the sparsity of fluid can mean that it may remain undetected until the baby is delivered. Extreme vigilance is therefore required in labouring patients thought to have no amniotic fluid. In the Dublin trial such patients were excluded, and continuously monitored. [2]

(b) MSAF in the presence of an abnormal fetal heart rate pattern

The presence of MSAF without an abnormal fetal heart rate pattern does not appear to jeopardize fetal outcome, but when late decelerations are present the risk of meconium aspiration seems to be enhanced and the neonatal outcome may be prejudiced [20].

91.3.2 INTERMITTENT AUSCULTATION OF THE FETAL HEART RATE

In the early part of the nineteeth century, when instrumentation was developed to listen to the adult heart, it became obvious that the fetal heart could also be auscultated. Different stethoscopes were pioneered to ascertain the presence of the fetal heart pulsation and so confirm fetal life. Pinard's stethoscopes evolved in 1876 and is still commonly used in obstetric practice throughout the world. In the last decade, in which substantial technological advances have been made in the development of lightweight equipment, many midwives have changed to auscultation with a portable battery-operated hand-held doptone instrument which is easier to use and more reliable in the detection of the sounds.

From the turn of this century until the widespread use of electronic fetal heart rate monitoring in the late 1970s, the term 'fetal distress' implied meconium stained liquor or an auscultatory abnormality of the heart rate. An irregular fetal heart rate, or one above 160 or less than 100–120 beats/min, was considered to signify distress. These findings, although fairly insensitive, were significant and associated on occasions with the birth of an asphyxiated or stillborn infant.

Auscultation is usually performed for 60 seconds once every 15 minutes between contractions, when the fetal heart pulsations are more audible, and the rate is averaged over the sampling period. During the second stage auscultation is usually undertaken between each contraction when possible because of the greater likelihood of fetal bradycardia. The disadvantages of intermittent auscultation are that small changes in the rate may not be detected, no information is obtained on variability or on the rate during contractions, a significant counting error may occur and overall only 3% of the information is available from the short counting time. There are no published studies which have demonstrated an improvement in fetal outcome from intermittent auscultation.

91.3.3 CONTINUOUS FETAL HEART RATE MONITORING

Following Hon's [21] original report on the electronic evaluation of the fetal heart rate in 1958, continuous monitoring became accepted into routine clinical practice and by the late 1970s many obstetricians considered that all labours should be managed in this way. The transition appeared logical because more information was being obtained which, it was assumed, could only be for the better. Research was also undertaken into those new patterns of fetal heart rate change which were uncovered, and a better understanding of the fetal responses to hypoxia resulted. However, the technique was introduced and adopted into routine practice before it was subjected to scrutiny by randomized controlled trials to evaluate its effectiveness in improving neonatal outcome and subsequent development.

No obstetrician doubts that an ominous intrapartum cardiotocograph (CTG) may be associated with the birth of an asphyxiated neonate, who may subsequently show signs of cerebral palsy. However, intrapartum asphyxia accounts for not more than 10% of cases of cerebral palsy and there has been no decrease in the incidence of cerebral palsy since the introduction of fetal monitoring [22]. In addition, there are serious difficulties in quantifying the degree of abnormality of a CTG [23] and there is no clear association or prediction between an abnormal CTG and subsequent developmental handicap [24]. The abnormal CTG may be the end-result of an hypoxic insult which may have predated the onset of labour. The best chance of a normal outcome for the fetus is a normal CTG during labour. This reflects a resilient fetus who can sustain transient impairment of oxygen delivery during contractions and whom the obstetrician can confidently predict will be born in good condition.

The practising obstetrician has to deliver intrapartum care utilizing this technique to the best of his or her ability. Recognition of the abnormal CTG is paramount in avoiding litigation. Experienced clinicians and academics will debate the degree of abnormality but failure to act appropriately is not acceptable. Careful, patient and vigilant interpretation is necessary in all cases, at all hours. The resident obstetrician must be able to describe and interpret the CTG, to evaluate likely causes of the abnormality and to institute the appropriate management.

(a) Description and interpretation of the cardiotocogram

The CTG is only a small part of intrapartum care and the condition of the mother and the progress of labour are also important to note. To assess an abnormal pattern, the whole trace from the beginning should be considered to assess the segment causing concern. Thus an impression is obtained of the development of any fetal heart rate abnormality and subtle changes will not be missed. Sometimes the pattern defies the descriptive guidelines. The classification described by Hon in 1963 [25] has stood the test of time and best approximates the pathophysiology. Consideration should be given to the **baseline** features (rate and variability) and **periodic** changes (accelerations and decelerations).

Baseline features

The **normal** fetal heart rate is between 110 and 150 beats/min and has a variability of 5–15 beats per minute. The rate is regulated by the autonomic nervous system [26]: a preponderance of sympathetic neuronal activity causes an increase in rate and the converse occurs with parasympathetic dominance which is more noticeable as pregnancy advances, when a gradual decrease in rate is normally seen.

Although this definition of normal rate has been stipulated by the International Federation of Obstetrics and Gynaecology (FIGO) [27], it should not be accepted over-rigidly. Gradual changes in rate may occur during labour within this normal range, which may imply abnormality. For example, a progressive rise in rate from 110 to 160 beats/min signifies the development of a tachycardia which the complacent observer may not detect. Such subtle changes are of particular concern when variability is lost and decelerations subsequently appear.

A **bradycardia** is defined as a rate less than 110 beats/min. Some define 120 beats/min as the lower limit of normal. Once more, the important consideration is the evolution of the bradycardia, whatever lower limit is utilized. Four types of bradycardia can be distinguished, as follows.

1. Physiological. This term is used when the rate is between 100 and 110 beats/min and remains in this range with normal variability. It is more commonly seen in the post-term fetus when there is increased vagal tone.
2. Intermittent. A bradycardia which lasts for 2–10 minutes is the most common type found in clinical practice. It normally occurs as an isolated event and can equally effectively be described as a 'prolonged bradycardia' or 'prolonged deceleration', although decelerations are best defined when the change in rate lasts less than 2 minutes. Intermittent bradycardias result from baroreceptor and/or chemoreceptor reflexes which are triggered by changes in blood pressure and oxygen tension, respectively. The clinical causes of such intermittent and sudden bradycardias are:
   (a) Uterine hypertonicity, usually due to overdosage with oxytocin or prostaglandin;
   (b) Occult maternal vena caval and/or aortic arterial occlusion, as seen in patients when in the dorsal position and more common in those with epidural anaesthesia;
   (c) intrauterine cord compression or, less commonly, overt cord prolapse.
3. Terminal. Such a bradycardia is usually preceded by a grossly abnormal fetal heart rate pattern which has features pathognomonic of hypoxia. The chronic, severe hypoxia produces the bradycardia by direct myocardial suppression [28]. The initial bradycardia usually evolves over a minute or two but there follows a progressive diminution in rate over 10–20 minutes until cardiac arrest occurs (Figure 91.2). This pattern is seen when major intrapartum placental abruption occurs. The clinical features may not be obvious, in that there may only be slight revealed

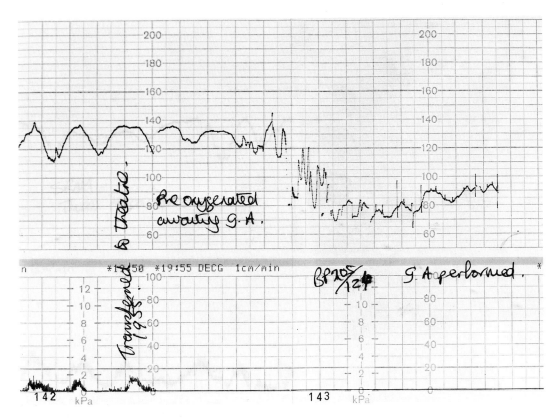

Figure 91.2   A terminal bradycardia preceded by an ominous fetal heart rate pattern. Emergency caesarean section failed to save this baby.

bleeding and the pain may be masked by labour contractions. When a terminal bradycardia develops there is little time to save the baby, and perinatal death is not unusual.
4. Congenital heart block. A constant rate of less than 100 beats/min usually signifies congenital heart block, the rate typically being around 60 beats/min. In these circumstances the fetus is not hypoxic but the heart rate response to hypoxia will be compromised.

A **tachycardia** occurs when the fetal heart rate is more than 150 beats/min. There are three principal causes, as follows.

1. Maternal pyrexia. This is the most common cause and need not be associated with fetal hypoxia, but a compromised neonate may result if the tachycardia is prolonged and the fetus becomes infected.
2. Fetal hypoxia. In the absence of maternal pyrexia, the development of a tachycardia usually signifies progressive fetal hypoxia. This is due to vagal inhibition and release of catecholamines from the adrenal medulla. If reduced variability and late or severe variable decelerations subsequently develop and are sustained, then immediate delivery must be considered because such a pattern signifies unequivocal fetal hypoxia.

3. Maternal ketoacidosis. In the diabetic patient, a fetal tachycardia will occur in the presence of ketoacidosis. Correction of the ketoacidosis will result in a return of the fetal heart rate to a normal rate. Immediate delivery is not always indicated and control of the maternal diabetes is paramount.

Variability in the baseline rate of 5–15 beats/min is normal and less than 5 beats/min is regarded as abnormal. The early reports on fetal heart rate patterns distinguished short-term and long-term variability but in clinical practice such subdivision is unnecessary. Normal fetal heart rate variability reflects a responsive autonomic nervous system which may be depressed by hypoxia with resultant loss of variability [29]. However, the following should all be considered.

1. Physiological sleep. The fetus normally has a 20–40-minute sleep–wake cycle in which it alternates between being inactive without movement and active with movement. During the sleep phase, there is reduced variability.
2. Maternal sedation. Drugs with sedative properties given to the mother during labour have the same effect on the fetus and cause reduced variability. Typical examples are pethidine, diamorphine, diazepam and chlormethiazole.
3. Hypoxia. This must be considered when there is

persistently reduced variability or other fetal heart rate abnormalities, such as changes in the baseline rate and/or decelerations.

Periodic features

These are decelerations or accelerations of brief duration [25], 2 minutes being a useful upper limit. **Accelerations** are alterations in the fetal heart rate of more than 15 beats/min in response to uterine contractions and may also occur with movements of the fetus. They indicate a responsive, intact central system and are associated with a normal outcome. Accelerations sometimes immediately precede variable decelerations and, in such instances, evaluation of the deceleration pattern is the priority.

Decelerations are classified according to their temporal relationship to uterine contractions and are termed variable, early or late.

1. Variable. This type of deceleration pattern is the most common and is due to cord compression. Vagal stimulation occurs, probably due to a baroreceptor reflex but the mechanism is not clear and hypoxia may be responsible [30]. The shape of the decelerations, as the name implies, is variable and their onset, in relationship to the onset of the contractions, is variable. Undoubtedly the onset of some of the decelerations will be late and this frequently leads to misinterpretation. An additional clue is the sudden drop in the heart rate over a couple of seconds to the nadir, with an equally rapid recovery to the baseline.

   There are three useful checks which should be used to assess the severity of this type of deceleration pattern. Firstly, does the baseline rate show features of compromise such as a tachycardia or loss of variability? Secondly, does Goodlin's rule of 60 [31] apply? This refers to a deceleration pattern where the drop from the baseline rate is more than 60 beats/min, the nadir is below 60 beats/min and the duration is greater than 60 seconds. If these criteria are met then fetal acidosis is likely to develop if the pattern persists. Cerebral blood flow ceases when the rate falls below 60 beats/min. A third check is to assess the recovery to the baseline rate. A slow recovery implies a 'late' component to the deceleration pattern and is of more concern.

   A mild variable deceleration pattern with a normal baseline rate showing good variability can simply be observed. Changing maternal position to alleviate possible cord compression may help. Excessive uterine activity may be a contributing factor and intravenous oxytocin dosage should be reduced if appropriate. If there is a tachycardia and the rule of 60 pertains, then a vaginal examination is required to assess cervical dilatation and exclude occult cord prolapse. If delivery is not imminent, then fetal blood sampling is required to assess acid–base status. This will require repetition, depending on the fetal heart rate pattern and progress of labour.

2. Early. This type of deceleration is uncommon. Early decelerations occur following head compression which results in an increase in intracranial pressure and a decrease in carotid blood flow activating the vagus, probably as a result of pressure change [32]. They have an open V shape and their onset is always simultaneous with the onset of a contraction. Their shape is virtually the same with each contraction, which they mirror in timing, and they are rarely more than 20 beats below the baseline rate in the first stage of labour. They are not associated with fetal compromise and no specific action is required. It is imperative to distinguish them from late decelerations.

3. Late. It has been demonstrated in monkeys that hypoxia is the essential component causing late decelerations [33]. They are also vagally mediated but are due to chemoreceptor rather than baroreceptor activity [34]. After a contraction, poorly oxygenated blood returns from the placenta via the umbilical arteries and the heart to the arch of the aorta and the carotid arteries where the chemoreceptors are located. The onset of these decelerations is therefore persistently late in relationship to the onset of the contractions and the fall to the nadir is gradual, as is the return to the baseline. The depth or amplitude of the decelerations may be deceivingly shallow, varying between 20 and 60 beats/min and usually related to the intensity of the contractions. Such a shallow deceleration pattern appears visually innocuous and may be misinterpreted or continue unrecognized by the novice. They are frequently associated with reduced variability (Figure 91.3) and a progressive tachycardia which help interpretation of the deceleration pattern. Vigilance to their appearance is necessary at all times because they are due to hypoxia which will cause acidosis and tissue damage. Whether fetal blood acid–base assessment is prudent, or expedient delivery more appropriate, depends on the exact clinical circumstances, degree of abnormality and persistence of the abnormal pattern.

91.3.4 FETAL SCALP BLOOD ACID–BASE ASSESSMENT

Fetal scalp blood sampling to assess acid–base status was first described by Saling in [35] 1968 in Berlin and was introduced independently of continuous electronic fetal heart rate monitoring. Although not published, the

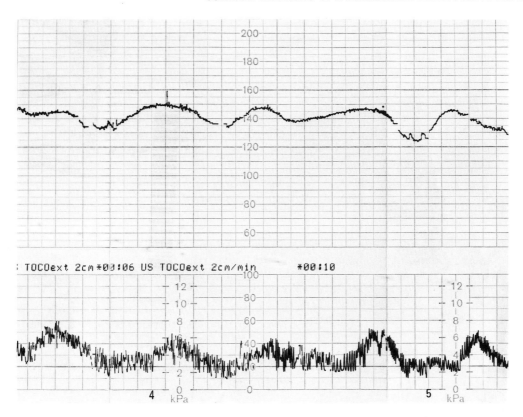

Figure 91.3 Late decelerations in association with a reduced variability.

early workers must have found the specificity for each test was good but the sensitivity poor and it became obvious that the combination of both tests would improve diagnostic precision.

Randomized controlled trials have subsequently shown that continuous fetal heart rate monitoring combined with acid–base assessment is associated with a reduced risk of neonatal convulsions compared with intermittent auscultation alone. Continuous fetal heart rate monitoring, used alone, is associated with a higher caesarean section rate than when used with fetal scalp blood pH measurement but a difference in the asphyxia rate has never been shown [1]. Therefore to maintain a respectable rate for caesarean section the evidence overwhelmingly shows that electronic fetal heart rate monitoring should be used in conjunction with fetal scalp blood sampling. The two are complementary, the scalp blood pH measurement acting as the final arbiter.

In the modern labour ward, fetal scalp blood sampling is used to evaluate the significance of a suspicious CTG. Familiarity with the measurement equipment and precise technique are essential to ensure the accuracy of results [36]. The interpretation of the results depends on a clear understanding of the principles of fetal acid–base biochemistry.

(a) Biochemical principles of fetal acid–base assessment

The maintenance of an optimal pH is essential for cellullar metabolism, which produces the energy necessary for survival. Under normal circumstances, the fetal acid–base status is determined by that of the mother. When uteroplacental insufficiency occurs, gaseous exchange is impaired, resulting in hypoxia and carbon dioxide retention in the fetus. The carbon dioxide combines with water and is converted within the erythrocytes to carbonic acid, which immediately dissociates to hydrogen and bicarbonate ions. As a consequence of the hypoxia, glycogen and glucose are broken down anaerobically to lactic acid for energy rather than aerobically via the citrate cycle to carbon dioxide and water. The buffer bases become saturated: a base deficit and acidosis result. In the human fetus it appears that the acidosis due to hypoxia is mixed, having both respiratory and metabolic components and being caused by a simultaneous accumulation of carbon dioxide and lactate [37].

All the fetal acid–base parameters (P_{O_2}, P_{CO_2}, pH, bicarbonate, base deficit, base deficit of the extracellular fluid, lactate) have been evaluated and correlated with fetal heart rate patterns and condition at birth

[38]. Lactate and pH are the best indicators of hypoxia. The measurement of pH has become the most widely used due to easy availability of blood gas and pH analysers. Lactate measurement is equally good [39] and may replace pH if recently improved assay techniques become widespread [40].

The lower limit for a normal fetal scalp blood pH is widely accepted as 7.25 [35,41]; 7.20–7.25 is regarded as preacidotic and 7.20 is frankly abnormal. The upper limit for normal lactate il 3.0 mmol/l and the preacidotic range 3.0–3.5 mmol/l [36]. The upper limit of the normal range for Pco$_2$ and the lower limit for base deficit are 8 kPa (60 mmHg) and −8 mmol/l, respectively [41].

(b) Clinical aspects of fetal blood sampling (FBS)

When there is uncertainty about fetal well-being from a suspicious CTG then FBS should be undertaken. Suggested indications for FBS are given in Table 91.2; each indication should be considered according to the clinical circumstances. As previously stated, the pattern may be so ominous that FBS is inappropriate and superfluous to management.

The values obtained from FBS relate only to the acid–base status at the time of sampling. The subsequent fetal heart rate pattern must be assessed so that guidance to the frequency of sampling is obtained. An improvement in the fetal heart rate pattern is reassuring but if it deteriorates then further acidosis is likely, and if it remains unchanged then further sampling may be necessary. FBS should be repeated to evaluate the significance of persistent moderate or severe variable decelerations. Acidosis will inevitably develop in the presence of persistent late decelerations but, if they occur intermittently or with less than 30% of contractions, this is less likely and evaluation of acid–base status is necessary.

The temporal development of acidosis is difficult to delineate because oxygen deprivation to the human fetus is usually subacute and intermittent, unless there is cord prolapse or abruption. Acute anoxia in newborn animals has been shown to result in a fall in pH from 7.4 to 7.0 within 10–20 minutes, and death usually occurs at pH levels below 6.8 [42,43]. The interval

between consecutive scalp samples rarely needs to be less than 30 minutes, and in any case this is the usual minimum time required for preparation, sampling and analysis.

When values of less than 7.25 are obtained then immediate delivery is usually required. If the value is unexpected and does not appear to equate with the degree of fetal heart rate abnormality, a repeat sample will be necessary. Another useful check is measurement of maternal venous pH to exclude an infusion acidosis from mother to fetus. In addition, the maternal value is a good control for checking the accuracy of the pH analyser. Maternal–fetal pH values of more than 0.20 indicate fetal acidaemia [44] and values of 0.15–0.20 are in the preacidaemic range.

Maternal alkalosis as a result of overbreathing can cause a falsely elevated fetal pH (false-negative). In addition, prolonged exposure of a fetal blood sample to air results in loss of carbon dioxide and elevation of pH. On the other hand, maternal acidosis can cause a falsely low fetal pH (infusion acidosis) which appears to be harmless to the fetus. Other causes of false-positive values are local stasis of blood due to large caput succedaneum, too much pressure from the endoscope, or contamination of the fetal blood sample with amniotic fluid.

91.3.5 INTERMEDIATE METHODS

Many women understandably object to being connected to a fetal heart rate monitor throughout labour, principally because they are immobilized. Transmission of the fetal heart rate signal from either an internal electrode, or preferably an external transducer, to the monitor by radio waves (telemetry) allows mobility in the patient who requires to be monitored. The great dilemma is what degree of monitoring is necessary for the low risk patient.

The fetal heart rate admission test appears to be a good adjudicator of whether continous fetal heart rate monitoring should be implemented or not and detects ominous patterns which would be missed by intermittent auscultation [45]. To be absolutely certain that fetal distress is not developing, it is necessary to repeat the tracing at regular intervals. One problem is the non-reactive pattern. Simply to prolong the observation period is sufficient in the majority and accelerations should appear within 40 minutes. Another alternative for the impatient observer is to alarm the resting fetus with a blast of sound (acoustic stimulation) [40].

FBS is highly invasive for the mother and also uncomfortable for the operator. To reduce the need for FBS, stimulation tests appear to have a place in management. In addition to acoustic stimulation, pinching the scalp of the fetus with an Allis tissue

---

Table 91.2 Indications for fetal blood sampling

Fetal heart rate
Change in the baseline rate
Unaccountable and persistent loss of variability
Moderate or severe variable decelerations
Late decelerations with less than 30% contractions
Mixed patterns
Appearance of meconium and associated fetal heart
 rate abnormality

forceps produces an acceleration of the fetal heart rate in the non-acidotic fetus [47].

Research into alternative methods of detecting the hypoxic fetus are still required because of the imprecision of current methods.

91.4 Futuristic methods of intrapartum fetal surveillance

91.4.1 FETAL ELECTROCARDIOGRAPHIC WAVEFORM

Many of the problems of fetal electrocardiographic signal processing and analysis have been overcome in the last decade with the advent of microprocessing and microcomputer technology, such that on-line objective analysis of the fetal electrocardiogram can be undertaken from a fetal scalp electrode.

Changes in the PR/RR and the ST waveform have the potential of distinguishing the well-oxygenated from the hypoxic fetus. The PR interval has a positive correlation with the RR interval which becomes negative when the fetus is stressed, probably as a result of catecholamines. An increase in the ST segment and T wave develops when anaerobic metabolism occurs due to hypoxia in the myocardium. This change can be expressed as a ratio of T wave height to QRS height (T : QRS ratio) [48].

The results of a recently reported randomized trial [49] have shown that the use of ST waveform analysis in conjunction with fetal heart rate monitoring reduced the incidence of operative delivery for fetal distress from 9.6% to 4.4% compared with fetal heart rate monitoring without ST analysis. FBS was used in both arms of the trial. On review of the CTG patterns the operative rate for fetal distress was only significantly lower among those with normal or intermediate patterns. There was no difference between the two methods when the fetal heart rate was classified as abnormal. It seems strange that 29% of the operative deliveries for 'fetal distress' in the fetal heart rate only group were carried out when the fetal heart rate was normal.

The addition of scalp pH to fetal heart rate monitoring lowers the operative delivery rate and a further reduction with the addition of ST waveform analysis is a welcome finding. It has been suggested that the need for FBS will be reduced when an abnormal CTG has a normal ST waveform [49,50]. A concern is the poor correlation between the ST waveform and other indices of fetal oxygenation: the ST waveform is poor in the detection of fetal acidaemia compared with fetal heart rate patterns [51] and has no clear relationship with fetal heart rate abnormalities or with umbilical arterial pH [52]. It appears that its main contribution to

intrapartum monitoring will be to reduce the operative delivery rate rather than detect the hypoxic fetus.

91.4.2 SYSTOLIC TIME INTERVALS

These are indicators of myocardial function. The two most sensitive are the pre-ejection period (PEP), from the onset of the Q wave to aortic valve opening, and the ventricular ejection time (VET), from opening to closure of the aortic valves. The PEP is an indicator of myocardial contractility and the VET reflects peripheral resistance. There are many physiological variables which cause these to change but there is firm evidence to suggest that changes occur with progressive hypoxia and the development of acidosis [53]. Substantial technological development is required to ensure accurate and continuous measurement so that further evaluation can be undertaken.

91.4.3 CONTINUOUS MONITORING OF FETAL BLOOD GAS AND ACID–BASE STATUS

Individual electrodes have been developed to measure fetal scalp tissue pH and transcutaneous Po_2 or Pco_2 continuously during labour [36]. In addition, continuous simultaneous recording of Pco_2 and pH using separate electrodes has been undertaken [54], and simultaneous Po_2 and Pco_2 have been measured by mass spectrometry [55]. As can be imagined, there are substantial difficulties in maintaining adequate contact with the fetal scalp, and amniotic fluid, blood, fetal hair and caput formation are impediments to accurate measurement.

The most recent innovation is the continuous measurement of fetal oxygen saturation (So_2) by pulse oximetry [56]. Initial reports were disappointing but a modification of the oximeter for fetal use has revealed a reasonable correlation between oximetry readings and both oxygen saturation and pH of the umbilical vein [57]. Fetal So_2, rather than Po_2, is a better parameter to measure. (The opposite is true in the adult.) This is because, firstly, the fetus has a relatively narrow range of Po_2 and small changes in Po_2, from only 10 to 30 mmHg, result in large changes in So_2 from 20 to 80%; and, second, there is a shift in the oxygen dissociation curve when fetal acidosis develops such that a high Po_2 may exist in the presence of a low So_2.

91.5 Conclusions

The development of significant intrapartum fetal hypoxia and acidosis are relatively rare events but, if undetected, significant morbidity and mortality can result. The difficulties are that each fetus will tolerate the stress of labour to a different extent and our current methods of monitoring result in overtreatment and misinterpretation. Research must be supported to evaluate more effective methods of intrapartum monitoring and to ensure the safe management of the mother and birth of a lively baby.

References

1. Grant, A. (1992) Monitoring the fetus during labour, in *Effective Care in Pregnancy and Childbirth*, vol. 1 (eds I. Chalmers, M. Enkin and M.J.N.C. Keirse, Oxford University Press, Oxford, pp. 846–82.
2. MacDonald, D., Grant, A., Sheridan-Pereira, M. *et al.* (1985) The Dublin randomized controlled trial of intrapartum fetal heart-rate monitoring. *Am. J. Obstet. Gynecol.*, 152, 524–39.
3. Minchom, P., Niswander, K., Chalmers, I. *et al.* (1987) Antecedents and outcome of very early neonatal seizures in infants born at or after term. *Br. J. Obstet. Gynaecol.*, 94, 431–39.
4. Little, W.J. (1861) On the influence of abnormal parturition, difficult labour, premature birth and asphyxia neonatorum on the mental and physical condition of the child especially in relation to deformities. *Lancet*, 11, 378–80.
5. Myers, R.E. (1972) Two patterns of perinatal brain damage and their conditions of occurrence. *Am. J. Obstet. Gynecol.*, 112, 246–76.
6. Brann, A.W. and Myers, R.E. (1974) Central nervous system findings in the newborn monkey following severe *in utero* partial asphyxia. *Neurology*, 25, 69–75.
7. Anderson, J.M., Brown, J.K. and Cockburn, F. (1974) On the role of disseminated intravascular coagulation in the pathology of birth asphyxia. *Dev. Med. Child Neurol.*, 16, 581–91.
8. Myers, R.E. and Yamaguchi, M. (1976) Effects of serum glucose concentration on brain response to circulatory arrest. *J. Neuropathol. Exp. Neurol.*, 35, 301.
9. Yamaguchi, M. and Myers, R.E. (1976) Comparison of brain biochemical changes produces by anoxia and hypoxia. *J. Neuropathol. Exp. Neurol.*, 35, 302
10. Johnson, P. (1991) Fetal distress or physiological response and adaption, in *Fetal Monitoring* (ed. J.A.D. Spencer), Oxford University Press, Oxford, pp. 28–33.
11. Lilienfeld, A.M. and Parkhurst, E. (1951) A study of the association of factors of pregnancy and parturition with development of cerebral palsy *Am. J. Hyg.*, 53, 262–82.
12. James, L.S., Weisbrot, I.M., Price, C.E. *et al* (1958) The acid–base status of human infants in relation to birth asphyxia and the onset of respiration. *J. Paediatr.*, 52, 379–94.
13. Dennis, J., Johnson, A., Mutch, L. *et al.* (1989) Acid base status at birth and neurodevelopmental outcome at four and a half years. *Am. J. Obstet. Gynecol.*, 161, 213–20.
14. Dijxhoorn, M.J., Visser, G.H.A., Fidler, V.J. *et al.* (1986) Apgar score, meconium and acidaemia at birth in relation to neonatal neurological morbidity in term infants. *Br. J. Obstet. Gynaecol.*, 83, 217–22.
15. Van Liere, E.J. (1942) *Anoxia: its Effects on the Body*, University of Chicago Press, Chicago, p. 169
16. Desmond, M., Moore, J., Lindley, H.E. and Brown, C.A. (1957) Meconium staining of the amniotic fluid. *Obstet. Gynecol.*, 9, 91–103.
17. Hon, E.H. (1962) Electronic evaluation of the fetal heart rate. VI Fetal distress – a working hypothesis. *Am. J. Obstet. Gynecol.*, 83, 333–53.
18. Boylan, P. (1987) Intrapartum fetal monitoring. *Baillière's Clin Obstet. Gynaecol.*, 1, 73–95.
19. O'Driscoll K.M., Coughlan, M., Fenton, V. and Skelly, M. (1977) Active management of labour: care of the fetus. *BMJ*, ii, 1451–43.
20. Miller, F.C., Sack, D.A., Yeh, S.Y. *et al.* (1975) Significance of meconium during labour. Am. J. Obstet. Gynecol., 122, 573–80.
21. Hon, E.H. (1958). The electronic evaluation of the fetal heart rate. Preliminary report. *Am. J. Obstet. Gynecol.*, 75 1215–30.
22. Lamb, B. and Lang, R. (1992) Aetiology of cerebral palsy. *Br. J. Obstet. Gynaecol.*, 99, 176–78.
23. Nielsen, P.V., Stigsby, B., Nickelson, C. and Nim, J. (1987) Intra- and Inter-observer variability in the assesment of intrapartum cardiotocograms. *Acta Obstet. Gynecol. Scand.*, 66, 421–24.
24. Nelson, K. (1988) What proportion of cerebral palsy is related to birth asphyxia? *J. Pediatr.*, 112, 572–74.
25. Hon, E.H. (1963) The classification of fetal heart rate. *Obstet. Gynecol.*, 22, 137–47.
26. Martin, C.B. (1978) Regulation of the fetal heart rate and genesis of FHR patterns. *Semin. Perinatol.*, 12, 131–46.
27. FIGO (1987) Guidelines for the use of fetal monitoring. *Int. J. Gynaecol. Obstet.*, 93, 314–21.
28. Hon, E.H. (1974) Additional observations on 'pathologic' bradycardia. *Am. J. Obstet. Gynecol.*, 118, 428–41
29. Paul, R.H., Suidan, A.K., Yeh, S.Y. *et al.* (1975) Clinical fetal monitoring, VII. The evaluation and significance of intrapartum baseline FHR variability. *Am. J. Obstet. Gynecol.*, 123, 206–10.
30. Lee, S.T. and Hon, E.H. (1963) Fetal haemodynamic response to umbilical cord compression. *Obstet. Gynecol.*, 22, 553–62.
31. Parer, J.T. (1983) *Handbook of Fetal Heart Rate Monitoring*, W.B. Saunders, Philadelphia, p. 99.
32. Paul, W.M., Quilligan, E.J. and MacLaughlan, T. (1964) Cardiovascular phenomena associated with fetal head compression. *Am. J. Obstet. Gynecol.*, 82, 824–26.
33. James, L.S., Morishima, H.O., Daniel, S.S. *et al.* (1972) Mechanism of late decelerations of the fetal heart rate. *Am. J. Obstet. Gynecol.*, 113, 578–82.
34. Parer, J.T., Krueger, T.R. and Harris, J.L. (1980) Fetal oxygen consumption and mechanisms of heart rate response during artificially produced late decelerations of fetal heart rate in sheep. *Am. J. Obstet. Gynecol.*, 136, 478–82.
35. Saling, E. (1968) *Foetal and Neonatal Hypoxia*, Arnold London.
36. Smith, N.C. (1987) Assessment of fetal acid–base status. *Baillière's Clin. Obstet. Gynaecol.*, 1, 97–109.
37. Smith, N.C., Soutter, W.P. and Sharp, F. (1986) Observations on the evolution of human fetal acidosis, in *Fetal and Neonatal Physiological Measurements* (ed. P. Rolfe), Butterworth, London, pp. 124–29.
38. Smith, N.C. (1983) Fetal scalp blood lactate as an indicator of hypoxia during labour. Aberdeen University, MD thesis.
39. Smith, N.C., Soutter, W.P. and Sharp, F. (1983) Fetal scalp blood lactate as an indicator of intrapartum hypoxia. *Br. J. Obstet. Gynaecol.*, 90, 821–31.
40. Nordstrom, L., Persson, B., Shimojo, N. and Westgren, M. (1992) Fetal scalp and umbilical artery blood lactate measured with a new test strip method. *Br. J. Obstet. Gynaecol.*, 99, 307–309.
41. Lumley, J., McKinnon, L. and Wood, C. (1971) Lack of agreement on normal values for fetal scalp blood. *J. Obstet. Gynaecol. Br. Commonw.*, 78, 13–21
42. Myers, R.E. (1977) Experimental models of perinatal brain damage: relevance to human pathology, in *Intrauterine Asphyxia and the Developing Brain* (ed. L. Gluck), Year Book Medical, London, p. 42.
43. Shelley, H.J. (1969) The metabolic response of the fetus to hypoxia. *J. Obstet. Gynaecol. Br. Commonw.*, 76, 1–15.
44. Rooth, G., McBride, R. and Ivy, B.J. (1973) Fetal and maternal pH differences, a basis for common normal values. *Acta Obstet. Gynecol. Scand.*, 52, 47–50.
45. Ingemarsson, I., Arulkumaran, S., Ingemarsson, E. *et al.* (1986) Admission test: a screening test for fetal distress in labor. *Obstet. Gynecol.*, 68, 800–806.
46. Smith, C.V., Phelan, J.P., Platt, L.D. *et al.* (1986) Fetal acoustic stimulation testing. II. A randomized clinical comparison with the non-stress test. *Am. J. Obstet. Gynecol.*, 155, 131–34.
47. Clark, S.L., Gimovsky, M.L. and Miller, F.C. (1984) The scalp stimulation test: a clinical alternative to fetal blood sampling. *Am. J. Obstet. Gynecol.*, 148, 274–77.
48. Greene, K.R. (1987) The ECG waveform. *Baillère's Clin. Obstet. Gynaecol.*, 1, 131–55.
49. Westgate, J., Harris, M., Curnow, J.S.H. and Greene, K.R. (1992) Randomised trial of cardiotocography alone or with ST waveform analysis for intrapartum monitoring. *Lancet*, 340, 194–98.
50. Johansen, R.B., Rice, C., Shokr, A. *et al.* (1992) ST-waveform analysis of the fetal electrocardiagram could reduce fetal blood sampling. *Br. J. Obstet. Gynaecol.*, 99, 167–68.
51. MacLachlan, N.A., Spencer, J.A.D., Harding, K. and Arulkumaran S. (1992) Fetal acidaemia, the cardiotocograph and the T/QRS ratio of the fetal ECG in labour. *Br. J. Obstet. Gynaecol.*, 99, 26–31.
52. Murphy, K.W., Russell, V. and Johnson, P. (1992) Clinical assessment of fetal electrocardiogram monitoring in labour. *Br. J. Obstet. Gynaecol.*, 99, 32–37.
53. Raymond, S.P.W. and Whitfield, C.R. (1987) Systolic time intervals of the fetal cardiac cycle. *Baillère's Clin. Obstet. Gynaecol.*, 1, 185–201.
54. Nickelsen, C., Thomsen, S.G. and Weber, T. (1985) Continuous acid–base assessment of the human fetus during labour by tissue pH and transcutaneous carbon dioxide monitoring. *Br. J. Obstet. Gynaecol.*, 92, 220–25.
55. Sykes, G.S., Molloy, P.M., Wollner, J.C. *et al.* (1984) Continuous, noninvasive measurement of fetal oxygen and carbon dioxide levels in labor by mass spectrometry. *Am. J. Obstet. Gynecol.*, 150, 847–58.
56. Gardosi, J., Carter, M. and Becket, T. (1989) Continous intrapartum monitoring of fetal oxygen saturation. *Lancet*, ii, 692–93.
57. McNamara, H., Chung, D.C., Lilford, R. and Johnson, N. (1992) Do fetal pulse oximetry readings at delivery correlate with cord blood oxygenation and acidaemia? *Br. J. Obstet. Gynaecol.*, 99, 735–38.

92 DELIVERY ROOM CARE AND NEONATAL RESUSCITATION

P. Dennery and D.K. Stevenson

92.1 Etiology of asphyxia in the newborn

Perinatal asphyxia and birth injuries are important factors associated with neurologic and intellectual impairment in the pediatric population [1]. This association has been considered since 1861 when Little [2] correlated neurologic problems in infants with perinatal events. Since then, it has become evident that despite adequate intrapartum monitoring, some factors that contribute to neurologic injuries will not be recognized [3]. The incidence of perinatal asphyxia associated with encephalopathy is roughly 6 per 1000. Asphyxia, by definition, implies diminished gas exchange between the maternal and fetal circulation, resulting in increased carbon dioxide and decreased oxygen and pH values in fetal blood [4]. This can be of maternal, placental or fetal origin. Precipitating maternal causes are many and include decreased maternal oxygen and decreased uteroplacental blood flow caused by hypertension, hypotension, uterine hyperactivity or uterine abnormalities. Some placental causes are due to maternal hypertension, placental anomalies such as placenta previa, vasa previa, abruptio placenta or abnormal insertion of the umbilical cord [5]. Cord prolapse, cord compression, single umbilical artery and true knots in the cord can also lead to asphyxia. Fetal causes of asphyxia include hemolysis and fetal–maternal hemorrhage [6] (Chapters 21 and 91).

92.2 Pathophysiology of hypoxic–ischemic encephalopathy

92.1 BIOCHEMICAL CHANGES

Hypoxic-ischemic encephalopathy resulting from asphyxia is a well-recognized syndrome which is the most common cause of neurologic impairment and seizures in the neonatal period. The chemical changes result from the conversion of aerobic oxidation of glucose to anaerobic glycolysis, and accumulation of lactic acid [7]. Biochemical alterations noted in hypoxic–ischemic encephalopathy occur in the first 20–30 minutes after the insult [8]. There are shifts of ion gradients, increased extracellular potassium level, decreased sodium and calcium level extracellularly and contraction of the extracellular volume [9]. Lactic acid accumulates with increased glycolysis and glycogenolysis; brain glucose and glycogen levels decrease within 5 minutes [7]. Although the brain can use ketone bodies as substrate, it is unlikely that this occurs under conditions of hypoxia and glycogen depletion [10, 11].

After an asphyxial event, excitatory amino acids increase in the extracellular fluid [12,13]. Glutamic acid is taken up by specific brain cell receptors and mediates calcium influx into the cells with subsequent formation of toxic by-products [14,15]. Free fatty acids rise and arachidonic acid accumulates [16,17]. The latter is metabolized to prostaglandins and leukotrienes by cyclo-oxygenase and lipoxygenase enzyme systems. The resultant metabolites can lead to the production of free radicals that mediate brain cell damage and death [17]. They can alter oxygen consumption mechanisms and cerebral blood flow as well [18]. Inhibitory molecules such as γ-aminobutyric acid (GABA) and alanine levels also increase markedly in the brain [19]. In the first 10–30 minutes after injury, ATP levels decrease as observed by phosphorous nuclear magnetic resonance spectroscopy (NMRS) [17,20]. Cerebral blood flow increases and there is a loss of autoregulation shortly after perinatal asphyxia [21]. This reflects the body's attempt to continue to deliver oxygen preferentially to the brain (Chapters 21, 30 and 44).

92.2.2 HISTOLOGIC CHANGES

(a) Fullterm infants

On gross pathology, lesions associated with neonatal hypoxic–ischemic encephalopathy range from cortical

Diseases of the Fetus and Newborn, 2nd edn, Edited by G.B. Reed, A.E. Claireaux and F. Cockburn. Published in 1995 by Chapman & Hall, London. ISBN 0 412 39160 0

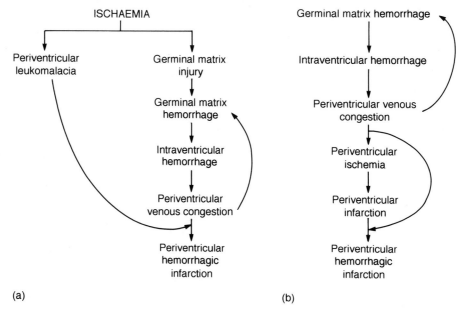

(a)   (b)

Figure 92.1 Proposed mechanism for pathogenesis of hemorrhagic intracerebral involvement with major intraventricular hemorrhage. (a) Ischemia leading to periventricular leukomalacia is an important initial event. (b) Major intraventricular hemorrhage is the important initial event. (Reproduced with permission from Volpe, J.J. (1987) Intracranial hemorrhage of the premature infant, in *Neurology of the Newborn*, 2nd edn, W.B. Saunders, Philadelphia, p. 336.)

infarctions resulting from arterial or venous occlusion, necrosis of nuclei, brain-stem necrosis, cerebral necrosis, intraventricular hemorrhage or white matter degeneration. Later on in the course of the disease, cystic changes gradually develop, especially in the caudate and putamen. The basal ganglia and thalamus develop a chronic lesion termed status marmoratus [22]. Brain-stem injury occurs usually with acute hypotension [23]. Neurons in the pons and Purkinje cells of the cerebellum are particularly vulnerable. Glial fatty metamorphosis, astrocytosis or necrosis of the white matter can be observed [24] (Chapter 91, p. 1352).

(b)   Preterm infants

The most common findings in preterm infants are periventricular or intraventricular hemorrhage and periventricular leukomalacia or white matter disease [25,26] (Figure 92.1). Intraventricular hemorrhage arises from the germinal matrix in the lateral ventricle. Because of impaired autoregulation, changes in systemic blood pressure and increasing central venous pressure, the germinal matrix capillary endothelium leaks, resulting in blood collection in the ventricle [23]. Intraventricular hemorrhage can spread through the ventricular system, and clot formation can impair cerebral spinal fluid egress. Hydrocephalus occasionally results in obstruction of the aqueduct or the foramina [25,26]. Possible consequences of intraventricular hemorrhage are destruction of the germinal matrix and periventricular hemorrhagic infarction in 15% of the

cases. The latter is an asymmetric, often extensive, lesion that results from hemorrhagic venous obstruction and infarction of brain tissue. It usually occurs on the side where the intraventricular hemorrhage is largest [27,28]. Periventricular leukomalacia results from a different process. The lesion is usually symmetric, non-hemorrhagic and has a predilection for the periventricular arterial border zones [27,28]. Another rarer complication of intraventricular hemorrhage is pontine necrosis. Death usually occurs secondary to respiratory failure [29]. In term infants intraventricular hemorrhage can occur, but it usually originates from the choroid plexus. It can be a consequence of trauma, although many of the cases show no identifiable etiology [30].

92.3   Pathophysiology of asphyxia

The goals of delivery room care and resuscitation of the newborn are to ensure survival of the infant and prevent hypoxic–ischemic encephalopathy and its consequences. This requires a knowledge of the pathophysiology of asphyxia and factors that may adversely affect these processes.

92.3.1   FETAL CIRCULATION

There is a substantial gradient between oxygen levels of maternal uterine arterial blood and fetus umbilical venous blood through the placenta but the fetal hemoglobin has higher affinity for oxygen than does

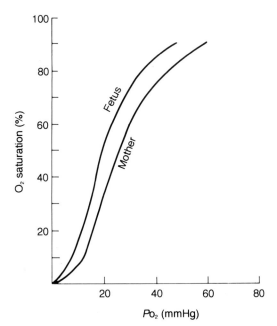

Figure 92.2 The oxyhemoglobin dissociation curves of maternal and fetal human blood at pH 7.4 and 37°C. (Reproduced with permission from Meschia, G. (1989) *Maternal Fetal Medicine: Principal and Practice*, W.B. Saunders, Philadelphia, p. 309.)

maternal hemoglobin [31]. This results in fetal blood becoming more saturated than maternal blood at a given Po_2 (Figure 92.2). Despite this, there is still less oxygen in fetal blood. The fetus, therefore, must compensate for this by preferentially providing blood flow to vital organs such as the heart and brain. This is partially done by increasing the cardiac output. The fetal heart rate is much higher than the adult heart rate, resulting in a fetal cardiac output which is double that of adults [32]. The capacity of the fetus to withstand asphyxia depends on the capacity of the cardiovascular system to maintain or increase organ perfusion and oxygen delivery to the heart and brain [33]. When the fetal arterial Po_2 decreases, the cardiac output is redistributed, and oxygen delivery becomes insufficient to meet the needs of the less vital organs.

92.3.2 ANIMAL MODELS

Most of the information on the pathophysiology of asphyxia is determined through animal experimentation for obvious ethical reasons [34–37]. Since there is great variability between species and their response to asphyxia, it is difficult to make generalizations concerning human neonates. The closest primate model, the rhesus monkey, probably reflects patterns in human fetuses. Several studies conducted by Dawes and others in the late 1960s gave us some insight as to the functioning of asphyxiated rhesus monkeys. The fetuses

were delivered by cesarean section after placement of catheters in fetal vessels. The head was immediately covered with a saline-filled bag to prevent air breathing during gasping. At delivery, the umbilical cord was immediately tied. The monkeys were subjected to longer and longer periods of asphyxia and then subsequently resuscitated. Within the first minute of asphyxia, rapid gasps occurred shortly after the onset of asphyxia, accompanied by muscular effort. The heart rate dropped considerably, but was still above 100. After 4–5 minutes, small spontaneous gasps were replaced by more deep spontaneous gasps that gradually became weaker, with a last gasp after approximately 8 minutes of total asphyxia. After this period, the monkeys were unable to gasp and death occurred. The longer the delay in initiating the resuscitation measures after the last gasp, the longer the time for resumption of breathing movements. During asphyxia, pH dropped, Pco_2 rose and Po_2 fell to virtually zero in 10 minutes. Levels of blood lactic acid rose rapidly with asphyxia. The human fetus or newborn may tolerate greater amounts of asphyxia than the rhesus monkey without developing brain damage, and the time to the last gasp is probably longer than in the monkey. Also, fetal hypoxia is usually incomplete and intermittent, therefore it is difficult to estimate the actual time course of asphyxia and the subsequent outcome [38].

Hypoxia and asphyxia lead to decreased cardiac function, myocardial necrosis [39] and depressed responsiveness to norepinephrine [40]. There is also a correlation between cardiac glycogen stores and the length of time fetal animals can survive anoxia.

Fetuses and newborns can survive longer periods of anoxia than adults, in part due to the greater reliance of the cardiac muscle on energy derived from glycolytic mechanisms [41–43]. The newborn also has a relatively immature brain with a lower resting metabolism than those of adults, which have the ability to utilize stored glycogen and is more efficient at mobilizing available energy [42,43]. There is also possible shunting of blood flow to critical areas of the brain and brain stem [44]. This can improve survival from asphyxia. Nevertheless, these mechanisms can be overcome with severe insults.

92.4 Neonatal resuscitation

92.4.1 IMMEDIATE MANAGEMENT

Anticipation is the essential tool in preparing for neonatal resuscitation [45]. Assessment of maternal problems such as premature labor [46], premature rupture of membranes [47], oligohydramnios, intrauterine growth retardation [48–51], presence of meconium-stained amniotic fluid [45], postdate pregnancy [52] severe eclampsia, vaginal bleeding [53] and maternal diabetes [54] can help suggest some fetal abnormality and potential for poor outcome. A low or elevated fetal heart rate [53] and decreased scalp pH can also help us recognize infants who are at risk for asphyxia. Trained personnel should be available for resuscitation 24 hours a day at any hospital offering delivery services since unexpected problems occur at a fair frequency [55–57]. The concept of a resuscitation team is helpful and can significantly impact on neonatal outcome and survival [58]. The composition of this team may vary from hospital to hospital [59]. There should be at least two members of the team able to provide endotracheal intubation [60], assisted ventilation, umbilical catheterization and drug administration as required. A resuscitation cart containing all the necessary drugs and equipment should be available in or adjacent to the delivery room for ready access. Use of charts that outline resuscitation procedures have been shown to be helpful [61]. The team members should observe the infant for tone, color, heart rate, respiratory efforts and response to stimulation in the first seconds of life [57]. Apgar scores should be assessed at 1 minute and 5 minutes, and then every 5 minutes thereafter until the infant achieves two consecutive scores of more than 8 [62].

The alphabetic mnemonic ABCDE depicts the areas of importance in neonatal resuscitation, namely, airway, breathing, circulation, drugs, environment and evaluation [63,64]. The infant should immediately be placed on a radiant warmer and dried to prevent hypothemia because the latter leads to increased metabolic requirements and impaired cardiac performance [65]. Airway patency should be provided by positioning the head in the 'sniffing position', i.e. with slight extension of the neck and jaw to open the airway. If this is insufficient for spontaneous respiration, endotracheal intubation should be performed until spontaneous respiration occurs. The heart rate should be auscultated or the pulse palpated. If it is less than 100 beats/min, circulation should be supported by immediate initiation of external cardiac compressions. If there is not prompt recovery of heart rate, color and respiratory effort, drug administration is usually the last resort. Oxygen should be used to maintain adequate Pa_{O_2}; glucose should be administered immediately. Drugs used during neonatal resuscitation mainly help glucose homeostasis, correct acidosis, enhance cardiac output and increase heart rate [62]. Glucose is the major energy substrate of infants, and is utilized rapidly, therefore it should be administered to prevent hypoglycemia and possibly prevent brain injury [11]. Oxygen corrects tissue hypoxia in many conditions. If there is cyanotic congenital heart disease, it will not help since there is fixed right-to-left shunting [66]. Acidemia can be corrected by bicarbonate infusion, but one should ensure that there is adequate ventilation so as not to increase carbon dioxide content

of the blood. Overcorrection of the pH should be not be attempted since this may impair oxygen hemoglobin dissociation and lead to metabolic alkalosis and subsequent inactivation of catecholamines [62,63]. Rapid administration of bicarbonate to correct acidosis may also lead to intraventricular hemorrhage [67].

In order to enhance cardiac output and provide adequate cerebral systemic circulation, several agents can be used. Since the newborn infant increases cardiac output primarily by increasing heart rate [32], ionotropic agents improve the cardiac output dramatically. Epinephrine is one such agent. It can be instilled intravenously or intratracheally in infants with bradycardia or asystole [62,63,68]. Atropine is used in bradycadia and may be useful in asystole refractory to epinephrine and calcium [62,63,68]. Cardioversion and defibrillation can be used when there is an electromechanical dissociation or ventricular fibrillation [62]. Drugs to improve myocardial function may help in cases of sepsis, metabolic derangements or other intrinsic disorders of the myocardium. Calcium can increase heart rate, increase cardiac contractility and improve blood pressure in the infants [69,70]. The opiate antagonist, naloxone, has been tried in the pharmacologic management of asphyxia and was shown to have no benefit and potentially harmful side-effects [71]. The ventricles of neonates are less compliant than those of adults, therefore cardiac output will not increase significantly with vascular volume expansion [72]. Nevertheless, it is important to achieve normovolemia in these infants. Crystalloid (albumin, fresh frozen plasma, cryoprecipitate) and colloid solutions (physiological saline) can be used to improve systemic volume.

92.4.2 LONG-TERM MANAGEMENT

After the initial resuscitation, infants that are profoundly asphyxiated will require long-term extended management. This includes artificial assisted ventilation to maintain adequate oxygenation and ventilation and sustaining cardiac output with ionotropic drug infusions, such as dopamine and dobutamine [66,68]. Afterload reduction can be achieved by the use of nitroprusside [73]. Anemia can be corrected with packed red blood cell transfusions. Infants with refractory hypoxemia should be evaluated further [66,68]. The hyperoxia test involves administering 100% oxygen to infants and monitoring Pa_{O_2} levels pre- and postductally. If the preductal oxygen is much higher than the postductal oxygen, this reflects a right-to-left shunt. This could mean that hypoxia is secondary to pulmonary hypertension or congenital heart disease. To help differentiate the two entities, a hyperventilation test is then conducted. Hyperventilation is initiated as well as administration of 100% oxygen. If the Pa_{O_2} is above 100 mmHg (13.3 kPa), pulmonary hypertension

Table 92.1 Evaluation of the neonate with hypotonic hypoxemia

Test	Result	Probable diagnosis	Potential causes of error	Additional studies
Hyperoxia test	$Pa_{O_2} > 150$ mmHg (19.95 kPa)	Pulmonary parenchymal disease	Reactive pulmonary hypertension	Consider preductal and postductal Pa_{O_2} or echocardiography
	Pa_{O_2} 100–150 mmHg (13.30–19.95 kPa)		All diagnoses possible	
	$Pa_{O_2} < 100$ mmHg (13.3 kPa)	Right to left shunting	Severe pulmonary parenchymal disease	Compare preductal and postductal Pa_{O_2} and consider trial of continuous positive airway pressure
Preductal and postductal Pa_{O_2}	Preductal < postductal	Transposition of great arteries	Venous preductal sample	Echocardiogram
	Preductal = postductal	Intracardiac or intrapulmonary right to left shunting	May result from cardiac disease, severe parenchymal disease or severe pulmonary hypertension	Hyperventilation–hyperoxia test, echocardiogram, electrocardiogram
	Preductal > postductal	Ductal right to left shunting	Must distinguish pulmonary hypertension from reduced left ventricular output	Hyperventilation–hyperoxia test, assess systemic blood pressure and cardiac output
Hyperventilation–hyperoxia test	$Pa_{O_2} > 100$ mmHg (13.3 kPa)	Pulmonary hypertension	Hypoplastic left heart, interrupted aortic arch with ventricular septal defect, total anomalous pulmonary venous return	Consider echocardiogram
	$Pa_{O_2} < 100$ mmHg (13.3 kPa)	Fixed right to left shunting	Must distinguish heart disease from intrapulmonary shunting	Echocardiogram, electrocardiogram

Source: reproduced with permission from Stevenson, D.K. and Benitz, W.E. (1987) A practical approach to diagnosis and immediate care of the cyanotic neonate. *Clin. Pediatr.*, **26**, 325.

is usually suspected. If there is a Pa_{O_2} of less than 100 mmHg (13.3 kPa), then one must be concerned with a fixed right-to-left shunt, as in cyanotic congenital heart disease (Table 92.1). The tests described above may help the physician reach a diagnosis, but do not always differentiate between pulmonary and cardiac disease. Asphyxiated infants should also be fluid restricted in the event of renal failure. This measure is also useful in preventing cerebral edema. It has been shown that oliguria associated with asphyxia correlates with poor neurologic outcome [74–76].

92.5 Neurodevelopmental outcome in neonatal asphyxia

92.5.1 APGAR SCORES AS PREDICTORS OF OUTCOME

In 1953, Virginia Apgar [77] first described a method of evaluation of newborn infants (Table 92.2). This system was used to identify infants who were depressed and required resuscitative efforts. Although it was not intended to be used as a tool for predicting outcome and subsequent neurologic damage, it has been utilized in this manner by the National Collaborative Perinatal Project of the National Institutes of Health for Neurologic Disease and Stroke (NCPP) [78]. Although imperfect, the Apgar score has remained the standard by which neonates are evaluated after birth. There is no good correlation of long-term neurologic outcome with low Apgar scores at 1, 5 and 10 minutes [79], but correlation improves after 15–20 minutes if the Apgar score is less than 4 [80]. Infants who were essentially stillborn (Apgar scores < 3 at 10 minutes) and resuscitated have a very poor outcome and most die [81]. If one uses an Apgar score of less than 7 at 5 minutes to indicate asphyxia, the incidence rises to almost 5%. Sykes and co-workers [82], and Silverman and associates [83] re-evaluated the use of the Apgar scores to assess whether this correlated with neonatal asphyxia.

Table 92.2 Apgar score

| Sign | Score | | |
	0	1	2
Heart rate	Absent	Below 100	Over 100
Respiratory effort	Absent	Weak, irregular	Good; crying
Muscle tone	Flaccid	Some flexion of extremities	Well flexed
Reflex irritability (catheter in nose or slap sole of foot)	No response	Grimace	Cry
Color	Pale	Blue	Completely pink

Source: reproduced with permission from Fischer, D.E. and Patton, J.B. (1986) Resuscitation of the newborn infant, in *Care of the High Risk Neonate*, W.B. Saunders, Philadelphia, p. 31.

An association between Apgar scores at 1 minute and significant acidosis did not exist. Sykes found that only 20% of neonates with Apgar scores of 6 or less had cord pH values of less than 7.1 [82]. Of infants whose cord pH value was 7.1 or less, 22% had Apgar scores of 6 or less. Levene, Kornberg and Williams [84] found that 23% of infants with asphyxial encephalopathy had unremarkable Apgar scores at 1 and 5 minutes. Therefore, low Apgar scores with little evidence of neurologic depression in the neonatal period are not associated with significant neurologic sequelae. Nelson and Ellenberg [85] attempted to correlate cerebral palsy with Apgar scores in term infants. They demonstrated that there was an increase in correlation with cerebral palsy when low Apgar scores persisted for more than 10 minutes. If the scores were 0–3 at 5 minutes, but increased to 4 by 10 minutes, the incidence of cerebral palsy was less than 1% in survivors. It was only when the score remained low (0–3) for 15 minutes more that the incidence of cerebral palsy increased significantly. On the other hand, 55% of patients who developed cerebral palsy had 1-minute Apgar scores of 7–10 and 73% of patients had Apgar scores of 7–10 at 5 minutes. The authors found that over two-thirds of the patients with cerebral palsy did not come from the group of infants who had been given the diagnosis of perinatal asphyxia according to Apgar scores of less than 7 at 5 minutes, and, in fact, over 97% of patients identified in the high-risk population group did not have cerebral palsy. Seidman and associates [86] assessed the value of low Apgar scores (< 7) at 1 and 5 minutes in predicting low intelligence (IQ scores) at 17 years of age. After controlling for confounding effects of perinatal and demographic factors, the sensitivity and positive predictive values of a low Apgar score at 5 minutes were 1.5 and 5%, respectively. Therefore, low Apgar scores are not very predictive of adverse neurologic outcome [85–88].

Obstetricians have used other means of assessing fetal well-being during the intrapartum period, and one of these is the biophysical profile [89] (Table 92.3). Infants with a profile score of 0 had 48% death rates. All survivors exhibited perinatal morbidity and the accuracy of biophysical profile scores of 0 with mortality and morbidity used as end-points was 100% [89]. This indicates that a very abnormal fetal biophysical profile is a perinatal emergency. Unfortunately, death or adverse outcome occurred despite aggressive intervention in children with low biophysical profile (Chapter 91).

92.5.2 MORBIDITY AND MORTALITY

Significant intrapartum asphyxia results in hypoxic–ischemic encephalopathy. Outcome is influenced by the severity of asphyxia and other factors such as racial and socioeconomic parameters. Hispanic and black infants have increased mortality secondary to asphyxia [90,91].

The onset of seizures before 48 hours usually reflects severe asphyxia [92]. Term or near-term infants have several degrees of encephalopathy dependent on the severity of asphyxia. Sarnat and Sarnat [93] developed an infant scoring system categorizing patients into three states of postasphyxial encephalopathy, as follows:

1. Mild: irritable, hyperactive reflexes, tachycardic, and poor sucking but no seizures, and a normal EEG.
2. Moderate: mild hypotonia, weak or incomplete reflexes, and focal or multifocal seizures.
3. Severe: stuporous, hypotonic, no suck, decerebrate posturing, with no Moro or tonic neck reflexes. Encephalographic pattern consistent with burst suppression or isopotential.

Using Sarnat's categories, Robertson and Finer [94] reported that infants with mild encephalopathy had no handicaps. Moderate encephalopathy was associated with 80% normal outcome, whereas severe encephalo-

Table 92.3 Biophysical profile scoring: management protocol

Score	Interpretation	Recommended management
10	Normal infant, low risk for chronic asphyxia	Repeat testing at weekly intervals. Repeat twice weekly in diabetic patients and patients ≥42 weeks gestation
8	Normal infant, low risk for chronic asphyxia	Repeat testing at weekly intervals. Repeat twice weekly in diabetic patients and patients ≥42 weeks. Oligohydramnios indication for delivery
6	Suspected chronic asphyxia	Repeat testing in 4–6 h. Deliver if oligohydramnios present.
4	Suspected chronic asphyxia	If ≥36 weeks and favorable, then deliver. If <36 weeks and L/S <2 repeat test in 24 h. If repeat score <4, deliver
0–2	Strong suspicion of chronic asphyxia	Extend testing time to 120 min. If persistent score ≤4 deliver, regardless of gestational age

L/S = amniotic fluid lecithin:sphingomyelin.
Source: reproduced with permission from Manning, F.A. (1990) Fetal biophysical assessment by ultrasound, in *Maternal–Fetal Medicine*, W.B. Saunders, Philadelphia, p. 359.

pathy was associated with a high proportion of deaths or handicaps.

Seizures occurring in the neonatal period (the first 2–3 days of life) correlate more strongly with long-term neurologic handicaps [95]. Ellenberg and Nelson [96] demonstrated that these infants are 15–17 times more likely to have neurologic sequelae than infants without seizures. Neonatal seizures occur in between 1 and 14 per 1000 livebirths. Over 16% of them occur in the first 48 hours of life, except when associated with bacterial meningitis [92,97]. The overall mortality associated with neonatal seizures varies from 9 to 35%. Neonatal seizures vary in their etiology (Table 92.4). Levine and Trounce [98] found that 53% of patients with neonatal seizures had a history of intrapartum or postnatal asphyxia.

Perinatal asphyxia can lead to cerebral palsy, but data suggest that cerebral palsy can occur without any evidence of perinatal problems [99,100]. In fact most patients with ataxia or hypotonic cerebral palsy have had prenatal rather than perinatal problems. Perinatal problems are usually manifested with spastic diplegia or quadriplegia [101]. There is usually an association with mental handicap and cerebral palsy in infants with intrapartum asphyxia. Several studies have shown that perinatal asphyxia is only responsible for about 10% of mild to moderate mental handicap [102]. In most patients, severe mental handicap occurs from other problems such as chromosomal abnormalities, biochemical inborn errors of metabolism and intrauterine infection [103]. Visual [104,105] and hearing impairments [105] can also result from asphyxia.

In premature infants, the diagnosis of hypoxic–ischemic encephalopathy and the subsequent neurologic problems resulting from this are more difficult to assess. It had previously been suggested that infants less than 1500 g be delivered by cesarean section to prevent perinatal asphyxia since they are less able to tolerate labor [106,107], but this is no longer recommended and has not been proven to be an effective means of reducing intrapartum asphyxia in these neonates unless there is entrapment of the head. Premature infants have complicating problems in the neonatal period that make it difficult to determine what role perinatal asphyxia played in the overall outcome. They are more at risk for adverse outcome due to postpartum events such as premature lung disease and intraventricular hemorrhage and these factors impact on subsequent neonatal outcome [106,108].

92.6 Methods of evaluation of hypoxic–ischemic encephalopathy and outcome

92.6.1 ELECTROENCEPHALOGRAPHY

Neonatal seizures are a common manifestation of hypoxic–ischemic encephalopathy [98]. The electroencephalogram (EEG) has been used to assess neonates for over 20 years [109]. It can be performed at the infant's bedside, and is non-invasive. An adequate study involves recording some active and sleep states in the infants. An interpretation of the recordings requires a skilled individual since the patterns may be subtle and complex. It is also known that prematures have different EEG patterns than do term infants [96,110]. The EEG is usually the most sensitive method of determining encephalopathy [95–113], although occasionally seizure activity on EEG is not associated with clinical manifestations or abnormalities [114]. Nevertheless it may be even more effective in predicting

Table 92.4 Etiology of neonatal seizures

Etiology	Comments
Hypoxic–ischemic encephalopathy	60% of all cases: both in fullterms and preterms
Intracranial hemorrhage	15% of all cases: subarachnoid in fullterm (infants appear well); intraventricular hemorrhage in preterm
Hypoglycemia	Usually in small-for-gestational age (SGA) and infants of diabetics (IDM); early onset
Hypocalcemia	Usually in low-birth-weight infants, SGA, or IDM; early onset
Intracranial infections	12% of all cases: group B streptococci, *Escherichia coli*, viruses (Coxsackie B, herpes)
Developmental defects	Cortical dysgenesis (lissencephaly, pachygyria, polymicrogyria)
Drug withdrawal	First 3 days of life, after passive addiction to opiates, barbiturates, alcohol
Drug intoxications	Local anesthetics: mepivacaine, lidocaine (lignocaine)
Hyponatremia	Associated with menengitis or HIE
Hypernatremia	Usually iatrogenic secondary to overcorrection
Hyperammonemia	Usually with organic acidemias
Pyridine deficiency	Onset in first few hours of life, occasionally *in utero*
Hypomagnesemia	–
Familial	Self-limited, benign course
Fifth day fits	Occurs in late part of first week of life; ?zinc deficiency
Unknown	Rare

outcome than a neurologic examination [115]. It is difficult to make prognostic statements with a single, even markedly abnormal EEG in term or premature infants [96]. Good prognosis is usually associated with an abnormality on EEG that results within 48 hours [111]. Therefore, electroencephalograms in the first 48 hours have less predictive values of long-term outcome than do tracings obtained at an older age [110]. In the first few hours of life, an EEG can be influenced by maternal anesthesia and drug ingestion [119]. An abnormal EEG pattern persisting unchanged for several weeks reflects an already established encephalopathy rather than a perinatally acquired process [117,118]. In a study conducted at Stanford University, neurologic follow-up at 2–3 years of age correlated with serial EEGs obtained at weekly intervals. All infants with at least one markedly abnormal EEG had neurologic sequelae or died. At least one moderately abnormal EEG was associated with a high proportion of abnormalities. If infants had two or more moderately abnormal tracings at weekly intervals, abnormal outcome was even more likely. Infants with normal EEGs were normal for the most part. Of the infants who died or were abnormal, the majority had acquired neurologic

syndromes that occurred after the last EEG was recorded [110]. The EEG provides valuable data for assessing critically ill infants who are at risk for hypoxic–ischemic injury.

92.6.2 OTHER METHODS OF EVALUATION

Other techniques are available to monitor brain function and these are variable in their applicability and predictability. Cerebral blood flow can be assessed by positron emission tomography (PET) which uses an emitting isotope and computer technology for scanning and reconstruction of two-dimensional images [119] or by Doppler [120,121]. Venous occlusion plethysmography [122,123] is used to estimate fetal cerebral blood flow on the basis of expansion of the neonatal skull after occlusion of the jugular veins. This may be hazardous in the critically ill child with limited ability to tolerate increased intracranial pressure [122,123]. Cerebral metabolism can be assessed by NMRS [124–127] and near infrared spectroscopy (NIRS) [127,128]. The former estimates energy reserves and pH of cells in the brain. This method requires transport of patients to a dedicated facility, and therefore is not ideal for critically ill infants. NIRS uses infrared lasers to measure hemoglobin A, both in its deoxygenated and oxygenated states, and cytochrome aa_3, an enzyme involved in phosphorylation of mitrochondria. It can be applied at the bedside, but is only a qualitative tool. Time of flight absorbance (TOFA) [129 and D.A. Benaron, M.A. Lenox and D.K. Stevenson, personal communication] can image the concentration and saturation of cytochrome and hemoglobin, as does NIRS. This is done through analysis of scattering of photons as they travel through tissue. It has the advantage of not requiring a pulse, thus it can be used in surgeries where patients are cooled to slow their metabolism. It is also a quantitative tool, unlike NIRS. All of these techniques hold promise, but further studies need to be conducted to determine the exact correlative values and applicability of these tools (Chapter 96).

92.6.2 BIOCHEMICAL MARKERS

Cord blood pH is a test done routinely to assess the severity of asphyxia. It correlates poorly with outcome [87,130] and Apgar scores [82]. It can be deceptive since infants with low cord pH often have normal Apgar scores [87]. Other biochemical markers of asphyxia are being investigated. Isoenzymes such as creatinine kinase (CK)-BB are elevated with severe asphyxia, and correlate with poor short-term neurologic outcome [131]. Hypoxanthine levels increase in asphyxial injury. Since this molecule is metabolized by xanthine oxidase, free radicals will be generated in this pathway, leading to tissue death; thus hypoxanthine levels can be correlated with degree of injury [132]. At the present time, no biochemical markers other than cord pH are used routinely by clinicians in the assessment of asphyxia.

In summary, the consequences of perinatal asphyxia are variable and several factors can be used to help determine which infants are more at risk for poor outcome. The EEG is often helpful in predicting outcome. Imaging studies which assess cerebral metabolism or cerebral blood flow and biochemical tests can help as well. The use of the Apgar score is limited since it is not a good predictive tool unless the Apgar score remains low (0–3) at 15 minutes of life. The impact of perinatal asphyxia on neonatal outcome is often greatly overestimated, placing our obstetrical colleagues at great liability [87,88].

References

1. Brann, Jr A.W. (1986) Hypoxic ischemic encephalopathy (asphyxia). *Pediatr. Clin. North Am.*, **33**, 451–64.
2. Little, W.J. (1861) On the influence of abnormal parturition, difficult labours, premature birth, and asphyxia neonatorum on the mental and physical condition of the child especially in relation to deformities. *Trans. Obstet. Soc. Lond.*, **62**, 293.
3. Paneth, N. and Stark, R.I. (1983) Cerebral palsy and mental retardation in relation to indicators of perinatal asphyxia. An epidemiological overview. *Am. J. Obstet. Gynecol.*, **147**, 960–66.
4. Menkes, J.H. (1989) Definition of perinatal asphyxia (letter). *J. Pediatr.*, **114**, 168.
5. Williams, L.J. and Lucci, A.P. (1990) Placental examination can help determine cause of brain damage in neonates. *Tex. Med.*, **86**, 33–38.
6. Brann, Jr A.W. and Cefalo, R.C. (1983) *Guidelines for Perinatal Care*, American Academy of Pediatrics, Elk Grove, IL, pp. 260–261.
7. Vannucci, R.C. and Duffy, T.E. (1976) Carbohydrate metabolism in fetal and neonatal rat brain during anoxia and recovery. *Am. J. Physiol.*, **230**, 1269–75.
8. Nicholson, C. (1980) Measurement of extracellular ions in the brain. *Trends Neurosci.*, **3**, 216–18.
9. Harris, R.J., Symon, L., Branston, N.M. *et al.* (1981) Changes in extracellular calcium activity in cerebral ischemia. *J. Cereb. Blood Flow Metab.*, **1**, 203–209.
10. Daniel, P., Love, E., Moorehouse, L. *et al.* (1971) Factors influencing utilization of ketone bodies by the brain in normal rats and rats with ketoacidosis. *Lancet*, **ii**, 637–38.
11. Hattori, H. and Wasterlain, C.G. (1990) Posthypoxic glucose supplement reduces hypoxic-ischemic brain damage in the neonatal rat. *Ann. Neurol.*, **28**, 122–28.
12. Dao, D.N., Ahdab, B.M. and Schor, N.F. (1991) Cerebellar glutamine synthetase in children after hypoxia or ischemia. *Stroke*, **22**, 1312–16.
13. Choi, D.W. and Rothman, S.M. (1990). The role of glutamate neurotoxicity in hypoxic-ischemic neuronal death. *Ann. Rev. Neurosci.*, **13**, 171–82.
14. Michaels, R.L. and Rothman, S.M. (1990) Glutamate neurotoxicity *in vitro*: antagonist pharmacology and intracellular calcium concentrations. *J. Neurosci.*, **10**, 283–92.
15. Rothman, S.M., Thurston, J.H. and Hauhart, R.E. (1987) Delayed neurotoxicity of excitatory amino acids *in vitro*. *Neuroscience*, **22**, 471–80.
16. Gardiner, M., Nilsson, B., Rehncrona, S. *et al.* (1981) Free fatty acids in the rat brain in moderate and severe hypoxia. *J. Neurochem.*, **36**, 1500–505.
17. Espinoza, M.I. and Parer, J.T. (1991) Mechanisms of asphyxial brain damage, and possible pharmacologic interventions, in the fetus. *Am. J. Obstet. Gynecol.*, **164**, 1582–89; discussion 1589–91.
18. Rosenberg, A.A., Murdaugh, E. and White, C.W. (1989) The role of oxygen free radicals in postasphyxia cerebral hypoperfusion in newborn lambs. *Pediatr. Res.*, **26**, 215–19.
19. Hagberg, H., Lehmann, A., Sanberg, M. *et al.* (1985) Ischemia induced shift of inhibitory and excitatory amino acids from intracellular compartments. *J. Cereb. Blood Flow Metab.*, **5**, 413–19.
20. Vannucci, R.C. and Duffy, T.E. (1977) Cerebral metabolism in newborn dogs during reversible asphyxia. *Ann. Neurol.*, **1**, 528–34.
21. Cheung, J.Y., Bonventre, J.V., Malis, C.O. *et al.* (1986) Calcium and ischemic injury. *N. Engl J. Med.*, **314**, 1670–76.
22. Malamud, N. and Hirano, A. (1974) *Atlas of Neuropathology*, University of California Press, Berkeley, pp. 1–462.
23. Gilles, F.H. (1969) Hypotensive brain stem necrosis: selective symmetrical necrosis of tegmental neuronal aggregates following cardiac arrest. *Arch. Pathol.*, **88**, 32–41.
24. Novotny, E.J.J. (1989) Hypoxic-ischemic encephalopathy, in *Fetal and Neonatal Brain Injury: Mechanisms, Management, and the Risk of Practice* (eds D.K. Stevenson and P. Sunshine), B.C. Decker, Philadelphia, pp. 113–22.
25. Dolfin, T., Skidmore, M.B., Fong, K.W. et al. (1983) Incidence, severity and timing of subependymal and intraventricular hemorrhage in preterm infants born in a perinatal unit as detected by serial real-time ultrasound. *Pediatrics*, **71**, 541–46.
26. Enzmann, D., Murphy-Irwin, K., Stevenson, D.K. *et al.* (1985) The natural history of subependymal germinal matrix hemorrhage. *Am. J. Perinatol.*, **2**, 123–33.
27. Volpe, J.J. (1989) Intraventricular hemorrhage and brain injury in the premature infant. Neuropathology and pathogenesis. *Clin. Perinatol.*, **16**, 361–86.
28. Volpe, J.J. (1989) Intraventricular hemorrhage in the premature infant – current concepts. Part I. *Ann. Neurol.*, **25**, 3–11.
29. Armstrong, D.L., Sauls, C.D. and Goddard-Finegold, J. (1987) Neuropathologic findings in short term survivors of intraventricular hemorrhage. *Am. J. Dis. Child.*, **141**, 617–21.
30. Fenichel, G.M., Webster, D.L. and Wang, W.K.T. (1984) Intracranial hemorrhage in the term newborn. *Arch. Neurol.*, **41**, 30–34.
31. Parer, J.T., Puttler, O.L., Freeman, R.K. (eds) (1974) *A Clinical Approach to Fetal Monitoring*, Berkeley Bioengineering, Berkeley, CA, Report No. 17.
32. Rudolph, A.M. and Heymann, M.A. (1970) Circulatory changes during growth in the fetal lamb. *Circ. Res.*, **26**, 289–99.
33. Block, B.S., Schlafer, D.H., Wentworth, R.A. *et al.* (1990) Intrauterine asphyxia and the breakdown of physiologic circulatory compensation in fetal sheep. *Am. J. Obstet. Gynecol.*, **162**, 1325–31.

34. Field, D.R., Parer, J.T., Auslender, R.A. *et al.* (1990) Cerebral oxygen consumption during asphyxia in fetal sheep. *J. Dev. Physiol.*, **14**, 131–37.
35. Dawes, G. (1968) *Foetal and Neonatal Physiology*, Yearbook Medical, Chicago, pp. 7–247.
36. Ment, L.R., Stewart, W.B., Gore, J.C. and Duncan, C.C. (1988) Beagle puppy model of perinatal asphyxia: alterations in cerebral blood flow and metabolism. *Pediatr. Neurol.*, **4**, 98–104.
37. Ment, L.R., Stewart, W.B., Petroff, O.A. *et al.* (1989) Beagle puppy model of perinatal asphyxia: blockade of excitatory neurotransmitters. *Pediatr. Neurol.*, **5**, 281–86.
38. Brann, A.W. (1981) *Neonatal Hypoxic Ischemic Encephalopathy. Perinatal Brain Insult.* Symposium on Perinatal and Developmental Medicine, vol. 17, Mead Johnson, Evansville, IN, p. 49.
39. Donnelly, W.H. (1987) Ischemic myocardial necrosis and papillary muscle dysfunction in infants and children. *Am. J. Cardiovasc. Pathol.*, **1**, 173–88.
40. Friedman, W.F. (1972) The intrinsic physiologic properties of the developing heart. *Prog. Cardiovasc. Dis.*, **15**, 87–111.
41. MacDonald, H., Mulligan, J., Allen, A. *et al.* (1980) Neonatal asphyxia. I. Relationship of obstetric and neonatal complications to neonatal mortality in 38 405 consecutive deliveries. *J. Pediatr.*, **96**, 898–902.
42. James, L. (1959) *Biochemical Aspects of Asphyxia at Birth in Adaptation to Extrauterine Life.* Report of the 31st Ross Conference on Pediatric Research, Ross Laboratories, Columbus, OH, pp. 66–71.
43. Jilek, L., Travnickova, E. and Projan, S. (1970) Characteristic metabolic and functional responses to oxygen deficiency in the central nervous system, in *Physiology of the Perinatal Period* (ed., U. Stave), Appleton-Century-Crofts, NY, pp. 967–1041.
44. Stewart, W.B. (1987) Blood flow and metabolism in the developing brain. *Semin. Perinatol.*, **11**, 112–16.
45. Coughtrey, H., Jeffery, H.E. Henderson, S.D. *et al.* (1991) Possible causes linking asphyxia, thick meconium and respiratory distress. *Aust. N.Z. J. Obstet. Gynaecol.*, **31**, 97–102.
46. Bowes, W.J. (1988) Clinical management of preterm delivery. *Clin. Obstet. Gynecol.*, **31**, 652–61.
47. Kilbride, H.W., Yeast, J.D. and Thibeault, D.W. (1989) Intrapartum and delivery room management of premature rupture of membranes complicated by oligohydramnios. *Clin. Perinatol.*, **16**, 863–88.
48. Schauseil, Z.U., Hamm, W. Stenzel, B. *et al.* (1989) Severe intra-uterine growth retardation: obstetrical management and follow up studies in children born between 1970 and 1985. *Eur. J. Obstet. Gynecol. Reprod. Biol.*, **30**, 1–9.
49. Laurin, J., Persson, P.H. and Polberger, S. (1987) Perinatal outcome in growth retarded pregnancies dated by ultrasound. *Acta Obstet. Gynecol. Scand.* **66**, 337–43.
50. Villar, J. de O.M., Kestler, E. Bolanos, F. *et al.* (1990) The differential neonatal morbidity of the intrauterine growth retardation syndrome. *Am. J. Obstet. Gynecol.*, **163**, 151–57.
51. Cnattingius, S. (1989) The small-for-gestational-age infant: obstetrical management and perinatal outcome. *Ups. J. Med. Sci.*, **94**, 55–65.
52. Mannino, F. (1988) Neonatal complications of postterm gestation. *J. Reprod. Med.*, **33**, 271–76.
53. Daga, A.S., Daga, S.R. and Patole, S.K. (1990) Risk assessment in birth asphyxia. *J. Trop. Pediatr.*, **36**, 34–39.
54. Mimouni, F., Miodovnik, M. Siddiqi, T.A. *et al.* (1988) Perinatal asphyxia in infants of insulin-dependent diabetic mothers. *J. Pediatr.*, **113**, 345–53.
55. Bailey, C. and Kattwinkel, J. (1990) Establishing a neonatal resuscitation team in community hospitals. *J. Perinatol.*, **10**, 294–300.
56. Moore, J.J., Andrews, L. Henderson, C. *et al.* (1989) Neonatal resuscitation in community hospitals. A regional-based, team-oriented training program coordinated by the tertiary center. *Am. J. Obstet. Gynecol.*, **161**, 849–55.
57. Permezel, J.M., Pepperell, R.J. and Kloss, M. (1987) Unexpected problems in patients selected for birthing unit delivery. *Aust. N.Z. J. Obstet. Gynaecol.*, **27**, 21–23.
58. Byrd, F.H. (1990) Early experience with the neonatal resuscitation program. *Neonatal Netw.*, **9**, 35–40.
59. Hanvey, L. (1988) Breathing new life into neonatal resuscitation guidelines. *Dimens. Health Serv.*, **65**, 8–9.
60. Daga, S.R., Fernandes, C.J. Soare, M. *et al.* (1991) Clinical profile of severe birth asphyxia. *Indian Pediatr.*, **28**, 485–88.
61. Roy, R.N. and Betheras, F.R. (1990) The Melbourne Chart – a logical guide to neonatal resuscitation. *Anaesth. Intensive Care*, **18**, 348–57.
62. Benitz, W.E., Frankel, L.R. and Stevenson, D.K. *et al.* (1989) Management of the depressed or neurologically dysfunctional infant. Immediate management, in *Fetal and Neonatal Brain Injury: Mechanisms, Management, and the Risks of Practice* (eds D.K. Stevenson and P. Sunshine), B.C. Decker, Philadelphia, pp. 94–103.
63. Benitz, W.E., Frankel, L.R. and Stevenson, D.K. (1986) Pharmacology of neonatal resuscitation and cardiopulmonary intensive care. Part I. Immediate resuscitation. *West. J. Med.*, **144**, 704–709.
64. McKlveen, R.E. and Ostheimer, G.W. (1987) Resuscitation of the newborn. *Clin. Obstet. Gynecol.*, **30**, 611–20.
65. Cui, J.J. (1991) (Desirable temperature in the operating room during neonatal resuscitation.) *Chung Hua Fu Chan Ko Tsa Chih*, **26**, 213–14, 250.
66. Benitz, W.E., Frankel, L.R. and Stevenson, D.K. (1989) Management of the depressed or neurologically dysfunctional infant. Extended management, in *Fetal and Neonatal Brain Injury: Mechanisms, Management, and the Risks of Practice* (eds D.K. Stevenson and P. Sunshine), B.C. Decker, Philadelphia, pp. 104–12.
67. Papile, L., Burnstein, J., Burnstein, R. *et al.* (1978) Relationship of intravenous sodium bicarbonate infusions and cerebrospinal intraventricular hemorrhage. *J. Pediatr.*, **93**, 834–36.
68. Zaritsky, A. and Chernow, B. (1984) Use of catecholamines in pediatrics. *J. Pediatr.*, **105**, 341–50.
69. Salsbury, D.J. and Brown, D.R. (1982) Effect of parental calcium treatment on blood pressure and heart rate in neonatal hypocalcemia. *Pediatrics*, **69**, 605–609.
70. Mirro, R. and Brown, D.J. (1984) Parenteral calcium treatment shortens the left ventricle systolic time intervals of hypocalcemic neonates. *Pediatr. Res.*, **18**, 71–73.
71. Chernick, V., Manfreda, J., De, B.V. *et al.* (1988) Clinical trial of naloxone in birth asphyxia. *J. Pediatr.*, **113**, 519–25.
72. Romero, T. and Fridman, W.F. (1979) Limited left ventricular response to volume overload in the neonatal period: a comparative study with the adult animal. *Pediatr. Res.*, **13**, 910–15.
73. Keeley, S.R. and Bohn, D.J. (1988) The use of inotropic and afterload-reducing agents in neonates. *Clin. Perinatol.*, **15**, 467–89.
74. Perlman, J.M. and Tack, E.D. (1988) Renal injury in the asphyxiated newborn infant: relationship to neurologic outcome. *J. Pediatr.*, **113**, 875–9.
75. Perlman, J.M. (1989) Systemic abnormalities in term infants following perinatal asphyxia: relevance to long-term neurologic outcome. *Clin. Perinatol.*, **16**, 475–84.
76. Jayashree, G., Dutta, A.K., Sarna, M.S. and Saili, A. (1991) Acute renal failure in asphyxiated newborns. *Indian Pediatr.*, **28**, 19–23.
77. Apgar, V. (1953) A proposal for a new method of evaluation of the newborn infant. *Curr. Res. Anaesth. Analg.*, **32**, 260–67.
78. Niswander, K.R. and Gordon, M. (1972) *Collaborative Perinatal Study of the National Institute for Neurological Disease and Stroke: the Women and their Pregnancies*, W.B. Saunders, Philadelphia, pp. 2–540.
79. Ruth, V.J. and Raivio, K.O. (1988) Perinatal brain damage: predictive value of metabolic acidosis and the Apgar score. *BMJ*, **297**, 24–27.
80. Odden, J.P. and Bratlid, D. (1990) (Neonatal asphyxia in full-term infants). *Tidsskr. Nor. Laegeforen.*, **110**, 602–605.
81. Jain, L., Ferre, C., Vidyasagar, D. *et al.* (1991) Cardiopulmonary resuscitation of apparently stillborn infants: survival and long-term outcome. *J. Pediatr.*, **118**, 778–82.
82. Sykes, G.S., Molloy, P.M., Johnson, P. *et al.* (1982) Do Apgar scores indicate asphyxia? *Lancet*, **i**, 494–96.
83. Silverman, F., Surdan, J., Wasserman, J. *et al.* (1985) The Apgar score: is it enough? *Obstet. Gynecol.*, **66**, 331–36.
84. Levene, H.L., Kornberg, J. and Williams, T.H.C. (1985) The incidence and severity of postasphyxial encephalopathy in full-term infants. *Early Hum. Dev.*, **11**, 21–26.
85. Nelson, K.B. and Ellenberg, J.H. (1984) Obstetric complications as risk factors for cerebral palsy or seizure disorders. *JAMA*. **251**, 1843–48.
86. Seidman, D.S., Paz, I., Laor, A. *et al.* (1991) Apgar scores and cognitive performance at 17 years of age. *Obstet. Gynecol.*, **77**, 875–78.
87. Giacoia, G.P. (1988) Low Apgar scores and birth asphyxia. Misconceptions that promote undeserved negligence suits. *Postgrad. Med.*, **84**, 77–82.
88. Nelson, K.B. and Leviton, A. (1991), How much of neonatal encephalopathy is due to birth asphyxia? *Am. J. Dis. Child.*, **145**, 1325–31.
89. Manning, F.A., Harman, C.R., Morrison, I. and Menticoglou, S. (1990) Fetal assessment based on fetal biophysical profile scoring. III. Positive predictive accuracy of the very abnormal test (biophysical profile score =0). *Am. J. Obstet. Gynecol.*, **162**, 398–402.
90. Binkin, N.J., Rust, K.R. and Williams, R.L. (1988) Racial differences in neonatal mortality. What causes of death explain the gap? *Am. J. Dis. Child.*, **142**, 434–40.
91. Langkamp, D.L. Foye, H.R. and Roghmann, K.J. (1990) Does limited access to NICU services account for higher neonatal mortality rates among blacks? *Am. J. Perinatol.*, **7**, 227–31.
92. Minchom, P., Niswander, K., Chalmers, I. *et al.* (1987) Antecedents and outcome of very early neonatal seizures in infants born at or after term. *Br. J. Obstet. Gynecol.*, **94**, 431–39.
93. Sarnat, H.B. and Sarnat, M.S. (1976) Neonatal encephalopathy following fetal distress. A clinical and electroencephalographic study. *Arch. Neurol.*, **33**, 696–705.
94. Robertson, C. and Finer, N. (1985) Term infants with hypoxic ischemic encephalopathy: outcome at 3–5 years. *Dev. Med. Child Neurol.*, **27**, 473–84.

95. Ellenberg, J.H. and Nelson, K.B. (1988) Cluster of perinatal events identifying infants at high risk for death or disability. *J. Pediatr.*, **113**, 546–52.

96. Tharp, B.R., Scher, M.S. and Clancy, R.R. (1989) Serial EEGs in normal and abnormal infants with birth weights less than 1200 grams – a prospective study with long term follow-up. *Neuropediatrics*, **20**, 64–72.

97. Grant, A. (1988) The relationship between obstetrically preventable intrapartum asphyxia, abnormal neonatal neurologic signs, and subsequent motor impairment in babies born at or near term, in *Perinatal Events and Brain Damage in Surviving Children* (eds F. Kubli, N. Patel, W. Schmidt and O. Linderkemp), Springer, Berlin, pp. 149–61.

98. Levine, M.I. and Trounce, J.Q. (1986) Cause of neonatal convulsions. Towards more precise diagnosis. *Arch. Dis. Child.*, **61**, 78–87.

99. Blair, E. and Stanley, F.J. (1988) Intrapartum asphyxia: a rare cause of cerebral palsy (published erratum appears in *J. Pediatr.*, **113**, 420). *J. Pediatr.*, **112**, 515–19.

100. Nelson, K.B. (1989) Relationship of intrapartum and delivery room events to long-term neurologic outcome. *Clin. Perinatol.*, **16**, 995–1007.

101. Holm, V. (1982) The causes of cerebral palsy – a contemporary perspective. *JAMA*, **247**, 1473–77.

102. Hagberg, B. and Kyllerman, M. (1983) Epidemiology and mental retardation – a Swedish survey. *Brain Dev.*, **5**, 441–49.

103. Nelson, K.B. and Ellenberg, J.H. (1986) Antecedents of cerebral palsy. Multivariate analysis of risk. *N. Engl. J. Med.*, **315**, 81–86.

104. Groenendaal, F., van Hof-van Duin, J., Baerts, W. and Fetter, W.P. (1989) Effects of perinatal hypoxia on visual development during the first year of (corrected) age. *Early Hum. Dev.*, **20**, 267–79.

105. Holst, K., Andersen, E., Philip, J., Henningsen, I. (1989) Antenatal and perinatal conditions correlated to handicap among 4-year-old children. *Am. J. Perinatol.*, **6**, 258–67.

106. Segerer, H., Landendorfer, W., Deeg, K.H. and Richter, K. (1988) (Reduction of cerebral hemorrhage and respiratory distress syndrome in premature infants by avoiding perinatal asphyxia.) *Monatsschr. Kinderheilkd.*, **136**, 176–80.

107. Voigt, H.J., Lang, N., Segerer, H. and Stehr, K. (1989) (Effect of obstetric-perinatal measures on mortality and early morbidity of premature infants weighing 500 to 1500 grams.) *Geburtshilfe Frauenheilkd.*, **49**, 720–27.

108. Zielonka, V.S. and Gmyrek, D. (1989) (Neuropsychiatric disorders in very-low-birthweight newborn infants (VLBW-infants) – before and after the introduction of modern perinatal medicine. 3. Discussion of trends in quality of survival (CNS morbidity) and conclusions.) *Kinderarztl. Prax.*, **57**, 371–79.

109. Donn, S.M., Goldstein, G.W. and Schork, M.A. (1988) Neonatal hypoxic-ischemic encephalopathy: current management practices. *J. Perinatol.*, **8**, 49–52.

110. Tharp, B.R. (1990) Electrophysiological brain maturation in premature infants: an historical perspective. *J. Clin. Neurophysiol.*, **7**, 302–14.

111. Andre, M., Matisse, N., Vert, P. and Debruille, C. (1988) Neonatal seizures – recent aspects. *Neuropediatrics*, **19**, 201–207.

112. Tudehope, D.I., Harris, A., Hawes, D. and Hayes, M. (1988) Clinical spectrum and outcome of neonatal convulsions. *Aust. Paediatr. J.*, **24**, 249–53.

113. Connell, J., Oozeer, R. de V.L., Dubowitz, L.M. and Dubowitz, V. (1989) Continuous EEG monitoring of neonatal seizures: diagnosis and prognostic considerations. *Arch. Dis. Child.*, **64**, 452–58.

114. Mizrahi, E.M. (1987) Neonatal seizures: problems in diagnosis and classification. *Epilepsia*, **28** (suppl. 1), S46–S5.

115. Mizrahi, E.M. (1989) Consensus and controversy in the clinical management of neonatal seizures. *Clin. Perinatol.*, **16**, 485–500.

116. Doberczak, T.M., Shanzer, S., Cutler, R. *et al.* (1988) One-year follow-up of infants with abstinence-associated seizures. *Arch. Neurol.*, **45**, 649–53.

117. Tharp, B.R. (1987) An overview of pediatric seizure disorders and epileptic syndromes. *Epilepsia*, **28** (suppl. 1), S36–45.

118. Tharp, B. (1989) Electroencephalographs in assessment of premature and full terms, in *Fetal and Neonatal Brain Injury: Mechanisms, Management, and the Risks of Practice* (eds D.K. Stevenson and P. Sunshine), B.C. Decker, Philadelphia, pp. 175–84.

119. Volpe, J.J., Herscovitch, P., Perlman, J.M. *et al.* (1983) Positron emission tomography in the newborn: extensive impairment of regional cerebral blood flow with intraventricular hemorrhage and hemorrhagic intracerebral involvement. *Pediatrics*, **72**, 589–601.

120. Anderson, J.C. and Mawk, J.R. (1988) Intracranial arterial duplex Doppler waveform analysis in infants (see comments). *Childs Nerv. Syst.*, **4**; 144–48.

121. Lingman, G. and Marsal, K. (1989) Noninvasive assessment of cranial blood circulation in the fetus. *Biol. Neonate*, **56**, 129–35.

122. Cross, K.W., Dear, P.R.F., Warner, R.M. *et al.* (1976) An attempt to measure cerebral blood flow in the newborn infant. *J. Physiol.*, **260**, 42P–43P.

123. Cooke, R.W.I. and Rolfe, P. (1979) Apparent cerebral blood flow in newborns with respiratory disease. *Dev. Med. Clin. Neurol.*, **21**, 154–60.

124. Azzopardi, D., Wyatt, J.S., Cady, E.B. *et al.* (1989) Prognosis of newborn infants with hypoxic-ischemic brain injury assessed by phosphorus magnetic resonance spectroscopy. *Pediatr. Res.*, **25**, 445–51.

125. Nalin, A., Frigieri, G., Caggia, P. and Vezzalini, S. (1989) State of the art of magnetic resonance (MR) in neonatal hypoxic-ischemic encephalopathy. *Childs Nerv. Syst.*, **5** 350–55.

126. Moorcraft, J., Bolas, N.M., Ives, N.K. *et al.* (1991) Spatially localized magnetic resonance spectroscopy of the brains of normal and asphyxiated newborns. *Pediatrics*, **87**, 273–82.

127. Wyatt, J.S, Edwards, A.D., Azzopardi, D. and Reynolds, E.O. (1989) Magnetic resonance and near infrared spectroscopy for investigation of perinatal hypoxic-ischaemic brain injury. *Arch. Dis. Child.*, **64**, 953–63.

128. Brazy, J.E. (1991) Near infrared spectroscopy. *Clin. Perinatol.*, **18**, 519–34.

129. Benaron, D.A., Benitz, W.E. and Ariagno, R.L. (1992) Noninvasive methods for estimating *in vivo* oxygenation. *Clin. Pediatr.*, **31**, 258–73.

130. Dixhoorn, M.J., Visser, G.H.A., Huisjes, H.J. *et al.* (1985) The relationship between umbilical pH values and neonatal neurological morbidity in full-term AFD infants. *Early Hum. Dev.*, **11**, 33–42.

131. De Praeter, C., Vanhaesebrouck, P., Govaert, P. *et al.* (1991) Creatine kinase isoenzyme BB concentrations in the cerebrospinal fluid of newborns: relationship to short-term outcome. *Pediatrics*, **88**, 1204–10.

132. Pietz, J., Guttenberg, N. and Gluck, L. (1988) Hypoxanthine: a marker for asphyxia. *Obstet. Gynecol.*, **72**, 762–66.

93 NEONATAL INTENSIVE CARE

I.A. Laing

93.1 Introduction

Neonatal units throughout the world must try to serve their individual communities according to their needs. Where infants are dying of hypothermia or malnutrition it is inappropriate to plan expensive programmes involving advanced technologies. The present author has recently visited a unit where replacement surfactant improves the immediate respiratory status of the preterm neonate, yet almost all such infants subsequently succumb from sepsis. Another unit has exceedingly poor handwashing facilities and yet has embarked on a controlled trial of intravenous immunoglobulin as prophylaxis against sepsis of the low-birth-weight infant. Too often a new technological advance may be pursued for its own sake without first considering whether this is the top priority for the community served. Too often the price is paid in long-term morbidity of the child. Too often follow-up facilities are inadequate, and clinical audit is impracticable or else the results are ignored. Anecdotal impressions of handicap rates gleaned from a hard-pressed outpatient clinic may be misleading, and should therefore be formalized statistically. Yet technological advances may bring opportunities to improve care for infants. The pursuit of lower mortality for the 26-week gestation infant may bring with it a lower morbidity for the child born at 30 weeks' gestation. In experienced hands the sophisticated ventilator may allow a 600 g infant to survive, but with risk of long-term handicap; yet such technical development may serve to reduce the prevalence of bronchopulmonary dysplasia in infants of birth weight 750–1500 g. The social needs of the powerless infant and the emotional needs of the highly stressed family have been given too little attention in the past. Such omissions are being corrected now, thanks largely to the demands of farsighted and determined parents.

93.2 Organization of neonatal services

Most attention in this chapter is given to neonatal units which serve urban communities in the developed world. Table 93.1 shows categories of infants requiring assistance as drawn up by the Working Group of the British Association of Perinatal Medicine 1992 [1].

During the planning of a new neonatal unit, due account must be taken of the population density and geographical area served. It has been recommended that there should be 1.5 maximal intensive care cots per thousand births [2,3] and five high dependency and special care cots per thousand births. The tertiary referral centre should provide all maximal intensive care cots for its catchment area, and take into account the high dependency and special care facilities available in neighbouring district general hospitals. A threat to the level 1 intensive care cots occurs when infants who no longer require full intensive care now have no 'step-down' facilities outwith the intensive care area, whether in the referral centre or in the district general hospital. The neonatal unit's intensive care cots are then occupied inappropriately and it ceases to function as a satisfactory referral centre. This can be overcome only by careful planning of staffing both in the referral centre and in the 'step-down' facilities, wherever they may be. Close co-operation between medical and nursing staff involves mutual understanding of problems. If geographically possible, this may be facilitated by outreach teaching from the referral centre, and by rotation of nursing/midwifery and junior medical staff between the units. Flexibility in allocation of regional resources may be enhanced by a single medical and nursing management structure for neonatal services whose executive operates by authority of a joint regional neonatology division. Cosmetic and functional unification can be more readily approached if there is a unified system of computerized medical records, accessible and retrievable audit data, guidelines to clinical

Diseases of the Fetus and Newborn, 2nd edn, Edited by G.B. Reed, A.E. Claireaux and F. Cockburn. Published in 1995 by Chapman & Hall, London. ISBN 0 412 39160 0

Table 93.1 Clinical categories of neonatal care*

Level 1 intensive care (maximal intensive care) should be provided for babies:

- Receiving assisted ventilation (including intermittent positive airway pressure, intermittent mandatory ventilation and constant positive airway pressure), and in the first 24 hours after its withdrawal
- Of less than 27 weeks' gestation for the first 48 hours after birth
- With birth weight of less than 1000 g for the first 48 hours after birth
- Who require major emergency surgery for the preoperative period and postoperatively for 48 hours
- On the day of death
- Being transported by a team including medical and nursing staff
- Who are receiving peritoneal dialysis
- Who require exchange transfusions complicated by other disease processes
- With severe respiratory disease in the first 48 hours of life requiring an FiO_2 of >0.6
- With recurrent apnoea needing frequent intervention, e.g. over five stimulations in 8 hours or resuscitation with intermittent positive pressure ventilation two or more times in 24 hours
- With significant requirements for circulatory support, e.g. inotropes, three or more infusions of colloid in 24 hours, or infusions of prostaglandins

Level 2 intensive care (high dependency intensive care) should be provided for babies:

- Requiring total parenteral nutrition
- Who are having convulsions
- Being transported by a trained skilled neonatal nurse alone
- With arterial line or chest drain
- With respiratory disease in the first 48 hours of life requiring an FiO_2 of 0.4–0.6
- With recurrent apnoea requiring stimulation up to five times in an 8-hour period or any resuscitation with intermittent positive pressure ventilation
- Who require an exchange transfusion alone
- Who are more than 48 hours postoperative and require complex nursing procedures
- With tracheostomy, for the first 2 weeks

Special care should be provided for babies:

- Requiring continuous monitoring of respiration or heart rate, or PO_2 by transcutaneous transducers
- Receiving additional oxygen
- With tracheostomy, after the first 2 weeks
- Being given intravenous glucose and electrolyte solutions
- Who are being tube fed
- Who have had minor surgery in the previous 24 hours
- Who require terminal care but not on the day of death
- Being barrier nursed
- Undergoing phototherapy
- Receiving special monitoring (e.g. frequent glucose or bilirubin estimations)
- Needing constant supervision (e.g. babies whose mothers are drug addicts)
- Being treated with antibiotics

---

* Note: US level III equals UK level I.

management which are widely agreed, and educational programmes available to all professional neonatal staff of the associated units.

93.3 Recent advances

93.3.1 REPLACEMENT SURFACTANT

There can be little doubt that the development of replacement surfactant has revolutionized the care of the preterm infant with respiratory distress syndrome (RDS). This condition is caused by a deficiency of specialized phospholipids and proteins in the lung of the premature infant. Successful therapeutic administration of intratracheal exogenous surfactant first took place in 1980 [4]. Since then a wide range of animal and artificial surfactants have been used in therapeutic trials (Chapter 95).

It is still unclear which infants should receive endogenous surfactant and when it should be given. Replacement surfactants can be given at the time of birth to 'at-risk' preterm infants as **prophylaxis** against the development of RDS. This raises the anxiety that many infants who would not have developed RDS are given an expensive drug unnecessarily, and in units which favour 'natural' surfactants it must be recognized that foreign (animal) proteins are being delivered into the infant's respiratory tree. There is, however, no evidence as yet that this policy results in any detrimental immune response. The alternative is to use replacement surfactant in a 'rescue' manner, treating the premature infant who is showing clinical signs of RDS and who is already receiving intermittent positive pressure ventilation therapy. In an increasingly finance-aware UK many units favour this latter approach.

Meta-analysis of clinical trials of surfactant therapy leave no doubt of its efficacy [5]. There is a 40% decrease in mortality in treated infants, and the risk of major complications such as pneumothorax is also reduced [6]. In infants of birth weight greater than 1250 g there may be a cost saving because of the resultant reduction in intensive care days. However the improved survival of the extremely low-birth-weight infant implies a successful but costly stay in hospital. This financial burden must be borne, since to withold a potentially life-saving drug has serious ethical implications. It is unclear at present how great will be the prevalence of chronic lung disease in our community as a result of this new population of graduates from our neonatal units.

The two most widely used replacement surfactants in the UK are Exosurf (an artificial surfactant) and Curosurf (a porcine surfactant). Exosurf is colfosceril palmitate and is supplied as a vial of white freeze-dried powder which is then mixed with sterile water to a white suspension containing no animal protein. A dosage of 5 ml/kg body weight is administered into the infant's distal trachea over several minutes via a side-arm of the endotracheal tube. Two doses 12 hours apart are commonly used. In December 1992 the OSIRIS Collaborative Group [7] reported that administration of the first dose of Exosurf at 2 hours of life reduced the risk of death, chronic dependence on oxygen, and pneumothorax when compared with initial treatment at 3 hours of life. There was no apparent advantage in administering a third or fourth dose of surfactant.

Curosurf is prepared from minced pig lungs and contains approximately 99% polar lipids and 1% low molecular weight hydrophobic proteins. A single dose of Curosurf reduces mortality in severe RDS by 40% and doubles the proportion of survivors without chronic lung disease. Results of a European multicentre randomized trial comparing high and low dose surfactant regimens for the treatment of RDS show that a regimen of 100 mg/kg initially, repeated at 12 and 24 hours as indicated, is as effective as higher dosage regimens [8]. There is no evidence yet to show whether a 'natural' or a 'synthetic' surfactant will provide a superior long-term outcome. Curosurf acts more rapidly and may dramatically improve the dynamic compliance of the chest of the infant with RDS.

93.3.2 EXTRACORPOREAL MEMBRANE OXYGENATION

While replacement surfactants have established themselves as major advances in the therapy of the newborn, extracorporeal membrane oxygenation (ECMO) has been much more controversial. It is estimated that approximately 200 mature newborn infants per year die in the UK because of acute respiratory failure, including infants with meconium aspiration syndrome, diaphragmatic hernia or persistent pulmonary hypertension of the newborn. Worldwide over 5000 infants have now been treated with ECMO and approximately 83% have survived. In venoarterial perfusion, cannulation of the right common carotid artery and the internal jugular vein allows desaturated blood to be channelled by mechanical pump to a membrane oxygenator and then returned to the central arterial circulation, thus oxygenating the infant without the requirement for high ventilator settings, and so minimizing barotrauma. In general ECMO is considered only for those infants of 34 weeks' gestation or more because in neonates born more prematurely there is difficult vascular access, and furthermore the need for anticoagulation during ECMO carries an increased risk of periventricular haemorrhage and consequent neurological damage [9]. The technique is labour intensive, expensive and not without major side-effects, including intracranial haemorrhage and sepsis. Nevertheless it is now widely used in the USA where the treatment is so entrenched that a randomized trial is no longer practicable. In the UK, however, a randomized trial, aiming to collect data from approximately 300 infants, has been embarked on, comparing the results of infants treated with ECMO in four established centres versus maximal conventional management in tertiary referral centres. The study aims to assess both clinical effectiveness, principally in terms of survival to 1 year of age without severe disability, and cost effectiveness.

Meanwhile ECMO threatens to be usurped by the discovery in animals and in human infants that inhaled nitric oxide causes decreased pulmonary pressure and vascular resistance, and dose-dependent increases in pulmonary blood flow, without affecting systemic arterial pressure [10]. It may be that several children in Boston, Massachusetts, have escaped undergoing ECMO because of their successful response to endothelin inhibition by inhaled nitric oxide. The current author predicts that this discovery will eventually dwarf ECMO as a therapeutic technique (Chapter 102).

93.3.3 ANALGESIA

When considering advances in neonatology it is tempting to dwell only on a new drug, a new machine or a new investigative technique. A new area of understanding is perhaps equally important, and the last 5 years have focused on the reality that newborn infants, however premature, feel pain, and that this sensation may impede recovery. Extreme hormonal and metabolic responses to stress are associated with increased morbidity and mortality in adults. In 1992 Anand and Hickey [11] investigated the responses of ill neonates to cardiac surgery, and showed that those who received deep anaesthesia (with sufentanil) had significantly reduced responses of β-endorphin, noradrenaline, adrenaline, glucagon, aldosterone, cortisol and other steroid hormones. The neonates who received lighter anaesthesia (with halothane plus morphine) showed marked hyperglycaemia and lactic acidaemia during surgery. The neonates treated with deep anaesthesia had a decreased incidence of sepsis, metabolic acidosis and disseminated intravascular coagulation, and also had fewer postoperative deaths.

In the human fetus, nociceptive pathways are well developed by late gestation, and cortical and subcortical centres for pain perception are present and functional by the time of birth [12]. Physiological responses to painful stimuli have now been shown to be even greater in the neonate than in adult subjects. Studies are currently being undertaken to establish whether analgesia and sedation in the neonatal unit, including during standard procedures such as intubation and intermittent positive pressure ventilation, may improve the outcome in terms of morbidity and mortality. It is attractive to suggest that an opiate infusion may cause an infant to synchronize spontaneous respiration with that imposed by the ventilator, and that this will reduce barotrauma, thus lessening the risk of pneumothorax and perhaps even chronic lung disease. Now that there is an appreciation of the infant's awareness of discomfort, humane considerations for the child must rank as one of the major neonatal advances of the decade.

93.4 Ethical decisions in the neonatal unit

The advent of ultrasound, amniocentesis and chorionic villus sampling has produced a new era in ethical decision-making. The identification of an abnormality during pregnancy may bring forward by several months the need to provide advice for a family. A team approach is mandatory and the subspecialists each bring their individual expertise to contribute to this process. As in the labour ward, the three categories of neonatal illness which most frequently cause distress in the neonatal unit are (1) extreme prematurity, (2) perinatal asphyxia, and (3) severe congenital abnormality.

93.4.1 EXTREME PREMATURITY

The advent of ventilators and intravenous nutrition designed for the newborn child provide means of life support. Now the child of 23 weeks' gestation may survive to go home [13], and the recent introduction of replacement surfactant (see above) has improved further the survival of very-low-birth-weight infants [14,15]. Severe neurological problems, including significant cerebral palsy, major seizure disorders, hydrocephalus, sensorineural loss (including blindness and deafness) and severe mental handicap, may occur in extremely low-birth weight infants: 26% of those survivors who weigh less than 800 g at birth, 17% of those weighing 750–1000 g and 11% of those weighing 1000–1500 g [16]. An effort to offer a practical guideline prompted Campbell [17] to suggest a 'cut-off' birth weight of 750 g, below which full resuscitative measures would not be offered without first discussing the hazards with the parents. Ten years on, should this guideline be altered, or do recent advances in the care of these infants compel the neonatologist to provide maximum intensive care for infants weighing 500 g at birth?

93.4.2 PERINATAL ASPHYXIA

Perinatal asphyxia provides equally challenging problems. Fullterm asphyxiated infants have a mortality of 10–20%. Those with mild encephalopathy are almost all normal at follow-up. Of those with moderate hypoxic ischaemic encephalopathy, 80% are normal on subsequent examinations. Almost all those with severe neonatal hypoxic ischaemic encephalopathy either die (50%) or have major neurological sequelae, including cerebral palsy, mental handicap, epilepsy or microcephaly [18]. It is exceedingly rare for even the most compromised neonates to fulfil criteria for determination of brain death as laid down by the American Academy of Pediatrics [19] (Chapter 92). Can these difficulties be resolved in the interests of infant and parents?

93.4.3 SEVERE CONGENITAL ABNORMALITY

The third category, severe congenital abnormality, may also be fraught with difficulties. Some are entirely incompatible with long-term survival, e.g. anencephaly. Others may have a prognosis of a few weeks or months of dependent life without apparent neurological or emotional development, e.g. trisomy 13 or 18. Some chromosomal disorders may have an uncertain prognosis, or may indeed show themselves uniquely in a particular patient or family [20]. Finally, children with Down's syndrome may live to adulthood but clinicians and ethicists still wrestle with the question of operative intervention for associated abnormalities such as atrioventricular canal defect or tracheo-oesophageal fistula. Each referral centre must now form its own care team which specializes in the care of the abnormal fetus. Regular meetings involving radiologist, obstetrician, neonatologist, geneticist, pathologist, paediatric surgeon and perinatal counsellor are of great benefit in pooling knowledge and in providing the nucleus of a perinatal care team (Chapter 90).

93.5 Formulation of a plan

All three of the above categories (extreme prematurity, perinatal asphyxia and congenital abnormality) present great difficulties to the neonatal unit staff, to the parents, and to their advisors and friends. However, guidelines can be offered and the following six steps may help to ensure that a mature plan emerges.

1. Document in the casenotes what is known, what can be discovered, and assess what is beyond current knowledge.
2. Document an assessment of probabilities including the likelihood and degree of anticipated brain damage or maldevelopment.
3. Ask: 'Is the child suffering?' How great is the price of continuing with invasive intensive care?
4. The members of staff most closely involved, once fully informed of the perceived problems, should meet to discuss all the details including the family situation. Particular attention is paid to the parents' current knowledge and their reactions to the severity of the child's illness.
5. If the staff unanimously believe, after prolonged consideration that it is in the child's interests to be managed with comfort measures only then a small number (preferably two) of the professional care team are chosen to present the facts and options to the parents. The responsible consultant paediatrician and an experienced nurse may be the best combination. The discussion *must* involve both parents if father and mother are still involved in the child's welfare. A sensitive balance must be struck such that discussions allow parents to participate actively in decision-making, yet they should be provided with recommendations which can help them.
6. Further discussions among staff members must follow to ensure that all interested parties are in accord with the emerging plan.

It is most frequently the experience of neonatal teams that the parents will accept the recommendation provided. Such acceptance may be immediate or delayed for some days. The parents' independent voice is essential, and the team must respect the possibility that the parents may disagree. If parents express the view that full intensive care should continue, this wish must be followed. An independent consultant opinion from a source not previously involved in the infant's

clinical care may be invaluable in providing further advice both to the neonatal unit staff and to the family.

93.5.1 GUIDED CONSENSUS

'Guided consensus' [21] does not mean that the consultant decides an infant's fate and the staff and family agree automatically. Nor should parents be provided with a summary of the facts and then allowed to decide on their infant's future without staff involvement. Guided consensus involves the appraisal of facts, the development of a plan considered by staff to be in the child's best interests, and the detailed discussion of both facts and plan with the parents. Provision of a careful recommendation by the staff puts the responsibility firmly with the neonatal unit, but allows the parents to feel deeply involved in their child's present and future care (Chapter 94).

93.6 Management of neonatal death

Neonatal death may ocasionally occur suddenly and unexpectedly: the term infant who is delivered apparently free of congenital abnormalities may collapse and die later in the first week of life due to hypoplasia of the left heart. More frequently neonatal death is predictable, involving an inexorable deterioration, and parents may even begin the grieving process before the death of their baby. In both situations the needs of the infant and parents are of paramount importance, not forgetting the real feelings of loss and sometimes guilt experienced by the staff. It is essential to recognize these normal feelings of family grief, and the sensitive nurturing of infant and family can evolve into dignity during the death of the infant, and gradual acceptance and adjustment to future life by the parents. Parents and influential groups such as the Stillbirth and Neonatal Death Society (SANDS) have taught professionals much of what is important in this field.

The needs of the dying infant are warmth, dignity and freedom from pain. Once the decision has been taken to reorient care to comfort measures only, the doctor and nurse discuss the following plans with the parents. An opiate infusion is commenced after a loading dose has ensured immediate relief from distress. All monitors are removed, and it is perfectly appropriate to do this in the presence of the parents who may wish to participate. It is common for them to wish to dress their infant even though assisted ventilation continues. The parents, sitting in a chair by the incubator side, may then cradle their infant while respiratory support is given to the child. Transfer to a private side room with sympathetic decor may be appropriate; oxygen cylinders are used as required. If the family wish, then a religious ceremony, including baptism if this has not happened previously, may be of great solace. Parents will later frequently say time was too short, and will seldom feel that they had too long with their dying infant. All relatives and supportive friends are encouraged to visit as the parents wish. Siblings of the dying infant may be most supportive, and contrary to many expectations are generally unafraid and are glad to handle and groom the infant, and may enjoy choosing last clothes and toys for the baby. Staff and family may take many photographs. Parents are warned that polaroid prints bleach over months and years and should therefore be copied on to more permanent film.

The timing of elective removal of the endotracheal tube will vary according to the needs of the family as perceived by the neonatal unit staff. It is the present author's view that the extubation should be carried out by the senior doctor present and only after ensuring that the infant's opiate infusion precludes any possible sensation of an asphyxiating death. Family intimacy is extremely important at this most sensitive stage, and the extubation may be carried out while the infant is in a parent's arms while the other parent lays a hand on the child's head. The moment of death may still be minutes or hours away, and the family continue to need emotional support throughout the remainder of the child's life, and during the hours thereafter.

Although other relatives and friends may occasionally have seen the infant in the neonatal unit, the parents will often wish to talk about the baby with the staff who were most involved in the child's care. The child's first name should invariably be used throughout this time. Both sad and happy times in the short course of the infant's life may be recalled. Parents often enjoy listening to their baby's heart beat through a stethoscope. Symbols of the child's life are important after death. A lock of hair, the identifying anklets and the named incubator card may be treasured memories. Hand and foot prints are appreciated, and become important mementos in future years [22]. After the infant's death is confirmed to the parents, they should be encouraged to stay with their child for as long as they wish – perhaps several hours on the day of death and a further visit on the following day, ideally in an area designed for this purpose. Parents should be encouraged to be responsible for funeral arrangements, with the guidance of staff. Each neonatal unit should have ready access to authorities who can advise about ceremonial rites and customs compatible with the law of the land of any religious persuasion.

93.7   Autopsy

At first thought the idea of asking the bereaved parents for permission to arrange an autopsy examination may seem like the final insult after the infant's death.

However if a senior doctor who is committed to inviting the family back for a detailed follow-up interview requests the post mortem for the purpose of discovering the fullest information for the family, it is likely that they will acquiesce, especially if the genetic implications are important, and especially if the parents themselves will receive a copy of the report. At follow-up, discussion of the report may even help the parents' grieving process. The results of such an independent examination may also be critical in providing the clinician with information that will allow a prediction of the likelihood of recurrence in a subsequent pregnancy (Chapters 26, 27 and 44).

93.8   Postbereavement care

About one month after the infant's death, an invitation is sent to the parents to return to the hospital to discuss their child's life and death. During this interview and perhaps at other meetings, some of which may be with an obstetrician or geneticist, there must be extended opportunities for the parents to discuss the neonatal course, the postmortem examination, any questions which arise, their feelings, their past and current state of grief, their support from family and community, and the implications for future pregnancies. 'How are you?' addressed to the parents is the question most needed and most frequently forgotten. The parents can be put in touch with other sources of help as they are judged to be necessary, including the general practitioner, health visitor, social worker, chaplain, SANDS, Compassionate Friends, or any other community facility known to the neonatal unit team. It may help to talk of their fears for the future – Christmas or other religious feast-days, anniversary of the child's birth and death, and the contemplation of a future pregnancy. How soon will appetites, including sexual, return?

There is no doubt that neonatal intensive care is stressful for the infant, the parents, the relatives, the visitors and of course the members of the neonatal unit. The staff and parents must be circumspect about how much intensive care an infant should endure. Relatives and friends will need help in their role of providing strength for the immediate family. Parents must be encouraged to talk, and to build confident relationships with the neonatal unit staff. Their needs at home, during travelling, and in their unsought-for life in the neonatal unit should be addressed whenever possible.

If the caring team are to survive the psychological pressures, adequate safety valves are necessary. Work rotas which allow them time for family, for relaxation, for study and for development are essential. A climate in the neonatal unit which allows trust to thrive is also necessary. This includes fresh cool water against the heat, a comfortable sitting area for moments of calm, and colleagues who can exchange advice and understanding. The perspectives may now be seen more clearly, but the challenges remain (Chapters 59 and 60).

93.9 Summary

Technological advances continue to expand the possibilities for care of the sick newborn infant. Replacement surfactants have undoubtedly improved dramatically the prognosis of the preterm infant with respiratory distress syndrome. Many other aspects of neonatal care have also seen recent advances. These advances may bring new challenges. Adequate skilled staffing is needed to fulfil the greater potential of the neonatal unit. Technological advances may bring about new problems in making the best clinical judgments on the patient's behalf. Ethical decisions which could not have been made immediately in the labour ward must be resolved over hours, days or weeks in the neonatal unit. Therapeutic advances might outstrip the unit's ability to look after the infant as a whole being, and only recently has there been full appreciation that the newborn infant feels pain and therefore needs analgesia in the operating room and in the newborn intensive care unit. In the event of a baby dying, members of the neonatal unit staff require to care for the entire family throughout the period of bereavement.

References

1. *Report of Working Group of the British Association of Perinatal Medicine on Categories of Babies Requiring Neonatal Care* (1992) British Paediatric Association, London.
2. Royal College of Physicians (1988) *Medical Care of the Newborn in England and Wales*, Royal College of Physicians, London.
3. Speidel, B. (1987) Paediatric facilities, in *Birth Place: Report of Confidential Enquiry into Facilities Available at the Place of Birth* (eds G. Chamberlain and P. Gunn), Wiley, Chichester, pp. 203–49.
4. Fujiwara, T., Chida, S., Watabo, Y. *et al.* (1980) Artificial surfactant therapy in hyaline membrane disease. *Lancet*, i, 55–59.
5. Soll, R.F. and McQueen, M.C. (1992) Respiratory distress syndrome, in *Effective Care of the Newborn Infant* (eds J.C. Sinclair and M.B. Bracken), Oxford University Press, Oxford, pp. 325–58.
6. Halliday, H.L. (1992) Other acute lung disorders, in *Effective Care of the Newborn Infant* (eds J.C. Sinclair and M.B. Bracken), Oxford University Press, Oxford, pp. 359–84.
7. OSIRIS Collaborative Group (1992) Early versus delayed neonatal administration of a synthetic surfactant – the judgment of OSIRIS. *Lancet*, ii, 1363–69.
8. Halliday, H.L., Tarnow-Mordi, W.O., Corcoran, J.D. *et al.* (1993) A multicentre randomised trial comparing high and low dose surfactant regimens for the treatment of respiratory distress syndrome (the Curosurf 4 trial). *Arch. Dis. Child.*, 69, 276–80.
9. Cilley, R.E., Zwischenberger, J.B., Andrews, A.F. *et al.* (1986) Intracranial haemorrhage during extracorporeal membrane oxygenation. *Pediatrics*, 78, 699–704.
10. Zayek, M., Cleveland, D. and Morin, F.C. (1992) *Treatment of Persistent Pulmonary Hypertension of the Newborn Lamb by Inhaled Nitric Oxide.* Proceedings of Hot Topics 92 in Neonatology. Washington, DC. Ross Laboratories, Columbus, OH, p. 96.
11. Anand, K.J.S. and Hickey, P.R. (1992) Halothane–morphine compared with high-dose sufentanil for anesthesia and postoperative analgesia in neonatal cardiac surgery. *N. Engl. J. Med.*, 326, 1–9.
12. Anand, K.J.S. and Hickey, P.R. (1987) Pain and its effects in the human neonate and fetus. *N. Engl. J. Med.*, 317, 1321–29.
13. Yu, V.Y.H., Loke, H.L., Bajuk, B. *et al.* (1986) Prognosis for infants born at 23 to 28 weeks' gestation. *BMJ*, 293, 1200–203.
14. Corbet, A.J., Bucciarelli, R., Goldman, S.A. *et al.* (1991) Decreased mortality in small premature infants treated at birth with a single dose of synthetic surfactant: a multicenter trial. *J. Pediatr.*, 118, 277–84.
15. Collaborative European Multicenter Study Group (1988) Surfactant replacement therapy for severe neonatal respiratory distress syndrome: an international randomized clinical trial. *Pediatrics*, 82, 683–91.
16. McCormick, M.C. (1991) Follow-up, in *Manual of Neonatal Care* (eds J. Cloherty and A.R. Stark), Little, Brown, Boston, pp. 588–94.
17. Campbell, A.G.M. (1982) Which infants should not receive intensive care? *Arch. Dis. Child.*, 57, 569–71.
18. Robertson, C. and Finer, N. (1985) Term infants with hypoxic ischaemic encephalopathy: outcome at 3–5 years. *Dev. Med. Child Neurol.*, 4, 473–84.
19. American Academy of Pediatrics (1987) Criteria for determination of brain death in the newborn. *Pediatrics*, 80, 298–300.
20. Laing, I.A., Lyall, E.G.H., Hendry, L.M. *et al.* (1991) Typus Edinburgensis explained. *Pediatrics*, 88, 151–54.
21. Laing, I.A. (1989) Withdrawing from invasive neonatal intensive care, in *Paediatric Forensic Medicine and Pathology* (ed. K. Mason), Chapman & Hall, London, pp. 131–40.
22. Stillbirth and Neonatal Death Society (1991) *Miscarriage, Stillbirth and Neonatal Death, Guidelines for Professionals*, SANDS, London.

94 ETHICS OF DELIVERY ROOM PRACTICE

A.G.M. Campbell

94.1 Introduction

The hospital delivery room is fertile ground for conflicts of opinion and misunderstandings that may adversely affect the standard of care. It is also the setting for a number of moral issues that can be complex and troubling for parents and staff. The birth of an eagerly awaited infant, usually an event to be celebrated, will be an occasion for shock, grief and frequently anger if the infant is seriously abnormal or damaged. As the parents begin to understand the full implications of this tragedy for infant and family, recriminations and a lasting sense of bitterness may follow. While most realize that 'these things happen' or that the outcome was inevitable, some may blame the doctors and nurses involved or question their clinical judgement, particularly if their attitude or conduct has been insensitive or unhelpful at a time when parents require particular understanding and support. The conduct of doctors and nurses in the often tense and anxious atmosphere that surrounds a complicated birth will do much to mitigate the distress of families bereaved in this way.

94.2 Communication

94.2.1 COMMUNICATION WITH COLLEAGUES

Perinatal care should imply good communication and teamwork among obstetricians, paediatricians and midwives in particular but other specialists like the obstetric anaesthetist may also be involved in difficult cases. The paediatrician (usually a neonatologist) has no direct responsibility for clinical management before birth, but it may be important for him or her to be aware of the progress of 'high-risk' pregnancies well in advance of delivery. Early discussions with the paediatrician should help the obstetrician to assess the potential risks and benefits of early delivery in situations where the fetus is thought to be in jeopardy. Early warning will also facilitate adequate preparations for immediate attention to the infant at birth and for any further care that may be necessary in the neonatal unit.

94.2.2 COMMUNICATION WITH PARENTS

There are circumstances when it will be important for the paediatrician to meet with the parents during a pregnancy to answer their questions about the baby and provide some reassurance about the problems that may be encountered after birth. A preliminary visit to the neonatal unit, if sensitively conducted, can help to reduce much of the apprehension and fear felt by parents when they first come face to face with the realities of neonatal intensive care and its bewildering technology. This is particularly important if serious fetal anomaly is diagnosed antenatally. In these circumstances it may be prudent to make advance arrangements for the infant to receive specialized surgical treatment, or it may be appropriate to seek the parents' views on withholding intensive care from birth.

94.3 The place of care

In deciding the most appropriate setting for birth, the obstetrician has to be concerned about the safety of the mother and infant. In discussing this with mothers, especially those whose pregnancies are thought to be at higher risk, it will be prudent to seek the advice of the neonatologist, so that the mother can be given all the information likely to be relevant to her baby before coming to an informed choice. With the heightened expectations of medical miracles in contemporary society, and the increasing complexities and demands of modern care, members of the perinatal team must base their advice firmly on what is best for mother and baby, not what is most convenient for them or the extended family, or what is most advantageous to their hospital or practices. For example, when a congenital abnormality best corrected by immediate skilled neo-

Diseases of the Fetus and Newborn, 2nd edn, Edited by G.B. Reed, A.E. Claireaux and F. Cockburn. Published in 1995 by Chapman & Hall, London. ISBN 0 412 39160 0

natal surgery is suspected it may be appropriate to arrange for the mother's confinement to take place at another hospital, a decision that is clearly in the infant's best interests but one that may require considerable professional honesty and humility.

94.4 The paediatrician in the delivery room

94.4.1 RESPONSIBILITY

A paediatrician should be available at the birth of any infant where abnormality or difficulties with resuscitation are anticipated. Obstetricians and paediatricians usually agree a list of conditions for which a member of the paediatric staff is expected to be present. The paediatrician will assume responsibility for the infant's care from birth and deal with any special problems that may arise. These might include attending to congenital abnormalities that have been identified by antenatal screening, deciding on the most appropriate type of resuscitation for an infant with asphyxia, or helping to establish effective breathing for the very tiny premature infant. While the presence of a paediatrician will usually be helpful, it is essential that he or she is adequately trained and experienced to perform the necessary tasks competently or is willing to seek immediate help. Otherwise the mutual respect and confidence that are essential for good working relationships may be lost. For example, if there is a problem with resuscitation, assistance should be obtained or accepted immediately from the obstetric anaesthetist who is often present for complicated deliveries, rather than persist with futile attempts at intubation in order not to 'lose face'. Conflicts of opinion and demarcation disputes about who is responsible for what must be settled elsewhere.

94.4.2 SHARED CARE

If an infant is stillborn, is abnormal, or is potentially damaged from a complication of the pregnancy, the family will seek an explanation of what went wrong and why. In these circumstances it is particularly important for the primarily responsible doctors, preferably the obstetrician and paediatrician in charge, to agree their respective responsibilities for seeing the parents and keeping them informed of the progress of events. Such discussions should not be delegated to junior staff, although their presence can be a valuable part of their training. It is always very difficult to convey bad news well but doing it sensitively and showing that you care deeply about what happened is an important part of being a good doctor. Opportunities must be provided for the parents, or sometimes other family members, to ask questions about the pregnancy, labour and delivery, and to keep them up to date with the neonatal care and the baby's progress. Just as it is important for the paediatrician to show interest and concern about the progress of the fetus before birth, it can be helpful and much appreciated if the obstetrician shows similar interest in the progress of the infant after birth.

94.5 Dilemmas of resuscitation and treatment

Silverman [1] has pointed out that it is only in relatively recent history that the salvage of all infants born alive has been seen by some as a desirable social goal. Modern perinatal care (and other factors such as improved maternal health and social circumstances) has led to greatly improved infant mortality and morbidity, and has brought great benefits to many families. At the same time there has been a growing realization that some infants who would have died several decades ago can now be helped to survive, but at a price. They may be left with grievous handicaps which result in incalculable human costs to themselves and their families, and cause a severe strain on the resources of the community health and social services.

When so much **can** now be done to save and prolong life for these infants, it is not surprising that some of the most controversial questions in perinatal medicine today relate to how much **should** be done and who should bear the ultimate responsibility for deciding when to stop? Should all infants be resuscitated and given life-sustaining treatment, or should such treatment be used selectively with some infants being 'allowed to die'? In other words, where should we 'draw the line' at resuscitation and the use of aggressive life-sustaining treatments? Are there any circumstances in which it is morally (or legally) right to withhold or withdraw treatment [2,3]?

94.5.1 'VIABILITY' AND EXTREME PREMATURITY

Neonatologists are optimistic about the prospects for most infants born between 25 and 28 weeks' gestational age or with corresponding birth weights between 700 and 1000 g. For this group there is also some evidence to justify the routine use of life-sustaining intensive care [4]. However, survival under 25 weeks' gestation is increasingly possible, a fact reflected in efforts to have 500 g (with the corresponding gestational age of 22 weeks) recognized as the lower limit for the collection of perinatal statistics, a change that should also result in achieving improved consistency in data collection from neonatal centres [5]. This changing perception of viability is also recognized in the recent amendments to the 1967 Abortion Act which now specifies 24 weeks as the upper limit for abortion but sensibly removes any upper limit for cases where severe fetal anomaly is detected or where there is substantial threat to the health of the mother.

Unfortunately, current data on survival following birth under 26 weeks indicate that the incidence of severe disability increases alarmingly with decreasing gestational age. Elsewhere the author has argued that intensive life-sustaining treatments such as mechanically assisted ventilation should not be continued routinely for infants weighing under 750 g until there has at least been an opportunity to discuss the various options for care and their implications for the baby with the parents [6]. It must be emphasized that such a weight criterion cannot be rigidly applied and that other factors, like gestational age, associated problems and even family circumstances will also need to be considered. With continuing improvements in the skills and technology of neonatal intensive care and the changing prognosis for premature infants that become apparent through ongoing data analysis, it is inevitable that criteria will change. Nevertheless, the principle of drawing a line at some point will remain valid, whatever the criteria.

94.5.2   THE PROCESS OF DECISION-MAKING

For the resuscitation and treatment dilemmas that arise in the newborn unit, it has been argued that decisions to withhold or withdraw life-sustaining treatment should be made by the responsible doctor(s) and the parents and that such fundamental decisions should only be reached by following a careful process of decision-making by which the infant's interests are seen to be protected [7]. It is well known that some parents abuse and exploit their children, but fortunately the vast majority can still be trusted to have the interests of their children at heart and are likely to be an infant's best advocates in any decision that affects his or her future. Abuses of this trust are most unlikely in the 'public' setting of a neonatal intensive care unit. But whatever the views of the parents, these must continue to be primarily 'medical decisions', and therefore the responsibility of the doctor in clinical charge. They will be shared and debated with medical and nursing colleagues, including those who will hold varying views on the 'rightness' and 'wrongness' of such decisions. It is also likely that both doctors and parents will seek further advice outside the neonatal unit. The doctor will consult with specialist colleagues and seek confirmation of the diagnosis and prognosis. The parents may seek the views of grandparents, and perhaps their family doctor or clergyman, before any final decision is made. Such an informal 'moral community' can ensure that such a poignant and tragic decision to allow an infant to die is not made arbitrarily or capriciously, but is truly family centred and likely to be the least detrimental of several unsatisfactory options for the individual infant and family [8]. In a modern pluralistic society it has to be recognized that there will be considerable national and cultural variations in these decisions and how they are reached. In some societies parents, while welcoming the sharing of information and the opportunity to express their views, still seem to prefer to leave much or even all of these decisions to doctors, trusting them to act in whatever way seems best for their baby.

94.5.3   DECISION-MAKING IN THE DELIVERY ROOM

This carefully considered process of decision-making requires time for establishing the diagnosis and prognosis, and for the staff and parents to reflect on the various treatment options available and their implications for the baby. It also implies that such considered judgements about the withholding or withdrawal of life-sustaining treatments should be made by senior members of staff. Thus, for several reasons, the delivery room is not an appropriate setting for such fundamental decisions which cannot be made in haste. First, it is often junior doctors who, for practical reasons, are given the responsibility of attending difficult births; second, the information on which to base a properly considered decision is not usually complete; and third, there usually is insufficient time or opportunity to discuss the issues fully with the parents. Moreover, they will still be shocked and in a highly emotional state which may affect their ability to think clearly and rationally about what is best for their baby.

In constructing delivery room protocols, it should be made clear that any liveborn infant of whatever gestational age or condition should be resuscitated, and this should include the use of intubation and assisted ventilation as necessary to establish and maintain effective breathing. In other words, at this time all the available resuscitative measures should not be denied to marginally viable infants or to abnormal infants. Subsequently, decisions to continue, withhold or withdraw certain treatments, **but not care**, may be appropriate but these should be reached in the neonatal unit in the carefully considered manner just described. This approach has been described as the 'individualized prognostic strategy' whereby maximum treatment is initiated for all infants to give them a 'trial of life', followed by the withholding or withdrawal of intensive treatment if further information and subsequent developments indicate that death or severe brain damage is the probable outcome [9].

An exception to the above general 'rule' may be

made with the antenatal diagnosis of a severely abnormal infant for whom abortion is not an option and postnatal intensive treatment is likely to be futile or particularly burdensome in terms of survival or in ensuring an acceptable or 'tolerable' quality of life. In such circumstances, any system of high quality perinatal care should require the involvement of a paediatrician in antenatal discussions with the parents about the appropriate care to be given to the infant after birth. For example, for a condition like anencephaly or other gross neurological anomalies, it might be agreed that vigorous resuscitation and other forms of life support will be withheld (unless it had been decided that temporary support would be provided pending use of the infant's organs for transplantation). It should not need emphasizing that such infants must not be abandoned to a corner of the labour ward but should be admitted to the neonatal unit and provided with the basic nursing care due to any infant, with treatment limited to that required to relieve distress or discomfort until death. The parents must be afforded privacy and support in helping to care for their dying infant during this sad period [10].

94.5.4   LEGAL IMPLICATIONS

I believe that the approach just described is not only consistent with good ethical practice but it may also protect doctors from accusations of acting illegally in allowing an infant to die. No matter how immature or how badly malformed, an infant who is alive at birth is due the full protection of the law. This protection also extends to deliberately aborted fetuses who show signs of life at birth, a problem described as 'the new neonatal dilemma [11]. Strict interpretation of the law means that the attending doctor has a duty of care to liveborn infants whatever the potential for severe handicap and whatever the wishes of the parents. Paediatricians acknowledge this but most believe that there are some circumstances in which it is morally correct to be selective in the use of life-saving or life-sustaining treatment. In other words they may draw the line at vigorously resuscitating or treating a gasping, hypoxic and acidotic infant of 550 g or an infant with a gross abnormality. 'The law', as reflected in some recent court decisions, also seems to take a sensitive and pragmatic view of these difficult cases and accepts that it may be prudent to be selective in certain circumstances, provided that there is supportive evidence that the doctor's action was within the boundaries of accepted medical practice. For example, in a recent Scottish case, the Sheriff took the view that a premature infant of just under 700 g, although alive at birth, was 'non-viable' [12]; and in a recent English case, the judge decided that the quality of life for a child with severe abnormalities and brain damage

would be so intolerable that 'treatment without which death would ensue, could be withheld even though the child was not dying' [13]. In the USA too, the courts have consistently supported families (or 'moral communities') in such ambiguous situations when treatment has been refused [14].

Although these cases provide some indication of how a court might react to the facts of an individual case brought to its attention, a neonatologist is still left in a position of some uncertainty about where the line of 'viability' or 'intolerable life' might be drawn in other circumstances. It is important, therefore, for junior staff to be made aware of the process of decision-making that they should follow. The facts must be carefully documented by the doctors involved so that their conduct will withstand medical, ethical and legal scrutiny.

No matter how carefully considered, there is always some uncertainty about these difficult decisions, but it is through such a process that uncertainty can be reduced to a minimum. If doctors or parents still feel ambivalent or unsure about the best course of action for the infant, or if there are any remaining doubts about the accuracy of the diagnosis or prognosis, they should err on the side of life. This means that doctors should continue or initiate all the treatments that would be appropriate for otherwise normal infants until the infant's condition or new information dictates a change of policy.

94.5.5   STATE INTERVENTION

In the USA, decision-making for severely handicapped infants has been complicated by Federal intervention [15]. A sequence of events beginning in the 1970s with open debate about these dilemmas in the medical and lay press led to heightened public concern about the plight of these babies. In early 1982, the publicity generated by media reaction to an apparent abuse of a handicapped infant's right to treatment was sufficient to stimulate the Federal authorities, already sympathetic to the 'pro-life' lobby, to introduce 'rules' specifically aimed at curbing the discretion traditionally afforded doctors and parents in deciding to withhold or withdraw treatment. In 1984 these controversial 'Baby Doe rules' were eventually incorporated as amendments to the Child Abuse Prevention and Treatment Act which brought failure to treat a handicapped infant within the meaning of child abuse and neglect, and required that any State receiving Federal funds for child protection must include the category of 'medical neglect'. No evidence was ever produced that there was widespread abuse of infants' rights by undertreatment before Baby Doe, but this example of Governmental intervention into medical decision-making has created a climate of considerable legal uncertainty in American neonatal units, to the extent that abuse by overtreatment is now a significant problem [16].

It is important to emphasize that Baby Doe did not alter the law relating to infants. Furthermore, the amendments note a number of exceptions to the requirement of providing 'medically indicated treatment' that are open to considerable variation in interpretation, thus still allowing considerable medical discretion. It is also important to emphasize that a doctor's conscientious decision to forgo treatment if he or she believes it is futile, harmful or disproportionately burdensome is legally defensible even in the face of parental objections [17].

One potentially useful outcome of the Baby Doe controversy was the establishment of infant care review committees in the major American hospitals to provide a broader forum for debate about neonatal policies and practices. If appropriately constituted and prepared to become familiar at first hand with individual families and the complex issues involved, they (or individual members) can be very helpful to the doctors, nurses and parents as they wrestle with these dilemmas. Unfortunately some committees have taken on (or have been delegated) the responsibility for making some difficult clinical decisions. This can have disastrous consequences if the interests of the infant become secondary, for example, to those of the hospital. The author believes that the patient's doctor should remain as the primary decision-maker and the leader of the 'moral community' embracing the infant and family. No matter how tempting it is for doctors to avoid the emotional hassle and potential legal vulnerability that may follow such decisions, abrogating responsibility to a committee devalues the role of the doctor in providing leadership in clinical care. This trend, if it continues, must eventually diminish respect for the physician as a responsible and capable moral agent who is expected and trusted to act in the best interests of the patient.

References

1. Silverman, W.A. (1981) Mismatched attitudes about neonatal death. *Hastings Center Report*, **11**, 12–16.
2. Whitelaw, A. (1986) Death as an option in neonatal intensive care. *Lancet*, ii, 328–31.
3. Campell, A.G.M. (1990) Withholding neonatal care: 1. A paediatrician's view, in *Philosophical Ethics in Reproductive Medicine* (eds D.R. Bromham, M.E. Dalton and J.C. Jackson), Manchester, Manchester University Press, Manchester, pp. 107–23.
4. Britton, S.B., Fitzhardinge, P.M. and Ashby, S. (1981) Is intensive care justified for infants weighing less than 801 gm at birth? *Journal of Pediatrics*, **99**, 937–43.
5. Chiswick, M.L. (1986) Commentary on current World Health Organisation definitions used in perinatal statistics. *Archives of Disease in Childhood*, **61**, 708–10.
6. Campbell, A.G.M. (1982) Which infants should not receive intensive care? *Archives of Disease in Childhood*, **57**, 569–71.
7. Campbell, A.G.M. (1989) Some ethical issues in neonatal care, in *Doctors' Decisions: Ethical Conflicts in Medical Practice* (eds G.R. Dunstan, and E.A. Shinebourne), Oxford University Press, Oxford, pp. 51–56.
8. Duff, R.S. and Campbell, A.G.M. (1987) Moral communities and tragic choices, in *Euthanasia and the Newborn: Conflicts Regarding Saving Lives* (eds R.C. McMillan, H.T. Engelhardt Jr, and S.F. Spicker), Reidel, Dordrecht, pp. 273–89.
9. Rhoden, N.K. (1986) Treating Baby Doe: the ethics of uncertainty. *Hastings Center Report*, **16**(4), 34–42.
10. Duff, R.S. and Campbell, A.G.M. (1976) On deciding the care of severely handicapped or dying persons: with particular reference to infants. *Pediatrics* **57**, 487–93.
11. Rhoden, N.K. (1984) The new neonatal dilemma: live births from late abortions. *Georgetown Law Journal*, **72**, 1451–509.
12. Brahams, D. (1988) No obligation to resuscitate a non-viable infant. *Lancet* i, 1176.
13. Anonymous (1992) News: Appeal Court supports doctors' decision not to treat. *BMJ*, **304**, 1527–28.
14. Holder, A. (1983) Parents, courts, and refusal of treatment. *Journal of Pediatrics*, **103**, 515–21.
15. Caplan, A.L., Blank, R.H. and Merrick, J.C. (1992) *Compelled Compassion: Government Intervention in the Treatment of Critically Ill Newborns*, Humana Press, Totowa, NJ.
16. Engelhardt Jr, H.T. (1989) Comments on the recommendations regarding Section 504 of the Rehabilitation Act of 1973 and the Child Abuse Amendments of 1984. *US Commission on Civil Rights: Medical Discrimination Against Children with Disabilities*, **447**, 158–65.
17. Paris, J.J., Crone, R.K. and Reardon, F. (1990) Physicians' refusal of requested treatment. The case of Baby LN. *New England Journal of Medicine*, **322**, 1012–14.

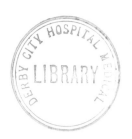

95 RESPIRATORY PROBLEMS IN THE PRETERM INFANT

R.L. Ariagno

95.1 Introduction

Since the recent clinical introduction of surfactant replacement therapy, the severity of respiratory distress syndrome (RDS) has decreased and the mortality due to RDS has dramatically fallen [1–14]. At first glance, apnea and RDS appear to be disparate topics. The causes of respiratory pattern abnormalities and respiratory insufficiency in the preterm infant are, however, usually multifactorial and often associated with respiratory and central nervous system immaturity. Surfactant deficiency associated with lung immaturity is clearly an important factor in respiratory insufficiency, but there are also many **non-surfactant** aspects which include lung structure and development, chest wall and diaphragm, upper airway function/patency, respiratory drive, temperature, cardiovascular immaturity, patent ductus arteriosus and transitional circulation, renal immaturity and the effect on fluid balance and lung water clearance. In this chapter the incidence, causes and measurement of apnea, a common clinical problem in the preterm infant, will be discussed and related to pulmonary insufficiency. The indications for and the clinical effects of endotracheal surfactant treatment will be discussed. Bronchopulmonary dysplasia, a complication seen in preterm infants with RDS who require oxygen and mechanical ventilation therapy, and the trend for decreased incidence and/or severity with surfactant therapy replacement will be briefly discussed. Although surfactant replacement therapy has had a dramatic affect on the severity of RDS, and mortality due to RDS, a reduction in the incidence of prematurity would have the greatest impact on complications associated with adaptation of the premature infant to extrauterine life.

95.2 Apnea

95.2.1 A BRIEF CLINICAL DESCRIPTION

Clinically significant apnea may be defined as respiratory pauses (central, obstructive or mixed) with durations of 20 seconds or longer, accompanied by bradycardia (i.e. heart rate less than 100 beats/min) and/or oxygen desaturation ($Sao2 < 95\%$) for ≥ 5 seconds. Short respiratory pauses (≤ 10 seconds) are commonly observed in preterm infants, coincident with a startle, movement, defecation or swallow. These short respiratory pauses are usually not associated with clinically significant oxygen desaturation or bradycardia. The most common form of apnea seen in the preterm infant is **central apnea** in which there is a failure of both respiratory effort and air movement. **Obstructive apnea** is defined by active respiratory effort with partial or complete blockage of air movement, and **mixed apnea** refers to that apnea in which, initially, there is a central event followed by an obstructive component.

Historically, a wide range of durations for abnormal or clinically significant apnea for the preterm infant have been proposed. These have ranged from ≥ 30 seconds in 1970 to the currently accepted ≥ 20 seconds or shorter durations if the apneic events are associated with bradycardia or cyanosis. The incidence of apnea increases with lower birth weight and lower gestational age and has been reported to occur in over 80% of infants born at less than 30 weeks' gestation, 50% of infants at 30–31 weeks, 14% at 32–33 weeks and 7% at 34–35 weeks' gestation [15,16]. In a study of 249 infants with clinical apnea, the onset was within 48 hours of birth in 77% of cases. Apneic events usually occur in the first week of life unless the infant has RDS and requires oxygen supplementation and mechanical ventilation support. When the total duration of respiratory pauses in two comparable groups of preterm infants with or without RDS over the first week of life were examined, a greater mean duration of pause was found in the non-RDS infant group [17] (Figure 95.1). Often, apnea in the preterm infant is 'idiopathic' and related primarily to factors associated with prematurity at birth and failure of extrauterine adaptation. Although there is a close relationship between gestational age, postnatal maturation and the resolution of

Diseases of the Fetus and Newborn, 2nd edn, Edited by G.B. Reed, A.E. Claireaux and F. Cockburn. Published in 1995 by Chapman & Hall, London. ISBN 0 412 39160 0

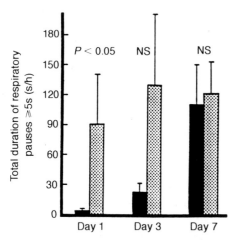

Figure 95.1 A comparison of the total duration of respiratory pauses ≥5 seconds between infants with (black bars) and without (shaded bars) respiratory distress syndrome (RDS). Note the earlier incidence of apnea in the first day of life in the non-RDS infant. (Reproduced with permission from Carlo *et al.* [17].)

disease, spongiform degeneration is seen in brain-stem areas associated with regulation of ventilation, including the nucleus reticularis and nucleus gigantocellularis. These pathologic lesions may affect central respiratory drive and respiratory pattern and increase the occurrence of apnea.

95.2.2 CHEMORECEPTOR RESPONSES

Henderson-Smart, Pettigrew and Campbell [21] assessed brain-stem conduction times with auditory evoked responses and determined that infants who had a history of apnea had longer conduction times compared with matched premature infants without apnea. This is indirect evidence that infants with apnea have brain-stem immaturity and suggests that stability of central respiratory drive may improve as dendritic and other synaptic interconnections multiply in the maturing brain. Ventilatory responses to increased inspired carbon dioxide, which predominantly reflect central respiratory chemoreceptor activity, are less well developed in infants ≤ 33 weeks' gestation and in infants

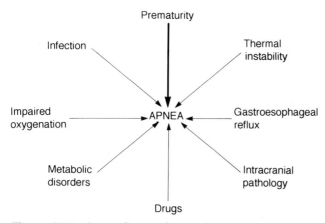

Figure 95.2 Some diverse factors known to precipitate development of apneic episodes in preterm infants. (Reproduced with permission from Martin, Miller and Carlo [18].)

apnea, other major factors influencing apnea include perinatal asphyxia, infection, temperature, hypoglycemia, seizures and intracranial hemorrhage, all of which are more common in the most immature infants [18] (Figure 95.2). In some cases an underlying specific neuropathology can be identified [19]. Infants who have disorders which affect the brain stem may present with apnea and have neuropathologic lesions which include olivopontocerebellar atrophy, myotonic dystrophy and syringobulbia, as well as brain-stem infarction due to asphyxia. Adickes, Buehler and Sange [20] described a family in which three of six siblings (between 18 and 26 months of age) presented with sleep apnea and subsequently died of Leigh's disease (subacute necrotizing encephalomyelopathy). In this

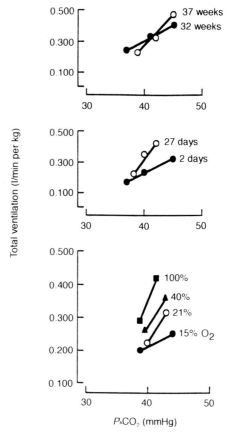

Figure 95.3 The relationship between ventilatory sensitivity to carbon dioxide and gestational age (top), postnatal age (middle) and the concentration of inspired oxygen (bottom) (see text for discussion). (Reproduced with permission from Rigatto, Brady and Verduzco [23] and Rigatto, Verduzco and Cates [24].)

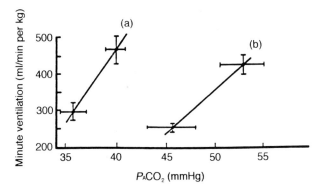

Figure 95.4 Comparison of CO_2 sensitivity (obtained from ventilatory responses to changing alveolar P_{CO_2} (P_{ACO_2})) in preterm infants (b) with and (a) without apnea. Note a decreased ventilatory response and higher P_{ACO_2} threshold (47 versus 36 at 300 ml/min per kg) in the apneic group. Difference in slope, $P < 0.001$. (Reproduced with permission from Gerhardt and Bancalari [27].)

who are less than 3 weeks' postnatal age. The ventilatory response [22–26], using a steady-state normoxic carbon dioxide (CO_2) challenge, was decreased in the 32-week gestation infant compared with a 37-week infant (Figure 95.3 upper panel). Furthermore, the response at 27 versus 2 days postnatal age shows an increase in the slope (sensitivity) (Figure 95.3 middle panel); the lower panel (Figure 95.3) shows the effects of inspired oxygen on the ventilatory responses to CO_2. There was no augmentation in the ventilation response when hypoxia (15% O_2) and hypercapnia were combined. The greatest increase in ventilation occurred when the CO_2 challenge was presented in a 100% O_2 ambient environment. A significantly lower slope was observed in the apneic group (Figure 95.4) [27,28]. In the preterm infant the inhalation of low oxygen (15%) produces an immediate increase in ventilation at 1 minute after exposure, followed by a decrease later at 5 minutes. This response is in contrast to the adult subject who has a sustained increase in ventilation. This late decrease in ventilation may be due to depression of central respiratory neurons. Infants with borderline oxygenation at baseline, therefore, are more prone to develop apnea [22–26].

95.2.3 UPPER AIRWAY

A simple congenital problem such as choanal stenosis or atresia can cause apnea even in the fullterm neonate. Patency of the extrathoracic airway is actively modulated by the upper airway muscles, which have increased tone during inspiration, in synchrony with contraction of diaphragm and chest wall muscles. When these events are not in synchrony, the negative intraluminal pressure generated during inspiration can cause collapse of the compliant pharynx [29]. Many

upper airway muscles, including the ala nasi, laryngeal abductor and the pharyngeal abductor muscles, affect the patency of the extrathoracic airway. Failure of the genioglossus activation has most often been implicated in obstructive apnea in both adults and infants. Genioglossus activation which opens the airway has been shown to be curtailed for about 1 minute following hypercapnia, with reinstitution occurring only after a CO_2 threshold of 45 mmHg was achieved [30]. This restriction of an upper airway muscle's tonic response demonstrates how airway patency in the preterm infant can be unstable.

Reflexes originating from the upper airway can affect the pattern of respiration in infants and play a crucial role in both causing as well as leading to the termination of the apnea. The walls of the nasal cavity, nasopharynx, oropharynx and larynx contain sensory inputs which can respond to both mechanical [31] and chemical stimuli [32]. These afferent stimuli travel through cranial nerves, V, VI, IX, X, and XII and can have a powerful effect on respiratory rate and rhythm, heart rate and vascular resistance. Responses of the upper airway to sensory input change significantly with postnatal maturation. In newborn rabbits, mechanical stimulation to the external nares can cause fatal apnea [33]. In human infants, apneic responses have been elicited by changes in the luminal pressure within the nasopharynx, or by stimulation of chemoreceptors near the larynx and hypopharynx. It is well known that topical anesthesia of the mucous membranes within the upper airway inhibits normal airway reflex responses to pressure and can lead to pharyngeal obstruction.

Mennon, Shefft and Thach [34] have described apnea associated with regurgitation of gastric contents into the upper airway of human infants. This acidic stimulus caused both apnea and swallowing through excitation of chemoreceptors in the laryngeal area. Thach [35] found that swallows were much more common during apnea than in comparable periods of uninterrupted sleep, suggesting that there is an association between idiopathic apnea of prematurity and inhibitory reflexes arising within the upper airway. The introduction of saline boluses into the oropharynx during sleep resulted in both central and obstructive apneic episodes. This work suggests that an accumulation of saliva in the pharynx may lead to an adaptive apneic response and swallowing responses mediated through a chemoreceptor reflex.

95.2.4 PERIODIC BREATHING

Periodic breathing is a common breathing pattern in preterm infants which should be differentiated from apnea. It is well known that hypoxia can often stimulate periodic breathing, and methylxanthine treatment (caffeine and theophylline) or 1% CO_2 can

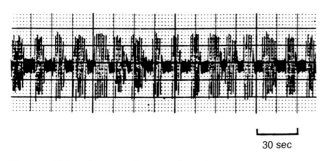

Figure 95.5 A typical example of periodic breathing. (Reproduced with permission from Glotzbach and Ariagno [36].)

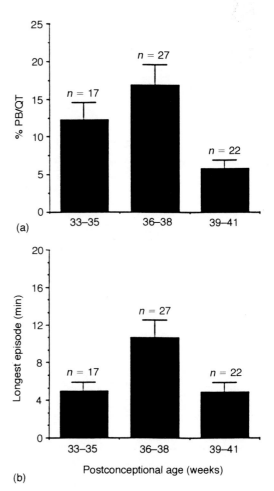

Figure 95.6 Changes in two measures of periodic breathing (PB) obtained from 24-hour pneumograms at three different postconceptional age groups in preterm infants. Values are mean ± SEM. (a) There is a significant reduction in the percentage PB during quiet time (QT) at 39–41 weeks compared with both 33–35 ($P = 0.024$) and 36–38 ($P = 0.004$) weeks. (b) The longest episode of PB was decreased at 33–35 ($P = 0.044$) and 39–41 ($P = 0.031$) compared to 36–38 weeks. (Reproduced with permission from Glotzbach and Ariagno [36].)

decrease the amount. Periodic breathing is frequently defined as three or more respiratory pauses ≥ 3 seconds duration with intervening periods of respiration of < 20 seconds (Figure 95.5) The amount of periodic breathing and the length of the periodic breathing cycles usually decrease with increasing postconceptional age (Figure 95.6) [36,37]. The incidence of periodic breathing is usually < 1% by 52 weeks postconceptional age. In most circumstances, periodic breathing is a benign phenomenon that occurs as an irregular or regular pattern seen most frequently during rapid eye movement (REM) sleep. No significant correlation has been observed between the amount of periodic breathing and the occurrence of prolonged apnea (Figure 95.7) [36–38]. Barrington and Finer [39] recently examined the temporal relationship between prolonged apnea (i.e. apnea > 15 seconds with concurrent hypoxia and bradycardia) and periodic breathing in preterm infants and found that of 116 apneic periods, 1% occurred within 2 minutes of periodic breathing episodes. Furthermore, the postconceptional ages of maximum propensity for prolonged apnea and for periodic breathing did not overlap, leading them to conclude that periodic breathing was not a precursor of prolonged apnea, and the mechanisms underlying prolonged apnea and periodic breathing are different.

95.2.5 MANAGEMENT OF APNEA

In most intensive care nurseries, electronic apnea, cardiac and oxygen saturation monitoring is routine in the care of preterm infants. Alarms for apnea are set at 15–20 seconds to allow timely intervention (before the infant becomes cyanotic, limp or unresponsive), which is generally gentle tactile stimulation to arouse the infant. Further intervention such as oxygen supplementation or assisted ventilation may be instituted if needed. If there is a specific etiology, e.g. sepsis or respiratory failure and hypoxia, successful treatment of the precipitating condition may resolve the apnea problem.

Oscillating waterbeds [40] have been shown to stimulate respiration through non-specific sensory input from the vestibular system. The most common therapy for idiopathic apnea is the administration of methylxanthines, which enhance respiratory drive [41–44]. Clinical trials have confirmed the efficacy of methylxanthines in reducing severe apneas. The resting heart rate may also be increased with methylxanthine therapy and the bradycardia component associated with the apneic events diminished. Approximately 25% of infants, particularly very-low-birth-weight infants <1200 g, may not respond to methylxanthine therapy and may require mechanical ventilator support. Methylxanthines have also been helpful in the weaning of premature

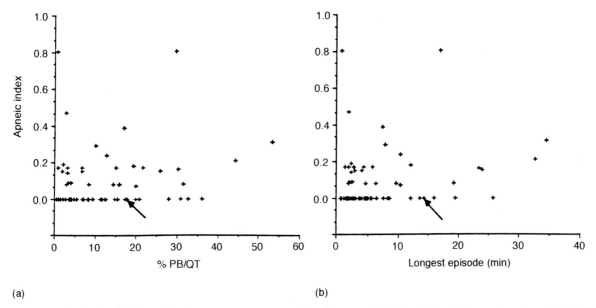

Figure 95.7 The lack of relationship between percentage of both (a) periodic breathing during quiet time (%PB/QT) and (b) longest episode of PB with an apneic index [(number of central apneas > 15 s) × 100]. The arrow highlights values from a single sudden infant death syndrome (SIDS) victim. (Reproduced with permission from Glotzbach and Ariagno [36].)

infants from mechanical ventilation prior to extubation by stimulating respiration and decreasing the amount of postextubation apnea. Close attention to plasma concentrations is essential to maintain therapeutic levels (theophylline range from 5 to 15 μmg/ml and 8–20 μmg/ml for caffeine) and to avoid toxicity. More recently, doxapram has been used as a respiratory stimulant [45]. The disadvantage of this medication is that it must be used parenterally since it has a variable absorption rate when given orally.

Continuous positive airway pressure (CPAP) at 2–5 cm H_2O delivered by nasal prongs, nasal mask or face mask has been effective in the treatment of apnea and in the support of infants who are extubated and weaned from mechanical ventilation. The beneficial effects of CPAP may be due to maintaining lung inflation, stabilization of the chest wall and improved oxygenation. CPAP is most helpful in the management of mixed and obstructive apnea but is less effective with central apnea (Figure 95.8) [46].

In summary, apnea can be treated most effectively if it can be associated with a specific diagnosis. In many cases of apnea of prematurity, simple measures (i.e. tactile stimulation) are adequate treatment until the infant matures. When the apnea is severe and recurrent, mechanical ventilator support is the appropriate treat-

ment until the infant recovers. With current management of apnea in the modern intensive care nursery the degree of asphyxia and related morbidity due to apnea can be minimized [47].

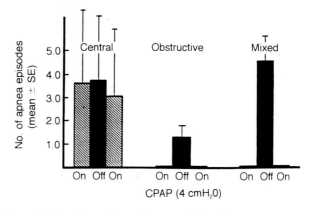

Figure 95.8 Effect of continuous positive airway pressure on number of apneic episodes ≥10 seconds in ten preterm infants. Mixed and obstructive apneas decreased significantly during CPAP treatment; however, no effect on central apnea was noted. (Reproduced with permission from Miller, Carlo and Martin [46].)

95.3 Respiratory distress syndrome

95.3.1 A BRIEF CLINICAL DESCRIPTION

RDS, historically referred to as hyaline membrane disease, occurs after the onset of breathing in preterm infants who are immature and have respiratory failure. Although the cause is multifactoral, pulmonary surfactant insufficiency is a major factor. It is estimated that approximately 40 000 cases of RDS occur annually in the USA. The incidence is 10–15% in low-birth-weight infants (< 2.5 kg). The incidence of RDS is inversely proportional to gestational age and occurs in approximately 70% of infants of 29 weeks' gestation and declining to near 0 by 39 weeks' gestation. Birth by cesarean section without labor, male gender and Caucasian ethnicity are associated with an increased incidence of RDS. The incidence of RDS is higher when there is gestational diabetes or in insulin-dependent mothers without vascular disease [48–51]. The most common etiology of respiratory failure in the preterm infant is, however, RDS; Table 95.1 shows a more comprehensive list of possible causes.

RDS is characterized by respiratory insufficiency and failure that starts at birth and progresses to maximum severity by 1–2 days after birth [50–52]. Recovery of the surfactant system usually occurs in 3–5 days and may lead to complete recovery from RDS except in the more immature infants who have multiple factors, such as morphologic lung immaturity, patent ductus arteriosus, apnea or an acquired lung injury, which may prolong their course of mechanical ventilator support. The maturation of the pulmonary surfactant system is delayed in infants of diabetic mothers and there may be a delayed appearance of phosphatidyl glycerol, which is an important stabilizing component of surfactant. Characteristically, infants with RDS are hypoxic at birth, have poor respiratory effort and poor breath sounds as well as a ground-glass pattern on a chest radiograph which is consistent with diffuse atelectasis.

Table 95.1 Differential diagnosis of respiratory distress syndrome

A. Pulmonary causes of respiratory distress in the newborn

 1. Developmental
     (a) posterior choanal atresia
     (b) laryngeal webs or cyst, vocal fold paralysis
     (c) tracheal stenosis
     (d) laryngotracheal malacia
     (e) cystic adenomatoid malformation of the lung
     (f) congenital lobar emphysema
     (g) congenital hypoplastic lung
     (h) congenital agenesis of the lung
 2. Congenital bacterial or viral pneumonia
 3. Aspiration syndrome
     (a) meconium aspiration (uncommon in preterm <34 weeks' gestation)
     (b) thick mucus aspiration
     (c) blood or amniotic fluid aspiration
 4. Pneumothorax and pneumomediastinum
 5. Transient tachypnea of the newborn (usually in fullterm infants)
 6. Chylothorax
 7. Wilson–Mikity syndrome – etiology unclear; cystic lung changes compatible with bronchopulmonary dysplasia; onset in first week but not immediately following birth
 8. Pulmonary hemorrhage
 9. Congenital pulmonary lymphangiectasia
10. Pulmonary morphologic immaturity

B. Extrapulmonary causes of respiratory distress in the newborn

 1. Tracheo-esophageal fistula
 2. Diaphragmatic hernia
 3. Muscular weakness
     (a) amyotonia congenita
     (b) myasthenia gravis
 4. Phrenic nerve injury or paralysis
 5. Depressant drugs, such as meperidine
 6. Central nervous system pathology, such as cerebral hemorrhage, meningoencephalitis or subdural hematoma
 7. Congenital heart disease with congestive heart failure or pulmonary edema

Table 95.2 Hyaline membrane disease [After Ref. 53 with permission]

Epidemiology

Worldwide	Second-born twin at greater risk
Predisposed by cesarean section without labor	Premature rupture of membranes
	Intrauterine growth retardation
Perinatal asphyxia predisposes	Maternal 'stress' spares
Male > female	Maternal diabetes predisposes if <37 weeks
Caucasian > Black	Maternal hemorrage predisposes

Clinical signs

Onset near the time of birth	Fine inspiratory rales
Retractions and tachypnea	Hypothermia
Expiratory grunt	Peripheral edema
Cyanosis	Pulmonary edema
Systemic hypotension	
Characteristic chest film	
Course to death or improvement 3–5 days	

Pathophysiology

Reduced lung compliance	If hypotensive and hypoxic, poor peripheral perfusion, poor renal perfusion, mycoardial malfunction
Reduced functional residual capacity	
Poor lung distensibility	
Poor alveolar stability	Patent ductus arteriosus contributes
Right-to-left shunts	
Reduced effective pulmonary blood flow	

Pathobiochemistry

Respiratory acidosis	Decreased total serum proteins
Decreased saturated phospholipids	Decreased fibrinolysins
Low amniotic fluid L/S ratio	Low thyroxine levels
Low surfactant associated proteins	

Pathology

Atelectasis	Osmiophilic lamellar bodies decreased early, increased later
Injury to epithelial cells, edema	
Membrane contains fibrin and cellular products	
No tubular myelin	

Etiology

Surfactant deficiency during disease	Probable inadequate hormonal (corticoid) stimulus *in utero*
	Dipalmitoyl lecithin synthesis impaired and/or destruction increased
	Autonomic dysfunction

Prevention

Prenatal glucocorticoids for >24 hours
Surfactant replacement before 1–2 hours

The epidemiology, pathophysiology, pathobiochemistry and pathologic findings of RDS are summarized in Table 95.2. Approximately 20% of RDS survivors will experience a prolonged course of ventilation resulting in a lung injury pattern that has been described as bronchopulmonary dysplasia [54] and can last for months or years, usually improving by 2 years of age [55–58]. Pathologic reports of infants with bronchopulmonary dysplasia at 3 years of age show marked alterations in lung morphology and development, suggesting that complete resolution and attainment of normal lung development may not occur [59,60].

95.3.2 PULMONARY SURFACTANT

Pulmonary surfactant (Figure 95.9), which decreases the surface forces at the air–liquid interface, is a prerequisite for successful adaptation to air breathing, and is found in all air-breathing vertebrates studied, including animals as phylogenetically ancient as the lungfish. The major component of surfactant is phosphatidylcholine. Pulmonary surfactant, a complex lipid–protein mixture, is produced primarily by the type 2 epithelial cells lining the alveoli. Reduction in surface tension is achieved by the absorption of the phospholipids

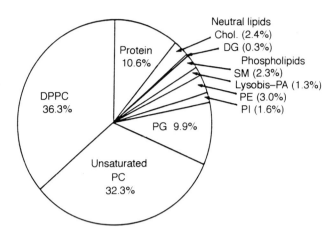

Figure 95.9 Composition of bovine pulmonary surfactant obtained from lung lavage. Components are expressed as percentage weight (% wt). Chol = cholesterol; DG = diacylglycerol; SM = sphingomyelin; PA = phosphatidic acid; PE = phosphatidylethanolamine; PI = phosphatidylinositol; PG = phosphatidylglycerol; PC = phosphatidylcholine; DPPC = dipalmitoylphosphatidylcholine. (Reproduced with permission from Possmayer *et al.* [61].)

(primarily the phosphatidylcholine and phosphotidylglycerol) to the extracellular alveolar surface. Phospholipid molecules form a tightly packed monolayer at the surface and counteract the surface tension forces generated by water molecules at the air–liquid interface. The properties of rapid surface absorption and stability during dynamic compression are conferred by surfactant associated apoproteins A, B, and C. Apoprotein A (SPA) (a glycoprotein of 26 000–35 000 daltons) may be important in host defense. Apoprotein B (SPB) a small (8000 daltons) hydrophobic polypeptide alters the surfactant lipid structure to enhance the surface properties. Apoprotein C (SPC) is the most highly hydrophobic protein (3800 daltons) isolated from pulmonary surfactant. SPC alone imparts surfactant-like properties to synthetic phospholipids and a mixture of SPB and C enhances the rate of absorption of surfactant phospholipids and confers important surfactant-like properties to the lipids. Like SPB, addition of SPC peptides to phospholipid vesicles enhances surfactant production by type 2 epithelial cells *in vitro*. In summary, the primary role of surfactant in pulmonary physiology is to **reduce surface tension and thereby improve compliance, decrease the work of breathing, increase alveolar stability** and to **improve alveolar recruitment** [50,52,62,63].

Although the emphasis has been placed on the lack of surfactant which may contribute to respiratory failure in a preterm infant, there are several non-surfactant factors which should be mentioned briefly. Among these factors are limited alveolar development, instability of and increased compliance of the chest wall, immaturity of the diaphragm and poor maintenance of upper airway patency. Other factors include left-to-right patent ductus arteriosus shunting, cardiovascular immaturity, transitional circulation, central nervous system immaturity, respiratory drive, thermoregulation, renal immaturity, fluid balance and lung water clearance. All of these factors, from multiple systems, may contribute to the respiratory failure seen in immature preterm infants. A common clinical response of the preterm infant who develops respiratory failure and hypoxia is apnea (Chapter 32).

95.3.3 PATENT DUCTUS ARTERIOSUS

The identification and management of a clinically significant patent ductus arteriosus (PDA) shunt is an important problem in the preterm infant who can have increased pulmonary blood flow from a left-to-right shunt and develop congestive heart failure and pulmonary edema. Like RDS, the incidence of the clinically significant PDA shunt leading to pulmonary edema and congestive heart failure is increased in the immature infant. The presence of a left-to-right shunt or bidirectional shunt from the aorta to the pulmonary artery through the ductus arteriosus is also common in the normal term neonate at birth. However, the PDA usually constricts and closes within the first few days of life. The magnitude of the left-to-right shunt is determined by the pulmonary artery/systemic arterial resistance ratio and the size of the ductus arteriosus. The approximate incidence of a prolonged ductus patency in preterm infants is 85% in infants < 1000 g, 50% in 1000-1500 g infants 25% in the 1500-2000 g birth weight infants. PDA management and detection in modern newborn intensive care nurseries is aided by two-dimensional echocardiography which allows estimation of the size and the direction of the shunt. Since the introduction of surfactant replacement for the treatment of the respiratory failure due to RDS, the incidence of PDA shunting has increased as a result of improved lung inflation and a decrease in the peripheral vascular resistance after surfactant therapy [64] (Chapter 103).

95.3.4 MANAGEMENT OF RESPIRATORY DISTRESS SYNDROME

(a) Respiratory distress syndrome

The diagnosis of RDS may be predicted if the prenatal amniotic fluid lecithin : sphingomyelin (L/S) ratio is < 2, or if phosphotidyl glycerol is decreased or absent [65]. At the time of birth, the infant with RDS is usually cyanotic in room air, has intercostal and sternal retractions, has poor breath sounds, and may have a reflex expiratory 'grunt' (produced by partial closure of the glottis) associated with a positive pressure at end expiration (an attempt to physiologically achieve positive end expiratory lung distension) in response to atelectasis. Initial treatment includes maintaining an optimal (37°C) body temperature, supplemental oxygen therapy, providing manual positive pressure ventilation and, if necessary, intubation and support with mechanical ventilation. Venous and/or arterial umbilical lines are usually placed to sample arterial blood gasses as well as to provide fluids and other medications such as antibiotics until infection is ruled out. The warming environment during resuscitation and management is servocontrolled by setting the controlling limit of the skin temperature probe at the euthermic core temperature (36.3–37.5°C) to maintain the infant at a normal core body temperature.

(b) Surfactant

In recent years, controlled trials of several surfactant replacement therapies (human, bovine and synthetic) have been shown to improve survival and to reduce morbidity in preterm infants with RDS [1–13,66–73] (Table 95.3). Treatment is recommended in two scenarios: first, in which surfactant is introduced into the endotracheal tube and insufflated into the lung before the infant begins to breath; or second, given shortly after the infant shows evidence of respiratory failure and has chest radiograph findings characteristic of RDS. Repeat treatment may be given every 6–12 hours if the infant continues to have respiratory failure. The total number of doses ranges from one to several. The optimal number of doses is currently under investigation, but bedside management is based on the clinician's best judgement on a case by case basis. There

are no contraindications for surfactant treatment except for adequate resuscitation and stabilization before adding the stress of intratracheal surfactant. Careful attention during dosing requires monitoring of heart rate, oxygen saturation and ventilation. The side-effects are infrequent if the dosing, usually 5 ml/kg per dose is given slowly to avoid airway occlusion, bradycardia and oxygen desaturation. The position of the endotracheal tube is also very important to avoid unilateral insufflation of the surfactant into the right or left bronchus and lung. Under these circumstances, overinflation of the treated lung may occur, with under-inflation and atelectasis of the contralateral untreated lung. The appropriate maneuver under these circumstances is to position the infant with the overinflated side down to allow the untreated lung to inflate. Before giving the next dose of surfactant, the position of the endotracheal tube should be confirmed with a chest radiograph and bedside auscultation of the lungs to verify equal breath sounds. It should also be kept in mind that positioning the infant during dosing will affect the endotracheal tube position, e.g. neck flexion can advance the tube towards the carina. Autoimmune responses are avoided with artificial surfactants; however, no adverse effects have been observed with use of animal or human surfactants. Clinical improvement in gas exchange is usually seen within 2 hours of treatment, followed by an improvement in pulmonary mechanics by 1–3 days [75]. Although surfactant replacement appears to decrease the severity of respiratory failure, PDA closure may be delayed, and close monitoring of ductus status is recommended. If the PDA causes a significant left-to-right shunt and exacerbation of lung dysfunction, pharmacologic therapy (indomethacin) or surgical closure of the ductus may be

Table 95.3 Surfactants used in replacement therapy [After Ref. 74 with permission]

Surfactant	Origin	Reference
Surfactant from amniotic fluid		
Human surfactant	Gradient isolated fraction of amniotic fluid surfactant	Hallman et al. [66]
Extracts of natural surfactant		
Surfactant-TA	Organic solvent extract of minced cow lungs fortified with lipids	Fujiwara et al. [69]
Bovine lung surfactant extract (BLSE)	Organic solvent extract of cow lung lavage	Enhorning et al. [68]
Calf lung surfactant extract (CLSE)	Organic solvent extract of calf lung lavage	Shapiro et al. [2]
Infasurf	Organic solvent extract of calf lung lavage	Kwong et al. [1]
Curosurf	Organic solvent extracted and chromatographically purified preparation from minced cow or pig lungs	Noack et al. [71]
Survanta	Surfactant-TA modified for better dispersion and storage	Soll et al. [72]
Surfactants containing no protein		
ALEC	DPPC:PG, 7:3	Morley et al. [70]
Exosurf	DPPC plus tyloxapol and hexadecanol, two spreading agents	Durand et al. [67]

DPPC = dipalmitoylphosphatidylcholine.

required to improve the infant's respiratory failure [76,77].

(c) Bronchopulmonary dysplasia (Chapters 30 and 44)

Bronchopulmonary dysplasia was originally described by Northway, Rosan and Porter [54] as a complication of RDS in babies who were treated with oxygen and mechanical ventilation. The incidence of bronchopulmonary dysplasia is highest in the lowest birth-weight infants who are immature and is usually not seen in term infants. The cause of bronchopulmonary dysplasia is multifactorial: it is primarily related to immaturity, and results from oxygen toxicity and barotrauma associated with mechanical ventilation, inadequate nutrition and limited antioxidant pulmonary defenses usually seen in the critically ill preterm infant. The incidence of bronchopulmonary dysplasia in the very-low-birth-weight infant (< 1200 g) may not have changed with surfactant replacement therapy, which may be explained in part by the fact that surfactant treatment may not influence immaturity of the lung alveolar development. Infants with bronchopulmonary dysplasia generally have prolonged chronic respiratory failure accompanied by hypoxemia in 21% O_2 and CO_2 retention. There may be chronic lung changes and limitation in the potential for pulmonary development which may be life long, at least in some infants. Surfactant replacement therapy and new ventilation strategies may lessen the severity and may decrease the incidence of bronchopulmonary dysplasia [57,58].

In summary, it is noteworthy that infant mortality has declined significantly from 1989 to 1990. The provisional rate for 1990 reported by Wegman [14] is 9.1 per 1000 livebirths, which is the lowest ever recorded in the USA and is due primarily to the decline in mortality from RDS. Surfactant therapy has been identified as the most important factor leading to the decrease in severity of respiratory failure and mortality. Prenatal therapies which can influence lung surfactant maturation are reviewed in Chapter 89. Since the advent of postnatal surfactant therapy, some perinatologists have overlooked the importance of prenatal glucocorticoid [78] and thyrotropin releasing hormone treatment, which have been shown to decrease the incidence and/or the severity of RDS and to reduce the mortality due to RDS when used in combination with surfactant replacement therapy. Although these are exciting advances in newborn medicine, there is an obvious consensus that public health measures, which may reduce the incidence of premature infant birth, would have the greatest impact on infant mortality and complications associated with adaptation of the premature infant to extrauterine life.

References

1. Kwong, M.S., Egan, E.A., Notter, R.H. and Shapiro, D.L. (1985) Double-blind clinical trial of calf lung surfactant extract for the prevention of hyaline membrane disease in extremely premature infants. *Pediatrics*, 76, 585–92.
2. Shapiro, D.L., Notter, R.H., Morin III, F.C. *et al.* (1985) Double blind, randomized trial of a calf lung surfactant extract administered at birth to very premature infants for prevention of respiratory distress syndrome. *Pediatrics*, 76, 593–99.
3. Merritt, T.A. Hallman, M., Bloom, B.T. *et al.* (1986) Prophylactic treatment of very premature infants with human surfactant. *N. Engl. J. Med.*, 315, 785–90.
4. Raju, T.N.K., Vidyasagar, D., Bhat, R. *et al.* (1987) Double-blind controlled trial of single dose treatment with bovine surfactant in severe hyaline membrane disease. *Lancet*, i, 651–56.
5. Horbar, J.D., Soll, R.F., Sutherland, J.M., *et al.* (1989) A multicenter randomized placebo-controlled trial of surfactant therapy for respiratory distress syndrome. *N. Engl. J. Med.*, 320, 959–65.
6. Lang, M.J., Hall, R.T., Reddy, N.S. *et al.* (1990) A controlled trial of human surfactant replacement therapy for severe respiratory distress syndrome in very low birth weight infants. *J. Pediatr.*, 116, 295–300.
7. Hoekstra, R.E., Jackson, J.C., Myers, T.F. *et al.* (1991) Improved neonatal survival following multiple doses of bovine surfactant in very premature neonates at risk for respiratory distress syndrome. *Pediatrics*, 88, 10–18.
8. Liechty, E.A., Donovan, E., Purohit, D. *et al.* (1991) Reduction of neonatal mortality after multiple doses of bovine surfactant in low birthweight neonates with respiratory distress syndrome. *Pediatrics*, 88, 19–28.
9. Long, W., Thompson, T., Sundell, H. *et al.* (1991) Effects of two rescue doses of synthetic surfactant on mortality rate and survival without bronchopulmonary dysplasia in 700–1300 gm infants with respiratory distress syndrome. *J. Pediatr.* 118, 595–605.
10. Bose, C., Corbet, A., Bose, G. *et al.* (1990) Improved outcome at 28 days of age for very low birthweight infants treated with a single dose of a synthetic surfactant. *J. Pediatr.*, 117, 947–53.
11. Corbet, A.J., Goldman, S.A., Lombardy, L. *et al* (1991) Decreased mortality in small premature infants treated at birth with a single dose of synthetic surfactant: a multicenter trial. *J. Pediatr.*, 118, 277–84.
12. Long, W.A., Corbet, A., Cotton, R. *et al.* (1991) A controlled trial of synthetic surfactant in infants weighing 1250 grams or more with the American Exosurf Neonatal Study Group I and the Canadian Exosurf Neonatal Study Group. *N. Engl. J. Med.*, 325, 1696–703.
13. Stevenson, D.K., Walther, F., Long, W. *et al.* (1992) Controlled trial of a single dose of synthetic surfactant at birth in premature infants weighing 500 to 699 grams. *J. Pediatr.*, 120, S3–12.
14. Wegman, M.E. (1992) Annual summary of vital statistics – 1991. *Pediatrics*, 88, 1081–92.
15. Lee, D., Caces, R., Kwiatkowski, K. *et al.* (1987) Developmental study on types and frequency distribution of short apneas (3 to 15 seconds) in term and preterm infants. *Pediatr. Res.*, 22, 344–49.
16. Hoppenbrouwers, T., Hodgman, J.E., Harper, R.M. *et al.* (1977) Polygraphic studies of normal infants during the first six months of life. III. Incidence of apnea and periodic breathing. *Pediatrics*, 60, 418–25.
17. Carlo, W.A., Martin, R.J., Versteegh, F.G.A. *et al.* (1982) The effect of respiratory distress syndrome on chest wall movements and respiratory pauses in preterm infants. *Am. Rev. Resp. Dis.*, 126, 103–107.
18. Martin, R.J., Miller, M.J. and Carlo, W.A. (1986) Pathogenesis of apnea in preterm infants. *J. Pediatr.*, 109, 733–41.
19. Brazy, J.E., Kinney, H.C. and Oakes, W.J. (1987) Central nervous system structure lesions causing apnea at birth. *J. Pediatr.*, 11, 163–75.
20. Adickes, E.D., Buehler, B.A. and Sange, W.G. (1986) Familial lethal sleep apnea. *Hum. Genet.*, 73, 39–43.
21. Henderson-Smart, D.J., Pettigrew, A.G. and Campbell, D.J. (1983) Clinical apnea and brainstem neural function in preterm infants. *N. Engl. J. Med.*, 308, 353–57.
22. Ariagno, R.L. (1979) Development of respiratory control, in *Advances in Perinatal Neurology*, vol. I (eds R. Korobkin and C. Guillemenault), Spectrum, New York, pp. 249–80.
23. Rigatto, H., Brady, J. and Verduzco, R.T. (1975) Chemoreceptor reflexes in preterm infants. II. The effect of gestational and postnatal age on the ventilatory response to inhaled carbon dioxide. *Pediatrics*, 55, 614–20.
24. Rigatto, H., Verduzco, R.T. and Cates, D.B. (1975) Effects of O_2 on the ventilatory response to CO_2 in preterm infants. *J. Appl. Physiol.*, 39, 896–96.
25. Frantz III, I.D., Adler, S.M., Thach, B.T. *et al.* (1976) Maturational effects on respiratory responses to inhaled carbon dioxide in premature infants. *J. Appl. Physiol.*, 41, 41–5.
26. Rigatto, H. (1992) Maturation of breathing control in the fetus and newborn infant, in *Respiratory Control Disorders in Infants and Children* (eds R.C. Beckerman, R.T. Brouillette and C.E. Hunt), Williams & Wilkins, Baltimore, MD, pp. 61–75.
27. Gerhardt, T. and Bancalari, T. (1984) Apnea of prematurity: lung function and regulation of breathing. *Pediatrics*, 74, 58–62.

28. Durand, M., Cabal, L.A. and Gonzalez, F. *et al.* (1986) Ventilatory control and carbon dioxide response in preterm infants with idiopathic apnea. *Am. J. Dis. Child.*, **139**, 717–20.

29. Abu-Osba, Y.K., Mathew, O.P. and Thach, B.T. (1981) An animal model for airway sensory deprivation producing obstructive apnea with postmortem findings of sudden infant death syndrome. *Pediatrics*, **68**, 796–801.

30. Carlo, W.A., Martin, R.J. and Difiore, J.M. (1988) Differences in the CO_2 threshold of respiratory muscles of preterm infants. *J. Appl. Physiol.*, **65**, 2434–39.

31. Nail, B.S., Sterling, G.M. and Widdicombe, J.G. (1969) Epipharyngeal receptors responding to mechanical stimulation. *J. Physiol.*, **204**, 91–98.

32. Lawson, E.E. (1981) Prolonged central respiratory inhibition following reflex induced apnea. *J. Appl. Physiol.*, **50**, 874–79.

33. Teitelbaum, H.A. and Ries, F.A. (1935) A study of the comparative physiology of the glossopharyngeal nerve–respiratory reflex in the rabbit, cat and dog. *Am. J. Physiol.*, **112**, 684–89.

34. Mennon, A.P., Schefft, G.L. and Thach, B.T. (1985) Apnea associated with regurgitation in infants. *J. Pediatr.*, **106**, 625–29.

35. Thach, B.T. (1983) The role of pharyngeal airway obstruction in prolonging infantile apneic spells, in *Sudden Infant Death Syndrome* (eds J.T. Tilden, L.M. Roeder and A. Steinschneider), Academic Press, New York, pp. 279–92.

36. Glotzbach, S.F. and Ariagno, R.L. (1992) Periodic Breathing, In *Respiratory Control Disorders in Infants and Children* (eds R.C. Beekerman, R.T. Brovillette and C.E. Hunt), Williams & Wilkins, Baltimore, MD, pp. 142–60.

37. Glotzbach, S.F., Baldwin, R.B., Lederer, N.E. *et al.* (1989) Periodic breathing in preterm infants: incidence and characteristics. *Pediatrics*, **84**, 785–92.

38. Glotzbach, S.T., Taasey, P.A., Baldwin, R.B. and Ariagno, R.L. (1989) Periodic breathing cycle duration in preterm infants. *Pediatr. Res.*, **25**, 258–61.

39. Barrington, K.J. and Finer, N.N. (1990) Periodic breathing and apnea in preterm infants. *Pediatr. Res.*, **27**, 118–21.

40. Korner, A.F., Guilleminault, C., Van den Hoed, J. and Baldwin, R.B. (1978) Reduction of sleep apnea and bradycardia in preterm infants in oscillating waterbeds: a controlled polygraphic study. *Pediatrics*, **61**, 528–33.

41. Aranda, J.V., Turmen, T., Davis, J. *et al.* (1983) Effect of caffeine on control of breathing in infantile apnea. *J. Pediatr.*, **103**, 975–79.

42. Gerhardt, T., McCarthy, J., Bancalari, E. (1979) Effect of aminophylline on respiratory center activity and metabolic rate in premature infants with idiopathic apnea. *Pediatrics*, **63**, 537–42.

43. Eldrige, F.L., Millhorn, D.E., Waldropt, T.G. *et al.* (1983) Mechanism of respiratory effects of methylxanthines. *Respir. Physiol.*, **53**, 239–69.

44. Darnall Jr, R.A. (1985) Aminophylline reduces hypoxic ventilatory depression: possible role of adenosine. *Pediatr. Res.*, **19**, 706–10.

45. Barrington, K.J., Finer, N.N. and Peters, K.L. (1986) Physiologic effects of doxapram in idiopathic apnea of prematurity. *J. Pediatr.*, **108**, 124–29.

46. Miller, M.J., Carlo, W.A. and Martin, R.J. (1985) Continuous positive airway pressure selectively reduces obstructive apnea in preterm infants. *J. Pediatr.*, **106**, 91–94.

47. Ariagno, R.L. (1988) Management of apnea in the ICN graduate, in *Pediatric Care of the ICN Graduate* (ed. R.A. Ballard), W.B. Saunders, Philadelphia, pp. 264–80.

48. Robert, M.F., Neff, R.K., Hubbell, J.P. *et al.* (1976) Association between maternal diabetes and the respiratory distress syndrome in the newborn. *N. Engl. J. Med.*, **294**, 357–60.

49. Usher, R.H., Allen, A.C. and McLean, F.H. (1971) Risk of respiratory distress syndrome related to gestational age, route of delivery and maternal diabetes. *Am. J. Obstet. Gynecol.*, **111**, 826–32.

50. Farrell, P.M. and Avery, M.E. (1975) State of the art: hyaline membrane disease. *Am. Rev. Respir. Dis.*, **111**, 657–88.

51. Farrell, P.M. and Wood, R.E. (1976) Epidemiology of hyaline membrane disease in the United States: analysis of national mortality statistics. *Pediatrics*, **58**, 167–76.

52. Avery, M.E. and Mead, J. (1959) Surface properties in relation to atelectasis and hyaline membrane disease. *Am. J. Dis. Child.*, **97**, 517–23.

53. Hansen, T. and Corbett, A. (1984) Disorders of the transition, in *Diseases of the Fetus and Newborn* (eds H.W. Taeusch, R.A. Ballard and M.E. Avery), W.B. Saunders, Philadelphia, p. 498.

54. Northway, W.H., Rosan, R.G. and Porter, D.Y. (1967) Improved prognosis of infants mechanically ventilated for hyaline membrane disease. *N. Engl. J. Med.*, **276**, 357–68.

55. Groothuis, J.R. and Rosenberg, A.A. (1987) Home oxygen promotes weight gain in infants with bronchopulmonary dysplasia. *Am. J. Dis. Child.*, **19**, 992–95.

56. Sauve, R.S., McMillan, D.D., Mitchell, I. *et al.* (1989) Home oxygen therapy. Outcome of infants discharged from NICU on continuous treatment. *Clin. Pediatr.*, **28**, 113–18.

57. Bancalari, E. and Stocker, J.T. (1988) *Bronchopulmonary Dysplasia*, Hemisphere, Washington, DC.

58. Merritt, T.A., Northway Jr, W.H. and Boynton, B.R. (1988) *Bronchopulmonary Dysplasia*, Blackwell Scientific, Boston.

59. Sobonya, R.E., Logvinoff, M.M., Taussig, L.M. and Theriault, A. (1982) Morphometric analysis of the lung in prolonged bronchopulmonary dysplasia. *Pediatr. Res.*, **16**, 969–72.

60. Stocker, J.T. (1986) Pathologic features of long-standing 'healed' bronchopulmonary dysplasia: a study of 28 3 to 30-month old infants. *Hum. Pathol.*, **17**, 943–61.

61. Possmayer, F., Yu, S.-H., Weber, J.M. and Harding, P.G.R. (1984) Pulmonary surfactant. *Can. J. Biochem. Cell Biol.*, **62**, 1121–33.

62. Harwood, J.L. (1987) Lung surfactant. *Prog. Lipid Res.*, **26**, 211–56.

63. Wisett, J.A. (1992) Composition of pulmonary surfactants, lipids and proteins, in *Fetal and Neonatal Physiology*, vol. II (eds R.A. Polin and W.W. Fry), WB Saunders Co., Philadelphia, pp. 941–48.

64. Heldt, G.P., Pesonen, E., Merritt, T.A. *et al.* (1989) Closure of the ductus arteriosus and mechanics of breathing in preterm infants after surfactant replacement therapy. *Pediatr. Res.*, **25**, 305–10.

65. Gluck, L. and Kulovich, M.V. (1973), Lecithin–sphingomyelin ratios in amniotic fluid in normal and abnormal pregnancy. *Am. J. Obstet. Gynecol.*, **115**, 539–46.

66. Hallman, M., Merritt, T.T., Jarvenpaa, A.L. *et al.* (1985) Exogenous human surfactant for treatment of severe respiratory distress syndrome: a randomized prospective clinical trial. *J. Pediatr.*, **106**, 963–69

67. Durand, D.J., Clyman, R.I., Heymann, M.A. *et al.* (1985) Effects of a protein-free, synthetic surfactant on survival and pulmonary function in preterm lambs. *J. Pediatr.*, **107**, 775–79.

68. Enhorning, G., Shennan, A., Dunn, M. *et al.* (1985) Prevention of neonatal respiratory distress syndrome by tracheal instillation of surfactant: randomized clinical trial. *Pediatrics*, **76**, 145–53.

69. Fujiwara, T., Maeta, H., Chida, S. *et al.* (1980) Artificial surfactant therapy in hyaline membrane disease. *Lancet*, i., 55–59.

70. Morley, C.J., Bangham, A.D., Miller, N. *et al.* (1981) Dry artificial surfactant and its effect on very premature babies. *Lancet*, i, 64–70

71. Noack, G., Berggren, P., Curstedt, T. *et al.* (1987) Severe neonatal respiratory distress syndrome treated with the isolated phospholipid fraction of natural surfactant. *Acta Paediatr. Scand.*, **76**, 697–705.

72. Soll, R.F., Hoekstra, R.E., Fangman, J.J. *et al.* (1990) Multicenter trial of single-dose modified bovine surfactant extract (Survanta) for prevention of respiratory distress syndrome. *Pediatrics*, **85**, 1092–102.

73. Shapiro, D.L. and Notter, R.H. (eds) (1989) *Surfactant Replacement Therapy*, Alan R. Liss, New York.

74. Shapiro, D.L. (1992) Surfactant therapy, in *Fetal and Neonatal Physiology*, vol. II (eds R.A. Polin and W.W. Fox), W.B. Saunders, Philadelphia, pp. 1007–13

75. Armsby, D.H., Bellon, G., Carlisle, K. *et al.* (1992) Delayed compliance increase in infants with respiratory distress syndrome following synthetic surfactant. *Pediatr. Pulmonol.*, **14**, 206–13.

76. Gersony, W.M., Peckham, G.J., Ellison, R.C. *et al.* (1983) Effects of indomethacin in premature infants with patent ductus arteriosus: results of a national collaborative study. *J. Pediatr.*, **102**, 895–906.

77. Jacob, J., Gluck, L., DiSessa, T. *et al.* (1980) The contribution of patent ductus arteriosus in the neonate with severe RDS. *J. Pediatr.*, **96**, 79–87.

78. OSIRIS Collaborative Group (1992) Early vs. delayed neonatal administration of a synthetic surfactant – the judgement of OSIRIS (Open study of infants at high risk of or with respiratory insufficiency – the role of surfactant). *Lancet*, **340**, 1363–69.

96 NEONATAL CEREBROVASCULAR MONITORING

M. Levene

96.1 Introduction

Complications affecting the neonatal brain are the most common causes of long-term disability in surviving babies. Due to rapid changes in developmental anatomy and physiological control systems within the central nervous system between 24 weeks and fullterm, the type of cerebral pathology sustained by neonates varies with gestational age. Recent technological advances have allowed the application of highly sophisticated monitoring techniques to the developing brain. Indeed, some of these techniques have been developed especially to study the human newborn brain during life.

A clear understanding of these techniques is important so that clinicians can evaluate the published data and in particular weigh any potential hazards of the techniques against the advantages of the information that is obtained from them. The data accumulated by these techniques can be used in two ways. In the first, the monitoring technique may be used further to unravel the intricacies of cerebral pathophysiology with the aim of eventually modifying treatment based on improved understanding as to how injury occurs. The equipment, which may be very expensive or bulky and limited to a few highly specialized centres, may also be used to calibrate more clinically acceptable monitoring tools. The second stage in development of these monitoring techniques is to use them in clinical practice to improve or rationalize clinical management. A number of techniques lie somewhere between these two extremes as their clinical role remains to be defined (Chapter 92).

96.2 Imaging

There are three techniques available for imaging the neonatal brain, ultrasound, computed tomography (CT) and magnetic resonance imaging (MRI). These are reviewed in detail elsewhere [1]; they make use of entirely different physical properties and consequently

Table 96.1 Comparison of three imaging techniques used in the neonatal period

	Ultrasound	CT	MRI
Portability	++	−	−
Need for sedation	−	+	+
Radiation	−	+	−
Detection of pathology:			
in premature infants	++	+	+
in mature infants	+	++	+++
Cost	+	++	++++

images produced by them can show considerable variation in the detection of pathology. Table 96.1 compares some of these important features.

96.2.1 ULTRASOUND

Real-time ultrasound is now widely used in most neonatal units for imaging the neonatal brain. Images are obtained by a 5- or 7-MHz transducer placed over the anterior fontanelle and images can be obtained until approximately 6 months of age when the anterior fontanelle becomes too small to obtain good quality images. Real-time ultrasound machines are portable and the infant can be scanned within the intensive care environment. Ultrasound is most sensitive in the diagnosis of periventricular haemorrhage, which occurs in about 50% of very premature infants. It is also reasonably sensitive in the diagnosis of periventricular leucomalacia, an ischaemic condition that occurs in approximately 10–20% of premature infants. In the most severe form of periventricular leucomalacia, cavities develop in the white matter and are easily detected using ultrasound once the lesion exceeds 1 mm in diameter.

96.2.2 COMPUTED TOMOGRAPHY

This was the first technique used to detect intracranial haemorrhage in the preterm infant but is the least

Diseases of the Fetus and Newborn, 2nd edn, Edited by G.B. Reed, A.E. Claireaux and F. Cockburn. Published in 1995 by Chapman & Hall, London. ISBN 0 412 39160 0

valuable imaging modality currently available. The baby must be moved from the intensive care incubator to the CT facility and is exposed to X irradiation. Anatomical delineation is good, but MRI (see below) gives the same quality of image as well as additional information not obtained by CT. If MRI is not available, CT imaging may detect important pathology in the fullterm infant that is not detected by ultrasound examination.

96.2.3 MAGNETIC RESONANCE IMAGING

This very sophisticated technique requires the patient to lie motionless within a strong magnetic field. A radio-frequency impulse is applied to the brain by a special coil lying over the organ, producing a perturbation in hydrogen nuclei. The relaxation of these nuclei can be detected and an image generated. This technique requires a very expensive facility and the baby must be moved to it, but it is non-invasive and not associated with ionizing radiation. In addition, the technique is unique in giving information on myelination, but as the neonate has little myelin formation at early stages of development this is not particularly useful. Another advantage of MRI is that images can be generated in multiple planes including axial, coronal or sagittal.

96.3 Assessment of cerebral haemodynamics

The two major forms of cerebral pathology that occur in the term brain, periventricular haemorrhage and periventricular leucomalacia, are thought to be due to changes in cerebral blood flow. Periventricular haemorrhage arises as the result of hyperfusion through the germinal matrix, although the subsequent parenchymal injury may be associated with low flow in the affected hemisphere. Periventricular leucomalacia is a condition that occurs in a watershed distribution of the cerebral white matter as the result of cerebral underperfusion. The most common brain injury in term infants, and which causes irreversible injury, is hypoxic–ischaemic encephalopathy, also known as birth asphyxia. This condition most commonly arises as the result of intrapartum asphyxia and the baby is born in poor condition and may develop multiorgan complications, including cerebral dysfunction. There is considerable evidence that the progression to irreversible brain damage is associated with changes of blood flow in the cerebral microvasculature which may be associated in the early stages with impaired cerebral perfusion and later with cerebral hyperperfusion. It is clear that the major forms of brain injury occurring in the perinatal period are associated with changes in cerebral blood flow and measurement of this variable in newborn

infants may be fundamental to further understanding the pathophysiology and the development of therapeutic interventions (Chapters 21, 30 and 44).

96.3.1 DOPPLER

Doppler ultrasound measures the velocity of blood cells within vessels. The physics of this technique is discussed elsewhere [2]. In order for velocity to be measured, the angle of insonation (the difference between the direction of the ultrasound wave and the vessel) must be known. If the angle cannot be measured but is known to be low (<15°), or if the angle is fixed between repeated measurements then it is assumed that changes in cerebral blood flow (CBF) velocity can be measured. If the angle is not known, or if the angle varies between examinations, an angle-independent formula has been used. This is referred to as either the Pourcelot resistance index (PRI) or the pulsatility index. The PRI is calculated as:

$$PRI = \frac{S - D}{S}$$

where S is the maximum systolic frequency and D is the maximum diastolic frequency. Much of the early Doppler work in the newborn used the PRI, which has been described as reflecting changes in cerebral vascular resistance.

Another assumption which is fundamental to the Doppler technique is that there is no change in the cross-sectional diameter of the vessel either during the cardiac cycle or under changing physiological conditions. Unfortunately, there is now considerable evidence that this does not hold under all circumstances.

It is important to stress that CBF velocity is not the same measurement as CBF. CBF is the product of CBF velocity and the cross-sectional diameter of the insonated vessel. As it is not possible to measure the cross-sectional diameter of the intracranial vessels accurately, CBF remains an elusive measurement.

Despite all these methodological pitfalls Doppler has been quite extensively evaluated as a clinical tool in the neonatal period. The main areas where it is considered to be of some clinical value are as follows.

(a) Hypoxic–ischaemic encephalopathy

It has been shown that infants who have suffered moderate or severe hypoxic–ischaemic encephalopathy may show a consistent abnormality detected by Doppler ultrasound [3,4]. There is a progressive fall in the PRI [3] and a related increase in CBF velocity [4], although these changes are not seen until the second 24 hours after birth. Follow-up studies have shown that these abnormalities are associated with a poor prognosis for intact survival [4]. The cause of these Doppler changes is probably related to vasoparalysis of the cerebral arterioles and appears to represent a state of irreversible vascular injury.

(b) Prediction of haemorrhage or ischaemic lesions

The absolute value of CBF velocity has been measured in a group of very premature infants to assess whether low or high velocities predict these lesions. No correlation between velocity and eventual pathology could be established [5]. It has recently been shown that the majority of premature infants show a regular cycling pattern of CBF velocity with changes in absolute velocity of the order of 70% over the course of 1 minute [6]. As the standard deviation of velocity measurements are so high it is therefore unlikely that Doppler will be able to detect relatively small changes in velocity which may precede periventricular haemorrhage or leucomalacia. It has been suggested that CBF velocity may predict outcome in a population of premature infants. Van Bel and colleagues [7] found that children with a disability at 2 years of age had significantly higher pulsatility indices than children who had a more normal outcome.

(c) Posthaemorrhagic hydrocephalus

This condition occurs in about 10–15% of infants with intracranial haemorrhage. Treatment is by medication (acetazolamide, glycerol) and intermittent drainage of cerebrospinal fluid at lumbar puncture or from a ventricular access device or shunting. The timing of treatment is controversial and Doppler has been assessed for its ability to predict elevated intracranial pressure. It has been shown that in older infants who have a blocked shunt Doppler assessment indicates those children who are developing significantly raised pressure [8]. Doppler has recently been assessed as an instrument for determining which infants require treatment. Unfortunately, Doppler ultrasound is a very poor predictor of raised intracranial pressure (ICP) and its role in this respect is very limited [9].

96.3.2 FICK'S PRINCIPLE

The measurement of inflow and outflow of an inert tracer into the brain can be utilized to measure CBF by application of Fick's principle. This states that the change of the mean tracer concentration in a tissue equals the product of the perfusion rate and the arteriovenous concentration difference. Nitrous oxide was originally used in the Kety–Schmidt method. This has only rarely been utilized in the newborn as a catheter has to be advanced to the jugular bulb to measure the concentration of nitrous oxide in cerebral venous blood and this severely limits the value of this technique. Other tracers have been used in measure-

ment of CBF in the newborn, particularly radioactive xenon and oxyhaemoglobin.

96.3.3 RADIOACTIVE TECHNIQUES

A variety of radioactive tracers has been used in neonates to assess cerebral haemodynamics, including ^{133}Xe, ^{99m}Tc in single photon emission computed tomography (SPECT) and ^{15}O or ^{11}C in positron emission tomography (PET). Only the xenon technique allows quantification of cerebral blood flow, although the last two methods may give important information on qualitative regional CBF.

Xenon is a freely diffusible inert tracer which can be given to the baby either intra-arterially, intravenously or by inhalation. The intravenous route is the most widely used method in the newborn: γ emissions can be detected over the head by a scintillator and the input function of γ irradiation measured by another scintillator over the anterior chest wall. Clearance of γ emissions is measured for 15 minutes after injection. If the brain–blood partition coefficient for the newborn brain is known, then using a mathematical deconvolution technique, an estimate of global CBF can be calculated [10]. Using ^{133}Xe, estimates of mean CBF in mechanically ventilated newborn infants have been reported to be 10 ml/100 g per min [11]. They also showed that there was a significant increase in CBF with increasing postnatal age over the first 48 hours and the CBF tended to increase with increasing mean arterial blood pressure. Babies who subsequently developed severe intracranial pressure had significantly lower CBF than those infants with a normal outcome.

Xenon-133 appears to give the most reliable estimate of global CBF in the ill newborn infant, but this technique is limited by the exposure of the infant to radiation. For obvious reasons there are no data from healthy newborn infants.

96.3.4 NEAR INFRARED SPECTROSCOPY

Light in the near infrared range penetrates tissues far better than visible light and a number of intracerebral substances absorb light in this wavelength, including oxyhaemoglobin, deoxyhaemoglobin and oxidized cytochrome aa_3. Near infrared light is applied to the head by an optode attached to the skin and an identical optode opposite the first measures the number of photons that penetrate between the transmitting and receiving optodes [12]. The technique can also be used in reflectance mode. This procedure is now possible as a bedside technique and may be used routinely on the newborn unit.

Measured changes in oxyhaemoglobin and deoxyhaemoglobin can be processed to derive cerebral blood volume and CBF. In order to do this it is necessary to provoke a small change in arterial oxygen saturation by reducing the inspired oxygen concentration [12]. This is difficult to do if the baby is breathing air, and limits the value of this technique.

The method for measuring CBF is ingenious and depends on the use of a small injection of oxyhaemoglobin into the cerebral circulation [13]. The rate of arrival and departure can be measured by an oxyhaemoglobin clip and the relative changes in oxyhaemoglobin and deoxyhaemoglobin can be measured by the near infrared spectroscopy (NIRS) signal. Using Fick's principle, CBF can be calculated. Assessment of CBF using NIRS depends on a number of assumptions which have been reasonably well validated; Skov, Pryds and Greisen [14] have shown that there is a reasonably good agreement ($r^2 = 0.84$) between assessment of CBF using ^{133}Xe and NIRS. NIRS has shown that indomethacin reduces the median values of CBF from 23 ml/100 g per min to 9 ml/100 g per min [13]. Although NIRS may give quantitative measurements of cerebral energy state, there are as yet no good data to show that cerebral metabolism can be quantified.

96.4 Measurement of intracranial pressure

Measurement of ICP may be of value in two clinical situations. The first is in babies who develop posthaemorrhagic ventricular dilatation and the second is in babies who may develop cerebral oedema as a result of hypoxic–ischaemic encephalopathy. ICP may be assessed by palpation of the anterior fontanelle. Measurement of pressure by devices attached to the anterior fontanelle has been attempted for a number of years. There are many different instruments but most have the inherent disadvantage of unreliability in the measurement of actual or true ICP. The reason for this is that changes in the application pressure when the device is attached to the fontanelle alters the registered pressure [15]. Attempts have been made to overcome this by new designs, but transfontanelle devices have not become widely used as clinical tools.

The alternative technique is the insertion of a pressure transducer or fluid-filled catheter into an intracerebral space. Neurosurgical bolts, which screw into the skull and measure extradural or subarachnoid pressure, are unacceptable because the newborn skull is too thin to support their insertion. Levene [16] has developed a percutaneously placed cannula for the measurement of subarachnoid pressure which can be inserted at the cotside in term infants with birth asphyxia. This appears to be a safe and reliable method for measuring ICP. Normal ICP in neonates ranges from 0 to 5 mmHg and Levene et al. [17] have reported pressures up to 30 mmHg in some severely asphyxiated infants. Unfortunately, in only 9% of asphyxiated babies can measurement of ICP possibly alter the outcome [17] and the impetus to measure pressure for clinical reasons in these infants has diminished.

In the preterm infant with ventricular dilatation, in whom measurement of ICP is necessary to decide whether treatment is required, most neonatologists rely on the measurement of an opening pressure at lumbar puncture or at ventricular tap. In babies with a ventricular reservoir in situ, ICP can be measured readily by placing a needle into the reservoir and attaching the line to a continuous recording chart recorder.

96.5 Neurophysiology

Small electrical potentials generated by neurons may be detected, amplified and recorded from the central nervous system and have been used to assess function in the developing brain. These techniques depend on recording potentials from the cerebral cortex, known as electroencephalography (EEG), or potentials that arise following stimulation of a particular sensory input, such as auditory, visual or sensory. These latter techniques involve computed averaging of many responses from repeated stimuli to enhance the evoked potentials and average out random potentials. These techniques have been used to detect cerebral injury and a predisposition to subsequent disability.

96.5.1 ELECTROENCEPHALOGRAPHY

EEG is a widely used technique in adult and paediatric neurology. Its role has been limited in the neonatal period because of the limitation of a full array of electrode positions, the bulkiness of the equipment and the hostile electrical environment present in many neonatal intensive care units. Recently, the development of portable and reliable techniques for continuously recording EEG activity, or a function of it (referred to as cerebral function monitoring), has widened the scope of this technique in the neonatal period, particularly in infants requiring intensive care.

The Oxford Medilog continuous four-channel EEG recorder has been quite widely evaluated in the neonatal unit for monitoring of neonatal seizures and assessing response to anticonvulsants [18–20]. This records the EEG on to a 24-hour audiotape which can then be played back and analysed. Using this technique, Connell et al. [19] reported electroconvulsive seizures to occur in 25% of high-risk neonates receiving intensive care. Of infants with EEG evidence of seizures, 42% showed no clinical signs and in only 22% did clinical seizures occur simultaneously with EEG seizure activity. In a subsequent paper Connell et al. [20] showed that the main anticonvulsants used in the neonatal period had little effect on seizure control.

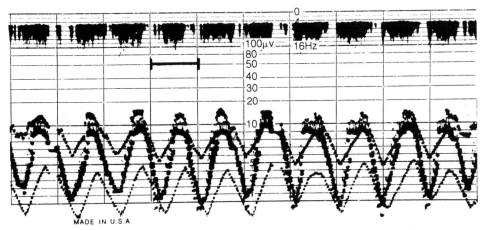

Figure 96.1   Cerebral function monitor trace showing repeated regular seizure activity lasting for approximately 30 seconds and repeated every minute.

Of 31 infants treated for EEG seizure activity, only two had a complete response and a further six had an equivocal response.

The Oxford Medilog system requires expertise in interpretation of the recorded traces and, as there is no readily available on-line system for displaying the signals, attempts have been made to modify and simplify the signal so that a compressed 'cerebral function monitor' trace can be displayed at the cotside. An increase in cerebral activity has been shown to occur with increasing gestational age and sleep–wake cycling can be readily recognized [21]. Abnormalities in the background trace as well as seizure activity can be recognized [22]. Figure 96.1 shows an example of repeated seizures recognized on continuous cerebral function monitor tracing (CFM).

Although cerebral function monitoring is a convenient method for monitoring a modified EEG signal, it may not detect short-lived seizures lasting 10 seconds or less and it is sensitive to movement artefact, which makes interpetation difficult. Some commercially available cerebral function monitors have preset filters which remove many of the high- and low-frequency signals normally found in the neonatal EEG.

96.5.2   AUDITORY BRAIN-STEM RESPONSE

The auditory brain-stem response (ABR) is also referred to as the brain-stem evoked response (BSER) and records the brain stem potentials generated following stimulation of the auditory nerve. The stimulus is produced by a repetitive click stimulus at about 10/second using a small microphone by the baby's ear. The response is recorded from scalp electrodes and consists of seven small positive waves, known conventially by the Roman numerals I to VII. These responses are collected, computer averaged and displayed on an oscilloscope. The response can be quantified by measur-

ing latency (duration of time from stimulus and any particular peak or interpeak interval) and amplitude of various waves. The latency is prolonged in preterm infants compared with term and shortens further up to 2 years of age.

The ABR may be used clinically to assess hearing and is used to quantify hearing impairment in preterm and term infants [23] and conductive causes may be distinguished from neural causes. The ABR has also been used to assess neurological function in the newborn by investigating the interpeak latency.

96.5.3   VISUAL EVOKED POTENTIAL

The stimulus used is a flashing stroboscopic light or light emitting diodes which may be built into goggles that the baby wears. The response is measured by a number of scalp electrodes and the potentials computer averaged. The visual evoked potential (VEP) shows maturation with increasing gestational age, with shortening of the latency and a more complex waveform shape. Changes in the VEP have been shown to be associated with acute haemorrhagic or ischaemic lesions in the premature neonatal brain, although these tend to mature and normalize with increasing postnatal age. Unfortunately, the VEP is relatively non-specific for visual impairment when used in the newborn period [24].

96.5.4   SOMATOSENSORY EVOKED POTENTIAL

The sensory stimulus is produced by electrical stimulation over a mixed sensory/motor nerve. The median or posterior tibial nerves are the most commonly tested. The stimulus current is increased until a twitch occurs. The responses are collected from electrodes placed over the cervical spine and scalp. Like the ABR and VEP, the somatosensory evoked potential (SEP) waveform varies

Table 96.2 Suggested protocol for routine ultrasound brain scanning

Indication	Frequency of scans
Ventilated infants ≤28 weeks	Twice weekly
Infants ≤34 weeks' gestation	Once at the end of first week
Infants with intracranial haemorrhage	Weekly until ventricular size stable
Infants outwith above indications but who develop overt clinical neurological abnormalities	At the time of neurological abnormalities
An infant with a rapidly growing head	When problem recognized
Dysmorphic babies with possible congenital brain abnormalities	At birth

with maturity and reaches adult values by 8 years. The SEP has been evaluated in preterm infants with cranial ultrasound abnormalities by stimulating the posterior tibial nerve [25]. This demonstrated that infants with ultrasound abnormalities showed consistent differences on the SEP compared with those with normal scans. These changes appeared to correlate with early neurodevelopmental outcome. Term infants have also been studied following birth asphyxia and show consistent abnormalities in the waveform which correlate with adverse outcome [26].

96.6 Practical monitoring techniques in clinical practice

The main role of these techniques in clinical practice is in imaging the neonatal brain. This is most conveniently done by using real-time ultrasonography. It is appropriate for every neonatal intensive care unit to have its own dedicated machine available for imaging 24 hours a day. Intraventricular haemorrhage occurs most frequently in the first 3 days after premature birth and the most likely consequence of this which may require intervention is posthaemorrhagic hydrocephalus. For routine purposes it is only necessary to scan prematurely born infants (<35 weeks) once at the end of the first week of life and if the scan shows intraventricular haemorrhage then repeated scans at weekly intervals will detect increasing ventricular size. A scan at the end of the first week may also pick up echodensities due to periventricular leucomalacia, but there is at present no effective therapeutic intervention in these cases, other than considering withdrawal of ventilatory care. It has been shown that the most sensitive method for the detection of those infants at highest risk of adverse neurodevelopmental outcome is a late cerebral scan. This is best done at 40 weeks' postconceptional age or immediately before discharge, depending on which comes first. Table 96.2 lists the

indications and recommended timing for routine ultrasound scans.

As indicated above, although ultrasound scans are a good screening test, they are not the best technique for picking up certain forms of pathology, particularly in term babies. All mature infants with persistent clinical neurological abnormalities should undergo CT or MRI of the brain. Suspected or actual congenital anomalies of the brain are best analysed by MRI.

Doppler has a clinical role in assessing mature newborn infants who have suffered significant birth asphyxia. The low PRI or high cerebral blood flow velocity does seem to be very sensitive and specific for outcome and this will aid clinical management.

The role of neonatal EEG is less clear. It is recognized that clinical detection of fits is very non-specific for electroconvulsive seizures, but there is no evidence that detection of subclinical seizures is of benefit. Electroconvulsive seizures may not respond to anticonvulsants and there is very little data to suggest that detection of these fits improves outcome. Nevertheless, as many critically ill infants are pharmacologically paralysed to facilitate mechanical ventilation, a case can be made for the monitoring of these infants with a CFM in order to recognize those with neurological problems who may be at greatest risk of adverse outcome. Further work must be done to design a robust and reliable neonatal CFM.

The role of neurophysiological techniques in clinical practice is very limited. Access to a good neurophysiological laboratory is of value for assessing those infants at high risk of hearing impairment in whom ABR will determine a significant deficit. It is rarely necessary to do this in a sick infant and it is probably best for the infant to be taken to the neurophysiology department for the ABR to be done.

In conclusion, several monitoring techniques aid clinical management, but these must never replace careful clinical judgement. Investigations may give misleading results and high technology will never take the place of the thoughtful clinician.

References

1. Haddad, J., Christmann, D. and Messer, J. (eds) (1991) *Imaging Techniques of the CNS of the Neonates*, Springer, Berlin.
2. Evans, D.H., McDicken, W.N., Skidmore, R. and Woodcock, J.P. (1989) *Doppler Ultrasound. Physics, Instrumentation and Clinical Applications*. Wiley, Chichester.
3. Archer, L.N.J., Levene, M.I. and Evans, D.H. (1986) Cerebral artery Doppler ultrasonography for prediction of outcome after perinatal asphyxia. *Lancet*, ii, 1116–18.
4. Levene, M.I., Fenton, A.C., Evans, D.H. *et al.* (1989) Severe birth asphyxia and abnormal cerebral blood flow velocity. *Dev. Med. Child Neurol.*, 31, 427–34.
5. Shortland, D.B., Levene, M., Archer, L.N.J. *et al.* (1990) Cerebral blood flow velocity recordings and the prediction of intracranial haemorrhage and ischaemia. *J. Perinat. Med.*, 18, 411–18.
6. Anthony, M.Y., Evans, D.H. and Levene, M.I. (1991) Cyclical variations in cerebral blood flow velocity. *Arch. Dis. Child.*, 66, 12–16.
7. Van Bel, F., Den Ouden, L., Van de Bor, M. *et al.* (1989) Cerebral blood-

flow velocity during the first week of life of preterm infants and neurodevelopment at two years. *Dev. Med. Child Neurol.*, **31**, 320–28.

8. Quinn, M.W. and Pople, I.K. (1992) Middle cerebral artery pulsatility in children with blocked cerebrospinal fluid shunts. *J. Neurol. Neurosurg. Psychiatry*, **55**, 325–27.

9. Quinn, M.W., Ando, Y. and Levene, M.I. (1992) Cerebral artery and venous flow velocity changes in post-haemorrhagic ventricular dilatation and hydrocephalus. *Dev. Med. Child Neurol.*, **34**, 863–69.

10. Greisen, G. (1988) Methods for assessing cerebral blood flow, in *Fetal and Neonatal Neurology and Neurosurgery* (eds M.I. Levene, M.J. Bennett and J. Punt), Churchill Livinstone, Edinburgh, pp. 151–61.

11. Pryds, O., Greisen, G., Lou, H. and Friis-Hansen, B. (1989) Heterogeneity of cerebral vasoreactivity in preterm infants supported by mechanical ventilation. *J. Pediatr.*, **115**, 638–45.

12. Wyatt, J.S., Edwards, A.D., Azzopardi, D. and Reynolds, E.O.R. (1989) Magnetic resonance and near infrared spectroscopy for investigation of perinatal hypoxic-ischaemic brain injury. *Arch. Dis. Child.*, **64**, 953–63.

13. Edwards, A.D., Wyatt, J.S., Richardson, C. *et al.* (1988) Cotside measurement of cerebral blood flow in ill newborn infants by near infrared spectroscopy. *Lancet*, **ii**, 770–71.

14. Skov, L., Pryds, O. and Greisen, G. (1991) Estimating cerebral blood flow in newborn infants: comparison of near infrared spectroscopy and ^{133}Xe clearance. *Pediatr. Res.*, **30**, 570–73.

15. Horbar, J.D., Yeager, S., Philip, A.G.S. and Lucey, J.F. (1980) Effect of application force on noninvasive measurements of intracranial pressure. *Pediatrics*, **66**, 455–57.

16. Levene, M.I. and Evans, D.H. (1985) The medical management of raised intracranial pressure following severe birth asphyxia. *Arch. Dis. Child.*, **60**, 12–16.

17. Levene, M.I., Evans, D.H., Forde, A. and Archer, L.N.J. (1987) Value of intracranial pressure monitoring of asphyxiated newborn infants. *Dev. Med. Child Neurol.*, **29**, 311–19.

18. Eyre, J.A., Oozeer, R.C. and Wilkinson, A.R. (1983) Diagnosis of neonatal seizure by continuous recording and rapid analysis of the electroencephalogram. *Arch. Dis. Child.*, **58**, 785–90.

19. Connell, J., Oozeer, R., De Vries, L. *et al.* (1989) Continuous EEG monitoring of neonatal seizures: diagnostic and prognostic considerations. *Arch. Dis. Child.*, **64**, 452–58.

20. Connell, J., Oozeer, R., De Vries, L. *et al.* (1989) Clinical and EEG response to anticonvulsants in neonatal seizures. *Arch. Dis. Child.*, **64**, 459–64.

21. Thornberg, E. and Thiringer, K. (1990) Normal pattern of the cerebral function monitor trace in term and preterm neonates. *Acta Paediatr. Scand.*, **79**, 20–25.

22. Hellstrom-Westas, L., Rosen, I. and Svenningsen, N.W. (1991) Cerebral function monitoring during the first week of life in extremely small low birthweight (ESLBW) infants. *Neuropediatrics*, **22**, 27–32.

23. Lary, S., Briassoulis, G., De Vries, L. *et al.* (1985) Hearing threshold in preterm and term infants by auditory brainstem response. *J. Pediatr.*, **107**, 593–99.

24. Mushin, J. (1988) Visual evoked potentials, in *Fetal and Neonatal Neurology and Neurosurgery* (eds M.I. Levene, M.J. Bennett and J. Punt), Churchill Livingstone, Edinburgh, pp. 206–12.

25. Klimach, V.J. and Cooke, R.W.I. (1988) Short-latency cortical somatosensory evoked responses of preterm infants with ultrasound abnormality of the brain. *Dev. Med. Child Neurol.*, **30**, 215–21.

26. Willis, J., Duncan, M.C. and Bell, R. (1987) Short-latency somatosensory evoked potentials in perinatal asphyxia. *Pediatr. Neurol.*, **3**, 203–207.

97 NEONATAL METABOLISM

F. Cockburn

97.1 Introduction

The normal term breast-fed human infant unaffected by maternal drugs and toxins and without damage during delivery quickly returns to the anabolic state of the fetus *in utero*. Failure to achieve anabolism within a few days of birth can result in a cessation of cell division and cell development which may have long-term effects on the infant's function and adult health. The term infant, maintained in a benign environment (indoors and well insulated by subcutaneous fat and clothing) is rarely cold stressed. Heat production during the first day after birth is fuelled almost entirely from glycogen and fat reserves because very little colostrum is ingested during that period. Where cold stress is applied, thermogenesis is predominantly non-shivering in type, and increase in the metabolism of brown adipose tissue accounts almost entirely for the increased heat production [1–4]. The metabolic adaptations which occur between fetal and neonatal life are of considerable magnitude. During late gestation fetal energy demands are small and the conservation of energy by the fetus is necessary for normal fetal growth and development. At birth near maximal rates of metabolic activity are necessary to establish breathing and maintain body temperature, which are important for infant survival and subsequent feeding behaviour and growth [5]. Maternal metabolic and hormonal environment has a large influence on nutrient partitioning and energy supply to the growing fetus [6]. Maternal homoeostatic mechanisms also regulate fetal temperature [7]. Maintenance of relatively low metabolic activity rates in the fetus is necessary for the promotion of fetal growth and the development of episodic functioning and entrainments such as fetal breathing and normal diurnal variations. There are a number of placental inhibitory factors, such as prostaglandin E_2, which inhibit the release of energy from brown adipose tissue and other fat stores [8]. Low rates of sympathetic nervous system activity and triiodothyronine production are dominant factors regulating metabolic rate during neonatal life. There is increasing evidence indicating that changes in sympathetic nervous activity and thyroid status during and following birth, together with the removal of placental and fetal inhibitory factors, are important in the regulation of neonatal metabolism and subsequent infant growth [9].

In the first few days, while breast feeding is being established, some human infant nutrient reserves are mobilized to maintain cell division and growth in most major organs. For the infant born preterm it is almost impossible to prevent disruption of genetically predetermined programmes of cellular divisions, growth, maturation and activities. The more immature the infant at birth the more difficult it is to ensure adequate nutrition. The consequences of such impaired tissue growth might well be disordered central nervous function in childhood and disordered cardiovascular function in later life. The preterm infant has a lack of nutritional reserve and immaturity of organ function, whereas in many instances the light-for-dates infant is born mature but lacks nutritional reserve.

There are inherited metabolic disorders described for nearly every metabolic process known to humans. Some already compromise the fetus before birth, some present in the newborn and others may take decades before they become manifest. Congenital malformations such as the masculinization of the female genitalia in congenital adrenal hyperplasia may give forewarning of a neonatal salt-losing crisis but many inherited metabolic disorders present with few if any diagnostic features. In this chapter only this last category of inherited metabolic defect will be described (Chapter 98).

97.2 Anabolism

The normal state of the embryo, fetus and newborn human infant is an anabolic state. An adequate supply of all essential nutrient materials, together with normal enzymatic and hormonal control, should ensure that most newborn infants sustain an anabolic state. Table 97.1 gives some relative compositions of infants born at 22, 26 and 29 weeks' gestation weighing 500–1500 g

Diseases of the Fetus and Newborn, 2nd edn, Edited by G.B. Reed, A.E. Claireaux and F. Cockburn. Published in 1995 by Chapman & Hall, London. ISBN 0 412 39160 0

Table 97.1 Relative body compositions of human infants born preterm and at term [After Ref. 10]

Gestational age (week)	22	26	29	40
Weight (g)	500	1000	1500	3500
Water (g)	433	850	1240	2380
Fat (g)	6	23	60	525
Carbohydrate (g)	2	5	15	34
Protein (g)	36	85	125	390

and a 3.5 kg infant born at 40 weeks' gestation. Virtually all of the fat, carbohydrate and protein of the preterm infant is structural, whereas in the term infant there is reserve glycogen, fat and other nutrients [1]. Once the oxygen requirements have been met the next immediate need for survival is an adequate supply of water. It has been calculated that a 1000 g preterm infant might survive 3–4 days, a term infant 30 days and an adult 90 days if supplied with water alone. In starvation states a minimal energy expenditure of about 75 kcal/kg (0.32 MJ) per 24 hours is necessary to maintain life. In the absence of fresh nutrient supply, tissue protein breakdown must commence within hours and cellular division and therefore growth must cease. In the preterm infant there is virtually no reserve of free amino acids and when new functional peptides and proteins, such as hormones and enzymes, have to be manufactured they can only be obtained at the expense of the structural proteins in the infant's organs, such as muscle and liver. At the same time there will be breakdown of structural lipid and carbohydrate. The relative excess of water, particularly extracellular water in preterm as compared with term infants, confers no protection against dehydration since the obligatory daily turnover of water is equal to 15–20% of the total body water pool. Table 97.2 shows the mineral content of a 26-week infant expressed in terms of fat-free body tissue compared with the composition at term [10]. The distribution of minerals between those found at 26 weeks and at 40 weeks alters as the ratio between

Table 97.2 Mineral content of preterm infants born at 26 and 34 weeks' gestation compared with that of a 40-week infant [After Ref. 10]

	Gestation (weeks)		
Minerals[a]	26	34	40
Sodium (mmol)	94	200	286
Potassium (mmol)	42	108	185
Chloride (mmol)	68	139	192
Calcium (g)	6.3	19	33.6
Phosphorus (g)	3.9	11.9	19.6
Magnesium (g)	0.2	0.58	0.91
Iron (mg)	65	200	229
Copper (mg)	3.4	8.8	16.4
Zinc (mg)	20	40	70

[a] Minerals are expressed in terms of fat-free body tissue.

intracellular and extracellular fluid alters, and different tissues have differing contents of minerals, e.g. high concentrations of calcium, phosphorus, magnesium, zinc and sodium in bone, and high concentrations of copper and iron in liver. The quantities of chromium, selenium, sulphur, molybdenum, manganese, cobalt, iodine and fluorine also increase with maturation and these elements are known to be involved in normal infant metabolic processes. Deficiences of iodine, for example, can severely affect thyroxine and triiodothyronine function. The fetal and neonatal concentrations of water-soluble and fat-soluble vitamins are dealt with in Chapter 81.

97.3 Catabolism

After birth, heat production by brown adipose tissue and hepatic triiodothyronine synthesis is stimulated and there is a transition from a net anabolic to a catabolic state as the glycogen and lipid reserves are mobilized to meet the required three to fourfold increase in metabolic rate [1]. The extent of these adaptations is strongly influenced by the state of maternal nutrition in late pregnancy and by the maturity of the infant at birth. Human infants are entirely dependent on non-shivering thermogenesis in order to increase metabolic rate at birth, although this process takes several hours to become fully effective [1,11]. The extent to which infants are capable of maintaining body temperature is influenced by the immediate postpartum environment. Infants kept in skin-to-skin contact with the mother have axillary, interscapula and skin temperatures 0.3–1.0°C above those placed in a cot [12], and delivery by caesarean section results in lower body temperatures than in those delivered vaginally [13]. Such differences in thermoregulatory ability may be related to the sensitivity of brown adipose tissue to β-adrenergic stimulation and to the plasma concentrations of thyroid hormones [6]. The extent to which the infant can survive without an adequate early exogenous source of food is dependent upon the maturity of the infant at birth and the level of endogenous energy stores. Exogenous nutritional requirements are met through the process of suckling.

97.4 Infant feeding

To achieve the satisfactory establishment of feeding, an intact brain stem is essential. Most of the reflexes which subserve feeding are regulated through the brain stem and ensure normal rooting, suckling and the co-ordination of swallowing, gag and the other reflexes necessary to ensure the transmission of food from the mother's breast to the infant gastrointestinal tract. There are major changes in gut structure and function and in intermediary metabolism after term birth [14].

In altricial species milk is not only a source of nutrition but is essential to ensure gastrointestinal development [15]. Gut hormones act as mediators of the postnatal effects of enteral feeding. There are multiple gut hormone surges associated with bolus enteral feeds where some plasma hormone concentrations reach values exceeding those found in adults. Enteral glucagon and gastrin probably induce gut growth and proliferation of gut mucosa, while increasing circulating motilin and neurotensin stimulate gut motility. Gastric inhibitory peptide enhances insulin release and glucose tolerance. Glucagon secretion probably switches on the activity and synthesis of hepatic enzymes, including phospho-enol pyruvate carboxykinase and enzymes essential for gluconeogenesis. Ingestion of human milk results in a different neuroendocrine response to that obtained in formula-fed infants. Preterm infants fed by continuous infusion into the stomach or duodenum have blunted or absent gut peptide release, as do infants fed parenterally. Bolus ingestion of human colostrum and milk is probably important in the promotion of normal gut growth and function [14].

There are many factors present in human milk, including hormones and growth promoting factors, which may well be essential for normal human gut growth and development. Hormones reported to be present in human milk include oestrogens, progestogens, thyroxine, insulin, thyroid-stimulating hormone, luteinizing hormone releasing hormone, thyrotrophin-releasing hormone, adrenocorticotrophic hormone, prolactin, calcitonin, melatonin and prostaglandins. Growth promoting factors found in human milk include epidermal growth factor and insulin-like growth factor 1. Epidermal growth factor is present in human milk in concentrations many times greater than in plasma and probably accounts for over 70% of the mitogenic activity of human milk on cultured human fibroblasts [16].

In addition to these nutrient promoting and controlling factors, human colostrum and milk contain macrophages, T and B lymphocytes, polymorphonuclear leucocytes and other factors which protect the newborn against infection. It is difficult to differentiate 'simple' nutrients from the many cellular and complex chemical substances ingested by the newborn infant, which, after fulfilling their function, may well be used as a source of energy or indeed as elements for new tissue synthesis. The heat production of the newborn infant in an ambient temperature of 32–38°C is about 6.9 kJ/h per kg. The respiratory quotient during the first 24 hours varies between 0.85 in the first 2 hours and 0.80 by the end of 24 hours [1]. Infants consume about 70 ml/kg of colostrum during the first day after birth. Exposure to air temperatures of 15°C has produced a recorded rate of heat production of 19 kJ/h per kg [17]. The energy obtained from the colostrum cannot meet the basic

energy requirement of the infant in the first 24 hours, never mind that associated with cooling. Hence the need for the reserves of fat and glycogen.

After birth, colostrum provides 100 mg secretory IgA per millimetre which gives mucous membrane and intestinal mucosa protection. This secretory IgA contains specific immunoglobulin determined by the type of micro-organisms to which the mother had been exposed in her life [18–20]. Other protective materials identified in colostrum and milk include complement, lysozyme, lactoferrin, lactoperoxidase and fatty acids, particularly linoleic, lauric and palmitoleic acids [21]. Despite the existence of these multiple mechanisms which control microbial populations at mucosal surfaces, the mucous membranes remain an important portal of entry for infection. Bifidobacteria which colonize the small intestine of breast-fed human infants are encouraged by the presence of a bifidus factor found in human milk [22]. There are many active enzymes present in human milk some of which, like amylase, may be predominantly protective and others, such as lipases, which predigest the triglyceride and other lipids in human milk as they are being swallowed by the infant.

Modified cow milk preparations and 'milks' of vegetable origin can contain none of these living and bioactive substances but do provide the inert elements of nutrition. These elements have to be synthesized into peptides, proteins, enzymes, hormones, etc. and this requires the enzyme systems as well as the substrate necessary for their synthesis. The newborn human infant and particularly the preterm infant may have enzyme systems which are absent or inadequate for these purposes. In spite of this, when preterm and term infants are given complete parenteral nutrition with virtually no living or bioactive substance present, anabolism and tissue growth can be achieved [23]. There is no doubt that the mother's own milk, including the 'preterm milk' of mothers delivering before term, provides nutrient advantages to the human infant. The infant born preterm is an unphysiological creature and there may well be advantage in providing complementary milk either in the form of concentrated human milk or synthetic formula with increased concentrations of protein, energy, sodium, calcium, phosphorus, magnesium, copper, zinc and vitamins. Clinical trial data have indicated a number of potential advantages and disadvantages of currently available diets, including faster weight gain, length gain, brain growth and a reduced incidence of metabolic bone disease, jaundice, hyponatraemia, anaemia, vitamin deficiencies and metabolic upsets in the preterm human infant [24–26]. Many data pertaining to growth and development published in the paediatric literature during the past 50 years have been based on populations containing a varying percentage of breast-fed and bottle-fed infants.

Many infant formulae fed during this time had a high protein content. Recent results from the DARLING Study indicate that formula feeding is not advantageous as the extra protein consumed is offset by an increase in energy expenditure, decreased efficiency of nitrogen utilization and an increase in fat deposition, as well as imposing a greater metabolic stress on the liver and kidneys [27,28]. These differences in tissue content and metabolic adaptation between breast-fed and formula-fed infants are in part mediated by altered endocrine responses to feeding, e.g. the different amino acid content of formula stimulates insulin secretion and increases the molar insulin/glucagon ratio and causes an enhanced rate of lipid deposition [29,30]

97.4.1 GLUCOSE METABOLISM

Glucose is the major substrate for carbohydrate metabolism in the newborn infant. The infant plasma concentration at birth depends on factors such as the timing of the last maternal meal, the duration of labour, the route of delivery and any intravenous fluid administered to the mother. After normal delivery the plasma glucose concentration declines to approximately 50 mg/dl by 2 hours of age but equilibrates at approximately 70 mg/dl by 72 hours after birth [31]. In the term infant a plasma glucose concentration of less than 30 mg/dl on the first day of life and less than 40 mg/dl on the second day are the limits set for the definition of hypoglycaemia in the term infant [32]. Values for hypoglycaemia in the preterm infant should be no different from those given for the term infant [33]. Hyperglycaemia is defined as a concentration of more than 125 mg/dl [34].

Physical signs of neonatal hypoglycaemia are an apathetic weak cry, recurrent apnoeic attacks, cardiac arrest, generalized multifocal seizures, cyanosis, hypothermia, muscular hypotonia, jitteriness, lethargy and occasionally tachypnoea. Failure to correct perinatal hypoglycaemia can have adverse affects on subsequent intellectual development. Preterm infants and infants who are small for their gestational age have increased frequency of hypoglycaemia. Infants experiencing perinatal hypoxaemia, cold-stressed infants and infants with neonatal sepsis and congenital heart disease, with or without congestive heart failure, are also subject to hypoglycaemia. Hypoglycaemia is also a feature of infants with hyperinsulinaemia related to maternal hyperglycaemia or to maternal alcohol consumption but it may also be due to the hyperinsulinism associated with haemolytic diseases, pancreatic nesidioblastosis, pancreatic islet cell adenomata and the Beckwith–Wiedemann syndrome. Type 1 glycogen storage disease (glucose-6-phosphatase deficiency) is an autosomal recessive genetic defect which presents with severe hypoglycaemia and hepatomegaly, and fructose-l, 6-diphosphatase deficiency is also associated with hypoglycaemia [35–38].

Galactosaemia is a recessively inherited condition usually due to a defect in galactose-l-phosphate uridyltransferase but may be due to kinase and epimerase defects. In the more common transferase defect there can be severe hypoglycaemia with convulsions and hepatocellular jaundice. Exclusion of milk and milk products (lactose) is essential to prevent further tissue, particularly brain tissue, damage. Hereditary fructose tolerance will not become evident until sucrose or other fructose-containing sugars are added to the diet. Maternal chlorpropamide ingestion has been reported to result in postnatal hypoglycaemia, as have thiazide diuretics [39–40]. Hypoglycaemia is also found in individuals sensitive to the amino acid leucine, in whom there is increased insulin release after ingestion of milk [41]. Lethal hypoglycaemia has been reported in the child with a deficiency of 3-hydroxy-3-methylglutaryl coenzyme A lyase [42]. Hypoglycaemia is also found in children with adrenocortical failure, as in congenital adrenal hyperplasia [43].

Neonatal hyperglycaemia presents with failure to thrive and dehydration, usually in a markedly small for gestational age infant. Probably the major cause of hyperglycaemia in the newborn period at present is secondary to the use of parenteral nutrition. The amount of dextrose infusion should be reduced if the hyperglycaemia is due to this. Exogenous insulin to maintain euglycaemia may be required in occasional infants. Many of the small for gestational age infants with hyperglycaemia 'lose' their hyperinsulinaemia over the first 5–6 weeks of life. Many of these infants develop true diabetes in later life.

Hormonal regulation of glucose homoeostasis is largely controlled by the relative concentrations of insulin and glucagon but there can be major influences of other contrainsulin hormones relative to the quantity of available insulin [44]. Glucocorticoids and insulin mediate the glycogen accumulation rate during fetal life and although muscle glycogenolysis supplies lactate, which is subsequently oxidized by neonatal tissue to act as a substrate until glucose and ketones are available, liver glycogenolysis and gluconeogenesis are switched on to maintain euglycaemia postnatally. Noradrenaline is a very active contra-insulin hormone which can result in rapid fluctuations in circulating glucose concentrations. Hepatic fetal receptors for the hormones of glucose homoeostasis may also regulate the response of fetal and neonatal tissues to the actions of insulin, glucagon and noradrenaline [45]. In the term infant the gluconeogenic pathway can be demonstrated 6 hours after birth but in the infant born preterm there is sometimes difficulty in demonstrating activity in this pathway [46]. It has been estimated that about half of the glucose produced in gluconeogenic activities is oxidized and about one-third is recycled. The remaining 20% represents local oxidation of tissue glycogen stores [47]. Glucose is the major substrate for brain metabolism, although ketones, glycerol and lactate can have a lesser role. Hypoxia and circulatory failure can result in a switch to an anaerobic metabolism and a 'wasteful' use of available glucose and tissue accumulation of lactate. If this process or hypoglycaemia and metabolic acidaemia persists for any length of time there can be permanent neurological damage.

97.4.2 PROTEIN METABOLISM

The total protein content of a 20-week fetus is about 8.5% of the body weight, whereas at birth this percentage is about 11%. In the adult human 17.5% of the body weight is protein. Nearly half of the protein in the adult is contained in skeletal striated muscle but in the 1.5 kg preterm infant only 20% of the total body mass is muscle tissue. There is virtually no reserve of free amino acid and in the absence of a supply of amino acids tissue protein breakdown must commence. Protein synthesis takes place in the cell cytoplasm from the component amino acids and is an energy consuming process controlled by the DNA template and messenger RNA. The energy requirement for protein synthesis is considerable. Synthesis of one peptide bond requires four high energy bonds from ATP and GTP respectively. One mole of glucose is known to yield 38 moles of high energy phosphate under aerobic conditions and 2 moles of high energy phosphate under anaerobic conditions. Based on an energy need of 6 moles ATP for the incorporation of 1 mole amino acid into a polypeptide chain the theoretical value for the cost of protein gain would be 1 kcal/g. Methods for establishing the true metabolic cost of protein synthesis have not yet been established. In very-low-birth-weight infants up to 70% of the absorbed amino acids are used for protein synthesis and the remaining 30% are oxidized for energy. It is likely that a similar amount of ATP would be required to process the protein degradation which occurs as part of normal development. The availability of substrate for protein synthesis in the form of amino acids, glucose, fatty acids and glycerol will also affect the ability to synthesis and degrade protein. Substrate supply by the enteral route does not normally meet these requirements until the end of the first week of postnatal life in the term infant. The hormonal disequilibrium caused by stress with increased circulating concentrations of catecholamines, glucocorticosteroids and growth hormone with their anti-insulin effects inhibit protein synthesis and tend to promote gluconeogenesis. In stress situations there is increased renal nitrogen excretion. Glucocorticosteroids and glucagon stimulate the synthesis of acute phase protein in the liver whilst inhibiting protein synthesis in muscle. Attempts to increase the amino acid intake of preterm infants in order to achieve the intrauterine growth rate may result in amino acid overload and potentially toxic concentrations of some amino acids. Casein-predominant formulas contain relatively high amounts of tyrosine, phenylalanine and methionine and can give rise to concentrations of these amino acids potentially toxic to the developing brain.

Whereas in fetal life the basic building blocks are supplied from the placenta directly to the fetus, after birth the newborn infant has to digest milk proteins enzymatically into resorbable amino acids and oligopeptides. This requires protelytic enzymes in the stomach and pancreas as well as the intestinal brush border. The relatively high concentration of free amino acids and peptides in human milk probably enhances the release of gastrin and cholecystokinin which promote the release of proteolytic enzymes [48]. The passage of heterologous food proteins such as β-lactoglobulin through the mucosal wall during early postnatal life may induce hypersensitization to cow's milk. Soy proteins may also induce allergic features in atopic infants through a similar process. In addition to the eight amino acids considered essential for the adult (tryptophan, phenylalanine, leucine, isoleucine, threonine, methionine, lysine and valine), quantities of cystine, taurine, histidine and arginine may need to be given to immature infants to ensure optimal protein synthetic rates. In the growing fetus, infant and child essential and non-essential amino acids are required for the synthesis of new tissue and its seems inappropriate not to supply a completely balanced input of essential and non-essential amino acids.

97.4.3 LIPID METABOLISM

Mature human milk has a fat content of 3.5–4.5%. This fat is contained within membrane-enclosed milk fat globules with the core of the globule comprised of triglycerides and the membrane composed of phospholipids, cholesterol and proteins. The packaging of the triglyceride within the globule permits dispersion of the lipids in the aqueous environment of milk and protects them from hydrolysis by milk lipases [49–51]. There are changes in milk fat content and composition during lactation. In colostrum secreted during the first 3 days post partum the total fat content is approximately 2%, whereas in mature milk the value increases up to 4.5% [52]. Phospholipids and cholesterol are in higher concentration in colostrum than in mature human milk. Medium chain fatty acids comprise approximately 10% of the total fatty acids in mature milk. Saturated fatty acids constitute 42% and unsaturated 57% of the total lipid in human milk. Essential fatty acid concentrations are greater in colostrum and transitional milk than in mature milk. Long chain polyunsaturated fatty acids derived from linoleic acid and from linolenic acid are in significantly greater concentration in colostrum and in preterm mothers' milk than in the mature milk of mothers with term infants. The major differences between human milk and infant formulae are the absence of long chain unsaturated fatty acids in formulae and the presence of only traces of cholesterol compared with the higher concentrations of both in human milk. Milk fat composition can be affected by the maternal diet. In women consuming large amounts of hydrogenated fat in margarines the milk trace fatty acid content increases markedly [53]. Maternal hyperlipaemia, cystic fibrosis and diabetes can all markedly affect the quantity and quality of fat in human milk. A high fish diet, as in the Inuit, will increase the concentration of docosahexaenoic acid (DHA) content. More than 95% of dietary fat, including that in human milk and infant formula, is triglyceride. Digestion and absorption of dietary fat involves:

1. a luminal phase of solubilization and hydrolysis of triglycerides to free fatty acids, monoglycerides and glycerol prior to their uptake by intestinal mucosa;
2. a mucosal phase which involves the re-esterification of fatty acids to form triglycerides that are incorporated into chylomicrons and very-low-density lipoproteins (VLDL) before their release from the mucosal cell into the blood via the lymphatics;
3. a transport and delivery phase during which the fatty acids within chylomicrons and VLDL are taken up by individual tissues for their metabolic needs.

Ketone bodies produced during fatty acid catabolism are important metabolites for the infant. Acetate is metabolized by the mitochondria and energy is released. Ketone bodies can provide a major source of energy for the developing brain in many species, including humans, and there is considerable activity of the enzymes which convert ketone bodies to acetyl-coA in newborn infant tissues.

97.4.4 DIETARY FATS AND TISSUE PHOSPHOLIPIDS

In mammals membrane lipids are mainly phosphoglycerols and unesterified cholesterols. In neuronal membranes there are also sphingomyelins (phosphosphingolipids and cerebrosides) and glycosphingolipids, where the phospholipids are sphingosine (an amino alcohol) based rather than glycerol based (phosphoglycerols). Phospholipids are amphilic (like both water and lipid) because they have chemical groupings at one end which are hydrophilic (like water) and at the other end hydrophobic (dislike water). This property makes these molecules have the unique ability to permit interactions between the wide range of water-soluble and fat-soluble substances whilst limiting movement of water and other substances between the outside and inside of the membrane, whether it is a cell membrane or an intracellular membrane, e.g. mitochondrial. Membrane lipid provides a flexible and adaptable structure into which are inserted proteins and glycoproteins such as enzymes, transmembrane transporter proteins or receptors, for example, for hormones, growth factors and antigens. Ethylenic double bonds in mono- and polyunsaturated fatty acids provide a site of chemical reactivity. Saturated fatty acids and those containing *trans* double bonds tend to adopt a straighter and more rigid configuration. Thus membranes with higher concentrations of *cis* double bonds are more flexible and more permeable. Membrane thickness, elasticity, porosity and ability to support or transmit other molecules also depend on the organic bases such as choline, ethanolamine, serine or inositol which are attached to the phosphoglycerides. There is no known control mechanism for the determination of the siting and type of phospholipid in the lipid bilayers of membranes. Whereas protein synthesis will cease if essential amino acid supplies are deficient, incorporation of fatty acids into membrane phospholipids will proceed and it would appear that the next nearest available fatty acid will be substituted, thus altering the properties and fluidity of that membrane. Stability of mammalian membranes is crucially dependent upon the presence of longer chain polyunsaturated fatty acids [54]. In fatty acid deficiency states essential fatty acids of the ω-3 and ω-6 series are replaced by non-essential fatty acids of the ω-9 family. The membrane becomes metabolically unstable and more permeable to water. Where there is a deficiency of ω-3 series alone then ω-6 fatty acids may substitute for them. Neuronal and retinal membranes have a highly selective uptake and esterification of polyunsaturated fatty acids. After birth neuronal membranes and photoreceptor cells derive most of their high phospholipid DHA ($C_{22:6}$,ω-3) content from diet and liver synthesis rather than from neuronal synthesis. Most of this DHA is incorporated in the form of phosphatidylethanolamine and phosphatidylserine. The retina has extracellular and intracellular DHA binding proteins and a high affinity DHA acyl-CoA synthetase [5]. Neither the liver nor the retinal and neuronal cells can synthesize DHA if there is inadequate precursor essential fatty acid (α-linolenic acid) or if the elongases, desaturases, synthetases and acyl-transferases are not yet activated or inactivated. When human milk is consumed a supply of ready-synthesized DHA and arachidonic acid (AA) is available. Many infant formulae contain little or no DHA or AA and in some there is insufficient essential fatty acid precursor to allow for their synthesis. Evidence from animal studies suggests that retinal function and learning ability are permanently impaired if there is a failure in the accumulation of sufficient DHA during development [56–58].

Low-birth-weight infants, whether born preterm, light for date or both, are the most vulnerable to the effects of fatty acid deficiency states [59,60]. A significant reduction in cerebral cortex DHA in both term and preterm infants fed on artificial formulae compared with those fed human milk has recently been described [61]. Phosphatidylethanolamine in the cerebral cortex of breast-fed infants contained significantly more DHA than formula-fed infants and the deficiency in the ω-3 series in the brain phospholipids was substituted by the ω-6 series so that the total ω-6 fatty acid content in the formula-fed infants' brains exceeds that in the breast-fed infants. Similar findings were demonstrated for phosphatidylserine. In preterm infants the brain contains more ω-9 series fatty acids, probably indicating a deficiency of both the long chain polyunsaturated fatty acids of the ω-3 and ω-6 series (J. Farquharson et al., unpublished data). Preterm infants fed artificial formulae supplemented with DHA have improvements in their visual acuity and in their perception, memory, learning, problem solving, vocalization, early verbal communication and abstract thinking [62]. There is an urgent need for further research into the short-term and long-term consequences of the feeding of artificial formulae, whether milk or vegetable based, to human infants. All mothers should be encouraged to feed their babies naturally.

97.5   Clinical features of inherited metabolic diseases in the newborn

Inherited metabolic diseases are individually rare but have been described as affecting virtually every metabolic process known to man. Thus, collectively, inborn errors of metabolism have become a major cause of neonatal pathology. The incidence may well be underestimated as diagnostic errors are frequent [3,4]. Every newborn with unexplained neurological deterioration, ketosis, metabolic acidosis or hypoglycaemia should be suspected of having an inherited metabolic error of intermediary metabolism (Table 97.3). A high index of suspicion and rapid diagnosis can prevent death and severe neurological damage in a significant number of affected infants and will ensure adequate prenatal diagnosis in subsequent pregnancies. The newborn human infant has a limited repertoire of response to severe illness, whether caused by overwhelming infections or metabolic defects. Most inborn errors of intermediary metabolism fall into two categories: 'intoxications' and 'energy deficiencies'.

Intoxications are secondary to an accumulation of toxic compounds, such as branched chain ketoacids in maple syrup urine disease, most organic acidurias, urea cycle defects, galactosaemia, fructosaemia and tyrosinaemia. The clinical features (vomiting, lethargy, coma,

Table 97.3   Neonatal neurological distress [After Ref. 63]

Energy deficiencies
Respiratory chain disorders
Peroxisomal disorders
Fatty acid oxidation disorders

Neurotransmitter defects
Glycine (non-ketotic hyperglycinaemia, D-glycericaciduria)
GABA (transaminase, 4-hydroxybutyric aciduria)
Dopa, serotonin (biopterin synthesis deficiencies)

Disturbed metabolism of complex lipids
Plasmalogen (peroxisomal disorders)
Acylcholesterol, dolichol
Mevalonic, 3-hydroxyglutaconic acidurias
3-Ketothiolase deficiency

Intracellular vitamin disturbances
Folic acid, vitamins B_{12}, B_6, etc.

Metals
Molybdenum (sulphite oxidase deficiency)
Copper (Menkes' disease)

Others

Table 97.4   Initial investigations [After Ref. 63]

Urine	Smell
	Acetone
	Reducing substances
	Ketoacids (dinitrophenylhydrazine test)
	Sulphites (Sulfitest, Merck)
	pH
Blood	Blood cell count
	Electrolytes (look for anion gap)
	Calcium
	Glucose
	Blood gases (pH, P_{CO_2}, HCO_3, P_{O_2})
	Ammonia
	Lactic acid, pyruvic acid
	3-Hydroxybutyrate, acetoacetate
	Uric acid
Store at $-20°C$	Urine (as much as possible)
	Heparinized plasma, 2–5 ml)
	Do not freeze whole blood!
	CSF, 0.5–1.0 ml
Miscellaneous	EEG, bacteriological samples, chest radiograph, lumbar puncture, cardiac echography, cerebral ultrasonogram

liver failure, acidosis, ketosis, hyperammonaemia) are common to most of these conditions. Treatment has to be aimed initially at removal of the toxic metabolites by peritoneal or haemodialysis, exchange transfusion and special diets.

Energy deficiencies are due, in part at least, to a deficiency of energy production or a defect in utilization. Defects of gluconeogenesis, congenital lactic acidaemias (pyruvate carboxylase and dehydrogenase deficiencies), fatty acid oxidation defects, disorders of the mitochondrial respiratory chain and disorders of peroxisomal metabolism belong to this group. Clinical features common in this group include severe hypotonia, cardiomyopathy, failure to thrive, circulatory collapse, sudden infant death and hyperlactic acidaemia. There may also be congenital malformations such as absent corpus callosum and cerebral malformations with congenital lactic acidaemia and facial and bone anomalies with peroxisomal defects. There can be overlapping of the clinical features between the toxic and energy deficient disorders when there is accumulation of toxic compounds in addition to a deficiency of energy production. A third category of clinical presentation is with hypoglycaemia and liver dysfunction. Convulsions and hepatomegaly with ketosis and lactic acidosis are the usual presenting features. The main diseases in this group are the glycogen storage diseases. Table 97.4 gives a list of initial investigations which can help categorize the metabolic disorders. More specialized investigations such as amino and organic acid analyses can then be arranged. If the child dies it is important to have obtained urine, plasma, white cell DNA, fibroblast culture and muscle and liver biopsy, stored deep frozen. Subsequent analyses may help determine the nature of the metabolic defect and allow proper genetic counselling to be given to the family (Chapters 61, 63, 74 and 77).

References

1. Mellor, D.J. and Cockburn, F. (1986) Comparison of energy metabolism in the newborn infant, piglet and lamb. *Q. J. Exp. Physiol.*, 71, 361–79.
2. Heim, T. (1983) Energy and lipid requirements of the fetus and preterm infant. *J. Pediatr. Gastroenterol. Nutr.*, 2 (suppl. 1), S16–41.
3. Saint, L., Smith, M. and Hartmann, P.E. (1984) The yield and nutrient content of colostrum and milk of women from giving birth to one month post-partum. *Br. J. Nutr.*, 52, 87–95.
4. Bruck, K. (1961) Temperature regulation in the newborn infant. *Biol. Neonate*, 3, 65–119.
5. Jansen, A.H. and Chiernick, V. (1991) Fetal breathing and development of control of breathing. *J. Appl. Physiol.*, 70, 1431–46.
6. Symonds, M.E. and Lomax, M.A. (1992) Maternal and environmental influences on thermo-regulation in the neonate. *Proc. Nutr. Soc.*, 51, 165–72.
7. Gluckman, P.D., Gunn, T.R., Johnston, B.M. and Quinn, J.P. (1984) Manipulation of the temperature of the fetal lamb *in utero*, in *Animal Models in Fetal Medicine* (ed. P.W. Nathanielsz), Perinatology Press, New York, pp. 37–56.
8. Gunn, T.R., Ball, K.T. and Gluckman, P.D. (1993) Withdrawal of placental prostaglandins permits thermogenic responses in fetal sheep brown adipose tissue. *J. Appl. Physiol.*, 74, 998–1004.
9. Symonds, M.E., Clarke, L. and Lomax, M.A. (1994) The regulation of neonatal metabolism and growth, in *Early Fetal Growth and Development*, Proceedings of the 27th Study Group of the Royal College of Obstetricians and Gynaecologists (eds R.H.T. Ward, S.K. Smith and D. Donnai), RCOG Press, London, pp. 407–19.
10. Widdowson, E.M. and Dickerson, J.W.T. (1964) Mineral metabolism, in *Chemical Composition of the Body*, vol. 2A (eds C.L. Connor and F. Browner), Academic Press, New York, pp. 1–247.
11. Smales, O.R.C. and Kime, R. (1978) Thermal regulation in babies immediately after birth. *Arch. Dis. Child.*, 53, 58–61.
12. Christensson, K., Siles, C., Moreno, L. *et al.* (1992) Temperature, metabolic adaptation and crying in healthy full-term newborns cared for skin-to-skin or in a cot. *Acta Paediatr.*, 81, 488–93.
13. Christensson, K., Siles, C., Carbera, T. *et al.* (1993) Lower body temperatures in infants delivered by caesarean section than in vaginally delivered infants. *Acta Paediatr.*, 82, 128–31.
14. Aynsley-Green, A. (1988) The adaptation of the human neonate to extra uterine nutrition; a pre-requisite for postnatal growth, in *Fetal and Neonatal Growth* (ed. F. Cockburn), Wiley, Chichester, pp. 153–93.
15. Weaver, L.T. (1992) Breast and gut: the relationship between lactating mammary function and neonatal gastrointestinal function. *Proc. Nutr. Soc.*, 51, 155–63.
16. Read, L.C. (1988) Milk growth factors, in *Fetal and Neonatal Growth* (ed. F. Cockburn), Wiley, Chichester, pp. 131–152.
17. Adamsons, K., Gandy, G.M. and James, L.S. (1965) The influence of thermal factors upon oxygen consumption of the newborn human infant. *J. Pediatr.*, 66, 495–508.
18. Allardyce, R.A., Shearman, D.J.C, McClelland, D.B.L. *et al.* (1974) Appearance of specific colostrum antibodies after clinical infection with *Salmonella typhimurium*. *BMJ*, iii, 307–309.
19. Goldblum, R.M., Ahlstedt, S. Carlsson, B. *et al.* (1975) Antibody-forming cells in human colostrum after oral immunisation. *Nature*, 257, 797–98.
20. Ogra, P.L. and Dayton, D.H. (1990) *Immunology of Breast Milk*, Raven Press, New York.
21. Goldman, A.S., Garza, C., Nichols, B.L. and Goldblum, R.M. (1982) Immunologic factors in human milk during the first year of lactation. *J. Pediatr.*, 100, 563–67.
22. Beerens, H., Romond, C. and Neut, C. (1980) Influence of breast-feeding on the bifid flora of the newborn intestine. *Am. J. Clin. Nutr.*, 33 (suppl.), 2434–39.
23. Cockburn, F. (1976) The place of parenteral nutrition in the preterm infant. *Curr. Med. Res. Opin.*, 4 (Suppl. 1); 90–99.
24. Wharton, B.A. (1987) *Nutrition and Feeding of Preterm Infants*, Blackwell Scientific, Oxford.
25. Lucas, A. (1987) Does diet in preterm infants influence clinical outcome? *Biol. Neonate*, 52 (suppl. 1), 14.
26. Cockburn, F. (1983) Milk composition – the infant human diet. *Proc. Nutr. Soc.*, 42, 361–73.
27. Heinig, M.J., Nommsen, L.A. and Peerson, J.M. *et al.* (1993) Energy and protein intakes of breast-fed and formula-fed infants during the first year of life and their association with growth velocity: the DARLING study. *Am. J. Clin. Nutr.*, 58, 152–61.
28. Whyte, R.K. and Bayley, H.S. (1990) Energy metabolism of the newborn infant, in *Advances in Nutritional Research*, vol. 8 (ed. H.H. Draper), Plenum Press, New York, pp. 79–108.
29. Salmenpera, L., Perheentupa, J., Silmes, M.A. *et al.* (1988) Effects of feeding regimen on blood glucose levels and plasma concentrations of pancreatic hormones and gut regulatory peptide at 9 months of age: comparison between infants fed with milk formula and infants exclusively breast-fed from birth. *J. Pediatr. Gastroenterol. Nutr.*, 7, 651–56.
30. Girard, J., Ferre, P., Pegorier, J.P. and Duee, P.H. (1992) Adaptations of glucose and fatty acid metabolism during perinatal period and suckling–weaning transition. *Physiol. Rev.*, 72, 507–62.
31. Cornblath, M. and Schwartz, R. (1976) *Disorders of Carbohydrate Metabolism in Infancy*, 2nd edn, W.B. Saunders, Philadelphia.
32. Heck, L.J. and Erenberg, A. (1987) Serum glucose levels in the term neonate during the first 48 hours of life. *Pediatrics*, 110, 119–22.
33. Koh, T.H., Aynsley-Green, A., Tarbit, M. *et al.* (1988) Neural dysfunction and hypoglycaemia. *Arch. Dis. Child.*, 63, 1353–58.
34. Pildes, R.S. (1986) Neonatal hyperglycemia. *J. Pediatr.*, 109, 905–907.
35. Hers, H.G., Van Hoof, F. and de Barsy, T. (1989) Glycogen storage diseases, in *The Metabolic Basis of Inherited Disease* (eds C.R. Scriver, A.L. Beaudet, W.S. Sly and D. Valle), McGraw-Hill, New York, pp. 425–52.
36. Pagliara, A.S., Karl, I.E., Keating, J.P. *et al.* (1972) Hepatic fructose-1,6-diphosphatase deficiency, a cause of lactic acidosis and hypoglycaemia in infancy. *J. Clin. Invest.*, 51, 2115–23.
37. Rawleson, M.I., Mukle, A.W. and Zigrang, W.D. (1979) Hypoglycemia and lactate acidosis associated with fructose-1,6-diphosphatase deficiency. *J. Pediatr.*, 94, 933–36.
38. Vidnes, J. and Sovic, O. (1976) Gluconeogenesis in infancy and childhood; deficiency of the extra mitochondrial form of hepatic phosphoenol pyruvate carboxykinase in a case of persistent neonatal hypoglycaemia. *Acta Paediatr.*, 65, 307–12.
39. Zucker, P. and Simon, G. (1968) Prolonged symptomatic neonatal hypoglycemia associated with maternal chlorpropamide therapy. *Pediatrics*, 42, 824–25.
40. Senior, B., Slone, D., Shapiro, S. *et al.* (1976) Benzothiadiazides and neonatal hypoglycemia. *Lancet*, ii, 377.
41. Brownere, R.E. and Young, R.B. (1970) Possible role for the exocrine pancreas in the pathogenesis of neonatal leucine sensitive hypoglycemia. *Am. J. Dig. Dis.*, 15, 65–72.
42. Schutgens, R.B.H., Heymans, H., Ketel, A. *et al.* (1979) Lethal hypoglycaemia in a child with a deficiency of 3-hydroxy-3-methyl glutaryl co-enzyme A lyase. *J. Pediatr.*, 94, 89–91.

43. Actavia-Loria, E., Chaussain, J.L., Bogneres, P.F. *et al.* (1986) Frequency of hypoglycaemia in children with adrenal insufficiency. *Acta Endocrinol. Suppl.*, **279**, 275–78.
44. Mayor, F. and Cuezva, J.M. (1985) Hormonal and metabolic changes in the perinatal period. *Biol. Neonate*, **48**, 185–96.
45. Menon, R.K. and Sperling, M.A. (1988) Carbohydrate metabolism. *Semin. Perinatol.*, **12**, 157–62.
46. Frazer, T.E., Karl, I.E., Hillman, L.S. *et al.* (1981) Direct measurement of gluconeogenesis from (2,3-¹³C) alanine in the human neonate. *Am. J. Physiol.*, **240**, E615–21.
47. Denne, S.C. and Kalhan, S.C. (1986) Glucose carbon recycling and oxidation in human newborns. *Am. J. Physiol.*, **251**, E71–77.
48. Matthews, D.E. (1983) Protein digestion and absorption, in: *Nutritional Adaptation of the Intestinal Tract of the Newborn* (eds N. Kretschner and A. Minkowski), Raven Press, New York, pp. 73–91.
49. Hamosh, M., Bitman, J., Wood, D.L. *et al.* (1985) Lipids in milk and the first steps in their digestion. *Paediatrics*, **75** (suppl.), 146–50.
50. Mehta, N.R., Jones, J.B. and Hamosh, M. (1992) Lipases in human milk; ontogeny and physiologic significance. *J. Pediatr. Gastroenterol. Nutr.*, **1**, 317–26.
51. Hamosh, M. (1981) Physiological role of human milk lipases, in *Gastrointestinal Development and Infant Nutrition* (ed. E. Lebenthal), Raven Press, New York, pp. 473–82.
52. Bitman, J., Wood, D.L., Hamosh, M. *et al.* (1983) Comparison of the lipid composition of breast milk from mothers of term and preterm infants. *Am. J. Clin. Nutr.*, **38**, 300–12.
53. Chappell, J.E., Clandinin, M.T. and Kearney-Volpi, C. (1985) Trace fatty acids in human milk lipids: influence of maternal diet and weight loss. *Am. J. Clin. Nutr.*, **42**, 49–56.
54. Stubbs, C.D. and Smith, A.D. (1990) Essential fatty acids in membrane; physical properties and function. *Biochem. Soc. Trans.*, **18**, 779–81.
55. Bazaan, N.G. (1989) Lipid-derived metabolites as possible retina messengers: arachidonic, leucotrienes, eicosanoids and platelet activating factor, in *Extracellular and Intracellular Messengers in the Vertebrate Retina* (eds D.A. Reburn and H.P. Morales), Alan R. Liss, New York, pp. 269–300.
56. Sinclair, A.J. and Crawford, M.A. (1973) The effect of a low fat maternal diet on neonatal rats. *Br. J. Nutr.*, **29**, 127–37.
57. Yamamoto, N., Saitoh, M., Moriuchi, A. *et al.* (1987) Effect of dietary β-linolenate/linoliate balance on brain lipid composition and learning ability in rats. *J. Lipid Res.*, **28**, 144–51.
58. Neuringer, M., Anderson, E.J. and Connor, W.E. (1988) The essentiality of n-3 fatty acids for the development and function of the retina and brain. *Am. Rev. Nutr.*, **8**, 517–41.
59. Carlson, S.E., Rhodes, P.G. and Ferguson, M.G. (1986) Docosahexaenoic acid status of preterm infants at birth following feeding with human milk or formula. *Am. J. Clin. Nutr.*, **44**, 798–804.
60. Uauy, R., Treen, M. and Hoffman, D. (1989) Essential fatty acid metabolism and requirements during development. *Semin. Perinatol.*, **13**, 118–30.
61. Farquharson, J., Cockburn, F., Patrick, W.A. *et al.* (1992) Infant cerebral cortex phospolipid fatty acid composition and diet. *Lancet*, **340**, 810–13.
62. Carlson, S.E. (1994) Long chain fatty acids and visual and cognitive development of preterm infants. *E. J. Nutr.* (in press).
63. Saudubray, J.M., Ogier, H., Donnefont, J.P. *et al.* (1989) Clinical approach to inherited metabolic diseases in the neonatal period: a 20-year survey. *J. Inherited Metab. Dis.*, **12** (suppl. 1), 25–41.
64. Scriver, C.R., Beaudet, A.L., Sly, W.S. and Valle, D. (eds) (1989) *The Metabolic Basis of Inherited Diseases*, 6th edn, McGraw-Hill, New York.

98 NEONATAL PARENTERAL NUTRITION

J.A. Kerner Jr

98.1 Introduction

Optimal nutritional support is critical in the management of the ever increasing number of surviving small premature infants [1]. Although it is important to ensure that the infant receives an adequate caloric intake, the capacity of the very-low-birth-weight (VLBW) infant to digest, absorb and metabolize enteral nutrients is limited. In addition, these infants often have other major difficulties, such as respiratory distress, cardiovascular instability, hemorrhagic diatheses and a relatively immature renal system. The challenge of providing ideal nutrition for low-birth-weight infants is to satisfy their growth needs in the face of physiologic and biologic immaturity [2].

To provide proper nutrition to the premature infant, one must have an understanding of the biochemical and physiologic processes that occur during development of the gastrointestinal tract. By 28 weeks of gestation the morphologic development of the gastrointestinal tract in humans is nearly complete, yet as an organ of nutrition, the gut is functionally immature. Details of gastrointestinal tract development have been described previously [3–5] and have been summarized [6] recently (Table 98.1). Further, complications due to the incomplete development of the gastrointestinal tract in the low-birth-weight infant have been delineated superbly by Sunshine (Table 98.2).

The association of necrotizing enterocolitis (NEC) with early enteral feeding of such infants has also discouraged aggressive attempts to feed them orally. Parental nutrition (PN) appears to be an attractive alternative which enables the neonatologist to advance oral feedings very slowly, allowing the gastrointestinal tract to adapt gradually to extrauterine life, while continuing to provide adequate nutrition. The historical overview of PN in the neonate has been reviewed previously [2,7].

98.2 Indications

Although PN is potentially life-saving therapy and is now an accepted practice, increasing experience has demonstrated metabolic, mechanical, and infectious complications. Therefore, candidates for PN should be selected carefully and the indications considered diligently. The principle indications for the use of PN in neonates are shown in Table 98.3. Even 2–3 days without adequate nutritional intake for VLBW infants is an indication for PN, since in this short time depletion of their limited endogenous stores can occur. There is rapid deposition of body fat that occurs during late fetal development [8]. The 1000 g infant only has fat stores of about 1% body weight, or about 10 g. The total endogenous nutrient stores of the 1000 g infant are sufficient to support survival without exogenous nutrients for approximately 5 days [9].

PN is not indicated in patients with adequate intestinal function in whom nutrition may be maintained by oral, tube or gastrostomy feeding [10]. PN is also contradicted during:

- acute metabolic derangements;
- acute hemodynamic instability;
- surgical operations, since the nutrient solutions may be used inadvertently for fluid resuscitation [11].

Relative contraindications to PN are intended use for less than 5 days and the probability that a patient will die imminently because of his or her underlying disease [12].

Infants receiving central vein TPN retain nitrogen and grow as well as normal infants fed either human milk or standard formulas. TPN has been directly credited with improving the survival of infants with gastrointestinal tract anomalies. No controlled studies have examined the efficacy of TPN in infants who require intestinal tract surgery, but data from other sources overwhelmingly argue in its favor. In these gastrointestinal disorders, the congenital anomalies

Diseases of the Fetus and Newborn, 2nd edn, Edited by G.B. Reed, A.E. Claireaux and F. Cockburn. Published in 1995 by Chapman & Hall, London. ISBN 0 412 39160 0

Table 98.1 Development of the human gastrointestinal tract [After Ref. 6]

Age (weeks)	Crown–rump length (mm)	Stage of development
2.5	1.5	Gut not distinct from yolk sac
3.5	2.5	Foregut and hindgut present; yolk sac broadly attached at midgut; liver bud present; mesenteries forming
4	5.0	Intestine present as a single tube from mouth to cloaca; esophagus and stomach distinct; liver cords, ducts and gallbladder forming; omental bursa forming; pancreatic buds appear as outpouching of gut
5–6	8.0–12.0	Intestine elongates into a loop and duodenum begins to rotate under superior mesenteric artery; stomach rotates; parotid and submandibular buds appear; cloaca elongates and septum forms to divide cloaca
7	17.0	Circular muscle layer present; duodenum temporarily occluded; intestinal loops herniate into cord; villi begin to develop; pancreatic anlagen fuse
8	23	Villi lined by single layer of cells; small intestine coiling within cord; taste buds appear; microvilli short, thick, and irregularly spaced; lysosomal enzymes detected; cloacal membrane, which sealed the rectum, begins to disappear
9–10	30–40	Auerbach's plexus appears; intestine re-enters abdominal cavity; crypts of Lieberkühn develop; active transport of glucose appears aerobically and anaerobically; dipeptidases present; microvilli of enterocytes more regular and glycocalyx present; mitochondria numerous below microvilli
12	56	Parietal cells present in stomach; muscular layers of intestine present; alkaline phosphatase and disaccharidases detectable; active transport of amino acid present; mature taste buds present; enterochromaffin cells appear; pancreatic islet cells appear; bile secretions begin; colonic haustra appear; coelomic extension into umbilical cord obliterated; meconium first detected in ileum
13–14	78–90	Meissner's plexus appears; circular folds appear; peristalsis detected; lysosomes detected ultrastructurally
16	112	Pancreatic lipase and tryptic activity detected; lymphopoiesis present; peptic activity present; swallowing evident – 2–7 ml/24 h;
20	160	Peyer's patches present; muscularis mucosae present; mesenteric attachments complete; zymogen granules present and well developed in pancreas (22 weeks); intestine has lost ability to transport glucose anaerobically
24	200	Paneth's cells appear; maltase, sucrase and alkaline phosphatase very active; ganglion cells detected throughout small and large intestine and in the rectum; amylase activity present in intestine
28	240	Enterokinase activity increases; esophageal glands present; frequency and intensity of duodenal peristaltic contractions increasing
32	270	Lactase activity increases; hydrochloric acid found in stomach
34	290–300	Sucking and swallowing become coordinated; esophageal peristalsis rapid, non-segmental contraction occurs; small intestinal motility becomes co-ordinated
36–38	320–350	Maturity of gastrointestinal tract achieved

prevent the use of the alimentary tract. TPN fills the patient's nutritional needs until recuperation from the corrective surgical procedure is complete.

Heird and Winters [13] studied 21 infants with surgical gastrointestinal disorders for at least 12 months after the operation; all received TPN. At follow-up, 15 (71%) of the patients had normal gastrointestinal function, two (10%) had special dietary requirements, and the remaining four (19%) had died. The results of this study were dramatic because, before the advent of TPN, this group of patients would have had an extremely high death rate. Dudrick, Copeland and MacFadyen [14] described infants who received TPN following surgery for ruptured omphalocele or gastroschisis. None of their patients died. Without TPN, they would have predicted the death of 60–80% of the patients! Other investigators have found similar posit-

ive responses to the use of TPN in major gastrointestinal tract surgery.

In the short bowel syndrome, PN has been a major factor in the maintenance of appropriate nutrition while the intestine is adapting to massive resection [15]. Since the advent of PN as supportive therapy, survival with normal growth is now possible with as little as 11 cm of jejunoileal intestine with an intact ileocecal valve and as little as 25 cm of jejunoileal intestine without an ileocecal valve [16].

98.2.1 LOW-BIRTH-WEIGHT INFANTS

Low-birth-weight infants probably constitute the largest group of pediatric patients who receive parenteral nutrients [17]. In a review by Moyer-Mileur and Chan [18], parenteral feeds in VLBW infants requiring

Table 98.2 Complications due to the incomplete development of the gastrointestinal tract in the low-birth-weight infant [After Ref. 6]

Incomplete development of motility
  Poor coordination of sucking and swallowing
  Aberrant esophageal motility
  Biphasic esophageal peristalsis
  Decreased or absent lower esophageal sphincter
    pressure
  Delayed gastric emptying time
  Poorly co-ordinated motility of the small and large
    intestine
    Stasis
    Dilation
    Impaired blood supply
    Functional obstruction

Delayed ability to regenerate new epithelial cells
  Decreased rates of proliferation
  Decreased cellular migration rates
  Shallow crypts
  Shortened villi
  Decreased mitotic indices

Inadequate host resistance factors
  Decreased gastric acidity
  Decreased concentrations of immunoglobulins in lamina
    propria and intestinal secretions
  Impaired humoral and cellular response to infection

Inadequate digestion of nutrients
  Decreased digestion of protein
    Decreased activity of enterokinase
    Trypsin activity low prior to 28 weeks' gestation
    Decreased concentration of gastric hydrochloric acid
      and pepsinogen
  Decreased digestion of carbohydrates
    Decreased hydrolysis of lactose
    Decreased ability to transport glucose actively
    Decreased activity of pancreatic amylase
  Decreased digestion of lipids
    Decreased production and reabsorption of bile
      acids
    Decreased activity of pancreatic lipase

Increased incidence of other problems that may indirectly
  lead to poor gastrointestinal function
  Hyaline membrane disease
  Intraventricular hemorrhage
  Patent ductus arteriosus
  Hypoxemic ischemic states

Table 98.3 Indications for parenteral nutrition in neonates

Surgical gastrointestinal disorders (gastroschisis, omphalocele, tracheo-esophageal fistula, multiple intestinal atresias, meconium ileus and peritonitis, malrotation and volvulus, Hirschsprung's disease with enterocolitis, diaphragmatic hernia)

Short bowel syndrome

Serious acute alimentary diseases (necrotizing enterocolitis)

Acute renal failure

Meconium ileus

Respiratory distress syndrome

Intensive care of low-birth-weight infants

Neonatal asphyxia

Rare disorders (chylothorax and chylous ascites, idiopathic intestinal pseudo-obstruction, congenital villous atrophy)

assisted ventilation for more than 6 days led to a decrease in the percentage of weight loss from birth weight and a lesser amount of time required for recovery of birth weight than in those fed enterally or by a combination of enteral and parenteral feeds. Furthermore, a delay in enteral feeds increased the tolerance to subsequent enteral feeds in these infants. Tolerance was defined as absence of residuals, abdominal distension, or guaiac-positive, reducing substance-positive stools [18]. Another retrospective study presented conflicting data regarding the benefits and risks of parenteral nutrition [19].

Limited data exist on the potential benefit of PN in the treatment of preterm infants. A controlled study [20] of peripheral TPN composed of casein hydrolysate, dextrose and soybean emulsion in 40 premature infants with respiratory distress syndrome showed that TPN neither favorably altered the clinical course of the syndrome nor worsened an infant's pulmonary status. Among infants weighing less than 1500 g, those who received TPN had a greater survival rate than did the control group (71% versus 37%).

Yu and co-workers [21] performed a controlled trial of TPN on 34 preterm infants with birth weights of less than 1200 g. Infants in the TPN group had a greater mean daily weight gain in the second week of life and regained birth weight sooner than did control infants. Four in the milk-fed control group developed NEC, whereas none did in the TPN group.

The result of a study conducted by the author's group [22] of 40 infants who weighed less than 1500 g at birth were in agreement with the two aforementioned controlled studies. No increased risk in using peripheral PN was found as compared with conventional feeding techniques; also comparable growth was found in the two groups, with significantly increased skinfold thickness values in the peripheral PN group compared with the conventional feeding group.

A classic study that remains a model for nutritional support in the VLBW infant was performed by Cashore, Sedaghatian and Usher [23]. They described 23 infants weighing less than 1500 g in whom peripheral PN was begun on day 2 of life to supplement enteral feedings, thus allowing for adequate nutrition while avoiding overtaxing the immature gastrointestinal tract. These infants regained their birth weight by the age of 8–12 days and achieved growth rates that approximated intrauterine rates of growth. Interestingly, infants weighing less than 1000 g were still not

Table 98.4 Total daily parenteral nutrition intake for infants weighing less than 1500 g [After Ref. 23]

Age (days)	Volume (ml/kg)	Fat (g/kg)	Protein (g/kg)	Carbo-hydrates (g/kg)	Calories (per kg)
1	65.0	0.0	0.0	6.5	26.0
2	100.0	2.0	2.0	8.0	60.0
3	115.0	2.5	2.0	9.0	71.0
4	125.0	3.0	2.5	9.5	81.0
5+	140.0	3.5	3.0	10.5	93.0

taking all their nutrients enterally by 25 days of age. The regimen used in this study is shown in Table 98.4.

A survey [24] of 269 neonatal intensive care units showed that TPN was used exclusively during the first week of life in 80% of infants weighing 1000 g or less at birth. The others received a combination of parenteral and enteral feedings in the first week. As a general rule we, like Adamkin [25], begin PN by 72 hours of age in neonates with a birth weight of less than 1000 g in whom respiratory disease and intestinal hypomotility limit the safety of feedings in the first 1–2 weeks of life. In addition, preterm infants, especially those who have respiratory distress syndrome and are incapable of full oral feeds, often receive PN because of their extremely limited substrate reserve, very rapid growth rate and perceived susceptibility to irreversible brain damage secondary to malnutrition [26].

98.2.2 ASPHYXIATED INFANTS

In an asphyxiated infant, in addition to the complications due to incomplete development of the gastrointestinal tract, there is a superimposed insult to the gut from the asphyxia itself.

Most centers do not enterally feed an asphyxiated infant for the first 5 days to 2 weeks after the insult. This practice is extrapolated from animal data on cellular proliferation and migration. The intestinal mucosa of newborn and suckling rats has a very slow rate of cellular proliferation and migration compared with that of adult animals [27]. Although the turnover of intestinal epithelia in the adult jejunum is 48–72 hours, the rate in the 10-day-old animal is at least twice that long and in the 2- to 3-day-old animal it may be even longer [28]. In a study by Sunshine and colleagues [29] in the adult animal, labeled cells reached the tips of the villi within 48 hours. During the same period of time the labeled cells had migrated only one-eighth to one-quarter the length of the villi in the suckling animal. There are indications that this same slower rate of turnover of intestinal epithelia exists in the newborn human [30].

Asphyxia *per se* may cause significant injury to the gastrointestinal tract. Further, asphyxia may predispose

an infant to develop NEC. Coupled with asphyxia, feeding the premature infant poses a significant risk for the development of neonatal NEC.

98.2.3 NECROTIZING ENTEROCOLITIS

Because approximately 95% of patients with NEC have been fed, many nurseries have attempted to prevent the disease by delaying enteral feedings. Brown and Sweet [31] have employed a regimen of prolonged periods of bowel rest following patient exposure to any risk factors that may lead to poor bowel perfusion, to allow for recovery of the intestinal mucosa, while supplying all nutrients by the parenteral route. After a variable period of time (5–10 days), rigorous attention is paid to a slow progressive feeding regimen for these patients, with careful examination of gastric residua and reducing substances in the stool. By strict adherence to this regimen, they have shown marked reduction and almost elimination of NEC in their institution.

The downside of prolonged periods of bowel rest is that bowel maturation may be delayed. There is evidence that enteral feeding may be the critical element that triggers postnatal gut maturation through release of gut peptide hormones [32]. Recent research in our laboratory confirms that intestinal development is arrested when animals receive TPN with no enteral nutrients but that resumption of intestinal maturation occurs on reintroduction of intraluminal nutrients [33]. A comprehensive discussion of nutritional support in NEC is available to the reader [34]; also please see Chapters 35 and 104 in this text for further insight into NEC.

98.3 Route of administration

Ziegler and co-workers [35] compared the complication rates of children receiving nutrition via central and peripheral veins; their findings are summarized in Table 98.5. Although infectious complications occurred in

Table 98.5 Complications of total parenteral nutrition [After Ref. 35]

	Central vein	Peripheral vein
No. of patients	200	385
Mean duration (days)	33.7	11.4
Total days of therapy	6629	4389
Gained or maintained weight (%)	82.5	63.0
Number of complications		
Infectious	21	0
Administration	7	32
Metabolic	12	3
Complication rate		
Total complications	40 (20.0%)	35 (9.1%)
Per patient day (%)	0.604	0.797

approximately 10% of the central-vein group and in none of the peripheral-vein group, morbidity related to the administration of solution (primarily in the form of soft-tissue sloughs) was more prevalent in the peripheral-vein group. Complications such as pleural effusions and thrombosis occurred in the central-vein group. The overall complication rate was higher in the central-vein group (20% versus 9.08% in the peripheral-vein group). However, when total days of therapy are considered in the complication incidence, a daily complication rate is not different between the two groups.

The authors of this study acknowledge that the problem of venous accessibility is a deterrent to central venous nutrition in small infants. Their experience with percutaneous subclavian vein cannulation suggests that this technique is safe, allows repeated cannulation of the central venous system and can be used in infants weighing as little as 600 g. Their data imply that **caloric need** is the primary determining factor for selecting the route of nutritional support. Peripheral-vein nutrient solutions are less calorically dense than central-vein solutions; therefore, centrally alimented patients may receive more calories and gain more weight on a daily basis. Further, with frequent peripheral-vein infiltrations the number of calories actually infused is often less than ordered (if the patient is ordered to receive 100 kcal/kg over 24 hours and the intravenous line is out 30% of the time, the patient only receives 70 kcal/kg per day). Since peripheral PN regimens maintain existing body composition, this routine of delivery is a reasonable choice for a normally nourished infant who is likely to tolerate an adequate enteral regimen in less than 2 weeks. Central PN is a more reasonable choice for infants, regardless of initial nutritional status, who will be intolerant of enteral feedings for longer than 2 weeks. It is difficult to maintain peripheral PN for more than 2 weeks; normal growth, rather than simply maintaining existing body composition, can be achieved with central but not peripheral PN [17].

98.3.1 UMBILICAL ARTERY CATHETERS

In some nurseries umbilical arterial (UA) catheters are used for infusing parenteral nutrition. Few studies exist regarding the safety of this practice. Yu *et al.* [21] studied 34 infants with birth weight less than 1200 g and randomly assigned them to TPN via UA catheters or enteral feeds. The TPN group had better nitrogen balance, weight gain, less NEC and unchanged mortality compared with the enterally fed group. No data on catheter-related complications were presented, although bacterial or fungal septicemia did not occur in either group in the study period [21].

Higgs and co-workers [36] described a controlled trial of TPN versus formula feeding by continuous nasogastric drip. The study included 86 infants weighing from 500 to 1500 g. The TPN, including glucose, amino acids and fat emulsion, was administered by umbilical artery catheter for the first 2 weeks of life. There was no difference in neonatal morbidity or mortality between the two groups. Specifically, there was no difference in septicemia, although four of the 43 TPN babies had 'catheter problems', described in the text only as 'blockage' of the catheter.

Hall and Rhodes [37] delivered TPN to 80 infants by UA lines and to nine infants by indwelling umbilical venous catheters; these 89 infants were all 'high-risk' infants unable to tolerate enteral feedings. Results were compared with those for 23 infants with tunneled jugular catheters for chronic medical or surgical problems preventing use of the gastrointestinal tract. All infants studied ranged in weight from approximately 1000 to 2500 g. As in the study of Higgs *et al.*, Hall and Rhodes found that morbidity, mortality and the common complications, such as infection and thrombosis, were similar in both groups [37].

Hall and Rhodes concluded that TPN by indwelling umbilical catheters presents no greater risk than infusion through tunneled jugular catheters. However, careful analysis of the authors' data raises questions about their conclusions. According to the authors, 'six deaths may have been catheter related' [37]. Five of those deaths occurred in the umbilical artery catheter group; death resulted from the thrombosis of the aorta in one patient, candidal septicemia in two, streptococcal septicemia in one and enterococcal septicemia in one. One death occurred in the jugular venous catheter group, with right atrial thrombosis, superior vena cava syndrome and *Staphylococcus epidermidis* on blood culture.

Merritt [38] cautions against the use of umbilical arterial catheters for TPN, as this practice is associated with a high incidence of arterial thrombosis. Dr Arnold Coran, a pediatric surgeon, strongly recommends that PN **not** be given through either umbilical arteries or umbilical veins [39]. PN through umbilical veins causes phlebitis, which may lead to venous thrombosis and portal hypertension. He is especially concerned about infusing PN solutions into a UA line, since this practice can lead to thrombosis of the aorta or iliac vessels. Furthermore, severe damage to an artery can occur without being recognized. There may even be thrombosis of the aorta without recognition. Only over an extensive period of time will the side-effects of UA catheter use – such as inappropriate growth of one limb [39] – be known. Although the first three studies described earlier all claimed there were no short-term complications, they did not address the problem of long-term complications.

Coran states that if PN is required and peripheral

veins are not usable, or if peripheral vein delivery is inadequate to provide necessary calories, he would consider percutaneous subclavian vein catheterization, which he can perform successfully even in a 900-g infant [39].

Like Coran and Merritt, the author's group is reluctant to use umbilical catheters for the infusion of parenteral nutrients. An attempt is made to provide needed calories by peripheral vein. If more calories are needed or if PN must be provided for longer than 2 weeks, a central venous line is placed [40].

A recent retrospective review [41] compared TPN via umbilical catheters versus central lines in 48 neonates (birth weight 1.7±0.58 kg). There was no difference in infection rate between the two groups when adjustment was made for the number of days of catheter life. Transient hypertension occurred in two (4%) of the UA catheter group and in one (3.8%) of the central catheter group. There was one aortic thrombus noted on autopsy in the UA catheter group. There was one vegetation on the tricuspid valve in the central catheter group. They concluded that UA catheters are a reasonable route for PN solutions. As nurseries become more comfortable with percutaneous central lines [42,43], hopefully UA catheters will be used less frequently to provide nutrition.

98.4   Requirements

98.4.1   CALORIES (ENERGY)

In a controlled trial [44] of 14 preterm appropriate-for-gestational-age infants, two isocaloric intravenous feeding regimens were compared. Each provided 60 kcal/kg per day, one via glucose alone and the other via glucose plus 2.5 g/kg per day of crystalline amino acids. Infants on the glucose-only regimen had a negative mean nitrogen balance, whereas those fed glucose plus amino acids had a positive balance. There was no significant weight gain in either group. Of interest was the development of essential fatty acid deficiency in infants receiving glucose plus amino acids, but not in those receiving glucose alone.

In a study of preterm infants, Zlotkin, Bryan and Anderson [45] found that intravenous intakes of 70–90 kcal/kg per day resulted in weight gain, and that energy intakes providing more than 70 kcal/kg per day (including intakes of 2.7–3.5 g/kg per day of protein) resulted in nitrogen accretion and growth rates similar to *in utero* values. They reported greater nitrogen retention in infants receiving amino acid intakes of 3 or 4 g/kg per day with a concomitant energy intake of 80 versus 50 kcal/kg per day. In contrast, Pineault *et al.* [46] observed a minimal effect of an energy intake of 80 versus 60 kcal/kg per day on nitrogen retention of low-birth-weight infants receiving 2.7 g/kg per day

of amino acids. These two pieces of data suggest that 2.7 g/kg per day of amino acids is reasonably well utilized, although perhaps not maximally utilized if accompanied by an energy intake of 60 kcal/kg per day, whereas an amino acid intake of 3 g/kg per day is not [9]. In addition, earlier studies of adults suggested that additional stresses such as sepsis would increase caloric requirements by as much as 40%. More recent work [47], however, has questioned such an increase, and it is probable that severe stress does not increase requirements by any more than 10–15%. The effect of stresses like sepsis on caloric requirements in preterm infants has not been critically studied. As in adults admitted to the intensive care unit and confined to their beds, preterm infants' requirements for energy and physical activity may be reduced and hence may balance with the increased needs due to the stress condition [26].

It has been shown that portable indirect calorimetry (measurement of oxygen consumption and carbon dioxide production) gives a precise and easily taken measurement of resting energy expenditure in the malnourished pregnant patient [48]. Studies of infants have been offered as arguments that indirect calorimetry provides a more accurate basis for calculating daily caloric needs than other clinical estimations [49–51]. The technology for providing indirect calorimetry in neonates has advanced dramatically, now allowing measurement even of infants on respirators. The cost of such equipment and the staff required to run the machine and interpret the results, however, prevent its routine use. More studies are needed to discover whether the use of indirect calorimetry significantly improves patient morbidity and mortality.

Fluid restrictions secondary to severe respiratory, cardiac or renal disease may prevent the delivery of adequate calories, even if the calories are given by central PN.

Balanced PN, including both fat and carbohydrate (as non-nitrogen calories), is the ideal regimen, especially for respiratory conditions (e.g. hyaline membrane disease). Such a regimen decreases the respiratory quotient, prevents excessive fluid administration, and may help to avoid fatty infiltration of the liver. In addition, since equivalent nitrogen retention has been demonstrated with glucose versus glucose plus lipid as the non-nitrogen source [52], the latter is preferred since the development of essential fatty acid deficiency is prevented.

One may also calculate caloric requirements using published formulas. Many centers use the Harris–Benedict equations to determine basal energy expenditure (BEE) for children over 10 years of age [53]. A newer equation has been developed for infants [54]: $\text{kcal}/24\text{ h} = 22.10 + (31.05 \times W) + (1.16 \times H)$, where W = weight in kilograms and H = height in centimeters.

There are significant differences between caloric requirements for the first and second week of life. In a neutral thermal environment in the first week of life the small premature infant has a low, near-fetal, metabolic rate of 35–40 kcal/kg per day; in the second week the metabolic rate increases to about 50–55 kcal/kg per day, as additional energy is required for tissue synthesis [55]. There are few data regarding energy dynamics in the extremely low-birth-weight infants (< 1000 g). Van Aerde [56] recommends 60–70 kcal/kg per day and 2 g/kg per day of protein by 72 hours of age for the extremely low-birth-weight infant. Detailed discussions of energy metabolism in the neonate are available to the interested reader [56–58].

98.4.2 FLUIDS

Preterm infants have unique fluid requirements [2,59–62]. Factors that increase or decrease requirements are shown in Table 98.6. Further, excess fluid intake (> 150 ml/kg per day) in low-birth-weight infants may be associated with patent ductus arteriosus, bronchopulmonary dysplasia, NEC and intraventricular hemorrhage. During PN, in order to provide adequate calories, fluids are given in excess of maintenance, especially if using peripheral PN [7]. General guidelines for fluid management in neonatal TPN are readily available [2,7,59–62].

98.4.3 CARBOHYDRATE

The major source of non-protein calories in PN is dextrose (D-glucose), which is provided in the monohydrate form for intravenous use, reducing its caloric yield to 3.4 kcal/g rather than the 4 kcal/g of enteral

Table 98.6 Water requirements in premature infants [After Ref. 62]

Factors increasing requirements
Radiant warmers
Conventional single-walled incubators
Phototherapy
An ambient temperature above the neutral thermal range
Respiratory distress
Any hypermetabolic problem
Elevated body temperature
Furosemide (frusemide) treatment
Diarrhea
Glycosuria (with associated osmotic diuresis)
Intravenous alimentation

Factors decreasing requirements
Heat shields
Thermal blankets
Double-walled incubators
Placing the infant in relatively high humidity
Use of warm humidified air via endotracheal tube
Renal oliguria

glucose or other carbohydrates. Dextrose contributes the majority of the osmolality of the PN solution. With peripheral PN, concentrations of dextrose above 10% are associated with an increased incidence of phlebitis (secondary to increased osmolarity) and thus a decreased 'lifespan' of peripheral lines. Carbohydrates are initiated in a slow, stepwise fashion to allow an appropriate response of endogenous insulin and thus to prevent glucosuria (and subsequent osmotic diuresis). Specific guidelines for advancing glucose infusions have been described elsewhere [63,64]. Solutions containing greater than 20% glucose at 150 ml/kg per day may contribute to hepatic steatosis [65]. Glucose as the sole calorie source leads to greater water retention than when combined with intravenous lipids [66]. As mentioned previously, a balanced TPN solution, including both carbohydrate and fat (as non-nitrogen calories) may avoid (1) fatty infiltration of the liver, (2) water retention, and (3) worsening already severe respiratory compromise: in acutely ill ventilator-dependent patients, carbon dioxide production has been shown to be significantly higher with glucose as the entire source of non-protein calories than when fat emulsion provides some of the total caloric load [67].

Small premature infants have a poor glucose tolerance in the first days of life, and hyperglycemia (serum glucose more than 125 mg/dl) occurs frequently. Dextrose infusions are well tolerated by the neonate if the initial rate of administration does not exceed the hepatic rate of glucose production (6–8 mg/kg per min). The premature infant may develop hyperglycemia even at lower rates of infusion [60]. An infusion rate of 7.5 mg/kg per min is equivalent to 11.3% dextrose at 96 ml/kg per day or 7.5% dextrose at 144 ml/kg per day [68].

Insulin is usually not given to permature infants because of reports of highly variable responses: some infants have developed profound hypoglycemia with minuscule insulin doses, and others have had no response. Vaucher and colleagues [69] suggested a possible benefit from continuous insulin infusion (through addition to the reservoir of the intravenous infusion set). Although the number of subjects was quite small, the researchers did document increased weight gain and increased tolerance of intravenous glucose in extremely premature hyperglycemic infants who received continuous insulin infusion. Theoretical considerations and practical limitations, such as the infiltration of peripheral intravenous lines, caused one reviewer to recommend the restriction of insulin use of this kind to investigative studies only [70].

Continuous insulin infusion by pump has recently been shown to be of potential benefit to VLBW [71,72] and extremely low-birth-weight infants [73–75]. The data all show improved glucose tolerance with subsequent weight gain using insulin therapy. The lack of understanding of the composition of the weight gain or of other outcome variables related to insulin use argues for further study of this therapy before it is recommended routinely.

98.4.4   PROTEIN

Preterm neonates given 2.5–3.5 g/kg per day of protein and approximately 80 kcal/kg per day achieve nitrogen retention at levels that approximate intrauterine nitrogen retention [45]. However, intakes greater than 2.5–3.0 g/kg per day may result in azotemia, especially in low-birth-weight infants [17].

Until recently, no marketed amino acid solution appeared ideal for neonatal or pediatric use. The major solutions available were designed according to the requirements of normal, orally fed adult subjects and not infants and growing children. These solutions produce weight gain and positive nitrogen balance in the stable neonate or infant when adequate non-protein calories are also provided. However, use of these solutions leads to high plasma concentrations of amino acids such as methionine, glycine and phenylalanine (a cause for concern regarding safety) and to low plasma concentrations of amino acids such as the branched chain amino acids, tyrosine and cysteine (the basis of concern regarding efficacy) [76].

Heird and Malloy [77] found that free amino acid patterns of brain tissue from beagle puppies that received TPN were grossly abnormal compared with those of suckled puppies. Brain weight and protein content of the TPN puppies were lower than those of controls. The abnormal free amino acid patterns of the TPN puppy brains reflected plasma amino acid levels. These findings led to the idea that completely normal plasma amino acid patterns should be an end-point for defining amino acid solutions used for TPN in neonates and infants.

Extensive research led to the production of a new parenteral formula, TrophAmine (McGaw, Irvine, CA), which normalizes amino acid levels within the target range recommended by Wu, Edwards and Storm [78] (the values of 2-hour postprandial plasma amino acid concentrations in healthy, normal growing 30-day-old breast-fed term infants). TrophAmine is unique in that it provides the essential amino acids (including taurine, tyrosine and histidine) in adequate amounts as judged by the normalized plasma amino acid profile, as well as providing aspartic acid, glutamic acid and the dicarboxylic acids at appropriate levels.

TrophAmine outperformed Freamine III (a **standard** amino acid solution) in a comparison study [79] in 25 neonates requiring gastrointestinal tract surgery. Both groups were supplemented with 100 mg/kg per day L-cysteine hydrochloride. The TrophAmine group had significantly greater weight gain and nitrogen retention plus plasma amino acid concentrations within the postprandial neonatal target range [78]. Levels of methionine, glycine and phenylalanine were above and tyrosine was below the range when Freamine III was used. There was no difference in serum albumin or direct bilirubin levels between the two groups.

An uncontrolled non-blind multicenter study [80] of the clinical, nutritional and biochemical effects of intravenous administration of TrophAmine with a cysteine additive was conducted in 40 infants and children receiving only TPN. Subjects ranged from 2.0 to 12.6 kg in weight. Each received 2.5 g/kg per day of TrophAmine, 1.0 mmol/kg per day of L-cysteine hydrochloride, and approximately 110 kcal/kg per day of nonprotein calories. The subjects gained approximately 11 g/kg per day, and all were in positive nitrogen balance and had normalization of the plasma amino acid profile without adverse effects. Serial γ-glutamyl transpeptidase (GGTP) values actually declined during the course of the study. Only one of the 31 subjects who received TPN for more than 10 days had an increase in direct bilirubin, despite a predicted incidence of cholestasis of 30–50%. TrophAmine has recently been shown to be equally efficacious in preterm infants [81]. The distinct decrease in cholestatic tendency with TrophAmine may be due to the presence in the solution of taurine, which results in 'normal' plasma levels of taurine. Taurine deficiency has been proposed as a possible cause of cholestasis in patients receiving TPN for a prolonged period [82]. Overall imbalance of amino acids or toxicity of one or more amino acids elevated in plasma may also be responsible for hepatic dysfunction and cholestasis [83]. Thus, the normalization of plasma amino acids during PN, as demonstrated in this study, appears to be a desirable goal.

Abbott Laboratories released Aminosyn-PF in hopes of producing a product comparable to TrophAmine. TrophAmine contains 60% essential amino acids while Aminosyn-PF contains 50% essential amino acids. One investigator's results ($n=23$), as part of a larger multicenter study, suggested improved nitrogen balance and better levels of methionine and tyrosine in the TrophAmine group [84]. An initial report from the rest of the multicenter group [85], where $n=87$, demonstrated similar nitrogen balance and weight gain in both groups. The first published paper comparing the two groups comes from the latter group ($n=44$) showing weight gain of nearly 15 g/kg per day for both solutions, with no differences in nitrogen balance or retention between the two groups [86]. Both formulas contain supplemental **taurine**, based on data showing a potentially deleterious effect of taurine deficiency on the developing brain and retina [87].

(a) Cysteine

Cysteine is considered an indispensable amino acid for infants since hepatic cystathionase activity is absent or low until some time after term birth (cystathionase converts methionine to cysteine); in addition, removal of cysteine from an otherwise adequate diet inhibits the rate of weight gain and nitrogen retention. Enterally fed infants do not have a major problem since human milk and infant formulas contain cysteine. Because cysteine is unstable and cystine is only sparingly soluble in aqueous solution, parenteral amino acid solutions previously did not contain cysteine. Infants receiving TPN have low plasma cysteine levels; further, nitrogen retention is usually lower than in infants receiving the same nitrogen intake enterally. Cysteine hydrochloride can be added to TPN but within 24 hours approximately 50% of it complexes with glucose to form D-glucocysteine. Previous studies of cysteine supplementation of TPN failed to show improvement in growth or nitrogen retention, which might have been because the regimens used were also deficient in tyrosine. Kashyap, Abildskov and Heird [88] recently showed that supplementation of TPN with cysteine HCl (where the amino acid solution was TrophAmine, which contains tyrosine), either by admixture or piggyback, resulted in cysteine retention, higher plasma cysteine concentrations, possible improved nitrogen retention, and increased acidosis – requiring increased acetate to offset. In neonates, we start at 0.5 g/kg per day of amino acids and increase by 0.5 g/kg per day until we reach our desired goal. The development of amino acid solutions **specific** to the needs of neonates may ultimately allow adequate growth to be maintained with protein and calorie intakes at lower amounts than have been previously described. In a preliminary study, Helms *et al.* [89] reported positive nitrogen balance (greater than 200 mg/kg per day) and weight gain (greater than 10 g/kg per day) with low doses of TrophAmine (2 g/kg per day) with fewer calories (50 kcal/kg per day) in preterm infants receiving PN. In the past, these results were achievable only with high calorie and standard protein intakes.

(b) Calorie-to-nitrogen ratio

To promote efficient net protein utilization (i.e. not to use the protein source exclusively as an energy source), approximately 150–200 non-protein calories are required per gram of nitrogen:

1. Nitrogen content (g) $= \dfrac{\text{protein (g)}}{6.25}$.
2. 1 g protein contains 0.16 g nitrogen.

3. Therefore, 24–32 non-nitrogen calories must be supplied per gram of protein infused to yield a proper ratio of 150–200:1

(a) $\dfrac{\text{Non-nitrogen calories}}{\text{N(g)}} = \dfrac{24}{0.16} = \dfrac{150}{1}$;

$$\dfrac{32}{0.16} = \dfrac{200}{1}$$

(b) If 2 g/kg per day of protein as amino acids is supplied, then 48–64 kcal/kg per day of non-nitrogen calories must be supplied to ensure adequate protein utilization.

(c) If 2.5 g/kg per day of protein is supplied, then 60–70 kcal/kg per day of non-nitrogen calories must be supplied.

98.4.5 FAT

Intravenous fat (IVF) has become an integral part of the PN regimen. It not only provides a concentrated isotonic source of calories (the 10% solution supplies 1.1 kcal/ml; the 20% solution supplies 2.0 kcal/ml) but also prevents or reverses essential fatty acid (EFA) deficiency. Patients who cannot tolerate large glucose loads can receive sufficient calories if IVF is added to the dextrose–amino acid regimen. The inclusion of fat with PN solutions infused through a peripheral vein can provide enough calories for growth in preterm neonates and infants who can tolerate fluid loads of 140 ml/kg per day [23]. In addition, continuous administration of IVF with the PN regimen prolongs the viability of peripheral intravenous lines in infants who may have limited venous access [90].

EFA deficiency has been produced inadvertently in hospitalized infants and adults who were receiving nothing by mouth and fat-free TPN. Biochemical evidence of EFA deficiency has been noted in the serum of neonates as early as 2 days after initiating fat-free TPN [91]. Biochemical evidence of deficiency precedes clinical signs of deficiency – reduced growth rate, flaky dry skin, poor hair growth, thrombocytopenia, increased susceptibility to infections and impaired wound healing [91,92]. EFA deficiency can be assessed by determination of the ratio of 5,8,11-eicosatrienoic to arachidonic acid (triene-to-tetraene ratio). A ratio greater than 0.4 is generally assumed to be an early indicator of EFA deficiency [92]. An initial report [93] of topically applied sunflower seed oil reversing biochemical and clinical EFA deficiency in two neonates on fat-free PN could not be duplicated in a later study of 15 neonates [94] or 28 surgical patients from newborn to 66 years of age [95].

Interestingly, 15 ml twice a day enterally of corn oil, sunflower oil or safflower oil provides as much linoleic acid as 150 ml of 10% IVF at less than 5% of the cost. Many PN patients not on complete bowel rest tolerate such a regimen [96].

EFA deficiency can be prevented by providing 2–4% of total calories as IVF (1–2% linoleic acid) – an IVF dose of 0.5–1.0 g/kg per day. Fat may frequently contribute 30–40% of total non-nitrogen calories, but should not exceed 60%. A suggested regimen for advancing IVF is shown in Table 98.7. IVF must be infused separately from any other PN solution, since these solutions may 'crack' (disturb) the fat emulsion. IVF may be infused with dextrose amino acid solutions using a Y connector near the infusion site and beyond (proximal to) the micropore filter. When administered in this way, the fat emulsion remains stable.

The rate of elimination and metabolic fate of IVF particles are the same as those of naturally occurring chylomicrons. Thus, clearance from the plasma is dependent upon the activity of lipoprotein lipase in the capillary endothelial cells, primarily in muscle and adipose tissue.

Lecithin-cholesterol acyl transferase (LCAT) catalyzes the synthesis of almost the entire cholesterol ester of circulating lipoproteins. LCAT acts exclusively in plasma, while lipoprotein lipase is active at the capillary wall and, under normal conditions, is completely absent from plasma. Low-birth-weight infants have lower levels of lipolytic enzymes (lipoprotein lipase) and LCAT than fullterm infants explaining, in part, why VLBW infants may develop hyperlipidemia with IVF doses >2 g/kg per day [7].

IVF should be infused over 24 hours whenever possible. Continuous IVF infusions (24 hours/day) are better tolerated than intermittent infusions (8 hours/day) by preterm infants [97]. Early studies argued against exceeding a rate of 0.15 g/kg per hour (3.6 g/kg per day) [92]. Slower infusion rates are required for small-for-gestational age (SGA) infants. Eighteen-hour infusions at a rate of 0.15 g/kg per hour with '6 hours off' to 'assure cyclical regeneration of the enzyme systems involved in lipid metabolism' has also been suggested, especially if the patients have hyperglycemia associated with IVF use [98]. Brans et al. [99] showed that intermittent infusions (over 18 hours) greatly increased the fluctuations of plasma lipids and tended to elicit higher concentrations than continuous infu-

sions (over 24 hours), especially at the higher daily rates of infusion. Infusion rates of 0.12 g/kg per hour or less resulted in less elevation of plasma lipid levels than rates of 0.17 g/kg per hour or more [99].

Linoleic acid was previously thought to be the only essential fatty acid. Although the essentiality of linolenic acid in man has not been established, its presence in certain mammalian tissue such as the brain has led some investigators to speculate that it might be essential, especially in the developing neonate. On the other hand, there is the possibility that too much linolenic acid inhibits the conversion of linoleic to arachidonic acid. These concerns led to the development of Liposyn II (Abbott Laboratories), a blend of safflower oil (0.1% linolenic acid) and soybean oil (8.0% linolenic acid).

Currently used intravenous fat products are shown in Table 98.8. One study did clearly demonstrate that hypertriglyceridemia was more common in preterm infants who receive safflower oil-based as opposed to soybean oil-based intravenous fat [100].

A recent study in neonates comparing Liposyn II and Intralipid found no difference in the incidence of hypertriglyceridemia between the two products [101]. Two recent studies in neonates show that the plasma fatty acid profiles in the two products are comparable [102,103].

For optimum oxidation of fatty acids, carnitine is necessary [92]. Solutions currently used for intravenous alimentation contain no carnitine, although they contain all the precursor material required for its endogenous production. Infants maintained on PN solutions have decreased total plasma carnitine levels. Decreased tissue carnitine levels have also been found in neonates receiving TPN for more than 15 days. A recent study examined infants receiving long-term PN who were given a supplement of oral L-carnitine (50 mmol/kg per day); these infants achieved normal carnitine levels [104]. Another study of neonates [105] showed that intravenous administration of L-carnitine supplements

Table 98.7 Use of intravenous fat

	Premature or SGA infants	Full term AGA infants
Initial dose (g/kg per day)	0.5	1.0
Increase daily dose by (g/kg per day)	0.5	0.5
Maximum dose (g/kg per day)	3.0	4.0

SGA = small for gestational age; AGA = appropriate for gestational age.

Table 98.8 Commercially available parenteral fat emulsions

Preparation	Manufacturer
Safflower/soybean	
Liposyn II	Abbott
Soybean	
Intralipid	Clintec Nutrition
Liposyn III	Abbott
NutriLipid	McGaw Laboratories
Soyacal	Alpha Therapeutic
Soybean/MCT	
Lipofundin[a]	Braun

[a] Available in Europe.

resulted in normal plasma carnitine levels and lower peak triglyceride levels following delivery of a fat bolus (suggesting an enhanced ability to utilize exogenous fat for energy). Since other studies of supplemental carnitine [106] have not shown significant improvement in metabolism of fat emulsions, further research is needed in this area.

Recent reports suggest the benefit of adding medium-chain triglycerides (MCT) to intravenous preparations over using long-chain triglycerides (LCT) alone. Fifty-one neonates received Lipofundin MCT/LCT (50% MCT, 50% LCT) (B. Braun Medical) or conventional IVF. IVF was given over 20 hours. Triglyceride and fatty acid levels were not significantly different in the two groups. After 6 days of IVF, mean plasma cholesterol was 100% higher in the group receiving conventional IVF [107]. A second study of neonates showed elevation of triglycerides and free fatty acids in the MCT/LCT group [108]. Further studies are needed to evaluate the MCT/LCT regimen.

Finally, Canadian investigators are concerned that preterm infants lack transplacental accretion for eicosapentaenoic acid (EPA) and docosahexaenoic acid (DHA). These fatty acids are essential for brain development but are not available in soybean-based IVF products. They designed a soy emulsion enriched with EPA and DHA and found no toxicity or biochemical abnormalities in piglets [109].

When there is a drastic need to restrict fluid volume (e.g. renal or cardiac compromise, chronic lung disease), 20% IVF is indicated. The dose should not exceed 0.15 g/kg per hour. Less increase of plasma lipids was caused by 4 g/kg per day of 20% IVF than 2 g/kg per day of 10% IVF [110]. In another study, hyperlipidemia in TPN with 10% IVF but not 20% IVF was caused by an increase in lipoprotein X [111]. Twenty per cent IVF has **twice** the amount of triglyceride (i.e. 20 g/dl) compared with the 10% IVF, while having the **same** amount of phospholipid (there is less phospholipid per gram of triglyceride in 20% solutions). Phospholipid is believed to inhibit lipoprotein lipase – the main enzyme responsible for IVF clearance. Given this knowledge, one can appreciate why 20% IVF is cleared more rapidly than 10% IVF.

98.4.6 ELECTROLYTES AND MINERALS

The ranges of recommended intakes of electrolytes and minerals for PN solutions in pediatrics [112] are shown in Table 98.9. Calcium and phosphorus requirements are much greater in preterm infants than in term infants or older children [113]. Recommendations for this unique group [114] are shown in Table 98.10. During the last 6–8 weeks of gestation, calcium and phosphorus are incorporated into the bone matrix. Thus, premature infants are at risk for developing rickets and

Table 98.9 Parenteral provision of electrolytes and minerals

Electrolytes and minerals	Daily amount	
Phosphate	0.5–2.0	mmol/kg
Sodium	2.0–4.0	mmol/kg
Potassium	2.0–3.0	mmol/kg
Chloride	2.0–3.0	mmol/kg
Acetate	1.0–4.0	mmol/kg
Magnesium	0.125–0.25	mmol/kg
Calcium gluconate[a]	50–500	mg/kg

[a] Gluconate is the recommended calcium salt for use in parenteral nutrition solutions. Calcium chloride dissociates more readily than calcium gluconate solutions and can lead to precipation problems with phosphate.

Table 98.10 Recommended intravenous intakes of calcium, phosphorus and magnesium [After Ref. 114]

Nutrient	Preterm infants[a]	Term infants	Children >1 year[b]
Ca (mg/l)	500–600	500–600	200–400
P (mg/l)	400–450	400–450	150–300
Mg (mg/l)	50–70	50–70	20–40

[a] To prevent Ca–P precipitation, intakes are described per liter, to prevent administration of high concentration of Ca and P, which may result if intakes are expressed per kilogram body weight and there is fluid restriction. These recommendations also assume an average fluid intake of ~120–150 ml/kg per day with 25 g amino acid/l of a pediatric amino acid solution. These dosage levels for preterm infants should only be given in central venous infusions.
[b] Requirements are less with advancing age: few data available.

Table 98.11 Normal serum phosphorus levels (mg/dl)

Premature infants	5.6–9.4
Term infants	5.0–8.9

Adapted from Kempe, C.H., Silver, H.K., O'Brien, D. and Fulginiti, V.A. (eds) (1987) *Current Pediatric Diagnosis and Treatment*, Appleton and Lange, Norwalk, 1128–36.

'handling' fractures. Radiographs should be periodically checked for evidence of early changes consistent with rickets. Calcium and phosphorus serum levels should be obtained weekly. The serum calcium level will be maintained at the expense of bone (demineralization), so a normal serum calcium does not necessarily mean that adequate amounts of calcium are being delivered. Serum phosphorus level does not fluctuate as rapidly and is a better indicator of total body stores (normal values [115] are shown in Table 98.11). Kovar, Mayne and Barltrop [116] suggest screening for rickets in preterm infants with plasma alkaline phosphatase: levels of up to five times the upper limit of the normal adult reference range are acceptable; a value of six times the upper limit of the adult reference range should prompt a radiograph to exclude rickets.

Calcium and phosphorus requirements for some patients may exceed the solubility of these two elements in PN solutions. This happens most frequently when patients are fluid restricted or have several other intravenous fluid lines. The maximum amounts of calcium and phosphorus that can be admixed in PN solutions are determined primarily by the pH of the solution, which in turn is determined by the amino acid product and concentration [117]. Currently there are two amino acid products on the market designed for use in infants which have a low enough pH to allow adequate amounts of calcium and phosphorus for growth. They are TrophAmine and Aminosyn PF. Of the other amino acid solutions designed for use in adults, Aminosyn has the lowest pH. Consult your pharmacy for information on institutional products and calcium phosphate precipitation curves.

Continuous infusion of calcium in the PN solution is preferable to bolus administration of calcium. With bolus administration, large amount of calcium are lost in the urine [118]. Also, the potential tissue damage from line infiltration is much greater with concentrated calcium given as a bolus than with dilute calcium as a continuous infusion.

When daily calcium and phosphorus requirements were infused in two separate alternating 12-hour infusions, there were alternating periods of high and low serum concentrations of calcium and phosphorus, depending on which solution was being infused [119]. Infusions of solutions containing both calcium and phosphorus resulted in stable calcium and phosphorus concentrations. Calcium concentrations of 50 mmol/l and phosphate concentrations of 20 mmol/l were compatible in solutions containing 2% TrophAmine, 10% dextrose, and 0.08% L-cysteine [120]. A subsequent study compared calcium–phosphorus solubility previously found with TrophAmine with results for similar Aminosyn PF solutions and showed that calcium–phosphorus solubility was less with Aminosyn PF [121].

The recommendations in Table 98.10 result in a calcium : phosphorus ratio of 1.3 : 1 by weight or 1 : 1 molar ratio. More recently, a higher, more physiologic ratio of 1.7 : 1 by weight (1.3 : 1 by molar ratio, similar to fetal mineral accretion ratio) allowed for the highest absolute retention of both minerals and came closest to published *in utero* accretion of calcium and phosphorus [122,123]. This successful ratio provided **76 mg/kg per day of calcium** and **45 mg/kg per day of phosphorus** using Aminosyn PF as the amino acid. Two promising studies suggest there may be an advantage of using calcium glycerophosphate versus conventional

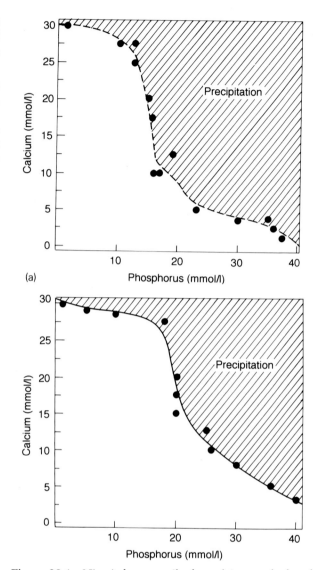

Figure 98.1 Ninetieth percentile for calcium and phosphorus precipitation in neonatal TPN solutions containing (a) 1% or (b) 2% amino acids. The measured calcium solubility after 24 hours is greater than 90% on the left side of the 90th percentile curve and less than 90% on the right side. (Reproduced with permission from Dunham [126].)

calcium gluconate because the former is more soluble [124,125]. Further studies are needed before such a change is made. Dunham *et al.* [126] have generated calcium and phosphorus precipitation curves for neonatal TPN, using TrophAmine, to guide pharmacists and clinicians in avoiding compounding TPN solutions that will precipitate (Figure 98.1).

Calcium phosphate is more soluble at cooler temperatures than at room or body temperature. Thus, serious concerns have been raised about the recent advocates for three-in-one infusates that contain glucose, amino acids and the lipid emulsion in the same bottle (or bag) with required electrolytes, minerals and vitamins. As these infusates must be administered without an in-line filter, the presence of lipid in the infusate obscures any visible precipitation that may occur, either on removal from refrigeration and warming prior to administration or during the time of infusion. Their use in low-birth-weight infants seems unwise, especially when efforts are being made to maximize calcium and phosphate intakes [9]. One retrospective review of three-in-one solutions in infants found such use safe, efficacious and cost effective for infants under 1 year of age [127].

The amino acid solutions compatible in three-in-one solutions are not those with the lowest pH values; in the Rollins et al. review [127], Travenol was the amino acid solution used – it does not even have the lowest pH of the adult standard solutions, Aminosyn does. Thus, maximal calcium and phosphorus levels cannot be achieved with three-in-one solutions and should not be used routinely in the neonate.

98.4.7 VITAMINS

A distinguished subcommittee has recently re-evaluated parenteral vitamin requirements [114]. The committee's major recommendations were as follows.

1. The initial guidelines for stable term infants and children in the 1975 American Medical Association (AMA) report appear adequate for the maintenance of blood levels of vitamins within acceptable ranges for short-term as well as long-term TPN.
2. MVI-Pediatric has been tested primarily in medically stable infants; children receiving oral supplements may need adjustments in the parenteral formulation.
3. There is an urgent need for a new formulation made specially for high-risk preterm infants.

Their specific recommendations for utilization of the existing vitamin preparation (1 vial of MVI-Pediatric per day for term infants and children and 40% of a vial per kilogram of body weight for preterm infants) and for a **new** formulation for preterm infants are both shown in Table 98.12.

Intravenous vitamins may be lost through adsorption to plastic TPN bags and tubing or through light exposure. Vitamin A, for instance, is lost primarily because of its adherence to intravenous tubing and secondarily because of its biodegradation in the presence of light [129]. Using radiolabeled vitamins, researchers found that only 31% of vitamin A, 68% of vitamin D and 64% of vitamin E were actually delivered to the patient over a period of 24 hours [130]. The problem of vitamin loss (e.g. retinol loss) during TPN appears much more severe in the management of VLBW infants because light intensity is higher in nurseries, and the TPN solution remains exposed to the administration tubing for longer periods of time [114].

The American Academy of Pediatrics (AAP) has suggested that safe and effective blood levels of vitamin

Table 98.12 Suggested intakes of parenteral vitamins in infants and children [After Ref. 114]

Vitamin	Term infants and children (dose per day)[a]	Preterm infants (dose/kg body wt) (maximum not to exceed term infant dose)	
		Current suggestions[b]	Best estimate for new formulation[c]
Lipid soluble			
A (μg)[d]	700.0	280.00	500.00
E (mg)[d]	7.0	2.80	2.80
K (μg)[d]	200.0	80.00	80.00
D (μg)[d]	10.0	4.00	4.00
(iu)	400.0	160.00	160.00
Water soluble			
Ascorbic acid (mg)	80.0	32.00	25.00
Thiamine (mg)	1.2	0.48	0.35
Riboflavin (mg)	1.4	0.56	0.15
Pyridoxine (mg)	1.0	0.40	0.18
Niacin (mg)	17.0	6.80	6.80
Pantothenate (mg)	5.0	2.00	2.00
Biotin (μg)	20.0	8.00	6.00
Folate (μg)	140.0	56.00	56.00
Vitamin B_{12} (μg)	1.0	0.40	0.30

[a] These guidelines for term infants and children are identical to those of the AMA (NAG) published in 1979. MVI-Pediatric (Armour)[e] meets these guidelines. Recent data indicate that 40 iu/kg per day of vitamin D (maximum of 400 iu per day) is adequate for term and preterm infants [128]. The higher dose of 160 iu/kg per day has not been associated with complications and maintains blood levels within the reference range for term infants fed orally. This dosage therefore appears acceptable until further studies using the lower dose formulation indicate its superiority.
[b] These represent a practical guide (40% of the currently available single-dose vial MVI-Pediatric (Armour)[e] formulation per kilogram of body weight), which will provide adequate levels of vitamins E, D and K but low levels of retinol and excess levels of most of the B vitamins. The maximum daily dose is one single-dose vial for any infant.
[c] Because of elevated levels of the water-soluble vitamins, the current proposal is to reduce the intake of water-soluble vitamins and increase retinol as described in the Committee's report.
[d] 700 μg RE (retinol equivalents) = 2300 international units (iu); 7 mg α-tocopherol = 7 iu; 10 μg vitamin D = 400 iu.
[e] Now produced by Asta.

E are between 1 and 2 mg/dl [131]. Vitamin E levels > 3.5 mg/dl have been associated with an increased incidence of NEC and sepsis. Forty per cent of a vial (2 ml = 2.8 mg α-tocopherol) per kilogram per day results in normal serum vitamin E levels within the range of 1.0–2.5 mg/dl [132]. Using this dosage of 2 ml MVI-Pediatric per kilogram (to a maximum of 5 ml) per day, infants with birth weights between 450 and 1360 g maintained adequate vitamin E levels [133]; this dose is recommended (Table 98.12). A recent study

[134] convincingly showed that the fluorescent method of measuring vitamin E is very inaccurate in patients receiving IVF. The method of choice for monitoring vitamin E levels in intensive care nurseries is by high-pressure liquid chromatography [134].

In addition, Greene et al. [135] have recently shown that extremely low-birth-weight infants (less than 1000 g) who receive TPN for 1 month show a progressive decline in serum retinol, with half of such infants showing levels below 10 μg/dl (the level believed to result in clinical manifestations of vitamin A deficiency). Their observation was of significant importance in light of two reports correlating a higher incidence of bronchopulmonary dysplasia with low plasma retinol levels [136,137]. Shenai et al. [138] subsequently performed a blind randomized trial to see if increased plasma retinol levels would alter the incidence or severity of bronchopulmonary dysplasia. The treatment group received approximately 400–450 μg/kg per day intramuscularly and an additional intravenous intake of 50–150 μg/kg per day for 4 weeks. The treatment group showed a significant increase in plasma retinol levels from 20.7 ± 0.9 to 34 ± 3.2 per deciliter. Additionally, the vitamin A-treated infants showed a significant reduction in the incidence of bronchopulmonary dysplasia compared with the control group [138]. In one study of VLBW infants, adding 40% of a vial (280 μg retinol) per kilogram body weight to the IVF emulsion [133] resulted in significant increases in plasma retinol levels. Such an approach helps to avoid loss of vitamin on to the plastic tubing. In Europe, fat-soluble vitamins have been added to IVF for years. The introduction of Vitalipid (Kabi-Vitrum, Stockholm) into North America could mimic the results above [56]. Vitalipid is an intravenous soybean oil emulsion containing vitamins A, D, E and K. A recent study concluded that mixing of multivitamins in dextrose–amino acid–electrolyte solutions results in poor delivery of vitamin A; this problem is improved by mixing the vitamin preparation in lipid [139].

98.4.8 TRACE ELEMENTS

An expert committee [114] has recently updated trace element recommendations for neonates (Table 98.13).

(a) Aluminum

Parenteral feeding solutions currently used for preterm infants are contaminated with aluminum. These infants have been shown to have increased aluminum concentrations in brain [140], bone [141] and liver [141]. Aluminum in bone may impair bone calcium uptake and may contribute to the pathogenesis of PN-related bone disease [141]. There is experimental evidence that aluminum can reduce bile flow in both rats and piglets, and possibly contribute to neonatal cholestasis [141]. Standards are being established for safe amounts of aluminum in intravenous nutrition products [142].

Table 98.13 Recommended intravenous intakes of trace elements[a] [After Ref. 114]

	Infants		Children (μ/kg per day) (maximum μg/day)
Element	Preterm[b] (μg/kg per day)	Term (μg/kg per day)	
Zinc	400.00	250 <3 months 100 >3 months	50.00 (5000)
Copper[c]	20.00	20.00	20.00 (300)
Selenium[d]	2.00	2.00	2.00 (30)
Chromium[d]	0.20	0.20	0.20 (5.0)
Manganese[c]	1.00	1.00	1.00 (50)
Molybdenum[d]	0.25	0.25	0.25 (5.0)
Iodide	1.00	1.00	1.00 (1.0)

[a] When TPN is only supplemental or limited to less than 4 weeks, only zinc (Zn) need be added. Thereafter, addition of the remaining elements is advisable.
[b] Available concentrations of molybdenum (Mo) and manganese (Mn) are such that dilution of the manufacturer's product may be necessary. Neotrace (Lyphomed Co, Rosemont, IL) contains a higher ratio of Mn to Zn than suggested in this table (i.e. Zn = 1.5 mg and Mn = 25 μg in each milliliter).
[c] Omit in patients with obstructive jaundice. (Manganese and copper are excreted primarily in bile.)
[d] Omit in patients with renal dysfunction.

98.4.9 ALBUMIN

The simultaneous administration of albumin with TPN in hypoalbuminemic adult and pediatric patients has been shown to produce a sustained increase in serum albumin levels [143]. Improved albumin levels lead to normalization of serum colloid osmotic pressures, improvement in gastrointestinal tolerance of enteral feedings, improved wound healing, decreased morbidity and mortality, and a decrease in length of hospital stay [143,144].

In a recent study of 24 neonates [144] with albumin < 3 g/dl, the study group (mean birth weight 1.26 ± 0.1 kg) received supplemental albumin infusions concurrently with their TPN. The study infants regained birth weight earlier than the control group, in addition to showing sustained increase in serum albumin concentration and increased mean arterial blood pressure. Slow albumin infusion (no more than 1 g/kg per day) had no adverse effect on the severity of their respiratory distress [144].

98.5 Initiating therapy

Ideally, prior to initiating PN, a complete nutritional assessment including anthropometric measurements should be carried out to determine the potential need for nutritional repletion and to estimate caloric requirements (which will help dictate the route of administration utilized). Nutritional assessment techniques have been reviewed elsewhere [145]. Skinfold thickness reference data are now available for preterm infants from 24 weeks of gestation onward [146]. Mid-arm circumference (MAC) data are also available for preterm infants [146–148]. Using the mid-arm circumference to head circumference (MAC/HC) provides a 'discriminative method for evaluation of intrauterine growth and a non-invasive technique for following somatic protein status in growing preterm infants' [147]. Preterm infants' anthropometric values have recently been summarized [149].

98.5.1 ORDER WRITING

We designed a preprinted PN order sheet to save time for both the house staff and pharmacy personnel. In addition, the order sheet serves to avoid errors of omission, ensuring that all necessary nutrients are ordered. The order sheet provides the necessary input for a computer program written by Nick MacKenzie MD [150]. Required input includes the patient's weight (kg), total fluid intake for the day (ml/kg per day), the amount of fat emulsion (g/kg per day), fat concentration (10 or 20%), fluid volumes contributed by other parenteral lines or enteral feeds, desired protein intake

via amino acids (g/kg per day) and the percentage concentration of dextrose. The doses of trace elements, vitamins and electrolytes are ordered in amounts per day or amounts per kilogram per day. The computer performs all necessary calculations (Figure 98.2). Protocol recommendations are provided in the right hand column of the order sheet for reference.

The output of the computer program includes:

1. TPN and fat emulsion bottle labels;
2. mixing instructions for the pharmacy with calcium phosphate precipitation curve data;
3. a detailed nutritional summary including calorie : nitrogen ratio, kilocalories per kilogram per day, and percentage of total calories given as fat.

The calcium–phosphate precipitation curve data and the calorie : nitrogen ratio are new modifications not available in the original program.

The use of the order sheet and computer program has saved approximately 20 minutes of physician time per patient per day, time that was previously spent doing tedious, error-prone manual calculations. An additional 20 minutes per patient per day of pharmacy time is saved. Calculation and labeling errors have been eliminated by using this program.

98.6 Complications

Patients receiving PN are at risk for developing technical, infectious and metabolic complications. These complications can be avoided or minimized only by regular monitoring, strict asepsis and a multidisciplinary nutrition support team including a physician, pharmacist, nutrition support nurse and nutritionist [151]. Complications are fewer when PN protocols are administered by those familiar with the technique [152].

98.6.1 TECHNICAL COMPLICATIONS

Possible complications at the time of the catheter insertion are depicted in Table 98.14. Complications related to ongoing use of the catheter are shown in Table 98.15.

Catheters placed with the tip lying in the right atrium are at risk for precipitating: (1) arrhythmias, and (2) atrial perforation with cardiac tamponade, occasionally with hydrothorax [153,154]. Mehta et al. [155] studied 42 newborns prospectively after Broviac catheter placement. The catheter tip, distal superior vena cava and right atrium were evaluated by weekly two-dimensional echocardiograms. Six infants (14%) had thrombus by echocardiographic examination after the catheter had been in place for a median of 7 weeks. Those with thrombus formation had significantly **lower** birth

LUCILE SALTER PACKARD
CHILDREN'S HOSPITAL AT STANFORD
725 Welch Road • Palo Alto • CA 94304

PHYSICIAN'S ORDERS FOR

PEDIATRIC PARENTERAL NUTRITION

Pharmacy: 497–8287

(addressograph stamp)

A. Please send TPN orders to the Pharmacy before 11:00 A.M. DAILY.
B. Order all additives on a 24-hours basis; i.e., mEq/Kg/day, mM/Kg/day, ml/day, ml/Kg/day.

PERIPHERAL ____ or CENTRAL ____ TPN LINE (check one)   Today's DATE _____
DUE DATE ____/____/____ TIME DUE _____(AM PM)   Today's WEIGHT _____ Kg
TOTAL FLUID INTAKE (ml/Kg/day) _____   Next Bottle # _____
AMOUNT OF FAT EMULSION (gm/Kg/day) _____   Fat Concentration ____ 10% ____ 20% (check one)

How many IV or IA lines exist which will not be used for TPN? _____

	Line		**Line**
Enter flow rates (ml/hr):	(1) _____	and % NaCl:	(1) _____
	(2) _____	(e.g., 0.45%)	(2) _____
	(3) _____		(3) _____

If taking enteral feeds, complete the following section (check one):

____ 1. Total fluids administered as parenteral and advancing enteral, i.e., "TPN + PO." (Additives are distributed assuming that the total fluids will be given parenterally)

____ 2. Total fluids administered as parenteral and fixed enteral. (Additives are distributed in parenteral fluids only; ignores electrolyte content of enteral fluids)

Enter Amount _____ (mls), Frequency: q ____ hrs, Calories/ml _____, Product Name _____

Enter AMINO ACIDS (gm/Kg/day) † _____ Enter DEXTROSE CONCENTRATION _____ %

TODAY'S ADDITIVES		**PROTOCOL RECOMMENDATION**
TRACE ELEMENTS AND VITAMINS:		
1. PEDIATRIC TRACE ELEMENTS	____ ml/Kg/day	0.2 ml /Kg/day (weight < 20 Kg)
2. ADULT TRACE ELEMENTS	____ ml/day	5 ml/day (weight > 20 Kg)
3. ZINC (additional)	____ mcg/Kg/day	100 mcg/Kg/day — Premies Only
4. PEDIATRIC M.V.I.	____ ml/day	2 ml/Kg/day — infants < 2.5 Kg
	____ ml/day	5 ml/day — infants > 2.5 Kg and Children up to 11 years of age
5. ADULT M.V.I. – 12 (or generic)	____ ml/day	10 ml/day — children > 11 yrs. of age
6. VITAMIN K	____ mg/day	0.5 mg/day — children > 11 yrs. of age
ELECTROLYTES AND MINERALS:		
1. PHOSPHATE*	____ nM/Kg/day	0.5–2 mM/Kg/day
2. SODIUM	____ mEq/Kg/day	2.4 mEq/Kg/day (Sodium from other IVs is included)
3. POTASSIUM	____ mEq/Kg/day	2–3 mEq/Kg/day
4. ACETATE*†	____ mEq/Kg/day	1–4 mEq/Kg/day
5. MAGNESIUM	____ mEq/Kg/day	0.25–0.5 mEq/Kg/day
6. CALCIUM GLUCONATE	____ MG/Kg/day	50–500 mg/Kg/day
7. HEPARIN	____ Units/ml	0.5–1 Unit/ml
8. INSULIN	____ Units/liter	
9. OTHER (specify)	____	
10. OTHER (specify)	____	

*NOTE: Balance of anions will be provided as chloride.

† Each 0.5 Gm/Kg/day of Amino Acid provides either 0.47 mEq/Kg/day of Acetate (TrophAmine) or 0.74 mEq/Kg/day of Acetate (Aminosyn)

_____ RN   _____ MD

Figure 98.2 Example of physician's order sheet for neonatal TPN.

Table 98.14 Possible complications at the time of catheter insertion

Pneumothorax	Catheter embolism
Hemothorax	Catheter malposition
Hydromediastinum	Thoracic duct laceration
Subclavian artery injury	Cardiac perforation and
Subclavian hematoma	tamponade
Innominate or subclavian vein	Brachial plexus injury
laceration	Horner's syndrome
Arteriovenous fistula	Phrenic nerve paralysis
Air embolism	Carotid artery injury

Table 98.15 Possible complications related to use of the catheter

Venous thrombosis
    Superior vena cava syndrome
    Pulmonary embolus

Catheter dislodgment

Perforation and/or infusion leaks (pericardial, pleural, mediastinal)

weight and gestational ages than those without thrombus. The catheter was removed with the first sign of thrombosis. There was no correlation of thrombosis with duration of catheter placement.

As mentioned previously, more nurseries are employing percutaneous central venous catheterization. Recently, 481 catheters placed percutaneously in a neonatal intensive care unit were followed over 3 years [156]. Fifty percent of the catheters were placed in infants weighing ≤1 kg. Mean catheter life was 13 days. Almost half were removed non-electively for leaking, clotting or suspicion of sepsis (6%); 1.3% were confirmed catheter sepsis. For catheter-related sepsis, three factors were important: prolonged catheter stay (3–5 weeks), *Staphylococcus epidermidis* and weight ≤1 kg [156]. These 'perc' lines result in lower complication rates than those reported with surgically placed central venous catheters.

98.6.2 CATHETER ASSOCIATED INFECTION

The major catheter-related complication is infection. Diagnosis and treatment of catheter sepsis has been discussed thoroughly elsewhere [7].

98.6.3 METABOLIC COMPLICATIONS

Potential metabolic complications in patients on PN are shown in Table 98.16. As Heird and Kashyap [9] have pointed out, these complications are of two general types: (1) those resulting from the patient's limited metabolic capacity for the various components of the PN infusate; and (2) those secondary to the PN infusate *per se*.

(a) Use of intravenous fat

If the IVF infusion exceeds its maximal clearance rate, hyperlipidemia occurs, which may then cause the potential complications shown in Table 98.17. Thus, careful monitoring of the use of IVF emulsions is essential.

Neither 'turbidity checks' nor nephelometry measurements (a more accurate measurement of plasma turbidity) have been shown to correlate well with elevated lipid levels [157,158]. One must, therefore, regularly monitor serum triglycerides, cholesterol and fatty acid/albumin molar ratios when using IVF.

Altered pulmonary function

Several investigators have demonstrated significant drops of Pao_2 without alteration in other pulmonary function tests after the administration of boluses of IVF to neonates [159,160]. McKeen, Brigham and Bowers [161] found that administering IVF doses of 0.25 g/kg per hour to sheep caused:

1. an increase in pulmonary artery pressure;
2. a decrease in arterial oxygen tension (Pao_2);
3. an increase in pulmonary lymphatic flow.

Identical findings have been described with doses of only 0.125 g/kg per hour [162].

The use of IVF in patients with pulmonary compromise has yielded conflicting results. Because fat emboli were found in pulmonary capillaries during post-mortem examinations of neonates who received Intralipid, the infusion of IVF in neonates was postulated to alter pulmonary function further [163]. Yet the fat deposition in the pulmonary microcirculation also occurred in babies who never received IVF [164]. Shroeder, Paust and Schmidt [165] found **no** pulmonary fat accumulation in 22 infants, 13 of whom received Intralipid, when lungs were fixed *in situ* immediately after death; they attributed the previous findings to artifact secondary to delayed fixation of the lungs. Yet, Shulman, Langston and Schanler [166] reviewed the histopathology and clinical course of 39 hospitalized infants who died during a 2-year period. Thirteen had received no IVF; 26 had received IVF. All 39 had lipid in pulmonary macrophages, chondrocytes and interstitial cells. However, the incidence of pulmonary vascular lipid deposition in the group given IVF was significantly greater than in the other group. The severity of pulmonary vascular lipid depositions in the IVF group correlated positively with the percentage of the infants' lives during which lipids were administered

Table 98.16 Potential metabolic complications of parenteral nutrition

Complication	Possible etiology
Disorders related to metabolic capacity of the patient	
Congestive heart failure and pulmonary edema	Excessively rapid infusion of the PN solution
Hyperglycemia (with resultant glucosuria, osmotic diuresis and possible dehydration)	Excessive intake (either excessive dextrose concentration or increased infusion rate) Change in metabolic state (e.g. sepsis, surgical stress, use of steroids) Common in low-birth-weight infants if dextrose load exceeds their ability to adapt
Hypoglycemia	Sudden cessation of infusate
Azotemia	Excessive administration of amino acids or protein hydrolysate (excessive nitrogen intake)
Electrolyte disorders Mineral disorders Vitamin disorders Trace element disorders	Excessive or inadequate intake
Essential fatty acid deficiency	Inadequate intake
Hyperlipidemia (increased triglycerides, cholesterol, and free fatty acids)	Excessive intake of intravenous fat emulsion
Disorders related to infusate components	
Metabolic acidosis	Use of hydrochloride salts of cationic amino acids
Hyperammonemia	Inadequate arginine intake, ? deficiencies of other urea cycle substrates, ? plasma amino acid imbalance, ? hepatic dysfunction
Abnormal plasma aminograms	Amino acid pattern of infusate
Miscellaneous	
Anemia	Failure to replace blood loss; iron deficiency; folic acid and vitamin B_{12} deficiency; copper deficiency
Demineralization of bone; rickets	Inadequate intake of calcium, inorganic phosphate and/or vitamin D
Hepatic disorders Cholestasis Biochemical and histopathologic abnormalities	Prematurity; malnutrition; sepsis; ? hepatotoxicity due to amino acid imbalance; exceeding non-nitrogen calorie : nitrogen ratio of 150 : 1 to 200 : 1, leading to excessive glycogen and/or fat deposition in the liver; decreased stimulation of bile flow; non-specific response to refeeding
Eosinophilia	Unknown

Modified from Heird, W.C. (1981) Total parenteral nutrition, in *Textbook of Gastroenterology and Nutrition in Infancy* (ed. E. Lebenthal) Raven Press, New York, p. 662.

Table 98.17 Potential hazards of the hyperlipidemia resulting from failure to 'clear' intravenous fat

Major
Impairment of pulmonary function
Deposition of pigmented material in macrophages (which may lead to diminished immune responsiveness)
Displacement of albumin-bound bilirubin by plasma free fatty acids (which may lead to kernicterus)

Minor
Possible risk of coronary artery disease
Fat overload syndrome (hyperlipemia, fever, lethargy, liver damage, coagulation disorders) encountered infrequently in infants and children.

and with mean intake; there was no correlation with the peak serum triglyceride level or the frequency of elevated triglycerides [166]. Experimental animal studies have shown that lipid-induced hypoxemia can be prevented with indomethacin [161]. Interestingly, Hageman *et al.* [167] noted that in rabbits there were no blood gas or prostaglandin changes in lipid-infused normal animals. However, when the rabbits' lungs were damaged with oleic acid and then infused with IVF, significant deterioration in gas exchange occurred. Furthermore, these changes were blocked by indomethacin (implying prostaglandin-mediated effects of IVF). Brans *et al.* [168] found that oxygen diffusion in the lungs of premature infants was not affected by the infusion of up to 4 g/kg per day of Intralipid over 24 hours. A recent study [169] was quite disturbing. Forty-two neonates (less than 1750 g birth weight) were randomly assigned to PN with or without IVF for 5 days in the first week of life. Chronic lung disease increased in duration and tended to be more severe after lipid administration. Five IVF patients developed stage 3 bronchopulmonary dysplasia versus none of the control group. Seven IVF infants were discharged home on oxygen versus none in the control group. Other centers have administered IVF in similar manner in the first week of life (beginning at 0.5 g/kg per day, increasing to a maximum of 2.5 g/kg per day) without reporting such findings. Further, many centers avoid IVF during the first week of life in low-birth-weight infants owing to hyperbilirubinemia. In two subsequent studies (one starting IVF on the first day of life [170] and one starting IVF on day 4 [171]), the adverse effects seen by Hammerman and Aramburo [169] did not occur. Gilbertson et al. [170] concluded that when given at rates not exceeding 0.15 g/kg per hour, sick VLBW infants can tolerate IVF with stepwise dose increases from the first day of life without increased incidence of adverse effects. In the Adamkin, Radmacher and Klingbeil [171] study, doses were similar to those in the Gilbertson study – 0.5–3.0 g/kg per day IVF; mean free fatty acid:albumin molar ratio was <1.0 at all doses (maximum ratio = 3.0). Interestingly, in the Adamkin study [171] 5% of patients had triglycerides > 200 mg/dl. A third study [172], using a LCT/MCT mix, also demonstrated no adverse effects of starting IVF on day 3 (at 1 g/kg per day) to a maximum of 3 g/kg per day. There was a marked increase in free fatty acid levels in the MCT/LCT group but the fraction of unbound (free) bilirubin was significantly less in this group. A significant increase in cholesterol occurred only in the MCT/LCT group.

Risk of kernicterus

There has been concern that liberation of free fatty acids during hydrolysis of IVF might displace albumin-bound bilirubin. If infants are icteric, the use of IVF emulsions has been considered hazardous if, indeed, unbound or free bilirubin might potentially increase the risk of kernicterus. Andrew, Chan and Schiff [173] recommended that a safe method for monitoring and preventing such complications would be to maintain a free fatty acid : serum albumin molar ratio (FA : SA) at 6 or less. Using a simplified method to measure the FA : SA, we found that in preterm infants receiving 0.5–3.3 g/kg day of continuous IVF infusions in the second week of life, the mean ratio was only 1.1, range 0–5 [174]. If, on the other hand, bolus infusions are utilized or if IVF is administered in the first week of life, the FA : SA might exceed 6 [173] and such infants might be at risk. Premature infants can have FA : SA

ratios greater than 10 [97]. Spear et al. [175] studied 20 premature infants (26–37 weeks of gestational age) given 1, 2 and 3 g/kg IVF over 15 hours on successive days. Infants of less than 30 weeks of gestation had significant increases in FA : SA with each increase in lipid dose, whereas infants greater than 30 weeks tolerated the IVF without increase in FA : SA. Infants whose FA : SA was greater than 4.0 were significantly more premature; such elevations occurred at both 2 and 3 g/kg per day. One gram per kilogram per day IVF over 15 hours resulted in minimal risk of decreased bilirubin binding [175]. Therefore, in icteric infants, it is crucial to monitor the FA : SA if they are receiving IVF. The American Academy of Pediatrics recommends that infants with bilirubin levels of 8–10 mg/dl (assuming an albumin concentration of 2.5–3.0 mg/dl) should receive **only** the amount of IVF required to meet essential fatty acid requirements (0.5–1.0 g/kg per day) [6].

Sepsis

A 1984 study [177] confirms previous observations that septic infants can develop significant elevations in triglyceride levels. A sudden rise in triglycerides not associated with an increase in IVF dose should make caregivers suspicious of sepsis. Dahlstrom and co-workers [178] also argue that the dose of IVF be lowered during acute illness. In a 1-year prospective study of 15 children on home TPN, they noted that acutely sick children had significantly increased serum triglyceride levels and prolonged prothrombin and partial thromboplastin values compared with times when they were well.

Thrombocytopenia

There is a reluctance to use IVF in patients with low platelet counts, based on reports of varying degrees of thrombocytopenia with earlier IVF preparations and on one case report with Intralipid. Many anecdotal reports of thrombocytopenia may well be secondary to an underlying condition (e.g sepsis) rather than to IVF. Cohen, Dahms and Hays [179] could not implicate IVF as a cause of thrombocytopenia in any of the 128 patients studied. In addition, ten of the patients had established thrombocytopenia secondary to sepsis or bone marrow suppression by cancer chemotherapy. In all ten, platelet counts actually rose with IVF use, concomitant with the improvement of the septicemia state or marrow recovery after cessation of chemotherapy. Interestingly, TPN **without** IVF may lead to EFA deficiency, which in turn may cause thrombocytopenia and platelet dysfunction. A study in ill neonates also failed to document any association between IVF and thrombocytopenia [180]. Goulet et al. [181] have the only recent documented association of IVF with thrombocytopenia. Seven patients on home TPN receiving 1–2 g per 24 hours over 3–18 months developed recurrent thrombocytopenia. Platelet life span was reduced. Sea-blue histiocytes containing granulations and hemophagocytosis were seen on bone marrow smears. Scans taken after injection of autologous erythrocytes labeled with ^{99m}Tc showed bone marrow sequestration of these cells. The authors concluded that long-term IVF administration induces hyperactivation of the monocyte–macrophage system [181]. Finally, Herson and colleagues [182] investigated bleeding time, platelet count and aggregation in ten neonates of 28–40 weeks' gestation, receiving 1 g/kg per day of Intralipid over 16 hours; no adverse effects were found.

Recommendations

- Patients receiving IVF should have laboratory specimens for total bilirubin, sodium and calcium ultracentrifuged to avoid spurious laboratory values.
- All patients receiving IVF should have triglyceride and cholesterol determinations at least weekly. If either value is elevated, the IVF dose should be adjusted appropriately.
- A serum triglyceride level should be obtained 24 hours after any increase in IVF dose to be sure that the patient can tolerate this new dose.
- A sudden elevation in triglyceride level at an IVF dose previously tolerated should raise the suspicion of sepsis.
- A determination of the FA : SA should be performed twice weekly on infants with any elevation of indirect bilirubin who are receiving IVF. Ideally, the FA : SA should be kept below 4 (the level at which no free bilirubin is generated in a number of *in vitro* studies).
- Any infant with respiratory or cardiac disease should have frequent monitoring of Pa_{O2} or transcutaneous oxygen and any fall in this value should result in an appropriate decrease in the IVF dose.
- We attempt to keep the serum triglyceride below 150 mg/dl (our laboratory normal values: 30–200 mg/dl), the cholesterol below 250 mg/dl (normal: 120–280 mg/dl) and the FA : SA below 4.
- Monitor platelet count and prothrombin time weekly during hospitalizations.

(b) Osteopenia of prematurity

Premature infants are subject to a unique condition, 'osteopenia of prematurity' or 'rickets of prematurity', a frequently occurring but poorly defined metabolic bone disease associated with decreased bone mineralization. In most cases, decreased bone mineralization is subclinical; this condition is diagnosed only after the development of bone fractures or overt rickets [183]. Experts now believe that a deficiency of calcium and phosphorus is more likely than a defect in vitamin D metabolism to be the cause of osteopenia in preterm infants [184]. Kovar, Mayne and Barltrop [116], as described earlier, suggest screening for rickets in preterm infants with plasma alkaline phosphatase: levels of up to five times the upper limit of the normal adult reference range are acceptable; a value of six times the upper limit of the adult reference range should prompt a radiograph to exclude rickets. Serial infant-adapted photon absorptiometry can help physicians follow the bone mineral content of preterm infants; unfortunately, this study is not routinely available. Two recent papers provide excellent reviews of osteopenia/metabolic bone disease [185,186].

(c) Hepatic dysfunction

Hepatic dysfunction remains one of the most common and most serious complications of TPN. Cholestasis is especially prevalent in very premature infants and in infants on TPN for longer than 2 weeks. The administration of 50 mg/kg per day of metronidazole for 3 weeks prevented the elevation of transaminases during TPN in neonates, suggesting the possible involvement of intestinal anaerobic flora in the pathogenesis of TPN-associated liver dysfunction [187]. Likewise, a study using prophylactic gentamicin in preterm neonates <1500 g showed such treatment may have a protective effect against TPN-induced cholestasis [188].

Hepatomegaly with mild elevation of serum transaminases in the absence of cholestasis may result from hepatic accumulation of lipid or glycogen secondary to either excess carbohydrate calories or an inappropriate non-nitrogen calorie : nitrogen ratio. Fatty infiltration of the liver as a result of excessive caloric intake is readily reversible in nearly all instances by reduction of total calories administered and, if necessary, alteration of the non-nitrogen calorie-to-nitrogen ratio [189].

Abnormal liver function tests are not uncommon in patients on PN for long periods of time. Those with chronic intestinal conditions complicated by infection or bacterial overgrowth are particularly susceptible to hepatic complications. In most of these patients, elevated liver enzymes improve with the initiation of partial enteral alimentation [189].

A small percentage of infants and children go on to develop chronic liver disease associated with poor growth [190] and even cirrhosis and hepatic failure [191]. A recent follow-up study of patients on long-term PN documented a wide variety of complications, but all of them except liver dysfunction proved to be temporary [192]. In this series, 57.6% of the children showed liver dysfunction during PN, and some of them

Table 98.18(a) Metabolic monitoring during peripheral or central parenteral nutrition – initial period[a]

| | Frequency per week | | | | |
Parameter	Stanford University USA	Miller Children's USA[c]	Columbia University USA[d]	Adelaide Children's Australia[e]	Hospital for Sick Children London, England[f]
Growth variables					
Weight	7	7	7	2	7
Length	1	1	1	–	1
Head circumference	1	–	1	Q 2 weeks	–
Anthropometrics[b]	Q 2 weeks	prn	–	–	–
Calorie/protein intakes	7	7	–	–	–
Nursing					
Intake/output	Q shift	Q shift	–	–	–
Urine specific gravity	Q shift	Q shift	–	2/day	–
Urine glucose	2–6/day	Q 4 hours	2–6/day	2/day	–
Urine electrolytes	–	–	–	Daily	–
Metabolic variables					
Electrolytes (Na, K, Cl, CO_2)	7	7	3–4	7	7
Ca, Mg, phosphate	2	7	2	7	2
Albumin	1	1	1	1	2
Transferrin+/or prealbumin	1	1	–	–	–
Liver function tests	1	1	1	1	2
Hemoglobin or hematocrit	1	–	2	2	2
Platelet count	1	–	–	2	2
Prothrombin time	1	–	–	1	–
Serum glucose	–	7	–	–	7
Blood urea nitrogen	7	7	2	–	–
Triglycerides	7	7	–	7	–
Plasma turbidity	–	–	–	–	7
Copper/zinc	Monthly	–	–	–	1
Folate/B_{12}	Monthly	–	–	Q 2 weeks	–
Blood NH_3	–	–	–	–	–
Screening for signs of infection					
WBC and differential	prn	–	prn	–	2
Cultures	prn	–	prn	–	–
Clinical observation (activity, temperature, etc.)	7	–	7	–	–

See footnote to Table 98.18(b) for key.

showed long-term abnormalities after its cessation. Significantly less serious liver disease is being documented in recent years due to more appropriate amino acid solutions (especially for neonates) and due to the initiation of enteral feeding earlier (stimulating bile flow).

Recommendations

If the serum glutamic oxaloacetic transaminase (SGOT; now known as aspartate transaminase or AST) or serum glutamic–pyruvic transaminase (SGPT; now known as alanine transaminase or ALT) rise in association with a normal or nearly normal direct bilirubin and alkaline phosphatase, check the total caloric intake and the calorie : nitrogen ratio. Reduce the caloric intake and/or decrease the non-nitrogen calorie : nitrogen ratio, which ideally should be 150–200 : 1.

Monitor for early evidence of cholestasis: use either the GGTP, 5′-nucleotidase or serum bile acids, or, if these tests are not easily obtainable, measure the direct or conjugated bilirubin on a weekly basis.

Table 98.18(b) Metabolic monitoring during peripheral or central parenteral nutrition – later period (when the patient is in a metabolic steady state)

Parameter	Frequency per week					
	Stanford University USA	Miller Children's USA[c]	Columbia University USA[d]	Adelaide Children's Australia[e]	Hospital for Sick Children London, England[f]	Alder Hey Children's Liverpool, England[g]
Growth variables						
Weight	7	7	7	2	7	–
Length	1	1	1	–	1	–
Head circumference	1	–	1	Q 2 weeks	–	–
Anthropometrics	Q 2 weeks	prn	–	–	–	–
Calorie/protein intakes	7	prn (as adjustments made)	–	–	–	–
Nursing						
Intake/output	Q shift	Q shift	–	–	–	–
Urine specific gravity	Q shift	Q shift	–	7	–	–
Urine glucose	Q shift	Q shift	2/day	7	–	–
Urine electrolytes	–	–	–	1	–	–
Metabolic variables						
Electrolytes (Na, K, Cl, CO_2)	1–2	1–2	1	2	2	1
Ca, Mg, phosphate	1	1	1	2	1	1
Albumin	1	1	1	1	1	1
Transferrin and/or prealbumin	1	1	–	–	–	1
Liver function tests	1	1	1	1	1	1
Hemoglobin or hematocrit	1	1	1	1	1	1
Platelet count	1	–	–	1	1	1
Prothrombin time	1	–	–	1	–	Monthly
Serum glucose	–	1	–	–	2	–
Blood urea nitrogen/creatinine	1	1	1	2	–	–
Triglycerides	1	1	–	1	–	1
Plasma turbidity	–	–	–	–	2	–
Copper/zinc	Monthly	–	–	Q 2 weeks	Q 2 weeks	Monthly
Folate/B_{12}	Monthly	–	–	Q 2 weeks	–	Monthly
Blood NH_3	1	1	–	–	–	–
C-reactive protein	–	–	–	–	–	1
Serum iron	–	–	–	–	–	Monthly
Amino acid profile	–	–	–	–	–	Monthly
Carnitine	–	–	–	–	–	Monthly
Selenium/peroxidase	Q 3 monthly	–	–	–	–	Q 3 monthly
Ferritin/thyroxine	–	–	–	–	–	Q 3 monthly
Screening for infection						
WBC with differential	prn	–	prn	–	1	–
Cultures	prn	prn	prn	–	–	–
Clinical observation	7	–	7	–	–	–

[a] Usually takes 1 week; the time during which full caloric intake is being achieved; any time of suspected or actual metabolic instability (e.g. postoperative period, presence of infection).
[b] Triceps skinfold thickness (TSF); mid-upper arm circumference (MAC).
[c] Pediatric Parenteral Nutrition Guideline, July 1988, Miller Children's Hospital, Long Beach, California
[d] Heird, W. (1987) Total parenteral nutrition and enteral feeding, in *Pediatric Nutrition: Theory and Practice* (eds R.J. Grand, J.L. Sutphen and W.H. Dietz) Butterworth, Boston, p.75b.
[e] Kingsley Coulthard, Chief Pharmacist (personal communication, 1989).
[f] Booth, I.W. and Shaw, V. (1988) Parenteral nutrition, in *Harries' Pediatric Gastroenterology*, Churchill Livingstone, Edinburgh, p.567.
[g] Tony Nunn, Chief Pharmacist (personal communication, 1989).

(d) Increased risk of gallstones

Long-term administration of PN increases the risk of gallstones in patients of all ages [193–199]; children with ileal disease or bowel resection are at particularly high risk [198]. In one adult series, there was a twofold increase in gallbladder disease in patients who received no oral intake during PN as opposed to those who had oral supplementation in addition to PN [197]; the gallbladder disease appears to be secondary, at least in part, to bile stasis.

Clinically, gallbladder disease can be detected by the demonstration of 'sludge' or a stone (or stones) in a patient with liver function tests consistent with cholestasis. Messing *et al.* [196] demonstrated 'sludge' in 6% of cases in the first 3 weeks of TPN; the incidence increases to 50% between the fourth and sixth weeks and reaches 100% after 6 weeks.

Roslyn *et al.* [198] recommend periodic ultrasonography in children on prolonged PN, especially if they have an ileal resection or underlying ileal disease. They advise clinicians to suspect cholecystitis in any child on TPN who complains of abdominal pain.

A review [200] of 246 infants and children receiving PN for more than 4 weeks revealed significant biliary disease. In 68 who died there were postmortem or ultrasound studies available in 16; of the 178 survivors, 68 had adequate abdominal ultrasonographic findings. Eleven of the 84 patients studied had cholelithiasis. Six required cholecystectomy for relief of chronic abdominal pain, pancreatitis or empyema of the gallbladder. One had cholecystotomy. Two of the remaining four are asymptomatic; one has abdominal colic, and one expired of hepatic insufficiency related to PN. The authors recommend routine abdominal ultrasonography for those on PN for longer than 30 days as well as for any patient on PN who presents with abdominal pain. They argue for early elective cholecystectomy for PN-associated cholelithiasis, but many centers elect to watch asymptomatic patients, and several have actually described spontaneous resolution of stones. Forty-two infants receiving furosemide (study group) and 44 patients not receiving the drug were compared while receiving TPN [201]. The incidence of gallstones in the study group was 21% (compared with 2% in controls). When followed over 1 year, the gallstones did not resolve. Furosemide, either independently or in conjunction with the use of TPN, predisposes to the development of gallstones.

It is of interest that two cases of gallstones have been described in infants after extracorporeal membrane oxygenation (ECMO) [202]. TPN, prolonged fasting and the use of diuretics all contribute to stone formation, but the hemolysis during ECMO may be particularly important in these patients. Gallstones should be considered in any post-ECMO child with abdominal complaints or jaundice.

98.7   Monitoring

Our suggested schedule for monitoring patients while on PN is shown in Table 98.18, where a comparison is given of the author's monitoring regimen with other regimens in the USA and worldwide.

98.8   Summary

Parenteral nutrition remains a therapy in evolution. Since the publication of *Manual of Pediatric Parenteral Nutrition* [203], a new technology for the provision of continuous insulin to VLBW infants has appeared. New amino acid solutions (e.g. TrophAmine, Aminosyn PF) have been designed for the preterm infant. A new fat emulsion has been released (Liposyn II), and fat emulsions containing MCT oil have been released in Europe. A new pediatric multivitamin (MVI-Pediatric) has also been released. A recent revision of AMA expert guidelines has been published on the use of vitamins, trace elements, calcium, phosphorus and magnesium. Oral and intravenous preparations of L-carnitine have become available. New technology to help access caloric needs better has been designed [204]. Standards for nutritional support in hospitalized pediatric patients have been established [205]. Finally, alternative routines of nutrient delivery are being considered [206,207]. The practitioner is strongly urged to keep up with the latest literature so that his or her patients may continue to receive state-of-the-art care.

References

1. Committee on Nutrition (1985) Nutritional needs of low-birthweight infants. *Pediatrics*, 75, 976–86.
2. Pittard, W.B. and Levkoff, A.H. (1988) Parenteral nutrition for the neonate, in *Nutrition During Infancy* (eds R.C. Tsang and B.L. Nichols), Hanley & Belfus, Philadelphia, pp. 327–39.
3. Grand, R.J., Watkins, J.B. and Torti, F.M. (1976) Development of the human gastrointestinal tract. *Gastroenterology*, 70, 790–810.
4. Lebenthal, E. and Lee, P.C. (1983) Interactions of determinants in the ontogeny of the gastrointestinal tract: a unified concept. *Pediatr. Res.*, 17, 19–24.
5. Milla, P.J. (1984) Development of intestinal structure and function, in *Neonatal Gastroenterology – Contemporary Issues* (eds M.S. Tanner and R.J. Stocks), Intercept, Newcastle upon Tyne, pp. 1–20.
6. Sunshine, P. (1990) Fetal gastrointestinal physiology, in *Assessment and Care of the Fetus: Physiological, Clinical, and Medicolegal Principles* (eds R.D. Eden and F.H. Boehm), Appleton & Lange, East Norwalk, CT, pp. 93–112.
7. Kerner, Jr, J.A. (1991) Parenteral nutrition, in *Pediatric Gastrointestinal Disease* (eds W.A. Walker *et al.*), B.C. Decker, Philadelphia, pp. 1645–75.
8. Warner, B.W. (1992) Parenteral nutrition in the pediatric patient, in *Total Parenteral Nutrition*, 2nd edn (ed. J. Fisher), Little, Brown, Boston, pp. 299–322.
9. Heird, W.C. and Kashyap, S. (1991) Intravenous feeding, in *Neonatal Nutrition and Metabolism* (ed. W.W. Hay Jr), Mosby Yearbook, St Louis, pp. 237–59.
10. Booth, I.W. and Shaw, V. (1988) Parenteral nutrition, in *Harries' Pediatric Gastroenterology*, 2nd edn (eds P.J. Milla and D.R.R. Muller), Churchill Livingstone, Edinburgh, pp. 558–83.

11. Ramanujam, T.M. (1989) *Parenteral Nutrition in Infants and Children*, V.V. Publishers, Madras, India, pp. 9–12.
12. Weinsier, R.L., Heimburger, D.C. and Butterworth, C.E. (1989) *Handbook of Clinical Nutrition*, Mosby, St Louis, pp. 221–42.
13. Heird, W.C. and Winters, R.W. (1975) Total parenteral nutrition: the state of the art. *J. Pediatr.*, 86, 2–16.
14. Dudrick, S.J., Copeland, E.M. III and MacFadyen, B.V. (1975) Long-term parenteral nutrition: its current status. *Hosp. Pract.*, 10, 47–58.
15. Kerner Jr, J.A., Hartman, G.E. and Sunshine, P. (1985) The medical and surgical management of infants with the short bowel syndrome. *J. Perinatol.*, 5, 13–18.
16. Dorney, S.F.A., Ament, M.E., Berquist, W.E. *et al.* (1985) Improved survival in very short small bowel of infancy with use of long-term parenteral nutrition. *J. Pediatr.*, 107, 521–25.
17. Heird, W.C. (1987) Parenteral nutrition, in *Pediatric Nutrition* (eds R.J. Grand, J.L. Sutphen and W.H. Dietz), Butterworth, Boston, pp. 747–61.
18. Moyer-Mileur, L. and Chan, G.M. (1986) Nutritional support of very-low-birth-weight infants requiring prolonged assisted ventilation. *Am. J. Dis. Child.*, 140, 929–32.
19. Unger, A., Goetzman, B.W., Chan, C. *et al.* (1986) Nutritional practices and outcome of extremely premature infants. *Am. J. Dis. Child.*, 140, 1027–33.
20. Gunn, T., Reaman, G. and Outerbridge E.W. (1978) Peripheral total parenteral nutrition for premature infants with the respiratory distress syndrome: a controlled study. *J. Pediatr.*, 92, 608–13.
21. Yu, V.Y.H., James, B., Hendry, P. *et al.* (1979) Total parenteral nutrition in very-low-birth-weight infants: a controlled trial. *Arch. Dis. Child.*, 54, 653–61.
22. Kerner, J.A., Hattner, J.A.T., Trautman, M.S. *et al.* (1988) Postnatal somatic growth in very-low-birth-weight infants on peripheral parenteral nutrition. *J. Pediatr. Perinat. Nutr.*, 2, 27–34.
23. Cashore, W.J., Sedaghatian, M.R. and Usher, R.H. (1975) Nutritional supplements with intravenously administered lipid, protein hydrolysate, and glucose in small premature infants. *Pediatrics*, 56, 8–16.
24. Churella, H.R., Bachhuber, B.S. and MacLean, W.C. (1985) Survey: methods of feeding low-birth-weight infants. *Pediatrics*, 76, 243–49.
25. Adamkin, D.A. (1986) Nutrition in very very-low-birth-weight infants. *Clin. Perinatol.*, 13, 419–43.
26. Zlotkin, S.H., Stallings, V.A. and Pencharz, P.B. (1985) Total parenteral nutrition in children. *Pediatr. Clin. North Am.*, 32, 381–400.
27. Koldovsky, O., Sunshine, P. and Kretchmer, N. (1966) Cellular migration of intestinal epithelia in suckling and weaned rats. *Nature*, 212, 1389–90.
28. Herbst, J.J. and Sunshine, P. (1969) Postnatal development of the small intestine of the rat. *Pediatr. Res.*, 3, 27–33.
29. Sunshine, P., Herbst, J.J., Koldovsky, O. *et al.* (1971) Adaptation of the gastrointestinal tract to extrauterine life. *Ann. N. Y. Acad. Sci.*, 176, 16–29.
30. Herbst, J.J., Sunshine, P. and Kretchmer, N. (1969) Intestinal malabsorption in infancy and childhood. *Adv. Pediatr.*, 16, 11–64.
31. Brown, E. and Sweet, A. (1982) Neonatal necrotizing enterocolitis. *Pediatr. Clin. North Am.*, 29, 114–70.
32. Aynsley-Green, A. (1985) Metabolic and endocrine interrelation in the human fetus and neonate. *Am. J. Clin. Nutr.*, 41, 399–417.
33. Feng, J.J., Kwong, L.K., Kerner, J.A. *et al.* (1987) Resumption of intestinal maturation upon reintroduction of intraluminal nutrients: functional and biochemical correlations. *Clin. Res.*, 35, 228A.
34. Malkani, A., and Kerner Jr, J.A. (1989) Nutritional management, in *Fetal and Neonatal Brain Injury* (eds D.K. Stevenson and P. Sunshine), B.C. Decker, Toronto, pp. 159–72.
35. Ziegler, M., Jakobowski, D., Hoelzer, D. *et al.* (1980) Route of pediatric parenteral nutrition: proposed criteria revision. *J. Pediatr. Surg.*, 15, 472–76.
36. Higgs, S.C., Malan, A.F., Heese, H. De V. *et al.* (1974) A comparison of oral feeding and total parenteral nutrition in infants of very-low-birth-weight. *S. Afr. Med. J.*, 48, 2169–73.
37. Hall, R.T. and Rhodes, R.G. (1976) Total parenteral alimentation via indwelling umbilical catheters in the newborn period. *Arch. Dis. Child.*, 51, 929–34.
38. Merritt, R.J. (1981) Neonatal nutritional support. *Clin. Consul. Nutr. Support*, 1, 5–10.
39. Coran, A.G. (1981) Parenteral nutritional support of the neonate. *Tele Session (a group telephone workshop), New York*: Tele Session Corporation, August 17, 1981.
40. Kerner Jr, J.A. (1983) The use of umbilical catheters for parenteral nutrition, in *Manual of Pediatric Parenteral Nutrition* (ed J.A. Kerner, Jr), Wiley, New York, pp. 303–306.
41. Kanarek, K.S., Kuznicki, M.B. and Blair, R.C. (1991) Infusion of total parenteral nutrition via the umbilical artery. *JPEN*, 15, 71–74.
42. Nakamura, K.T., Sato, Y. and Erenberg A. (1990) Evaluation of a percutaneously placed 27-gauge central venous catheter in neonates weighing less than 1200 grams. *JPEN*, 14, 295–99.
43. Abdulla, F., Dietrich, K.A. and Pramanik, A.K. (1990) Percutaneous femoral venous catheterization in preterm neonates. *J. Pediatr.*, 117, 788–91.
44. Anderson, T.L. Muttart, C.R., Bieber, M.A. *et al.* (1979) A controlled trial of glucose versus glucose and amino acids in premature infants. *J. Pediatr.*, 94, 947–51.
45. Zlotkin, S.H., Bryan, M.H. and Anderson, C.H. (1981) Intravenous nitrogen and energy intakes required to duplicate *in utero* nitrogen accretion in prematurely born human infants. *J. Pediatr.*, 99, 115–20.
46. Pineault, M., Chessex, P., Bisaillon, S. *et al.* (1988) Total parenteral nutrition in the newborn infant: impact of the quality of infused energy on nitrogen metabolism. *Am. J. Clin. Nutr.*, 47, 298–304.
47. Baker, J.P., Detsky, A.S., Stewart, S. *et al.* (1984) Randomized trial of total parenteral nutrition in critically ill patients: metabolic effects of varying glucose–lipid ratios as the energy source. *Gastroenterology*, 87, 53–59.
48. Landon, M.B., Gabbe, S.G. and Mullen, J.L. (1986) Total parenteral nutrition during pregnancy. *Clin. Perinatol.*, 13, 57–72.
49. Mendeloff, E., Wesley, J.R., Dechert, R. *et al.* (1986) Comparison of measured resting energy expenditure versus estimated resting expenditure in infants. *JPEN*, 10 (suppl.), 6s.
50. Schafer, L., Wesley, J.R., Tse, Y. *et al.* (1986) Effects of necrotizing enterocolitis (NEC) on calculation of resting energy expenditure (REE) in infants with gastroschisis. *JPEN*, 10 (suppl.), 6s.
51. Dechert, R.E. Wesley, J.R., Schafer, L.E. *et al.* (1988) A water-sealed indirect calorimeter for measurement of oxygen consumption (VO_2), carbon dioxide production (VCO_2) and energy expenditure in infants. JPEN, 12, 256–59.
52. Rubecz, I., Mestyan, J., Varga, P. *et al.* (1981) Energy metabolism, substrate utilization, and nitrogen balance in parenterally fed postoperative neonates and infants. *J. Pediatr.*, 98, 42–46.
53. Wheeler, N. (1984) Parenteral nutrition, in *Manual of Pediatric Nutrition* (eds D.G. Kelts and R.D. Jones), Little, Brown, Boston, pp. 151–65.
54. Caldwell, M.D. and Kennedy, C.C. (1981) Normal nutritional requirements. *Surg. Clin. North Am.*, 61, 491–98.
55. Chessex, P., Reichman, B.L., Verellen, G.J.E. *et al.* (1981) Influence of postnatal age, energy intake, and weight gain or energy metabolism in the very-low-birth-weight infant. *J. Pediatr.*, 99, 761–66.
56. Van Aerde, J. (1992) Parenteral nutrition, in *Neonatal–Perinatal Medicine: Diseases of the Fetus and Infant*, 5th edn. (eds A.A. Fanaroff and R.J. Martin), Mosby Yearbook, St Louis, pp. 496–526.
57. Van Aerde, J.E.E. (1990) Energy balance in the extremely-low-birth-weight infant: how important is it and how can it be maintained? *The Micropremie: The Next Frontier*, Report of the 99th Ross Conference on Pediatric Research, Ross Laboratories, Columbus, OH, pp. 93–103.
58. Reichman, B., Chessex, P., Putet, G. *et al.* (1981) Diet, fat accretion, and growth in premature infants. *N. Engl. J. Med.*, 305, 1495–1500.
59. Adamkin, D.H. (1986) Total parenteral nutrition in hyaline membrane disease, in *Total Parenteral Nutrition: Indications, Utilization, Complications, and Pathophysiologic Considerations* (ed. E. Lebenthal), Raven Press, New York, pp. 305–18
60. Pereira, G.R. and Glassman, M. (1986) Parenteral nutrition in the neonate, in *Parenteral Nutrition*, vol. 28, Clinical Nutrition (eds J.L. Rombeau and M.D. Caldwell), W.B. Saunders, Philadelphia, pp. 702–20.
61. Hay Jr, W.W. (1986) Justification for total parenteral nutrition in premature and compromised newborn, in *Total Parenteral Nutrition: Indications, Utilization, Complications, and Pathophysiologic Considerations* (ed. E. Lebenthal), Raven Press, New York, pp. 277–303.
62. Kerner Jr, J.A. (1983) Fluid requirements, in *Manual of Pediatric Parenteral Nutrition* (ed J.A. Kerner Jr), Wiley, New York, pp. 69–77.
63. Kerner Jr, J.A. (1983) Carbohydrate requirements, in *Manual of Pediatric Parenteral Nutrition* (ed J.A. Kerner Jr), Wiley, New York, pp. 79–88.
64. Committee on Nutrition, American Academy of Pediatrics (1985) Parenteral nutrition, in *Pediatric Nutrition Handbook*, edn (eds G.B. Forbes and C.W. Woodruff), American Academy of Pediatrics, EIK Grove Village, IL, p. 154.
65. Committee on Nutrition, American Academy of Pediatrics (1983) Commentary on parenteral nutrition. *Pediatrics*, 71, 547–52.
66. Macfie, J., Smith, R.C. and Hill, G.L. (1981) Glucose or fat as a non-protein energy source? A controlled clinical trial in gastroenterological patients requiring intravenous nutrition. *Gastroenterology*, 80, 103–107.
67. Askanazi, J., Nordenstrom, J., Rosenbaum, S.L. *et al.* (1981) Nutrition for the patient with respiratory failure: glucose vs fat. *Anesthesiology*, 54, 373–77.
68. Yu, V.Y.H., James, B.E., Hendry, P.G. *et al.* (1979) Glucose tolerance in very-low-birth-weight infants. *Aust. Paediatr. J.*, 15, 147–51.
69. Vaucher, Y.E., Walson, P.D. and Morrow, G. (1982) Continuous insulin infusion in hyperglycemic, very-low-birth-weight infants. *J. Pediatr. Gastroenterol. Nutr.*, 1, 211–17.
70. Schwartz, R. (1982) Should exogenous insulin be given to very-low-birth-weight infants? *J. Pediatr. Gastroenterol. Nutr.*, 1, 287–88.
71. Ostertag, S.G., Jovanovic, L., Lewis, B. *et al.* (1986) Insulin pump therapy in the very-low-birth-weight infant. *Pediatrics*, 78, 625–30.
72. Heron, P. and Bourchier, D. (1988) Insulin infusions in infants of birthweight less than 1250 g and with glucose intolerance. *Aust. Paediatr. J.*, 24, 362–65.

73. Binder, N.D., Raschko, P.K., Benda, G.I. *et al.* (1989) Insulin infusion with parenteral nutrition in extremely-low-birth-weight infants with hypoglycemia. *J. Pediatr.*, 114, 273–80.

74. Collins, J.W., Hoppe, M., Brown, K. *et al.* (1991) A controlled trial of insulin infusion and parenteral nutrition in extremely-low-birth-weight infants with glucose intolerance. *J. Pediatr.*, 118, 921–27.

75. Kanarek, K.S., Santeiro, M.L. and Malone, J.I. (1991) Continuous infusion of insulin in hyperglycemic low-birth-weight infants receiving parenteral nutrition with and without lipid emulsion. *JPEN*, 15, 417–20.

76. Winters, R.W., Heird, W.C. and Dell, R.B. *et al.* (1977) Plasma amino acids in infants receiving parenteral nutrition in *Clinical Nutrition Update: Amino Acids* (eds H.L. Greene, M.A. Holliday and H. Munro), American Medical Association, Chicago, pp. 147–54.

77. Heird, W.C. and Malloy, M.H. (1979) Brain composition of beagle puppies receiving total parenteral nutrition, in *Nutrition and Metabolism of the Fetus and Infant* (ed.V. Itka), Nijhoff, The Hague, p. 365.

78. Wu, P.Y.K., Edwards, N.B. and Storm, M.C. (1986) Characterization of the plasma amino acid pattern of normal term breast-fed infants. *J. Pediatr.*, 109, 347–49.

79. Helms, R.A., Christensen, M.L. and Mauer, E.C. *et al.* (1987) Comparison of a pediatric versus standard amino acid formulation in preterm neonates requiring parenteral nutrition. *J. Pediatr.*, 110, 466–70.

80. Heird, W.C., Dell, R.B and Helms, R.A. *et al.* (1987) Amino acid mixture designed to maintain normal plasma amino acid patterns in infants and children requiring parenteral nutrition. *Pediatrics*, 80, 401–408.

81. Heird, W.C., Hay, W. and Helms, R.A. *et al.* (1988) Pediatric parenteral amino acid mixture in low-birth-weight infants. *Pediatrics*, 81, 41–50.

82. Cooper, A., Betts, J.M. and Pereira, G.R. (1984) Taurine deficiency in the severe hepatic dysfunction complicating total parenteral nutrition. *J. Pediatr. Surg.*, 19 462–66.

83. Kerner Jr, J.A. (1983) Metabolic complications, in *Manual of Pediatric Parenteral Nutrition* (ed. J.A. Kerner Jr), Wiley, New York, pp. 199–215.

84. Helms, R.A., Johnson, M.R. and Christensen, M.L. *et al.* (1988) Evaluation of two pediatric amino acid formulations (abstract). *JPEN*, 12, 4.

85. Adamkin, D.H., McClead, R., and Marchildon, M. *et al.* (1989) Multicenter comparative evaluation of Aminosyn-PF (A) and Troph-Amine (T) in preterm infants (abstract). *JPEN*, 13, 18.

86. Adamkin, D.H., McClead Jr, R.E. and Desai, N.S. *et al.* (1991) Comparison of two neonatal intravenous amino acid formulations in preterm infants: a multicenter study. *J. Perinatol.*, 11, 375–82.

87. Zelikovic I., Chesney, R.W., Friedman, A.L. *et al.* (1990) Taurine depletion in very-low-birth-weight infants receiving prolonged total parenteral nutrition: role of renal immaturity. *J. Pediatr.*, 116, 301–306.

88. Kashyap, S., Abildskov, K. and Heird, W.C. (1992) Cyst(e)ine supplementation of very-low-birth-weight infants receiving parenteral nutrition. *Pediatr. Res.*, 31, 290A.

89. Helms, R.A., Johnson, M.R., Christensen, M.L. and Fernandes, E. (1987) Altered caloric and protein requirements in neonates receiving a pediatric amino acid formulation. *Pediatr. Res.*, 21, 429 (abstract).

90. Phelps, S.J., Cochran, E.C. and Kamper, C.A. (1987) Peripheral venous line infiltration in infants receiving 10% dextrose, 10% dextrose/amino acids, 10% dextrose/amino acids/fat emulsion (abstract). *Pediatr. Res.*, 21, 67A.

91. Friedman, Z., Danon, A., Stahlman, M.T. *et al.* (1976) Rapid onset of essential fatty acid deficiency in the newborn. *Pediatrics*, 58, 640–49.

92. Kerner Jr, J.A. (1983) Fat requirements, in *Manual of Pediatric Parenteral Nutrition* (ed. J.A. Kerner Jr) Wiley, New York, pp. 103–27.

93. Friedman, Z., Shochat, S.J., Maisels, J.M. *et al.* (1976) Correction of essential fatty acid deficiency in newborn infants by cutaneous application of sunflower seed oil. *Pediatrics*, 58, 650–54.

94. Hunt, C.E., Engel, R.R., Modler, S. *et al.* (1978) Essential fatty acid deficiency in neonates: inability to reverse deficiency by topical applications of EFA-rich oils. *J. Pediatr.*, 92, 603–607.

95. O'Neill, J.A., Caldwell, M.D. and Meng, H.C. (1977) Essential fatty acid deficiency in surgical patients. *Ann. Surg.*, 185, 535–42.

96. Pelham, L.D. (1981) Rational use of intravenous fat emulsions. *Am. J. Hosp. Pharm.*, 38, 198–208.

97. Kao, L.C., Cheng, M.H. and Warburton, D. (1984) Triglycerides, free fatty acids, free fatty acids/albumin molar ratio, and cholesterol levels in serum of neonates receiving long-term lipid infusions: controlled trial of continuous and intermittent regimen. *J. Pediatr.*, 104, 429–35.

98. Das, J.B., Joshi, I.D. and Philippart, A.I. (1980) Depression of glucose utilization by Intralipid in the post-traumatic period: an experimental study. *J. Pediatr. Surg.*, 15, 739–45.

99. Brans, Y.W., Andrews, D.S., Carrillo, D.W. *et al.* (1988) Tolerance of fat emulsions in very-low-birth-weight infants. *Am. J. Dis. Child.*, 142, 145–52.

100. Cooke, R.J. and Burckhart, G.J. (1983) Hypertriglyceridemia during the intravenous infusion of a safflower-oil based fat emulsion. *J. Pediatr.*, 103, 959–61.

101. Nizar, L., Vyhmeister, N., Fisher, L. *et al.* (1990) The risk of hypertriglyceridemia increases with the duration of intravenous fat administration (abstract). *Clin. Res.*, 38, 191A.

102. Grill, B., Yoon, S., Fisher, L. *et al.* (1990) Prospective comparison of two intravenous lipid emulsions in premature infants: effects on plasma fatty acids, abstract. *JPEN*, 14, 115 (abstract).

103. Malkani, A., Abraham, S., Hartman, G. *et al.* (1990) Evaluation of a new fat emulsion (Liposyn II) in neonates (abstract). *Clin. Res.*, 38, 190A.

104. Helms, R.A., Whitington, P.F., Mauer, E.C. *et al.* (1986) Enhanced lipid utilization in infants receiving oral L-carnitine during long-term parenteral nutrition. *J. Pediatr.*, 109, 984–88.

105. Helms, R.A., Borum, P.R., Hay, W.W. *et al.* (1987) Intravenous (IV) carnitine during parenteral nutrition (PN) in neonates. *JPEN*, 11 (suppl. 95), 9 (abstract).

106. Stahl, G.E., Spear, M.L. and Hamosh, M. (1986) Intravenous administration of lipid emulsions to premature infants. *Clin. Perinatol.*, 13, 133–62.

107. Lima, L.A.M., Murphy, J.F., Stansbie, D. *et al.* (1988) Neonatal parenteral nutrition with a fat emulsion containing medium chain triglycerides. *Acta Paediatr. Scand.*, 77, 332–39.

108. Bientz, J., Frey, A., Schirardin, H. *et al.* (1988) Medium chain triglycerides in parenteral nutrition in the newborn: a short-term clinical trial. *Infusionstherapie*, 15, 96–99.

109. Van Aerde, J. and Chan, G. (1989) Eicosapentaenoic (EPA) and docosahexanoic acid (DHA)-enriched intravenous (IV) fat emulsions for the neonate (abstract). *Clin. Res.*, 37, 209 (abstract).

110. Haumont, D., Richelle, M., Dahlan, W. *et al.* (1989) Four g/kg/day Intralipid (IL) increases plasma lipids less than 2 g of 10% (abstract). *JPEN*, 13, 5S.

111. Tashiro, T., Sanada, M., Mashima, Y. *et al.* (1989) Lipoprotein metabolism during TPN with Intralipid 10% vs 20% (abstract). *JPEN*, 13, 7S.

112. Poole, R.L. (1983) Electrolyte and mineral requirements, in *Manual of Pediatric Parenteral Nutrition* (ed. J.A. Kerner Jr), Wiley, New York, pp. 129–36.

113. Vileisis, R.A. (1987) Effect of phosphorus intake in total parenteral nutrition infusates in premature neonates. *J. Pediatr.*, 110, 586–90.

114. Greene, H.L., Hambidge, K.M., Schanler, R. *et al.* (1988) Guidelines for the use of vitamins, trace elements, calcium, magnesium and phosphorus in infants and children receiving total parenteral nutrition: report of the subcommittee on pediatric parenteral nutrient requirements from the committee on clinical practice issues of the American Society for Clinical Nutrition. *Am. J. Clin. Nutr.*, 48, 1324–42.

115. O'Brien, D. and Hammond, K.B. (1978) Normal laboratory values, in *Current Pediatric Diagnosis and Treatment* (eds C.H. Kempe, H.K. Silver and D. O'Brien), Lange Medical, Los Altos, pp. 1045.

116. Kovar, I., Mayne, P. and Barltrop, D. (1982) Plasma alkaline phosphatase activity: a screening test for rickets in preterm neonates. *Lancet*, i, 308–10.

117. Poole, R.L., Rupp, C.A. and Kerner, J.A. (1983) Calcium and phosphorus in neonatal TPN solutions. *JPEN*, 7, 358–60.

118. Goldsmith, M.A., Bhatia, S.S. and Kanto Jr, W.P. *et al.* (1981) Gluconate calcium therapy and neonatal hypercalciuria. *Am. J. Dis. Child.*, 135, 538–43.

119. Kimura, S., Nose, O. and Seino, Y. (1986) Effects of alternate and simultaneous administration of calcium and phosphorus on calcium metabolism in children receiving total nutrition. *JPEN*, 10, 513–16.

120. Fitzgerald, K.A. and McKay, M.W. (1986) Calcium and phosphate solubility in neonatal parenteral nutrient solutions containing Troph-Amine. *Am. J. Hosp. Pharm.*, 43, 88–93.

121. Fitzgerald, K.A. and McKay, M.W. (1987) Calcium and phosphate solubility in neonatal parenteral nutrient solutions containing Aminosyn PF. *Am. J. Hosp. Pharm.*, 44, 1396–1400.

122. Pelegano, J.F., Rowe, J.C., Carey, D.E. *et al.* (1989) Simultaneous infusion of calcium and phosphorus in parenteral nutrition for premature infants: use of physiologic calcium/phosphorus ratio. *J. Pediatr.*, 114, 115–9.

123. Pelegano, J.F., Rowe, J.C., Carey, D.E. *et al.* (1991) Effect of calcium/phosphorus ratio on mineral retention in parenterally fed premature infants. *J. Pediatr. Gastroenterol. Nutr.*, 12, 351–55.

124. Hanning, R.M., Atkinson, S.A. and Whyte, R.K. (1991) Efficacy of calcium glycerophosphate vs conventional mineral salts for total parenteral nutrition in low-birth-weight infants: a randomized clinical trial. *Am. J. Clin. Nutr.*, 54, 903–908.

125. Hanning, R.M., Mitchell, M.K. and Atkinson, S.A. (1989) *In vitro* solubility of calcium glycerophosphate versus conventional mineral salts in pediatric parenteral nutrition solution. *J. Pediatr. Gastroenterol. Nutr.*, 9, 67–72.

126. Dunham, B., Marcuard, S., Khazanie, P.G. *et al.* (1991) The solubility of calcium and phosphorus in neonatal total parenteral nutrition solutions. *JPEN*, 15, 608–11.

127. Rollins, C.J., Elsberry, V.A., Pollack, K.A. *et al.* (1990) Three-in-one parenteral nutrition: a safe and economical method of nutritional support for infants. *JPEN*, 14, 290–94.

128. Koo, W.K., Tsang, R.C., Succo, P.P. *et al.* (1987) Vitamin D requirements in infants receiving parenteral nutrition. *JPEN*, **11**, 172–77.

129. Shenai, J.P., Stahlman, M.T. and Chytil, F. (1981) Vitamin A delivery from parenteral alimentation solution. *J. Pediatr.*, **99**, 661–63.

130. Gillis, J., Jones, G. and Pencharz, P. (1983) Delivery of vitamins A, D, and E in parenteral nutrition solutions. *JPEN*, **7**, 11–14.

131. Polland, R.L. (1986) Vitamin E: what should we do? *Pediatrics*, **77**, 787–88.

132. Phillips, B., Franck, L.S. and Greene, H.L. (1987) Vitamin E levels in premature infants during and after intravenous multivitamin supplementation. *Pediatrics*, **80**, 680–83.

133. Baeckert, P.A., Greene, H.L., Fritz, I. *et al.* (1988) Vitamin concentrations in very low birth weight infants given vitamins intravenously in a lipid emulsion: measurement of vitamins A, D, and E and riboflavin. *J. Pediatr.*, **113**, 1057–65.

134. Henton, D.H., Merritt, R.J. and Hack, S. (1992) Vitamin E measurement in patients receiving intravenous lipid emulsions. *JPEN*, **16**, 133–35.

135. Greene, H.L., Phillips, B.L., Franck, L. *et al.* (1987) Persistently low blood retinol levels during and after parenteral feeding of very low birth weight infants – examination of losses into IV administration sets and a method of prevention by addition to a lipid emulsion. *Pediatrics*, **79**, 894–900.

136. Hustead, V.A., Gutcher, G.R., Anderson, S.A., *et al.* (1984) Relationship of vitamin A (retinol) status to lung disease in the preterm infant. *J. Pediatr.*, **105**, 610–5.

137. Shenai, J.P., Chytil, F. and Stahlman, M.T. (1985) Vitamin A status of neonates with bronchopulmonary dysplasia. *Pediatr. Res.*, **19**, 185–87.

138. Shenai, J.P., Kennedy, K.A., Chytil, F. *et al.* (1987) Clinical trial of vitamin A supplementation in infants susceptible to broncho-pulmonary dysplasia. *J. Pediatr.*, **111**, 269–77.

139. Thomas, D.G., James, S.L., Fudge, A. *et al.* (1991) Delivery of vitamin A from parenteral nutrition solutions in neonates. *J. Paediatr. Child Health*, **27**, 180–83.

140. Bishop, N.J., Robinson, M.J., Lendon, M. *et al.* (1989) Increased concentration of aluminum in the brain of a parenterally fed preterm infant. *Arch. Dis. Child.*, **64**, 1316–17.

141. Klein, G.L. (1989) Aluminum in parenteral products: medical perspective on large and small volume parenterals. *J. Parenter. Sci. Tech.*, **43**, 120–24.

142. ASCN/ASPEN Working Group on Standards for Aluminum Content of Parenteral Nutrition Solutions. (1991) Parenteral drug products containing aluminum as an ingredient or a contaminant: response to Food and Drug Administration notice of intent and request for information. *JPEN*, **15**, 194–98.

143. Cochran, E.B. and Hogue, S.L. (1991) Prediction of serum albumin concentration after albumin supplementation in pediatric patients receiving parenteral nutrition. *Clin. Pharm.*, **10**, 704–706.

144. Kanarek, K.S., Williams, P.R. and Blair, C. (1992) Concurrent administration of albumin with total parenteral nutrition in sick newborn infants. *JPEN*, **16**, 49–53.

145. Hattner, J.A.T. and Kerner Jr, J.A. (1983) Nutritional assessment of the pediatric patient, in *Manual of Pediatric Parenteral Nutrition* (ed. J.A. Kerner, Jr) Wiley New York, pp. 19–60.

146. Vaucher, Y.E., Harrison, G.G., Udall, J.N. *et al.* (1984) Skinfold thickness in North American infants 24–41 weeks gestation. *Hum. Biol.*, **56**, 713–31.

147. Sasanow, S.R., Georgieff, M.K. and Pereira, G.R. (1986) Mid-arm circumference and mid-arm/head circumference ratios: standard curves for anthropometric assessment of neonatal status. *J. Pediatr.*, **109**, 311–15.

148. Georgieff, M.K., Sasanow, S.R., Mammel, M.C. *et al.* (1986) Mid-arm circumference and mid-arm/head circumference ratios: for identification of symptomatic LGA, AGA, and SGA newborn infants. *J. Pediatr.*, **109**, 316–21.

149. Kerner, Jr J.A. and Poole, R.L. (1992) Metabolic monitoring and nutritional assessment, in *Intravenous Feeding of the Neonate* (eds V.Y.H. Yu and R.A. MacMahon), Edward Arnold, London, pp. 207–33.

150. MacKenzie, N. (1983) TPN PGM: a computer program to help provide PN in pediatric patients, in *Manual of Pediatric Parental Nutrition* (ed. J.A. Kerner Jr), Wiley, New York, pp. 345–57.

151. Poole, R.L. and Kerner Jr, J.A. (1983) The nutrition support team, in *Manual of Pediatric Parenteral Nutrition* (ed. J.A. Kerner Jr), Wiley New York, pp. 281–84.

152. Nehme, A.L. (1980) Nutritional support of the hospitalized patient. The team concept. *JAMA*, **243**, 1906–908.

153. Rogers, B.B., Berns, S.D., Maynard, E.C. *et al.* (1990) Pericardial tamponade secondary to central venous catherization and hyperalimentation in a very-low-birthweight-infant. *Pediat. Pathol.*, **10**, 819–23.

154. Giacoia, G.P. (1991) Cardiac tamponade and hydrothorax as complications of central venous parenteral nutrition in infants. *JPEN*, **15**, 110–13.

155. Mehta, S. Connors Jr, A.F., Danish E.H. and Grisoni, E. (1992) Central venous catheters and risk of thrombosis in newborns. *J. Pediatr. Surg.*, **27**, 18–22.

156. Chathas, M.K., Paton, J.B. and Fisher, D.E. (1990) Percutaneous central

157. Schreiner, R.L., Glick, M.R., Nordschow, C.D. *et al.* (1979) An evaluation of methods to monitor infants receiving intravenous lipids. *J. Pediatr.*, **94**, 197–200.

158. D'Harlingue A.D., Hopper, A.O., Stevenson, D.K. *et al.* (1983) Limited value of nephelometry in monitoring the administration of intravenous fat in neonates. *JPEN*, **7**, 55–58.

159. Pereira, G.R., Fox, W.W., Stanley, C.A. *et al.* (1980) Decreased oxygenation and hyperlipemia during intravenous fat infusions in premature infants. *Pediatrics*, **66**, 26–30.

160. Sun, S.C., Ventura, C. and Verasestakul, S. (1978) Effect of Intralipid®-induced lipemia on the arterial oxygen tension in preterm infants. *Resuscitation*, **6**, 265–70.

161. McKeen, C.R., Brigham, K.L. and Bowers, R.E. (1978) Pulmonary vascular effects of fat emulsion infusion in unanesthetized sheep. *J. Clin. Invest.*, **61**, 1291–97.

162. Teague, W.G., Braun, D., Goldberg, R.B. *et al.* (1984) Intravenous lipid infusion increases lung fluid filtration in lambs (abstract). *Pediatr. Res.*, **18**, 313.

163. Barson, A.J., Chiswick, M.L. and Doig, M.C. (1978) Fat embolism in infancy after intravenous fat infusions. *Arch. Dis. Child.*, **53**, 218–23.

164. Hertel, J., Tystrup, I. and Andersen, G.E. (1982) Intravascular fat accumulation after Intralipid® infusion in the very-low-birth-weight infant. *J. Pediatr.*, **100**, 975–76.

165. Shroeder, H., Paust, H. and Schmidt, R. (1984) Pulmonary fat embolism after Intralipid® therapy – a post-mortem artifact? *Acta Paediatr. Scand.*, **73**, 461–64.

166. Shulman, R.J., Langston, C. and Schanler, R.J. (1987) Pulmonary vascular lipid deposition after administration of intravenous fat to infants. *Pediatrics*, **79**, 99–102.

167. Hageman, J., McCulloch, K., Gora, P. *et al.* (1983) Intralipid® alterations in pulmonary prostaglandin metabolism and gas exchange. *Crit. Care Med.*, **11**, 794–98.

168. Brans, Y.W., Dutton, E.B., Andrew, D.S. *et al.* (1986) Fat emulsion tolerance in very-low-birth-weigh neonates: effect on diffusion of oxygen in the lungs and on blood pH. *Pediatrics*, **78**, 79–84.

169. Hammerman, C. and Aramburo, M.J. (1988) Decreased lipid intake reduces morbidity in sick premature neonates. *J. Pediatr.*, **113**, 1083–88.

170. Gilbertson, N., Zovar, I.Z., Cox, D.J. *et al.* (1991) Introduction of intravenous lipid administration on the first day of life in the very-low-birth-weight infant. *J. Pediatr.*, **119**, 615–23.

171. Adamkin, D.H., Radmacher, P.G. and Klingbeil, R.L. (1992) Use of intravenous lipid and hyperbilirubinemia in the first week. *J. Pediatr. Gastroenterol. Nutr.*, **14**, 135–39.

172. Rubin, M., Harell, D., Naor, N. *et al.* (1991) Lipid infusion with different triglyceride cores (long-chain vs. medium-chain/long-chain triglycerides): effect on plasma lipids and bilirubin binding in premature infants. *JPEN*, **15**, 642–46.

173. Andrew, G., Chan, G. and Schiff, D. (1976) Lipid metabolism in the neonate. II. The effect of Intralipid® on bilirubin binding *in vitro* and *in vivo*. *J. Pediatr.*, **88**, 279–84.

174. Kerner Jr, J.A., Cassani, C., Hurwitz, R. *et al.* (1981) Monitoring intravenous fat emulsions in neonates with fatty acid/serum albumin molar ratio. *JPEN*, **5**, 517–18.

175. Spear, M.L., Stahl, G.E., Paul, M.H. *et al.* (1985) The effect of fifteen hour fat infusions of varying dosage on bilirubin binding to albumin. *JPEN*, **9**, 144–47.

176. American Academy of Pediatrics, Committee on Nutrition (1981) Use of intravenous fat emulsions in pediatric patients. *Pediatrics*, **68**, 738–43.

177. Park, W., Paust, H. and Schroder H. (1984) Lipid infusion in premature infants suffering from sepsis. *JPEN*, **8**, 290–92.

178. Dahlstrom, K.A., Goulet, O.J., Roberts, R.L. *et al.* (1988) Lipid tolerance in children receiving long-term parenteral nutrition: a biochemical and immunologic study. *J. Pediatr.*, **113**, 985–90.

179. Cohen, I.T., Dahms, B. and Hays, D.M. (1977) Peripheral total parenteral nutrition employing a lipid emulsion (Intralipid®): complications encountered in pediatric patients. *J. Pediatr. Surg.*, **12**, 837–45.

180. Stern, S.T. and Christensen, R.D. (1985) Intralipid® and thrombocytopenia in ill neonates (abstract). *Clin. Res.*, **33**, 134.

181. Goulet, O., Girot, R., Maier-Redelsperger, M. *et al.* (1986) Hematologic disorders following prolonged use of intravenous fat emulsions in children. *JPEN*, **10**, 284–88.

182. Herson, V.C., Block, C., Einsenfeld, L. *et al.* (1989) Effects of intravenous fat emulsion on neonatal neutrophil and platelet function. *JPEN*, **13**, 620–22.

183. Greer, F.R., Steichen, J.J. and Tsang, R.C. (1982) Effects of increased calcium, phosphorus, and vitamin D intake on bone mineralization in very-low-birth-weight infants fed formulas with Polycose and medium-chain triglycerides. *J. Pediatr.*, **100**, 951–55.

184. Tsang, R.C. (1983) The quandary of vitamin D in the newborn infant. *Lancet*, **i**, 1370–72.

venous catheterization – three years experience in a neonatal intensive care unit. *Am. J. Dis. Child.*, **144**, 1246–50.

185. Koo, W.W.K. (1992) Parenteral nutrition-related bone disease. *JPEN*, **16**, 386–94.

186. Senterre, J. (1991) Osteopenia versus rickets in premature infants, in *Rickets* (ed. F.H. Glorieux), Nestle Nutrition Workshop Series, vol. 21, Vevey/Raven Press, New York, pp. 145–54.

187. Kubota, A., Okada, A., Imura, K. *et al.* (1990) The effect of metronidazole on TPN-associated liver dysfunction in neonates. *J. Pediatr. Surg. J.*, **25**, 618–21.

188. Spurr, S.G., Grylack, L.J. and Mehta, N.R. (1989) Hyperalimentation-associated neonatal cholestasis: effect of oral gentamicin. *JPEN*, **13**, 633–36.

189. Thaler, M.M. (1982) Liver dysfunction and disease associated with total parenteral alimentation, in *ASPEN 6th Clinical Congress*, American Society for Parenteral and Enteral Nutrition, San Francisco, p.67.

190. Marino, L., Hack, M. and Dahms, B. (1981) Two year follow-up: growth and neonatal PN-associated liver disease. *JPEN*, **5**, 569 (abstract).

191. Hodes, J.E., Grosfeld, J.L., Weber, T.R. *et al.* (1982) Hepatic failure in infants on total parenteral nutrition (TPN): clinical and histopathologic observations. *J. Pediatr. Surg.*, **17**, 463–68.

192. Suita, S., Ikeda, K., Nagasaki, A. *et al.* (1982) Follow-up studies of the children treated with long-term intravenous nutrition (IVN) during the neonatal period. *J. Pediatr. Surg.*, **17**, 37–42.

193. Boyle, R.J., Sumner, T.E. and Volberg, F.M. (1983) Cholelithiasis in a 3-week-old small premature infant. *Pediatrics*, **71**, 967–69.

194. Callahan, J., Haller, J.O., Caccirelli, A.A. *et al.* (1982) Cholelithiasis in infants: association with total parenteral nutrition and furosemide. *Radiology*, **143**, 437–39.

195. Holzbach, R.T. (1983) Gallbladder stasis: consequence of long-term parenteral hyperalimentation and risk factor for cholelithiasis. *Gastroenterology*, **84**, 1055–58.

196. Messing, B., Bories, C., Kunstlinger, F. *et al.* (1983) Does total parenteral nutrition induce gallbladder sludge formation and lithiasis? *Gastroenterology*, **84**, 1012–19.

197. Roslyn, J.J., Pitt, H.A., Mann, L.L. *et al.* (1983) Gallbladder disease in patients on long-term parenteral nutrition. *Gastroenterology*, **84**, 148–54.

198. Roslyn, J.J., Berquist, W.E., Pitt, H.A. *et al.* (1983) Increased risk of gallstones in children receiving total parenteral nutrition. *Pediatrics*, **71**, 784–89.

199. Whitington, P.F. and Black, D.D. (1980) Cholelithiasis in premature infants treated with parenteral nutrition and furosemide. *J. Pediatr.*, **97**, 647–49.

200. King, D.R., Ginn-Pease, M.E., Lloyd, T.V. *et al.* (1987) Parenteral nutrition with associated cholelithiasis: another iatrogenic disease of infants and children. *J. Pediatr. Surg.*, **22**, 593–96.

201. Randall, L.H., Shaddy, R.E., Sturtevant, J.E. *et al.* (1992) Cholelithiasis in infants receiving furosemide: a prospective study of the incidence and one-year follow-up. *J. Perinatol.*, **12**, 107–11.

202. Almond, P.S., Adolph, V.R., Steiner, R. *et al.* (1992) Calculous disease of the biliary tract in infants after neonatal extra corporeal membrane oxygenation. *J. Perinatol.*, **12**, 18–20.

203. Kerner Jr, J.A. (ed.) (1983) *Manual of Pediatric Parenteral Nutrition*, Wiley, New York.

204. Foster, G.D., Knox, L.S., Dempsey, D.T. *et al.* (1987) Caloric requirements for total parenteral nutrition. *J. Am. Coll. Nutr.*, **6**, 231–53.

205. American Society for Parenteral and Enteral Nutrition (1989) Standards for nutrition support – hospitalized pediatric patients. *Nutr. Clin. Pract.*, **4**, 33–37.

206. Wenner Jr, W.J. and Kerner Jr, J.A. (1986) The addition of amino acids to the peritoneal dialysate in acute renal failure. *J. Perinatol.*, **6**, 342–43.

207. Merritt, R.J., Atkinson, J.B., Whalen, T.V. *et al.* (1988) Partial peritoneal alimentation in an infant. *JPEN*, **12**, 621–25.

99 NEONATAL BACTERIAL AND VIRAL SEPSIS

C. Sabella and C.G. Prober

99.1 Introduction

Approximately 10% of liveborn infants contract an infection in the neonatal period [1]. The relative immunodeficient state of neonates and the increasing survival of progressively more premature infants contribute to this high risk of infection. When compared with older children and adults, neonates have less effective neutrophil function, lower antibody levels and natural killer cell activity and abnormal T-cell function and cytokine regulation. These defects are most profound in preterm infants. In addition, high-risk neonates are often subjected to indwelling intravascular catheters, surgical procedures, prolonged mechanical ventilation, total parenteral nutrition and broad-spectrum antibiotics, all of which further increase their risk of infection.

'Neonatal sepsis' refers to a bloodstream infection affecting infants during the first month of life. While these infections may be caused by a wide variety of bacterial and viral pathogens, the clinical syndromes that result are similar.

99.2 Bacterial sepsis

The overall incidence of neonatal bacterial sepsis is estimated to be between 1 and 5 per 1000 live births [2]. Although these infections primarily involve the bloodstream, 25–30% of neonates with bacterial sepsis also develop meningitis [3].

Classically, neonatal bacterial sepsis is divided into early-onset and late-onset forms. Infants with early-onset sepsis become ill before 5 days of age and usually have a history of maternal obstetrical complications. These infections invariably result from vertical transmission of organisms colonizing the maternal genital or gastrointestinal tracts. Infants with late-onset sepsis develop symptoms at or beyond 5 days of age. Some of these infants have been born after an uneventful labor and delivery and have had no evident problems in the postnatal period. Following hospital discharge they develop sepsis, often accompanied by purulent meningitis. The source of infection in theses infants is not clear. Other infants with late-onset sepsis have remained in the hospital after premature delivery. They contract a nosocomial infection [4].

99.2.1 RISK FACTORS

Risk factors for bacterial sepsis can be separated into those associated with the pregnancy and delivery, and those associated with being cared for in an intensive care environment (Table 99.1).

Infants with early-onset sepsis commonly have a history of one or more risk factors associated with pregnancy and delivery. Premature, low-birth-weight infants appear to be at highest risk; they have a 4–25-fold higher incidence of early-onset sepsis than fullterm normal birth-weight infants [5]. Other risk factors associated with early-onset sepsis include maternal peripartum fever, prolonged interval after rupture of membranes (>24 hours) and depressed respiratory function at birth requiring intubation and resuscitation [2,5].

Most infants with late-onset sepsis, especially low-birth-weight infants, acquire their infections nosocomially. These neonates undergo invasive procedures

Table 99.1 Risk factors associated with bacterial sepsis

Gestational factors
Prematurity and low birth weight
Maternal peripartum fever
Prolonged interval after rupture of membranes (>24 hours)
Depressed respiratory function at birth

Nursery factors
Invasive procedures
Mechanical ventilation
Indwelling intravascular catheters
Total parenteral nutrition
Widespread use of broad-spectrum antibiotics

Diseases of the Fetus and Newborn, 2nd edn, Edited by G.B. Reed, A.E. Claireaux and F. Cockburn. Published in 1995 by Chapman & Hall, London. ISBN 0 412 39160 0

and demand intensive respiratory and nutritional support, enabling pathogens to invade the host and establish infection. In addition, the extensive use of broad-spectrum antibiotics in the nursery facilitates proliferation of resistant strains with subsequent invasion of the host.

99.2.2 ETIOLOGY/BACTERIOLOGY

The relative frequencies of bacterial pathogens causing neonatal sepsis are dependent upon the time of onset of infection (Table 99.2).

Despite geographic differences, group B streptococci and *Escherichia coli* are currently the most common organisms causing early-onset sepsis [6,7]. At Yale University, between 1979 and 1988, GBS and *E. coli* accounted for 55% and 14% of all cases of early-onset sepsis, respectively [6]. In West Germany, *E. coli* and other Gram-negative bacilli are more common causes of early-onset sepsis than GBS [8].

The most common causes of late-onset sepsis currently include coagulase-negative staphylococci, Gram-negative bacilli, *Staphylococcus aureus* and enterococci [6] These organisms reflect the increasing incidence of nosocomial infections and the change in the population at risk. In a recent Centers for Disease Control surveillance study, coagulase-negative staphylococci, rarely a cause of sepsis in the past, accounted for 31% of all neonatal intensive care unit nosocomial infections [9].

Group B streptococci and *Listeria monocytogenes* are important causes of late-onset sepsis that is not nosocomially acquired.

99.2.3 CLINICAL MANIFESTATIONS

The clinical features of neonatal sepsis are subtle and non-specific. Respiratory distress, lethargy, fever, hypothermia, apnea, jaundice, feeding intolerance and

Table 99.2 Etiology of neonatal bacterial sepsis[a]

Early-onset sepsis
Group B streptococci
E. coli
L. monocytogenes
Streptococci (other than group B streptococci)
S. aureus
Haemophilus influenzae

Late-onset sepsis
Coagulase-negative staphylococci
Gram-negative bacilli (*E. coli*, *Klebsiella* sp., *Enterobacter* sp., *Pseudomonas* sp.)
S. aureus
Enterococci
Group B streptococci
L. monocytogenes

[a] In approximate order of relative frequency.

tachycardia are common. Features of neonatal meningitis are often indistinguishable from those of sepsis. It is important to stress that non-infectious illnesses in the neonate have similar clinical features. Furthermore, most neonatal pathogens produce similar clinical syndromes.

(a) Group B streptococci

Group B streptococci are common causes of both early-onset and late-onset sepsis, affecting 1.3–3.7 and 1–1.8 per 1000 livebirths, respectively [10–12]. The incidence of early-onset disease is 10–15 times higher in premature infants than in term neonates [12,13].

These organisms are frequent inhabitants of the lower gastrointestinal and genital tracts of women; the colonization rate in pregnant women is about 35% [10,14]. Most infants with early-onset group B streptococci sepsis acquire the organism from the maternal genital tract [11,12,14]. Although 30–70% of group B streptococci-colonized pregnant mothers will transmit the organism to their infants, only 1–2% of these infants will develop early-onset group B streptococci sepsis [11,12,14]. This risk increases dramatically, however, if any high-risk gestational factors are present (Table 99.1) [12,13,14,16].

Ninety per cent of infants with early-onset group B streptococci sepsis have their onset of disease within 24 hours of birth; respiratory signs, including apnea, grunting respirations, tachypnea and cyanosis, are the most common presenting features [17]. Hypotension and septic shock occur in 25% of these infants, while meningitis is present in 15–30% [17]. Chest radiography in those infants with pulmonary involvement is indistinguishable from hyaline membrane disease or other bacterial infections [13,18]. The case-fatality rate of early-onset group B streptococci disease ranges from 10 to 50%, with the lower rates being observed in the most recent analyses [10,11,17].

Late-onset group B streptococci sepsis usually affects term infants, between 1 and 12 weeks of age, who have had an unremarkable early neonatal history. These infants most commonly present with meningitis and bacteremia; respiratory findings are rare [17]. The case-fatality rate of late-onset sepsis ranges from 0 to 5% [11,17]. However, permanent neurological sequelae are present in 25–50% of survivors of meningitis [19–21].

(b) E. coli

Neonatal sepsis caused by *E. coli* affects approximately 1 of every 1000 livebirths [22]. Most cases of *E. coli* sepsis present during the first days of life.

The K1 capsular antigen of *E. coli* is closely

associated with neonatal infections, especially meningitis; 75% of cases of meningitis are associated with this marker of virulence [23–25].

Vertical transmission from mother to infant during or just prior to delivery appears to be the major route by which infants acquire *E. coli* [24]. Horizontal transmission in the nursery may also occur, but this is much less frequent [24]. Although 200–300 infants per 1000 livebirths become colonized with *E. coli*, only 1 of these 200–300 infants will have invasive disease [26]. In comparison, 1 in 100–200 neonates colonized with group B streptococci contract infection. Infants with galactosemia are particularly susceptible to *E. coli* sepsis [27].

The clinical features of sepsis and meningitis caused by *E. coli* are similar to those caused by other bacterial pathogens. However, unlike meningitis caused by Gram-positive organisms, where organisms are rapidly cleared from the cerebrospinal fluid (CSF), the CSF of patients with meningitis caused by *E. coli* is not usually sterilized for 3–4 days [28]. The case-fatality rate for neonatal *E. coli* sepsis and meningitis is 15–25%, but significant neurologic sequelae develop in 30–50% of survivors [29].

(c) *Listeria monocytogenes*

L. monocytogenes is a Gram-positive bacillus occasionally associated with neonatal sepsis. Although this organism is a relatively rare cause of sporadic neonatal disease, since 1983 it has been associated with four food-borne outbreaks of perinatal disease which have resulted in substantial mortality and morbidity [30–33].

Early-onset and late-onset forms of infection have been described. Infants with early-onset disease are infected *in utero*, either transplacentally or as a result of ascending transmission [34]. Mothers of these infants have usually experienced an influenza-like illness, representing maternal listeriosis, during the third trimester of pregnancy. Late-onset disease affects fullterm products of uncomplicated pregnancies.

Pneumonia, septicemia and occasionally meningitis are the hallmarks of early-onset listeriosis [34,35]. Widespread microabscesses, seen as discrete pustular lesions on the skin and pharynx, may accompany severe disease [36]. These can serve as early clues to diagnosis. An elevated blood monocyte count is present in about 50% of bacteremic neonates, although monocytes are not typically found in the CSF of those with meningitis [37].

Infants with late-onset disease typically present between the first and sixth week of life with meningitis [36].

The mortality rate of early-onset listeriosis approaches 30% while that of late-onset disease is about 10% [35]. Survivors generally have a lower rate of long-term sequelae than infants with neonatal meningitis due to other organisms [37].

(d) Nosocomial infections

Nosocomial infections in intensive care nurseries account for substantial mortality and morbidity [38–40]. A recent study from Toronto reported a rate of 14 nosocomial infections per 100 neonatal intensive care unit admissions [41].

Low birth weight is the most important risk factor for these infections. In one study, infants with a birth weight < 1500 g had a 14% risk of developing a nosocomial infection as compared with a 3% risk for infants with a birth weight > 1500 g [40].

Bacteremia accounts for about one-fifth of nosocomial infections and coagulate-negative staphylococci are responsible for about one-third of these infections [9].

99.2.4 DIAGNOSIS

Isolation of an organism from the blood or CSF provides definitive evidence of bacterial sepsis. Bacterial growth is evident within 48 hours in the majority of blood cultures taken from infants ultimately proven to have bacterial sepsis [42,43].

Although rapid diagnostic tests such as latex particle agglutination to detect group B streptococci and *E. coli* antigens have been developed, their utility is limited by low sensitivity and specificity.

Since 25–30% of neonates with bacterial sepsis also will have meningitis, a lumbar puncture is indicated whenever sepsis is documented. Furthermore, even in the absence of positive blood cultures, examination of the CSF should be strongly considered when sepsis is suspected. Fifteen percent of neonates with meningitis will have a positive CSF culture despite negative blood cultures [44].

Hematologic findings often accompanying bacterial sepsis include an elevated ratio of immature neutrophils to total neutrophils (>0.2), neutropenia, an elevated total neutrophil count and thrombocytopenia [45,46].

99.2.5 THERAPY

Supportive management, including ventilatory assistance, early treatment of shock with fluids and vasopressors, and seizure control is critical.

Because of the subtle signs and rapid progression of disease, antibiotics should be considered whenever an infant develops signs and symptoms consistent with infection.

Antimicrobial therapy for early-onset disease must include coverage for group B streptococci, *E coli* and *L. monocytogenes*. A combination of a penicillin (e.g.

ampicillin) and an aminoglycoside (e.g. gentamicin) provides such coverage. Therapy for late-onset sepsis must consider the likely nosocomial nature of the infection. Thus, the combination of vancomycin and a third-generation cephalosporin to provide coverage for coagulase-negative staphylococci and Gram-negative pathogens is reasonable. Once culture and sensitivity results are available, the antimicrobial regimen should be re-evaluated.

Penicillin or ampicillin remains the drug of choice for group B streptococci and *L. monocytogenes* infections and an aminoglycoside is often also used because the β-lactam antibiotic and aminoglycosides act synergistically against these organisms.

The aminoglycosides have excellent activity against *E. coli* and most other Gram-negative bacilli. Although third-generation cephalosporins are also active against these organisms and penetrate the CSF better than aminoglycosides, these agents have not proven to be more efficacious than aminoglycosides.

The duration of antimicrobial therapy for bacterial sepsis has been arbitrarily defined: 10–14 days for sepsis and 21 days for neonatal meningitis are common recommendations [2].

The potential benefits of intravenous immune globulin and granulocyte transfusions as adjunctive therapies for neonatal sepsis are currently under investigation [47].

99.2.6 PREVENTION

The majority of preventive efforts have focused on group B streptococcal infections. The efficacy of maternal chemoprophylaxis in preventing group B streptococci sepsis in infants born to high-risk parturients has been demonstrated [48]. Experts currently recommend intrapartum chemoprophylaxis for women who are colonized with group B streptococci during the third trimester of pregnancy and have one or more of the following risk factors: preterm delivery, premature rupture of membranes, chorioamnionitis, rupture of membranes >18 hours prior to delivery, maternal fever or multiple births [10].

Maternal immunoprophylaxis with a type III group B streptococcal capsular polysaccharide vaccine is currently under investigation [49].

99.3 Viral sepsis

The neonate is highly susceptible to infection with a wide variety of viral agents. These agents may exert their effects *in utero* (congenital infection), at the time of birth (natal infection) or after birth but during the neonatal period (postnatal infection).

The manifestations of congenital infections are usually present at birth and suggest a chronic infection.

Typical findings include intrauterine growth retardation, microcephaly, hepatosplenomegaly, congenital defects and chorioretinitis.

The manifestations of natal and postnatal viral infections are usually evident several days to weeks after birth and may resemble those of bacterial sepsis. Because of their ability to mimic bacterial sepsis, those viruses that cause natal and postnatal infections will be reviewed.

99.3.1 HERPES SIMPLEX VIRUS

Neonatal herpes simplex virus (HSV) infections are the most feared consequence of gestational genital HSV infections. They may mimic neonatal bacterial infections, often delaying prompt diagnosis. Despite effective antiviral therapy, the morbidity and mortality rates for these infections remain high.

The incidence of neonatal HSV infections is 1 in 3500–7500 livebirths, and apparently rising [50]. Most neonates acquire the virus from an infected maternal genital tract at the time of delivery. This can occur following either a primary or recurrent maternal genital HSV infection. The transmission rate is estimated to be 35–50% when the mother is experiencing a primary infection and <5% during a recurrent infection [51–53]. The higher transmission rate following primary maternal infection may be a consequence of the high titer of virus in the genital tract and the usual involvement of the cervix with primary infections and the lack of transplacental antibody.

Because of a high prevalence of 'silent' maternal HSV infection, most infants exposed to HSV at delivery are born to asymptomatic women who have no past history of genital HSV infection [54,55]. Because HSV-2 accounts for 85% of primary and 99% of recurrent maternal HSV infections it also is the type responsible for most cases of neonatal HSV infections [54].

Neonatal HSV infections can be separated into three clinical forms: (1) disseminated disease, (2) central nervous system (CNS) disease, and (3) localized cutaneous disease involving the skin, eye and/or oral mucosa (SEM) (Table 99.3). SEM disease currently accounts for 43% of all neonatal HSV infections, while disseminated and CNS disease account for 23% and 34%, respectively [56,57].

Infants with disseminated disease usually present during the first week of life with non-specific symptomatology. Irritability, temperature instability, apnea, jaundice, hepatosplenomegaly, disseminated intravascular coagulation, overwhelming hepatic failure, seizures and shock are common features. A vesicular rash occurs in 80% of neonates but is often absent at the time of presentation [56,58]. Encephalitis occurs in 60–75% of patients with this form of disease. Without

Table 99.3 Neonatal herpes simplex (HSV-1 and HSV-2) disease

Clinical form	Relative frequency (%)	Average age at presentation (weeks after birth)	Clinical manifestations	Mortality rate with antiviral therapy (%)[a]
Disseminated	23	1	Irritability; temperature instability; apnea; seizures; shock; disseminated intravascular coagulation; vesicular rash in 80%	57
CNS	34	2–4	Seizures; fever; lethargy, vesicular rash in 60%	15
SEM	43	1–2	Vesicles on skin and mucous membranes; ocular involvement in 10–15%	0

[a] Acyclovir or vidarabine therapy (see text).

antiviral therapy, the mortality rate for this form of disease is 70% and half the survivors will have long-term sequelae [54]. Even with antiviral therapy, the mortality rate is >50% and the morbidity rate about 40% [57,59].

Neonates with CNS disease typically present between the second and fourth week of life, usually with lethargy, fever, seizures, CSF pleocytosis and elevated CSF protein. Only 60% have skin vesicles at any time during the disease course [56,58]. With antiviral therapy the mortality rate is 15%, but two-thirds of the survivors have long-term neurologic sequelae, often of a profound nature [57,59].

Neonates with SEM disease usually present at 1–2 weeks of age with vesicular lesions, occurring singly or in clusters, on an erythematous base. Ocular involvement, in the form of keratitis, conjunctivitis or chorioretinitis occurs in 10–15% of these infants. SEM disease has the best prognosis; infants treated early in their course with antiviral therapy uniformly survive, usually without sequelae [57,59]. If untreated, SEM disease progresses to the disseminated and CNS forms of disease, and assumes the mortality rates associated with those forms of disease.

The diagnosis of HSV infections is difficult, especially in the absence of vesicular lesions. A high clinical suspicion is mandatory, given the non-specific nature of the illness.

Viral culture provides the most sensitive method of making the diagnosis. The virus may be isolated from cutaneous lesions, the nasopharynx, CSF, conjunctiva, urine and/or the maternal genital tract. When cutaneous lesions are present, a direct fluorescent antibody test can play a critical diagnostic role. This test is designed to detect viral antigens on infected cells taken directly from lesions. In contrast to cytologic evaluations, this test has excellent sensitivity and specificity [60,61].

Vidarabine (Ara-A) was the first antiviral agent to have demonstrable efficacy in the treatment of neonatal

HSV infections [62]. A recently completed double-blind study involving 210 infants compared vidarabine with acyclovir for the treatment of neonatal HSV disease [57]. No significant differences in outcome were found between infants who received either drug. However, because of its ease of administration and safety profile when compared to vidarabine, acyclovir is recommended as the drug of choice for neonatal HSV infections [57]. It must be stressed that even with appropriate antiviral therapy the mortality and morbidity rates for these infections remain high. Improved diagnostic techniques and more effective therapeutic strategies need to be evaluated.

99.3.2 ENTEROVIRUSES

While these viruses commonly cause benign febrile illnesses in older infants and children, they tend to cause more severe infections in neonates. Echoviruses 9, 11, 30 and Coxsackie B viruses are currently the most common enteroviruses causing neonatal disease [63].

These viruses are transmitted by fecal–oral and oro-oral routes. Although transplacental spread may occur, enteroviral infection during the birth process is the most likely route of transmission [63]. Transmission from nursery personnel to infants also may occur [63]. In temperate climates, enteroviral infections are most common in the summer and fall.

Although enteroviruses can cause mild non-specific neonatal disease, 20% of infections are severe and life threatening [64]. Fever, feeding intolerance, abdominal distension and irritability are the usual presenting features [65]. Diarrhea, vomiting, shock, disseminated intravascular coagulation, hepatomegaly, jaundice and apnea may follow. A macular or maculopapular rash accompanies this syndrome in 40% of cases, but petechial and vesicular exanthems have also been described [65]. Hepatitis, myocarditis and meningoencephalitis also may accompany these illnesses.

Differentiating between enteroviral and bacterial infections is often difficult. Laboratory parameters are not helpful. A maternal history of a recent febrile viral-like illness, lack of obstetrical complications, a predilection for summer and fall and the presence of hepatitis and/or myocarditis all favor the diagnosis of enteroviral infection.

Isolation of the virus from the nasopharynx, throat, stool, blood, urine and/or CSF confirms the diagnosis.

Unfortunately, there is currently no specific therapy for these infections and infants with myocarditis, encephalitis and/or liver involvement have a grave prognosis [63].

99.3.3 CYTOMEGALOVIRUS

Perinatally and postnatally acquired cytomegalovirus (CMV) infections occasionally result in a sepsis-like syndrome. Infants can become infected with CMV during passage through the maternal genital tract, via breast milk or via blood transfusions.

Although 4–20% of all infants are perinatally infected with CMV, the vast majority of term healthy infants remain asymptomatic. Premature and ill full-term neonates may however develop a syndrome of hepatosplenomegaly, gray pallor, septic appearance, deteriorating respiratory function, thrombocytopenia, neutropenia, lymphocytosis and hemolytic anemia [66–69]. Low-birth-weight infants born to CMV negative mothers, who receive blood transfusions from one or more seropositive donors, are at highest risk [67,70,71]. This syndrome can be prevented by the exclusive use of CMV seronegative donor blood, which eliminates the acquisition of the virus [69].

99.3.4 RESPIRATORY VIRUSES

Respiratory viruses, especially influenza and respiratory syncytial virus, have occasionally been associated with nosocomial infection in neonates [72,73]. These infections often result in non-specific symptomatology: apnea, lethargy and poor feeding being common manifestations.

Although many of these infections are self-limited, fatal neonatal infections have been reported [74].

Antiviral therapy with aerosolized ribavirin has recently been shown to be effective for infants who require mechanical ventilation because of severe respiratory syncytial virus infections [75].

References

1. Ingall, D. (1990) Symposium on perinatal infectious diseases: update, 1990. *Pediatr. Infect. Dis. J.*, 9, 761–84.
2. Klein, J.O. and Marcy, S.M. (1990) Bacterial sepsis and meningitis, in *Infectious Diseases of the Fetus and Newborn Infant*, 3rd edn (eds J.S. Remington and J.O. Klein), W.B. Saunders, Philadelphia, pp. 601–56.
3. Siegel, J.D. and McCracken, G.H. (1981) Sepsis neonatorum. *N. Engl J. Med.*, 304, 642–47.
4. Baker, C.J, Rench, M.A., Noya, F.J.D. and Garcia-Prats, J.A. (1990) Role of intravenous immunoglobulin in prevention of late-onset infection in low-birth-weight neonates. *Rev. Infect. Dis.*, 12, S463–69.
5. Boyer, K.M., Gadzak, C.A., Burd, L.I. et al. (1983) Selective intrapartum chemoprophylaxis of neonatal group B streptococcal early-onset disease. I. Epidemiologic rationale. *J. Infect. Dis.*, 148, 795–801.
6. Gladstone, I.M., Ehrenkranz, R.A., Edberg, S.C. and Baltimore, R.S. (1990) A ten-year review of neonatal sepsis and comparison with the previous fifty-year experience. *Pediatr. Infect. Dis. J.*, 9, 819–25.
7. Hall, R.T., Kurth, C.G. and Hall, S.L. (1987) Ten-year survey of positive blood cultures among admissions to neonatal intensive care unit. *J. Perinatol.*, 7, 122–26.
8. Speer, C.P., Hauptmann, D., Stubbe, P. and Gahr, M. (1985) Neonatal septicemia and meningitis in Gottingen, West Germany. *Pediatr. Infect. Dis. J.*, 4, 36–41.
9. Jarvis, W.R. (1987) Epidemiology of nosocomial infections in pediatric patients. *Pediatr. Infect. Dis. J.*, 6, 344–51.
10. Committee on Infectious Diseases and Committee on Fetus and Newborn (1992) Guidelines for prevention of group B streptococcal (GBS) infection by chemoprophylaxis. *Pediatrics*, 90, 775–78.
11. Dillon, H.C., Khare, S. and Gray, B.M. (1987) Group B streptococcal carriage and disease: a 6-year prospective study. *J. Pediatr.*, 110, 31–36.
12. Pass, M.A., Gray, B.M., Khare, S. and Dillon, H.C. (1979) Prospective studies of group B streptococcal infections in infants. *J. Pediatr.*, 95, 437–43.
13. Vollman, J.H., Smith, W.L., Ballard, E.T. and Light I.J. (1976) Early onset group B streptococcal disease: clinical, roentgenographic, and pathologic features. *J. Pediatr.*, 89, 199–203.
14. Boyer, K.M., Gadzala, C.A., Kelly, P.D. et al. (1983) Selective intrapartum chemoprophylaxis of neonatal group B streptococcal early-onset disease. II. Predictive value of prenatal cultures. *J. Infect. Dis.*, 148, 802–809.
15. Aber, R.C., Allen, N., Howell, J.T. et al. (1976) Nosocomial transmission of group B streptococci. *Pediatrics*, 58, 346–53.
16. Faro, S. (1981) Group B beta-hemolytic streptococci and puerperal infections. *Am. J. Obstet. Gynecol.*, 139, 686–89.
17. Yagupsky, P., Menegus, M.A. and Powell, K.R. (1991) The changing spectrum of group B streptococcal disease in infants: an eleven-year experience in a tertiary care hospital. *Pediatr. Infect. Dis. J.*, 10, 801–808.
18. Leonidas, J.C., Hall, R.T., Beatty, E.C. and Fellows, R.A. (1977) Radiographic findings in early onset neonatal group B streptococcal septicemia. *Pediatrics*, 59, 1006–11.
19. Chin, K.C. and Fitzhardinge, P.M. (1985) Sequelae of early-onset group B hemolytic streptococcal neonatal meningitis. *J. Pediatr.*, 106, 819–22.
20. Edwards, M.S., Rench, M.A., Haffar, A.A.M. et al. (1985) Long-term sequelae of group B streptococcal meningitis in infants. *J. Pediatr.*, 106, 717–22.
21. Wald, E.R., Bergman, I., Taylor, H.G. et al. (1986) Long-term outcome of group B streptococcal meningitis. *Pediatrics*, 77, 217–21.
22. Howard, J.B. and McCracken, G.H. (1974) The spectrum of group B streptococcal infections in infancy. *Am. J. Dis. Child.*, 128, 815–18.
23. Robbins, J.B., McCracken, G.H., Gotschlich, E.C. et al. (1974) *Escherichia coli* K1 capsular polysaccharide associated with neonatal meningitis. *N. Engl. J. Med.*, 290, 1216–20.
24. Sarff, L.D., McCracken, G.H., Schiffer, M.S., Glode, M.P. et al. (1975) Epidemiology of *Escherichia coli* Ki in healthy and diseased newborns. *Lancet*, i, 1099–104.
25. Mulder, C.J.J., Alphen, L.V. and Zanen, H.C. (1984) Neonatal meningitis caused by *Escherichia coli* in The Netherlands. *J. Infect. Dis.*, 150, 935–40.
26. McCracken, G.H. and Freij, B.J. (1987) Infectious diseases of the fetus and newborn, in *Textbook of Pediatric Infectious Diseases*, 2nd edn (eds R.D. Feigin and J.D. Cherry), W.B. Saunders, Philadelphia, pp. 940–1007.
27. Levy, H.L., Sepe, S.J., Shih, V.E. et al. (1977) Sepsis due to *Escherichia coli* in neonates with galactosemia. *N. Engl. J. Med.*, 297, 823–25.
28. McCracken, G.H. (1972) The rate of bacteriolgic response to antimicrobial therapy in neonatal meningitis. *Am. J. Dis. Child.*, 123, 547–53.
29. McCracken, G.H., Mize, S.G. and Threlkeld, N. (1980) Intraventricular therapy in Gram-negative bacillary meningitis of infancy. *Lancet*, i, 787–91.
30. Schelch, W.F., Lavigne, P.M., Bortolussi, R.A. et al. (1983) Epidemic listeriosis – evidence for transmission by food. *N. Engl. J. Med.*, 308, 202–206.
31. Fleming, D.W., Cochi, S.L., MacDonald, K.L. et al. (1985) Pasteurized milk as a vehicle of infection in an outbreak of listeriosis. *N. Engl. J. Med.*, 312, 404–407.
32. Linnan, M.J., Mascola, L., Lou, X.D. et al. (1988) Epidemic listeriosis associated with Mexican-style cheese. *N. Engl. J. Med.*, 319, 823–28.
33. Bula, C., Bille, J., Mean, F. et al. (1988) Epidemic food-borne listeriosis in western Switzerland: I. Description of the 58 adult cases. In *Abstracts of the 28th Interscience Conference on Antimicrobial Agents and Chemotherapy*, Los Angeles, American Society for Microbiology, Washington, DC, 305, 1106.

34. Lennon, D., Lewis, B., Mantell, C. *et al.* (1984) Epidemic perinatal listeriosis. *Pediatr. Infect. Dis.*, **3**, 303–34.
35. Ahlfors, C.E., Goetzman, B.W., Halsted, C.C. *et al.* (1977) Neonatal listeriosis. *Am. J. Dis. Child.*, **131**, 404–408.
36. Bortolussi, R. and Seeliger, H.P.R. (1990) Listeriosis, in *Infectious Diseases of the Fetus and Newborn Infant*, 3rd edn (eds J.S. Remington and J.O. Klein), W.B. Saunders, Philadelphia, pp. 812–33.
37. Visintine, K.M., Oleske, J.M. and Nahmia, A.J. (1977) *Listeria monocytogenes* infection in infants and children. *Am. J. Dis. Child.*, **131**, 393–97.
38. Hemming, V.G., Overall, J.C. and Britt, M.R. (1976) Nosocomial infections in a newborn intensive-care unit. *N. Engl J. Med.*, **294**, 1310–16.
39. LaGamma, E.F., Drusin, L.M., Mackles, A.W. *et al.* (1983) Neonatal infections. An important determinant of late NICU mortality in infants less than 1000 g at birth. *Am. J. Dis. Child.*, **137**, 838–41.
40. Goldman, D.A., Durbin, W.A. and Freeman, J. (1981) Nosocomial infections in a neonatal intensive care unit. *J. Infect. Dis.*, **5**, 449–59.
41. Ford-Jones, E.L., Mindorff, C.M., Langley, J.M. *et al.* (1989) Epidemiologic study of 4684 hospital-acquired infections in pediatric patients. *Pediatr. Infect. Dis. J.*, **8**, 668–75.
42. Pichichero, M.E. and Todd, J.K. (1979) Detection of neonatal bacteremia. *J. Pediatr.*, **94**, 958–60.
43. Rowley, A.H. and Wald, E.R. (1986) Incubation period necessary to detect bacteremia in neonates. *Pediatr. Infect. Dis.*, **5**, 590–91.
44. Visser, V.E. and Hall, R.T. (1980) Lumbar puncture in the evaluation of suspected neonatal sepsis. *J. Pediatr.*, **96**, 1063–67.
45. Manroe, B.L., Rosenfeld, C.R., Weinberg, A.G. and Browne, R. (1977) The differential leukocyte count in the assessment and outcome of early-onset neonatal group B streptococcal disease. *J. Pediatr.*, **91**, 632–7.
46. Spector, S.A., Ticknor, W. and Grossman, M. (1981) Study of the usefulness of clinical and hematologic findings in the diagnosis of neonatal bacterial infections. *Clin. Pediatr.*, **20**, 385–92.
47. Cairo, M.S., Worcester, C.C., Rucker, R.W. *et al.* (1992) Randomized trial of granulocyte transfusions versus intravenous immune globulin therapy for neonatal neutropenia and sepsis. *J. Pediatr.*, **120**, 281–85.
48. Boyer, K.M. and Gotoff, S.P. (1986) Prevention of early-onset neonatal group B streptococcal disease with selective intrapartum chemoprophylaxis. *N. Engl. J. Med.*, **314**, 1665–69.
49. Baker, C.J., Rench, M.A., Edwards, M.S. *et al.* (1988) Immunization of pregnant women with a polysaccharide vaccine of group B streptococci. *N. Engl. J. Med.*, **319**, 1180–85.
50. Sullivan-Bolyai, J., Hull, H.F., Wilson, C. and Corey, L. (1983) Neonatal herpes simplex virus infection in King County, Washington. *JAMA*, **250**, 3059–62.
51. Prober, C.G., Sullender, W.M., Yasukawa, L.L. *et al.* (1987) Low risk of herpes simplex virus infections in neonates exposed to the virus at the time of vaginal delivery to mothers with recurrent genital herpes simplex virus infections. *N. Engl. J. Med.*, **316**, 240–44.
52. Brown, Z.A., Vontner, L.A., Benedetti, J. *et al.* (1987) Effects on infants of a first episode of genital herpes during pregnancy. *N. Engl. J. Med.*, **317**, 1246–51.
53. Brown, Z.A., Benedetti, J., Ashley, R. *et al.* (1991) Neonatal herpes simplex virus infection in relation to asymptomatic maternal infection at the time of labor. *N. Engl. J. Med.*, **324**, 1247–52.
54. Whitley, R.J., Nahmias, A.J., Visintine, A.M. *et al.* (1980) The natural history of herpes simplex virus infection of mother and newborn. *Pediatrics*, **66**, 489–94.
55. Prober, C.G., Hensleigh, P.A., Boucher, F.D. *et al.* (1988) Use of routine viral cultures at delivery to identify neonates exposed to herpes simplex virus. *N. Engl. J. Med.*, **318**, 887–91.
56. Whitley, R.J., Corey, L., Arvin, A. *et al.* (1988) Changing presentation of herpes simplex virus infection in neonates. *J. Infect. Dis.*, **158**, 109–16.
57. Whitley, R., Arvin, A., Prober, C. *et al.* (1991) A controlled trial comparing vidarabine with acyclovir in neonatal herpes simplex virus infection. *N. Engl. J. Med.*, **324**, 444–49.
58. Arvin, A.M., Yeager, A.S., Bruhn, F.W. and Grossman, M. (1982) Neonatal herpes simplex infection in the absence of mucocutaneous lesions. *J. Pediatr.*, **100**, 715–21.
59. Whitley, R., Arvin, A., Prober, C. *et al.* (1991) Predictors of morbidity and mortality in neonates with herpes simplex virus infections. *N. Engl. J. Med.*, **324**, 450–54.
60. Goldstein, L.C., Corey, L., McDougall, J.K. *et al.* (1983) Monoclonal antibodies to herpes simplex viruses: use of antigenic typing and rapid diagnosis. *J. Infect. Dis.*, **147**, 829–37.
61. Volpi, A., Lakeman, A.D., Pereira, L. and Stagno, S. (1983) Monoclonal antibodies for rapid diagnosis and typing of genital herpes infections during pregnancy. *Am. J. Obstet. Gynecol.*, **146**, 813–15.
62. Whitley, R.J., Nahmias, A.J. and Soong, S-J. *et al.* (1980) Vidarabine therapy of neonatal herpes simplex virus infection. *Pediatrics*, **66**, 495–501.
63. Cherry, J.D. (1990) Enteroviruses, in *Infectious Diseases of the Fetus and Newborn Infant*. 3rd edn (eds J.S. Remington and J.O. Klein), W.B. Saunders, Philadelphia, pp. 325–66.
64. Morens, D.M. (1978) Enteroviral disease in early infancy. *J. Pediatr.*, **92**, 374–77.
65. Lake, A.M., Lauer, B.A., Clark, J.C. *et al.* (1976) Enterovirus infections in neonates. *J. Pediatr.*, **89**, 787–91.
66. Yeager, A.S., Palumbo, P.E. and Malachowski, N. *et al.* (1983) Sequelae of maternally derived cytomegalovirus infections in premature infants. *J. Pediatr.*, **102**, 918–22.
67. Adler, S.P. (1983) Transfusion-associated cytomegalovirus infections. *Rev. Infect. Dis.*, **5**, 977–93.
68. Ballard, R.A., Drew, L., Hufnagle, K.G. and Riedel, P.A. (1979) Acquired cytomegalovirus infection in preterm infants. *Am. J. Dis. Child.*, **133**, 482–85.
69. Yeager, A.S., Grumet, F.C., Hafleigh, E.B. *et al.* (1981) Prevention of transfusion-acquired cytomegalovirus infections in newborn infants. *J. Pediatr.*, **98**, 281–87.
70. Yeager, A.S. (1974) Transfusion-acquired cytomegalovirus infection in newborn infants. *Am. J. Dis. Child.*, **128**, 478–83.
71. Adler, S.P., Chandrika, T., Lawrence, L. and Baggett, J. (1983) Cytomegalovirus infections in neonates acquired by blood transfusions. *Pediatr. Infect. Dis.*, **2**, 114–18.
72. Meibalane, R., Sedmak, G.V., Sasidharan, P. *et al.* (1977) Outbreak of influenza in a neonatal intensive care unit. *J. Pediatr.*, **91**, 974–76.
73. Hall, C.B., Kopelman, A.E., Douglas, G. *et al.* (1979) Neonatal respiratory syncytial virus infection. *N. Engl. J. Med.*, **300**, 393–96.
74. Joshi, V.V., Escobar, M.R., Stewart, L. and Bates, R.D. (1973) Fatal influenza A₂ viral pneumonia in a newborn infant. *Am. J. Dis. Child.*, **126**, 839–40.
75. Smith, D.W., Frankel, L.R., Mathers, L.H. *et al.* (1991) A controlled trial of aerosolized ribavirin in infants receiving mechanical ventilation for severe respiratory syncytial virus infection. *N. Engl. J. Med.*, **325**, 24–29.

100 MANAGEMENT OF NEONATAL HEMOLYTIC HYPERBILIRUBINEMIA

P. Dennery and D.K. Stevenson

100.1 Bilirubin metabolism and physiology

100.1.1 OVERVIEW OF BILIRUBIN METABOLIC PATHWAY (Figure 100.1)

Bilirubin is derived primarily through the breakdown of heme, from senescent red blood cells (80–90%); it can also originate from myoglobin, cytochromes and other hemoproteins [1–3]. Heme is degraded by the action of heme oxygenase and biliverdin reductase to form bilirubin. The first step of the process is an energy requiring rate-limiting step involving nicotinamide adenine dinucleotide phosphate (NADPH) and cytochrome *c* (P450) reductase. In the process, molecular oxygen is utilized, the iron in heme is reduced to its ferrous state and biliverdin is formed as well as equimolar amounts of carbon monoxide (CO), which is excreted unchanged by the lung [4]. Biliverdin is a green pigment that is further degraded through the action of biliverdin reductase with NADPH to form bilirubin [5]. Bilirubin, which is insoluble in water, is then circulated and bound at a 1:1 ratio to albumin. There is a second binding site for bilirubin binding, but it is much weaker [6]. The albumin–bilirubin complex goes to the liver where it is taken up by the hepatocyte. Bilirubin enters the liver by a carrier mediated process utilizing ligandin (Y protein) [7] as well as Z protein, another cytoplasmic carrier which binds bilirubin with lower affinity [8]. Hepatocytes transform bilirubin through conjugation [8]. This process involves two molecules of glucuronic acid added to bilirubin in a two-step process resulting in bilirubin diglucuronide, through the action of uridine diphosphoglucuronyl (UDP-glucuronyl) transferase. The conjugated bilirubin is then excreted in the bile at approximately 100-fold greater concentration than hepatocyte bilirubin. Conjugated bilirubin is relatively unstable and can be readily transformed to unconjugated bilirubin under the influence of alkaline conditions in the duodenum or

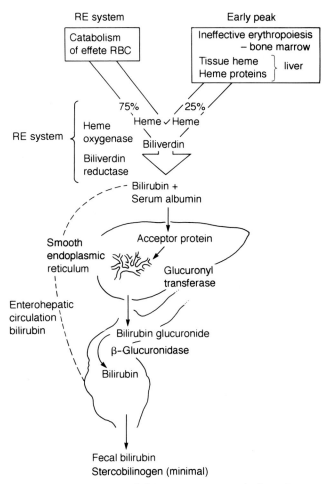

Figure 100.1 Neonatal bile pigment metabolism RE = reticuloendothelial; RBC = red blood cell. (Reproduced with permission from Maisels, J.J. (1972) *Neonatal Jaundice: Pathophysiology and Management*, J.B. Lippincott, Philadelphia, p. 541.)

jejunum or through the enzyme β-glucuronidase found in the mucosa. This new unconjugated bilirubin can then be reabsorbed across the intestinal mucosa and

Diseases of the Fetus and Newborn, 2nd edn, Edited by G.B. Reed, A.E. Claireaux and F. Cockburn. Published in 1995 by Chapman & Hall, London. ISBN 0 412 39160 0

Table 100.1 Causes of pathologic indirect neonatal hyperbilirubinemia

Disorder	Clinical conditions
Production	Isoimmunization: Rh, ABO, minor blood groups
	Erythrocyte biochemical defect: glucose-6-phosphate dehydrogenase, pyruvate kinase, hexokinase, porphyria
	Structural abnormalities of red blood cells: hereditary spherocytosis, elliptocytosis
	Infection: bacterial, viral, protozoal[a]
	Sequestered blood: subdural hematoma, cephalohematoma, ecchymoses, hemangiomas
	Polycythemia: maternal–fetal or fetal transfusion delayed cord clamping
	Other: infants of diabetic mothers
	obstructive jaundice[b]
	galactosemia[a]
	hemolysis (disseminated intravascular coagulation, vitamin K deficiency)
Uptake	Gilbert's syndrome
	Hypothyroidism[a]
	Galactosemia[a]
Conjugation	Crigler–Najjar syndromes (types I and II)
	Transient familial neonatal hyperbilirubinemia
	Galactosemia, hypothyroidism
Excretion	Galactosemia
	Hypothyroidism
Enterohepatic circulation	Breast milk jaundice (early–late onset)
	Starvation
	Pyloric stenosis
	Intestinal obstruction

[a] Mixed jaundice.
[b] Secondary to increased hemolysis due to red blood cell injury in the liver.

returned via the portal circulation to the liver [9,10]. In adults, it appears that 25% of the total bilirubin excreted into the intestine is reabsorbed as unconjugated bilirubin [11].

100.1.2 PHYSIOLOGIC JAUNDICE

Newborns usually show a progressive rise in serum unconjugated bilirubin in the first few days of life to a peak of approximately 6–9 mg/dl at 3 days of life, followed by a rapid decline to less than 2 mg/dl by the second week of life. This is referred to as physiologic jaundice. It results from an increase load of bilirubin to the liver, decreased hepatic uptake, a transient deficiency of hepatic bilirubin glucuronyl transferase activity and excretion of bilirubin [12,13]. The reason why infants have an increased load of bilirubin is that there is a decreased red blood cell life span and increased enteric reabsorption of bilirubin compared with adults [12,13]. Premature infants have more severe physiologic jaundice than do fullterm infants.

Mean peak concentration reaches approximately 12 mg/dl by the fifth day of life with a slower decline to normal values [14]. There are many conditions associated with increased bilirubin production beyond what could be referred to as physiologic jaundice (Table 100.1). In these cases the term 'pathologic hyperbilirubinemia' is used.

100.2 Historical perspective of hemolytic disease and its management

100.2.1 BACKGROUND

Hemolytic disease of the newborn, erythroblastosis fetalis, is caused by transplacental passage of maternal antibodies which react with fetal red blood cells. In most instances the mother has become immunized by fetal red cell antigens from previous pregancies, abortion, amniocentesis or blood transfusion. With the subsequent pregnancy a disruption of the red blood cells of the fetus by maternal antibodies causes severe hemolytic anemia in the newborn, with associated morbidity or mortality [15]. ABO blood typing incompatibility can lead to moderate or severe hemolytic anemia, but usually these infants present with early severe jaundice and rarely show signs of fetal hemolysis [16].

The most common cause of erythroblastosis fetalis is rhesus (Rh) immunization. This disease has been recognized as far back as 400 BC when Hippocrates described a syndrome similar to hydrops fetalis. Thereafter, there were many reports of this condition without any real understanding of the etiology. It was not until 1939 that Levine and Stetson [17] described the Rh system, and in 1946 Coombs [18] developed antiglobulin tests for the detection of antibody-coated red blood cells.

The first attempt at therapy for Rh hemolytic disease was in the early 1950s when Diamond, Allen and Thomas [19] described the first exchange transfusion through an umbilical venous catheter. In 1956, Bevis [20] reported changes in amniotic fluid bilirubin with severe disease. Lilley in 1963 [21] performed the first intrauterine transfusion in the fetal peritoneal cavity in an attempt to remedy severe fetal hemolytic anemia. In the mid-1960s two groups perfected the use of Rh antiglobulin immunization (Rhogam) which helped prevent Rh sensitization in many women [22,23]. Before the advent of immunization with Rhogam, erythroblastosis fetalis was observed in 1% of all pregnancies. Since the increased use of Rhogam from the late 1960s there has been a marked decrease in the condition [24,25]. Nevertheless, there are still women who were previously immunized and are still in their childbearing years and newly immunized pregnancies occur due to failure to administer Rhogam after delivery, abortion, amniocentesis or chorionic villus sampling [24,26]. Before the late 1940s, when there was no effective treatment for this condition, 20% of the affected infants were stillborn. Another 50% died in the neonatal period or suffered significant brain damage associated with the development of kernicterus [27], a condition characterized by motor abnormalities, hearing loss [28] and staining of the basal ganglia on pathologic examination [29]. Since 1981, direct intravascular fetal blood transfusion via fetoscopy has been performed in cases of severe erythroblastosis fetalis [30].

100.2.2 INTRAUTERINE MANAGEMENT OF ERYTHROBLASTOSIS FETALIS

Present day management of erythroblastosis fetalis starts early in pregnancy. In the first, immunized pregnancy, serial antibody determination showing a rise in antibody titer can indicate that the fetus of an Rh-negative mother is Rh positive. These titers are repeated frequently until a critical titer is reached [15,24,31,32]. In pregnancies where the mother had previously been immunized, antibody titers may not be valid and if the titer is high initially, it may fall. Therefore, one needs to resort immediately to amniotic fluid analysis to assess fetal well-being. Amniocentesis is usually performed at about 28 weeks' gestation and is repeated at regular intervals until delivery. A spectrophotometric scan of the amniotic fluid is performed to assess the quantity of bilirubin present. Based on the values noted in the subsequent amniocentesis and studies of fetal well-being, the need for intrauterine transfusion well as the need for early delivery can be assessed [15]. Most affected infants are delivered before term, usually as soon as fetal maturity is established. The absorbance (optical density) of amniotic fluid is plotted against wavelength to determine the magnitude of deviation from normal. The deviation in absorbance at 450 nm (ΔA_{450}) is an indication of the absorbance of unconjugated bilirubin pigment. Liley [33], who initially performed the first intrauterine transfusion, constructed a graph plotting maturity in weeks against change in ΔA_{450} and derived the probability of various grades of affliction expected in any given case. The graph is subdivided into three zones. Zone 1, the low zone, indicates an unaffected or mildly affected fetus. The upper zones reflect more severe disease. Zone 3 indicates a severely affected fetus. This graph was constructed based on a single amniotic fluid specimen (Figure 100.2a). Queenan and Goestchel [31] plotted serial determinations of ΔA_{450} with moderately affected, mildly affected and unaffected fetuses and showed that infants who died had increasing trends or a horizontal trend in ΔA_{450} as the pregnancy progressed (Figure 100.2b) (Chapter 84).

100.2.3 CLINICAL AND PATHOLOGIC PRESENTATION OF ERYTHROBLASTOSIS FETALIS

The fetus with erythroblastosis may present with mild to severe anemia or even hydrops fetalis and intrauterine death. Once the infant is born he or she may not appear icteric because the placenta is rather efficient at transferring unconjugated bilirubin, but jaundice may appear shortly thereafter and progress rapidly to reach concentrations as high as 40 mg/dl unless therapy is instituted. Most of the bilirubin present is in the unconjugated form. Without therapy many of these infants would go on to develop kernicterus, a condition seen much more frequently in infants with severe hemolytic disease than in infants with jaundice caused by other etiologies [34–36]. Bilirubin encephalopathy leads to yellow staining and necrosis of neurones in the

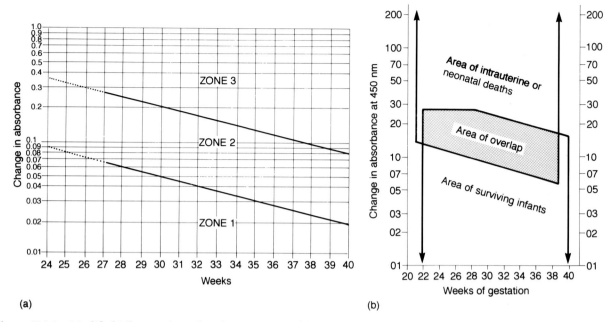

Figure 100.2 Modified Liley graph used to detect severity of fetal hemolysis. The dotted line represents a linear extrapolation from the original Liley data shown in the solid line. (Reproduced with permission from Liley (1963) *Am. J. Obstet. Gynecol.* 86, 492.) (b) Distribution of amniotic fluid values from surviving infants and those with intrauterine and neonatal death. (Reproduced with permission from Queenan, J.T. (1977) *Modern Management of the Rh Problem*, 2nd edn, Harper & Row, New York, p. 57.)

hippocampus, subthalamic nuclei, cerebellum and basal ganglia. The cerebral cortex is generally spared. Only the unconjugated bilirubin enters the neurones, and on autopsy one can see gross yellow staining of brain tissue. On microscopic examination, there are shrunken neurones with decreased Nissl bodies, eosinophilic cytoplasm, gliosis and eccentric swollen nuclei which later become pyknotic. Electron microscopy reveals mitochondrial and endoplasmic swelling, membrane damage and degeneration of nerve endings. Late changes seen with kernicterus include gliosis, neuronal loss in the basal ganglia and subthalamic nuclei, demyelinization in the globus pallidus and degeneration of the dentate fascia [37,38]. Hyperbilirubinemia can also lead to deposition of bilirubin in the liver, kidney, heart, adrenal gland, lung and brain [37,39], although it does not appear to correlate with functional injury in these organs [39] (Chapters 39, 80 and 84).

100.3 Postnatal management of erythroblastosis fetalis

100.3.1 EXCHANGE TRANSFUSIONS

Fortunately, methods exist for therapy of neonatal hemolytic disease. The standard care includes photo-therapy and exchange transfusion. The latter can prevent kernicterus and correct the anemia of erythro-

blastosis fetalis [40]. In this technique, the infant's circulating blood volume is replaced with donor blood in an amount equivalent to two times the infant's blood volume (160 mg/kg body weight). This is not a procedure without risk but can lead to a reduction of serum bilirubin concentration. It usually involves a push–pull technique consisting of withdrawing blood, usually from an umbilical artery catheter, and replacing it either through the same line or through a peripheral intravenous line [41]. This is done in small aliquots, not to exceed 10% of the total volume of blood, and takes an hour or two to complete. Whole or reconstituted anticoagulated blood with normal pH is used. In the past, administration of salt-poor albumin to infants prior to exchange transfusion was advocated but this is no longer recommended since it can lead to further displacement of bilirubin [42]. Exchange transfusion is relatively safe in experienced hands but it still carries a risk of mortality of 0.1–1% and significant morbidity, especially in premature infants [43,44]. Some of the complications of exchange transfusion are electrolyte abnormalities, hypoglycemia, hypocalcemia, thrombus formation, embolization, development of necrotizing enterocolitis, risk of infection from blood products, cardiopulmonary arrest and occasionally death [44,45]. It is usually used in infants with rapidly increasing bilirubin levels, a bilirubin of greater 20 mg/dl or occasionally at lower values in infants who have suffered acidosis, asphyxia or have a hemolytic anemia.

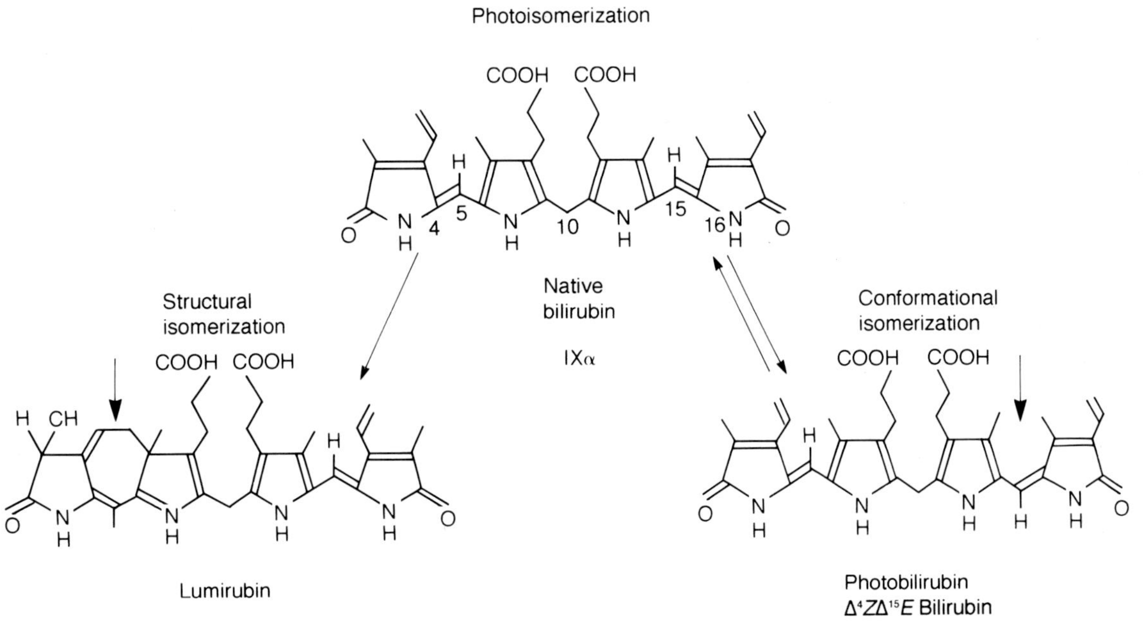

Figure 100.3 The photoisomerized conversion of bilirubin IX-α(Z,Z) to water-soluble bilirubin IX-α(Z,E) and lumirubin. (Reproduced with permission from Polan, R.L. and Ostrea Jr, E.M. (1986) *Neonatal Hyperbilirubinemia: Care of the High Risk Neonate*, 3rd end, W.B. Saunders, Philadelphia, pp. 239–261.)

100.3.2 PHOTOTHERAPY

(a) Mechanism of action

Since 1958, phototherapy has been the method of choice for treating neonatal jaundice. It was first described by Cremer, Perryman and Richards [46] in 1958 and has since been used and shown to be safe and efficacious with no serious long-term side-effects [47]. Usually phototherapy is begun at levels of bilirubin that are 5 mg/dl below exchange levels for a given infant. Some centers use phototherapy prophylactically in very-low-birth-weight infants [48].

Phototherapy works by three proposed mechanisms of action: (1) photo-oxidation, (2) structural isomerization, and (3) configurational isomerization [49–51]. Photo-oxidation involves the reaction of bilirubin with singlet oxygen leading to colorless non-reactive products that are readily excretable [52]. This mechanism has been shown to play a minor role in phototherapy [50]. Configurational isomerization involves changes in the spiral rings in the bilirubin molecule (Figure 100.3). Native bilirubin is usually in a 5Z–15Z configuration. When illuminated, bilirubin undergoes isomerization to an E form and this can lead to several different isomers, 5E–15Z, 5Z–15E or 5E–15E. E isomers are more polar than Z isomers and can be rapidly taken up by the liver and transported into the bile. This is an unstable reaction and the more soluble isomers can be rapidly converted back to native bilirubin [53–55]. This mechanism is felt to be an important pathway of bilirubin degradation by light. The third pathway involves the formation of lumirubin (Figure 100.3). This molecule results from intramolecular cyclization of the bilirubin molecule at the third carbon leading to a more polar compound [55,56]. This is felt to be the primary degradation product of bilirubin by light. This compound is formed maximally at wavelengths of 420–480 nm with a peak at 450 nm and is formed in direct proportion to the intensity of light.

(b) Clinical application

Phototherapy is usually applied in the nursery by placing a panel of eight fluorescent lights above an unclothed infant, lying in an open bassinet or an incubator. The radiance achieved is usually between 7 and 12 μW/cm^2 per nm [50]. Various types of lamp have been employed including white [57,58], blue [59], green [60–62] and halogen lights [63] as well as super blue lights [50], which have been shown to have the most optimal wavelength for bilirubin degradation. Unfortunately super blue lights are very difficult to work with since they require the use of special protective glasses and can make the nursing staff feel nauseated and dizzy [50]. Recently, fiberoptic blankets have become available for phototherapy [64–67]. When phototherapy is instituted, the infants wear protective shields over the eyes (except with fiberoptic blankets) to prevent any potential retinal damage from the light [68], although it is still debated whether this truly happens [69]. Fluids are also increased to compensate for water loss through the skin or the intestines

[70,71]. Some of the side-effects of phototherapy are loose stools [70], overheating [72], tanning [73], rash [72] and the 'bronze baby syndrome' [74,75]. This last disorder causes the skin to become brown after institution of phototherapy. In a large proportion of the patients, conjugated hyperbilirubinemia was noted. It is not known what causes the bronzed pigment seen in these infants, and it is felt that this may be a benign condition, purely cosmetic in nature, but there is still concern that there may be some liver toxicity associated with this condition [74]. There are also concerns about potential DNA damage with phototherapy [76,77] but this has not been demonstrated in vivo [78]. A contraindication to phototherapy is congenital erythropoietic porphyria because this disorder is characterized by hemolysis and bullous lesions when patients are exposed to light at wavelengths between 400 and 500 nm [79,80].

100.3.3 PHARMACOLOGIC AGENTS IN THE TREATMENT OF NEONATAL HYPERBILIRUBINEMIA

(a) Phenobarbital

Other modes of therapy exist for the management of hyperbilirubinemia. Phenobarbital (phenobarbitone) has been administered antenatally and postnatally with variable results [81–83]. The most efficient time of administration is prior to delivery since phenobarbital has a long half-life [84]. It is a potentially addicting drug and may lead to sedation, therefore its use should be limited to populations where there is a high risk of neonatal jaundice or where there may not be access to phototherapy.

(b) Metalloporphyrins

More recently other means of pharmacological intervention have been tried. For example, metalloporphyrins, structural analogs of the heme molecule and competitive inhibitors of the enzyme heme oxygenase, have been advocated for use in the therapy of neonatal jaundice [85–88]. One such compound, tin protoporphyrin, has been used in a clinical trial in Greek infants and was shown to be successful in reducing levels of unconjugated bilirubin [86]. The major drawback of these compounds is that some of them are photoreactive, and tin protoporphyrin is such an agent [89–91]. In fact, several studies showed tin protoporphyrin mediated mortality of neonatal rats exposed to light within a relatively short time (12 hours) [89,90]. There have been no cases of human mortality reported. In the clinical trial conducted by Kappas et al. [86], some of the infants developed rashes that disappeared once phototherapy was discontinued. Other less photosensitizing compounds exist, such as zinc protoporphyrin, zinc mesoporphyrin and chromium compounds [91–93]. These can competitively inhibit heme oxygenase without leading to phototoxic reactions. Presently, these compounds are not in use clinically but there is promise of potential use in the near future after appropriate laboratory and clinical trials are conducted.

(c) Newer modalities

Another pharmacological agent considered in the treatment of neonatal jaundice is bilirubin oxidase [94–98]. This enzyme degrades bilirubin to various water-soluble pigments and can be used in an extracorporeal filter system [97], given intravenously [95,96] or orally [94]. It is of relatively low efficiency and potential side-effects need to be investigated. Lastly, albeit most unconventional, is the use of Chinese medicinal herbs to decrease unconjugated hyperbilirubinemia [99–103]. Several reports in the Chinese literature describe the use of these compounds. There are no reports of trials conducted in the USA.

At the present time management of the hemolytic hyperbilirubinemia consists of prenatal diagnosis and potentially prenatal intervention (Chapter 84). Phototherapy, phenobarbital use and exchange transfusion are the only therapeutic modalities currently available for postnatal management of jaundice.

100.4 Outcome of erythroblastosis fetalis

Today we are able to prevent new cases of isoimmunization and identify pregnancies at risk and treat in utero if necessary. Neonatal care with exchange transfusion and phototherapy optimize neonatal outcome. Perinatal mortality secondary to erythroblastosis fetalis is now 8–9% of Rh-immunized patients [15].

References

1. Robinson, S.H. (1968) The origins of bilirubinemia. N. Engl. J. Med., 279, 143–49.
2. Schmid, R. and McDonagh, A.F. (1979) Formation and metabolism of bile pigments in vivo, in The Porphyrins (ed. D. Dolphin), Academic Press, New York, pp. 258–93.
3. Maines, M.D. (1988) Heme oxygenase: function, multiplicity, regulatory mechanisms and clinical applications. FASEB J., 2, 2557–68.
4. Tenhunen, R., Marver, H.S. and Schmid, R. (1969) Microsomal heme oxygenase. J. Biol. Chem., 244, 6388–94.
5. Yoshida, T. and Kikuchi, G. (1978) Features of the reaction of heme degradation catalyzed by the reconstituted microsomal heme oxygenase system. J. Biol. Chem., 253, 4230–36.
6. Brodersen, R. (1980) Binding of bilirubin to albumin. CRC Crit. Rev. Clin. Lab. Sci., 11, 305–99.
7. Wolkoff, A.W., Goresky, C., Sellin, J. et al. (1979) Role of lingandin in transfer of bilirubin from plasma to liver. Am. J. Physiol., 236, E638–48.
8. Wolkoff, A.W., Ketley, J.N., Waggoner, J.G. et al. (1978) Hepatic accumulation and intracellular binding of conjugated bilirubin. J. Clin. Invest., 61, 142–49.
9. Poland, R.L. and Odell, G.B. (1971) Physiologic jaundice: the enterohepatic circulation of bilirubin. N. Engl. J. Med., 284, 1–6.
10. Corongiu, B. and Roth, M. (1990) (Metabolism of bile pigments in the intestine.) Ann. Biol. Clin. (Paris), 48, 9–15.

11. Gartner, L.M. and Lee, K.S. (1987) Jaundice and liver disease, in *Diseases of the Fetus and Infant* (eds A.A. Fanaroff and R.J. Martin), Mosby, St Louis, pp. 946–65.
12. Cashore, W.J. and Stern, L. (1982) Neonatal hyperbilirubinemia. *Pediatr. Clin. North Am.*, 29, 1191–203.
13. Maisels, M.J. (1988) Neonatal jaundice. *Semin. Liver Dis.*, 8, 148–62.
14. Tan, K.L. (1987) Neonatal jaundice in 'healthy' very low birthweight infants. *Aust. Paediatr. J.*, 23, 185–88.
15. Queenan, J.T. (1987) Erythroblastosis fetalis, in *Diseases of the Fetus and Infant* (eds Fanaroff, A.A. and Martin, R.J.), Mosby, St Louis, pp. 53–62.
16. Han, P., Kiruba, R., Ong, R. et al. (1988) Haemolytic disease due to ABO incompatibility: incidence and value of screening in an Asian population. *Aust. Paediatr. J.*, 24, 35–38.
17. Levine, P. and Stetson, R.E. (1939) Unusual causes of intragroup agglutination. *JAMA*, 113, 126–27.
18. Coombs, R.R.A., Mourant, A.E. and Race, R.R. (1947) A new test for the detection of weak or incomplete Rh agglutinins. *J. Pathol. Bacteriol.*, 59, 105–11.
19. Diamond, L.K., Allen Jr, F.H. and Thomas, Jr W.O. (1951) Erythroblastosis fetalis: VII. Treatment with exchange transfusion. *N. Engl. J. Med.*, 244, 39–49.
20. Bevis, D.C.A. (1956) Blood pigments in haemolytic disease of the newborn. *J. Obstet. Gynaecol. Br. Empire*, 63, 68–75.
21. Liley, A.W. (1963) Intrauterine transfusion of the fetus in hemolytic disease. *BMJ*, 2, 1107–109
22. Finn, R., Clarke, C.A., Donohoe W. et al. (1961) Experimental studies on the prevention of Rh haemolytic disease. *BMJ*, i, 1486–90.
23. Freda, V.J., Gorman, J.G. and Polack, W. (1963) Successful prevention of experimental Rh sensitization in man with an anti-Rh gamma-2-globulin antibody preparation: a preliminary report. *Transfusion*, 4, 26–32.
24. Bowman, J.M. (1978) The management of Rh-isoimmunization. *Obstet. Gynecol.*, 52, 1–16.
25. Freda, V.J., Gorman, J.G., Pollack W. et al. (1975) Prevention of Rh hemolytic disease – 10 year clinical experience with Rh immune globulin. *N. Engl. J. Med.*, 292, 1014–1016.
26. Bowman, J.M. and Pollock, J.M. (1978) Antenatal Rh prophylaxis: 28 week gestation service program. *Can. Med. Assoc. J.*, 118, 622–360.
27. Potter, E.L. (1948) Reproductive histories of 322 mothers of infants with erythroblastosis. *Pediatrics*, 2, 369–80.
28. Connolly, A.M. and Volpe, J.J. (1990) Clinical features of bilirubin encephalopathy. *Clin. Perinatol.*, 17, 371–79.
29. Schmorl, G. (1903) Zur Kenntis des Icterus neonatorum. *Verh. Dtsch. Ges. Pathol.*, 6, 109–15.
30. Rodeck, C.H., Holman, C.A., Karicki, J. et al. (1981) Direct intravascular fetal blood transfusion by fetoscopy in severe isoimmunization. *Lancet*, i, 625–27.
31. Queenan, J.T. and Goetschel, E. (1968) Amniotic fluid analysis for erythroblastosis fetalis. *Obstet. Gynecol.*, 32, 120–33.
32. American College of Obstericians and Gynecologists (1990) Management of Isoimmunization in Pregnancy. *Tech. Bull.*, no. 148, pp. 1–6.
33. Liley, A.W. (1961) Liquor amnii analysis in the management of pregnancy complicated by Rhesus sensitization. *Am. J. Obstet. Gynecol.*, 82, 1359–70.
34. Cashore, W.J. (1990) The neurotoxicity of bilirubin. *Clin. Perinatol.*, 17, 437–47.
35. Hsia, D.Y-Y., Allen, F.H., Gellis, S.S. and Diamond, L.K. (1952) Erythroblastosis fetalis. VIII. Studies of serum bilirubin in relation to kernicterus. *N. Engl. J. Med.*, 247, 668–71.
36. Mollison, P.L. and Cutbush, M. (1954) Haemolytic disease of the newborn, in *Recent Advances in Pediatrics* (ed. D. Gairdner), Blakinston, New York, pp. 110–32.
37. Turkel, S.B. (1990) Autopsy findings associated with neonatal hyperbilirubinemia *Clin. Perinatol.*, 117, 381–96.
38. Haymaker, W., Margoles, C., Pentshew, A. et al. (1961) Pathology of kernicterus and posticteric encephalopathy: presentation of 97 cases, with consideration of pathogenesis and etiology, in *Kernicterus and its Importance in Cerebral Palsy*, C.C. Thomas, Springfield, IL, pp. 21–28.
39. Turkel, S.B. and Mapp, J.R. (1983) A ten-year retrospective study of pink and yellow neonatal hyaline membrane disease. *Pediatrics*, 72, 170–75.
40. Wennberg, R.P., Depp, R. and Weinrichs, W.L. (1978) Indications for early exchange transfusion in patients with erythroblastosis fetalis. *J. Pediatr.*, 92, 789–92.
41. Edwards, M.C. and Fletcher, M.A. (1983) Exchange transfusion, in *Atlas of Procedures in Neonatology* (eds M.A. Fletcher, M.G. McDonald and G.B. Avery), J.B. Lippincott, Philadelphia, pp. 313–26.
42. Chan, G. and Schiff, D. (1976) Variance in albumin loading in exchange transfusions. *J. Pediatr.*, 88, 609–13.
43. Panagoponlos, G., Valaes, T. and Doxiadis, S.A. (1969) Morbidity and mortality related to exchange transfusion. *J. Pediatr.*, 74, 247–54.
44. Dikshit, S.K. and Gupta, P.K. (1989) Exchange transfusion in neonatal hyperbilirubinemia. *Indian Pediatr.*, 26, 1139–45.
45. Paul, S.S., Thomas, V. and Singh, D. (1988) Outcome of neonatal hyperbilirubinemia managed with exchange transfusion. *Indian Pediatr.*, 25, 765–69.
46. Cremer, R.J., Perryman, P.W. and Richards, D.H. (1958) Influence of light on the hyperbilirubinaemia of infants. *Lancet*, i, 1094–97.
47. Scheidt, P.C., Bryla, D.A., Nelson, K.B. et al. (1990) Phototherapy for neonatal hyperbilirubinemia: six-year follow-up of the National Institute of Child Health and Human Development clinical trial. *Pediatrics*, 85, 455–63.
48. Ramagnoli, G., Polidori, G., Catalbi, L. et al. (1979) Phototherapy-induced hypocalcemia. *J. Pediatr.*, 94, 815–16.
49. Ennever, J.F. (1988) Phototherapy for neonatal jaundice. *Photochem. Photobiol.*, 47, 871–6.
50. Ennever, J.F. (1990) Blue light, green light, white light, more light: treatment of neonatal jaundice. *Clin. Perinatol.*, 17, 467–81.
51. Brown, A.K. and McDonagh, A.F. (1980) *Phototherapy for Neonatal Hyperbilirubinemia: Efficacy, Mechanism, and Toxicity.* Year Book Medical, Chicago, pp. 341–89.
52. Lightner, D.A., Linnane, W.P.I. and Ahlfors, C.E. (1984) Bilirubin photooxidation products in the urine of jaundiced infants receiving phototherapy. *Pediatr. Res.*, 19, 696–799.
53. Lightner, D.A., Wooldridge, T.A. and McDonagh, A.F. (1989) Configurational isomerization of bilirubin and the mechanism of jaundice phototherapy. *Biochem. Biophys. Res. Commun.*, 86, 235–43.
54. Ennever, J.F., Costarino, A.T., Polin, R.A. and Speck, W.T. (1987) Rapid clearance of a structural isomer of bilirubin during phototherapy. *J. Clin. Invest.*, 79, 1674–78.
55. Ennever, J.F. and Dresing, T.J. (1991) Quantum yields for the cyclization and configurational isomerization of 4E,15Z-bilirubin. *Photochem. Photobiol.*, 53, 25–32.
56. McDonagh, A.F., Palma, L.A. and Lightner, D.A. (1982) Phototherapy for neonatal jaundice: stereospecific and regioselective photoisomerization of bilirubin bound to human serum albumin and NMR characterization of intramolecular cyclized photoproducts. *J. Am. Chem. Soc.*, 104, 6867–69.
57. Tan, K.L. (1989) Efficacy of fluorescent daylight, blue, and green lamps in the management of nonhemolytic hyperbilirubinemia. *J. Pediatr.*, 114, 132–37.
58. Tan, K.L. and Boey, K.W. (1989) Clinical experience with phototherapy. *Ann. Acad. Med. Singapore*, 18, 43–48
59. McDonagh, A.F. and Lightner, D.A. (1985) 'Like a shrivelled blood orange' – bilirubin, jaundice, and phototherapy. *Pediatrics*, 75, 443–55.
60. Ennever, J.F. (1986) Phototherapy in a new light. *Pediatr. Clin. North Am.*, 33, 603–20.
61. Eidelman, A.L. and Schimmel, M.S. (1989) Phototherapy – 1988. A green light for a new approach? *J. Perinatol.*, 9, 69–71.
62. Ayyash, H., Hadjigeorgiou, M., Sofatzis, J. and Chatziioannou, A. (1987) Green light phototherapy in newborn infants with ABO hemolytic disease. *J. Pediatr.*, 111, 882–87.
63. Eggert, P., Stick, C. and Swalve, S. (1988) On the efficacy of various irradiation regimens in phototherapy of neonatal hyperbilirubinaemia. *Eur. J. Pediatr.*, 147, 525–28.
64. Gale, R., Dranitzki, Z., Dollberg, S. and Stevenson, D.K. (1990) A randomized, controlled application of the Wallaby phototherapy system compared with standard phototherapy. *J. Perinatol.*, 10, 239–42.
65. McFadden, E.A. (1991) The Wallaby Phototherapy System: a new approach to phototherapy. *J. Pediatr. Nurs.*, 6, 206–208.
66. Murphy, M.R. and Oellrich, R.G. (1990) A new method of phototherapy: nursing perspectives. *J. Perinatol.*, 10, 249–51.
67. Rosenfeld, W., Twist, P. and Concepcion, L. (1990) A new device for phototherapy treatment of jaundiced infants. *J. Perinatol.*, 10, 243–48.
68. Messner, K.H. (1978) Light toxicity to newborn retina (abstract). *Pediatr. Res.*, 12, 530.
69. Moseley, M.J. and Fielder, A.R. (1988) Phototherapy: an ocular hazard revisited. *Arch. Dis. Child.*, 63, 886–87.
70. Oh, W. and Karecki, H. (1972) Phototherapy and insensible water loss in the newborn infant. *Am. J. Dis. Child.*, 124, 230–32.
71. Wu, P.Y.K. and Hodgman, J.E. (1974) Insensible water loss in preterm infants: changes with postnatal development and non-ionizing radiant energy. *Pediatrics*, 54, 704–712.
72. Bell, E.F., Neidich, G.A., Cashore, W.J. and Oh, W. (1979) Combined effect of radiant warmer and phototherapy on insensible water loss in low birth weight infants. *J. Pediatr.*, 94, 810–13.
73. Woody, N.C. and Brodkey, M.J. (1973) Tanning from phototherapy for neonatal jaundice. *J. Pediatr.*, 82, 1042–1743.
74. Clark, C.F., Torii, S., Hamamoto, Y. and Kaito, H. (1976) The 'bronze' baby syndrome: post mortem data. *J. Pediatr.*, 88, 461–64.
75. Kopelman, A.E., Brown, R.S. and Odell, G.B. (1972) The 'bronze' baby syndrome: a complication of phototherapy. *J. Pediatr.*, 81, 466–72.
76. Tyrell, R.M. and Keyse, S.M. (1990) New trends in photobiology. The interaction of UVA radiation with cultured cells. *J. Photochem. Photobiol. [B]*, 4, 349–61.
77. Anderson, R.R. and Parrish, J.A. (1991) The optics of human skin. *J. Invest. Dermatol.*, 77, 13–19.
78. Bradley, M.O. and Sharkey, N.A. (1977) Mutagenicity and toxicity of

visible fluorescent light to cultured mammalian cells. *Nature*, **266**, 724–26.

79. Elder, G.H. (1990) The cutaneous porphyrias. *Semin. Dermatol.*, 63–9.
80. Murphy, G.M., Hawk, J.L., Nicholson, D.C. and Magnus, I.A. (1987) Congenital erythropoietic porphyria (Gunther disease). *Clin. Exp. Dermatol.*, **12**, 61–65.
81. Blackburn, M.G., Orzalesi, M.M. and Pigram, P. (1972) The combined effect of phototherapy and phenobarbital on serum bilirubin levels of premature infants. *Pediatrics*, **49**, 110–12.
82. Halpin, T.F., Jones, A.R., Bishop, H.L. *et al.* (1972) Prophylaxis of neonatal hyperbilirubinemia with phenobarbital. *Obstet. Gynecol.*, **40**, 85–90.
83. Valaes, T., Kipouros, K., Petmezaki, S. *et al.* (1980) Effectiveness and safety of prenatal phenobarbital for the prevention of neonatal jaundice. *Pediatr. Res.*, **14**, 947–52.
84. Kurata, N., Yoshida, T., Kuroiwa, Y. *et al.* (1989) Long-term effects of phenobarbital on rat liver microsomal drug-metabolizing enzymes and heme-metabolizing enzyme. *Res. Commun. Chem. Pathol. Pharmacol.*, **65**, 161–79.
85. Drummond, G.S. and Kappas, A. (1986) Sn-protoporphyrin inhibition of fetal and neonatal brain heme oxygenase. Transplacental passage of the metalloporphyrin and prenatal suppression of hyperbilirubinemia in the newborn animal. *J. Clin. Invest.*, **77**, 971–76.
86. Kappas, A., Drummond, G.S., Manola, T. *et al.* (1988). Sn-protoporphyrin use in the management of hyperbilirubinemia in term newborns with direct Coombs-positive ABO incompatibility. *Pediatrics*, **81**, 485–97.
87. Valaes, T.N. and Harvey, W.K. (1990) Pharmacologic approaches to the prevention and treatment of neonatal hyperbilirubinemia. *Clin. Perinatol.*, **17**, 245–73.
88. Vreman, H.J., Hintz, S.R., Kim, C.B. *et al.* (1988) Effects of oral administration of tin and zinc protoporphyrin on neonatal and adult rat tissue heme oxygenase activity. *J. Pediatr. Gastroenterol. Nutr.*, **7**, 902–906.
89. Hintz, S.R., Vreman, H.J. and Stevenson, D.K. (1990) Mortality of metalloporphyrin-treated neonatal rats after light exposure. *Dev. Pharmacol. Ther.*, **14**, 187–92.
90. Keino, H., Nagae, H., Mimura, S. *et al.* (1990) Dangerous effects of tin-protoporphyrin plus photoirradiation on neonatal rats. *Eur. J. Pediatr.*, **149**, 278–79.

91. Scott, J., Quirke, J.M., Vreman, H.J. *et al.* (1990) Metalloporphyrin phototoxicity. *J. Photochem. Photobiol. Biol.*, **7**, 149–57.
92. Vreman, H.J., Gillman, M.J. and Stevenson, D.K. (1989) *In vitro* inhibition of adult rat intestinal heme oxygenase by metalloporphyrins. *Pediatr. Res.*, **26**, 362–65.
93. Stevenson, D.K., Rodgers, P.A. and Vreman, H.J. (1989) The use of metalloporphyrins for the chemoprevention of neonatal jaundice. *Am. J. Dis. Child.*, **143**, 353–56
94. Johnson, L., Dworancsky, R. and Jenkins, D. (1989) Bilirubin oxidase (BOX) feeding at various time intervals and enzyme concentrations in infant Gunn rats. *Pediatr. Res.*, **25**, 116A.
95. Kimura, M., Matsumura, Y., Miyauchi, Y. and Maeda, H. (1988) A new tactic for the treatment of jaundice: an injectable polymer-conjugated bilirubin oxidase. *Proc. Soc. Exp. Biol. Med.*, **188**, 364–69.
96. Kimura, M. (1990) Enzymatic removal of bilirubin toxicity by bilirubin oxidase *in vitro* and excretion of degradation products *in vivo*. *Proc. Soc. Exp. Biol. Med.*, **195**, 646–69.
97. Mullon, C.J., Tosone, C.M. and Langer, R. (1989) Simulation of bilirubin detoxification in the newborn using an extracorporeal bilirubin oxidase reactor (published erratum appears in Pediatr. Res. (1990) 27, 117). *Pediatr. Res.*, **26**, 452–57.
98. Sugi, K., Inoue, M. and Morino, Y. (1989) Degradation of plasma bilirubin by a bilirubin oxidase derivative which has a relatively long half-life in the circulation. *Biochim. Biophys. Acta*, **991**, 405–409.
99. Cui, N.Q., Wu, X.Z. and Zheng, X.L. (1989) (Effect of li dan ling in decreasing jaundice and improving liver function in patients with obstructive jaundice). *Chung Hsi I Chieh Ho Tsa Chih*, **9**, 137–40.
100. Chen, H.Y. (1987) Artemisia composita for the prevention and treatment of neonatal hemolysis and hyperbilirubinemia. *J. Tradit. Chin. Med.*, **7**, 105–108.
101. Cheng, Y.Y., Chan, Y.S., Chuang, K.F. and Chang, H.M. (1985) (Active principle in a capillaris compound in the treatment of experimental acute jaundice in rats). *Chung Hsi I Chieh Ho Tsa Chih*, **5**, 356–60.
102. Wang, C.B., Ge, A.P., Song, W.Y. *et al.* (1987) The jaundice-suppressing effect of blood-cooling, circulation-invigorating, viscera-dredging and cholagogic Chinese herbs in the treatment of hepatitis. *J. Tradit. Chin. Med.*, **7**, 248–50.
103. Shi, Y.M., Shen, Y.J., Fu, M.D. and Lu, Y. (1989) The therapeutic efficacy of the choleretic mixture against the infantile hepatitis syndrome. *J. Tradit. Chin. Med.*, **9**, 103–105.

101 NEONATAL OBSTRUCTIVE UROPATHY

B. Blyth and J.W. Duckett Jr

101.1 Renal development and sonographic evaluation

In the fifth week of gestation the ureteric bud develops a posterior diverticulum of the mesonephric duct at the level of the second sacral vertebra [1]. The ureteric bud penetrates the adjacent renal blastema inducing the formation of the metanephric kidney, and forms the urinary collecting system, including the ureter, renal pelvis, calyces and collecting ducts. Urine formation begins at approximately 10 weeks of gestation [1] although some tubular absorptive functions can be demonstrated at 8 weeks of gestation [2].

Maternal fetal ultrasound by an experienced operator can identify 90% of fetal kidneys by 17 weeks' gestation [3]. The kidney is surrounded by highly echogenic fat and the characteristic appearance of the medullary pyramids separate from the renal cortical tissue assists in identification. The fetal bladder is visualized by 15–18 weeks between the bony landmarks of the ischial and iliac ossification centers, the ureters are not normally visualized unless dilated. Even in the hands of an experienced operator false results, both negative and positive, occur in 15–20% of studies. Repeated, studies are therefore mandatory before drawing significant conclusions. The urinary tract malformations are particularly evident because the fluid-filled masses are easily detected by sonography. In addition, when decreased fetal urine production results in oligohydramnios, ultrasound evaluation is often recommended, with the further detection of renal abnormalities.

It is believed that many of the prenatal urinary dilatations represent ureteral distension in response to the high fetal flow rate. Glomerular filtration in the fetus parallels the renal blood flow, and this gradually increases in proportion to kidney growth and weight, but the glomerular filtration rate is relatively low compared with that of an infant. The rate of urine output in the fetus is however high, due to the low rate of tubular reabsorption, which leads to a hypotonic urine with a high sodium content [4]. Indeed at term the urinary flow rate in the fetus approaches 15–18 ml/kg per h [5], nearly 20 times that of the full-term neonate. While the high urine flow does contribute to the ureteral distension that is commonly observed *in utero*, this dilatation can be markedly accentuated by the presence of any transient or persisting urinary tract obstruction.

The best evidence for transient ureteral obstruction is the description of the ureterovesical membrane, first described by Chwalla in 1927 [6], and confirmed subsequently (summarized by Alcaraz *et al.* in 1991 [7]). The membrane appears between days 35 and 37 of gestation and disappears between days 43 and 49 [7]. The purpose of this membrane – whether it simply relates to the resorption of the common nephric duct into the urogenital sinus, or whether it provides a protective mechanism from the excretions of the developing metanephros before the rupture of the cloacal membrane – is not clear.

In the embryogenesis of the ureter the initial tubular lumen of the ureteric bud becomes solidified, followed by ureteral lengthening and later recanalization [8,9]. This obstruction develops after day 37, beginning in the midureter and extending in either direction so that by day 39 there is total blockade of the ureter. Recanalization begins in the middle portion of the ureter and extends proximally and distally, with the most proximal, ureteropelvic junction, and distal, ureterovesical junction, segments being last to recanalize [9]. This is completed by 41 days of pregnancy.

The hypothesis that the ureteral dilatation observed clinically is related to transient obstruction *in utero* that has resolved by the time of birth does have some embryological support, which appears stronger for the narrow segments at the ends of the ureter. It can be postulated that where there is a delay in the rupture of Chwallas' membrane or in the recanalization of the ureter, the early onset of urine production may result in

Diseases of the Fetus and Newborn, 2nd edn, Edited by G.B. Reed, A.E. Claireaux and F. Cockburn. Published in 1995 by Chapman & Hall, London. ISBN 0 412 39160 0

distension of the upper urinary tract. This has been observed experimentally in rats where a deficiency of vitamin A or of pteroylglutamate delayed the resorption of the ureterovesical membrane, resulting in a megaureter [10,11].

There is less supportive evidence for a similar mechanism producing a transient obstruction at the ureteropelvic junction, but it is feasible that a non-distensible primary defect in the smooth muscle at the uteropelvic junction could function in the same manner.

101.2 Incidence of neonatal hydronephrosis

Hydronephrosis is the most commonly detected congenital condition that is observed by prenatal ultrasound and represents 50% of all abnormalities. The incidence of hydronephrosis varies in each study depending upon the criteria selected and the timing of the ultrasound. It is calculated that the incidence of detectable urinary dilatation *in utero* is 1 per 100 pregnancies but, of these, the order of significant uropathy is 1 per 500 [12]. This is similar to the incidence of congenital hydronephrosis, being 0.17% of pregnancies in a Swedish study [13]. In a well-designed population study at Stoke-on-Trent, 6892 pregnant women, representing 99% of the pregnant population in the district, were scanned at 28 weeks' gestation [14]. Hydronephrosis was found in 1.4% prenatally, and confirmed postnatally in 0.65%.

The degree of hydronephrosis will vary according to the stage of pregnancy and the underlying etiology. As the majority of hydronephrosis detected *in utero* represents physiologic dilatation it is mild, as illustrated in Figure 101.1. The majority of cases of hydronephrosis detected prenatally will resolve either before the end of pregnancy or in the first year of life [15]. Other causes of hydronephrosis included in the differential diagnosis are listed in Table 101.1.

101.3 Postnatal evaluation of neonatal hydronephrosis

The initial assessment of a neonate with prenatally identified hydronephrosis will consist of an ultrasound within the first 2 days of birth, although this must be expedited where the anticipated nature of the lesion is posterior urethral valves. If the initial ultrasound is negative, and was performed within 48 hours of birth, it should be repeated at 3–4 weeks of age. Well-documented cases of pathology have been missed where neonatal oliguria has masked a moderately obstructed lesion [16].

Where the initial evaluation reveals bilateral hydronephrosis, or unilateral hydronephrosis in a single

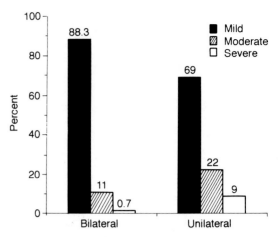

Figure 101.1 Degree of hydronephrosis detected on prenatal ultrasound in 274 fetuses. Hydronephrosis was graded by pelvic diameter, taking into account gestational age: at 15–20 weeks, mild <7 mm, moderate >7 mm; 20–30 weeks, mild <8 mm, moderate 9–15 mm, severe >15 mm; >30 weeks, mild <10 mm, moderate 11–15 mm, severe >15 mm. (Departments of Obstetrics and Gynecology, Brigham and Women's Hospital, and Division of Urology, The Children's Hospital, Boston, MA, unpublished data.)

Table 101.1 Differential diagnosis of suspected hydronephrosis detected by fetal ultrasound

Physiologic hydronephrosis
Ureteropelvic junction obstruction
Congenital obstructed megaureter
Congenital non-obstructed megaureter
Multicystic kidney
Ectopic ureter
Ureterocele
Vesicoureteral reflux
Prune-belly syndrome
Posterior urethral valves
Megacalycosis
Simple renal cyst
Urachal cyst
Ovarian cyst
Hydrocolpos
Sacrococcygeal teratoma
Bowel duplication
Duodenal atresia
Anterior meningocele

functioning kidney, an assessment of the renal reserve must be made. If there is a decrease in the thickness of the renal parenchyma, or areas of cystic dysplasia appear present, it is necessary to monitor the serum creatinine and expedite evaluation of obstructive lesions that will require early intervention. Where hydronephrosis is unilateral, or if bilateral is less marked, a diagnostic algorithm as outlined in Figure 100.2 is followed.

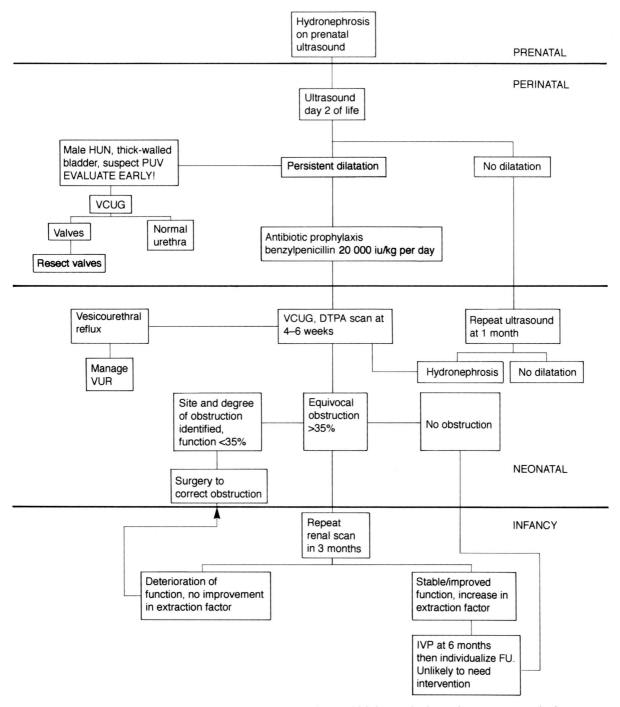

Figure 101.2 Algorithm for neonatal evaluation of unilateral or mild bilateral hydronephrosis. HUN = hydroureteronephrosis; PUV = posterior urethral valves; VCUG = voiding cystourethrogram; VUR = vesicoureteral reflux; IVP = intravenous pyelogram; FU = follow-up.

The upper urinary tract in prenatally detected hydronephrosis is rarely completely obstructed. Such rare cases, where total obstruction is present, result in a kidney devoid of function, with the association of severe cystic dysplasia of the nephrogenic tissue. Most often the upper urinary tract is dilated as a consequence of partial obstruction during embryological development. At the time of birth such transient partial obstruction may no longer be present, and here urinary tract obstruction cannot be precisely defined. Urinary tract obstruction has therefore been characterized as any restriction to urinary outflow that, left untreated, will cause progressive renal deterioration [17].

Current imaging techniques do not provide a reliable indicator of ureteral obstruction, each technique having its deficiencies.

101.3.1 ULTRASONOGRAPHY

This is the mainstay of screening and in the hands of an experienced ultrasonographer can provide an excellent morphological evaluation. The degree of hydronephrosis and caliectasis can be seen, together with the renal size, parenchymal thickness and some subjective assessment of cortical texture. The presence of cortical cysts, calcifications and corticomedullary junctions can be noted. The presence and morphology of the contralateral kidney, and importantly the distal ureters, must be evaluated. A careful evaluation can rule out distal ureteral dilatation, eliminating the necessity of a contrast study of the ureter. Where hydronephrosis is present it is useful to measure the anteroposterior diameter of the renal pelvis. Where this is greater than 15 mm there is a greater likelihood of requiring surgery to correct a ureteropelvic junction obstruction [18,19].

101.3.2 VOIDING CYSTOURETHROGRAM

This is indicated in all cases of hydronephrosis. Vesicoureteral reflux coexists with ureteropelvic junction obstruction in 14% of patients [20], and in 14% coexists with obstruction at the ureterovesical junction [21]. It is present in many ureteral duplication anomalies, with ectopic ureters and ureteroceles. Reflux without other associated anomalies may also be responsible for antenatally detected hydronephrosis.

101.3.3 DIURETIC RENOGRAM

This has now become the most widely used technique for assessing the function and drainage of kidneys in the presence of hydronephrosis. It involves the injection of a radioisotope and the monitoring of its passage through the upper urinary tract with a γ-camera–computer system. The early uptake of the tracer by a kidney can be measured and is indicative of separate renal function [22], while the washout from the kidney, augmented by the administration of a diuretic, is evaluated and plotted by the computer. The pattern of tracer excretion is evaluated and can reflect the presence of obstruction in the collecting system [23].

The most widely used agent is technetium-99m diethylenetriaminepenta-acetic acid (^{99m}Tc-DTPA). This tracer is excreted by glomerular filtration and is not secreted or reabsorbed by the renal tubules. It emits a 140-keV γ-ray which is optimal for imaging and does not emit β particles. A newer agent that has entered clinical practice is ^{99m}Tc-mercaptoacetyltriglycine (MAG$_3$). This isotope is cleared by the kidney in a similar manner to ^{131}I-o-iodohippurate (^{131}I-Hippuran) and offers enhanced visual and analog images over ^{99m}Tc-DTPA. Its cost, however, is significantly greater than that of DTPA.

The technique and standardization of the diuretic renogram varies from one institution to another. Variables include oral hydration versus intravenous hydration, the dosage and timing of administration of diuretic, the requirement for bladder catheterization, and the method of calculation of the clearance after the administration of diuretic. False-positives in interpretation may occur when the immature neonatal kidney fails to respond to diuretic, or the patient is dehydrated, when the bladder is distended or when the pelvis is significantly dilated, all factors often present in the neonate. Thus the half-life is of debatable value in the infant with hydronephrosis.

101.3.4 EXCRETORY UROGRAPHY

The excretory urogram has been the traditional method of evaluating hydronephrosis, but has significant limitations in the neonate. Gaseous distension of the intestine limits the detail of the radiological images, which is further impaired in children with poorly functioning kidneys or extremely dilated pelves. The excretory urogram still has a place in assessing ureteral anatomy, but is more satisfactorily performed in the older infant. Here it still has a useful role in distinguishing the extrarenal pelvis without calyceal dilatation requiring no further evaluation from the mild ureteropelvic junction obstruction.

101.3.5 WHITAKER TEST

The anterograde pressure–flow study was introduced by Whitaker in 1973 [24] as a technique for assessing and quantifying obstruction in hydronephrotic kidneys. This test involves the percutaneous puncture of the renal pelvis with two needles, one to perfuse the pelvis, simulating a diuresis, the second to record pressure. This test assumes that obstruction produces a constant restriction to outflow that necessitates elevated pressures to transport urine at high flow rates. Unfortunately not all obstructions are constant. Koff et al. [25]; have characterized the volume-dependent changes in pressure and classified patterns of pressure–exit flow curves as simple or complex. Where there was a severe intrinsic ureteropelvic junction obstruction a simple linear relation existed between pressure and flow. Here the Whitaker test was unequivocal. However when there was extrinsic obstruction a complex non-linear curve existed where the rate of increase in exit flow did not keep pace with the increase in pressure: it either plateaued or decreased. Here the type of pressure–flow curve indicated that the resistance was variable and was dependent on pelvic volume. This points out the fundamental failure of the Whitaker test, which is non-diagnostic in this situation. The Whitaker measurement records the response of the renal pelvis to distension, which does not truly define obstruction [25]. This is why the test has proved limited in the complex clinical situation where combinations of intrinsic and extrinsic factors contribute to the anatomy of the ureteropelvic junction and its radiologic appearance [26]. The Whitaker test is also non-physiologic in the neonate where the high flows employed greatly exceed the normal urine flow [27]. There is also some morbidity in performing this evaluation in the neonate, with adverse effects upon a subsequent pyeloplasty [28].

10.3.6 ANTIBIOTIC PROPHYLAXIS

All infants with prenatally detected hydronephrosis that is confirmed postnatally must be placed on antibiotic prophylaxis pending the outcome of further evaluation. In the neonate benzylpenicillin (called penicillin G) administered orally, 20 000 iu/kg, has the best spectrum against urinary pathogens encountered in the perinatal period, and high concentrations are achieved in the urine. Where benzylpenicillin cannot be obtained phenoxymethylpenicillin (pencillin V) is an alternative. It has twice the oral absorption of benzylpencillin but similar excretion and high urinary concentrations. Beyond 8 weeks of age in the term infant this can be replaced with trimethoprim–sulfamethoxazole (cotrimoxazole), which achieves high urinary concentrations with few side-effects. Nitrofurantoin is another excellent antibiotic for prophylaxis in urinary tract infections. There is limited experience in its use in the neonate. It is excreted unchanged in the urine and only accumulates with impaired renal function, when it can induce peripheral neuropathies; it has also been associated with hemolytic anemia.

101.4 Indications for prenatal urological intervention

Prenatal intervention is contemplated with the presentation of a fetus with sonographically detected bilateral hydronephrosis and a degree of oligohydramnios. The potential benefit from intervention is the prevention of further deterioration in renal or pulmonary impairment, yet it remains to be proven that this can be achieved. It is thus rare that prenatal intervention for hydronephrosis will be indicated. Glick et al. [29] have proposed criteria for intervention, as listed in Table 101.2, and in such cases where prenatal intervention is indicated it should only be undertaken in an experienced institution under approved protocols. Techniques for prenatal intervention involve both the percutaneous placement of shunts to divert the urine

Table 101.2 Prenatal intervention for hydronephrosis

Indications
Presumed obstructive hydronephrosis, persistent or progressive, bilateral or in a solitary unit
Oligohydramnios
Otherwise healthy fetus without severe structural or karyotypic abnormalities
Adequate fetal renal functional indices (urine output >2 ml/h, Na+ <100 mmol/l, Cl− <90, osmolality <210 mosmol/kg H$_2$O)
Without overt renal dysplasia (minimal echogenicity, hydronephrosis proportional to lower tracts)
Adequate informed consent

Contradictions
Presence of associated severe anomalies
Chromosomal abnormalities
Unilateral hydronephrosis with an adequately functioning contralateral kidney
Bilateral hydronephrosis without oligohydramnios
Severely dysplastic kidneys
Evidence of urethral atresia
Presence of a normal twin

from the dilated urinary tract into the amniotic cavity, and open fetal surgery where a cutaneous diversion of the urine is performed.

101.5 Indications for postnatal intervention

Surgery is indicated in all cases of infravesical obstruction, with either ablation of valves where the urethra is negotiable with an infant cystoscope, or a vesicostomy where the urethra is not patent, or inadequate to accommodate the pediatric cystoscope.

101.5.1 URETEROPELVIC JUNCTION OBSTRUCTION

Indications for surgery where hydronephrosis is associated with narrowing of the ureteropelvic junction or ureterovesical junction are more controversial. Once a ureteropelvic junction obstruction has been defined, prompt intervention is appropriate to relieve the obstruction as, at any age, ongoing ureteral obstruction is detrimental to the kidney. In the neonatal period early relief of obstruction maximizes functional renal development and increases the ultimate number of perfused and filtering nephrons [30]. The ongoing debate in the management of neonatal ureteropelvic junction obstruction is the definition of when significant obstruction is present.

In the neonate it is insufficient to rely on a morphological appearance of a dilated renal pelvis from excretory urography or ultrasonography to proceed to surgical correction. Diuretic renography, as outlined, has its limitations in the diagnosis of obstruction in the infant. The most useful measure in diuretic renography is the estimate of individual renal function either from the percentage uptake of isotope in the first minutes after injection [22] or the differential uptake between the two kidneys when one appears to be normal. This is considered significant when less than 30% [31] (normal = 50%), 35% [32] or 40% [33]. The percentage function is usually correlated with the half-life washout from the dilated collecting system [31] but the renogram is only useful in the neonate when the two kidneys can be compared [34]. The washout curve is influenced by the hydration, renal function, the volume and contractility of the renal pelvis, the timing of administration of diuretic and the severity of the outflow obstruction. These factors therefore have to be considered when evaluating the renal scan in the neonate as they too can significantly affect the washout curve, whether or not any obstruction is present. For this reason a reliance on the half-life of the diuretic washout curve is not a valid single indicator to proceed to surgery, especially in the neonate.

Surgery is therefore recommended in the neonatal period for those infants with the morphological appearance of ureteropelvic junction obstruction on ultrasound or excretory urography, with no evidence of distal ureteral distension, in whom the renal function is depressed below 35% of total renal function. Those with function better than 35% are followed with repeat scans at 3–6-month and 12-month intervals and surgery is indicated only when there is clear deterioration in renal function. In those cases where follow-up renal scans are suggestive of deterioration in renal function an excretory urogram defining calyceal anatomy assists in identifying obstruction. Using these criteria in 35 infants with apparent uteropelvic junction obstruction where the initial differential function was greater than 35%, managed recently at the Children's Hospital of Philadelphia [35], 85% have been followed without surgery. The indications for surgery in the six (15%) were decreasing function (4), recurrent urinary tract infections (1) and symptoms of renal colic (1). The eventual differential renal function achieved in this group of 35 patients was no different from a group of 12 patients with >35% function who had previously undergone early pyeloplasty [35].

In the newborn period there is a significant increase in the glomerular filtration rate [4,36] as illustrated in Figure 101.3, and this increase has been noted to occur in the majority of infants with partial ureteral obstruction secondary to narrowing at the ureteropelvic junction. Koff [37] has followed ten patients in whom the mean starting differential function was 25% and all have improved to better than 40% differential function with serial observation. It has been a failure to consider the rapid increase in the glomerular filtration rate that occurs in the neonate, and which then plateaus after 2

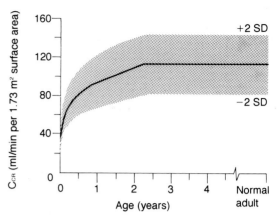

Figure 101.3 Normal glomerular filtration rate measured by endogenous creatinine clearance (C_{CR}) in relation to age. Mean ± two standard deviations are demonstrated. (Reprinted with permission from McRory, W. (1972) *Developmental Nephrology*, Harvard University Press, Cambridge, MA, p. 98.)

years of age, that has resulted in the promotion of early intervention in the past.

In a review by Mayor *et al.* [38] the renal function of 24 infants with hydronephrosis who underwent surgery were compared, based on the age at time of surgery. The youngest patients showed the greatest increase in glomerular filtration rate following surgery, which is actually equivalent to that expected in a normal young infant undergoing transitional nephrological changes and does not support early intervention. King *et al.* [39] reported on 11 patients (<3 months of age) who underwent pyeloplasty, and compared the relative increase in renal function with that of older patients also undergoing pyeloplasty. The mean increase in relative function was 18.9% in the younger patients, compared with an increase of only 4.6% in the older group. However the final relative functional values of 36.5% and 32.5% are not significantly different. The larger increase noted in the younger group is again only the result of the expected maturation in renal function with age.

Where there is relative renal function >35% at the initial renal scanning, these patients are followed on antibiotic prophylaxis, according to the flowchart in Figure 101.2. Serial studies are mandatory as several studies have indicated that approximately 20% of the group are at risk of deterioration in renal function and will require surgery [18,19,35,40].

101.5.2 URETEROVESICAL JUNCTION OBSTRUCTION

Similar recommendations are made for the infant detected with hydronephrosis secondary to a narrowing at the ureterovesical junction, the primary obstructive megaureter. Here impressive dilatation of the distal ureter in may cases has not been associated with any demonstrable loss of renal function, and when followed serially the dilatation resolves significantly. In a series of 34 renal units associated with primary obstructive megaureter detected by prenatal ultrasound only (6%) required surgery for diminishing renal function and most showed decreased dilatation on sequential evaluation [41]. Surgery in the absence of symptoms is therefore only recommended when the relative renal function is reduced (<35%).

101.5.3   OTHER CAUSES

Surgery is indicated for all other obstructive causes of neonatal hydronephrosis. Where a ureterocele is present, the best initial management is endoscopic incision [42]. With the diagnosis of an obstructed ectopic ureter a number of options are present, depending upon the degree of function in the associated renal unit, the size of the ureter and the presence of vesicoureteral reflux. When hydronephrosis is related to a neurogenic bladder or prune-belly syndrome it is necessary to establish that bladder emptying is adequate and usually surgery is not required. When vesicoureteral reflux is present, antibiotic prophylaxis is the initial management, while multicystic kidneys do not benefit from antibiotic prophylaxis and are followed by serial ultrasound.

101.6   Summary

Dilatation of the urinary tract is detected in 1% of pregnancies. This is most often physiologic in nature, reflecting the high urinary flow rate in the fetus. Transient narrowings of the urinary tract do occur during embryological development, and when these narrowings persist or the resolution of these is delayed, significant dilatation of the urinary tract results.

At birth, the neonate in whom hydronephrosis was detected prenatally is evaluated and placed on antibiotic prophylaxis. A stepwise protocol utilizing current imaging techniques is followed to determine if significant urinary obstruction is present. When obstruction is diagnosed, corrective surgery is indicated. The indications for prenatal intervention are rare.

References

1. Cook, W.A. and Stephens, F.D. (1988) Pathoembryology of the urinary tract, in *Urologic Surgery in Neonates and Young Infants* (ed. L.R. King), W.B. Saunders, Philadelphia. pp. 1–23.
2. Lauriola, L., Tallini, G., Sentinelli, S. and Massi, G. (1986) Protein absorption by tubular mesonephric and metanephric structures in the human embryo. *Cell Tissue Res.*, **246**, 77–80.
3. Lawson, T.L., Foley, W.D., Berland, L.L. and Clark, K.E. (1981) Ultrasonic evaluation of fetal kidneys: analysis of normal size and frequency of visualization as related to stage of pregnancy. *Radiology*, **138**, 153–56.
4. Chevalier, R.L. (1989) Perinatal renal development and physiology. *AUA Update Series*, **VIII**, 58–63.
5. Rabinowitz, R., Peters, M.T. and Vyas, S. (1989) Measurement of fetal urine production in normal pregnancy by real time ultrasonography. *Am. J. Obset. Gynecol.*, **161**, 1264–66.
6. Chwalla, R. (1927) Uber die Entwicklung der Harnblase und det Primaren der Menschen mit besonderer Berucksichtigung der Art und Weise, in der sich die Uretern von der Urnierengangen trennen, nebst Bemerkungen uber die Entwicklung der Mullerschen Gange und des Mastdarms. *Z. Anat. Entw. Gesch.*, **83**, 615–19.
7. Alcaraz, A., Vinaixa, F., Tejedo-Mateu, A. *et al.* (1991) Obstruction and recanalization of the ureter during embryonic development. *J. Urol.*, **145**, 410–16.
8. Ludwig, E. (1957) Embryologische Beobachtungen und den Hanoorganem des Mans und des Goldhamster. *Acta Anat.*, **29**, 1–4.
9. Ruano-Gil, D., Coca-Payeras, A. and Tejedo-Maten, A. (1975) Obstruction and normal recanalization of the ureter in human embroyo: its relation to congenital ureteric obstruction. *Eur. Urol.*, **1**, 287–93.
10. Wilson, J.G. and Warkany, J. (1948) Malformation in the genitourinary tract induced by vitamin A deficiency. *Am. J. Anat.*, **83**, 357–61.
11. Monie, I.W., Nelson, M.M. and Evans, H.M. (1957) Abnormalities of the urinary system of rat embryos resulting from transitory deficiencies of pteroil-glutamic acid during gestation. *Anat. Res.*, **127**, 711–15.
12. Thomas, D.F.M. (1990) Fetal uropathy: review. *Br. J. Urol.*, **66**, 225–31.
13. Helin, I. and Persson, P. (1986) Prenatal diagnosis of urinary tract abnormalities by ultrasound. *Pediatrics*, **78**, 879–82.
14. Livera, L.N., Brookfield, D.S.K., Egginton, J.A. and Hawnaur, J.M. (1989) Antenatal ultrasonography to detect fetal renal abnormalities: a prospective screening programme. *BMJ*, **298**, 1421–23.
15. Mandell, J., Blyth, B.R., Peters, C.A. *et al.* (1991) Structural genitourinary defects detected in utero. *Radiology*, **178**, 193–96.
16. Dejter, S.W.J. and Gibbons, M.D. (1989) The fate of infant kidneys with fetal hydronephrosis but initially normal postnatal sonography. *J. Urol.*, **2**, 661–62.
17. Koff, S.A. (1987) Problematic ureteropelvic junction obstruction. *J. Urol.*, **138**, 390.
18. Homsy, Y.L., Saad, F., Laberge, I. *et al.* (1990) Transitional hydronephrosis of the newborn and infant. *J. Urol.*, **144**, 579–83.
19. Ransley, P.G., Dhillon, H.K., Gordon, I. *et al.* (1990) The postnatal management of hydronephrosis by prenatal ultrasound. *J. Urol.*, **144**, 584–87.
20. Hollowell, J.G., Altman, H.G., Snyder III, H.M. and Duckett, J.W. (1989) Coexisting ureteropelvic junction obstruction and vesicoureteral reflux: diagnostic and therapeutic implications. *J. Urol.*, **142**, 490–93.
21. Weiss, R.M. and Lytton, B. (1974) Vesicoureteral reflux and distal ureteral obstruction. *J. Urol.*, **111**, 245–49.
22. Heyman, S. and Duckett, J.W. (1988) Extraction factor: an estimate of single kidney function in children during routine radionucleotide renography with 99m technetium diethylenetriaminepentacetic acid. *J. Urol.*, **140**, 780–83.
23. Kass, E.J. and Majd, M. (1985) Evaluation and management of upper urinary tract obstruction in infancy and childhood. *Urol. Clin. North Am.*, **12**, 133–41.
24. Whitaker, R.H. (1973) Methods of assessing obstruction in dilated ureters. *Br. J. Urol.*, **45**, 15–22.
25. Koff, S.A., Hayden, L.J., Cirulli, C. and Shore, R. (1986) Pathophysiology of ureteroplevic junction obstruction: experimental and clinical observations. *J. Urol.*, **136**, 336–38.
26. Floyd, J.W. and Hendren, W.H. (1990) Reoperative pyeloplasty: experience with 22 cases. *J. Urol.*, **143**, 275A.
27. Dhillon, H.K., Gordon, I., Ransley, P.G. and Duffy, P.G. (1990) *The Antegrade Pressure Perfusion Study in Infants with Prenatally Diagnosed Hydronephrosis*, American Academy of Pediatrics, Boston, MA.
28. Hanna, M.K. and Glick, R.U. (1988) Ureteropelvic junction obstruction during the first year of life. *Urology*, **31**, 41–45.
29. Glick, P.L., Harrison, M.R. and Golbus, M.S. (1985) Management of the fetus with congenital hydronephrosis. II: Prognostic criteria and selection for treatment. *J. Pediatr. Surg.*, **20**, 376–87.
30. Chevalier, R.L. and El Dahr, S. (1988) The case for early relief of obstruction in young infants, in *Urological Surgery in Neonates and Young Infants* (ed. L.R. King), W.B. Saunders, Philadelphia, pp. 95–118.
31. Kass, E.J. and Fink-Bennett, D. (1990) Radioisotopic evaluation of dilated urinary tract. *Urol. Clin. North Am.*, **17**, 273–89.
32. Cartwright, P.C., Snyder, H.M. and Duckett, J.W. (1991) The case for functional assessment of apparent UPJ obstruction. *Dialog. Pediatr. Urol.*, **14**, 4–5.
33. Ransley, P. and Manzoni, G.A. (1985) Extended role of DTPA scan in assessing function and UPJ obstruction in neonate. *Dialog. Pediatr. Urol.*, **8**, 6–7.
34. Homsy, Y.L. and Koff, S.A. (1988) Problems in the diagnosis of obstruction in the neonate, in *Urological Surgery in Neonates and Young Infants* (ed. L. King), W.B. Saunders, Philadelphia, pp. 77–94.
35. Cartwright, P.C., Duckett, J.W., Snyder, H.M. *et al.* (1992) Managing

apparent ureteropelvic junction obstruction in the newborn. *J. Urol.*, **148**, 1224–28.

36. Guignard, J.P. (1982) Renal function in the newborn infant. *Pediatr. Clin. North Am.*, **29**, 777–90.
37. Koff, S.A. (1991) Neonatal UPJ obstructions: current controversies. *Dialog. Pediatr. Urol.*, **14**, 6–8.
38. Mayor, G., Genton, N., Torrado, A. and Guignard, J.-P. (1975) Renal function in obstructive nephropathy: long-term effect of reconstructive surgery. *Pediatrics*, **56**, 740–47.

39. King, L.R., Coughlin, P.W., Bloch, E.C. *et al.* (1984) The case for immediate pyeloplasty in the neonate with ureteropelvic junction obstruction. *J. Urol.*, **132**, 725–28.
40. Johnson, H.W., Gleave, M., Coleman, G.U. *et al.* (1987) Neonatal renomegaly. *J. Urol.*, **138**, 1023–26.
41. Keating, M.A., Escala, J., Snyder III, H.M. *et al.* (1989) Changing concepts in managment of primary obstructive megaureter. *J. Urol.*, **142**, 636–40.
42. Blyth, B., Passerini-Glazel, G., Camuffo, G. *et al.* (1992) Endoscopic incision of ureteroceles: intravesical vs ectopic. *J. Urol.*, **149**, 556–60.

102 EXTRACORPOREAL MEMBRANE OXYGENATION

W.D. Rhine

102.1 History of cardiopulmonary bypass in neonates

The use of a membrane oxygenator within a cardiopulmonary bypass circuit is referred to as extracorporeal membrane oxygenation (ECMO). The development of cardiopulmonary bypass followed the understanding of cardiac and pulmonary physiology, complemented by knowledge of hematology and an ability to inhibit coagulation. Dr Gibbon transferred laboratory development of cardiopulmonary bypass techniques to the clinical arena with the first intraoperative use of bypass for repair of an atrial septal defect in 1953 [1]. This oxygenator worked by passing blood over vertical steel screens. Although effective for gas exchange, the large gas–blood surface area interface leads to hemolysis, thrombocytopenia and marked consumption of coagulation factors. More recent hollow-fiber oxygenators, able to provide operative cardiopulmonary bypass for several hours, are too blood destructive to provide support for days to weeks. The design of a membrane oxygenator in 1956 by Clowes, Hopkins and Neville [2] and its subsequent modification into a coiled cylinder shape by Kolobow and Bowman in the 1960s [3], introduced a means of providing efficient gas exchange, and hence cardiopulmonary support for longer periods.

When first tried in premature neonates in the 1960s and early 1970s, ECMO provided adequate cardiovascular support and gas exchange; but these babies succumbed from hemorrhagic complications. ECMO was also used in adults but was found not to improve survival in a multicenter, prospective randomized trial of adult patients with acute respiratory distress syndrome [4]. The first neonate to survive with ECMO was treated in 1975 [5]. ECMO techniques became further refined along with more widespread distribution of ECMO equipment and expertise. In the 1980s, two prospective, randomized studies supported the premise that ECMO resulted in improved survival rates when compared with conventional therapy for neonatal respiratory failure [6,7]. However, these trials have been criticized for their novel statistical methodologies [8–10]. Currently, more than 80 ECMO centers in the USA place over 1000 neonates on bypass annually. A prospective, randomized trial of ECMO versus conventional therapy is under way in the UK.

102.2 Indications

102.2.1 GENERAL PRINCIPLES

ECMO has been recommended for use in term and near-term newborns with a *reversible* respiratory or cardiac disease process, who have greater than an estimated 60–80% risk of dying with conventional ventilation and 'maximal medical therapy'. In these patients, ECMO should improve survival rates, and should also:

1. provide adequate oxygenation and ventilation to prevent hypoxic–ischemic tissue and organ injury;
2. allow for reduction of ventilator settings to reduce barotrauma and oxygen toxicity.

The latter contributes to more rapid pulmonary recovery and repair. ECMO has also been utilized as a bridge to lung or heart transplant in newborns with irreversible underlying disease processes. The definition of maximal medical therapy varies among institutions and individual physicians [11], and may include hyperventilation [12], 'gentle' ventilation or non-hyperventilation [13,14], high-frequency ventilation [15,16], negative-pressure ventilation [17], pressor support, e.g. dopamine or tolazoline, as well as surfactant replacement therapy [18]. Inhaled nitric oxide may soon be included as pre-ECMO therapy as it is a powerful, locally acting pulmonary vasodilator [19].

ECMO should be instituted before permanent hypoxic or ischemic injury occurs, especially to the

Diseases of the Fetus and Newborn, 2nd edn, Edited by G.B. Reed, A.E. Claireaux and F. Cockburn. Published in 1995 by Chapman & Hall, London. ISBN 0 412 39160 0

brain. Prematurity with gestation less than 34 weeks is usually considered a relative contraindication for ECMO as there may be too great a risk of intracranial hemorrhage during bypass [20]. Whenever possible, a cranial ultrasound is performed on the potential ECMO candidate to rule out the presence of intracranial hemorrhage. A patient with a small, grade I intracranial hemorrhage may be considered for ECMO, with appropriate understanding that extension of the hemorrhage may occur. Most centers prefer ECMO candidates to have been ventilated at high pressure and oxygen concentration for less than 7–10 days; otherwise there is a high likelihood of fibrotic, irreversible lung injury. Prior to ECMO, a hematologic work-up is performed to ensure that any coagulopathy is treated aggressively before or during bypass to reduce risk of hemorrhage.

102.2.2 NEONATAL DIAGNOSES

The most common neonatal diagnoses treated by ECMO can be divided into medical versus surgical or anatomical disease processes. Medical diagnoses include meconium aspiration syndrome, persistent pulmonary hypertension, severe hyaline membrane disease, pneumonia and sepsis. It is important to remember that pulmonary hypertension may not be the primary underlying pathologic process, but instead may accompany other disease such as meconium aspiration syndrome, or may be secondary to pneumonia or hyaline membrane disease. Persistent pulmonary hypertension of the newborn may result from *in utero* hypoxic or ischemic stress that leads to a relative overproliferation of the smooth muscle of the pulmonary vasculature [21]. The stressed fetus is then less likely to tolerate labor and delivery, leading to a higher incidence of meconium passage and aspiration. Severe hyaline membrane disease may be seen in the near-term infant, 34–36 weeks of gestation, especially in the presence of maternal diabetes. Respiratory failure may also be caused or exacerbated by pulmonary hemorrhage or air leak. The barotrauma of mechanical ventilation at high pressures to treat respiratory failure may lead to pneumothorax or other air leak, and may also contribute to increased pulmonary vascular resistance.

Congenital diaphragmatic hernia is the primary neonatal surgical disease treated by ECMO, which has played a significant role in lowering the mortality from this disease [22]. ECMO may be used either before hernia repair for stabilization and resolution of the persistent pulmonary hypertension that accompanies severe congenital diaphragmatic hernia, or it may be used after repair in patients not responding to maximal conventional therapy.

ECMO has also been used in neonates with congenital heart disease [23,24]. Most ECMO candidates have echocardiography performed before bypass so that any cardiac anomalies may be identified. Some congenital heart disease diagnoses, particularly anomalous pulmonary veins, may be difficult to identify by echocardiogram, or may be so severe that ECMO is needed for preoperative stabilization. More commonly, ECMO is necessary for congenital heart disease postoperatively, for either low cardiac output or pulmonary vasoreactive crisis.

ECMO can serve as a life-sustaining bridge to transplantion in otherwise lethal congenital pulmonary or cardiac disease. The first neonatal lung transplantation was performed in a patient with pulmonary hypertension associated with an abnormal pulmonary vasculature, who failed to wean off ECMO bypass despite 28 days of therapy [25]. Lung transplants after ECMO have also been performed for severe congenital diaphragmatic hernia [26] and pulmonary lymphangiectasia. Similarly, ECMO bypass may be used to support neonates with inoperable congenital heart disease while awaiting transplant.

102.2.3 RESPIRATORY FAILURE CRITERIA

Several criteria have been proposed as measurements of respiratory failure [27–29]. Oxygenation index (OI) (mean airway pressure $\times$ FiO_2(%)/post-ductal PO_2), when > 35–60, has been associated with a high mortality rate and has the advantage of reflecting the degree of ventilator pressure support. Other measurements of respiratory failure assume high ventilator settings, e.g. FiO_2 of 100%, and mean airway pressure over 15–18 cmH_2O. The alveolar–arterial PO_2 difference, when greater than 615–630 mmHg (82–84 kPa) for several hours, also has been found to correlate with poor outcome with conventional therapy [28]. Other criteria used by ECMO centers include postductal PaO_2 alone, barotrauma and acidosis. In patients with congenital diaphragmatic hernia, Bohn *et al.* [30] found survival to correlate with the ventilatory index (mean airway pressure $\times$ ventilator rate) and $PaCO_2$; however, these criteria have recently been challenged with the advent of ECMO [31]. Individual ECMO centers are recommended to conduct chart reviews from term and near-term neonates with respiratory failure from the era just before ECMO availability to determine the best predictor of mortality in their patient population. These 'objective' criteria may be influenced by the timing of blood gas analysis and may not necessarily reflect the lability of the patient's condition, e.g. when a patient requires frequent hand-bagging to achieve adequate oxygenation. There is an acknowledged limitation to retrospective analysis, given recent therapeutic advances in neonatology including high-frequency ventilation and surfactant replacement.

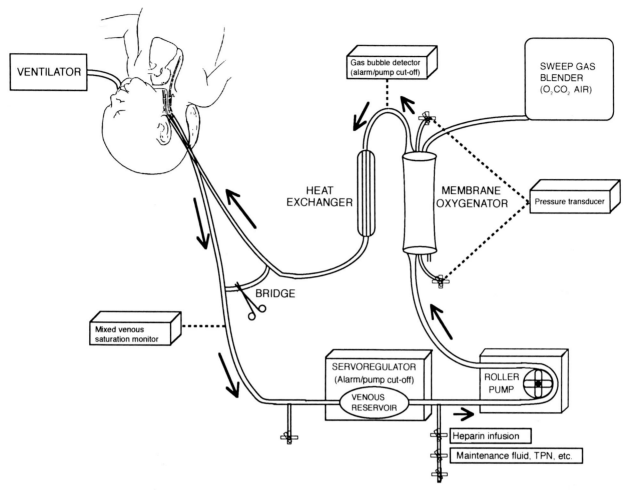

Figure 102.1 Basic venoarterial ECMO circuit. Optional equipment connects to circuit with dashed lines. TPN = total parenteral nutrition.

102.3 Techniques of ECMO bypass

102.3.1 VENOARTERIAL BYPASS

Until recently, virtually all neonatal ECMO entailed venoarterial bypass. A typical venoarterial ECMO circuit is depicted in Figure 102.1, but ECMO centers have their individual modifications. To achieve bypass, catheters between 8 and 14 Fr gauge are placed by sterile surgical technique, via an incision in the right neck, into the carotid artery and the jugular vein. The arterial catheter is positioned with the distal end near the arch of the aorta; the venous catheter tip should lie in the right atrium. The catheters are then connected to the previously prepared ECMO circuit. This circuit is prepared by flushing with carbon dioxide, which dissolves more readily than room air, and then priming with crystalloid. Albumin is added to the priming solution to coat the plastic in a process known as 'passivation'. Passivation decreases deposition of plasma proteins on to the tubing and oxygenator. To

finish the circuit preparation, blood is added to the ECMO circuit while the crystalloid is drained out.

During bypass, blood drains via the venous catheter by gravity into a venous reservoir or bladder. This bladder serves as a bubble trap, as well as an indicator of adequate vascular volume by virtue of placement within a servoregulator. Blood is drawn from the bladder by a roller pump. If the pump draws blood from the bladder faster than venous drainage from the patient, the bladder starts to collapse, stopping the pump and triggering an audible alarm. This bladder servoregulation prevents cavitation of gas due to excessive negative pressure, and eliminates the possibility of exsanguination from a circuit leak. A similar servoregulatory system can be implemented using pressure measurements from the circuit just before the bladder [32]. Alternatively, a centrifugal pump may be used instead of a roller pump, which obviates the need for a bladder [33].

Blood passes from the pump into the membrane oxygenator. The oxygenator (Figure 102.2) consists of

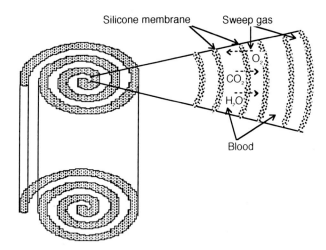

Silicone membrane   Sweep gas

O$_2$

CO$_2$

H$_2$O

Blood

Figure 102.2 Coiled membrane oxygenator. Sweep gas, comprising oxygen, carbon dioxide and nitrogen, passes inside the membrane envelope. Blood passes outside the envelope through the interstices between layers. Diffusion of gas occurs passively through the silicone membrane.

an envelope of silicon rubber containing an oxygen-rich, carbon dioxide-poor gas phase, which is constantly replenished by an entering sweep gas. Oxygen passively diffuses from a high concentration within the gas phase, across the membrane and into the blood. Similarly, carbon dioxide diffuses out of the blood into the sweep gas. Sweep gas flow rate and concentration of oxygen and carbon dioxide are controlled before entering the oxygenator.

The now oxygenated blood then passes through a heat exchanger of stainless steel tubing surrounded by a jacket of warm water. Warming the blood is necessary to prevent excess conductive heat loss from the extracorporeal circuit. Finally, the oxygenated blood returns to the patient via the arterial catheter. Near the catheters lies a section of tubing which serves as a 'bridge' between the venous and arterial sides of the circuit; this bridge is normally clamped during the ECMO run.

Many possible monitoring and safety devices can be attached to the ECMO circuit. An in-line mixed venous saturation monitor can provide continuous readout of this important marker of tissue oxygenation. Alternatively, in-line cells are available for constant analysis of blood gases (Po_2, Pco_2 and pH) from the venous and arterial limbs of the circuit. Pressure can be transduced to ensure that there is not excessive negative pressure pre-pump, nor excessive positive pressure post-pump as might occur from arterial catheter occlusion. Ultrasonic flow probes may be used to corroborate true circuit flow, which may vary from the set pump flow if tubing is underoccluded. Bubble detectors may be used to stop the pump if gas bubbles are passing through the arterial limb of the circuit. In-line filters are available to decrease emboli passage into the patient.

Once ECMO is initiated, bypass flow rates are increased to 80–120 ml/kg per min, which usually provides adequate oxygen delivery as well as blood pressure support. The ventilator can be reduced to 'rest' settings, generally with Fio_2 21–30%, a rate of 10–20 breaths/min and low peak inspiratory pressures (15–25 cmH$_2$O 47–2.45 kPa). Peak end-expiratory pressure (PEEP) may also be reduced to 4–6 cmH$_2$O (392–588 Pa), although higher PEEP, 10–14 cmH$_2$O (0.98–1.37 kPa), may decrease the extent of lung atelectasis and the duration of bypass [34]. Inotrope support is quickly discontinued; indeed, there is often a need to treat hypertension during the first few days of bypass.

Physical examination and serial radiographs demonstrate significant lung atelectasis within hours of bypass initiation [35]. After 3–4 days of bypass, lung re-expansion often occurs, even at low rest ventilator settings, due to improved lung compliance. Bypass flow can then be weaned over the next 24–72 hours, while following arterial and venous blood gases. The ventilator settings may be increased modestly to facilitate weaning and discontinuation of bypass. ECMO circuit flow should not be reduced below 50 ml/min as significant circuit clotting may occur, with an increased risk of emboli passage to the patient. To see how well a patient does off bypass without removing the circuit and the catheters, the catheters can be clamped and flow can be maintained through the now-unclamped bridge. Alternatively, if the patient tolerates idling at a low flow rate of 50–80 ml/min for several hours, bypass can usually be discontinued. To achieve this, the catheters are removed in a sterile decannulation procedure.

The median length of ECMO bypass is 5.5 days, with a range from 3 to 8 days for most medical diagnoses, and a slightly longer average run of 5 to 14 days for patients with congenital diaphragmatic hernia. ECMO has successfully supported newborns for several weeks, which may be necessary as a bridge to lung or heart transplantation. Although more resource intensive than conventional therapy, ECMO has been shown to reduce overall costs and length of hospital stay in newborns with respiratory failure [36]. The establishment of an ECMO team requires commitment and cooperation from medical and surgical staff, nurses, respiratory therapists, perfusionists, transfusion services and radiology.

To decrease clot formation on ECMO, a continuous heparin infusion of 20–50 units/kg per hour is administered, titrating to bedside measurement of whole blood activated clotting time (ACT). While ACT measurement depends in part upon equipment and methodology [37], most centers aim for ACT to be between 160 and 240 seconds during ECMO bypass. Coagulation studies may have to include measurement of fibrinogen, reptilase or heparinase-treated ACT, and factor levels to look for disseminated intravascular coagulation and depletion of clotting factors. There is a slow consumption of platelets by the ECMO circuit, necessitating regular transfusion of 1–2 units/day for most patients. To optimize oxygen delivery, the hematocrit is usually kept at 40–50%. Bleeding from operative sites, including the cannulation incision, may be treated by electrocautery or by application of topical fibrin glue, comprising cryoprecipitate and thrombin [38]. Excessive bleeding may be treated by decreasing the heparin infusion to maintain lower ACTs. Bleeding complications may also be lowered in high-risk neonates (with sepsis, disseminated intravascular coagulation, acidosis or prematurity) by administration of the fibrinolysis inhibitor aminocaproic acid [39]. The ECMO circuit slowly develops thrombi within the bladder, oxygenator and tubing; this may necessitate a circuit change after 5–10 days of bypass.

102.3.2 VENOVENOUS BYPASS

Venovenous ECMO was first described using a jugular venous drainage catheter, with return of oxygenated blood to a catheter entering the femoral vein [40,41], however the rate of femoral venous obstructive complications was prohibitively high in neonates. To circumvent this problem, Bartlett developed a double-lumen 14-Fr gauge catheter for neonatal venovenous ECMO [42]. This catheter, entering the right jugular vein and with its tip in the right atrium, can be used to provide ECMO to infants with adequate cardiac function. Blood enters through the larger drainage lumen, passes through the ECMO circuit, and oxygenated blood returns to the right atrium via the smaller-diameter lumen. The recirculation of a significant portion of the oxygenated blood back into the drainage lumen decreases the relative efficiency of oxygen delivery compared with venoarterial ECMO at the same circuit flow. To maintain adequate oxygenation, the ventilator may have to be adjusted to higher settings than normally used in venoarterial ECMO. Furthermore, as oxygen delivery is now dependent upon the baby's own cardiac output, continuation of inotropes, such as dopamine, is often necessary. If there is inadequate oxygen delivery or deteriorating cardiac output, as might be demonstrated by metabolic acidosis, a catheter may be placed in the carotid artery and appropriate connections made to the circuit, converting immediately from venovenous to venoarterial ECMO.

ECMO run lengths are similar in venovenous and venoarterial ECMO. When a patient has improved and circuit flow has been weaned, by removing the sweep gas source the venovenous ECMO circuit no longer provides any oxygenation or ventilation. The patient's ventilator can be adjusted to see if this trial 'off' is tolerated and whether decannulation should occur. Removal of the sweep gas during venoarterial ECMO leads to an obligate right-to-left shunt of venous, desaturated blood, so this is not used during weaning trials.

102.4 Physiology of ECMO bypass

102.4.1 VENOARTERIAL BYPASS

Management of the patient on bypass demands recognition of how physiology is either supplemented or perturbated by ECMO. In venoarterial ECMO, oxygen delivery will primarily depend upon bypass flow rate and hemoglobin concentration, as postoxygenator oxygen saturation is virtually 100%. The best indicator of tissue oxygenation will be mixed venous saturation. Due to the increased solubility of carbon dioxide, ventilation depends primarily on sweep gas flow and carbon dioxide concentration, and to a lesser extent is affected by ECMO circuit flow.

Venoarterial ECMO may cause a relative dampening of the blood pressure waveform, as the heart is being denied a significant preload volume. In approximately 5–10% of venoarterial ECMO patients, there is marked, albeit transient impairment of ventricular function, referred to as 'cardiac stun' [43,44]. This is postulated to reflect changes in preload and afterload in hearts with underlying hypoxic-ischemic injury, combined with coronary blood being less well saturated as it is supplied from the left ventricle [45]. Poor cardiac function may cause systemic arterial Po_2 to rise, as arterial flow will be increasingly dominated by ECMO bypass flow. As cardiac output increases, there is a paradoxical lowering of arterial Po_2, as a greater contribution is coming from less well-oxygenated blood from the patient's own cardiorespiratory circulation.

Neonates on ECMO receive intravenous fluids, usually at 80–120 ml/kg per day, with initiation of hyperalimentation possible when urine output is adequate and serum electrolytes are relatively stable. Diuretic therapy is typically provided to augment urine output, to remove excess fluid present from pre-ECMO volume support and to decrease accompanying edema exacerbated by capillary leak. Weight on bypass usually increases 5–30% above birth weight, representing an increase in both total body water and extracellular fluid [46]. Plasma renin levels are elevated, but this elevation is not associated with the hypertension found in ECMO patients [47]. For excessive weight gain and/or poor renal function, hemofiltration or hemodialysis circuits are easily appended on to the ECMO circuit [48]. Enteral feeds are usually not given as there may be underlying ischemic injury to the gut and intestinal perfusion may be suboptimal while the infant is on bypass. Antacid therapy may be necessary to prevent gastric stress ulceration and bleeding. After bypass, advancement to full enteral feeds may take 1–3 weeks beyond extubation.

During venoarterial ECMO the anterior and posterior communicating arteries deliver flow to the right cerebral hemisphere [49,50]. The left external carotid artery also serves as a collateral to the right internal carotid circulation [51]. Increased mean velocity and decreased pulsatility occurs in left carotid arterial flow, which reflects increased systemic diastolic blood pressure, the dampened pulsatility of blood pressure on ECMO, and the effect on cerebral vascular tone of changes in P_{CO_2} [49–51]. Cranial ultrasonography is followed at least daily to rule out significant intracranial hemorrhage. Neonatal ECMO patients are sedated with narcotics, midazolam and/or chloral hydrate to minimize movement and prevent catheter displacement or decannulation. The pharmacokinetics of fentanyl are affected by binding to the membrane oxygenator [52,53].

102.4.2 VENOVENOUS BYPASS

Although oxygen delivery is usually quite adequate during venovenous bypass, two factors limit venovenous circuit flow rates. Because the percentage of recirculation increases with flow, flow rates higher than 400 ml/min offer little, if any, additional oxygen delivery to the patient, and may decrease effectiveness of bypass. In addition, the relatively small return lumen of the catheter leads to elevated circuit pressures and increased hemolysis at high venovenous bypass flow rates. The blood pressure waveform is not dampened by venovenous ECMO. Any in-line measurement of venous saturation will overestimate true mixed saturation due to recirculation. Therefore, more reliance is placed upon the patient's saturation and blood gases. Oxygenation may be improved by changing circuit flow, minor repositioning of the catheter to reduce recirculation, optimizing hemoglobin concentration, or increasing ventilator settings. In extreme cases, oxygen consumption may be lowered by paralysis or modest hypothermia. If the above measures are inadequate to provide adequate oxygen delivery, conversion to venoarterial ECMO may be necessary. Fluid management and hematologic and sedation issues are comparable in venovenous and venoarterial ECMO.

102.5 Outcome

Appropriate application of ECMO depends on a thorough understanding of the risks, benefits and outcome of its use. A database reflecting the American and international experience of ECMO patients is available from the Extracorporeal Life Support Organization (ELSO) [54]. Careful records of indications, complications and survival outcome of ECMO in neonates, older children and adults are maintained in great detail by ELSO.

102.5.1 MORTALITY

Table 102.1 shows that the survival rate for neonatal ECMO patients with respiratory disease has remained over 80% for the last 5000 patients [55]. Survival rates can also be separated by primary diagnosis as shown in Table 102.2. Medical diagnoses fare better than surgical diagnoses (congenital diaphragmatic hernia, congenital heart disease) in neonates placed on ECMO. This is most likely due to increased hemorrhagic complications in the surgical ECMO patient; furthermore, in patients with congenital diaphragmatic hernia ECMO may help reverse persistent pulmonary hypertension, but there may remain significant pulmonary hypoplasia. Of the over 1000 neonatal patients treated with venovenous ECMO, 90% have survived. This may reflect less severe underlying pulmonary disease compared with concurrent or historical venoarterial ECMO patients.

Table 102.1 Neonatal ECMO patients with respiratory disease, including those with congenital diaphragmatic hernia [After Ref. 55]

Year	Total cases	No. of survivors	Survival (%)
1973–86	811	647	80
1987	647	555	86
1988	1006	825	82
1989	1114	912	82
1990	1336	1079	81
1991	1396	1128	81
1992	1472	1163	79
1993	1234	990	80

Table 102.2 Neonatal cases by diagnoses [After Ref. 55]

Primary diagnosis	Total	No. survivors	Survival (%)
Meconium aspiration syndrome	3395	3173	93
Pneumonia/sepsis	1431	1091	76
Respiratory distress syndrome/hyaline membrane disease	1051	879	84
Persistent pulmonary hypertension/persistent fetal circulation	1209	1008	83
Air leak syndrome	43	31	72
Congenital diaphragmatic hernia	1808	1057	58
Cardiac (neonatal and pediatric patients)	1222	537	44
Other	321	250	78

102.5.2 MORBIDITY

Complications related to ECMO are primarily: (1) hematologic; (2) infectious; (3) mechanical; and (4) circulatory. Hematologic problems include hemorrhage, such as intracranial or operative site bleeding, and hemolysis, caused by pump pressure and turbulent flow within the circuit. Excessive hemolysis, reflected by elevated plasma free hemoglobin, may lead to hyperbilirubinemia or cholestasis [56,57]. The ECMO patient remains on broad-spectrum antibiotics, yet is at increased risk for nosocomial infection, e.g. from *Candida albicans* or coagulase-negative staphylococci, caused by repeated blood sampling, and drug and fluid administration during bypass. Blood products are needed to prime the circuit, and multiple transfusions are necessary to maintain adequate hematocrit, platelet count and coagulation factors. With multiple donor exposures comes the risk of transfusion-related infection, including viral hepatitis and human immunodeficiency virus. Mechanical and electrical problems with tubing, connections, pump, servoregulator and oxygenator rarely necessitate cessation of ECMO, although bypass may have to be discontinued temporarily for troubleshooting and repairs. Oxygenator function may be impaired by excessive water in the gas phase, by clot formation in the blood phase, or by bleeding across a leak in the membrane.

Although the circulatory insult of carotid artery and jugular vein ligation is apparent for ECMO, the long-term consequences of vessel ligation are uncertain. After carotid artery ligation, sufficient collateral arterial circulation patterns quickly evolve in the neonate on ECMO. Venovenous ECMO obviates the need for carotid artery ligation. Approximately 25% of ECMO centers in the USA routinely attempt carotid artery repair after ECMO in selected patients. The potential benefits of this include re-establishment of right-sided carotid flow; the potential complications of reperfusion or embolic injury appear to be quite rare. A more common problem is stenosis at the site of repair; whether a stenotic vessel is better or worse than a ligated one remains to be seen. Post-ECMO studies have demonstrated symmetric cerebral blood flow after venoarterial ECMO, with or without right carotid artery repair [58]. Ligation of the jugular vein may increase cerebral venous resistance and thereby lower cerebral perfusion pressure.

Other morbidity is less related to ECMO and more related to underlying disease processes. Given the severity of the disease processes leading to ECMO, it is not surprising that 12–38% of ECMO patients have bronchopulmonary dysplasia or chronic lung disease [59–61]. One study showed 62% of ECMO survivors had a serious respiratory illness, and 25% required admission for such illness during the first year of life

[62]. Somatic growth is normal in 75–90% of ECMO patients, except for those with congenital diaphramatic hernia. In this population, growth failure was noted in 42–57% during the first 3 years of life, along with a high incidence of gastro-esophageal reflux [63].

102.5.3 NEURODEVELOPMENTAL FOLLOW-UP

ECMO centers follow the long-term neurodevelopment of ECMO survivors. It is impossible to attribute abnormal outcome to ECMO alone as there is no control group for these patients who have failed other conventional therapies. There are only historical controls [64], or else concurrent, 'near-miss' patients who presumably were less ill, having survived without ECMO. Furthermore, neurological injury in the ECMO patient may arise:

1. prenatally, with onset of asphyxia or intrauterine stress;
2. post partum, pre-ECMO – from hypoxia, ischemia, infection or secondary to intensive care intervention, such as decreased cerebral perfusion associated with hyperventilation;
3. during ECMO – with bypass-related risks of vessel ligation and intracranial hemorrhage or infarct;
4. after bypass.

Major neuroradiographic abnormalities, best delineated by computed tomography or magnetic resonance imaging, have been reported in 10–52% of ECMO patients [65,66]. The incidence of intracranial hemorrhage is reported to be 16–19% [55,67], with no consistent predilection noted for bleeding to occur on the side of vessel cannulation and ligation [67–69]. The other neuroradiographic abnormalities seen in ECMO patients are infarcts, atrophy, enlarged subarachnoid space and ventriculomegaly. Venovenous bypass appears to cause no more neuroradiographic abnormalities than venoarterial ECMO [70]. The incidence of seizures in neonatal ECMO patients is approximately 13% [55], with subsequent epilepsy estimated to be 2–3% in survivors. Sensorineuronal hearing loss has been reported in 4–21% of ECMO patients [61,62]. This rate is comparable with that in patients with persistent pulmonary hypertension treated with mechanical ventilation [71].

Of ECMO survivors between 1 and 3 years of age, 57–75% have normal development testing by measurements such as the Bayley Scales of Infant Development. Only 10–18% of this population have moderate to severe neurologic abnormalities [60–62]. As over 90% of neonates who have received ECMO are currently less than 7 years old, there are limited data regarding follow-up beyond this time frame. Hofkosh et al. [61] found nine of ten school-aged ECMO patients to have normal developmental outcome, with two of these having behavioral problems. Schumacher *et al.* [62] found 15 of 80 (19%) of ECMO graduates between 1 and 7 years of age to have either a moderate-to-severe neurologic abnormality or a mental developmental index/IQ score 2 standard deviations below the norm. A recent study of 34 ECMO survivors between 3 and 5 years old showed normal mean Stanford–Binet IQ scores, with only three patients scoring less than 85 [72]. Eight children had language problems and two had attention deficit disorders. Another study of 42 neonatal patients at age 5 showed significant gross motor delay in five (12%), focal neurologic abnormality in two (5%) and mild hypotonia in three (7%) [73]. Also in this population, 23 (55%) had either language, learning or attention deficit disorder, 15 (36%) had behavioral problems and six (14%) were felt to have a major handicapping condition.

102.6   Future modifications and application of extracorporeal membrane life support

An increasing number of ECMO centers are using an additional jugular venous catheter introduced via the right neck incision, placed in a cephalad direction with the tip in the jugular bulb. This cephalad drainage supplements the drainage from the right atrium. This cephalad catheter serves to decrease right-sided cerebral venous congestion, and should therefore improve cerebral perfusion. Early studies suggest that the use of a cephalad catheter may decrease the incidence of intracranial hemorrhage. During venovenous ECMO the cephalad catheter offers the additional advantage that its contribution to venous drainage is not recirculated, compared with that drained by the double-lumen catheter. Decreasing the percentage of recirculation leads to more efficient oxygen delivery at a given circuit flow rate. Currently, only 14-Fr gauge venovenous catheters are available, limiting this form of ECMO bypass to neonates weighing between 3.0 and 4.2 kg. Development and release of other sizes of venovenous catheters, in conjunction with the use of a cephalad catheter, should make venovenous bypass available to a wider weight range of neonates. An alternate method of providing venovenous ECMO is the use of tidal, or to-and-fro, flow through a single lumen venous catheter [74,75].

The recent development of heparin-bonded ECMO tubing and circuit components should lower the incidence of hemorrhagic complications [76,77]. An alternate approach to reducing systemic anticoagulation is the placement of a filter bonded with heparinase in the efferent, return limb of the circuit [78,79]. Premature infants may be considered for ECMO if the risk of intracranial hemorrhage is significantly decreased by technical advances such as heparin-bonded circuits and

cephalad jugular catherization. The extreme application of ECMO as an artificial placenta has been limited to the laboratory setting [80,81]. Improvement in heart and lung transplantation techniques and outcome may force an increased need for ECMO to serve as a life-sustaining bridge. As the risks and complication rate from ECMO decrease, the challenge will be to evaluate the appropriateness of ECMO versus other therapies, comparing mortality, morbidity and long-term neurodevelopmental outcome.

References

1. Hill, J.D. and Gibbon Jr, J.H. (1982) The development of the first successful heart lung machine. *Ann. Thorac. Surg.*, **34**, 337–41.
2. Clowes Jr, G.H.A., Hopkins, A.L. and Neville, W.E. (1956) An artificial lung dependent upon diffusion of oxygen and carbon dioxide through plastic membranes. *J. Thorac. Surg.*, **32**, 630–37.
3. Kolobow, T. and Bowman, R.L. (1963) Construction and evaluation of an alveolar membrane artificial heart lung. *Trans. Am. Soc. Artif. Intern. Organs*, **9**, 238–43.
4. Zapol, W.M., Snider, M.T., Hill, J.D. *et al.* (1979) Extracorporeal membrane oxygenation in severe acute respiratory failure: a randomized prospective study. *JAMA*, **242**, 2193–96.
5. Bartlett, R.H., Gazzaniga, A.B., Jefferies, M.R. *et al.* (1976) Extracorporeal circulation (ECMO) in neonatal respiratory failure. *Trans. Am. Soc. Artif. Intern. Organs.*, **22**, 80–93.
6. Bartlett, R.H., Roloff, D.W., Cornell, R.G. *et al.* (1985) Extracorporeal circulation in neonatal respiratory failure: a prospective randomized study. *Pediatrics*, **76**, 479–87.
7. O'Rourke, P.P., Crone, R.K., Vacanti, J.P. *et al.* (1989) Extracorporeal membrane oxygenation and conventional medical therapy in neonates with persistent pulmonary hypertension of the newborn: a prospective randomized study. *Pediatrics*, **84**, 957–63.
8. Paneth, N. and Wallenstein, S. (1985) Extracorporeal membrane oxygenation and the play the winner rule (commentary). *Pediatrics*, **76**, 622–23.
9. Meinert, C.L. (1990) Extracorporeal membrane oxygenation trials (commentary). *Pediatrics*, **85**, 365–66.
10. Chalmers, T.C. (1990) A belated randomized control trial (commentary). *Pediatrics*, **85**, 366–69.
11. Weigel, T.J. and Hageman, J.R. (1990) National survey of diagnosis and management of persistent pulmonary hypertension of the newborn. *J. Perinatol.*, **10**, 369–75.
12. Duara, S., Gewitz, M.H. and Fox, W.W. (1984) Use of mechanical ventilation for clinical management of persistent pulmonary hypertension of the newborn. *Clin. Perinatol.*, **11**, 641–52.
13. Wung, J.T., James, L.S., Kilchevsky, E. and James, E. (1985) Management of infants with severe respiratory failure and persistence of the fetal circulation without hyperventilation. *Pediatrics*, **76**, 488–94.
14. Dworetz, A.R., Moya, F.R., Sabo, B. *et al.* (1989) Survival of infants with persistent pulmonary hypertension without extracorporeal membrane oxygenation. *Pediatrics*, **84**, 1–6.
15. Cornish, J.D., Gerstmann, D.R., Clark, R.H. *et al.* (1987) Extracorporeal membrane oxygenation and high-frequency oscillatory ventilation: potential therapeutic relationships. *Crit. Care Med.*, **15**, 831–34.
16. Baumgart, S., Hirschl, R.B., Butler, S.Z. *et al.* (1992) Diagnosis-related criteria in the consideration of extracorporeal membrane oxygenation in neonates previously treated with high-frequency jet ventilation. *Pediatrics*, **89**, 491–4.
17. Sills, J.H., Cvetnic, W.G. and Pietz, J. (1989) Continuous negative pressure in the treatment of infants with pulmonary hypertension and respiratory failure. *J. Perinatol.*, **9**, 43–48.
18. Lotze, A., Knight, G.R., Bulas, D.I. *et al.* (1992) Survanta treatment of term infants in respiratory failure on ECMO: improved pulmonary outcome. *Pediatr. Res.*, **31**, 315A.
19. Frostell, C., Fratacci, M.D., Wain, J.C. *et al.* (1991) Inhaled nitric oxide. A selective pulmonary vasodilator reversing hypoxic pulmonary vasoconstriction. *Circulation*, **83**, 2038–47.
20. Bui, K.C., LaClair, P., Vanderferhove, J. and Bartlett, R.H. (1991) ECMO in premature infants: review of factors associated with mortality. *Trans. Am. Soc. Artif. Intern. Organs*, **37**, 54–59.
21. Heymann, M.A. and Soifer, S.J. (1990) Persistent pulmonary hypertension of the newborn, in *The Pulmonary Circulation: Normal and Abnormal* (ed. A.F. Fishman), University of Pennsylvania Press, Philadelphia, pp. 371–84.
22. Atkinson, J.B., Ford, E.G., Humphries, B. *et al.* (1991) The impact of extracoporeal membrane support in the treatment of congenital diaphragmatic hernia. *J. Pediatr. Surg.*, **26**, 791–93.

23. Hunkeler, N.M., Canter, C.E., Donze, A. and Spray, T.L. (1992) Extracorporeal life support in cyanotic congenital heart disease before cardiovascular operation. *Am. J. Cardiol.*, **69**, 790–93.

24. Meliones, J.N., Custer, J.R., Snedecor, S. *et al.* (1991) Extracorporeal life support for cardiac assist in pediatric patients. Review of ELSO Registry data. *Circulation*, **84** (suppl. 5), III-168–72.

25. Van Meurs K.P., Rhine, W.D., Sheehan, A.M. *et al.* (1991) Lobar lung transplantation in a neonate after ECMO treatment failure. *Seventh Annual Children's Hospital National Medical Center ECMO Symposium*, p. 94.

26. Van Meurs, K.P., Rhine, W.D., Benitz, W.E. *et al.* (1994) Lobar lung transplantation as a treatment for congenital diaphragmatic hernia. *J. Pediatr. Surg.* (in press).

27. Payne, N.R., Kriesmer, P., Mammel, M. and Meyer, C.L. (1991) Comparison of six ECMO selection criteria and analysis of factors influencing their accuracy. *Pediatr. Pulmonol.*, **11**, 223–32.

28. Beck, R., Anderson, K.D., Pearson, G.D. *et al.* (1986) Criteria for extracorporeal membrane oxygenation in a population of infants with persistent pulmonary hypertension of the newborn. *J. Pediatr. Surg.*, **21**, 297–302.

29. Cole, C.H., Jillson, E. and Kessler, D. (1988) ECMO: regional evaluation of need and applicability of selection criteria. *Am. J. Dis. Child.*, **142**, 1320–24.

30. Bohn, D., Tamura, M., Perrin, D. *et al.* (1987) Ventilatory predictors of pulmonary hypoplasia in congenital diaphragmatic hernia, confirmed by morphologic assessment. *J. Pediatr.*, **111**, 423–31.

31. Van Meurs, K.P., Newman, K.D., Anderson, K.D. and Short, B.L. (1990) Effect of extracoproreal membrane oxygenation on survival of infants with congenital diaphragmatic hernia. *J. Pediatr.*, **117**, 954–60.

32. Atkinson, J.B., Emerson, P., Wheaton, R. and Bowman, C.M. (1989) A simplified method for autoregulation of blood flow in the extracorporeal membrane oxygenation circuit. *J. Pediatr. Surg.*, **24**, 251–52.

33. Green T.P., Kriesmer, P., Steinhorn, R.H. *et al.* (1991) Comparison of pressure–volume–flow relationships in centrifugal and roller pump extracorporeal membrane oxygenation systems for neonates. *Trans. Am. Soc. Artif. Intern. Organs.*, **37**, 572–76.

34. Keszler, M., Ryckman, F.C., McDonald Jr, J.V. *et al.* (1992) A prospective, multicenter, randomized study of high versus low positive end-expiratory pressure during extracorporeal membrane oxygenation. *J. Pediatr.*, **120**, 107–13.

35. Taylor, G.A., Short, B.L. and Kriesmer, P. (1986) Extracopreal membrane oxygenation: radiographic appearance of the neonatal chest. *AJR*, **146**, 1257–60.

36. Pearson, G.D. and Short, B.L. (1987) An economic analysis of extracorporeal membrane oxygenation. *J. Intensive Care Med.*, **2**, 116–20.

37. Uden D.L., Payne, N.R., Kriesmer, P.J. and Cipolle, R.J. (1989) Procedural variables which effect activated clotting test results during extracorporeal membrane oxygenation therapy. *Crit. Care Med.*, **17**, 1048–51.

38. Moront, M.G., Katz, N.M., O'Connell, J. and Hoy, G.R. (1988) The use of topical fibrin glue at cannulation sites in neonates. *Surg. Gynecol. Obstet.*, **166**, 358–59.

39. Wilson, J.M., Bower, L.K., Fackler, J.C. *et al.* (1993) Aminocaproic acid decreases the incidence of intracranial hemorrhage and other hemorrhagic complications of ECMO. *J. Pediatr. Surg.*, **28**, 536–40.

40. Andrews, A.F., Klein, M.D., Toomasian, J.M. *et al.* (1983) Venovenous extracorporeal membrane oxygenation in neonates with respiratory failure. *J. Pediatr. Surg.*, **18**, 339–46.

41. Klein, M.D., Andrews, A.F., Wesley, J.R. *et al.* (1984) Venovenous perfusion in ECMO for newborn respiratory insufficiency. *Ann. Surg.*, **201**, 520–26.

42. Anderson, H.L., Otsu, T., Chapman, R.A. and Bartlett, R.H. (1989) Venovenous extracoporeal life support in neonates using a double lumen catheter. *Trans. Am. Soc. Artif. Intern. Organs.*, **35**, 650–53.

43. Hirschl, R.B., Heiss, K.F. and Bartlett, R.H. (1992) Severe myocardial dysfunction during extracorporeal membrane oxygenation. *J. Pediatr. Surg.*, **27**, 48–53.

44. Martin, G.R., Short, B.L., Abbott, C. and O'Brien, A.M. (1991) Cardiac stun in infants undergoing extracorporeal membrane oxygenation. *J. Thorac. Cardiovasc. Surg.*, **101**, 607–11.

45. Kinsells, J.P., Gerstmann, D.R. and Rosenberg, A.A. (1992) The effect of extracorporeal membrane oxygenation on coronary perfusion and regional blood flow distribution. *Pediatr. Res.*, **31**, 80–84.

46. Anderson, H.L., Coran, A.G., Drongowski, R.A. *et al.* (1992) Extracellular fluid and total body water changes in neonates undergoing extracorporeal membrane oxygenation. *J. Pediatr. Surg.*, **27**, 1003–8.

47. Boedy, R.F., Goldberg, A.K., Howell Jr, C.G. *et al.* (1990) Incidence of hypertension in infants on extracorporeal membrane oxygenation. *J. Pediatr. Surg.*, **25**, 258–61.

48. Yorgin, P.D., Kirpekar, R. and Rhine W.D. (1992) Placement alternatives for hemofiltration in extracorporeal membrane (ECMO) circuits. *ASIAO Trans.*, **38**, 801–803.

49. Taylor, G.A., Short, B.L., Glass, P. and Ichord, R. (1988) Cerebral hemodynamics in infants undergoing extracorporeal membrane oxygenation: further observations. *Radiology*, **168**, 163–67.

50. Mitchell, D.G., Merton, D.A., Graziani, L.J. *et al.* (1990) Right carotid artery ligation in neonates; classification of collateral flow with color Doppler imaging. *Radiology*, **175**, 117–23.

51. Lohrer, R.M., Bejar, R.F., Simko, A.J. *et al.* (1992) Internal carotid artery blood flow velocities before, during, and after extracorporeal membrane oxygenation. *Am. J. Dis. Child.*, **146**, 201–7.

52. Arnold, J.H., Truog, R.D., Scavone, J.M. and Fenton, T. (1991) Changes in the pharmacodynamic response to fentanyl in neonates during continuous infusion. *J. Pediatr.*, **119**, 639–43.

53. Rosen, D., Rosen, K., Davidson, B. *et al.* (1988) Fentanyl uptake by the Scimed membrane oxygenator. *J. Cardiothorac. Anesth.*, **2**, 619–26.

54. Stolar, C.J.H., Snedecor, S.M. and Bartlett, R.H. (1991) Extracorporeal membrane oxygenation and neonatal respiratory failure: experience from the Extracorporeal Life Support Organization. *J. Pediatr. Surg.*, **26**, 563–71.

55. Data from Neonatal ECMO Registry of the Extracorporeal Life Support Organization (ELSO), Ann Arbor, Michigan, July, 1994.

56. Steinhorn, R.H., Isham–Schopf, B., Smith, C. and Green, T.P. (1989) Hemolysis during long-term extracorporeal membrane oxygenation. *J. Pediatr.*, **115**, 625–30.

57. Shneider, B., Maller, E., VanMarter, L. and O'Rourke, P.P. (1989) Cholestasis in infants supported with extracorporeal membrane oxygenation. *J. Pediatr.*, **115**, 462–65.

58. Perlman, J.M. and Altman, D.I. (1992) Symmetric cerebral blood flow in newborns who have undergone successful extracorporeal membrane oxygenation. *Pediatrics*, **89**, 235–39.

59. Schwendeman, C.A., Clark, R.H., Yoder, B.A. *et al.* (1992) Frequency of chronic lung disease in infants with severe respiratory failure treated with high-frequency ventilation and/or extracorporeal membrane oxygenation. *Crit. Care Med.*, **20**, 372–77.

60. Glass, P., Miller, M. and Short, B. (1989) Morbidity for survivors of extracorporeal membrane oxygenation: neurodevelopmental outcome at 1 year of age. *Pediatrics*, **83**, 72–78.

61. Hofkosh, D, Thompson, A.E., Nozza, R.J. *et al.* (1991) Ten years of extracorporeal membrane oxygenation: neurodevelopmental outcome. *Pediatrics*, **87**, 549–55.

62. Schumacher, R.E., Palmer, T.W., Roloff, D.W. *et al.* (1991) Follow-up of infants treated with extracorporeal membrane oxygenation for newborn respiratory failure. *Pediatrics*, **87**, 451–57.

63. Van Meurs, K.P., Robbins, S.T., Karr, S.S. *et al.* (1991) Congenital diaphragmatic hernia: long-term outcome of ECM-treated survivors. *Pediatr. Res.*, **29**, 269A.

64. Sell, E.J., Gaines, J.A., Gluckman, C. and Williams, E. (1985) Persistent fetal circulation. *Am. J. Dis. Child.*, **139**, 25–28.

65. Griffin, P.M., Minifee, P.K., Landry, S.H. *et al.* (1992) Neurodevelopmental outcome in neonates after extracorporeal membrane oxygenation: cranial magnetic resonance imaging and ultrasonography correlation. *J. Pediatr. Surg.*, **27**, 33–35.

66. Sell, L.L., Cullen, M.L., Whittelesey, G.C. *et al.* (1986) Hemorrhagic complications during extracorporeal membrane oxygenation: prevention and treatment. *J. Pediatr. Surg.*, **21**, 1087–91.

67. Bulas, D.I. Short, B.L., Taylor, G.A. and Fitz, C.R. (1992) Intracranial abnormalities in infants treated with extracorporeal membrane oxygenation: update on US and CT imaging. *Pediatr. Res.*, **31**, 243A.

68. Schumacher, R.E., Barks, J.D.E., Johnston, M.V. *et al.* (1988) Right-sided brain lesions in infants following extracorporeal membrane oxygenation. *J. Pediatr.*, **113**, 110–13.

69. Mendoza, J.C., Shearer, L.L and Cook, L.L. (1991) Lateralization of brain lesions following extracoporeal membrane oxygenation. *Pediatrics*, **88**, 1004–1009.

70. Nguyen, H.T., Benitz, W.E., Rhine, W.D. *et al.* (1994) Intracranial abnormalities and neurodevelopmental status after veno-venous extracorporeal membrane oxygenation. *J. Pediatr.* (in press).

71. Walton, J.P. and Hendricks-Munoz, K. (1991) Profile and stability of sensorineuronal hearing loss in persistent pulmonary hypertension of the newborn. *J. Speech. Hear. Res.*, **34**, 1362–70.

72. Stewart, D.L, Reese, A.H., Wilkerson, S.A. and Cook, L.N. (1992) Neurodevelopmental outcome of extracoporeal life support (ECLS) patients at 3, 4, or 5 year follow-up. *Pediatr. Res.*, **31**, 261A.

73. Rajasingham, S., Glass, P., Civitello, L. and Short, B. (1992) Neuromotor morbidity at age 5 among 42 ECMO treated neonates. *Pediatr. Res.*, **31**, 257A.

74. Chevalier, J.Y., Durandy, Y., Batisse, A.M. *et al.* (1990) Preliminary report: extracorporeal lung support for neonatal acute respiratory failure. *Lancet*, **335**, 1364–66.

75. Tsuno, K., Terasaki, H., Tsutsumi, R. *et al.* (1989) To-and-fro venovenous extracorporeal lung assist for newborns with severe respiratory distress. *Intensive Care Med.*, **15**, 269–71.

76. Toomasian, J.M., Hsu, L.C., Hirschl, R.B. *et al.* (1988) Evaluation of Duraflow II heparin coating in prolonged extracorporeal membrane oxygenation. *Trans. Am. Soc. Artif. Intern. Organs*, **34**, 410–14.

77. Rossaint, R., Slama, K., Lewandowski, K. *et al.* (1992) Extracorporeal lung assist with heparin-coated systems. *Int. J. Artif. Organs*, **15**, 29–34.

78. Klein, M.D., Arensman, R.M., Weber, T.R. *et al.* (1988) Pediatric ECMO: directions for new developments. *Trans. Am. Soc. Artif. Intern. Organs*, **34**, 978–85.

79. Langer, R., Lindhardt, R.J., Joffberg, S. *et al.* (1982) An enzymatic system for removing heparin in extracorporeal therapy. *Science*, **217**, 261–63.

80. Kuwabara, Y., Okai, T., Kozuma, S. *et al.* (1989) Artificial placenta: long-term extrauterine incubation of isolated goat fetuses. *Artif. Organs*, **13**, 527–31.

81. Unno, N., Kuwabara, Y., Shinozuka, N. *et al.* (1990) Development of artificial placenta oxygen metabolism of isolated goat fetuses with umbilical arteriovenous extracorporeal membrane oxygenation. *Fetal Diagn. Ther.*, **5**, 189–95.

103 SURGICAL CORRECTION AND TRANSPLANTATION IN THE MANAGEMENT OF CONGENITAL HEART DISEASE IN THE NEONATE

D. Bernstein

103.1 Introduction

The surgical management of neonates with congenital heart disease has undergone a major revolution over the last decade [1]. Advances in cardiovascular surgical techniques have brought about a change in orientation from palliation towards primary repair in all but the most complex congenital heart lesions. This has resulted in a major change in the role of the neonatologist in the management of these infants. Whereas the focus of neonatal care had previously been primarily on medical management, e.g. limitation of pulmonary blood flow in left-to-right shunt lesions, improvement of arterial oxygen saturation in cyanotic lesions and optimization of growth, the focus has now moved more in the direction of perioperative care. Palliation and long-term medical management are now reserved for only the most complex congenital heart lesions and for premature infants, although cardiovascular surgeons have now begun to focus on extending primary repair to even the smallest prematures [2]. The role of the neonatologist in postoperative management has been expanded further as extracorporeal membrane oxygenation (ECMO) has found a role in providing temporary support for infants who cannot be weaned from cardiopulmonary bypass after complex cardiac repairs [3].

For those infants with complex congenital heart lesions for whom repair is not possible or extremely risky, cardiac transplantation has now become an acceptable option. Following the first neonatal heart transplantation for hypoplastic left heart syndrome in 1986 [4], major centers have demonstrated medium-term results that have compared favorably with the best results in older children and in adults. It is still a matter of controversy, however, whether there are any specific advantages in neonatal transplantation because of the immunological immaturity of the newborn.

103.2 Non-complex congential heart lesions

103.2.1 PATENT DUCTUS ARTERIOSUS

The incidence of patent ductus arteriosus (PDA) increases with decreasing gestational age. In infants close to term the incidence is approximately 20%, whereas at 28–30 weeks gestational age the incidence rises to approximately 75% [5]. A PDA may present a major hemodynamic stress to the immature cardiovascular system. The immature myocardium is less able to compensate for the volume load imposed by a ductal-level left-to-right shunt. Thus, in the premature infant, a PDA can lead to a worsening of the severity of the respiratory distress syndrome and its sequelae and lengthen the requirement for mechanical ventilation [6]. A PDA can also increase the risk for intracranial hemorrhage, necrotizing enterocolitis and apnea of prematurity. Use of indomethacin in the symptomatic premature with a PDA is routine and is effective in closing the ductus arteriosus in approximately 75% of patients, although a second course of therapy or surgery may be needed in 25% of these patients [7]. In neonates with contraindications to indomethacin (severe hemodynamic compromise, renal dysfunction, low platelet count) and in those who have failed indomethacin treatment, surgical intervention is curative and very low risk. Many centers perform surgical closure directly in the nursery, eliminating the potential

Diseases of the Fetus and Newborn, 2nd edn, Edited by G.B. Reed, A.E. Claireaux and F. Cockburn. Published in 1995 by Chapman & Hall, London. ISBN 0 412 39160 0

risks inherent in transportation of an unstable infant to the operating room. Prophylactic administration of indomethacin to very small premature infants who are asymptomatic to prevent problems associated with a PDA is still controversial [8].

103.2.2 VENTRICULAR SEPTAL DEFECT

In the full-term infant, pulmonary vascular resistance remains elevated during the first weeks of life, thus most left-to-right shunt lesions do not present with congestive heart failure in the immediate neonatal period. When heart failure does present in the full term neonate with a vertricular septal defect (VSD), the presence of additional lesions, especially left-sided obstructions such as coarctation of the aorta, must be ruled out. In the premature infant, however, pulmonary vascular resistance may drop more rapidly due to a less-developed pulmonary vascular smooth muscle bed. In these infants, symptoms of overcirculation may develop earlier and exacerbate concomitant respiratory distress syndrome. Another common manifestation of left-to-right shunts in both premature and full term infants is failure to thrive.

In the past, most neonates with VSDs underwent pulmonary arterial banding to decrease pulmonary blood flow and protect against pulmonary vascular disease. Banding allowed these infants to grow until they could be more safely repaired, usually at around 1 year of age. Surgical advances over the last decade have resulted in the ability to close most VSDs in the fullterm neonate primarily, thus eliminating the need for repeat surgery [9]. Banding is now reserved for small premature infants, for those with associated lesions such as coarctation of the aorta, and for infants with muscular VSDs (often multiple) which are difficult to reach via the standard surgical approach (trans-tricuspid valve). Eventually, non-surgical transcatheter closure of apical muscular VSDs using an occlusion device may be common practice.

102.2.3 COARCTATION OF THE AORTA

The presentation of coarctation of the aorta in the newborn period varies with the severity of the lesion and its proximal extension [10]. When coarctation is severe (near interruption), descending aortic blood flow is derived almost entirely from the right ventricle via the ductus arteriosus. These infants present with differential cyanosis: the upper extremities are pink and the lower extremities are blue. When the ductus begins to close in the first few days of life, these infants develop respiratory distress and lower extremity hypoperfusion, progressing to acidosis and shock. Coarctation of the aorta may also be associated with various degrees of hypoplasia of the transverse aortic arch: generally, the

more severe the hypoplasia, the earlier and more severe the symptoms. Coarctation of the aorta may be of a milder form, and this is usually in the immediate juxtaductal area. These infants may be minimally symptomatic or asymptomatic and diagnosis in the immediate newborn period may be difficult if the ductus arteriosus is still patent, as the aortic end of the ductus acts to widen the coarctated area and attenuate the obstruction.

Surgical management of coarctation of the aorta in the newborn period has in the past been associated with a high incidence of recoarctation, ranging from 7 to 60%. Several modifications of the repair method have been tried with varying success, e.g. patch aortoplasty and subclavian flap aortoplasty. Recent experience suggests that improved results may be obtained by anastomosing the descending aorta end-to-side with an angled incision along the inferior aspect of the transverse aorta. This widens the suture line, which is the potential site for residual coarctation. Balloon angioplasty has been used successfully in native coarctation of the aorta, although this procedure is still controversial because of concern over the risk of aneurysm development and the higher rate of femoral arterial complications in smaller infants [11].

103.3 Complex congenital heart lesions

Most complex congenital heart lesions present with symptoms in the immediate neonatal period. For purposes of classification and for understanding pathophysiology, these lesions are divided into two categories: cyanotic and acyanotic. It is beyond the scope of the present text to discuss all varieties of complex congenital heart lesions. Instead a select group of lesions will be presented, focusing on those for which therapeutic options have undergone the most dramatic changes during the last decade.

103.3.1 *d*-TRANSPOSITION OF THE GREAT VESSELS

Starting in the early 1960s, the atrial switch operation (Mustard or Senning repair) became widely available for patients with simple *d*-transposition of the great vessels. Infants with *d*-transposition were initially palliated with a Rashkind balloon atrial septostomy, which increased mixing of systemic and pulmonary venous returns, and allowed these infants to survive until surgical repair could be accomplished, usually at between 1 and 3 years of age. In the early 1980s, it was shown that the atrial switch procedure could be performed in the first 3 months of life with no increased short-term sequelae, reducing the detrimental effects of chronic cyanosis on growth and development [12]. However, late problems with the atrial switch procedure were a persistent problem despite surgical modifications. These included superior and inferior vena caval obstruction, pulmonary venous obstruction, arrhythmia, atrioventricular valve regurgitation and late failure of the systemic right ventricle [13,14].

In 1976, Jatene described a successful new method for performing an arterial switch procedure. This technique includes division of the great vessels, switching of the aorta and pulmonary artery to their proper locations, and reimplantation of the coronary arteries from the aortic root into the pulmonary root or 'neoaorta' [15]. The advantage of this technique was the avoidance of direct suturing of the coronary arteries by removing them together with a button of aortic wall and anastomosing these buttons into openings made at the base of the pulmonary artery. This procedure has now become the standard operation for neonates with simple d-transposition of the great vessels.

The physiological changes induced by the transitional circulation drastically affect the timing of the arterial switch operation. In the normally connected heart, pulmonary vascular resistance falls over the first few weeks of life, resulting in decreased pressure in the right ventricle and thinning of the right ventricular wall. Concurrently, the left ventricle, which is connected to the high resistance systemic circulation, is exposed to higher systemic arterial pressure and its mass increases. In contrast, in the patient with d-transposition, the left ventricle is connected to the pulmonary circulation, and thus left ventricular pressure and wall thickness decrease over the first weeks of life. If the arterial switch procedure is performed after left ventricular pressure and mass decline, usually after 2–3 weeks of age, the left ventricle will be unable to support systemic pressures and will fail. Initially, a pulmonary arterial band was placed to maintain systemic levels of pressure in the left ventricle, and the arterial switch procedure was performed on this 'prepared' left ventricle at between 6 and 12 months of age [16]. With increasing experience, the advantage of a single stage procedure in the immediate neonatal period was demonstrated [17]. The current management of d-transposition in many centers consists of echocardiographic diagnosis without cardiac catheterization or Rashkind balloon septostomy. Although definition of coronary arterial anatomy was considered important during the early days of this operation, currently all variations of coronary anatomy are considered switchable, although some patterns (single right coronary artery and inverted coronary arteries) carry an increased risk [18]. The patient is maintained on prostaglandin E_1 and an arterial switch procedure is performed within the first week to 10 days of life, before left ventricular pressures begin to fall. Balloon atrial septostomy is reserved for those neonates with poor pulmonary–systemic mixing who do not increase their saturations adequately in response to prostaglandin E_1 alone. In these cases,

septostomy may be performed in the catheterization laboratory or in the nursery under echocardiographic guidance [19].

Postoperative results of the arterial switch operation for simple d-transposition in the neonatal period show an early mortality of between 7 and 11% [18,20,21]. Intermediate-term results demonstrate a low incidence of serious complications. These include pulmonary stenosis, aortic regurgitation and occlusion of a coronary artery branch. Follow-up studies of clinical status and left ventricular function show evidence of excellent adaptation to the restoration of the left ventricle as the systemic ventricle [21,22].

103.3.2 SEVERE RIGHT-SIDED OBSTRUCTIVE LESIONS

Severe right-sided obstructive lesions presenting in the neonatal period include tricuspid atresia, pulmonary atresia with VSD, and pulmonary atresia with intact septum. The immediate physiologic consequences of these right-sided obstructions depends on the adequacy of pulmonary blood flow, whether maintained through a ventricular septal defect (in tricuspid atresia) or via a PDA (in pulmonary atresia). Neonates with severe tetralogy of Fallot also present with cyanosis early in the neonatal period and are pathophysiologically similar to those infants with pulmonary atresia and VSD. Initial surgical management in the neonatal period varies with the type of right-sided obstructive lesion and the degree of obstruction to pulmonary blood flow.

In patients with tricuspid atresia with large VSD and no pulmonary stenosis, a pulmonary arterial band may be necessary to limit pulmonary blood flow. Some patients, with moderate degrees of pulmonic stenosis, may be perfectly balanced between too much pulmonary blood flow (congestive heart failure) and too little (severe cyanosis) and not require any immediate surgical intervention. However, the VSD in these patients may close fairly rapidly, thus close follow-up is warranted and an arterial–pulmonary shunt is performed if cyanosis worsens. For patients with tricuspid atresia and severe pulmonary obstruction, an aortopulmonary shunt is performed in the neonatal period.

For patients with pulmonary atresia and intact septum, surgical treatment in the neonatal period usually consists of performing an aortopulmonary shunt, either a modified Blalock–Taussig shunt from subclavian artery to branch pulmonary artery or a central shunt from aorta to main pulmonary artery. In these patients, the size and morphology of the right ventricular chamber, the presence of a main pulmonary artery segment, and the size of the branch pulmonary arteries are all factors which affect the long-term prognosis. The presence of sinusoidal coronary vessels in the right ventricular myocardium, indicating a hypertensive right ventricular chamber, is usually a poor prognostic factor. Some centers perform, in addition to an aortopulmonary shunt, a transventricular pulmonary valvotomy in select patients with large right ventricular chambers (usually including both inlet and infundibular portions) and adequate-sized, confluent pulmonary arteries. When effective, pulmonary valvotomy may reduce right ventricular hypertension, optimize right ventricular growth and increase the probability of being able to perform a future biventricular repair [23,24].

The ultimate palliation for most of these infants with hypolastic right heart syndrome is one of several variations of the cavopulmonary shunt procedure [25,26]. This class of procedures has undergone many revisions since Glenn described the first clinical application of his superior vena cava–pulmonary anastomosis in 1958. Currently, a bidirectional Glenn procedure (anastomosis of the superior vena cava end-to-side with confluent pulmonary arteries) is often performed as a first stage once an infant outgrows an initial aortopulmonary shunt [27]. At a later age, complete separation of systemic venous and pulmonary venous returns is then accomplished by connecting the inferior vena cava directly to the pulmonary arteries by means of an intra-atrial baffle (cavopulmonary isolation or modified Fontan procedure).

The prognosis is poorest in patients with severe hypoplasia of the distal pulmonary arterial beds. Many of these patients cannot be adequately oxygenated by standard methodologies and often require ECMO. One new therapeutic modality for these infants with severe pulmonary hypoplasia is single lung or heart–lung transplantation. Early results with lung transplantation in the neonatal period are encouraging [28], however the long-term outlook remains uncertain, largely as a result of the risk of obliterative bronchiolitis, a form of chronic graft rejection. Because of the scarcity of heart–lung donors in the neonatal period, attempts have been made at partial lung transplantation, using a lobe from an older child, and thus increasing the potential donor pool.

103.3.3 EBSTEIN'S ANOMALY

Ebstein's anomaly of the tricuspid valve consists of a displacement of the tricuspid valve leaflets downwards into the right ventricular chamber below the tricuspid valve annulus. The leaflets are often dysplastic or hypoplastic and plastered to the endomyocardial surface. Ebstein's anomaly varies markedly in severity, with milder cases often going undetected until adulthood. However, the more severe varieties present with marked cyanosis and right ventricular failure in the newborn period. On echocardiogram the right atrium is huge and the right ventricular chamber small. Severe

tricuspid regurgitation is present. The pulmonary valve, although often morphologically normal, may appear not to open because the right ventricle cannot develop adequate pressure. Desaturation occurs because of right-to-left shunting at atrial level, either through a stretched foramen ovale or through an atrial septal defect. These infants are often ventilator and prostaglandin E_1 dependent. Previous attempts at medical management or aortopulmonary shunting have had very limited success, and mortality for infants presenting in the neonatal period has been as high as 75% [29]. In 1991, Starnes, Pitlick and Bernstein [30] decribed a procedure which has shown early promise in the management of these extremely ill infants. The tricuspid annulus is patched closed and an atrial septectomy is performed, essentially converting the Ebstein's anomaly into tricuspid atresia. Pulmonary blood flow is maintained by means of a centrally placed aortopulmonary shunt. The pulmonary valve is opened, if necessary, to allow coronary sinus blood to exit the right ventricle. This operation is followed at between 6 and 12 months by a bidirectional Glenn procedure, similar to those infants with congenital tricuspid atresia. The final stage, at approximately 2 years of age, is the cavopulmonary isolation modification of the Fontan procedure, anastomosing the inferior vena cava to the pulmonary arteries via an intra-atrial baffle.

103.3.4 HYPOPLASTIC LEFT HEART SYNDROME

Hypoplastic left heart syndrome refers to a diverse group of lesions involving hypoplasia of left-sided cardiac structures. In its most severe form, this syndrome consists of mitral stenosis or atresia, aplasia of the left ventricular chamber and atresia of the ascending aorta. Less severe varieties include aortic atresia in the presence of a well-formed left ventricular chamber, and left ventricular hypoplasia with a small ascending aorta. There are currently two surgical options available for the infant with hypoplastic left heart syndrome: the two- or three-stage Norwood procedure and cardiac transplantation. Because of the high risk of both options and the guarded long-term results, many cardiologists still believe that families of these infants should be offered the option of declining surgical intervention.

The Norwood procedure was described independently by Norwood, Kirklin and Sanders [31] and Doty et al. [32] in 1980. The first stage is a palliative procedure consisting of:

1. detachment of the proximal main pulmonary artery from the distal main pulmonary artery and its branches;
2. a transverse incision of the hypoplastic aortic arch;
3. anastomosis of the promixal main pulmonary artery

to the underside of the hypoplastic arch with augmentation by homograft material;

4. an aortopulmonary shunt from the aorta or subclavian artery to the branch pulmonary arteries;
5. an atrial septectomy.

This first stage establishes unimpeded systemic blood flow from the right ventricle via the 'neoaorta' and pulmonary blood flow via the aortopulmonary shunt. At between 3 and 12 months the second stage is performed consisting of an end-to-side shunt between the superior vena cava and the pulmonary arteries (bidirectional Glenn shunt), directing all upper body blood flow directly into the lungs. The third stage is performed at between 18 and 36 months and consists of anastomosing the inferior vena cava to the pulmonary arteries via an intra-atrial baffle (cavopulmonary isolation or modified Fontan procedure). The survival for the first stage repair in selected centers has been reported to be as high as 63–75% [33,34], although prospects for long-term survival are more guarded, ranging from 21% [35] to 61% [36]. The major drawback of the Norwood procedure is its reliance on the right ventricle as the systemic ventricular pump in combination with an eventual Fontan palliation. Long-term right ventricular failure and tricuspid regurgitation are thus potential limiting factors. Yet, as more experience is gained with this procedure and the management of its complications, the intermediate-term success rate has continued to improve.

The alternative, cardiac transplantation, has gained increasing acceptance as a treatment modality for the hypoplastic left heart syndrome. Following the initial report by Bailey and colleagues in 1986 [4], transplantation has produced excellent short and medium-term results for this group of patients [37]. The 1-year survival after infant heart transplantation is approximately 80%, with 5-year survival approximately 70%. However, donor availability remains a serious problem and some centers have reported a significant mortality for infants on the waiting list for transplantation [38].

As an alternative, in 1988 Stanford began a trial of offering a dual approach to treatment of the infant with the hypoplastic left heart syndrome. Newborns entering the program are evaluated as possible transplant candidates. This involves screening for additional serious congenital malformations, a social service evaluation, and a detailed discussion of all options with the family, including the option of not performing surgery but providing supportive care. If the patient is a suitable transplant candidate and the family consents, the infant is then placed on the waiting list for heart transplantation. If not a suitable candidate for transplantation, or if the family prefers surgical palliation, the infant undergoes the stage I Norwood procedure. If, while on the waiting list, the infant begins to show signs of hemodynamic decompensation due to pulmonary over-circulation, a trial of lowering the inspired oxygen concentration to 18–19% is attempted. If hemodynamic deterioration persists, a first stage Norwood procedure is performed. Additionally, if a suitable donor does not become available within a period of 3 weeks, the infant is then re-evaluated for features that would increase the risk of the Norwood procedure. If one of these high-risk conditions exists and the patient remains hemodynamically stable, the infant is kept on the waiting list for transplantation. However, if the infant is deemed a low-risk candidate, a Norwood procedure is performed. After the stage I Norwood procedure, the patient is re-evaluated by cardiac catheterization at approximately 6 and 12 months of age. If the patient is a good candidate for further palliation, management is directed towards stage II and III Norwood procedures. If the patient is a high-risk candidate for continued palliation because of right ventricular dysfunction, tricuspid valve regurgitation or pulmonary arterial abnormalities, he or she is listed for heart transplantation. The potential advantages of this approach are that it increases the transplant donor pool, decreases the number of potential recipients in the immediate neonatal period, and allows transplantation to be performed electively at a time when the patient is more hemodynamically stable. Given an unbiased presentation of the surgical options, approximately two-thirds of families have chosen the Norwood procedure initially, whereas one-third preferred transplantation. A few families have opted not to undergo any surgical treatment.

References

1. Turley, K., Mavroudis, C. and Ebert, P. (1982) Repair of congenital cardiac lesions during the first week of life. *Circulation*, 66 (suppl. I), I-214–19.
2. Hanley, F., Chang, A. and Wessel, D. (1992) Complex congenital heart lesions in low birth weight infants: surgical management and outcome. *Circulation*, 86 (suppl.I), I-359.
3. Meliones, J., Custer, J., Snedecor, S. *et al.* (1991) Extracorporeal life support for cardiac assist in pediatric patients: review of ESLO registry data. *Circulation*, 84 (suppl. III), III-168–72.
4. Bailey, L., Nehlsen-Cannarella, S.L., Doroshow, R.W. *et al.* (1986) Cardiac allotransplantation in newborns as therapy for hypoplastic left heart syndrome. *N. Engl. J. Med.*, 315, 949–51.
5. Siassi, B., Blanco, E., Cabol, L. and Coran, A. (1976) Incidence and clinical features of patent ductus arteriosus in low-birthweight infants. *Pediatrics*, 57, 347–51.
6. Dudell, G. and Gersony, W. (1984) Patent ductus arteriosus in neonates with severe respiratory distress. *J. Pediatr.*, 104, 915–20.
7. Gersony, W., Peckham, G., Ellison, R. *et al.* (1983) Effects of indomethacin in premature infants with patent ductus arteriosus: results of a national collaborative study. *J. Pediatr.*, 102, 895–906.
8. Mahoney, L., Carnero, V., Brett, C. *et al.* (1982) Prophylactic indomethacin therapy for patent ductus arteriosus in very-low-birth-weight infants. *N. Engl. J. Med.*, 306, 506–10.
9. Turley, K., Tucker, W. and Ebert, P. (1980) The changing role of palliative

procedures in the treatment of infants with congenital heart disease. *J. Thorac. Cardiovasc. Surg.*, **79**, 194–201.

10. Rudolph, A., Heymann, M. and Spitznas, R. (1972) Hemodynamic considerations in the development of narrowing of the aorta. *Am. J. Cardiol.*, **30**, 514–25.

11. Lock, J., Keane, J. and Fellows, K. (1987) *Diagnostic and Interventional Catheterization in Congenital Heart Disease*, Nijhoff, Boston, pp. 99–102.

12. Mahoney, L., Turley, K., Ebert, P. and Heyman, M. (1982) Long-term results after atrial repair of transposition of the great arteries in early infancy. *Circulation*, **66**, 253–58.

13. Clarkson, P., Barratt-Boyes, B. and Neutze, J. (1976) Late dysrhythmias and disturbances of conduction following Mustard's operation for complete transposition of the great arteries. *Circulation*, **53**, 519–24.

14. Graham, T., Atwood, G., Boucek, R. *et al.* (1975) Abnormalities of right ventricular function following Mustard's operation for transposition of the great arteries. *Circulation*, **52**, 678–84.

15. Jatene, A.D., Fontes, V., Souza, L. *et al.* (1976) Anatomic correction of transposition of the great vessels. *J.Thorac. Cardiovasc. Surg.*, **72**, 364–70.

16. Yacoub, M.H., Bernhard, A. and Lange, P. (1980) Clinical and hemodynamic results of the two-stage anatomic correction of simple transposition of the great arteries. *Circulation*, **62** (suppl. I), I-190–96.

17. Castañeda, A., Norwood, W., Jonas, R. *et al.* (1984) Transposition of the great arteries and intact ventricular septum: anatomical repair in the neonate. *Ann. Thorac. Surg.*, **38**, 438–43.

18. Mayer, J., Sanders, S., Jonas, R. *et al.* (1990) Coronary artery pattern and outcome of arterial switch operation for transposition of the great arteries. *Circulation*, **82** (suppl.IV), IV-139–45.

19. Lin, A.E., Di Sessa, T.G. and Williams, R.G. (1986) Balloon and blade atrial septostomy facilitated by two-dimensional echocardiography. *Am. J. Cardiol.*, **57**, 273–77.

20. Castañeda, A., Trusler, G., Paul, M. *et al.* (1988) The early results of treatment of simple transposition in current era. *J. Thorac. Cardiovasc. Surg.*, **95**, 14–28.

21. Losay, J., Planche, C., Gerardin, B. *et al.* (1990) Midterm surgical results of arterial switch operation for transposition of the great arteries with intact septum. *Circulation*, **82** (suppl. IV), IV-146–50.

22. Colan, S., Trowitzsch, E., Wernovsky, G. *et al.* (1988) Myocardial performance after arterial switch operation for transposition of the great arteries with intact ventricular septum. *Circulation*, **78**, 132–41.

23. Lewis, A., Wells, W. and Lindesmith, G. (1983) Evaluation and surgical treatment of pulmonary atresia and intact ventricular septum in infancy. *Circulation*, **67**, 1318–23.

24. Shaddy, R., Sturtevant, J., Judd, V. and McGough, E. (1990) Right Ventricular growth after transventricular pulmonary valvotomy and central aortopulmonary shunt for pulmonary atresia and intact ventricular septum. *Circulation*, **82** (suppl. IV), IV-157–63.

25. Castañeda, A. (1992) From Glenn to Fontan: a continuing evolution. *Circulation*, **86** (suppl. II), II-80–84.

26. Tursler, G., Williams, W., Cohen, A. *et al.* (1990) The cavopulmonary shunt: evolution of a concept. *Circulation*, **82** (suppl. IV), IV-131–38.

27. Bridges, N., Jonas, R., Mayer, J. *et al.* (1990) Bidirectional cavopulmonary anastomosis as interim palliation for high-risk Fontan candidates. *Circulation*, **82** (suppl. IV), IV-170–76.

28. Starnes, V., Oyer, P., Bernstein, D. *et al.* (1992) Heart, heart–lung, and lung transplantation in the first year of life. *Ann. Thorac. Surg.*, **53**, 306–10.

29. Watson, H. (1974) Natural history of Ebstein's anomaly of tricuspid valve in childhood and adolescence: an international cooperative study of 505 cases. *Br. Heart. J.*, **36**, 417–27.

30. Starnes, V., Pitlick, P., Bernstein, D. *et al.* (1991) Ebstein's anomaly appearing in the neonate: a new surgical approach. *J. Thorac. Cardiovasc. Surg.*, **101**, 1082–87.

31. Norwood, W., Kirklin, J. and Sanders, S. (1980) Hypoplastic left heart syndrome: experience with palliative surgery. *Am. J. Cardiol.*, **45**, 87–91.

32. Doty, B., Marvin, W., Scheiken, R. and Lauer, R. (1980) Hypoplastic left heart syndrome: successful palliation with a new operation. *J. Thorac. Cardiovasc. Surg.*, **80**, 148–52.

33. Murdison, K., Baffa, J., Farrell, P.J. *et al.* (1990) Hypoplastic left heart syndrome: outcome after initial reconstruction and before modified Fontan procedure. *Circulation*, **82** (suppl. IV), IV-199–207.

34. Starnes, V., Griffin, M., Pitlick, P. *et al.* (1992) Current approach to hypoplastic left heart syndrome: palliation, transplantation, or both. *J. Thorac. Cardiovasc. Surg.*, **103**, 189–95.

35. Meliones, J., Snider, A., Bove, E. *et al.* (1990) Longitudinal results after first-stage palliation for hypoplastic left heart syndrome. *Circulation*, **82** (suppl. IV), IV-151–56.

36. Barber, G., Murphy, J., Pigott, J. and Norwood, W. (1988) The evolving pattern of survival following palliative surgery for hypoplastic left heart syndrome. *J. Am. Coll. Cardiol.*, **2**, 139A.

37. Boucek, M. and Bernstein, D. (1993) Heart transplantation in infancy. *Prog. Pediatr. Cardiol.* (in press).

38. Dunn, J.M., Cavarochi, N.C., Balsara, R.K. *et al.* (1987) Pediatric heart transplantation at St Christopher's Hospital for Children. *J. Heart Transplant.*, **6**, 334–42.

104 NEONATAL NECROTIZING ENTEROCOLITIS

P.A.M. Raine

104.1 Incidence and aetiology

Neonatal necrotizing enterocolitis (NEC) can affect the intestine from stomach to rectum. Mucosal damage from ischaemia leads to necrosis with risks of transmural spread and gut perforation. It is a disease principally of premature infants [1] with an incidence of approximately 1% for proven NEC in babies under 1500 and 32 weeks' gestation [2,3]. Extensive epidemiological studies suggest an overall incidence of around 2.4 per 1000 livebirths [4]. Many possible risk factors have been cited, including ischaemia, intestinal bacteria (infection), enteral feeding, hypoxia, intravascular catheters, intestinal obstruction, congenital heart disease and drugs. Independent analysis of factors proves exceedingly difficult and a multifactorial aetiology appears likely. A 'unifying hypothesis' for the cause of NEC is elusive, but mucosal injury (vascular compromise), bacteria (infection) and a substrate (feed) in the bowel lumen are essential components [5,6].

Doppler studies in the fetus have shown that absence or reversal of end-diastolic flow in the umbilical artery is closely associated with subsequent susceptibility to NEC [7,8]. Intestinal ischaemia may result from the response to stress in which blood is preferentially shunted to the brain, heart and kidneys and away from the intestine – 'diving reflex' [9].

Enterobacteria [10,11] and clostridia [12] have been associated with an increased incidence of NEC; raised levels of anticlostridia toxin are found in sera. Overgrowth of bacteria and production of bacterial toxins may result from colonization of the gut due to parenteral feeding or antibiotic administration [13]. Oral vancomycin [14] and systemic vancomycin and aztreonam [11] have been shown to have preventive roles. Recently, mucormycosis (a fungal infection) has been reported in NEC-like presentation [15]. It has also been suggested that not only nosocomial hospital-specific infections but also more ubiquitous organisms may be involved when simultaneous outbreaks of NEC occur in separate units [16]. Epidemics are reported due to a variety of organisms and the possibility of a transmissble agent has been raised by reports of illness among intensive care unit personnel during NEC outbreaks [17].

Gut feeding is virtually a prerequisite for NEC. Early feeding with large volumes of formula increases the risks of NEC, especially in stressed babies [18]; delayed small volume feeds offer some protective effect.

The possibility of improving gut defences has been explored extensively [19]. Oral IgA administration reduces the incidence of NEC in premature babies [20]. The possibility that breast milk (containing IgA) offers similar immunoprotective benefit has been explored but the effect is not certain [21]. Attempts to enhance gastrointestinal maturity by steroid administration to mothers before delivery decreases the incidence of subsequent NEC in their offspring [21].

NEC may be related to other causes of bowel obstruction: small bowel atresia [22], gastroschisis [23,24], malrotation and anorectal malformations. It may present either before or after surgery. It is also associated with spina bifida [25] and congenital heart disease. In each of these conditions gut wall ischaemia and hypoxia may follow obstruction and distension.

104.2 Pathological features and pathogenesis

The lesions of NEC are patchy or continuous and can affect all parts of the gastrointestinal tract from stomach to rectum. The distal small bowel and colon (Figure 104.1) are most commonly involved. Mucosal ischaemia is associated with submucosal (intramural) gas collections – pneumatosis intestinalis (Figure 104.2).

Individual bubbles may coalesce to form larger gas collections and lead to complete sloughing of mucosa. The muscle layers may become ischaemic, with the appearance of perforating ulcers. Stasis in both venous

Diseases of the Fetus and Newborn, 2nd edn, Edited by G.B. Reed, A.E. Claireaux and F. Cockburn. Published in 1995 by Chapman & Hall, London. ISBN 0 412 39160 0

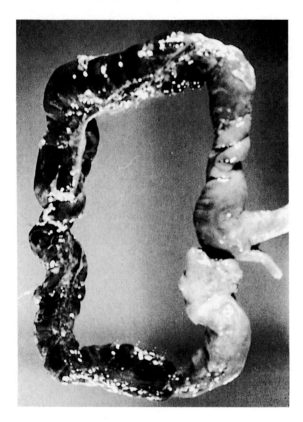

Figure 104.1 Necrosis of the colon.

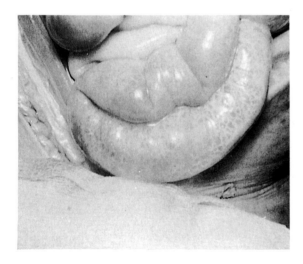

Figure 104.2 Pneumatosis intestinalis.

and arterial supply to the gut is an additional feature of ischaemia.

A prominent feature in the gut wall in NEC is coagulative necrosis related to ischaemia [26]. Reperfusion following hypoxia-ischaemia may increase this necrosis by the cytotoxic action of oxygen-free radicals [27]. Bacterial overgrowth may contribute to the

finding of hydrogen in the intramural gas bubbles [28]. Inflammatory and reparative processes are also seen in the gut wall, suggesting an evolving or ongoing process of some days' duration [26].

Platelet activating factor and tissue necrosis factor may be mediators in the production of NEC: levels of both are elevated in the disorder [29]. White cell depletion limits the damage due to hypotension and stress, suggesting that polymorphonuclear leucocytes have a harmful effect on the gut, especially when stimulated (Chapter 35).

104.3 Presentation

Systemic signs of the onset of NEC include brady-cardia, apnoeic episodes, decreased peripheral perfusion and poor skin colour with mottling. A persistent metabolic acidosis (arterial pH below 7.2) and hyponatraemia indicate clinical deterioration and developing sepsis. Thrombocytopenia is probably related to Gram-negative sepsis [30], and a positive blood culture is found in approximately one-third of cases of NEC [2]. A progressively falling platelet count correlates with the onset of necrosis/gangrene [31].

Stools positive for reducing substances due to decreased carbohydrate absorption may precede clinical evidence of NEC but passage of blood rectally heralds established changes. Bile vomiting occurs with ileus and obstruction. Abdominal signs include:

- tenderness;
- distension;
- redness of abdominal wall (cellulitis) and periumbil-ical flare;
- oedema of abdominal wall and labial/scrotal areas;
- abdominal wall crepitus due to palpable intramural gas bubbles;
- evidence of free intraperitoneal gas – absence of liver dullness;
- intra-abdominal mass/abscess.

Rectal examination (using an auriscope) may reveal inflamed mucosa.

The combination of gastric distension, paucity of bowel gas on radiograph, bowel wall oedema and bloody diarrhoea raise a strong suspicion of NEC [32]. Perforation is associated with a higher mortality (up to 40%); colonic perforation is generally more serious than small bowel perforation [33].

104.4 Diagnosis

The diagnosis may be strongly suspected on clinical grounds or clinical evidence of NEC may be minimal. The differential diagnosis includes other causes of gastrointestinal obstruction and bleeding, such as malrotation and volvulus, duplication cyst, meconium obstruction, atresia and Hirschsprung's disease.

104.4.1 PLAIN RADIOGRAPHY

Confirmation of the diagnosis of NEC may come from plain radiographic findings such as the following.

- Pneumatosis intestinalis [34] – ring or tramline sign of intramural gas seen end-on or side-on (Figure 104.3). It may also present a generalized appearance of gas bubbles in the bowel wall.
- Bowel loop distension suggesting partial obstruction, and static distended intestinal loops suggesting ischaemia.
- Gastric distension related to toxic dilatation or pyloric oedema.
- Gas in the intrahepatic portal vein seen as thin lucent lines in the uniform opacity of the liver – an ominous sign (Figure 104.4).
- Free intraperitoneal gas – passing over the liver in erect or decubitus views.
- Loculated intraperitoneal gas – beneath the liver or associated with intraperitoneal abscess.
- Gas-free appearance following sloughing of the

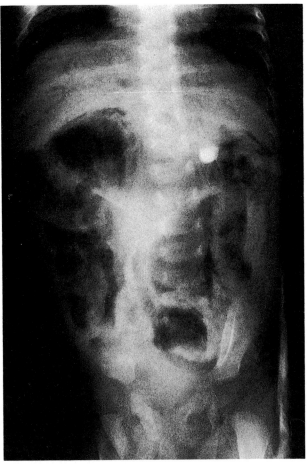

Figure 104.4 Plain abdominal radiograph showing pneumatosis intestinalis and intrahepatic portal vein gas.

mucosa and progressive oedema of the bowel or ascites.

104.4.2 BARIUM CONTRAST ENEMA

If the diagnosis remains uncertain a carefully screened barium enema may reveal the following characteristic appearances [35].

- An irregular, shaggy mucosal pattern (Figure 104.5).
- Spastic narrowing of an affected area.
- Intramural gas outlining barium.
- Stenosis or atresia secondary to established NEC.

A barium enema is especially important in exclusion of malrotation and volvulus and is useful in the diagnosis of early NEC. The technique has proved highly sensitive and specific in a large series of 126 neonates with ambiguous diagnosis of NEC [36]; no perforation occurred. Metrizamide, a water-soluble, non-ionic, contrast agent, has advantages if perforation

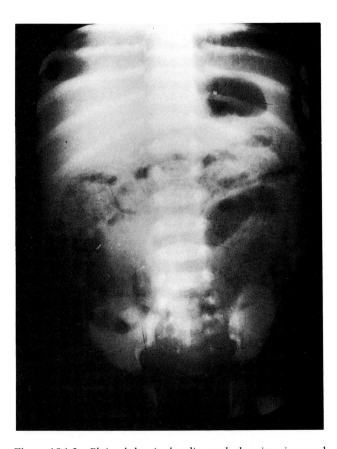

Figure 104.3 Plain abdominal radiograph showing rings and lines of intramural gas: pneumatosis intestinalis.

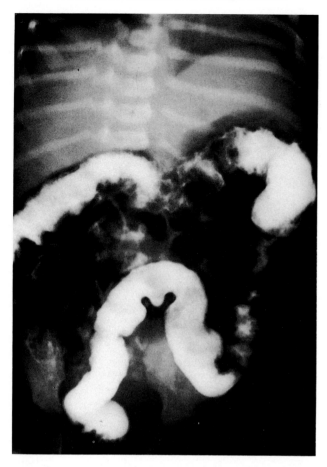

Figure 104.5 Barium enema in acute stage of NEC showing irregular mucosal outline and intramural gas.

is suspected as it is rapidly absorbed from the peritoneal cavity.

A segment of colonic narrowing seen on contrast enema is not necessarily evidence of incipient obstruction after NEC and does not constitute an indication for surgery [37].

104.4.3 NUCLEAR MEDICINE SCINTIGRAPHY

[^{99m}Tc]Pyrophosphate can be injected to define infarcted tissue [38] although false-positive and false-negative scans occur. Experimentally, [^{111}In]oxine-labelled leucocytes have been demonstrated to be taken up by ischaemic intestinal tissue [39].

104.4.4 OTHER DIAGNOSTIC METHODS

Ultrasonography and computed tomography have both been used to demonstrate portal vein gas in NEC. Magnetic resonance imaging has been shown to be helpful in detection of early NEC. Doppler flow studies of mesenteric and portal veins document reduced intestinal blood flow in established NEC. It is interesting that Doppler flow measurements in the superior

mesenteric artery may be increased at the time of appearance of symptoms of NEC, suggesting that ischaemia may not always be the primary insult [40].

104.5 Management

The diagnosis of NEC, either suspected or proven, requires immediate measures to support the infant and to arrest or limit progression of the disease. These measures include:

1. Cessation of oral feeds and passage of a nasogastric tube for gastric decompression;
2. Intravenous fluid administration using dextrose/saline or plasma to restore and maintain the circulating volume; parenteral feeding may be required through a peripheral vein site;
3. removal of umbilical artery or vein catheters which might further compromise the ischaemic process in the gut;
4. antibiotic therapy:
   (a) systemic antibiotic regimens using gentamicin/penicillin/metronidazole, cefotaxime/metronidazole or vancomycin/aztreonam [11];
   (b) oral antibiotics to decrease gut flora – neomycin, gentamicin or vancomycin [14];
5. correction of acidosis using intravenous 8.4% sodium bicarbonate or Tris buffer;
6. correction of hypoxaemia using enhanced Fio_2, endotracheal intubation and intermittent positive pressure ventilation;
7. correction of hypothermia by increasing the ambient temperature, swaddling and the use of a space-blanket;
8. correction of clotting disorders – fresh frozen plasma, platelet transfusion and specific clotting factor administration;
9. exchange blood transfusion – occasionally haemolysis may complicate NEC due to transfusion with blood products and activation of T-antigens, requiring exchange transfusion for their removal [41].

Repeated estimations of full blood count, clotting screen, serum electrolytes, and acid–base balance are important in assessing the effect of supportive therapy and defining the need to step up supportive therapy or consider surgical management. Repeated plain abdominal radiographs may show progression to more serious radiological signs of NEC (presence of free gas, increased intra-abdominal fluid, established intestinal obstruction or intrahepatic gas).

104.5.1 INDICATIONS FOR SURGICAL MANAGEMENT

The indications for surgical intervention cannot, in general, be regarded as absolute but must be interpreted in the light of the gestation, weight and fitness for surgery of the individual infant. However, surgery is usually indicated [42] in the following circumstances.

- Continuing deterioration despite maximum supportive therapy, as judged by low pH, thrombocytopenia, hypoxaemia and hyponatraemia.
- Evidence of perforation with pneumoperitoneum.
- Peritonitis and sepsis with abdominal wall inflammation.
- Intestinal obstruction with fixed dilated loops.
- Abdominal mass suggesting abscess or infarcted loops of intestine.

104.5.2 SURGICAL OPTIONS

The form of the surgical procedure depends on the fitness of the infant and the extent and site of the damaged bowel. A severely premature low-birth-weight infant with extensive NEC may only be able to tolerate a minimal procedure of peritoneal drainage. A relatively fit term baby with colonic disease may withstand a surgical procedure aimed at complete resection of infarcted bowel and restoration of continuity.

(a) Peritoneal drainage and lavage

In the very sick low-birth-weight preterm infant, perforation may be best managed by insertion of a peritoneal drain alone in the first instance [43–45]. A 12-Fr gauge infant chest drain or any form of Silastic cannula is inserted through a small stab incision lateral to the rectus muscle. It is usually passed horizontally beneath the anterior abdominal wall, with the infant in the supine position. The catheter is connected to a drainage system. Antibiotic solution (cefotaxime in physiological saline) can be infused with the intention of:

- keeping the cannula patent;
- irrigating the peritoneal cavity;
- directly combating peritoneal infection.

This regimen may result in:

- improvement in the general condition with resolution of NEC and recovery – subsequent strictures may require further attention;
- improvement in the general condition to a point where laparotomy becomes a safer option in dealing with the intestinal perforation, obstruction and peritoneal sepsis.

(b) Minimal laparotomy and defunctioning procedure

The peritoneal cavity is opened through a small incision with the aim of draining infected peritoneal fluid and

isolating a loop of intestine above the level of the NEC as a defunctioning ileostomy [46]. This may allow recovery from the acute episode of NEC but will require later surgery for resection of stenotic or atretic distal bowel and closure of the stoma.

(c) Laparotomy, resection of NEC and ileostomy/colostomy

A more extensive laparotomy incision is made in order to define and resect all the bowel affected by the NEC process [43]. Proximal and distal ostomies are then fashioned to defunction the residual bowel. Further surgery will be needed to restore continuity at a later date.

(d) Laparotomy, resection and primary bowel anastomosis

This procedure requires more extensive surgery but has the major advantage of restoring bowel continuity, avoiding the complications of ostomies and not requiring any further surgery. Good results have been reported from this procedure, provided the anastomosed bowel has normal viability [47].

(e) Second-look laparotomy

If at the initial laparotomy the NEC is so extensive that resection could not be considered without leaving a severely short gut, the possibility of closure and second-look laparotomy should be considered. Occasionally it transpires that with continued supportive therapy some areas of gut show improved viability and can be conserved at the second-look procedure.

104.6 Complications

104.6.1 FUNGAL SEPSIS

Fungal sepsis and colonization are relatively frequent in NEC and are probably related to multiple courses of antibiotics, long-term mechanical ventilation, impaired host defences and total parenteral nutrition [48]. Fungal sepsis is present in approximately 25% of cases of death resulting from NEC.

104.6.2 WOUND DEHISCENCE FOLLOWING SURGERY FOR NEC

Wound dehiscence is a particular problem due to prematurity and low birth weight, established sepsis, continuing abdominal distension and poor nutritional state of infants with NEC. Disruption of the wound may occur in up to 15% of cases and strategies using

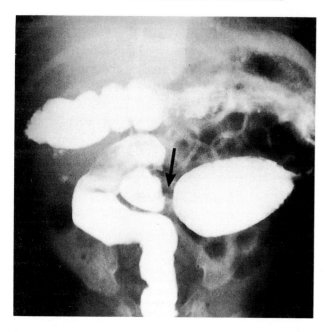

Figure 104.6 Barium enema 2 months after an episode of NEC showing sigmoid colon stricture (arrowed) and dilated proximal bowel.

silver-impregnated xenografts [49] have been developed to cope with this.

104.6.3 INTESTINAL STRICTURE

Intestinal stricture may follow either medical or surgical treatment and can occur in both the ileum and the colon (Figure 104.6). The incidence of stricture is approximately 25% [50,51] and a defined follow-up policy using a contrast enema is advisable [51,52]. Some strictures will resolve spontaneously and are presumed to be due to spasm at the time of the contrast examination. The extent of dilatation proximal to the stricture is an indication of the need for surgery [53]. The incidence of stricture in NEC is decreased following resection and primary anastomosis [54]. The complications of failure to recognize or delay in management of strictures include perforation, sepsis and death [50,55,56]. A scoring system based on clinical signs has been devised to predict the likelihood of stricture following NEC [57].

104.6.4 SHORT GUT SYNDROME

The short gut syndrome is a complication of excessive bowel resection in NEC but may be aggravated by poor mucosal absorption of the residual intestine. The management of short gut syndrome requires long-term parenteral therapy and possibly bowel transplantation.

104.6.5 MALABSORPTION

Malabsorption may follow NEC due to mucosal damage, leading to intolerance of feeds with intestinal hurry and diarrhoea. Gradual improvement usually occurs but the early management will include use of specially prepared, readily absorbed, premature infant feeding formulas.

104.6.6 PSEUDO-OBSTRUCTION

Continued evidence of intestinal obstruction and failure to thrive may present due to poor gut motility after NEC [57]. Further bowel resection in these circumstances carries the risk of short gut syndrome but prokinetic agents such as cisapride have been reported to improve motility [58].

104.7 Outcome

NEC continues to result in serious morbidity and mortality. However, the overall survival rate has been improved by increasingly intensive medical management with earlier recognition, altered feeding regimens, intravenous nutrition and antibiotic therapy and is now approximately 80% [34,59]. The mortality for surgically treated NEC is higher, at approximately 40% [42,48]. Poorer outcome from NEC can be related to low birth weight (less than 1500 g), bleeding disorders, thrombocytopenia, septicaemia and the need for surgical treatment [2]. Detailed analysis of various factors associated with NEC shows that blood pH, platelet count and the presence of congenital anomalies are of the greatest prognostic statistical significance and can be used to estimate the probability of death [60].

For survivors of NEC, the outcome is as good as for a group of infants with similar problems of prematurity but without NEC, and approximately 50% are completely normal at follow-up [5,61]. There is some evidence of delayed neurological problems in the long-term [61] and, for very-low-birth-weight babies, body weight and head circumference at 2 years follow-up are lower than for non-NEC babies [62].

References

1. Kliegman, R. and Walsh, M. (1987) Neonatal necrotizing enterocolitis: pathogenesis classification and spectrum of illness. *Current Problems in Paediatrics*, **17**, 215–88.
2. Palmer, S.R., Biffin, A. and Gamsu, H.R. (1989) Outcome of neonatal necrotizing enterocolitis: results of the BAPM/CDSC surveillance study, 1981–84. *Archives of Disease in Childhood*, **64**, 388–94.
3. Walther, F.J., Verloove-Van Horick, S.P., Brand, R. *et al.* (1989) A prospective survey of necrotizing enterocolitis in very low birthweight infants. *Paediatric and Perinatal Epidemiology*, **3**, 53–61.
4. Ryder, R.W., Shelton, J.D. and Guinan, M.E. (1980) Committee on necrotising enterocolitis. Necrotizing enterocolitis: a prospective multi centre investigation. *American Journal of Epidemiology*, **112**, 113–23.
5. Kosloske, A.M. (1990) A unifying hypothesis for pathogenesis and prevention of necrotizing enterocolitis. *Journal of Pediatrics*, **117**, 68–74.

6. Kliegman, R.M. (1990) Models of the pathogenesis of necrotizing enterocolitis. *Journal of Pediatrics*, **117**, 2–5.

7. Hackett, G.A., Campbell, S. and Gamsu, H. (1987) Doppler studies in the growth retarded fetus and prediction of neonatal nectrotizing enterocolitis, haemorrhage and neonatal morbidity. *BMJ*, **194**, 13–16.

8. Malcolm, G., Ellwood, D., Devonald, K. *et al.* (1991) Absent or reversed end diastolic flow velocity in the umbilical artery and necrotizing enterocolitis. *Archives of Disease in Childhood*, **66**, 805–807.

9. Scholander, P.F. (1963) The master switch of life. *Scientific American*, **209**, 92–105.

10. Hoy, C., Millar, M.R., MacKay, P. *et al.* (1990) Quantitative changes in faecal microflora preceding necrotizing enterocolitis in premature neonates. *Archives of Disease in Childhood*, **65**, 1057–59.

11. Millar, M.R., MacKay, P., Lavene, M. *et al.* (1992) Enterobacteriaceae and neonatal necrotizing enterocolitis. *Archives of Disease in Childhood*, **67** 53–56.

12. Gorham, P., Millar, M. and Godwin, P.G. (1988) Clostridial hand-carriage and neonatal necrotizing enterocolitis. *Journal of Hospital Infection*, **12**, 139–41.

13. Scheifele, D.W. (1990) Role of bacterial toxins in neonatal necrotizing enterocolitis. *Journal of Pediatrics*, **117**, 44–46

14. Ng, P.C., Dear, P.R. and Thomas, D.F. (1988) Oral vancomycin in prevention of necrotizing enterocolitis. *Archives of Disease in Childhood*, **63**, 1390–93.

15. Woodward, C., McTigue, C., Hogg, G. *et al* (1992) Mucormycosis of the neonatal gut: a new disease or variant of necrotizing enterocolitis? *Journal of Pediatric Surgery*, **27**, 737–40

16. Huppertz, H.I., Frauendienst, G., Doerck, M. *et al.* (1992) Necrotizing enterocolitis – A community-acquired infectious disease? *Lancet*, **339**, 241.

17. Rotbart, H. and Levin, M. (1983) How contagious is necrotizing enterocolitis? *Paediatric Infectious Diseases*, **2**, 406–13.

18. McKeown, R.E., Marsh, T.D., Amarnath, U. *et al.* (1991) Role of delayed feeding and of feeding increments in necrotizing enterocolitis. *Journal of Pediatrics*, **121**, 764–70.

19. Udall, J.N. (1990) Gastrointestinal host defense and necrotizing enterocolitis. *Journal of Pediatrics*, **117**, 33–43.

20. Eibl, M., Wolf, H., Furnkranz, H. *et al.* (1988) Prevention of necrotizing enterocolitis, in low birth weight infants by IgA–IgG feeding. *New England Journal of Medicine*, **319**, 1–7.

21. Kliegman, R.M. (1979) Neonatal necrotizing enterocolitis; implications for an infectious disease. *Pediatric Clinics of North America*, **26**, 327–44.

22. Lafferty, K., Brereton, R.J., and Wright, V.M.W. (1983) Necrotizing enterocolitis in small bowel atresia. *Zeitschrift für Kinderchirurgie*, **38**, 224–27.

23. Aaronson, I.A. and Eckstein, H.B. (1977) The role of silastic prosthesis in the management of gastroschisis. *Archives of Surgery*, **112**, 297–302.

24. Oldham, K.T., Koran, A.G. and Drongowski, R.A. *et al.* (1988) The development of necrotizing enterocolitis following repair of gastroschisis; a surprisingly high incidence. *Journal of Pediatric Surgery*, **23**, 945–49.

25. Irving, I.M. and Pabst, F. (1982) Neonatal necrotizing enterocolitis following surgery for spina bifida. *Zeitschrift für Kinderchirurgie*, **37**, 165–67.

26. Ballance, W.A., Dahms, B.B. and Shenker, N. *et al.* (1990) Pathology of neonatal necrotizing enterocolitis: a ten-year experience. *Journal of Pediatrics*, **117**, 6–13.

27. Parks, D.A., Bulkley, G.B. and Granger, D.N. (1983) Role of oxygen-derived free radicals in digestive tract diseases. *Surgery*, **94**, 414–22.

28. Engel, R.R. (1974) Studies of the gastrointestinal flora in necrotizing enterocolitis, in *Necrotizing Enterocolitis in the Newborn Infant*, Report of 68th Ross.Conference on Pediatric Research, Ross Laboratories, Columbus, OH, pp. 66–71.

29. Caplan, M.S. and Hsueh, W. (1990) Necrotizing enterocolitis, role of platelet activating factor, endotoxin, and tumour necrosis factor. *Journal of Pediatrics*, **117**, 47–51.

30. Rowe, M.I., Buckner, D.M. and Newmark, S. (1975) The early diagnosis of Gram negative septicaemia in the paediatric surgical patient. *Annals of Surgery*, **182**, 280–86.

31. O'Neill, J.A., Stahlman, M.T. and Meng, H.C. (1975) Necrotizing enterocolitis in the newborn. *Annals of Surgery*, **182**, 274–79.

32. Odita, J.C., Omene, J.A. and Okolo, A.A. (1987) Gastric distension in neonatal necrotizing enterocolitis. *Paediatric Radiology*, **17**, 202–205.

33. Dickens, St V., LeBouthillier, G., Luks, F.I. *et al.* (1992) Neonatal gastrointestinal perforations. *Journal of Pediatric Surgery*, **27**, 1340–42.

34. Grosfeld, J.L., Cheu, H., Schlatter, M. *et al.* (1991) Changing trends in necrotizing enterocolitis. *Annals of Surgery*, **214**, 300–306.

35. Negrette, J., Ziervogel, M.A. and Young, D.G. (1986) Barium enema examination in neohates with suspected necrotizing enterocolitis. *Zeitschrift für Kinderchirurgie*, **41**, 19–21.

36. Kao, S.C.S., Smith, W.L., Franken, E.A. *et al.* (1992) Contrast enema diagnosis of necrotizing enterocolitis. *Pediatric Radiology*, **22**, 115–17.

37. Dolan, P., Azmy, A.F., Young, D.G. *et al.* (1984) Necrotizing enterocolitis: experience with 54 neonates. *Scottish Medical Journal*, **29**, 166–70.

38. Caride, V.J., Touloukian, R.J., Ablow, R.C. *et al.* (1981) Abdominal and hepatic uptake of ^{99m}Tc-pyrophosphate in neonatal necrotizing enterocolitis. *Radiology*, **139**, 205–209.

39. DeAugustine, J., Kahlan, S. and Grisone, E. (1991) Indium 111 oxine-labelled leucocytes for early diagnosis of ischaemic enterocolitis. *Journal of Pediatric Surgery*, **26**, 1039–42.

40. Kempley, S.T. and Gamsu, H.R. (1992) Superior mesenteric artery blood flow velocity in necrotizing enterocolitis. *Archives of Disease in Childhood*, **67**, 793–96.

41. Squire, R., Kiely, E., Drake, D. *et al.* (1992) Intravascular haemolysis in association with necrotizing enterocolitis. *Journal of Pediatric Surgery*, **27**, 808–10.

42. Robertson, J.F.R., Azmy, A.F. and Young, D.G. (1987) Surgery for necrotizing enterocolitis. *British Journal of Surgery*, **74**, 387–89.

43. Dykes, E.H., Fitzgerald, R.J. and O'Donnell, B. (1989) Surgery for neonatal necrotizing enterocolitis in Ireland; 1980–85. *Intensive Care Medicine*, **15**, 24–26.

44. Ein, S.H., Shandling, B., Wesson, D. and Filler, R.M. (1990) A 13 year experience with peritoneal drainage under local anesthesia for necrotizing enterocolitis perforation. *Journal of Pediatric Surgery*, **25**, 1034–37.

45. Takamatsu, H., Akiyama, H., Ibara, S. *et al.* (1992) Treatment for necrotizing enterocolitis perforation in the extremely premature infant (weighing <1000 g). *Journal of Pediatric Surgery*, **27**, 741–43.

46. Legat, C. and Latour, J.P. (1989) Peritoneal drainage and ileostomy as a treatment for acute necrotizing enterocolitis. *Zeitschrift für Kinderchirurgie*, **44**, 315–16.

47. Griffiths, D.M., Forbes, D.A., Pemberton, P.J. *et al.* (1989) Primary anastomosis for necrotizing enterocolitis: a 12-year experience. *Journal of Pediatric Surgery*, **24**, 515–18.

48. Smith, S.D., Tagge, E.P., Miller, J. *et al.* (1990) The hidden mortality in surgically treated necrotizing enterocolitis: fungal sepsis. *Journal of Pediatric Surgery*, **25**, 1030–33.

49. Angel, C., Daw, S., Phillipe, P. *et al.* (1992) Pig in pouch: a technique for the management of complete wound dehiscence after laparotomy for neonatal necrotizing enterocolitis. *Journal of Pediatric Surgery*, **27**, 67–69.

50. Kosloske, A.M., Burstein, J. and Bartow, S.A. (1980) Intestinal obstruction due to colonic stricture following neonatal necrotizing enterocolitis. *Annals of Surgery*, **192**, 202–207.

51. Schwartz, M.Z., Hayden, C.K., Richardson, C.J. *et al.* (1982) A prospective evaluation of intestinal stenosis following necrotizing enterocolitis. *Journal of Pediatric Surgery*, **17**, 764–70.

52. Radhakrishman, J., Blechman, G., Shrader, C. *et al.* (1991) Colonic strictures following successful medical management of necrotizing enterocolitis: a prospective study evaluating early gastrointestinal contrast studies. *Journal of Pediatric Surgery*, **26**, 1043–46.

53. Tonkin, I.L.D., Bjelland, J.C., Hunter, T.B. *et al.* (1978) Spontaneous resolution of colonic strictures caused by necrotizing enterocolitis: therapeutic implications. *AJR*, **130**, 1077–81.

54. Harberg, F.J., McGill, C.W., Saleem, M.M. *et al.* (1983) Resection with primary anastomosis for necrotizing enterocolitis. *Journal of Pediatric Surgery*, **18**, 743–46.

55. Hartman, G.E., Drugas, G.T. and Schochat, S.J. (1988) Post-necrotizing enterocolitis strictures presenting with sepsis or perforation: risk of clinical observation. *Journal of Pediatric Surgery*, **23**, 562–66.

56. Kosloske, A.M. (1979) Necrotizing enterocolitis in the neonate. *Surgery, Gynecology and Obstetrics*, **148**, 259–69.

57. Evrard, J., Khamis, J., Rausin, L. *et al.* (1991) A scoring system in predicting the risk of intestinal stricture in necrotizing enterocolitis. *European Journal of Pediatrics*, **150**, 757–60.

58. Van Der Winden, J.M., Dassonville, M., Van-Der-Veken, E. *et al.* (1990) Post-necrotizing enterocolitis pseudo-obstruction treated with cisapride. *Zeitschrift für Kinderchirurgie*, **45**, 282–85.

59. Beasley, S.W., Auldist, A.W., Ramanujan, T.M. *et al.* (1986) The surgical management of necrotizing enterocolitis. *Pediatric Surgery International*, **1**, 210–17.

60. Dykes, E.H., Gilmour, W.H. and Azmy, A.F. (1985) Prediction of outcome following necrotizing enterocolitis in a neonatal surgical unit. *Journal of Pediatric Surgery*, **20**, 3–5.

61. Stevenson, D.K., Kerner, J.A., Malachowski, N. *et al.* (1980) Late morbidity among survivors of necrotizing enterocolitis. *Pediatrics*, **56**, 925–27.

62. Walsh, M.C., Kliegman, R.M. and Hack, M. (1989) Severity of necrotizing enterocolitis: influence on outcome at 2 years of age. *Pediatrics*, **84**, 808–14.

105 OMPHALOCELES AND GASTROSCHISIS

E. Sapin and F. Bargy

105.1 Pathobiology

105.1.1 DEFINITION OF TERMS

Gastroschisis is an intestinal herniation through a full-thickness defect of the anterior abdominal wall. This defect is situated in the immediate neighbourhood of a normally inserted umbilical cord, usually to the right of the umbilicus (95%), often with a skin-covered bridge between umbilical cord and wall defect. There is no sac covering the intestines, which are thickened, oedematous and covered by inflammatory exudates.

Omphalocele is a herniation of abdominal viscera into the umbilical cord. Abdominal contents remain in a membranous sac composed internally of peritoneum and externally of amnion but never of skin. The umbilical cord arises from the apex of the herniated sac. The size of the defect may range from a small one containing a bowel loop to a very large one containing most of the bowel organs.

A cephalic fold omphalocele is so called if it is primarily in the epigastrium or if any part of the sternum, ventral diaphragm, epicardium or heart is involved in the lesion. The pentalogy of Cantrell is the association of congenital defects involving all these structures [1].

A caudal fold omphalocele is the association of omphalocele with bladder exstrophy or cloaca or with hindgut agenesis.

A lateral fold omphalocele is the most common lesion, diagnosed when the omphalocele does not meet the criteria for cephalic or caudal fold types.

105.1.2 EMBRYOLOGY AND PATHOGENESIS

Major malformations and chromosomal anomalies are commonly associated with omphalocele but are rare with gastroschisis. The data suggest an acquired rather than a genetic aetiology for gastroschisis as compared with omphalocele. They are distinctly separate entities that have resulted from different events during the early stages of development [2]. The normal development of the anterior abdominal wall depends on the fusion of four ectomesodermic folds (cephalic, caudal and two laterals) [3,4].

Deficient morphogenesis of the somatopleure with abnormal development of the lateral folds before the end of the third week of embryonal life, preventing the later return of the midgut into the abdomen, leads to the formation of an isolated omphalocele. Failure of the cephalic or caudal fold to fuse with the other folds results respectively in cephalic or caudal fold omphalocele. The causal event of omphalocele occurs very early during embryogenesis, resulting in frequent association with major malformations.

Gastroschisis is a vascular accident occurring after intestinal return into the abdominal cavity. It results from vascular compromise of either the right umbilical vein or the omphalomesenteric artery. This infarcted area leads to a paraumbilical defect through which the bowel prolapses soon after, or later. Eviscerated bowel is often thickly matted, covered with a gelatinous matrix and apparently shortened. The aetiology of bowel damage has been a source of controversy for many years. Chemical peritonitis seems to be caused by the presence of irritant components of fetal urine in the amniotic fluid because of the increasing fetal renal function (with increasing concentrations of urea, creatinine and uric acid, and decreasing sodium levels and osmolality in the amniotic fluid). The high incidence of intestinal atresia encountered in association with gastroschisis may result from an ischemic injury to the territory of the superior mesenteric artery as an extensive disruption of the distal segment of the right omphalomesenteric artery, responsible for right-sided periumbilical ischaemia [5]. However, most authors consider intestinal atresia as an antenatal complication [6]. Small defects may predispose to strangulation of eviscerated bowel. The risk of infarction and atresia may be enhanced by oedema and swelling of the bowel,

Diseases of the Fetus and Newborn, 2nd edn, Edited by G.B. Reed, A.E. Claireaux and F. Cockburn. Published in 1995 by Chapman & Hall, London. ISBN 0 412 39160 0

resulting from its prolonged exposure to amniotic fluid and its lack of normal mesenteric attachment. If the accident occurred early enough in intrauterine life, this could result in an atretic segment of bowel. Most often it will result in motility and absorption disturbances. In omphalocele, the size of the defect is relatively large and the membranous sac protects the herniated bowel from contact with amniotic fluid. The intestine therefore remains morphologically and functionally normal.

105.2 Prenatal pathology

105.2.1 RELATIVE INCIDENCE AND ENVIRONMENTAL FACTORS

The exact incidence of major malformations associated with omphalocele is often underestimated because of fetal wastage. The true incidence of ventral wall defects may be higher than the birth prevalence noted among liveborn infants: 1/4000–1/5000 for omphalocele and 1/10 000–1/12 000 for gastroschisis. The advent of α-fetoprotein (AFP) screening and widespread use of prenatal ultrasonography confirms this impression. Furthermore, it seems that gastroschisis is more common than omphalocele and may be increasing in incidence, with an approximate 2 to 1 preponderance of gastroschisis over omphalocele in liveborn infants [7].

In literature reviews, the sex incidence in gastroschisis turns out to be exactly equal (male: female ratio: 1.17 in Carpenter *et al.* [8] and 1.03 in this series), whereas in omphalocele patients, males predominated slightly (sex ratio 1.27 in Carpenter *et al.* [8] but 0.79 in this series). The average maternal age for gastroschisis is younger than for omphalocele patients (22 versus 27 years in Moore and Nur [7], 22 versus 22.9 years in Carpenter *et al.* [8], 24.3 versus 29 years in this series).

105.2.2 OMPHALOCELE AND ASSOCIATED MALFORMATIONS

In cases of omphalocele, additional malformations are frequent, serious and generally multiple, whereas in cases of gastroschisis, they are often minor problems: jejunoileal and colic atresia may be regarded as antenatal complications. For all those abdominal wall defects, malrotation of the gut is the rule. Literature reviews have often reported a greater than 50% incidence of associated anomalies in infants with omphalocele (40–73%) [8–11]. The frequency of chromosomal aberrations has been reported to be as high as 35–58% [12,13]. The most frequent associated malformations reported in the literature are cardiac (30–40%), genitourinary (40%), gastrointestinal (20–30%), musculoskeletal (29%), central nervous system (6%) and miscellaneous (45%). Several patients have more than one anomaly. Chromosomal abnormalities are usually associated with multisystem malformations [9,14]. The specific seriousness of several associated anomalies is a main prenatal and postnatal prognostic factor. The likelihood of an underlying chromosomal defect with omphalocele increases with maternal age [11].

Familial cases of isolated omphalocele have been reported with sex-linked or autosomal patterns of inheritance [15,16]. For Moore and Nur [6], the geographical incidence of omphalocele syndromes (lower-midline syndrome, upper-midline syndrome or the Beckwith–Wiedemann syndrome) varies from a high of 40% in southern Europe to a low of 7–9% in the USA, Japan and Mexico, with intermediate levels (12–13%) in Scandinavia, northern Europe and Australia.

105.2.3 GASTROSCHISIS AND FETAL GROWTH

Intrauterine growth retardation (IUGR) is frequently encountered with gastroschisis. In the authors' experience, the birth weight was below the 10th centile of the normal range for gestation in 50 cases (69.5%), but in only 33.3% of omphalocele cases (Figure 105.1). Low serum albumin immunoglobulin G, transferrin and total serum proteins in infants with gastroschisis suggests that these infants have nutritional deprivation rather than a constitutionally determined limitation of growth. The prenatal intestinal damage may contribute to IUGR, mainly due to impairment of the trophic effect of amniotic fluid on fetal development [17–19]. Previous studies allowed the conclusion to be drawn that there is a fetal ingestion and metabolism of amniotic fluid protein [20–2] and carbohydrates [23]. This amniotic contribution to fetal growth normally increases with gestational age because of the gradual physiological development of intestinal function with age [24,25]. The increased rate of IUGR observed with gestational age in gastroschisis would support the hypothesis of intestinal damage responsibility (Figure 105.2).

105.3 Systemic and speciality pathology

105.3.1 BIOLOGICAL SCREENING

The advent of AFP screening and the increasing use of fetal sonography may allow greater prenatal detection of abdominal wall defects now and in the future. The maternal serum AFP (MSAFP) level has been shown to be elevated in abdominal wall defects. The test sensitivity is estimated to 0.75 and seems to be greater for gastroschisis than for omphalocele [26,27]: 77% versus 42% detection rate in the series by Mann *et al.* [12]

When an elevated maternal and amniotic AFP value

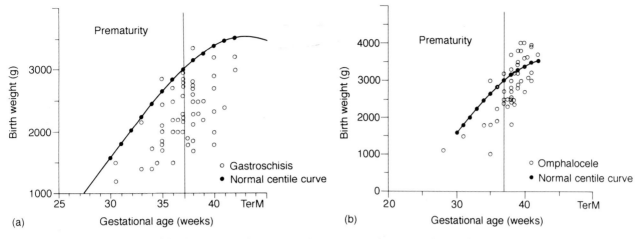

(a)

(b)

Figure 105.1 Distribution of birth weights of infants with (a) gastroschisis and (b) omphalocele.

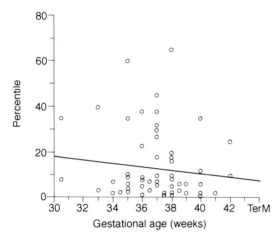

Figure 105.2 Gastroschisis: relative increases in growth retardation with gestational age.

is found, differential diagnosis should include neural tube defects, abdominal wall defects, sacrococcygeal teratoma, cystic hygromas and Rh isoimmunization. Acetyl cholinesterase band density ratios have been shown to differ between abdominal wall and open neural tube defects [28]. The combined measurements of AFP levels and acetyl cholinesterase ratio in amniotic fluid are highly reliable in detecting gastroschisis between 16 and 20 weeks of gestation.

105.3.2 RESEARCH

Hypoperistalsis after gastroschisis repair is related to intestinal damage observed initially. The pathophysiology of this process has been studied by histological examination of surgical material, at prenatal and postnatal human postmortem examination and by experimentation with animal models.

Histological examination of the intestine of gastroschisis patients revealed no evidence of histological

abnormalities in ganglion cells or in the myenteric nervous system [29]. The most consistent finding was the thickening peel in the serosal layer. Fibrous peel has been noted to begin at approximately 30 weeks' gestation and consists of type I collagen and fibrin. The peel dissolved after being repaired postnatally [30].

With the production of gastroschisis in the chick embryo by Klück *et al.* [31] and Tibboel *et al.* [32], bowel damage seems to be the result of a chemical peritonitis, most probably caused by the presence of irritant components of fetal urine in the amniotic fluid: bowel bathed in amniotic fluid alone, without exposure to allantoic contents, was normal. In fetal lambs, an experimental gastroschisis was created by Langer *et al.* at 80 days' gestation (term: 145 days), with or without a tie placed around the herniated bowel at the level of the abdominal wall. Near term, histology and *in vitro* bowel motility assays were studied: a fibrous peel was observed only in bowel exposed to amniotic fluid, with or without constriction. Lymphatic and venous dilatation, smooth muscle thickening and focal mucosal blunting were seen in bowel subjected to chronic obstruction by a constrictor regardless of whether it was exposed to amniotic fluid or not. Both constriction of the bowel and amniotic fluid exposure were associated with a decrease in motility.

105.4 Obstetric sonography

105.4.1 PRENATAL ULTRASONOGRAPHIC FEATURES

An abdominal wall defect can be identified *in utero* and adequately characterized. It can be noted incidentally during routine midgestation screening performed at 16–18 weeks, or because of maternal polyhydramnios or because of elevation in MSAFP. Detailed ultrasonography should therefore be performed to access the integrity of the anterior abdominal wall.

The sonographic differentiation between physiological herniation and pathological ventral wall defects may be very subtle, making definitive first-trimester diagnosis difficult. Although a very early tentative diagnosis might be possible at 8 or 9 weeks' gestation, the suspicion of ventral wall defect can be confirmed reliably only after 12 weeks' gestation [34,35]. Transvaginal ultrasonography may be helpful in difficult cases. The likelihood of major malformations and chromosomal abnormalities is as high as 82% among the cases of omphalocele diagnosed prenatally.

The overall accuracy of identifying gastroschisis and omphalocele was respectively 67% and 74.5% in the authors' experience, 65% versus 78% for gastroschisis in Roberts and Burge [36] and 64% versus 34% in Sermer et al. [37]. Failure to detect gastroschisis by antenatal ultrasound may be partly due to later perinatal onset. Indeed serial sonographic study has now shown that in gastroschisis cases evisceration can occur late [38].

105.4.2 ULTRASONOGRAPHIC DIFFERENTIATION BETWEEN OMPHALOCELE AND GASTROSCHISIS

Antenatal distinction between gastroschisis and omphalocele is critical because omphalocele is associated with a much greater incidence of major malformations [39]. In nearly all cases, ultrasonography is able to differentiate between them by distinguishing characteristics: location of the umbilical cord insertion, echogenicity of the contents of the protruding mass, and the presence or absence of a sac surrounding the mass (Figure 105.3).

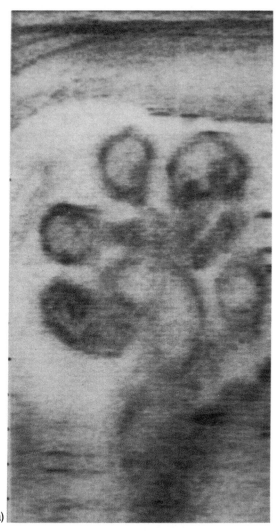
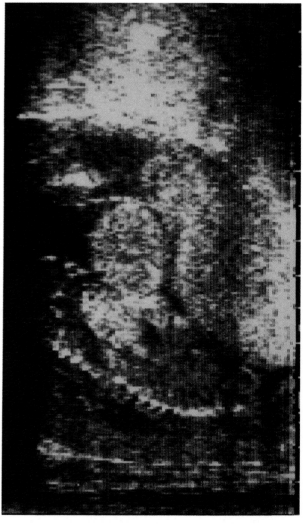

(a) (b)

Figure 105.3 Prenatal ultrasonographic features. (a) Gastroschisis: intestinal herniation with its cauliflower appearance; (b) giant omphalocele: with hepatic contents.

Omphalocele is a midline ventral defect with herniation of the intra-abdominal contents into the base of the umbilical cord. Herniated viscera are covered by a membranous sac and the umbilical cord insertion is at the apex of the herniated sac. A possible exception may be those cases of omphalocele in which rupture of the amnioperitoneal sac occurs *in utero*, an exceedingly rare complication. The presence of an associated malformation is in keeping with the diagnosis of omphalocele.

The ultrasonic image of a gastroschisis is of a mass adjacent to the anterior ventral wall, representing the herniated visceral organs and resulting typically in a cauliflower-like appearance. The intestines float freely within the amniotic cavity, characterized by bright bubble-like echoes produced by sound reflections of thickened bowel in the amniotic fluid. There is no covering membrane and the umbilical cord is normally connected to the abdominal wall, independent of the defect. The antenatal differential diagnosis should include ruptured omphalocele and amniotic band syndrome. The differential diagnosis with ruptured omphalocele may be very difficult but the normal umbilical cord insertion on the abdominal wall and the presence of bowel without liver in the protruding viscera without any other malformation allow the diagnosis of gastroschisis. The presence of associated asymmetrical limb defects and central nervous system deformities is a clue to the diagnosis of amniotic band syndrome.

105.4.3 COMPLETE CAREFUL SCANNING

After identification of a fetal abdominal wall defect, ultrasound should be used to determine the size of the lesion, abdominal transverse diameter and diameter of the defect. A small abdominal cavity measured by transverse abdominal diameter is a frequent finding. The size of the defect in omphalocele, associated with a relatively small peritoneal cavity, is predictive of outcome because giant omphalocele presents a more difficult surgical challenge, with a life-threatening prognosis. The identification of herniated organs in the omphalocele should be documented: extracoelomic small bowel is present in almost all cases, stomach in almost 50% and liver in 25%. In gastroschisis, the liver is rarely protruding. It is often difficult to measure precisely the size of the gastroschisis defect; in omphalocele it varies between 1.5 and 8 cm, with a mean of 3.5 cm [8]. Polyhydramnios can be observed in some cases of omphalocele, probably responsible for the increased incidence of premature labor.

When diagnosis of **omphalocele** is made, great attention has to be paid to detect associated malformations: fetal heart, diaphragm, bladder and kidneys, intracranial and spinal anatomy should be explored.

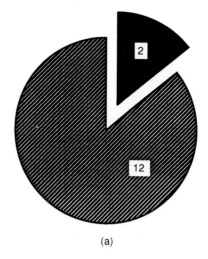

(a)

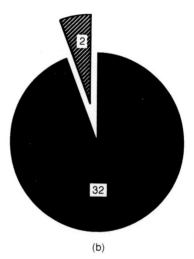

(b)

Figure 105.4 Relationship of omphalocele contents to chromosomal abnormalities. (a) Omphalocele with intracorporeal liver ($n = 14$); (b) omphalocele with extracorporeal liver ($n = 34$). ■ = No chromosomal anomaly; ▨ = chromosomal anomalies. (Additional findings reported by Nyberg *et al.* [42] and Benacerraf *et al.* [41].)

Beyond a careful scanning of the fetal anatomy, echocardiography and fetal karyotyping are mandatory. Indeed the mortality rate associated with omphalocele and cardiac defect is high (86% in the study by Sermer *et al.* [37]). In earlier antenatally diagnosed cases, the incidence of associated anomalies has been noted to be as high as 82% and association with autosomal trisomies (most often trisomy 18 or 13) about 10% [40]. The other most commonly associated malformations encountered are genitourinary (40%), cardiovascular (16–20%) and central nervous system (4%). The absence of liver in the defect may predict an abnormal karyotype even though fetuses with extracorporeal liver have normal karyotype [41,42] (Figure 105.4). Moore and Nur [7] have not documented a different incidence of associated anomalies according to the size of the defect. A pentalogy of Cantrell can be suspected in the presence of ectopia cordis, characterized on fetal ultrasonography by the protruding pulsating heart surrounded by amniotic fluid; it is sometimes possible to note that the apex of the heart deviates inferiorly and bulges under the skin of the chest, due to the sternal defect. An amniotic band syndrome should be suspected when omphalocele is associated with asymmetrical limb amputations and/or central nervous system or extremity deformities. Association of massive placental hydrops involving stem villi, omphalocele associated with visceromegaly and macroglossia and diploid DNA content may suggest possible Beckwith–Wiedeman syndrome in some cases; The antenatal suspicion of affected fetuses allows for clinical evaluation, discussion with parents and planning for neonatal care. Polyhydramnios is a frequent finding in Beckwith–Wiedeman syndrome [43].

In **gastroschisis** cases, neither the estimated size of the abdominal wall defect by sonography nor the known time of exposure to amniotic fluid can be correlated with the clinical outcome. However, it is possible to document the condition of the eviscerated intestine and therefore to predict the severity of intestinal damage: the presence of small bowel dilatation and mural thickening with a highly echogenic appearance have a high correlation with intestinal damage and poor clinical outcome; whereas the lack of these findings indicates a good prognosis [40,44–46]. In addition, measurement of both biparietal diameter and femur length allows detection of IUGR, which has been reported in up to 77% of infants [8]. Fetal abdominal circumference and uterine volume measurement may be ineffective in evaluating growth retardation in these cases.

In cases of omphalocele, more than low birth weight and prematurity, the most important prognostic indicator appears to be the presence of other anomalies. Antenatal monitoring of the patients should include serial ultrasound evaluations to monitor abdominal wall defects. In cases of omphalocele, they can decrease in size in proportion to fetal body size as gestation progresses [38]. In cases of gastroschisis, serial ultrasound monitoring is indicated to look for signs of intestinal obstruction and IUGR [45].

105.5 Goals of genetic screening and prenatal diagnosis

105.5.1 GENETIC SCREENING

Fetal karyotyping should be considered when the diagnosis of omphalocele by ultrasound is in doubt; it should be obtained from amniotic fluid amniocytes (amniocentesis), chorionic villi (placental biopsy) or fetal blood (percutaneous umbilical blood sampling or fetoscopy), depending upon the urgency of the diagnosis. Cordocentesis has the advantage of providing accurate results rapidly, thereby alleviating the parenteral anxiety associated with long delays in obtaining results. The incidence of chromosomal abnormalities such as trisomies 13 and 18 is 9% in the antenatally diagnosed cases reported by Nakayama *et al.* [38]; therefore risk factors statistically associated with chromosomal abnormalities are the absence of liver from the omphalocele sac, advanced maternal age (more than 33 years) and sonographically detectable concurrent malformations (48% versus 3% in Nicolaides, Rodeck and Gosden's series [13,41]. When an omphalocele is associated with a trisomy, great attention must be paid to excluding the possibility of a balanced translocation which increases the recurrence risk.

No routine amniocentesis and karyotype analysis is now performed in cases of gastroschisis.

105.5.2 PARENTAL COUNSELING

The parents should receive appropriate genetic and perinatal counselling based upon the antenatal findings. The management plan should take their wishes into consideration. Antenatal counselling allows the family to take informed decisions about abortion or continued antepartum follow-up. The occurrence of polyhydramnios may contribute to an increased risk of premature labor and delivery. Parents should be counselled about this possibility so that appropriate monitoring and therapeutic measures can be taken. *In utero* transfer can prevent complications of hypothermia and hypovolaemia with acidosis and bowel injury.

Therefore, the main goals of antenatal diagnosis of abdominal wall defects are to detect associated anomalies early, and, if the pregnancy is to continue, to deliver the child at a centre where appropriate postnatal care is available, to prevent iatrogenic injury during delivery and to time the delivery to prevent the development of bowel damage *in utero* [46].

105.6 Management of 'high-risk' fetus and newborn

105.6.1 FETAL MONITORING

When the antenatal diagnosis of abdominal wall defect is made, a complete evaluation should be undertaken according to the described guidelines. The frequency of concomitant abnormalities in omphalocele profoundly affects prognosis. Their detection is a major aim of antenatal diagnosis in this condition. Should the pregnancy continue, then the perinatal management will

Table 105.1 Fetuses and infants with abdominal wall defects seen between January 1982 and December 1991 at the Saint Vincent de Paul Children's Hospital

	Omphaloceles	Gastroschisis
No. cases	59	73
Sex ratio (M/F)	0.79	1.03
Average maternal age (years)	29±6	24±5
Prenatal diagnosis (%)	75	67
Prematurity rate (%)	17	38
IUGR rate (%)	33	70
Associated anomalies (%)	44	12
Meconium staining of amniotic fluid (%)	35	73
Mortality	16[a]	7[b]

[a] Prenatal 3; infants 13 (23%).
[b] Prenatal 2; infants 5 (7%).

consist of frequent antepartum fetal evaluation and caesarean section if fetal distress occurs. Careful monitoring for premature labour and for fetal growth should be carried out, then appropriate monitoring and therapeutic measures can be instituted. In gastroschisis the prematurity rate has been reported to be as high as 50% (Table 105.1). While monitoring those fetuses, attention must be directed to the possible complications occuring before birth, such as bowel obstruction, a very common event in gastroschisis, or rupture of the amnioperitoneal sac *in utero*, an exceedingly rare complication in omphalocele. In cases of gastroschisis, prenatal deaths have been reported in 12.5% in Kirk and Wah's series [46] and in 2.7% in this series. In cases of omphalocele, many deaths with chromosomal abnormalities or major associated malformations are today reported, due to elective termination of pregnancy, intrauterine or neonatal death.

105.6.2 ROUTE OF DELIVERY

In recent years the optimal mode of delivery of fetuses with an abdominal wall defect has been a subject of debate.

To avoid injury to the sac and its contents, patients with a large omphalocele with external protrusion of a large part of the liver may benefit from a caesarean section. However, in retrospective studies no increase in neonatal mortality and morbidity related to route of delivery has been reported. If the diagnosis of a ruptured omphalocele is made at or near term, delivery by caesarean section is to be recommended to minimize the risk of chemical peritonitis and the risk of delay of resumption of intestinal function after surgery.

Routine early delivery by caesarean section of all fetuses with gastroschisis is advocated to reduce the duration of exposure of the bowel to the irritant effects of amniotic fluid in the last trimester. Also, this

management may obtain a shorter period of dysmotility and malabsorption and greater ease of primary closure. Indeed, the morbidity associated with gastroschisis can largely be attributed to inflammatory damage to the bowel occurring after week 30 of gestation [47–49]. Furthermore, this damage might render intestine more susceptible to labour trauma [8]. Retrospective studies showed that caesarean section does not improve outcome in gastroschisis, perhaps because these studies have been biased in their evaluations (delay in repair, transport of the fetus.) [8,14,45,50,51]. If a correlation has been shown between prenatally detected small bowel dilatation and thickened and severe intestinal damage, these *in utero* measurements seem to be ineffective as indications for delivery intervention. Indeed, initial bowel dilatation may occur before a gestational age when lung maturity is achieved and the bowel is already beyond the point of salvage (one fetal death observed in the present series occurred at 30 weeks of gestation with findings of total intestinal necrosis *post mortem*). In keeping with most authors, the present authors did not advocate routine caesarean section. Nevertheless, recent data reported by Moore [48] with exceedingly short and uneventful follow-up after early scheduled caesarean section, may lead to changes in the current management.

105.6.3 NEONATAL MANAGEMENT

Delivery should preferably be performed in a tertiary care centre with appropriate surgical and paediatric back-up. Mortality is partly related to the clinical condition at the time of admission to the neonatal intensive care unit. Indeed, delay in treatment frequently results in hypothermia and fluid loss with acidosis, as well as increasing serosal oedema and the likelihood of intestinal necrosis [52]. Initial management can prevent these complications: improved temperature and fluid management, careful wound care with protection of the herniated bowel (slip into a bag), administration of antibiotics and speedy transfer to the operating room.

Fetal status during parturition is assessed by the presence or absence of meconium in amniotic fluid, electronic fetal heart rate monitoring and the 1- and 5-minute Apgar scores. Depressed 5-minute Apgar scores are found more frequently with omphalocele than with gastroschisis. Meconium-stained amniotic fluid is associated more often with gastroschisis than with omphalocele (62% versus 8% in Carpenter *et al.* [8] 73% versus 35% in the present experience, 65% and 75% respectively in Caniano, Brokaw and Ginn-Peare [53], and see Mercer *et al.* [54] for gastroschisis cases), but in cases of gastroschisis its presence is mainly due to bowel irritation. A subglottic aspiration of meconium has been reported in almost 30% of cases [53,54]. At

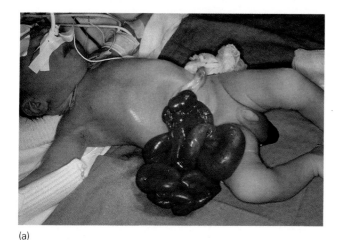

(a)

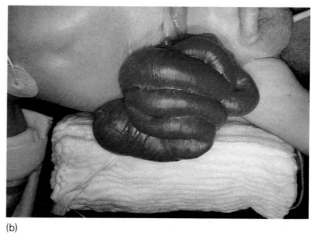

(b)

Figure 105.5 Gastroschisis. (a) Intestine quite free of peel; umbilical cord insertion is normal, to the left of the defect; (b) intestine thickly matted with proximal colon atresia.

birth, the proportion of infants with gastroschisis below the 10th birthweight percentile for gestational age is significantly greater than that of omphalocele cases (69.5% versus 33.3% in our series, 77% versus 20% in Carpenter *et al.* [8] (Figure 105.1). An increased prematurity rate was also noted (Table 105.1).

In gastroschisis, the herniated organs are mainly bowel loops; hepatic herniation is a very rare event. The length of intestine initially appears shortened with various degrees of peel (Figure 105.5). In omphalocele, the diameter of the defect ranges between 1.5 and 8 cm (mean 3.5±1.6 cm) (Figure 105.6). Extracoelomic content is small bowel in almost all cases, stomach in 47%, large bowel in 39% and liver in 24%. Additional malformations can be observed, especially in omphalocele cases: cephalic or caudal fold omphalocele, congenital heart lesions, genitourinary, musculoskeletal and neural abnormalities, and/or chromosomal trisomies. In cases of gastroschisis, the more frequently associated anomaly is undescended testis. Intestinal damage, multiple bowel atresia and *in utero* perforation of the small intestine are the common fetal bowel complications [7].

105.6.4 SURGICAL MANAGEMENT

Primary abdominal wall closure is aided by performing the operation early with thorough evacuation of meconium and manual stretching of the abdominal wall. Delays in surgical correction certainly make primary closure more difficult [52]. Intraoperative measurement of changes in intragastric pressure and/or central venous pressure can serve as a guide to the operative management of congenital abdominal wall defect [55]. If the bowel cannot be reduced immediately, a Silastic silo is constructed to cover the gut and reduction is gradually accomplished over several days, with removal

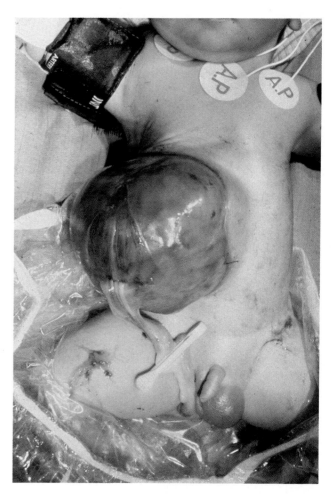

Figure 105.6 Giant omphalocele with hepatic and intestinal contents.

of the prosthesis wall as soon as possible to minimize septic complications [56] (Figure 105.7). This staged Silastic closure is used in cases of giant omphalocele with extracorporeal liver and in 20–40% of gastro-

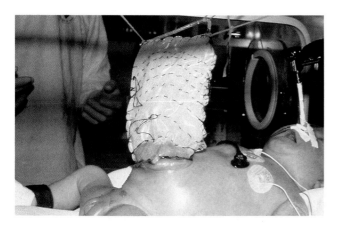

Figure 105.7 Giant omphalocele. Staged repair with a silastic chimney; gradual reduction allows complete abdominal closure and avoids excessive intra-abdominal pressure and respiratory disease.

schisis cases [51]. Nevertheless, primary fascial closure should be accomplished whenever it is possible to do so with reasonable effort. When intestinal atresia is encountered in gastroschisis, bowel resection and primary anastomosis can be performed; however, the anastomosis often fails to function. For this reason, resection and delayed anastomosis are recommended. The intestine appears nearly normal within 2–3 weeks of primary closure [38]. Re-exploration of the abdomen after initial abdominal closure, with or without jejunostomy or ileostomy, avoids extensive dissection and allows diagnosis and treatment of another, more distal atresia; the initially thick peel has resolved and the length of the intestine that has been difficult to appreciate at birth appears normal at the second operation [38]. In other series, treatment by the skin flap method, with secondary closure of the deliberately created abdominal hernia, or duraplastic enlargement of the anterior abdominal wall has been performed [57]. Nowadays, no prenatal experimental treatment has been attempted for abdominal wall defect. With hope of improvement in tocolysis and lack of adverse maternal effects, gastroschisis might in the future be an indication for early prenatal surgery to improve outcome.

105.6.5 FOLLOW-UP

Following initial surgical management, the infants are routinely started on a regimen of total parenteral nutrition; long-term hyperalimentation is instituted until the infant's gastrointestinal tract becomes functional. Ventilatory assistance with total paralysis is initially required.

Infants with gastroschisis are exposed to life-threatening complications: abdominal complications depending on pre-existing damage to the intestine and

on the increased intra-abdominal pressure resulting from closure. Intestinal ischaemia with prenatal loss of a large portion of the midgut, resulting in subsequent short gut syndrome, may be incompatible with life. Other complications encountered are necrotizing enterocolitis, bowel obstruction, aspiration pneumonia, intracranial haemorrhage and iatrogenic catheter-associated morbidity of total parenteral nutrition [58]. The mortality rate is today estimated at between 5 and 10% of livebirths (12.5% in Kirk and Wah's series [14], 6.8% in the present series, 4% in that of Crabbe et al. [51]). Prematurity, bowel infarction and sepsis are major causes of death in gastroschisis patients. The patients have an initial deficiency in the serum proteins, such as the γ-globulins and transferrin, necessary for defense against infection [59,60]. Postoperative intestinal ileus with absorption defect is prolonged [44,45,51].

The overall mortality rate of liveborn infants with omphalocele reported in the pediatric literature is between 20 and 50% [9,10]. Associated defects contributed heavily to neonatal morbidity among omphalocele cases [39]. Chromosomal abnormalities, ectopia cordis, pentalogy of Cantrell or extensive amniotic band syndrome have a poor prognosis for survival. Infants with Beckwith–Wiedeman syndrome have respiratory and feeding difficulties because of the large tongue and neonatal hypoglycaemia which have been implicated in the mild to moderate mental handicap noted in some of these infants. Malignant tumours have been reported in 10%. It is possible to expect a survival rate of 90% with isolated omphalocele. The morbidity is mainly related to the severity of the defect and the degree of prematurity. Giant omphalocele, even with herniation of the liver, presents a more difficult surgical challenge. Most common postoperative complications include sepsis, increased intra-abdominal pressure resulting from abdominal closure, aspiration pneumonia and iatrogenic ventilatory assistance-associated morbidity and total parenteral nutrition-associated liver disease and long hospital stay. Pulmonary insufficiency caused by narrow thoracic cage deformity and pulmonary hypoplasia may spoil the good outcome which can be anticipated in infants without associated anomalies.

Improvement in the care of babies born with omphalocele and gastroschisis would avoid many of the described intestinal and/or pulmonary sequelae and some degree of intellectual impairment reported by Berseth et al. [61]. That is the main goal of prenatal diagnosis of abdominal wall defects.

References

1. Cantrell, J.R., Haller, J.A., Ravitch, M.M. et al. (1958) A syndrome of congenital defects involving the abdominal wall, sternum, diaphragm, pericardium and heart. Surg. Gynecol. Obstet., 107, 602–14.

2. de Vries, P.A. (1980) The pathogenesis of gastroschisis and omphalocele. *J. Pediatr. Surg.*, **15**, 245–51.

3. Duhamel, B. (1963) Embryology of exomphalos and allied malformations. *Arch. Dis. Child.*, **38**, 142–47.

4. Gray, S.W. and Skandalakis, J.E. (1972) *Embryology for Surgeons*, W.B. Saunders, Philadelphia.

5. Hoyme, H.E., Jones, M.C. and Jones, K.J. (1983) Gastroschisis: abdominal wall disruption secondary to early gestational interruption of the omphalo-mesenteric artery. *Semin. Perinatol.*, **7**, 294–98.

6. Moore, T.C. and Nur, K. (1986) An international survey of gastroschisis and omphalocele (490 cases): I. Nature and distribution of additional malformations *Pediatr. Surg. Int.*, **1**, 46–50.

7. Moore, T.C. and Nur, K. (1986) An international survey of gastroschisis and omphalocele (490 cases); II. Relative incidence, pregnancy and environmental factors. *Pediatr. Surg. Int.*, **1**, 105–109.

8. Carpenter, M.W., Curci, M.R., Dibbins, A.W. and Haddow, J.E. (1984) Perinatal management of ventral wall defects. *Obstet. Gynecol.*, **64**, 646–51.

9. Yazbeck, S., Ndoye, M. and Khan, A.H. (1986) Omphalocele: a 25 years experience. *J. Pediatr. Surg.*, **21**, 761–63.

10. Knight, P.J., Sommer, A. and Clatworthy, H.W. (1981) Omphalocele: a prognostic classification. *J. Pediatr. Surg.*, **16**, 599–604.

11. Gilbert, W.M. and Nicolaides, K.H. (1987) Fetal omphalocele: associated malformations and chromosomal defects. *Obstet. Gynecol.*, **70**, 633–35.

12. Mann, L., Ferguson-Smith, H.A., Desai, M. *et al.* (1984) Prenatal assessment of anterior abdominal wall defects and their prognosis. *Prenat. Diagn.*, **4**, 427–35.

13. Nicolaides, K.H., Rodeck, C.H. and Gosden, C.M. (1986) Rapid karyotyping in non-lethal fetal malformations. *Lancet*, **i**, 283–86.

14. Kirk, E.P. and Wah, R.M. (1983) Obstetric management of the fetus with omphalocele or gastroschisis: a review and report of one hundred twelve cases. *Am. J. Obstet. Gynecol.*, **146**, 512–18.

15. Hershey, D.W., Haesslein, H.C., Marr, C.C. and Adkins, J.C. (1989) Familial abdominal wall defects. *Am. J. Med. Genet.*, **34**, 174–76.

16. Osuna, A. and Lindhan, S. (1976) Four cases of omphalocele in two generations of the same family. *Clin. Genet.*, **9**, 354–56.

17. Sapin, E., Kurzenne, J.Y., Bargy, F. and Hélardot P.G (1988) Laparoschisis hypotrophie et lésions intestinales. *Chir. Pédiatr.*, **29**, 1–6.

18. Jolleys, A. (1981) An examination of the birthweights of babies with some abnormalities of the alimentary tract. *J. Pediatr. Surg.*, **16**, 160–63.

19. Flake, A.W., Villa, R.L., Adzick, S.N. and Harrison, M.R. (1987) Transamniotic fetal feeding. II. A model of intrauterine growth retardation using the relationship of natural runting to uterine position. *J. Pediatr. Surg.*, **22**, 816–19.

20. Lev, R. and Orlic, D. (1972) Protein absorption by the intestine of the fetal rat *in utero*. *Science*, **177**, 522–23.

21. Pitkin, R.M. and Reynolds, W.A. (1975) Fetal ingestion and metabolism of amniotic fluid protein. *Am. J. Obstet. Gynecol.*, **123**, 356–63.

22. Gitlin, D., Kumate, J., Morales, C. *et al.* (1972) The turn-over of amniotic fluid protein in the human conceptus. *Am. J. Obstet. Gynecol.*, **113**, 632–45.

23. Charlton-Char, V. and Rudolph, A. (1979) Digestion and absorption of carbohydrates by the fetal lamb *in utero*. *Pediatr. Res.*, **13**, 1018–23.

24. Mulvihill, S.J., Stone, M.M., Debas, H.T. and Fonkalsrud, E.W. (1985) The role of amniotic fluid in fetal nutrition. *J. Pediatr. Surg.*, **20**, 668–72.

25. Mulvihill, S.J., Stone, M.M., Fonkalsrud, E.W. and Debas, H.T. (1986) Trophic effect of amniotic fluid on fetal gastro-intestinal development. *J. Surg. Res.*, **40**, 291–96.

26. Palomaki, G.E., Hill, L.E., Knight G.J. *et al.* (1988) Second-trimester maternal serum alpha-fetoprotein levels in pregnancies associated with gastroschisis and omphalocele. *Obstet. Gynecol.*, **71**, 906–909.

27. Glick, P.L., Polhson, E.C., Resta, R. *et al.* (1988) Maternal serum alphafetoprotein is a marker for fetal anomalies in pediatric surgery. *J. Pediatr. Surg.*, **23**, 16–20.

28. Goldfine, C., Miller, W.A. and Haddow, J.E. (1984) Amniotic fluid gel cholinesterase density ratios in fetal open defects of the neural tube and ventral wall. *Br. J. Obstet. Gynecol.*, **90**, 238–40.

29. Klück, P., Tibboel, D., Van Der Kamp, A.W.M. *et al.* (1984) The autonomous innervation of the bowel in gastroschisis: a histochemical study. *Ann. Paediatr. Surg.*, **1**, 117.

30. Amoury, R.A., Beatty, E.C., Wood, W.O. *et al.* (1988) Histology of the intestine in human gastroschisis – relationship to intestinal malfunction: dissolution of the 'peel' and its ultrastructural characteristics. *J. Pediatr. Surg.*, **23**, 950–56.

31. Klück, P., Tibboel, D., Van Der Kamp, A.W.M. *et al.* (1983) The effect of fetal urine on the development of the bowel in gastroschisis. *J. Pediatr. Surg.*, **18**, 47–50.

32. Tibboel, D., Vermey-Keers, C., Klück P. *et al.* (1986) The natural history of gastroschisis during fetal life: development of the fibrous coating on the bowel loops. *Teratology*, **33**, 367–72.

33. Langer, J.C., Longaker, M.T., Crombleholme, T.M. *et al.*. (1989) Etiology of intestinal damage in gastroschisis. I: Effects of amniotic fluid exposure and bowel constriction in a fetal lamb model. *J. Pediatr. Surg.*, **24**, 992–97.

34. Schmidt, W., Yarkoni, S., Crelin, E.S. and Hobbins, J.C. (1987) Sonographic visualization of physiologic anterior abdominal wall hernia in the first trimester. *Obstet. Gynecol.*, **69**, 911–15.

35. Curtis, J.A., and Watson, L. (1988) Sonographic diagnosis of omphalocele in the first trimester of fetal gestation. *J. Ultrasound. Med.*, **7**, 97–100.

36. Roberts, J.P. and Burge, D.M. (1990) Antenatal diagnosis of abdominal wall defects: a missed opportunity? *Arch. Dis. Child.*, **65** 687–89.

37. Sermer, M., Benzie, R.J., Pitson, L. *et al.* (1987) Prenatal diagnosis and management of congenital defects of the anterior abdominal wall. *Am. J. Obstet. Gynecol.*, **156**, 308–12.

38. Nakayama, D.K., Harrison, M.R., Gross, B.H. *et al.* (1984) Management of the fetus with an abdominal wall defect. *J. Pediatr. Surg.*, **19**, 408–13.

39. Vintzileos, A.M., Campbell, W.A., Nochimson, D.J. and Weinbaum, P.J. (1987) Antenatal evaluation and management of ultrasonically detected fetal anomalies. *Obstet. Gynecol.*, **69**, 640–60.

40. Langer, J.C. and Harrison, M.R. (1991) The fetus with abdominal wall defect, in *The Unborn Patient*, 2nd edn (eds M.R. Harrison, M.S. Golbus and R.A. Filly), W.B. Saunders, Philadelphia.

41. Benacerraf, B.R., Saltzman, D.H., Estrfoff, J.A. and Frigoletto, F.D. (1990) Abnormal karyotype of fetuses with omphalocele: prediction based on omphalocele contents. *Obstet. Gynecol.*, **75**, 317–19.

42. Nyberg, D., Fitzsimmons, J., Mack, L. *et al.* (1989) Chromosomal abnormalities in fetuses with omphalocele: significance of omphalocele contents. *J. Ultrasound Med.*, **8**, 299–308.

43. Nivelon-Chevallier, A., Mavel, A., Michiels, R. *et al.* (1983) Familial Beckwith–Wiedemann syndrome: prenatal echography, diagnosis and histologic confirmation. *J. Genet. Hum.*, **5**, 397–402.

44. Langer, J.C., Harrison, M.R., Adzick, N.S. *et al.* (1987) Perinatal management of the fetus with an abdominal wall defect. *Fetal Ther.*, **2**, 216–21.

45. Sapin, E., Lewin, F., Baron, J.M. *et al.* (1993) Prenatal diagnosis and management of gastroschisis. *Pediatr. Surg. Int.*, **8**, 31–33.

46. Bond, S.J., Harrison, M.R., Filly, R.A. *et al.* (1988) Severity of intestinal damage in gastroschisis: correlation with prenatal sonographic findings. *J. Pediatr. Surg.*, **23**, 520–21.

47. Fitzsimmons, J., Nyberg, D.A., Cyr, D.R. and Hatch, E. (1988) Perinatal management of gastroschisis. *Obstet. Gynecol.*, **71**, 910–13.

48. Moore, T.C. (1992) The role of labor in gastroschisis bowel thickening and prevention by elective preterm and pre-labor cesarean section. *Pediatr. Surg. Int.*, **7**, 256–59.

49. Lenke, R.R. and Hatch, E.I. (1986) Fetal gastroschisis: a preliminary report advocating the use of cesarean section. *Pediatr. Surg. Obstet. Gynecol.*, **67**, 395–98.

50. Bethel, C.A.I., Seashore, J.H. and Touluokian, R.J. (1989) Cesarean section does not improve outcome in gastroschisis. *J. Pediatr. Surg.*, **24**, 1–4.

51. Crabbe, C.G., Thomas, D.F.M., Beck, J.M. and Spicer, R.D. (1991) Prenatally diagnosed gastroschisis: a case for preterm delivery? *Pediatr. Surg. Int.*, **6**, 108–10.

52. Pokorny, W.J., Harberg, F.J. and McGill, C.W. (1981) Gastroschisis complicated by intestinal atresia. *J. Pediatr. Surg.*, **16**, 261–63.

53. Caniano, D.A., Brokaw, B, and Ginn-Pease, M.E. (1990) An individualized approach to the management of gastroschisis. *J. Pediatr. Surg.*, **25**, 297–300.

54. Mercer, S., Mercer, B., D'Alton, M.E.G. *et al.* (1988) Gastroschisis: ultrasonographic diagnosis, perinatal embryology, surgical and obstetric treatment and outcome. *Can. J. Surg.*, **31**, 25–26.

55. Wesley, J.R., Drongowski, R. and Coran, A.G. (1981) Intragastric pressure measurement: a guide for reduction and closure of the silastic chimney in omphalocele and gastroschisis. *J. Pediatr. Surg.*, **16**, 264–70.

56. Hallen, R.G. and Wrenn, E.L. (1969) Silon as a sac in the treatment of omphalocele and gastroschisis. *J. Pediatr. Surg.*, **4**, 3–8.

57. Klein, P., Hummer, H.P., Wellert, S. and Faber, T. (1991) Short-term and long-term problems after duraplastic enlargement of anterior abdominal wall. *Eur. J. Pediatr. Surg.*, **1**, 88–91.

58. Oldham, K.T., Coran, A.G., Drongowski, R.A. *et al.* (1988) The development of necrotizing enterocolitis following repair of gastroschisis: a surprisingly high incidence. *J. Pediat. Surg.*, **23**, 945–49.

59. Mabogunje, O.A. and Mahour, G.H. (1984) Omphalocele and gastroschisis; trends in survival across two decades. *Am. J. Surg.*, **148**, 680–86.

60. Gutenberger, J.E., Miller, D.L., Dibbins, A.W. and Gitlin, D. (1973) Hypogammaglobulinemia and hypoalbuminemia in neonates with ruptured omphaloceles and gastroschisis. *J. Pediat. Surg.*, **8**, 353–59.

61. Berseth, C.L., Malachowski, N., Cohn, R.B. *et al.* (1982) Longtitudinal growth and late morbidity of survivors of gastroschisis and omphalocele. *J. Pediatr. Gastroenterol. Nutr.*, **1**, 375–79.

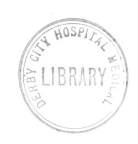

106 IMMUNOLOGICAL RECONSTITUTION OF PRIMARY IMMUNODEFICIENCIES IN THE NEONATAL PERIOD

R.U. Sorensen

106.1 Introduction

Several alternative strategies are available for the immunological reconstitution of primary immunodeficiency syndromes in neonates and young infants. These treatment modalities include the use of fetal lymphocyte progenitors, identical and haploidentical bone marrow transplantation, peripheral blood white cell transfusions, thymus transplants, the use of various cytokines, enzyme replacement therapy and gene therapy. Each of these methods has advantages and limitations which have to be analyzed in the context of the severity and pathogenesis of each congenital immunodeficiency syndrome.

The pathogenesis of all congenital immunodeficiency diseases includes the effect of the primary abnormality, plus the secondary effect of recurrent infections, malnutrition and possibly also malignancies and graft-versus-host disease (GVHD). Early diagnosis and treatment, before the onset of complications, is an important aspect of the effective management of congenital immunodeficiency diseases. Since an immunoglobulin or specific antibody deficiency is part of many congenital immunodeficiencies, IgG replacement therapy is an important adjunct to the management of these diseases. Passive IgG antibodies do not correct the primary defect, but protect against the damaging effect of infections. When blood transfusions are necessary in a patient with deficient cellular immunity, avoidance of graft-versus-host reactions caused by the transfusion of viable lymphocytes in blood products is crucial. GVHD can be very resistant to treatment, and it has the potential for endangering immunological reconstitution (Chapter 88).

106.2 Cell and tissue engraftment

The permanent engraftment of normal cells to provide the immunological functions which are defective is the optimal form of treatment for all immunodeficiency syndromes. The engraftment of normal cells in immunodeficiency syndromes is usually achieved without, or with only partial ablation of host hematopoietic cells. Consequently, various degrees of chimerism may exist. In split chimerism of lymphocyte subpopulations, T cells are of donor origin, and B cells are of host origin. Engrafted donor cells may enable host cells to normalize functions which are dependent on cell-to-cell collaboration.

The engraftment of foreign cells needs to be considered in the light of several crucial aspects concerning cell transplantation. Foremost are the degree of histocompatibility between the host and the donor, the degree of residual immunity present in the immunodeficient patient, and the need to engraft lymphocytes alone or in combination with other cell lines, e.g. platelets in the Wiskott–Aldrich syndrome, or all hematopoietic series after deep marrow ablation in hematologic malignancies.

Histocompatibility is the major determinant of the outcome of any cell transplant. In transplantation of immune cells, it determines both the acceptance of the transplant and the development of GVHD (Figure 106.1). Human leukocyte histocompatibility antigens (HLAs) are encoded by genes on the short arm of chromosome 6. They are grouped into major histocompatibility complexes (MHCs), each of which has several antigens. The full complement of histocompatibility antigens encoded in one chromosome is called a haplotype. Haplotypes are usually inherited in one block, unless crossovers occur within this region. Each

Diseases of the Fetus and Newborn, 2nd edn, Edited by G.B. Reed, A.E. Claireaux and F. Cockburn. Published in 1995 by Chapman & Hall, London. ISBN 0 412 39160 0

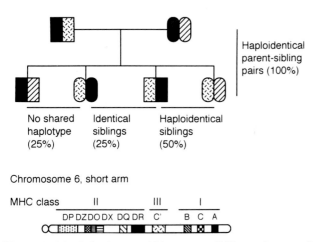

Figure 106.1 Inheritance of histocompatibility antigens and donor selection for allogeneic bone marrow transplantation. Each child inherits one haplotype, or complete set of major histocompatibility antigens, from each parent. There is a 25% chance for two siblings to inherit the same haplotype from each parent and to be identical. If only one haplotype is shared, the siblings are haploidentical. Histocompatibility antigens are grouped in major histocompatibility complexes (MHCs) I, II and III. In addition, there are many minor determinants which may account for differences between individuals who are identical for MHC I and MHC II.

antigen encoded by genes of both chromsomes is expressed on the surface of most nucleated cells, so that each cell will express two A, two B, and two DR antigens, as well as other major and minor histocompatibility antigens (Figure 106.2). Major histocompatibility antigens differ from minor histocompatibility antigens in that they elicit strong T-cell reactions without need for priming or *in vivo* immunization.

When all major and minor histocompatibility antigens are identical, as in monozygotic twins, donor and recipient are said to be syngeneic. In humans, most donor recipient pairs are allogeneic to one another, denoting that there usually are at least some differences, with the potential of causing graft rejections or GVHD. Cells which recognize and react against foreign HLAs are called alloreactive cells. There is a 25% chance that two siblings will be identical for A, B and DR antigens. Parents and their offspring, and 50% of sibling pairs, are haploidentical to each other, indicating that one haplotype will be identical, and the other will be different (Figure 106.2). The chances of identifying two unrelated individuals that are matched for A, B and DR antigens in the general population is very small, and depends on the frequency of the expression of given antigens in the population examined.

The development of tolerance to self HLAs, which occurs in the thymus, is another important aspect of cell transplantation (see also Chapter 88). In the thymus, T cells with receptors for self histocompatibility antigens are eliminated, and T cells which recognize foreign antigen presented in the context of self MHC I or II antigens are positively selected. Positive selection is probably a function of the epithelial cells of the thymus, while deletion of self-reacting T cells is more a function of marrow derived antigen-presenting cells [1]. Not all self antigens are present in the developing thymus, and additional mechanisms of peripheral tolerance are necessary for the control of mature T cells with self-reactive receptors [2]. Mature T cells do not return to the thymus, and their tolerance and recognition patterns cannot be changed through this mechanism. Therefore, there is a fundamental difference between transplantation of histocompatible

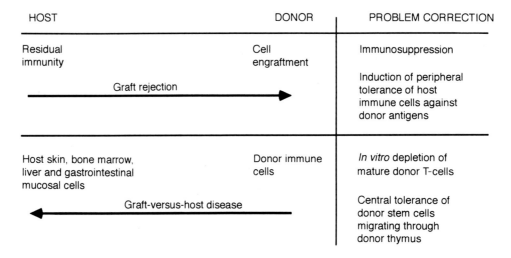

Figure 106.2 Allogeneic cell engraftment. Immunodeficient patients without residual cellular immunity will not reject a foreign graft. However, they are likely to develop a graft-versus-host disease if the mature, immunologically competent donor cells recognize different histocompatibility antigens on host cells. For patients with residual immunity, immunosuppression is usually necessary even when the donor is compatible for all major histocompatibility antigens.

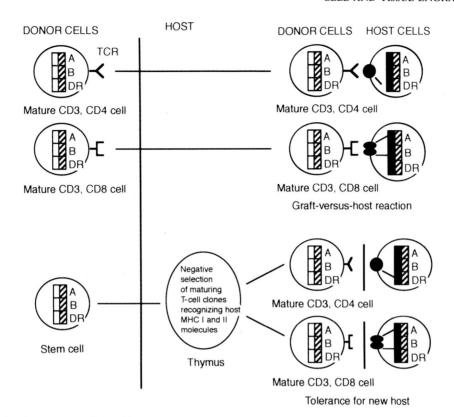

Figure 106.3 Role of mature T cells and hematopoietic stem cells in haploidentical bone marrow transplantation. The T-cell receptor (TCR) of mature T cells will recognize the non-identical histocompatibility antigen on host cells and cause graft-versus-host disease. CD4+ T-helper cells recognize class II molecules, and CD8+ T suppressor cells recognize class I histocompatibility antigens. Stem cells are selected in the host thymus, and those with TCRs capable of recognizing host histocompatibility antigens are eliminated.

cells from an HLA matched donor, and transplantation of partially HLA compatible or incompatible cells.

Transplantation of both mature T cells and stem cells from a compatible donor leads to engraftment of both types of cells. T cells play an important role in immunological reconstitution and probably also in the growth and engraftment of transplanted stem cells. In haploidentical or partially identical bone marrow transplantation, mature T cells can cause GVHD by reacting against different HLAs of the host (Figure 106.3). Due to CD4, T-helper and CD8, T-suppressor–cytotoxic cell collaboration, the graft-versus-host reaction is stronger when there are differences in both MHC class I and II antigens: class II antigens will be recognized by donor helper cells, which will enhance the reaction of cytotoxic cells directed against class I antigens.

In haploidentical bone marrow transplantation, mature T cells need to be depleted, and engraftment occurs from stem cells. These will migrate through the host thymus, and become tolerant to the host's HLAs if host antigen presenting cells are present. Interestingly, these cells will not be made tolerant for their own, donor HLAs, unless donor antigen presenting cells migrate and establish themselves in the host thymus, in

which case maturing T cells may become tolerant to both host and donor antigens [3]. When host antigen presenting cells are deficient in the thymus, tolerance to host antigens may fail and GVHD is more likely to occur even if no mature alloreactive T cells are transplanted. If no donor antigen presenting cells migrate to the thymus, it is possible that lack of tolerance of mature donor T cells to donor HLAs may hinder the engraftment of B lymphocytes (and also of antigen presenting cells) which express donor MHC class II antigens constitutively.

Donor stem cells migrating and maturing in the host thymus are also positively selected to recognize foreign antigen presented in the context of the host's MHC class I and II antigens (Figure 106.4). This is an important step which allows T cells of donor origin to interact with host antigen presenting cells and virally infected host cells. It is presently unclear if there is any restriction in the recognition of antigen in the context of MHC products which are different from those of the engrafted cells.

Stem cells obtained from unrelated fetal tissues are usually completely HLA incompatible. As in haploidentical bone marrow transplantation, stem cells are

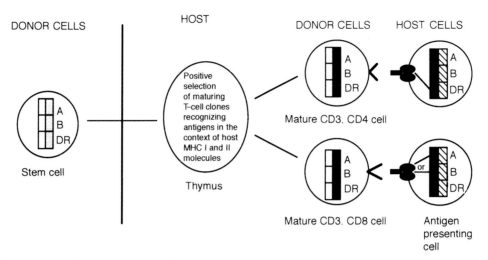

Figure 106.4 Recognition of antigen presented in the context of host histocompatibility antigens in haploidentical bone marrow transplantation. Donor stem cells that recognize antigen in the context of host histocompatibility antigens are positively selected for survival and export to peripheral lymphoid organs in the host thymus. The T-cell receptors of these cells are specific for the presented antigen, and not for the histocompatibility molecules without a foreign antigen.

more likely to become tolerant to different histocompatibility antigens than mature, post-thymic cells. These mature cells need to be eliminated from the sources of fetal tissue to avoid GVHD. There is limited experience to determine to what extent negative and positive selection in the host thymus is affected by the complete absence of HLA identity in these situations.

The rejection of transplanted cells by residual, mature T lymphocytes from the host poses a different problem. These host cells obviously cannot be educated in the donor thymus. Thus far, the approach has been to facilitate acceptance of donor cells using cytoreduction of the residual host immunity. This form of treatment is detrimental to the host, and may also be detrimental to the engraftment of donor cells. It is quite possible that recent results with the induction of peripheral tolerance of mature T cells to specific histocompatibility antigens will be used advantageously to overcome this problem in the future [4,5].

106.2.1 FETAL LYMPHOCYTE PROGENITORS

The earliest accessible fetal lymphocyte progenitors are found in the liver. As early as 1958, it was observed experimentally that hematopoietic liver cells from 2-week-old mouse fetuses reconstituted immunocompetence after transplantation into irradiated allogeneic hosts, while bone marrow or fetal liver cells obtained close to term caused GVHD [6]. Studies of human fetuses revealed that hematopoietic fetal liver cells obtained before 7.5 weeks do not react *in vitro* against allogeneic cells from adult donors [7]. Liver cells from older fetuses show some allogeneic responses even before migration to the thymus. However, these early allogeneic reactions do not appear to be due to

specific alloantigen recognition, which occurs only after maturation in the thymus [8].

Cells capable of specific recognition of different histocompatibility antigens were found in the thymus of a 12-week-old fetus, and in the spleen of a 15-week-old fetus. Only faint specific alloreactivity was found in the liver at later stages of fetal development, probably due to the presence of post-thymic cells in the liver. The information about absent or decreased alloreactivity in early liver cells was applied to the treatment of infants with severe combined immunodeficiency who did not have HLA-identical bone marrow donors [9–12]. However, in some patients GVHD developed after fetal liver cells obtained from fetuses as early as 4–5 weeks of gestation, before cell migration to the thymus [9,11]. Further understanding of the development of alloreactivity in fetal liver cells has been delayed by the restriction of the use of fetal tissue, and by the development of alternative sources of stem cells in bone marrow, cord blood and even peripheral blood (see later).

Liver cell transplants from 8–13-week-old fetuses given with simultaneous administrations of irradiated thymus tissue led to successful immunological reconstitution in some patients with severe combined immunodeficiency, despite the absence of any HLA identity [13]. The beneficial effect of combined fetal liver and thymus transplants may be particularly effective in some patients with severe combined immunodeficiency in whom both lymphoid stem cell and thymus functional defects are present [14]. Interestingly, in one patient receiving this form of treatment, T cells were shown to be of donor origin, while B cells were of host origin. Despite the differences in HLA antigens, cooperation between T cells and B cells appeared to be normal, and no graft-versus-host reaction occurred [15].

106.2.2 BONE MARROW TRANSPLANTATION

Bone marrow is an ideal source of cells for long-term reconstitution of immunodeficiency syndromes because of its richness in hematopoietic stem cells and the relative ease with which large amounts of cells can be harvested. In addition to stem cells, bone marrow samples contain abundant peripheral blood T lymphocytes which help rapid immunological reconstitution in HLA identical recipients and cause GVHD if they are not identical.

There are several sources of bone marrow for transplantation, as follows.

1. HLA matched donors. These are HLA identical twins or siblings, and also, occasionally, parents, grandparents or unrelated donors. HLA identical siblings are increasingly difficult to identify as the size of average sibships continues to decrease. In rare situations, when both parents share one haplotype, it is possible for one parent to be identical with the patient. In inbred families which share common haplotypes, even more distant relatives may be HLA identical [16].
2. Unrelated individuals may also share the same HLAs with a patient. These identical, unrelated donors are becoming available for some patients requiring bone marrow transplantation through the National Bone Marrow Registry [17]. Identical donors are very difficult to find for patients with less frequent HLAs, e.g. members of ethnic groups less intensively studied thus far.
3. Haploidentical donors, who share one haplotype with the recipient, are available whenever there is a parent, or in most instances of available siblings (Figure 106.1). Partially identical donors, who share several, but not all HLAs with the patient, can occasionally be found among family members. In haploidentical transplantation, GVHD will inevitably occur if T cells are not depleted from the bone marrow. Two approaches have been taken to prepare bone marrow for this form of transplantation.
   (a) Depletion of T lymphocytes using lectin columns. Lectins are plant glycoproteins known to react with receptors present on all T lymphocytes. These lectins can be immobilized within columns which allow the passage of cells. T lymphocytes with receptors for these lectins will be retained, while other cells flow through the column [18]. This treatment has been shown to eliminate over 99% of mature T lymphocytes, and all reactivity against allogeneic cells and mitogens [19].

   (b) Depletion of T cell with monoclonal antibodies. Depletion of T lymphocytes is achieved using monoclonal antibodies alone [20] or in combination with rosetting with sheep red cells [21].

Identical bone marrow transplantation for immunodeficiency diseases has a high success rate, although GVHD occurs in some cases. The results of haploidentical bone marrow transplantation are improving continually, as better methods to deplete mature T cells, and new strategies for the enhancement of engraftment are developed [22]. The use of T cell depleted haploidentical bone marrow has reduced the risk of GVHD [18,23,24]. However, engraftment of T lymphocytes is very slow and patients remain at risk for severe infections for several months. In addition, defective humoral immunity after haploidentical bone marrow transplantation may persist requiring long-term IgG replacement therapy [22,23,25].

106.2.3 PERIPHERAL BLOOD CELL TRANSFUSIONS

HLA compatible peripheral blood leukocyte transfusions can be used to reconstitute immunological function in patients with severe combined immunodeficiency. Although stem cells capable of reconstituting all hematologic cell lines can be found in peripheral blood [26], and particularly in cord blood [27], the immunological reconstitution is probably due to the engraftment of mature T lymphocytes. This possibility has been highlighted by an isolated instance in which peripheral blood leukocytes had to be substituted for bone marrow [16]. In this patient with severe combined immunodeficiency, rapid and persistent restoration of antibody and cell mediated immunity was seen after an infusion of compatible peripheral blood leukocytes. Donor lymphocytes were repeatedly demonstrated in the patient's peripheral blood, but not in the bone marrow. This patient has remained clinically well for 12 years after the leukocyte transfusion. Although it is possible that the long-term reconstitution was due to engraftment of peripheral blood stem cells, the positive role of mature cells in this patient's immunological reconstitution is evident.

106.2.4 THYMUS TRANSPLANTS

Thymus transplants alone have been used for immunological reconstitution of a few patients with the DiGeorge syndrome and various other cellular immunodeficiency syndromes [28]. In addition, fetal thymus transplantation has been used to enhance engraftment of fetal liver cells in severe combined immunodeficiency [13]. In patients with the DiGeorge syndrome, restoration of thymus function appears to enable the patients' own lymphoid precursor cells to undergo a normal development [29]. The role of thymus transplantation or of the administration of various thymic factors in patients with other forms of immunodeficiency is less clear. When thymus transplants are performed mainly to provide a hormonal environment with thymic hormones to provide T-cell maturation, the structure of engrafted thymus tissues may not be important. However, it has not been established if thymus cells injected intraperitoneally, subcutaneously or intramuscularly can provide the structure necessary to positively and negatively select maturing T cells derived from migrating stem cells. Recently, maturation and positive selection of immature, double-positive CD4 and CD8 positive cells using thymus stromal cell preparations was achieved *in vitro* [30], but it remains to be shown if this is sufficient to completely restore thymic function *in vivo*.

Two sources of thymus tissue have been used for thymus transplantation: portions of adult thymuses removed during cardiac surgery, and fetal thymuses. Adult thymuses are contaminated with mature, incompatible donor T cells capable of causing GVHD [31]. Long-term culture procedures used to decontaminate thymus tissue from mature T cells may also alter its functional capability. Since lymphocyte migration to the thymus occurs as early as week 10 of gestation, many fetal thymuses need to be irradiated to prevent GVHD, adding a potentially detrimental step in the use of this tissue [13].

Fetal thymus transplants have been successful in the reconstitution of some patients with the DiGeorge syndrome [32] and with the Nezelof syndrome [13]. Transplantation of fetal thymus tissue alone has had dismal results in patients with severe combined immunodeficiency [12]. Despite an initial report of successful reconstitution of a patient with severe combined immunodeficiency with cultured thymus epithelium [34], the development of fatal B-cell immunoblastic lymphomas in three patients has cast significant doubts on the safety of this procedure [35].

106.3 Cytokine therapy

Decreased interleukin-2 production has been described in patients with severe combined immunodeficiency syndromes including adenosine deaminase deficiency [36–40]. Selective interleukin-2 deficiency may lead to milder forms of cellular immunodeficiency [41]. Several patients with interleukin-2 deficiency have improved lymphocyte blastogenic responses upon addition of interleukin-2 *in vitro* [37–41]. Notably, therapy with recombinant interleukin-2 resulted in marked immunological and clinical improvement in one patient with severe combined immunodeficiency [39]. The long-term outcome of this therapy is not known.

Interferon-γ added *in vitro* to granulocytes and monocytes from patients with X-linked chronic granulomatous disease partially corrected the defective superoxide production in some patients [42]. A double-blind, placebo-controlled trial showed that the use of interferon-γ in patients with chronic granulomatous disease resulted in significantly fewer illnesses requiring hospitalization [43]. This result was observed despite the lack of significant changes in superoxide production by phagocytes, suggesting that the mechanisms of action, and the long-term effectiveness of interferon in this disease needs further study.

106.4 Enzyme replacement therapy

Enzyme replacement therapy has become available for patients with immunodeficiency due to adenosine deaminase (ADA) deficiency. This form of treatment was initially performed using red blood cell exchange transfusions [44]. Recently, the introduction of polyethyleneglycol treated ADA (PEG-ADA) has greatly simplified enzyme replacement. The PEG treatment of ADA increased the half-life of ADA from less than 30 minutes to 30 hours in mice and decreased the enzyme's immunogenicity, without altering the enzymatic activity [45]. In humans, PEG-ADA replacement therapy with 20–30 u/kg i.m., weekly resulted in correction of the metabolic abnormalities, followed by improvement in immune function and clinical status [46–48]. The reconstitution of immunological function from the patient's own stem cells is suggested by the increase in the size of the thymus shortly after initiation of enzyme replacement (Figure 106.5) [47,48].

The PEG-ADA experience has now been extended to 35 patients, including 25 treated for more than 1 year. Significant, though partial recovery of immune function is seen in most patients, but all treated patients have shown clinical improvement [48]. No adverse effects have been encountered. Neutralizing anti-ADA antibody formation occurred in two patients treated with PEG-ADA after 4 to 5 months of treatment. Induction of tolerance in one patient was achieved by stopping PEG-ADA therapy for 8 weeks, and then resuming the treatment by administering the PEG-ADA twice-weekly along with weekly intravenous immune globulin infusions and steroids for 4 months [49]. The second patient continues to receive two injections a week (M.S. Hershfield, personal comunication). PEG-ADA treatment has not been discontinued in any patient due to intolerance or lack of effectiveness. Its long-term effectiveness needs to be monitored as more experience with this treatment modality accumulates.

106.5 Gene therapy

Severe combined immunodeficiency due to ADA deficiency has been the first human disease targeted for

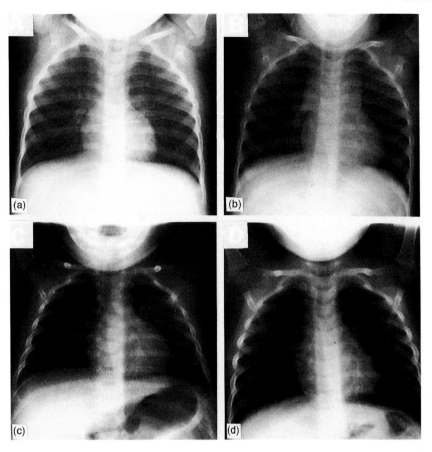

Figure 106.5 Thymus size 2 months after adenosine replacement therapy (upper panel) or identical bone marrow transplantation (lower panel). Before therapy (left), no thymus is visible in either patient with severe combined immunodeficiency. After correction of the biochemical abnormalities in adenosine deaminase deficiency, there is visible enlargement of this organ, probably due to a massive migration of stem cells to the thymus. With identical bone marrow transplantation, mature T lymphocytes in the transfused bone marrow bypass the thymus. A smaller amount of donor stem cells migrating through the host thymus does not lead to a visible enlargement of the thymus in most cases.

gene therapy. In this disease, adenosine deaminase deficiency leads to build-up of deoxyadenosine triphosphate (dATP) which is toxic to cells. Therefore, introduction of a functional human ADA gene expressing ADA activity could reverse the immunological disorder caused by ADA deficiency. This concept is reinforced by reappearance of functional lymphocytes with ADA enzyme replacement therapy. It is generally considered that introduction of the ADA gene into stem cells from the patient is more likely to produce adequate long-term results, while introduction of the gene into mature T cells may be limited by the life span of these cells. In general, however, various forms of gene transfer are more readily achieved with mature T cells. These cells are easily isolated in large quantities, and they can be induced to proliferate *in vitro*, facilitating gene transfer procedures. In contrast, stem cells constitute a very small percentage of bone marrow cells, and *in vitro* proliferation is difficult to achieve. To date, most human ADA cDNA insertions have been performed using retroviral vectors which insert ran-

domly into the genome, leaving the the mutant ADA genes intact. It has been proposed that true correction of specific mutations in the ADA genes of stem cells should involve homologous recombination using strategies that have been employed in developing gene knockouts [50].

Long-term expression of human ADA cDNA in multiple hematopoietic and lymphoid lineages after transplantation of retrovirally transfected marrow has been achieved in mice [51]. Large amounts of marrow were required in these experiments, and the patterns of tissue expression of ADA were variable. These experiments in mice are unlikely to be an adequate model for establishing procedures for stem cell ADA gene therapy in humans. Recently, long-term expression of human ADA was achieved in rhesus monkeys using a combination of vectors and enhancers to increase the chances of stable expression in stem cells [52]. Gene transfers of adenosine deaminase into human hematopoietic stem cells are in progress [53].

A proposal to introduce an ADA gene into mature T

cells was approved by the NIH Recombinant DNA Advisory Committe in July 1990, and the first treatment in a patient with severe combined immunodeficiency was started in September that year [54]. A second patient with a milder form of cellular immunodeficiency due to ADA deficiency [46] was started subsequently. Both patients had already shown significant improvement on enzyme replacement therapy [48], and have been maintained on enzyme replacement during and after the gene therapy experiments. It is presently unknown if cells now expressing the ADA gene will be able to expand sufficiently to maintain these patients' immunity, and if they will be able to provide sufficient enzyme activity to prevent the accumulation of toxic metabolites. Further patient enrolment into this protocol has been suspended until the success of gene therapy is evaluated after enzyme replacement is discontinued.

106.6 Treatment of specific immunodeficiency syndromes

Long-lasting reconstitution of immune function thus far has been achieved only with the engraftment of lymphocytic cells from different sources. All treatment forms with cytokines or enzymes are effective only as long as their administration is continued. Attempts to achieve similar long-lasting effects with gene therapy are in progress. A summary of the current treatment alternatives for some of the primary immunodeficiencies is shown in Table 106.1.

106.6.1 SEVERE COMBINED IMMUNODEFICIENCY DISEASES

Identical bone marrow transplantation is the treatment of choice of all forms of severe combined immunodeficiency syndrome. The early referral of patients with a family history of the syndrome, before development of complications, as well as the early recognition of sporadic cases significantly improves the outcome and reduces the cost of this procedure [55].

Partially identical bone marrow transplantation is indicated in severe combined immunodeficiency. Although this form of bone marrow treatment has made bone marrow transplantation available to many patients who do not have an identical donor, some patient groups do not respond as well as others.

Table 106.1 Treatment and immunological reconstitution of some congenital primary immunodeficiency syndromes

Deficiency	Treatment/reconstitution
Combined immunodeficiencies All forms (including leukocyte adherence deficiency)	Preferred: identical bone marrow transplantation from a related donor Alternative: haploidentical bone marrow transplantation; identical bone marrow transplantation, unrelated donor Experimental; fetal liver stem cells (plus fetal thymus?); identical, mature T cell infusion
Adenosine deaminase deficiency	Alternative: enzyme replacement Experimental: gene therapy
Interleukin-2 deficiency	Alternative: interleukin-2 replacement
Wiskott–Aldrich syndrome	Preferred: identical bone marrow transplantation, related or unrelated donor Alternative: identical bone marrow transplantation from unrelated donor
DiGeorge syndrome Partial	Observation only: frequent spontaneous improvement
Severe	Preferred: identical bone marrow transplantation, related or unrelated donor Experimental: thymic epithelium, thymic hormones
Chronic granulomatous disease	Preferred: cytochrome b production enhancement with interferon-γ Alternative: identical bone marrow transplantation

Patients with X-linked severe combined immuno-deficiency frequently have only their cellular immunity restored, but remain hypogammaglobulinemic and require long-term IgG replacement therapy [22]. In some series, the success rate of haploidentical bone marrow transplantation has been lower in patients with ADA deficiency than in patients with normal ADA activity [23,24], and antibody function in particular may be inadequate in patients receiving haploidentical bone marrow [56].

At the present time, enzyme replacement therapy and haploidentical bone marrow transplantation cannot be attempted simultaneously in the same patient. Since enzyme replacement is likely to produce a significant improvement in immune functions, it will jeopardize the engraftment of partially identical cells. Therefore, some authors recommend that a haploidentical trans-plantation should first be attempted, and enzyme replacement therapy used only if there is a failure in establishing a functional engraftment of normal cells [22]. Decisions regarding individual patients have to take into account the most recent results, including success rates and risks of both modalities of treatment, and also the feasibility of each treatment in the setting of the patient's care.

106.6.2 WISKOTT–ALDRICH SYNDROME

Both lymphocytes and platelets are affected in this disease, and bone marrow transplants provide stem cells capable of correcting both abnormalities. Since cel-lular immunity is only partially affected in the disease, cytoreductive treatments are required for acceptance of the graft [57]. While identical bone marrow trans-plantation from both related or unrelated donors has been successful [17], the use of haploidentical, T-cell depleted bone marrow in this disease is still experimental.

106.6.3 DiGEORGE SYNDROME

In this syndrome, lymphoid stem cells are not affected, but their maturation into functional T cells is hampered by the lack of a thymus. Immunological reconstitution is necessary only in patients with severe forms of the DiGeorge syndrome, where slow, spontaneous T-cell maturation due to residual thymus tissues is unlikely to occur. Bone marrow transplantation from an identical donor has been successful in some patients, probably because of the engraftment of mature T lymphocytes which no longer require a thymus [58,59]. Fetal thymus transplantation may be attempted when such tissues are available and no identical donor can be identified.

For the above immunodeficiency syndromes, as well as for many other syndromes not described here, new

therapeutic strategies are being developed. They all hinge on a better understanding of the pathophysiology of these immunodeficiencies. The experience which is accumulating with these different experiments of nature has been a driving force in the progress in our understanding of the developing human immune system.

References

1. Marrack, P., Lo, D. and Brinster, R. (1988) The effect of thymus environment on T cell development and tolerance. *Cell*, 53, 627–34.
2. Roser, B.J. (1989) Cellular mechanisms in neonatal and adult tolerance. *Immunol. Rev.*, 107, 179–85.
3. DeVillartay, J., Griscelli, C. and Fischer, A. (1986) Self tolerance to host and donor following HLA-mismatched bone marrow transplantation. *Eur. J. Immunol.*, 16, 117–22.
4. Maeda, T., Eto, M., Nishimura, Y. *et al.* (1993) Role of peripheral hemopoietic chimerism in achieving donor-specific tolerance in adult mice. *J. Immunol.*, 150, 753–62.
5. Sidhu, S., Deacock, S., Bal, V. *et al.* (1992) Human T cells cannot act as autonomous antigen-presenting cells, but induce tolerance in antigen-specific and alloreactive responder cells. *J. Exp. Med.*, 76, 875–80.
6. Uphoff, D.E. (1958) Preclusion of secondary phase of irradiation syndrome by inoculation of fetal hematopoietic tissue following lethal total-body X irradiation. *J. Natl Cancer Inst.*, 20, 625–32.
7. Sites, D.P., Carr, M.C. and Fudenberg, H.H. (1974) Ontogeny of cellular immunity in the human fetus. Development of responses to phytohemagg-lutinin and to allogeneic cells. *Cell. Immunol.*, 11, 257–71.
8. Asantila, T., Vahala, J. and Toivanen, P. (1974) Generation of functional diversity of T-cell receptors. *Immunogenetics*, 1, 407–15.
9. Buckley, R.H., Whisnant, J.K., Schiff, R.J. *et al.* (1976) Correction of severe combined immunodeficiency by fetal liver cells. *N. Engl J. Med.*, 294, 1076–81.
10. Keightley, R.G., Lawton, A.R., Cooper, M.D. and Yunis, E.J. (1975) Successful fetal liver transplant in a child with severe combined immuno-deficiency. *Lancet*, ii, 850–53.
11. Rieger, C.H., Lustig, J.V., Hirschhorn, R. and Rothberg, R.M. (1977) Reconstitution of T-cell function in severe combined immunodeficiency disease following transplantation of early embryonic liver cells. *J. Pediatr.*, 90, 707–12.
12. Touraine, J.-L., Griscelli, C., Vossen, J. *et al.* (1983) Fetal tissue transplantation for severe combined immunodeficiency: European exper-ience. *Tranplant. Proc.*, 15, 1427–30.
13. Royo, C. and Touraine, J.-L. (1990) Prenatal diagnosis and early treatment of immunodeficiencies in man, in *The Immunology of the Fetus* (ed. G. Chaouat), CRC Press, Boca Raton, FL, pp. 97–111.
14. Pahwa, R., Pahwa, S., Good, R.A. *et al.* (1977) Rationale for the use of fetal liver and thymus for immunological reconstitution of patients with variants of severe combined immunodeficiency. *Proc. Natl Acad. Sci. USA*, 74, 3002–3003.
15. Roncarolo, M.G., Touraine, J.L. and Banchereau, J. (1986) Cooperation between major histocompatibility complex mismatched mononuclear cells from a human chimera in the production of antigen-specific antibody. *J. Clin. Invest.*, 77, 673–80.
16. Polmar, S.H., Schacter, B.Z. and Sorensen, R.U. (1986) Long-term immunological reconstitution by peripheral blood leukocytes in severe combined immunodeficiency disease: implication for the role of mature lymphocytes in histocompatible bone marrow transplantation. *Clin. Exp. Immunol.*, 64, 518–25.
17. Kersey, J., Filipovich, A., McGleave, P. *et al.* (1993) Donor and host influences in bone marrow transplantation for immunodeficiency diseases and leukemia. *Semin. Hematol.*, 30, S105–109.
18. Reisner, Y., Kapoor, N., Kirkpatrick, D. *et al.* (1983) Transplantation for severe combined immunodeficiency with HLA-A, B, D, DR incompatible parental marrow cells fractionated by soybean agglutinin and sheep red blood cells. *Blood*, 61, 341–48.
19. Autran, B., Beuajean, F., Pillier, C. *et al.* (1987) T-cell depletion of bone marrow transplants: assessment of standard immunological methods of quantification. *Exp. Hematol.*, 15, 1121–27.
20. Parkman, R. (1986) Antibody-treated bone marrow transplantation for patients with severe combined immune deficiency. *Clin. Immunol. Immu-nopathol.*, 40, 142–46.
21. Morgan, M., Linch, D.C., Knott, L.T. and Sieff, D.C. (1986) Successful haploidentical mismatched bone marrow transplantation in severe com-

bined immunodeficiency: T cell removal using CAMPATH-1 monoclonal antibody and E-rosetting. *Br. J. Haematol.*, **62**, 421–30.

22. Buckley, R.H., Schiff, S.E., Schiff, R.I. *et al.* (1993) Haploidentical bone marrow stem cell transplantation in human severe combined immunodeficiency disease. *Semin. Hematol.*, **30**, S92–104.

23. O'Reilly, R.J., Keever, C.A., Small, T.N. and Brochstein, J. (1989) The use of HLA-non-identical T-cell-depleted marrow transplants for the correction of severe combined immunodeficiency disease. *Immunodefic. Rev.*, **1**, 273–309.

24. Fischer, A., Landais, P., Friedrich, W. *et al.* (1990) Clinical practice: European experience of bone-marrow transplantation for severe combined immunodeficiency. *Lancet*, **ii**, 850–54.

25. Wijnaendts, L., De Deist, F., Griscelli, C. and Fischer, A. (1989) Development of immunological function after bone marrow transplantation in 33 patients with severe combined immunodeficiency. *Blood*, **74**, 2212–19.

26. Henon, P.R., Butturini, A. and Gale, R.P. (1991) Blood-derived hematopoietic cell transplants: blood to blood? *Lancet*, **i**, 961–63.

27. Gluckman, E., Broxmeyer, H.E., Auerbach, A.D. *et al.* (1989) Hematologic reconstitution in a patient with Fanconi anemia by means of umbilical-cord from an HLA-identical sibling. *N. Engl. J. Med.*, **321**, 1174–78.

28. Stiehm, E.R. (ed.) (1989) *Immundeficiency Disorders: General Considerations*, 2nd edn, W.B. Saunders, Philadelphia, pp. 157–95.

29. Wara, D. and Ammann, A.J. (1976) Thymic cells and humoral factors as therapeutic agents. *Pediatrics*, **57**, 643–46.

30. Jenkinson, E.J., Anderson, G. and Owen, J.J.T. (1992) Studies on T cell maturation on defined thymic stromal cell population *in vitro*. *J. Exp. Med.*, **176**, 845–53.

31. Hong, R., Schulte-Wissermann, H. and Horowitz, S. (1979) Thymic transplantation for relief of immunodeficiency diseases. *Surg. Clin. North Am.*, **59**, 299–312.

32. Cleveland, W.W., Fogel, B.J., Brown, W.K. and Kay, H.E.M. (1968) Foetal thymic transplant in a case of DiGeorge's syndrome. *Lancet*, **ii**, 1211–14.

33. Shearer, W.T., Wedner, H.J., Strominger, D.B. *et al.* (1978) Successful transplantation of the thymus: Nezelof's syndrome. *Pediatrics*, **61**, 619–24.

34. Hong, R., Santosham, M., Schulte-Wisserman, H. *et al.* (1976) Reconstitution of T and B lymphocyte function in severe combined immunodeficiency disease following transplantation with thymic epithelium. *Lancet*, **ii**, 1270–72.

35. Borzy, M.S., Hong, R., Horowitz, S. *et al.* (1979) Fatal lymphoma after transplantation of cultured thymus in children with combined immunodeficiency disease. *N. Engl. J. Med.*, **301**, 565–68.

36. Chatila, T., Wong, R., Young, M. *et al.* (1989) An immunodeficiency characterized by defective signal transduction in T lymphocytes. *N. Engl. J. Med.*, **320**, 696–702.

37. Cowan, M.J., Smith, W. and Ammann, A.J. (1989) Interleukin 2 responsive lymphocytes in patients with adenosine deaminase deficiency. *Clin. Immunol. Immunopathol.*, **53** 59–67.

38. DiSanto, J.P., Keever, C.A., Small, T.N. *et al.* (1990) Absence of interleukin 2 production in a severe combined immunodeficiency syndrome with T cells. *J. Exp. Med.*, **171**, 1697–704.

39. Pahwa, R., Chatila, T., Pahwa, S. *et al.* (1989) Recombinant interleukin 2 therapy in severe combined immunodeficiency disease. *Proc. Natl Acad. Sci. USA*, **86**, 5069–73.

40. Weinberg, K. and Parkman, R. (1990) Severe combined immunodeficiency due to a specific defect in the production of interleukin-2. *N. Engl. J. Med.*, **322**, 1718–23.

41. Sorensen, R.U., Boehm, K.D., Kaplan, D. and Berger, M. (1992) Cryptococcal osteomyelitis and cellular immunodeficiency associated with interleukin-2 deficiency. *J. Pediatr.*, **121**, 873–79.

42. Ezekowits, R.A.B., Orkin, S.H. and Newburger, P.E. (1987) Recombinant interferon gamma augments phagocyte superoxide production and X-chronic granulomatous disease gene expression in X-linked variant chronic granulomatous disease. *J. Clin. Invest.*, **80**, 1009–16.

43. Gallin, J.I., Malech, H.L., Weening, R.S. *et al.* (1991) A controlled trial of interferon gamma to prevent infection in chronic granulomatous disease. *N.Engl. J. Med.*, **324**, 509–16.

44. Polmar, S.H., Stern, R.C., Schwartz, A.L. *et al.* (1976) Enzyme replacement therapy for adenosine deaminase deficiency and severe combined immunodeficiency. *N. Engl. J. Med.*, **295**, 1337–43.

45. Davis, S., Abuchowski, A., Park, Y.K. and Davis, F.F. (1981) Alteration of the cirulating life and antigenic properties of bovine adenosine deaminase in mice by attachment of polyethylene glycol. *Clin. Exp. Immunol.*, **46**, 649–52.

46. Levy, Y., Hershfield, S.M., Fernandez-Mejia, C. *et al.* (1988) Adenosine deaminase deficiency with late onset of recurrent infections: response to treatment with polyethylene glycol-modified adenosine deaminase. *J. Pediatr.*, **113**, 312–17.

47. Lahood, N.N., Hershfield, M.S., Leiva, L.E. and Sorensen, R.U. (1991) Recurrent infection, chronic diarrhea, and failure to thrive in a seven-month-old infant. *Ann. Allergy*, **67**, 389–93.

48. Hershfield, M.S., Chaffee, S. and Sorensen, R.U. (1993) Enzyme replacement therapy with PEG-ADA in adenosine deaminase deficiency: overview and case reports of three patients, including two now receiving gene therapy. *Pediatr. Res.*, **33**, S42–48.

49. Chaffee, S. and Hershfield, M.S. (1990) Immune response to polyethylene glycol-modified bovine adnosine deaminase (PEG-ADA) *Pediatr. Res.*, **27**, 155A.

50. Vega, M.A. (1992) Adenosine deaminase deficiency: a model for human somatic cell gene correction. *Biochem. Biophys. Acta*, **1138**, 253–60.

51. Lim, B., Apperley, J.F., Orkin, S.H. and Williams, D.A. (1989) Long-term expression of human adenosine deaminase in mice transplanted with retrovirus-infected hematopoietic stem cells. *Proc. Natl Acad. Sci. USA*, **86**, 8892–26.

52. van Beusechem, V.W., Kukler, A., Heidt, P.J. and Valerio, D. (1992) Long-term expression of human adenosine deaminase in rhesus monkeys transplanted with retrovirus-infected bone-marrow cells. *Proc. Natl Acad. Sci. USA*, **89**, 7640–44.

53. Curnoyer, D., Scarpa, M., Mitani, K. *et al.* (1991) Gene transfer of adenosine deaminase into primitive human hematopoietic progenitor cells. *Hum. Genet. Ther.*, **2**, 203–13.

54. Blaese, R.M. (1993) Development of gene therapy for immunodeficiency: adenosine deaminase deficiency. *Pediatr. Res.*, **33**, S49–55.

55. Sorensen, R.U., Strandjord, S.E. and Coccia, P.F. (1993) Outpatient bone marrow transplantation for severe combined immunodeficiency. *Lancet*, **i**, 52.

56. Ochs, H.D., Buckley, R.H., Kobayashi, R.H. *et al.* (1992) Antibody responses to bacteriophage φX174 in patients with adenosine deaminase deficiency. *Blood*, **80**, 1163–71.

57. Rim, I.J. and Rappeport, J.M. (1990) Bone marrow transplantation for the Wiskott–Aldrich syndrome. Long term follow-up. *Transplantation*, **50**, 617–20.

58. Goldsobel, A.B., Haas, A. and Stiehm, R.E. (1987) Bone marrow transplantation in the DiGeorge syndrome. *J. Pediatr.*, **111**, 40–44.

59. Borzy, M.S., Ridgway, D., Noya, F.J. and Shearer, W.T. (1989) Successful bone marrow transplantation with split lymphoid chimerism in DiGeorge syndrome. *J. Clin. Immunol.*, **19**, 386–92.

107 BASIC LABORATORY SUPPORT IN FETAL AND NEONATAL MEDICINE

J. Michaud

107.1 Introduction

In previous chapters we have been presented with a variety of molecular, cellular and organ developmental anomalies and acquired disorders. Too often, we are faced with a *fait accompli*; then, with fundamental and clinical research, we try to improve our understanding of the etiology and physiopathology of these conditions, in order to improve prevention, detection and eventual treatment. Often, we are faced with a 'high-risk' pregnancy, fetus and newborn. Beyond the clinical history and physical examination, the most effective environment is required to provide a quick and efficient investigation and treatment.

This environment is shaped by the type of institution. Early in this century, pediatric hospitals began emerging. In some regions, hospitals went beyond pediatric specialization, by merging obstetrical units with pediatric facilities. Our hospital represents such an association and has become, over the years, like other similar institutions, a referral center for prenatal evaluation and high-risk pregnancies.

This concept of tertiary care has led naturally to the formation of multidisciplinary prenatal diagnostic units, obstetrical units, intensive and intermediary neonatal intensive care units and a variety of pediatric functional units. The environment must deal with and resolve several problems in order to deliver high-quality investigation, care and therapy: transportation of pregnant mothers and of newborns, nursing, physical organization of the appropriate units, professional training and recruitment, quality control and assurance, pharmacotherapy, interaction with a suffering family and with referral institutions, education and bioethics.

A regional approach is thus highly desirable in order to enhance the quality of perinatal care and to further reduce perinatal morbidity and mortality. The institutions involved in such an approach have different characteristics and a system of designating three

levels of nursing has been used. The American Academy of Pediatrics' (AAP) and American College of Obstetricians and Gynecologists' (ACOG) *Guidelines for Perinatal Care* [1] describe the functions, facilities, equipment and personnel for each level.

In summary, level I nurseries provide:

1. routine care during normal pregnancies and identify high-risk pregnancies for referral to level II or level III centers prior to delivery;
2. supportive care of any problems occurring during labor and delivery, including the capacity of doing a cesarean section in 30 minutes;
3. routine resuscitation and stabilization of all newborns;
4. stabilization and proper support of any neonates or mother, including a transfer to level II or level III facilities.

In level II nurseries, in addition, there is support for relatively normal low-birth-weight newborns (1500–2500 g) and care for relatively common mild pregnancy complications. In level III nurseries there is complete neonatal intensive care and access to a wide range of pediatric, medical and surgical subspecialists and expertise for maternal intensive care.

In each level of care the most immediate environment for accurate investigation and therapeutic measures has to do with radiological investigations and laboratory support. The former was dealt with in previous chapters; therefore the focus in this chapter will be clinical laboratory medicine.

In their own environment, laboratories must face several challenges. Their physical organization is variable from one institution to another. One can find different types of configuration: dispersed, sectoral or urban. The first is most likely to be found in older and/ or very large institutions and requires a separate specimen access process, direction and management.

Diseases of the Fetus and Newborn, 2nd edn, Edited by G.B. Reed, A.E. Claireaux and F. Cockburn. Published in 1995 by Chapman & Hall, London. ISBN 0 412 39160 0

In the sectoral configuration, the administration, laboratory offices and accessioning are shared and the analyses are done in closely located but separate laboratories. In the urban configuration, the automated high volume and low cost testing is also centralized, while the low volume, high cost and specialized testing continues to be done in specific laboratories. The sectoral configuration and more certainly the urban one are the result of modern technologies and changing economic pressures. These configurations are likely to be found in more recently established institutions [2].

This era of rapid change is, for most institutions, a challenge for which there is no end in sight. For each level of care and each adopted technology, recruitment and training of technicians, residents, medical and administrative professionals, scheduling of urgent samples and of periods of coverage, quality control and assurance represent further challenges.

The challenge itself raises the following ethical questions: What is necessary? Do we have to do everything? Most industrialized nations now face these problems but are still able to resolve them; rationing, however, is around the corner. For developing countries, the goal is to attain the basic support that will allow decent care for as many babies as possible.

For pediatric critical care, four major components of general laboratory support have been identified: sampling, sample transportation, sample analysis and data reporting [3]. These components also apply to fetal and neonatal medicine. Except for a few specific comments, the following discussion excludes obstetrical units, where laboratory support is similar to most adult units, and the prenatal diagnostic units which have been addressed elsewhere.

107.2 Sampling

In fetal and neonatal medicine, the greatest difficulties and limitations come from the limited quantity of blood that can be drawn without inducing hypovolemia. Thus, even before sampling is done, perinatologists must carefully plan their investigations in order to avoid unnecessary repetitions in the sampling process. The sampling requires experienced personnel as it is a source of many potential errors (e.g. coagulation tests). In the author's center, biochemistry and hematology laboratories are in charge of the sampling in fetal and neonatal units. These laboratories have a specifically trained team that makes four regular rounds per day to each fetal and neonatal unit. These technicians are also available between rounds for emergencies and special requests. The regular rounds are made in co-ordination with medical activities so that the perinatologists will have seen the patients and the investigation plan will be known for every patient of the unit. This collaborative interaction is very important, for it allows

sampling in a predictable time and therefore enhances the prompt return of the team to the laboratory.

Limitations in the sampling quantity narrow the number of sampling techniques available, however. Disposable standardized depth lancets are used in almost all centers at the heel level, to retrieve the needed microliters of blood. This allows analyses of several blood constituents. In most types of physical configuration it is possible to share these samples among several laboratories in order to further limit the number of samples to be drawn.

Non-invasive technology is obviously a major goal in laboratory technology as it allows constant monitoring without the risk of hypovolemia. This technology is available for a number of analyses and involves several techniques from labsticks, for a variety of analyses, to cutaneous monitors, for various blood gas parameters or serum bilirubin.

Proper identification, precise requests, proper destination and pertinent clinical information are logical and compulsory requirements for any sample directed to a laboratory – more so for those directed to microbiology, virology, cytogenetics and anatomic pathology laboratories, because specimens are usually carried to the laboratory unit by the staff. At our center, for example, the teams in biochemistry and hematology responsible for sampling are on the spot to verify these data; we find this way of proceeding offers a great advantage in quality control activities.

In some centers, the bar code technology is now used to enhance the safety of patient identification [4]. This significantly reduces the risk of clerical errors and mismatch of specimens [5]. However, in the units under discussion, the test tubes are so small that one needs either to put them in larger containers or to apply special sticking flag labels, unless a micro bar code system has been designed. One thus avoids retranscription of information, which is a great source of errors.

10.3 Transportation of samples

This is a very important step in providing adequate turn-around time (TAT) [3,6]. The distance between the clinic units and the laboratories is a critical aspect of TAT [6], but the most essential is the care and importance given to this duty by the staff. We see a major advantage in this system by which laboratory teams are in charge of sampling as they also provide the support for sample transportation. Their laboratory training makes them aware of most pitfalls related to delays in transportation. Their daily contact with laboratory personnel allows immediate correction of any problem that may arise, either with the sampling procedures or the reception of samples in the laboratory.

Some centers have developed a vacuum tube system

as an alternative to manual transportation. The advantages are obvious because of the short transportation time. This system is also cost-effective if one considers the reduction in costs [3]. In some centers, however, the initial installation cost is not within the reach of available budgets. Also, some steps preceding the transportation (sampling, identification and preparation for transportation) or following it (laboratory reception and preparation for analyses) can also be responsible for delays as significant as the actual transportation time [6].

In our center, specimens obtained by cordocentesis are transported by the co-ordinating nurse. The nursing staff are in charge of transporting the umbilical cord blood samples from the obstetrics unit to the hematology and cytogenetic laboratories.

During the last decade, alternate site testing has been developed, also known as point-of-care testing, e.g. at the bedside, in doctors' offices or in unit-based or satellite laboratories.

Advances in technology and a policy to decrease the TAT are the two major factors, among others, leading to the decentralization of laboratory testing. This situation remains controversial for several reasons. Its implementation requires numerous criteria: central standards for validity and reliability of the results, fast and reliable instruments, cost-effectiveness and appropriate training for the personnel. To this day, the implementation of this type of testing has not always been preceded by a proper evaluation of a putative improvement in patient care. Also, the cost-effectiveness often remains elusive for several procedures [7,8].

The most important and critical element of out-of-laboratory testing is quality control and assurance. It is imperative to establish very strict written protocols, regular quality control testing (on every shift), external proficiency testing (main laboratory and outside centers) and an effective training program for the personnel. On top of these very important steps, it is mandatory to have identified one specific, responsible individual who will administer and supervise the whole process [8].

In hospital settings it is now generally accepted that satellite laboratories should be under the supervision of central laboratories [7,8]. For instance, as of 1991, the Canadian Council on Health Facilities accreditation requires that training and quality control and assurance be under the direct supervision of central laboratories.

So far, the impact of these new technologies in premature and neonatal critical care has not been as important as in pediatric or adult medicine, mainly because several highly variable parameters have to be taken into consideration; one, for example, is the influence of hematocrit on the blood glucose level [9].

Continuous blood gas monitoring is, however, a field where bedside testing is highly desirable, the technology of which is rapidly improving.

107.4 Sample analysis

In the last 20 years laboratory physicians have witnessed amazing improvements in technology and there is no indication that the future will be different [10]. Automation, automatic calibration, internal quality control, number of specimens analyzed, microprocessing, time-processing, computerization of all steps, comparative evaluation of computerized results, transmission of results and cost-effectiveness are some of the factors evaluated not only by companies which design such equipment but also by laboratory physicians and technicians in several centers throughout the Western World.

Because these technologies are primarily developed or calibrated for adults or older children, a few problems are related to neonatal samples. For example, red flags are often generated during blood cell count analysis, e.g. normoblasts. Albeit most of the time very safe, this step of laboratory support is preceded by processing of the samples, and the total number of those samples has a major impact on TAT. Also, for quality control purposes, the identification of specimens as received and as transferred for the automated step, the recognition of the type of analysis requested and the fragmentation and the orientation to the proper laboratory are sources of delays and errors. Procedures for these initial intralaboratory steps are crucial, have to be reviewed regularly, should be associated with proper training of secretarial and technical personnel and always have to be done while keeping in mind that the patient is the first beneficiary. Also, stat specimens (emergency requests) require special procedures and they should be treated as such, without disrupting other laboratory activities [3]. Special treatment varies according to the nature of the request and the internal physical organization of the laboratory.

If one excludes prenatal and postnatal investigations of specific inherited metabolic and genetic diseases and developmental defects, largely dealt with in previous chapters, one is left with a relatively standard set of tests. Although most of them have been mentioned or alluded to in previous sections of this book, one has to consider them in a perspective of availability and/or urgency (stat) in one's environment. The AAP–ACOG guidelines recommend that specific tests be made available in a specific time frame (TAT) for each level of nursery (Table 107.1) [11]. This is a minimal requirement which nevertheless allows very good support for each level of care.

The other major aspect of fetal and neonatal laboratory support, differentiating it from its adult counter-

Table 107.1 Perinatal care: laboratory microtechniques for each level of care as recommended by the AAP–ACOG [After Ref. 11]

	Level I	Level II	Level III
Within 15 minutes	Hematocrit	Blood gases, blood type and Rh	Levels I and II
Within 1 hour	Glucose, blood urea nitrogen, creatinine, blood gases, routine urinalysis	Level I plus: electrolytes, coagulation studies, blood available from type and screen program	Levels I and II plus: special blood and amniotic fluid tests
Within 1–6 hours	Complete blood count, platelet appearance on smear, blood chemistries, blood typed and cross-matched, Coombs' tests, bacterial smear	Level I plus: magnesium, urine electrolytes, hepatitis B surface antigen (6–12 h)	Levels I and II
Within 24–48 hours	Bacterial cultures and antibiotic sensitivity	Level I plus: metabolic screening	Levels I and II
Within hospital or facilities available	Viral cultures	Level I	Level I plus: laboratory facilities available
Radiography and ultrasound	Technicians on call 24 h/day available in 30 min; technicians experienced in performing abdominal pelvic, and obstetric ultrasound examinations; professional interpretation available on 24-h basis; portable radiographic and ultrasound equipment available to labor, delivery and nursery areas	Experienced radiology technicians immediately available in hospital; ultrasound on call; professional interpretation readily available; portable X-ray and ultrasound equipment available to labor, delivery and nursery areas	Level II plus: computed tomography; cardiac catheterization; sophisticated equipment for emergency gastrointestinal genitourinary or CNS studies available 24 h/day
Blood bank	Technicians on call 24 h/day, available on 30 min; performance of routine blood banking procedures	Experienced technicians immediately available in hospital for blood banking procedures and identification of irregular antibodies; blood component therapy readily available	Level II plus: resource center for network; direct line communications to labor, delivery and nursery areas

part, is the constant variation of normal reference values; numerous blood, plasma, serum, urine and cerebrospinal fluid values, ranging from the fetal period to the first few weeks of life, are given in Tables 107.3–107.16 at the end of the chapter. Many other books provide a wide range of laboratory values [12,13].

Normal pregnancy induces major physiological changes, including significant variations in several biochemical and hematologic values. This results, on computer-generated reports, in an increased number of 'so-called' abnormal results because reference ranges are usually those of normal non-pregnant women. As this topic is tangential to the focus of this chapter, the reader is referred to a recently published book reviewing and enlarging our knowledge on most routine hematological and biochemical laboratory data during normal pregnancy [14]

107.5 Selected specific analyses

Several tests are unique to the fetal and neonatal period. Their indications and interpretation were commented upon in previous chapters. For laboratories, most of them do not generate any special problems (α-fetoprotein, karyotypes, most viral studies including HIV-1, VDRL, TORCH, *Listeria moncytogenes*).

A few analyses, however, generate specific needs in the everyday management of laboratories.

Biochemistry At 24–28 weeks of gestation, a 50-g glucose tolerance test is done and insulinemia is evaluated for all pregnant mothers. This puts a heavy burden on laboratory facilities and, in our center, a special team is in charge of these tests. Complementary and follow-up studies are done if indicated. Reference values for blood glucose [15] and for insulin

Table 107.2 Indications for gross and microscopic placental examination [After Ref. 17]

Maternal conditions	Fetal and neonatal conditions
Diabetes mellitus (or glucose tolerance)	Stillbirth or perinatal death
Hypertension (pregnancy induced)	Multiple birth
Prematurity ($\leq$32 weeks' gestation)	Congenital abnormalities
Postmaturity (pregnancy >42 weeks)	Fetal growth retardation
Maternal history of reproductive failure	Prematurity ($\leq$32 weeks' gestation)
(defined as one or more previous	Hydrops
spontaneous abortions, stillbirths,	Meconium
neonatal deaths or premature births)	Admission to a neonatal intensive care unit
Oligohydramnios	Severe depression of the central nervous
Fever	system (Apgar score of 3 or less at 5
Infection	minutes)
Maternal history of substance abuse	Neurological problems, including seizures
Repetitive bleeding (other than minor	Suspected infection
spotting in the first trimester)	
Abruptio placentae	

[16] responses to glucose loads during pregnancy have been well documented.

Hematology   If samples are transported to this laboratory by the nursing staff, one nevertheless needs to set up a special team for coagulation tests as most potential errors occur at the time of sampling.

Microbiology   According to the level of care, minimal requirements are indicated in Table 107.1. The AAP–ACOG guidelines for perinatal care also cover several aspects of perinatal infections and infection control in the prenatal and neonatal periods [17]. If one excludes the source and types of samples submitted, there is no significant difference in handling and analyzing these specimens from those received from older babies or infants.

Microbiologists and virologists play a central role in the infection control committee and the establishment of policies related to surveillance of nosocomial infection and prevention and control of infections in all neonatal and obstetrical units.

Anatomic pathology   In the past, a number of new observations have been made from the morphological study of placentas, observations that could provide critical information for the care of neonates and mothers, for genetic counselling and for medicolegal litigation (Chapter 22). Consequently, it has even been proposed that all placentas should be examined by a pathologist [18].

In our center, a well-trained assistant pathologist describes the gross features and adequately samples these specimens. This is done under the supervision of the pathologist in charge. The histology is done by the pathologist. Formaldehyde-fixed specimens are stored for 1 month after the case is signed out.

If the histology cannot be done on all placentas, they should either be stored in a cold room for at least 1 week [19] and/or formaldehyde-fixed samples should be put aside for future reference, if needed, after

appropriate examination by the pathologist or an assistant [20]. This allows ample time for neonatalogists and pediatricians to signal problematic cases [19]. Nevertheless, most experts agree that a certain number of maternal, fetal and neonatal conditions call for a compulsory examination. A subcommittee of the College of American Pathologists' Placental Conference [21] provided a list of these conditions (Table 107.2)

In cases of stillbirth and early neonatal death, placentas should be examined during the autopsy, or the surgical pathology report should be included in the autopsy final conclusions with appropriate comments, if warranted. The etiologic evaluation of a stillbirth or neonatal death requires a multidisciplinary effort (Chapters 27 and 44).

When inborn errors of metabolism are suspected, frozen tissues from at least the liver and the brain are useful for biochemical and molecular analyses. All midtrimester spontaneous and induced abortions should be analyzed with the same care (Chapters 11–16).

With some variations, these steps have been included in the AAP–ACOG guidelines for perinatal care [22] and minimal requirements in case of perinatal death have been recommended by a British Joint Working Party [23]. This evaluation gains from being integrated in a regional strategy of perinatal care with a sufficient number of well-trained perinatal and pediatric pathologists [24].

107.6   Data reporting

In this era of technology and computerization, several laboratory instruments interface directly with the computerized medical charts located at the bedside or, at least, in the appropriate clinical units, in fetal and neonatal units. This integrated system is fast, precise and bypasses several verbal, secretarial and transcriptional steps [3] – all sources of errors and delays. It allows proper validation and 'signature' by the pathologists prior to the transmission of data. With an appropriate transmission system or interface, any physician can retrieve a specific result or profile, confidentiality being protected by selected passwords.

However, implementation of these systems is not yet widespread, computerization being sometimes operational in laboratories but not in individual units, or in some units but not in others. Fax transmission is an interesting solution as data can be transferred directly from the laboratory computers to any unit or medical office, thus again avoiding unnecessary transcription.

In some laboratories, however, one still has to rely on other less sophisticated tools. Telephone communication has numerous and well-identified problems [3] and has been largely replaced by fax transmission from the laboratory to the unit. This solution has largely ended the nightmare generated by the telephone system but a few problems remain: it requires substantial time for secretaries to transmit laboratory results best generated directly by the laboratory equipment, and it also requires substantial time for the unit staff to integrate the transmitted sheets to the patient's charts. Any inefficiency along the way impedes the process. This system does not in any way eliminate all telephone calls that one laboratory could receive.

107.7 Final considerations

Beyond the scientific aspects related to the laboratory disciplines mentioned throughout this book when dealing with specific diseases or developmental defects, previous topics surveyed so far concerning the basic laboratory support in neonatal medicine have to be put in context with two important activities which should never be neglected.

First, laboratory physicians and their assistants have to be good communicators. When our daily activities are reviewed in detail, it is obvious that much time is devoted to informing, giving advice, teaching, giving references, etc. Even physicians who are not working in university centers have to adopt similar behaviors.

In the laboratory, the emphasis is more on technology and quality control and assurance, not overlooking scientific meetings with colleagues and residents. Outside the laboratory, the range of transmitted information is much wider, ranging from explanations on how to read a new computerized result sheet to discussions on physiopathology for any given laboratory result. Overall, a lot of time is given to the explanation of the test. How is it done? With what frequency? How do I interpret it? What is its significance?

Second, physicians have to emphasize and see that all procedures are closely organized, supervised, modified and controlled along with the improvement of our scientific knowledge, technology and public needs. Thus, not surprisingly, during the last 15 years, laboratory direction and management has become a major concern for the continuing medical education activities of clinical pathology and laboratory medicine associations, for hospital directors and for accrediting organizations. Governmental regulations target this type of hospital activity more and more as it has a significant impact on the quality of health care and health costs. In the USA, the implementation of the Clinical Laboratory Improvement Amendments (CLIA) of 1988 is the result of several factors, but one of them was certainly the desire to improve the direction, management and implementation of quality control and quality assurance and the control of costs. Other countries are currently implementing similar measures. Excellent laboratory management is thus an indispensable requirement for high quality of health care at all levels.

Table 107.3 Normal hematologic values [After Ref. 25]

Value	Gestational age (weeks)		Full-term cord blood	Day 1	Day 3	Day 7	Day 14
	28	34					
Hb (g/dl)	14.5	15.0	16.8	18.4	17.8	17.0	16.8
Hematocrit (%)	45	47	53	58	55	54	52
Red cells (mm³)	4.0	4.4	5.25	5.8	5.6	5.2	5.1
MCV (μl³)	120	118	107	108	99	98	96
MCH (pg)	40	38	34	35	33	32.5	31.5
MCHC (%)	31	32	31.7	32.5	33	33	33
Reticulocytes (%)	5–10	3–10	3–7	3–7	1–3	0–1	0–1
Platelets (1000/mm³)			290	192	213	248	252

MCV = mean corpuscular volume; MCH = mean corpuscular hemoglobin; MCHC = mean corpuscular hemoglobin concentration.

Table 107.4 Hematological value in midtrimester cordocentesis samples [After Ref. 26]

Week of gestation	WBC (×10⁹/l)	Platelets (×10⁹/l)	RBC (×10¹²/l)	Hb (g/100 ml)	Ht (%)	MCV (fl)	MCH (pg)	MPHC (g/100 ml)	Red cell distribution width
18–20 (n = 25)	4.20±0.83	242.1±34.48	2.66±0.29	11.47±0.78	35.86±3.29	133.92±8.83	43.14±2.71	32±2.38	20.64±2.28
21–22 (n = 55)	4.19±0.84	258.2±53.65	2.96±0.26	12.28±0.89	38.53±3.21	130.06±6.17	41.39±3.32	31.73±2.78	20.15±1.92
23–25 (n = 61)	3.95±0.69	259.43±42.45	3.06±0.26	12.40±0.77	38.59±2.41	126.19±6.23	40.48±2.88	32.14±3.2	19.29±1.62
26–30 (n = 22)	4.44±0.85	253.54±36.6	3.52±0.32	13.35±1.17	41.54±3.31	118.17±5.75	37.94±3.67	32.15±3.55	18.35±1.67

Ht = hematocrit; MCV = mean corpuscular volume; MCH = mean corpuscular hemoglobin; MPHC = mean corpuscular hemoglobin concentration.
Studies performed with a Coulter S Plus 2.

Table 107.5 Midtrimester red cell and platelet values at cordocentesis [After Ref. 27]

	Gestational age (weeks)													
	15		16		17		18		19		20		21	
Hemoglobin (g/dl)	10.9	(0.7)	12.5	(0.8)	12.4	(0.9)	12.4	(1.2)	12.3	(1.2)	13.0	(1.1)	12.3	(0.8)
Total red cells (×10²²/liter)	2.43	(0.26)	2.68	(0.21)	2.74	(0.23)	2.77	(0.33)	2.92	(0.27)	3.12	(0.36)	3.07	(0.42)
Hematocrit (%)	35	(3.6)	38	(2.1)	37	(2.1)	37	(4.1)	38	(3.1)	39	(4.1)	37	(3.5)
Mean cell volume (fl)	143	(8)	143	(12)	137	(8)	135	(9)	129	(6)	126	(6)	123	(8)
Mean cell hemoglobin (pg)	45.4	(3.9)	46.6	(3.5)	45.4	(2.5)	44.7	(2.7)	42.5	(2.6)	41.8	(2.4)	40.6	(3.7)
Nucleated red cells (×10⁹/liter)	2.1	(0.8)	3.6	(1.8)	2.5	(0.9)	2.7	(2.2)	2.6	(1.7)	2.4	(1.2)	3.7	(0.8)
Reticulocytes (×10⁹/liter)	0.63	(0.15)	0.43	(0.07)	0.43	(0.08)	0.36	(0.09)	0.36	(0.01)	0.32	(0.17)	0.23	(0.08)
Platelets (×10⁹/liter)	190	(31)	208	(57)	202	(25)	192	(45)	211	(48)	170	(60)	223	(61)
Number of fetuses	6		5		16		18		29		12		13	

Values in parentheses are standard deviations.

Table 107.6 Leukocyte values (10³ cells/μl) in term and premature infants [After Ref. 28]

Age (hours)	Total white cell count	Neutrophils	Bands/ metamyelocytes	Lymphocytes	Monocytes	Eosinophils
Term infants						
0	10.0–26.0	5.0–13.0	0.4–1.8	3.5–8.5	0.7–1.5	0.2–2.0
12	13.5–31.0	9.0–18.0	0.4–2.0	3.0–7.0	1.0–2.0	0.2–2.0
72	5.0–14.5	2.0–7.0	0.2–0.4	2.0–5.0	0.5–1.0	0.2–1.0
144	6.0–14.5	2.0–6.0	0.2–0.5	3.0–6.0	0.7–1.2	0.2–0.8
Premature infants						
0	5.0–19.0	2.0–9.0	0.2–2.4	2.5–6.0	0.3–1.0	0.1–0.7
12	5.0–21.0	3.0–11.0	0.2–2.4	1.5–5.0	0.3–1.3	0.1–1.1
72	5.0–14.0	3.0–7.0	0.2–0.6	1.5–4.0	0.3–1.2	0.2–1.1
144	5.5–17.5	2.0–7.0	0.2–0.5	2.5–7.5	0.5–1.5	0.3–1.2

Table 107.7 Fetal platelet counts on blood obtained by cordocentesis [After Ref. 27]

Gestational age (weeks)	Platelets ($\times 10^9$ per litre)	
	Mean	SD
15	190	31
16	208	57
17	202	25
18	192	45
19	211	48
20	170	60
21	223	61

Table 107.8 Normal coagulation values [After Ref. 29]

Factor/measurement	Term infant	Preterm infant
Fibrinogen (mg%)	200–500	200–250
Factor II (%)	40	25
Factor V (%)	90	60–75
Factor VII (%)	50	35
Factor VIII (%)	100	80–100
Factor IX (%)	24–40	25–40
Factor X (%)	50–60	25–40
Factor XI (%)	30–40	25–40
Factor XII (%)	50–100	50–100
Factor XIII (titre)	1:16	1:8
Plasminogen	43	24
Antithrombin III	60	27
Partial thromboplastin time (s)	40–70	50–90
Prothrombin time (s)	12–18	14–20
Thrombin time (s)	12–16	13–20
α-Macroglobulin[a]	250	230
α-Antitrypsin[a]	100	90
Antithrombin[a]	12	12

[a] Plasma inhibitors of proteolytic enzymes.
See Chapter 82.

Table 107.9 Range of bone marrow differential counts in the neonatal period [After Ref. 13]

Cell type	Age		
	0–24 hours	7 days	1 month
Myeloblasts	0–2	0–3	0.4–1.9
Promyelocytes	0.5–6.0	0.5–7.0	1.0–2.5
Myelocytes	1–9	0.6–11	2.5–7.2
Metamyelocytes	4–19	2–30	3.1–9.1
Bands	10–30	13–43	17–32
Neutrophils	10–40	10–39	9–30
Eosinophils	1–3	1–3	2–5
Basophils	0.0–0.2	0.0–0.2	0.0–0.2
Red cell precursors	19–51	0–16	12–26
Lymphocytes	4–8	3.7–8.0	10–19
Monocytes	2–6	2.0–7.3	3–10
Plasma cells	–	–	0.0–0.2
Myeloid:erythroid ratio	1.5:1.0	6.5:1.0	2.9:1.0

Values are all percentages apart from the M:E ratio.

Table 107.10 Cord blood gas values in preterm and term infants delivered vaginally [After Ref. 30]

	Mean	SD	Percentiles			Mean	SD	Percentiles		
			5th	50th	95th			5th	50th	95th
Arterial										
P_{O_2}(mmHg)	19.1	9.1	8	18	33	18.4	8.2	9	17	32
P_{CO_2}(mmHg)	50.2	12.3	32	50	69.2	50.3	11.1	32	50	68
pH	7.28	0.089	7.14	7.29	7.4	7.27	0.069	7.15	7.28	7.38
BE (mmol/l)	−2.5	3	−7.6	−2.2	1.3	−2.7	2.8	−8.1	−2.3	0.9
HCO_3^-(mmol/l)	22.4	3.5	16	22.7	27.13	22	3.6	15.4	22.7	26.8
O_2 saturation (%)	25.1	17	5	22	59	23.3	16.2	5	19	57
O_2 content	4.8	3.24	0.97	4.2	11	4.6	3.2	1.1	3.8	11
Venous										
P_{O_2}(mmHg)	27.9	8.5	15	28	42	28.5	7.7	17	28	41
P_{CO_2}(mmHg)	41.7	10.1	28	41	57	40.7	7.9	29	40	53
pH	7.35	0.81	7.23	7.35	7.46	7.34	0.063	7.24	7.35	7.45
BE (mmol/l)	−2.1	2.2	−5.8	−1.9	0.7	−2.4	2	−6	−2.2	0.2
HCO_3^-(mmol/l)	21.8	2.6	17.4	22	25.4	21.4	2.5	17	21.7	24.9
O_2 saturation (%)	47.9	18.5	13.97	50.5	75.4	49.4	16.9	19.8	50.7	74.6
O_2 content	9.2	3.6	2.8	9.4	14.6	9.8	3.3	3.9	10	15.1

BE = base excess; HCO_3^- = bicarbonate.

Table 107.11 Predelivery and postdelivery cord blood gas values [After Ref. 31]

	pH	Pco$_2$ (mmHg)	Po$_2$ (mmHg)	Base excess (mmol/l)
Predelivery values	7.36±0.03	41.15±3.66	32.92±8.54	−0.79±1.19
Postdelivery values	7.31±0.04	46.29±5.71	26.97±4.43	−2.36±1.48

Table 107.12 Blood chemistry values in premature infants during the first 7 weeks of life (birth weight 1500–1750 g) [After Ref. 32]

	Age 1 week			Age 3 weeks			Age 5 weeks			Age 7 weeks		
Constituent	Mean	SD	Range	Mean	SD	Range	Mean	SD	Range	Mean	SD	Range
Na (mmol/l)	139.6	±3.2	133–146	136.3	±2.9	129–142	136.8	±2.5	133–148	137.2	±1.8	133–142
K (mmol/l)	5.6	±0.5	4.6–6.7	5.8	±0.6	4.5–7.1	5.5	±0.6	4.5–6.6	5.7	±0.5	4.6–7.1
Cl (mmol/l)	108.2	±3.7	100–117	108.3	±3.9	102–116	107.0	±3.5	100–115	107.0	±3.3	101–115
CO$_2$ (mmol/l)	20.3	±2.8	13.8–27.1	18.4	±3.5	12.4–26.2	20.4	±3.4	12.5–26.1	20.6	±3.1	13.7–26.9
Ca (mg/dl)	9.2	±1.1	6.1–11.6	9.6	±0.5	8.1–11.0	9.4	±0.5	8.6–10.5	9.5	±0.7	8.6–10.8
P (mg/dl)	7.6	±1.1	5.4–10.9	7.5	±0.7	6.2–8.7	7.0	±0.6	5.6–7.9	6.8	±0.8	4.2–8.2
BUN (mg/dl)	9.3	±5.2	3.1–25.5	13.3	±7.8	2.1–31.4	13.3	±7.1	2.0–26.5	13.4	±6.7	2.5–30.5
Total protein (g/dl)	5.49	±0.42	4.40–6.26	5.38	±0.48	4.28–6.70	4.98	±0.50	4.14–6.90	4.93	±0.61	4.02–5.86
Albumin (g/dl)	3.85	±0.30	3.28–4.50	3.92	±0.42	3.16–5.26	3.73	±0.34	3.20–4.34	3.89	±0.53	3.40–4.60
Globulin (g/dl)	1.58	±0.33	0.88–2.20	1.44	±0.63	0.62–2.90	1.17	±0.49	0.48–1.48	112	±0.33	0.5–2.60
Hb (g/dl)	17.8	±2.7	11.4–24.8	14.7	±2.1	9.0–19.4	11.5	±2.0	7.2–18.6	10.0	±1.3	7.5–13.9

Table 107.13 Reference serum amino acid concentration proposed as standards for neonates [After Ref. 33]

Amino acids	Breast-fed term infant	Cord blood
Isoleucine (μmol/l)	26–93	21–76
Leucine (μmol/l)	53–169	47–120
Lysine (μmol/l)	80–231	181–456
Methlonine (μmol/l)	22–50	8–42
Phenylalanine (μmol/l)	22–71	24–87
Threonine (μmol/l)	34–168	108–327
Tryptophan (μmol/l)	18–101	19–98
Valine (μmol/l)	88–222	98–276
Alanine (μmol/l)	125–647	186–494
Arginine (μmol/l)	42–148	28–162
Aspartic acid (μmol/l)	5–51	18–17
Glutamic acid (μmol/l)	24–243	92–57
Glycine (μmol/l)	77–376	123–312
Histidine (μmol/l)	34–119	42–136
Proline (μmol/l)	82–319	72–278
Serine (μmol/l)	0–326	57–174
Taurine (μmol/l)	1–167	41–461
Tyrosine (μmol/l)	38–119	34–83
Cystine (μmol/l)	35–132	4–37

Table 107.14 Urine amino acids in normal newborns [After Ref. 25]

Amino acid	Amount (μmol/day)
Cysteic acid	Trace–3.32
Phosphoethanolamine	Trace–8.86
Taurine	7.59–7.72
Hydroxyproline	0–9.81
Aspartic acid	Trace
Threonine	0.176–7.99
Serine	Trace–20.7
Glutamic acid	0–1.78
Proline	0–5.17
Glycine	0.176–65.3
Alanine	Trace–8.03
α-Aminoadipic acid	
α-Amino-n-butyric acid	0–0.47
Valine	0–7.76
Cystine	0–7.96
Methionine	Trace–0.892
Isoleucine	0–6.11
Tyrosine	0–1.11
Phenylalanine	0–1.66
β-Aminoisobutyric acid	0.264–7.34
Ethanolamine	Trace–79.9
Ornithine	Trace–0.554
Lysine	0.33–9.79
1-Methylhistidine	Trace–8.64
3-Methylhistidine	0.11–3.32
Garnosine	0.044–4.01
β-Aminobutyric acid	–
Cystathionine	–
Homocitrulline	–
Arginine	0.088–0.918
Histidine	Trace–7.04
Sarcosine	–
Leucine	Trace–0.918

Table 107.15 Cerebrospinal fluid values in very-low-birth-weight infants on basis of birth weight [After Ref. 25]

	≤1000 g		1001–1500 g	
	Mean ± SD	Range	Mean ± SD	Range
Birth weight (g)	763±115	550–980	1278±152	1020–1500
Gestational age (weeks)	26±1.3	24–28	29±1.4	27–33
Leukocytes/mm^3	4±3	0–14	6±9	0–44
Erythrocytes/mm^3	1027±3270	0–19 050	786±1879	0–9750
PMN leukocytes (%)	6±15	0–66	9±17	0–60
MN leukocytes (%)	86±30	34–100	85±28	13–100
Glucose (mg/dl)	61±34	29–217	59±21	31–109
Protein (mg/dl)	150±56	95–370	132±43	45–227

PMN = polymorphonuclear; MN = mononuclear.

Table 107.16 Cerebrospinal fluid values of healthy term newborns [After Ref. 25]

	Age			
	0–24 hours	1 day	7 days	>7 days
Color	Clear or xanthochromic	Clear or xanthochromic	Clear or xanthochromic	–
Red blood cells/mm^3	9 (0–1070)	23 (6–630)	3 (0–48)	–
Polymorphonuclear leukocytes/mm^3	3 (0–70)	7 (0–26)	2 (0–5)	–
Lymphocytes/mm^3	2 (0–20)	5 (0–16)	1 (0–4)	–
Proteins (mg/dl)	63 (32–240)	73 (40–148)	47 (27–65)	–
Glucose (mg/dl)	51 (32–78)	48 (38–64)	55 (48–62)	–
Lactate dehydrogenase (iu/l)	22–73	22–73	22–73	0–40

References

1. Freeman, R.K. and Poland, R.L. (eds) (1992) *Guidelines for Perinatal Care*, 3rd edn, American Academy of Pediatrics and American College of Obstetricians and Gynecologists, Elk Grove Village and Washington, DC.
2. Hardwick, D.F. and Morrison, J.I. (eds) (1990) *Directing the Clinical Laboratory*, Field & Wood, New York, pp. 172–78.
3. Fallon, K.D. (1989) Laboratory support for critical care areas, In *Textbook of Critical Care* (eds W.C. Shoemaker, S. Ayres, A. Grenvik *et al.*), W.B. Saunders, Philadelphia, pp. 269–72.
4. Titzer, L.L. and Jones R.W. (1988) Use of bar code labels on collection tubes for specimen management in the clinical laboratory. *Arch. Pathol. Lab. Med.*, **112**, 1200–1202.
5. Kasten, B.L. (1991) Bar code benefits. *CAP Today*, **5** 14, 61.
6. Cembrowski, G.S. and Steindel, S.J. (1990) Emergency Department turnaround time. Data Analysis and Critique. Q-Probes Short-Term Studies of the Laboratory's Role in Quality Care. *College of American Pathologists*, Northfield, IL 90-13A:1–15.
7. Check, W.A. (1993) How point-of-care is playing out. *CAP Today*, **7**, 1, 12–20.
8. Orgram, D. (1992) Out-of-laboratory testing. *Can. J. Med. Technol.*, **54** (suppl.), 1–17.
9. Kaplan, M., Blondheim, O. and Fidelman, A. (1990) Accuracy of glucose reflectance meters during the neonatal period. *J. Pediatr.*, **117**, 673–74.
10. Linder, J. (1992) Pathology patterns. Automation in pathology. *Am. J. Clin. Pathol.*, **98** (suppl. 1), 51–52.
11. Freeman, R.K. and Poland, R.L. (1992) *Guidelines for Perinatal Care*, 3rd edn, American Academy of Pediatrics and American College of Obstetricians and Gynecologists, Elk Grove Village and Washington, DC, pp. 238–39.
12. Meites, S. (ed.) (1989) *Pediatric Clinical Chemistry. Reference (Normal) Values*, 3rd edn, American Association for Clinical Chemistry Press, Washington, DC.
13. Hann, I.M., Gibson, B.E.S. and Letsky, E.A. (eds) (1991) *Fetal and Neonatal Haematology*, Baillière Tindall, London.
14. Lockitch, G. (ed.) (1993) *Handbook of Diagnostic Biochemistry and Hematology in Normal Pregnancy*, CRC Press, Boca Raton, FL.
15. Weiss, P.A.M. (1988) Gestational diabetes: a survey and the Graz approach to diagnosis and therapy, in *Gestational Diabetes* (eds P.A.M. Weiss and D.R. Cousteau), Springer, New York, pp., 1–12.
16. Kuhl, C. (1991) Insulin secretion and insulin resistance in pregnancy and GDM. *Diabetes*, **40** (suppl. 2), 18–24.
17. Freeman, R.K. and Poland, R.L. (eds) (1992) *Guidelines for Perinatal Care*, 3rd edn, American of Pediatrics and American College of Obstetricians and Gynecologists, Elk Grove Village and Washington, DC, pp. 117–75.
18. Salafia, C.M. and Vintzileos, A.M. (1990) Why all placentas should be examined by a pathologist in 1990. *Am. J. Obstet. Gynecol.*, **163**, 1282–93.
19. Altshuler, G. (1993) A conceptual approach to placental pathology and pregnancy outcome. *Semin. Diagn. Pathol.*, **10**, 204–21.
20. Baldwin, V.J. (1992) Placenta, in *Developmental Pathology of the Embryo and Fetus* (eds J.E. Dimmick and D.K. Kalousek), J.B. Lippincott, New York, pp. 271–319.
21. Travers, H., Schmidt, W.A. and Siegal G.P. (eds) (1991) College of American Pathologists Conference XIX on the Examination of the placenta. *Arch. Pathol. Lab. Med.*, **115**, 660–721.
22. Freeman, R.K. and Poland, R.L. (eds) (1992) *Guidelines for Perinatal Care*, 3rd edn, American Academy of Pediatrics and American College of Obstetricians and Gynecologists, Elk Grove Village and Washington, DC, pp. 216–18.
23. Stirrat, G.M., Wigglesworth, J., Berry, P.J. and Keeling, J. (1988) *Report on Fetal and Perinatal Pathology*, Royal College of Obstetricians and Gynecologists and Royal College of Pathologists, London, pp. 1–8.
24. Report of the Royal College of Pathology Working Party on Paediatric and Perinatal Pathology (1990) *Bull. R. Coll. Pathol.*, **69**, 10–13.
25. Klaus, M.H. and Fanaroff, A.A. (eds) (1982) *Care of the High-risk Neonate*, 4th edn, W.B. Saunders, Philadelphia.
26. Forestier, F., Daffos, F., Galactéros, F. *et al.* (1986) Pediatric research. *Int. Pediatr. Res. Found.*, **20**, 342–46.
27. Millar, D.S., Davis, L.R., Rodeck, C.H. *et al.* (1985) Normal blood cell values in the early mid-trimester fetus. *Prenat. Diagn.*, **5**, 367–73.

28. Oski, F. and Naiman, J. (1982) *Hematologic Problems in the Newborn*, W.B. Saunders, Philadelphia.
29. Halliday, H.L., McClure, G. and Reid, M. (eds) (1989) *Handbook of Neonatal Intensive Care*, 3rd edn, Baillière Tindall, London, p. 366.
30. Riley, R.J. and Johnson, J.W.C. (1993) Collecting and analyzing cord blood gases. *Clin. Obstet. Gynecol.*, 36, 13–23.
31. Khoury, A.D., Moretti, M.L., Barton, J.R. *et al.* (1991) Fetal blood sampling in patients undergoing elective cesarean section: a correlation with cord blood gas values obtained at delivery. *Am. J. Obstet. Gynecol.*, 165, 1026–29.
32. Thomas, J. and Reichelderfer, T. (1968) Premature infants: analysis of serum during the first seven weeks. *Clin. Chem.*, 14, 272.
33. Hanning, R.M. and Zlotkin, S.H. (1989) Amino-acid and protein of the neonates: effects of excess and deficiency. *Semin. Perinatol.*, 13, 131–41.

108 COMMENTS ON FETAL AND NEONATAL LABORATORY MEDICINE

G.B. Reed

Some prenatal samples require special laboratory handling and processing either 'in house' or at an outside referral centre. There are a number of *in utero* or at birth conditions, previously described, which are unique (Table 108.1). These uniques situations, samples and assays are listed and reviewed in Table 108.2. In these circumstances to make adequate use of the laboratory, clinicians and laboratorians should make prior consultations and plan the most appropriate options. The subjects are categorized as A, B and C:

A antenatal and neonatal conditions, *in utero* and at birth;

B unusual samples of blood, fluids, urine, cells and tissues obtained by special methods, e.g. chorionic villus sampling, cordocentesis or amniocentesis;

C assays unique to this age group, involving A and B, and which are done on small samples with micromethods; the 'normal' ranges need to be considered and it is important to interpret the results in terms of gestational age and/or body weight.

These diagnostic tests and/or evaluations of fetal and neonatal well-being are *not* screens. The results do not generally need confirmation, but may need a series of observations or results to establish or document 'well-being' or therapeutic effects. Clinicians must be aware of local or referral laboratory policies. Prior consultation is mandatory. Appropriate protocols must be followed if one wishes to receive a reliable result or interpretation. As Professor Michaud discussed in Chapter 107, this involves: (1) appropriate sampling technique; (2) optimal timing; (3) proper conditions for transport, receipt and logging (identification); and (4) appropriate 'in laboratory' handling, processing and reporting.

Two final points must be made. First, transfusion service and blood banks: appropriate methods should be available for small amounts of blood components to be used prenatally or in the neonatal intensive care unit; 'donor pools' from 'in house' staff or nurses should be avoided. Second, in a few large referral centers, tissue banks or fetal tissue banks are established and operating – hopefully under guidelines as strict as those that are applied to blood banks (Chapter 28).

References

MOLECULAR PATHOLOGY AND DIAGNOSTICS

Bernstram, V. (1992) *Guidebook of Gene Level Diagnostics in Clinical Practice*, CRC Press, Boca Raton, FL.

Brock, D. (1993) *Molecular Genetics for the Clinician*, Cambridge University Press, Cambridge.

Engle, L. (1993) The human genome project. *Arch. Pathol. Lab. Med.*, 117, 459–65.

Garvin, A., O'Leary, T., Bernstein, J. and Rosenberg, H. (eds) (1991 and 1992) *Pediatric Molecular Pathology*, vols 15,16, Krager, Basel; in *Perspect. Pediatr. Pathol.*, 15, 28–82, 83–105; in *Perspect. Pediatr. Pathol.*, 16, 7–26, 99–119.

Grody, W. (1993) Molecular genetics. *Arch Pathol. Lab. Med.*, 117, 459–65.

Michalopoulos, G. (1993) Meeting: pathology and molecular diagnostics: issues of structure and organization. *Am. J. Pathol.*, 142, 127–99.

Nakamura, R. (1993) Introduction: College of American Pathologists Conference XXIV on Molecular Pathology. *Arch. Pathol. Lab. Med.*, 117, 455–56 (Conference program: 457–58).

Stoler, M. (1993) *In situ* hybridization. *Arch. Pathol. Lab. Med.*, 17, 470–72.

FETAL MEDICINE: LABORATORY VALUES

For quick identification of specific tests/values: **hematology** (Daffos and Forrestier, 1990; Nicolaides and Snijders, 1992; Weiner, Sipes and Wenstrom, 1992); **urine** (Harrison and Filly, 1990; Cheng and Nicolaides, 1992); **hormones** (Economides and Nicolaides, 1990; Nicolaides and Snijders, 1992); **chemistries** (Soothill, Nicolaides and Rodeck, 1989; Economides and Nicolaides, 1990; Chatterjee, 1993; Nicolaides and Snijders, 1992; Economides *et al.*, 1993; Pardi *et al.*, 1993); **amniotic fluid** (Lockitch *et al.*, 1984; Brace and Wolf, 1989; Rodeck, Santolaya and Nicolini, 1990; Bowie *et al.*, 1991; Campbell *et al.*, 1992; Fryer *et al.*, 1993; Wathen *et al.*, **culture methods** (Gosden, 1992; Johnson and Miller, 1992).

Bowie, L., Shammo, J., Dohnal, J. *et al.* (1991) Lamellar body number density and the prediction of respiratory distress. *Am. J. Clin. Pathol.*, 95, 781–86.

Brace, R. and Wolf, E. (1989) Normal amniotic fluid volume changes throughout pregnancy. *Am. J. Obstet. Gynecol.*, 161, 382–88.

Campbell, J., Wathen, N., MacIntosh, N. *et al.* (1992) Biochemical composition of amniotic fluid and extraembryonic coelomic fluid in the first trimester of pregnancy. *Br. J. Obstet. Gynaecol.*, 99, 563–65.

Diseases of the Fetus and Newborn, 2nd edn, Edited by G.B. Reed, A.E. Claireaux and F. Cockburn. Published in 1995 by Chapman & Hall, London. ISBN 0 412 39160 0

Table 108.1 Conditions *in utero* and at birth

	Conditions	Tests
1.	**Anomalies**	AFP
	NTDs	Electrolytes, osmolarity
	Renal	Diuretic challenge
2.	**IUGR**	
	(FGR)	Lactate, Po_2, base excess
3.	**Lung maturity**	L/S ratio, SPA-D
	(via amniotic fluid)	Lamellar body count
4.	**Hydrops:** immune	ΔOD_{450}
	non-immune	TORCHS
	Hemolytic disorders	Chromosomes
	Anemia	Hemoglobinopathies
		Blood chemistries
5.	**Coagulopathies**	See Chapter 82
6.	**Sepsis:** TORCHS, AFIS	See Chapters 7, 18, 83
7.	**Metabolic**, endocrine, nutrition[a]	Appropriate chemical, vitamin or hormone level(s)
8.	**Inborn** errors of metabolism	Appropriate test(s)
		See Chapters 74, 77
9.	**Inborn** immune defects	Appropriate test(s)
		See Chapters 40, 106
10.	**Monitor** complications of fetal therapy	Appropriate test(s)
		See No.12
11.	**Specific**	NB screen
	Inborn errors of metabolism	See Chapters 61–63
	Chromosome syndrome(s)	US, Chapters 53, 61, 62
	Twins (zygosity)[b]	US, Chapter 55
12.	**Iatrogenic**	Appropriate tests and samples
		See Chapter 44
	Forensic	Appropriate tests and samples
		See Chapter 25
	Paternity	Appropriate tests and samples
13.	**Placenta**[b]	See Chapters 10, 22
	Amniotic fluid	See Chapters 69, 79
	Cord	See Chapter 67
	Membranes	See Chapter 22
	Yolk sac	See Chapters 10, 56
14.	**Transplantation**	See Chapters 88, 106
	Monitors	
	Also ECMO[c]	See Chapter 102
	TPN[a,c]	See Chapter 98
15.	**Teratogen**/mutagen	Screen, Chapter 6
	Substance abuse	Screen, Chapter 24
	TORCHS (maternal titers)	Screen, Chapters 7, 18, 83
16.	**Thoracic**, urological, gut and bowel surgery	See Part 6

AFIS = amniotic fluid infection syndrome; AFP = α-fetoprotein; Chromosomes = trisomy 13, 18, 21, others; ECMO = extracorporeal membrane oxygenation; IUGR = intrauterine growth retardation (fetal growth restriction); L/S = lecithin/sphingomyelin ratio; NB screen = newborn screen, e.g. thyroxine, thyroid stimulating hormone, galactosemia, phenylketonuria, etc. (Chapters 61–63); NTDs = neural tube disorders (anencephaly, spina bifida); ΔOD_{450} = amniotic fluid pigment, bilirubin, Rh; SPA-D = surfactant related lipoproteins A, B, C and D; TORCHS = toxoplasmosis, other (human immunodeficiency virus, hepatitis B virus), rubella, cytomegalovirus, herpes virus, syphilis; TPN = total parenteral nutrition (Chapter 98); Twins = diamniotic/dichorionic, monoamniotic/monochorionic, others (Chapters 16, 53); US = sonar, ultrasound.
[a] Overlap, 14, 16.
[b] Overlap, 7, 14.
[c] Overlap, 11, 13.

Table 108.2 Fetal–neonatal laboratory medicine

	Specimens	*Assay(s)*		*Discipline(s)*
1.	**Gametes** (male and female) (IVF)	X, Y		1, 2, 7
2.	**Pre-embryo** (INV) (IVF) to 14 days (see Chapter 64)	X-linked IEM		1, 2, 7
3.	**Coelomic fluid** (INV) (see Chapter 56)	–		1, 2, 3
4.	**Fetal 'cells' in maternal blood** (INV) RBC WBC, lymph Trophoblast elements (see Chapter 65)	X,Y IEM		1, 2, 3, 7
5.	**Chorionic villi** 10 weeks' cytotrophoblast (see Chapter 68)	IEM		1–7
6.	**Amniotic fluid** amniocytes fibroblast culture 12–16 weeks (see Chapters 69, 70)	AFP IEM X, Y Viral Bacterial	ΔOD_{450} ACHE L/S SPA-D Other	1–7
7.	**Fetal blood** 10 weeks (see Chapter 67)	IEM X, Y Viral	Other	1–7
8.	**Fetal tissue(s)** membranes placenta, cord, yolk sac (see Chapters 56, 70)	Specific indication(s)		Skin, liver, EM(8), cord, villi

ACHE = acetylcholine esterase; AFP = α-fetoprotein; IEM = inborn errors of metabolism; INV = investigational status; IVF = *in vitro* fertilization; L/S = lecithin/sphingomyelin ratio; ΔOD_{450} = amniotic fluid pigment, bilirubin, Rh; RBC, WBC, lymph = blood elements; SPA-D = surfactant related lipoproteins A, B, C and D; X, Y = chromosomes; 1 = cytogenetics and molecular cytogenetics (fluorescent *in situ* hybridization, Chapter 73); 2 = molecular and biochemical genetics (polymerase chain reaction, other); 3 = microbiology and virology; 4 = immunology, serology; 5 = hematology, oncology; 6 = metabolism, endocrinology, general chemistry, toxicology; 7 = DNA fingerprinting; 8 = anatomical pathology, electron microscopy (EM) and other techniques.

Chatterjee, M. (ed.) (1993) *Biochemical Monitoring of the Fetus*, Springer, New York.

Cheng, H. and Nicolaides, K. (1992) Renal and urinary tract abnormalities, in *Prenatal Diagnosis and Screening* (eds D. Brock, C. Rodeck and M. Ferguson-Smith), Churchill Livingstone, Edinburgh, pp. 257–70.

Daffos, F. and Forrestier, F. (1990) Fetal hematologic parameters, in *Hematologic Disorders in Maternal–Fetal Medicine* (eds M. Bern and F. Frigoletto), Wiley–Liss, New York, pp. 47–66.

Economides, D., Bowell, P., Sellinger, M. *et al.* (1993) Anti D concentration in fetal and maternal serum and amniotic fluid in rhesus allo-immunized pregnancies. *Br. J. Obstet. Gynaecol.*, **100**, 923–26.

Economides, D. and Nicolaides, K. (1990) Metabolic findings in small-for-gestational-age fetuses. *Contemp. Rev. Obstet. Gynaecol.*, **2**, 75–79.

Fryer, A., Jones, P., Strange, R. *et al.* (1993) Plasma protein levels in normal human fetuses. *Br. J. Obstet. Gynaecol.*, **100**, 850–55.

Gosden, C. (1992) Cell culture, in *Prenatal Diagnosis and Screening* (eds D. Brock, C. Rodeck and M. Ferguson-Smith) Churchill Livingstone, Edinburgh, pp. 85–98.

Harrison, M. and Filly, R. (1990) The fetus with obstructive uropathy, in *The Unborn Patient* 2nd edn (eds M. Harrison, M. Golbus and R. Filly) W.B. Saunders, Philadelphia, p. 375.

Johnson, M. and Miller, O. (1992) Cytogenetics, methodology, in *Reproductive Risks and Prenatal Diagnosis* (ed. M. Evans), Appleton & Lange, Norwalk, CT, p. 237–49.

Lockitch, G., Wittman, B., Mura, S. and Hawkley, L. (1984) Evaluation of the amniostat-FLM assay for assessment of fetal lung maturity. *Clin. Chem.*, **30**, 1233–37.

Makepeace, A., Fremont-Smith, F., Daily, M. and Carroll, M. (1931) The nature of the amniotic fluid. *Surg. Gynecol. Obstet.*, **53**, 635–44.

Nicolaides, K. and Snijders, R. (1992) Cordocentesis, in *Reproductive Risks and Prenatal Diagnosis* (ed. M. Evans), Appleton & Lange, Norwalk, CT, pp. 201–20.

Pardi, G., Cetin, I., Marconi, A. *et al.* (1993) Diagnostic values of blood sampling in fetuses with growth retardation. *N. Engl. J. Med.*, **328**, 692–96.

Rodeck, C., Santolaya, J. and Nicolini, U. (1990) The fetus with immune hydrops, in *The Unborn Patient* 2nd edn (eds M. Harrison, M. Golbus and R. Filly), W. B. Saunders, Philadelphia, pp. 215–27.

Soothill, P., Nicolaides, K. and Rodeck, C. (1989) Fetal blood gas and acid–base parameters, in *Fetal Medicine I* (ed. C. Rodeck), Blackwell Scientific, Oxford, pp. 57–89.

Wathen, N., Campbell, D., Kitau, M. and Chard, T. (1993) Alphafetoprotein levels in amniotic fluid from 8 to 18 weeks of pregnancy. *Br. J. Obstet. Gynaecol.*, **100**, 380–82.

Weiner, C., Sipes, S. and Wenstrom, K. (1992) The effect of fetal age upon normal fetal laboratory values and venous pressure. *Obstet. Gynecol.*, **79**, 713–18.

109 THE AUTOPSY AND PROTOCOLS

G.B. Reed and D.J. deSa

109.1 Introduction

This chapter falls into two parts: explanatory text followed by illustrative tables (Tables 109.1–109.10), figures (Figures 109.1–109.5) and protocols. Previous chapters (Chapters 25–27) have focused on specialty interests. This chapter repeats these concerns for the generalists, obstetricians, pediatricians and pathologists. It is prepared for those who work in large community hospitals with active maternity units where there is a need for a perinatal pathologist. If appropriate perinatal necropsies cannot be done at such centers, cases should be referred to a regional center where those with experience can perform appropriate investigations (again, please see Chapters 25–27).

Two principles are important. First, an autopsy is a medical consultation. Second, whoever is in charge of the perinatal pathology service must have the unqualified support of his or her department head and chairpersons in obstetrics and pediatrics. Without this multidisciplinary approach one's labors are lost, if not futile.

This book promotes the concept of a multidisciplinary approach to diseases of the fetus and newborn, and there is no reason why a 'team' cannot be formed from local talent in a given hospital or community. This presumes that a general pathologist is able and willing to co-ordinate the various disciplines and has some system of maintaining the continuity of information and reports which are necesary for family counseling and aftercare. This information is needed in order to provide optimal care to families 'at risk' for a recurrence of a poor pregnancy outcome.

109.1.1 THE NECROPSY

It is important to recognize that the underutilization of or reluctance to perform postmortem studies of antenatal deaths is based, in part, on expense (not budgeted for or a lack of resources) and on professionally chosen priorities. There are too few well-trained professionals in the field of antenatal pathology and even fewer recruits for the future. In any institution the evaluation of antenatal and neonatal deaths should include input from three departments: obstetrics, pediatrics and pathology. Since there is no 'routine' procedure for handling each case, each death can be evaluated using a 'tripod model'. The three legs of the tripod are (1) the mother, (2) the placenta, and (3) the conceptus. As in any branch of medicine an accurate history is essential. The availability of maternal and obstetrical records is crucial, and the identification and availability of all placentas for study is absolutely necessary. The conceptus, born dead or alive, should have a documented examination. A clinical summary (death note) addressed to pathology should be done. Ideally a member of the clinical service should be present at some stage of the postmortem examination. These practices can maintain good rapport and convey necessary information between both the prosector and the clinician. Without constant, cordial consultations between the clinical and pathology services the vagaries of each case may not be avoided. Too often clinicians justifiably complain that 'the pathologist did not examine the ...' or 'sections weren't taken of ...'. Such comments can be minimized if communications are optimal. Part of the traditional interprofessional friction that arises between clinician and pathologist is due to misunderstandings about the autopsy.

The autopsy is not only a procedure, it is also the first part of a series of post-mortem studies that may include any number of tests, consultations and analyses. All these data are evaluated before the pathogenesis can be outlined and the cause(s) for death can be determined. The end-results are a report which contains opinions, interpretations and diagnoses. Such pathology consultations may also include relevant

Diseases of the Fetus and Newborn, 2nd edn, Edited by G.B. Reed, A.E. Claireaux and F. Cockburn. Published in 1995 by Chapman & Hall, London. ISBN 0 412 39160 0

observations on management and discussions on how to improve diagnostic accuracy.

Many formulas have been devised to accommodate the volume of the necropsy workload while maintaining quality of histopathological investigations. In antenatal pathology a large number of deaths can be studied. The tripod model is one which may help prioritize individual cases. Another is to use a triage system similar to those described by others [1,2]. The triage system may reduce costs by prioritizing the cases in terms of the types and numbers of laboratory tests needed to complete a final study. None of the schemes such as the tripod model or triage system or others that I am aware of are foolproof or error free. It is the 'routine attitude' that leads to the incomplete report, lacking a vital confirmatory test, because the prosector did not think to obtain the sample and did not think to order the appropriate test.

Although a definite necropsy protocol, appropriate facilities and 'benign' supervision are essential for any efficient autopsy service, of equal importance are the quality of the staff and level of training of the professionals who do the actual work. It is not glamorous work and is very uncomfortable to some because it is often unpleasant to see a dead infant. Who are the professionals who will do this work? Currently pathology departments in the USA and elsewhere are deficient in antenatal and neonatal pathology training programs and trainees. As a career choice pathology is not popular and few recruits choose pediatric, much less antenatal pathology, as compared with general or surgical pathology. Because of this shortfall the bulk of antenatal and neonatal necropsies are done by general pathologists. These physicians' interests or experience in current obstetrics and pediatrics may be limited, and their available time to spend on such investigations may also be limited. At present it is not known how often general pathologists refer difficult cases to referral centers for a 'definitive work-up'. Some professional reluctance can be overcome if costs are controlled, if local medical interests are cultivated and if clinical (obstetrical and pediatric) encouragement is constant. A description of such a referral unit is given in Chapter 1. This sketch may belabor the problems: expenses, limited numbers of trained personnel and lack of basic protocols to enable one to carry out the necessary studies.

The following models are given as examples, and hopefully they will help others to think through their practice and to use these or other such examples to improve their existing autopsy service. Finally the 'methods and materials' section (sections 109.2.2–109.3.2) will not present details in the 'how to' manner, rather the reader will be referred to selected published references. Unfortunately these 'materials' are not neat

timed specimens, but are rare unique individuals derived from parents' blood and tears.

109.1.2 BACKGROUND

Appropriate signed witnessed permits are necessary, mediocolegally, in order to be able to examine specimens obtained from surgery and to perform a postmortem examination. One must understand and observe local medical regulations. Informed consent is implied, in the permits, and when special requests, restrictions or limitations are desired these should be documented on the permit and adhered to. Death certificates are usually completed and signed by the attending physician, and this is best done after the autopsy findings are known to the clinician. Prior to requesting autopsy permission from a member of the family, other than those deaths due to natural causes, all 'cases' should be reviewed and if necessary cleared with the coroner (medical examiner, procurator fiscal). Such cases include deaths soon after surgery, deaths of patients who have not recovered from anesthesia, deaths due to accidents (remote or recent) and sudden, unexpected, unexplained deaths. All these situations may be under the jurisdiction of the coroner (Chapter 25). Antenatal, perinatal and neonatal deaths present certain choices. Many cases can be handled as surgical specimens; such specimens include placentas, products of conception, spontaneous abortions and early stillbirths. Again, local regulations need to be observed; that is, when does a conceptus need to have a permit to be examined at an autopsy? Various jurisdictional time frames range from 20 to 28 weeks of gestational age (weeks of amenorrhea). If one assumes 20 weeks' gestation as the legal limit, then it follows that prior to 20 weeks the studies are handled as surgical reports, and after 20 weeks they are handled as autopsy reports. Additional permission should be obtained if tissues are to be used in research, treatment or transplantation. Informed consent is assumed, but permission should be documented when tissues or organs are donated (Chapter 28).

In practice, placentas are often examined independently of the conceptus (especially in postnatal deaths), and too often maternal histories are not a part of the surgical reports of products of conception, spontaneous abortion, etc. For this reason, we believe all obstetrical pathology studies (placentas, ectopic pregnancies, moles, products of conception, spontaneous abortions and early stillbirths) must include an abstract of the mother's history, and this document should be attached to the surgical pathology or autopsy report. All these reports can have the same accession number.

109.2 Organization of the pathology service

This combines (1) a multidisciplinary approach, and (2) an information processing system for an antenatal and neonatal surgical pathology and necropsy service.

109.2.1 MULTIDISCIPLINARY ORGANIZATION

In antenatal and neonatal medicine, three departments are involved in studying antenatal and neonatal morbidity and mortality: obstetrics, pediatrics and pathology. Although each department may have its traditional responsibilities, each unit should have certain mutual obligations not only to other departments served but also to the patients served. To provide optimal pathology and laboratory services there needs to be a fundamental agreement between departments, a multidisciplinary code, which recognizes that the practice of obstetrical and neonatal pathology is a vital element in the progress of their respective fields, in their educational programs and for the welfare of their patients.

Each department thus needs to make appropriate financial contributions and provide sufficient professional personnel to support the pathology services, to the degree that these 'external departments' utilize the laboratories. Without this interdisciplinary approach the quality and necessary documentations, investigations, consultations and appropriate counselling may not be attained. The commonly agreed goals of a multidisciplinary group need periodic monitoring.

Therefore, a good surgical pathology and autopsy service are dependent on continuous cordial clinical co-operation and pathology department credibility. These services are 'two-way' consultations. This two-way street concerns information which is obtained for the medical community, the public well-being and families who gave permission. Their 'gifts' provide for medical education and research. These gifts should be matched by an improvement in professional performance and achievement. To help improve performance, communication skills and co-operation among trainees in obstetrics, surgery, neonatology and pathology should be fostered. Such interplay provides information, complements training program goals and enhances the trainees' appreciation of the other person's job.

109.2.2 INFORMATION PROCESSING: GATHERING AND DISPENSING

Again, an interdepartmental philosophy should be promoted so that the exchange of current information regarding patients is efficient and accurate, while simultaneously maintaining respect for patient confidentiality. The information which needs to be collated and correlated by the prosector are:

A. maternal history
B. placental examination
C. conceptus ± history.

These are the three basic elements needed, whether the report is derived from a surgical specimen or a postmortem examination. This is the only proper way to study antenatal and neonatal material. Without this background information, reports become speculative, if not dangerous. For example, if the 'first time around' data or tissues are missed or reports are not evaluated properly the 'second time around' would not be anticipated or prevented. The second pregnancy could result in a second infant born with trisomy 21.

The following suggestions may enhance communications between departments.

- Prior to necropsy all records should be available to pathology.
- Death certificates should be completed after necropsy findings are known.
- Before requesting permission for a postmortem examination, all reportable cases (coroner or communicable diseases) should be promptly reported and cleared with the appropriate agency (done by the clinician and/or pathologist).
- All documents and specimens should be available for review and referral to other consultants or institutions.
- Written preliminary necropsy reports should be issued to the clinical service within 48 to 72 hours of the autopsy.
- A 'post-autopsy conference' should be scheduled when appropriate and agreeable to all parties, including the obstetrician, pediatrician and other involved clinicians.

By providing basic information to the clinician and family as soon as appropriate one can usually reduce unnecessary anxiety and confusion.

109.2.3 TRIAGE SYSTEM

Whether a surgical or necropsy report is required in a particular case is based on regulations, and is usually defined by the time when death occurred during gestation and beyond which point in time an autopsy is usually necessary. Most often this is 20–24–28 weeks of gestation. Before this time, surgical reports are done. In addition to gestational age, body weight and crown–heel length have been used as markers.

The merits of a triage system are equal to the care taken in evaluating the clinical history and diagnoses. 'New cases' can be evaluated by question and answer

('Q & A'). During the evaluation the extent of the investigations, documentations and tests needed can be anticipated by the prosector.

Using the 'Q & A' format a protocol can be selected. It cannot be emphasized enough that all cases studied need an abstract of the maternal history, which is attached to the placental, surgical or necropsy report. Whether one decides initially on a standard format is not as important as being flexible. During the course of a necropsy a discovery may require additions to the previously selected protocol or lead to more extensive investigations. Local resources and facilities may limit one's options. Can complex autopsy cases be referred to another institution? Possibly. Again, local regulations may or may not permit transport of bodies or tissues to another jurisdiction. The 'Q & A' format leads to categories and should allow one to select the appropriate protocol.

109.3   Procedures and documentation

109.3.1   GUIDELINES BEFORE, DURING AND AFTER NECROPSY

The section on triage used a 'Q & A' format to select the appropriate protocol. Simply, before 20 weeks consider surgical protocols and after 20 weeks employ the necropsy protocol. The performance of an autopsy should be planned. Simple guidelines are given for before, during and after completion of the necropsy.

The prosector's main concerns at outset are: to identify the purposes and goals of the investigation; to consider how much and what kind of data are needed; and to select the protocol which provides adequate and accurate documentation for that individual case. Each necropsy will present different questions, e.g. a 'tumor case' may be concerned with the amount of residual tumor. The procedures of any case sould be tailored to the information that is hoped to be gained from the autopsy.

(a)   Before necropsy

Organ procurement for transplantation should be arranged prior to autopsy. Photographs, radiographs, dermatoglyphics and other studies should be done beforehand. Toxicological, cell culture and microbiological cultures should be obtained prior to evisceration.

Body weight, length and other measurements should be recorded, and a detailed external examination of the face, habitus and surface anatomy made and recorded. Sketches or close-up photographs can be done with appropriate labels, dates and reference units in the photographic field. A facility and personnel exclusively devoted to postmortem photography and radiology is an ideal situation. Special radiological views are required for osteochondrodystrophies and some complex malformations (Chapters 27 and 43).

(b)   During necropsy

A senior pathologist should to be available, if not in attendance. The dissection technique should provide clean and bloodless fields. All external orifices should be evaluated for patency. Laryngoscopy can be done to detect foreign bodies in the upper airway. No facial or hand incisions should be made, nor should any be made on other regions which might be viewed later at a memorial service.

With the help of a trained assistant (denier) various procedures can be done rapidly, allowing information to be recorded as the observations are made. Care should be taken to demonstrate a pneumothorax and to record volumes of fluid or blood in body cavities. To maintain bloodless fields with each layer of tissue reflection, major arteries and veins should be tied proximal and distal to the point of section and then sectioned between the sutures (Table 109.4).

A sterile technique should be used to obtain any microbial culture of fluids or tissue samples. In the process of opening the chest and abdomen, the situs of the organs should be noted.

The heart should be opened *in situ* and not removed from the lungs. Care should be taken to rule out anomalous pulmonary venous return, aberrant coronaries, a patent ductus, a coarctation of the aorta, etc. Anomalous venous returns are most difficult to detect, especially those which are infradiaphragmatic.

Rokitansky's *en bloc* method is the preferred procedure for evisceration. The chest and abdomen are examined first, then the brain and spinal cord. Pelvic organ anomalies and fistulas should be ruled out before separating the various organs *in situ* or after evisceration. This is also true for the urinary tract: kidneys, ureters, urinary bladder and urethra. The gut, from esophagus to anus, should be opened with the minimum of 'washing' of the mucosa.

The following should be evaluated during dissection: anomalies of azygos vessels, diaphragmatic hernia or defects, tracheoesophageal fistula, laryngeal web, tracheomalacia, lobar sequestration, bowel atresia, volvulus or intussusception. Establish bile flow to the duodenum by pressing the gallbladder and watching the ampulla for flow of bile. Inspect external and internal genitalia.

(c)   After necropsy

Review the checklist which was prepared before starting the autopsy. The checklist is used to review gross findings after the post mortem is completed and before the body is removed from the dissecting table. Match the checklist and findings with clinical history and diagnoses. Insure all necessary samples are labeled and appropriately processed and stored. Review internal sufaces of the cranial and body cavities and sample skin, muscle and bone. When in doubt, document and take additional samples.

When in doubt, **do not dissect** unless a senior pathologist is in attendance. This is a major caution when examining complex urogenital or cardiac anomalies. **Do not cut.** Fix or refrigerate and review the complicated specimen the following day with others. Review worksheets for completeness and clarity. Inform the involved clinicians of your findings – at completion or early the following day.

109.3.2 PROTOCOLS

These are brief outlines which can be expanded and placed in a computer system for direct dictation or used as a written checklist. The protocols can then be transcribed on preprinted forms or produced by word processor. Examples of maternal, placental, surgical and necropsy protocols are given at the end of the chapter.

109.3.3 CONDITIONS REQUIRING DETAILED DOCUMENTATIONS OF EXTERNAL AND INTERNAL MORPHOLOGY

All anomalous conceptuses (whether a fetus or newborn) fall into this category. The details which need to be documented, both of the external and internal examinations, are commensurate with the complexity or rarity of an individual case (Chapters 26 and 29).

A brief series of examples is given. In the chapters on systemic pathology more examples are indicated. A few examples are conjoined twins, complex cardiovascular anomalies, uncommon chromosome syndromes and 'non-genetic syndromes' such as fetal alcohol syndrome, associations, etc.

(a) Genetic and dysmorphic conditions
(Chapters 26 and 27)

A number of textbooks and encyclopedias in print should be available for quick reference and should be familiar to the prosector [1,2–8]. A working knowledge of basic anthropomorphic measurements and nomenclature is needed [9–13]. This is especially true for facial defects. Two standard books on dysmorphology are those by Aase [12] and Goodman and Gorlin [13]. See references 1–19 for various ranges of measurements, anthropometric values, organ weights, body weight and length for gestational age.

These tables illustrate the appearance of ossification centers during gestation [3], foot length during ges-

tation [9,17], common anthropometric measurements of 'term' and 'preterm' infants [3,6,8–13] and pedigree symbols [11,12] for preparing genetic history which can be submitted with the protocols: placenta, maternal history and surgical or necropsy reports.

109.4 Tissue sampling

A standard systematic approach is helpful. Whatever system one uses, document the study case, label properly and use diagrams if necessary. Since fetal and neonatal tissues and organs are relatively small compared with adult specimens, several tissues usually can be included in one block. Transition zones can provide two or three tissue patterns in one section. Normal and abnormal tissue should be included in the same tissue sample, e.g. tumor plus adjacent normal tissue.

Tissue samples should be put in several fixatives if indicated, e.g. Bouin's, Zenker's, Jore's, formalin, glutaraldehyde. Tissues can also be 'snap' frozen to -20 or $-80°C$. Cryostat sections can be made and stored at the time of necropsy.

Fresh tissue should be kept in a tissue-culture holding medium (Hank's or media 199) if cell cultures or chromosome studies are desired. A rule of thumb is to 'oversample' and overstock: one does not have a second opportunity.

109.5 Brain and spinal cord (Chapter 30)

109.6 Heart and vascular system
(Chapter 31)

109.7 Conclusions

Most histopathology tissue reports that are concerned with tumor diagnosis include a comment on the degree of malignancy and prognosis. In making diagnoses for genetic disorders or pregnancy loss, a parallel approach should be considered when preparing an antenatal or neonatal pathology report. We propose advice be given in writing to the attending physician. In such a report a statement should address the genetic or reproductive risk; that is, what is the recurrence rate for the same condition or diagnosis happening in the next pregnancy? This probability can be expressed as a 'number' in terms of maternal risk (1:100 chances of a recurrence); or the future pregnancy should be screened or monitored since the risk is unknown or cannot be determined. Whether genetic counselling should or should not be offered to a couple or mother is a decision the family's doctor ought to make. Frederich Kraus cautions pathologists when they are dealing with tissue from reproductive failures to remember the 'clinical triangle' of father, mother and child. Each side of the biological triangle may need to be evaluated, particularly in cases of infertility or when recurrent pregnancy loss occurs [20] (Chapters 13 and 17).

In situations where the pathologist is uncertain about reproductive risks or implications, a clinical genetics consultation should be sought. The pathologist frequently needs to consult with experts and this activity provides continuous learning.

For those parents who have had a pregnancy loss or have chosen to have a termination of a pregnancy for an inherited disorder, Margaretha White-van Mourik and Michael Connor discuss the psychosocial support and the other needs of parents during bereavement in Chapter 60. Several groups in the UK and USA have published guidelines for parents and for professionals dealing with perinatal death and sequelae [21,22].

Several coding systems have been developed, such as ICD-9, SNOMED, etc. [23–26]. Buetow [27] has suggested a two-part death certificate: first, a clinical diagnosis is given as a cause of death, and, second, the autopsy results are documented as to the cause of death. This bicameral method, the author suggests, may improve the validity of perinatal statistics in terms of 'cause of death'.

As noted in Chapters 26 and 27, by Marvin Miller and Haynes Robinson, discuss the family's various needs to receive counsel and be informed about a pregnancy loss or neonatal death. After a period of grieving appropriate answers should be given to the family. Risks or implications for subsequent pregnancies should be spelled out. The information should be given in 'lay terms'. This information should allow couples to make informed decisions in the future. Such sessions, counseling and aftercare can be expedited when there is a clear, accurate and prompt pathology report available to all concerned [28,29].

If further information is needed by the pathologist, it can often be obtained from various 'on line' computer databases (see Further reading).

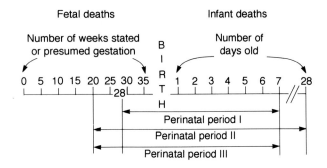

Figure 109.1 Classifications of perinatal mortality have been based on various criteria: obstetrical, pediatric, pathological and birth weight (BW) specific causes of death. 'Time' is based on menstrual weeks from the last menstrual period (LMP). Other terms used are conceptual or developmental age. First trimester terms are chemical or clinical pregnancy, blighted ova, spontaneous abortion or miscarriage. Embryonic period is from implantation to 8 weeks, <30 mm crown–rump length (CRL). Pre-viable fetus is <20 weeks, viable fetus is >20 weeks. Various classifications for abortion can be used. Products of conception are usually less than 12 weeks. A fetus is >8 weeks and >30 mm CRL. There are early, intermediate and late fetal deaths. Stillbirth = fetal death. There are antenatal deaths and intrapartum deaths. Term birth (259–294 days, 37–42 weeks, >2500 g BW). Preterm birth (<259 days) and low birth weight (<2500 g BW). Appropriate for gestational age (AGA) is used, e.g. 2500 g at 36 weeks, or small for gestational age (dates) (SGA) or large for gestational age (LGA). Post-term birth (>294 days, >42 weeks (post dates)). Other clinical terms: brain death and vegetative state. Perinatal morbidity, trends in . . . 'Causes' of death (mode of death): natural, accidental, suicide and homicide. Terms related to fetus or infant: abuse, neglect, feticide, neonaticide and infanticide.

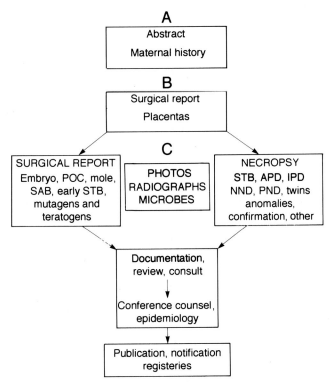

Figure 109.2 The ABCs of gathering and dispensing clinicopathological information. POC = products of conception; SAB = spontaneous abortion; STB = stillbirth; APD = antepartum death; IPD = intrapartum death, NND = neonatal death; PND = postnatal death.

Table 109.1 Multidisciplinary organization and interdepartmental information

I. Multidisciplinary approach and goals
   Obstetrics
   Pediatrics
   Pathology

II. Interdepartmental training programs
   Sonography, genetics, risk assessment
   Fetal medicine, intensive care nursery
   Laboratories, surgical pathology
   Autopsy service, molecular cytogenetics

III. Audit–monthly mortality and morbidity review
   Fetal treatment board

IV. Financial support – referral services

V. Reproductive medicine and developmental pathology programs linked to II

VI. Timely reports and post autopsy conferences
   Counseling and clinicopathological data linked to genetic, fetal and
   neonatal registries

Table 109.2 Triage 'Q&A': questions

Gestational age (weeks)	Conceptus	Mother
	1. **Age** 1,2,3 trimester Gestational age	1. Age ____ LMP ____ G___ P___ A___
<20	2. **<20 weeks** <30 mm: embryo (E) >30 mm: fetus (F) >30 mm: fetus (F) <450–500 g BW	2. **Other** Habitual abortion Lupus antibody Maternal/paternal HLA (see maternal abstract)
	3. **Recurrent abortion**: genetic, risks	3. **See no. 9 conceptus**
	4. **Preservation of tissue**: intact, fresh, macerated Sac ±E, ±F Normal, abnormal	4. At home delivery, transfer from another hospital after delivery records? placenta?
>20	5. **Multiple conceptuses**, A or B, vanishing	
	6. **Normal external features** (F, NB) AGA, SGA, LGA, IUGR	
<20>20	7. **Abnormal history, external features** (F, NB) US, PNDX or RX STB (FD), LB (NB) AGA, SGA, LGA, IUGR	
	8. **Any liveborn** S/P surgery, transplant, *in utero* RX Graduate NICU, <3 months SIDS, iatrogenic or forensic concerns	
	9. **History: 3rd trimester**, labor and delivery Placenta: abruptio, cervical competence, PROM, PTL; cord knots, compression, neck, Abn monitor, FHR, O$_2$ scalp, bleeding, fetal–maternal transfusion	

BW = birth weight; NB = newborn; AGA, SGA, LGA = *Appropriate, Small and Large for Gestational Age*, respectively; LMP = last menstrual period; G = gravida; P = parity; A = abortion; IUGR ; intrauterine growth retardation; US = ultrasound; PNDX, RX = parental diagnosis, treatment; STB = stillbirth; LB = livebirth; NICU = neonatal intensive care unit; SIDS = sudden infant death syndrome; PROM = premature rupture of membranes; PTL = premature labor; FHR = fetal heart rate; FD = fetal death; APD = antepartum death; IPD = intrapartum death.

Table 109.3 Triage 'Q&A': answers

Gestational age (weeks)	Answers	Protocol or report
	1. Placentas Regardless of gestational age	Surgical report
<20	2. POC, moles, embryos, SAB, early stillbirths	Surgical report
<20	3. STB, FD (APD, IPD) NND, PND: (a) normal: AGA, IUGR macerated, recurrent abortions (b) abnormal (as above): STB, FD, NND. Features: history, PNDX, PNRX, postnatal RX; iatrogenic/forensic issues; twins (concordance, zygosity); SIDS <3 months	Necropsy report see (4)
	4. Special examinations: (a) brain (b) heart (c) regional (d) dysmorphic (e) other	Detailed examinations See Table 109.10

POC = products of conception; SAB = spontaneous abortion; FD = fetal death; NND = neonatal death; PND = postnatal death; APD = antepartum death; IPD = intrapartum death; and see Table 109.2.
Posing the questions in Table 109.2 leads to a limited number of answers. The 'key' words are **age** (< or >20 weeks)? **Macerated or fresh? Normal or abnormal** history or external features? **Significant** placental or maternal factors? Most cases can then be categorized for study. These are our criteria and our subdivisions. There are other formats.

Table 109.4 Guidelines for internal examination

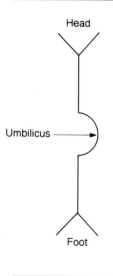

Examine the face and external genitalia carefully. Probe all external orifices for patency. Maintain bloodless fields. Use double 'Y' incision around the umbilicus. On entry determine situs, quantitate collections of air, blood and fluid. Obtain cultures sterilely. Ligate major vessels and rectum. Use Rokitansky *en bloc* evisceration. Rule out foreign body upper airway. Examine heart and lungs *in situ*, leave organs attached. Open gut from esophagus to rectum without 'washings'. Detach kidneys on sectioning if no hydronephrosis. Demonstrate bile flow. Rule out tracheoesophageal fistula, congenital diaphragmatic hernia, urogenital and colonic fistula, patent ductus, coarctation, a variety of abnormal venous returns. Rule out thrombi of major arteries and veins. Open skull using butterfly technique (below). Examine *in situ* the meninges, base, falx, tentorium. Remove from the anterior the spinal cord. Sample skin, muscle, bones.

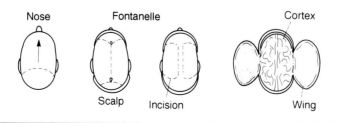

Table 109.5 Guide to fetal and placental growth

Placental weight[a] (g)	Placental weight[b] (g)	CH length[c] (cm)	Foot length[d] (mm)	BW[c] (g)	GA[c] (weeks)	Brain[c] (g)	Heart (g)	Lung R&L (g)	Liver (g)	Kidney R&L (g)	Adrenal R&L (g)	Spleen (g)	Thymus (g)
—	205	29	42	500	23	70	5	12	26	5	2.6	1	2
256	252	32	50	750	26	107	6	19	39	8	3.2	2	3
—	270	35	53	1000	27	143	8	24	47	10	3.5	3	4
—	306	38	57	1250	29	174	10	30	56	13	4.0	3.5	5
—	343	41	61	1500	31	219	11	34	65	15	4.5	5	6
362	360	43	63	1750	32	247	13	40	74	17	5.3	6	7
410	397	45	68	2000	34	281	15	44	82	19	5.3	7	8.0
453	433	46	74	2250	36	308	16	48	88	20	6.0	8.5	8.2
465	467	47	79	2500	38	339	18	48	105	23	7.1	9	8.3
—	480	49	81	2750	39	362	19	51	117	24	7.5	10	9.6

CH = crown–heel; BW = birth weight; GA = gestational age; R&L = right and left.
Data are expressed in rounded numbers.
[a] Grunenwald and Minh [14].
[b] Philippe [15].
[c] Grunenwald and Minh [16].
[d] Streeber [17] and Merlob, Sivan and Reisner [9].

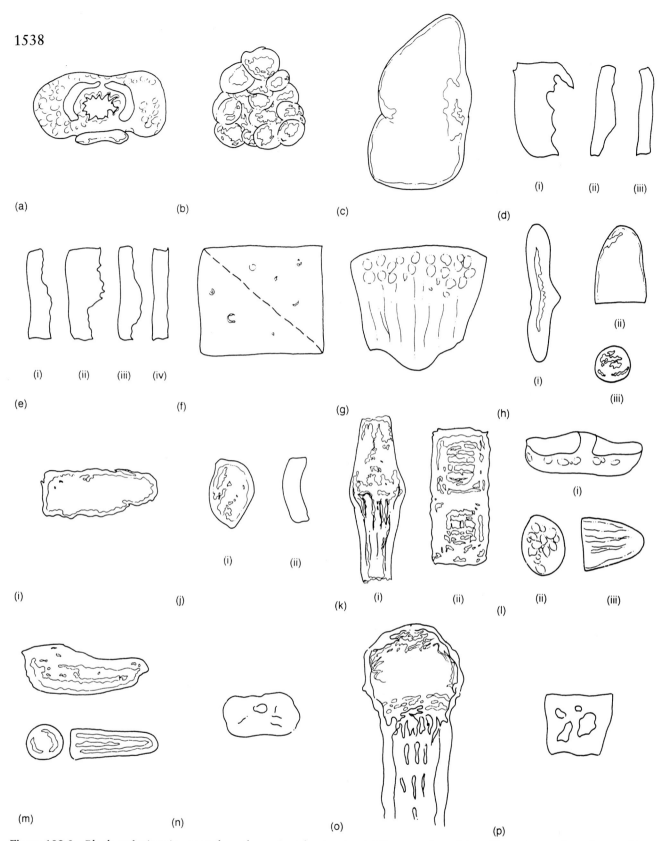

Figure 109.3 Block and trimming procedures for perinatal autopsies. (a) Cross-section of thyroid, trachea and esophagus; (b) thymus, longitudinal cut; (c) left lung, upper and lower lobes (special processing, see technician); (d) (i) right or left ventricle with valve; (ii) ductus, longitudinal cut; (iii) thoracic aorta; (e) block of gastrointestinal tract: (i) cardia; (ii) pylorus; (iii) cecum, i.e. ileocecal valve; (iv) colon, block on paper and trim after fixation; (f) liver: right ■ or left ▷ lobe; (g) kidney, longitudinal cut; (h) (i) adrenal; (ii) spleen; (iii) lymph node; (i) pancreas, longitudinal cut, body and tail; (j) gonad: (i) testes or ovary; (ii) urinary bladder; (k) (i) rib; (ii) vertebrae; (l) (i) skin (from umbilicus); (ii) and (iii) psoas muscle, cross and longitudinal cut; (m) uterus and/or appendix (tip longitudinal and cross-cut proximal); (n) prostate; (o) long bone, e.g. humerus; (p) mastoid bone; (q) optional – salivary gland, tongue, ureter, fallopian tube(s), breast tissue and other parts of skeletal system.

Table 109.6 Appearance of ossification centers *in utero*

Gestation (months)	Centres of ossification
1/2	Shaft of clavicle, mandible
2	Shafts of femur, humerus, radius, ulna, tibia and fibula, ilium
3	Ischium
4	Pubis
6	Talus, os calcis
7	Sternum: first part; toes, middle phalanx 2–4
8	Sternum: second part; toes, middle phalanx 5
Peripartum 9	Sternum; third part; epiphyses at knee: femur before tibia

Centers appear during months given (±1 month).
Reproduced with permission of R. Winters & J. Wiley Co., Chichester, UK.

Table 109.7 Foot length by week of gestation [After Ref. 17 with permission]

End of week	Mean foot length (mm)	Minimum foot length (mm)	Maximum foot length (mm)
8	4.2	3.8	4.6
9	4.6	4.2	5.0
10	5.5	5.0	6.0
11	6.9	6.0	7.8
12	9.1	7.5	10.8
13	11.4	9.8	13.0
14	14.0	12.5	15.5
15	16.8	15.2	18.5
16	19.9	18.2	21.6
17	23.0	21.0	25.0
18	26.8	24.8	28.8
19	30.7	28.5	33.0
20	33.3	31.0	35.7
21	35.2	32.5	38.0
22	39.5	36.0	43.0
23	42.2	39.0	45.5
24	45.2	42.0	48.5
25	47.7	44.5	51.0
26	50.2	47.0	53.5
27	52.7	49.0	56.5
28	55.2	51.5	59.0
29	57.0	53.0	61.0
30	59.2	55.5	63.0
31	61.2	57.5	65.0
32	63.0	59.0	67.0
33	65.0	61.0	69.0
34	68.2	64.0	72.5
35	70.5	66.0	75.0
36	73.5	69.0	78.0
37	76.5	72.0	81.0
38	78.5	74.0	83.0
39	81.0	76.0	86.0
40	82.5	77.5	87.5

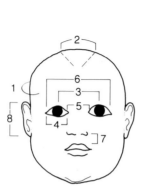
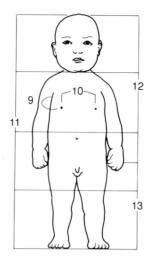

Table 109.8 Neonatal measurements

Measurement	Range (cm)	
	Term (38–40 weeks)	Preterm (32–33 weeks)
1. Head circumference	32–37	27–32
2. Anterior fontanelle $\left(\dfrac{L-W}{2}\right)$	0.7–3.7	–
3. Interpupillary distance	3.3–4.5	3.1–3.9
4. Palpebral fissure	1.5–2.1	1.3–1.6
5. Inner canthal distance	1.5–2.5	1.4–2.1
6. Outer canthal distance	5.3–7.3	3.9–5.1
7. Philtrum	0.5–1.2	0.5–0.9
8. Ear length	3–4.3	2.4–3.5
9. Chest circumference	28–38	23–29
10. Internipple distance[a]	6.5–10	5–6.5
11. Height	47–55	39–47
12. 13. Ratio $\dfrac{\text{upper body segment}}{\text{lower body segment}}$	1.7	–
14. Hand (palm to middle finger)	5.3–7.8	4.1–5.5
15. Ratio of middle finger to hand	0.38–0.48	0.38–0.5
16. Penis (pubic bone to tip of glans)	2.7–4.3	1.8–3.2

L = length; W = width.
[a] Internipple distance should not exceed 25% of chest circumference.

From Manchester [19] with permission.

Table 109.9 Major anthropometric measurements [After Ref. 9]

Name _____ _____   Gestational age (GA) _____ weeks

Sex _____   Postnatal age _____ days

Date _____   Birth weight _____ Per GA _____

	cm	Percentile		cm	Percentile
Head Normal/abnormal (N/A)			**Upper limb** N/A		
Occipito-frontal circumference	___	___	Total arm length	___	___
Anteroposterior diameter	___	___	Upper arm segment	___	___
Biparietal diameter	___	___	Lower arm segment	___	___
Length index	___	___	Upper segment index	___	___
Width index	___	___	Lower segment index	___	___
			Hand length	___	___
Eyes N/A			Middle finger length	___	___
Inner canthus	___	___	Middle finger index	___	___
Outer canthus	___	___			
Palpebral fissure	___	___	**Lower limb** N/A		
Interpupillary distance	___	___	Total lower limb length	___	___
			Lower segment	___	___
Ears N/A			Lower segment index	___	___
Ear length	___	___	Foot length	___	___
Ear above eyeline	___	___			
Percent of ear above eyeline	___	___	**Body length** N/A	___	___
Frankfort plane	___	___	Sitting length	___	___
			Sitting length index	___	___
Mouth N/A			Weight	___	___
Intercommissural distance	___	___			
Philtrum	___	___	**Genitalia**		
			Penile length	___	___
Chest N/A			Clitoral length	___	___
Circumference	___	___			
Internipple distance	___	___			
Internipple index	___	___			
Sternal index	___	___			
Torso length	___	___			
Torso index	___	___			

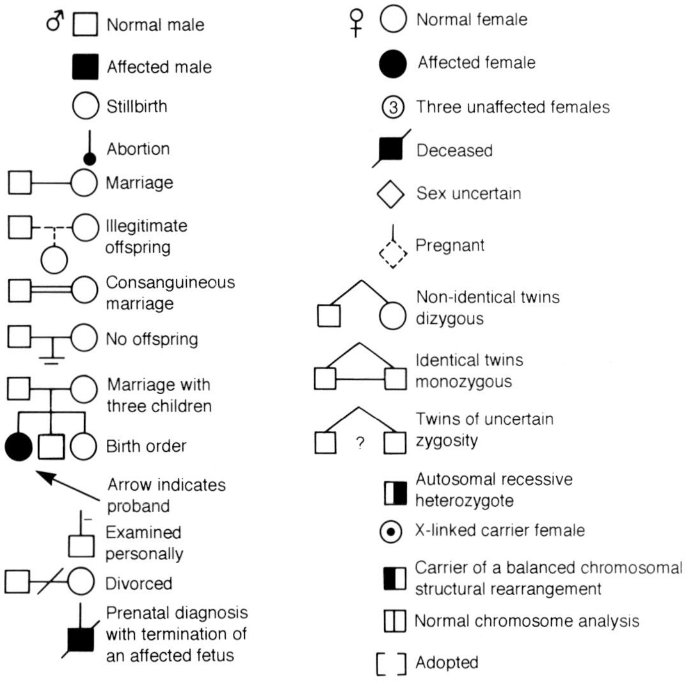

Figure 109.4 Family tree (pedigree): commonly used symbols.

1542

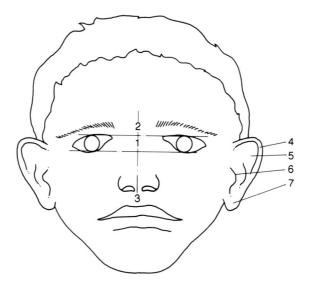

Figure 109.5 Terms used for the face. **Head shape:** sutures, fontanelles; hair pattern; eyebrows (synophrys); nose, tip, nares, ala, columella; philtrum (3); pupils, sclera, cornea; eye, anridia, inner (1) and outer (2) canthus, interpupillary distance; ear level, (4) helix, (5) antihelix, (6) tragus, (7) lobe (Frankfort plane); lips, vermillion, palate, tongue; chin, jaw, zygoma (mandible, maxilla); neck-web, goiter, cyst, pits, tags, pterygia; mouth size (intercommissural distance); measurements – biparietal diameter, head circumference.

Facial regions: brow, midface, cheeks, chin (malar, mandible); 1:1:1:eye|eye|eye|rule of one [12]; cataracts, coloboma.

Trunk, limbs: genitalia, skin; joints, digits, nails; sole, palm creases; body hair, distribution, absence; umbilicus, single umbilical artery; symmetry, absence; smaller or larger than normal (consider ±2 SD as within normal); terms (glossary, see Ref. 13).

Table 109.10 Special methods

Histochemistry
Fluorescent microscopy
Enzyme linked assays; radioimmunoassays
Autoradiography – radiolabelled *in situ* hybridization (ISH)
Electron microscopy: scanning, transmission
Serial section – three-dimensional reconstructions
Macro/microdissection – nerve fibers, renal tubules
Injected specimens – corrosion, cleared (prior staining)
Whole organ sections or whole body sections
In situ hybridization, fluorescent ISH – cytogenetics
Cell/tissue/organ culture; cell line; cell storage; cell or tissue bank
Karyotype preparation – standard, prophase, sperm, oocytes
Organ perfusion: lung, placenta, renal, liver, etc.
Extraction DNA, toxic substances; drugs from tissues, fluids, organs
Storage: biochemical samples, virology, serology, immunology, DNA bank
Other

| | Placenta Report | Page 1 of 1 |

PATH No.

Mother's Name _____ , _____

Med. Rec. No. _____

Dr. _____ Service _____   Date _____

Maternal: Age ____ G ____ P ____ A ____ LMP ____.

1.	Clinical diagnoses (codes) (see maternal abstract) Infant Med. Rec. No. _____	POC, Mole ____ SAB ____ STB ____ APD ____ IPD ____ NND____ PPND____ Other ____

Gross 2. review (1) (2) (3) (4)	Fresh ____ Fixed ____ Date deliv._____ Singleton, Multiple:** ____/____ (metric units) Cord Insertion _____ Number vessels _____ Cord Length _____ Knots ____ Hematoma ____ Membrane (roll) Color _____ Clear _____ Leading point ____ Yolk sac ____ Other ____ Placenta: Wt ____ W ____ L ____ Depth ____.	

Calcifications ____ Serial cuts ____ Cysts ____   Infarcts ____ Thrombi ____ Tumor _____

Other ____ Decidua ____ Attached clots ____   Constrictions of cord _____

Fetal surface: Bands _____ Cysts ____ Hemorrhage ____ Color ____ Clear _____

Nodules ____ Odor ____ Other ____. Abnormal lobation ____ Fenestra ____ Extra lobes ____

Increta, percreta, acreta, Circumvallate, marginate. Abnormal vessels ____ Insertions ____

Photos ____ Microbiology ____ Cytogenetics ____ Chemical ____ Other ____	**Twins? MA/MC; DA/MC; DA/DC; fused Vascular anastomoses

Microscopic 3. review	Microscopic: Normal/abnormal: Amnion, Chorion, Cord, Villi, Decidua (Primary, secondary, tertiary – arterioles – capillaries of villi) – Trophoblast, Cytotroph, Höfbauer & other cells, Collagen, fibrin, I.V.Space Abnormalities: Villitis, Tumor, Hydropic, C-Amnionitis, Other _____ (separate page)

Comment 4.	

Diagnoses 5. (code) placenta, cord and membranes	

Maternal History

Abstract

PATH No.

Name _____ , _____

Med. Rec. No. _____

Dr. _____ Service _____

Date _____

Synopsis	POC ____ SAB ____
	STB ____ FD ____ IPD ____
	NND ____
	Post ND ____ Twins+ ____
	Pl ____ Other ____
	Induced Abortion ____

1. Mother	Abstract ○
	Interview ○ Age ____ G ____ P ____ A ____ STB ____ Prev.Pregn. ____ If so (page 2) _____
	LMP ____ EDD ____ HT ____ WT ____ GAIN ____ BP ____ UA ____ G/P __/__ Smoker ____
	ETOH ____ Education ____ Ethnic ____ Occup ____ Gen.Health ____ Reg Med. ____ OTC ____
	Surgery ____

2. Father	Father Age ____ Smoker ____ ETOH ____ Recreation ____ Health ____ Occup ____ Ethnic ____
	>20/d >4 oz/d
	Siblings ____ Medications ____ Environmental exposures ____ Other ____

3. Maternal past history	PPD ____ HAV/HBV ____ Diabetes ____ TORCHS ____ STS/RPR/VDRL _____ UTI ____
	Radiation Exp. ____ Thryoid ____ DES ____ Epilepsy ____ Allergies ____ Asthma ____
	ABO/Rh ____ Anemia ____ FeRx ____ Immunizations ____ Foreign travel ____ Drug reactions ____
	Transfusions ____ Rhogam ____ Cardiac ____ Phlebitis ____ Accidents ____ Hospitalizations ____
	Serious injuries ____ Fractures ____ Illicit drug use ____ Consanguinity ____ Abuse ____
	Maternal drug screen ____ HIV ____ Past drug scene ____ Jaundice ____ Other ____

4. Family history	Genetic: Hemoglobinopathies ____ Metabolic ____ Familial ____ Neural tube ____ Crippled ____
	MR ____ Bleeding ____ Deaf or blind ____ Muscle disease ____ CF pancreas ____ Anemia ____
	Chromosome defects ____ Birth defects – both sides of family ____ Fits/seizures/spells ____
	Breakdown ____ Nervous disease ____ Blue baby ____ Infertile ____ Exposure toxins, pesticides,
	etc. ____ Breast cancer ____ Cancer ____ ↑ BP ____ Stroke ____ CAD ____ Die young ____
	Mental illness ____ TR-21 ____ Fragile X ____ DES ____ Hab.AB ____ STB ____ Lupus ____
	Any genetic diseases ____ Retarded – slow in school ____ Institutional care ____
	(see pedigree, separate page)

5. Gynecology	Normal ____ Abnormal ____ PAP smear ____ BCP ____ Other contraceptives ____ Menarche ____
	Days flow ____ Pads ____ Gyn. procedures ____ Infertile ____ STD ____ HCG ____ Risks ____
	Herpes ____ Venereal warts ____ Chlamydia ____ (over)

Name _____ Date _____ PATH No. _____ [box]

6. Previous pregnancies 2. Prior 3. "	SAB ____ STB ____ LB ____ NND ____ IND AB ____ PT ____ LBW ____ Ectopic ____ Multiple ____ 1. Date, EDC, GA, Labor time, Type deliv., Anesth., PTLRx, BW, Outcome _____ _____ _____ (If additional lines needed use separate page)
7. Antenatal studies	Dates/Place/Dr/Results (include DOB, date of test, lab.# and laboratory) MSAFP ____ AFAFP ____ Amniocentesis ____ FBS–PUBS ____ CVS ____ Other _____ HCG/UE3/ ____ BPP ____ Biometry ____ Doppler ____ Echo ____ Ultrasound(I–III) ____ Other ____ Laboratory data: Screen: ____ Biochemical ____ DNA ____ Cytogenetics ____ TVUS ____ Abdominal US ____ Stress tests ____ Cultures ____ L/S ratio ____ ΔOD_{450} ____ Other ____ (If additional lines needed use separate page)
8. Present pregnancy	Normal ____ Abnormal ____ 1,2,3rd trimesters. UTI ____ Bleeding ____ Spotting ____ N+V ____ Wt/gain ____ Proteinuria ____ ↑BP ____ Rash ____ Flu ____ Fever ____ Quickening ____ Fundal ht ____ FHR ____ Cervix ____ Discharge _____ Number prenatal visits ____ No. missed ____ OB/GP/RN ____ Midwife ____ Care provided ____ Any risks ____ Risk assessment ____ Protocol used ____ Nutrition ____ Eating habits ____ Bed rest ____ Labor and delivery – Transfer from another Facility _____ (see extra page) Labor and delivery – In House – In Home Dates ( ) Frequency contractions ____ Spontaneous ____ Induced ____ Labor (meds, anesthesia, other): ____/ROM/ _____ date _____ Length of labor _____ FHR ____ Mat BP ____ T ____ P ____ C/section _____ Delivery (mode) _____ /Presentation/_____ Date _____ Birth ____ Infant sex ____ BW ____ CHL ____ Apgar ____ 1 min ____ 5 min ____ Amount am. fluid ____ PROM ____ PTL ____ LBW ____ Meconium ____ Monitoring ____ Prolapse cord ____ Outcome ____ See Infant's chart ____. Placental time interval to deliver _____
	Infant No. [box] Placental No. [box]
9. Maternal summary diagnoses and codes	

1546

PATH No.

Mother's name _____

Med. Rec. No. _____

Dr. _____ Service _____

Mother's Age ____ LMP ____ G ____ P ____ A ____

Date _____

Maternal history abstract (see no. _____)
Clinical diagnosis

Placental report (see no. _____)
Clinical diagnosis

1.
Date delv. _____ Date rec'd _____

Type of specimen: EMBRYO ____ + Sac ____ No Sac ____

<20w GA _____   Fetus ____ ± Sac ____ Fragments ____ Placenta/intact ____ Fragments ____

Conceptual age ____   POC ____ Mole ____ SAB ____ Early STB ____

Developmental age ____   Gross normal ____ Abnormal ____ Other ____ Fresh ____ Fixed ____

Macerated ____

2.
PHOTOS _____   CH or CRL ____ BW ____ Foot L ____ Other ____

X-RAYS _____   Embryo: <8 w and <30 mm CR. Normal ____ Frag ____

MICROBIOLOGY____   G1 to GD4 ____ Specify _____

CYTOGENETICS ____   External and internal features

OTHER _____

(see next page)

---

3. FETUS: Organ wts (metric units)

	CNS	Heart	Lungs	Liver	Renal	Adrs	Thyrd	Spleen	Other	
[expected]	[ ]	[ ]	[ ]	[ ]	[ ]	[ ]	[ ]	[ ]	[ ]	[ ]

---

4. <u>External examination</u>: Normal ____ Symmetric ____ Fresh ____ Macerated ____ Fixed
Edema, hemorrhage, tears, maceration, dislocation, discoloration. Iatrogenic/traumatic lesions
Describe (separate page) abnormalities, fontanelles, sutures, scalp – (1) HEENT Neck-web, lids fused or not
(2) Chest/back (3) Abdomen/umbilicus (4) Perineum/genitalia (5) Limbs/hands/no. fingers ____ feet/nos. toes
____ (6) Hair/skin/nails (7) Other _____ Patent: choana, otic canal, urethra, oropharynx, anus
Palm/sole creases/prints ____

| Surgical Report |

5. <u>Internal Examination</u> (describe abnormal)/<u>Situs</u>, <u>fluid</u>, <u>air</u>, <u>blood</u> in abnormal locations

CNS – Meninges, tentorium, spinal cord. Chest – heart and lungs, great vessels

(Ductus, coarctation) IVC and SVC

Present/absent thyroid, thymus, TEF, CDH, cardiac defects, bronchial tree

Sections lung, liver, kidneys, spleen and adrenals. Thrombi – vessels

Bowel atresia or abnormalities. Any anomalies – absence of spleen, adrenals, ovaries, testes, uterus, vagina,

cervix, muscle, bone or skin

(see separate page)

6. <u>Microscopic evaluation – tissues sampled</u>

1. Brain (0–1), thyroid, larynx, thymus, tracheobronchial tree ____ R and L lungs ____ / ____

2. Heart (0–2): chambers, valves, aorta ____ R and L ventricles ____ / ____ Ductus _____

Diaphragm muscle, psoas, other ____ Ribs/sternum ____ Mediastinum ____ Lymph Nodes ____

Vertebrae ____ Marrow ____ Liver ____ Pancreas ____ Spleen ____ Mesentery _____

Various levels of the alimentary tract – Esoph: ____ Stom: ____ SM int: ____ LG int: ____

Adrenals ____ Ovary/testes ____ Kidneys ____ Ur. bladder _____

Prostate ____ Uterus/FT ____ Skin ____ Umbilical cord ____ Other _____

7. <u>Microscopic evaluation – general maturation</u>

See Brain cutting report: 0–1, Heart dissection report: 0–2

For complex anomalies use other: 0–3. Discussions should include level of development, clinicopathological

correlations and maternal/placental findings. Comments.

(see separate page)

8. <u>Diagnosis/Codes</u>

Necropsy Form

(Standard autopsy)

PATH No.

Mother's name _____

Med. Rec. No. _____

Dr. _____ Service _____ Patient's Name _____ Date _____

---

1. INFANT med. rec. no. (_____)

   Clinical diagnoses (codes)

   ____ induced, therapeutic AB

   STB ____ FD ____ APFD ____
   IPD ____ NND ____ Postnatal
   death ____ Other _____

2. MATERNAL abstract no. ____

3. PLACENTAL report no. ____

4. Photos ____ X-Rays ____ Microbiology ____ Chemical ____ Other ____

   Date of birth or delivery _____

   Singleton ____ Twin ____ Other ____ Fresh ____ Macerated ____ Fixed ____

5. GA ____ Sex ____ BW ____ CRL/CHL ____ Foot L ____ Other ____

   Metric units

External Symmetry R=L [expected]	CNS	Heart	Lungs	Liver	Renal	Adrs	Thyrd	Spleen	Other	
	[ ]	[ ]	[ ]	[ ]	[ ]	[ ]	[ ]	[ ]	[ ]	[ ]

6. General: Habitus ____ Normal ____ Abnormal ____ Discoloration ____ Hemorrhage ____ Edema ____
   (If abnormal describe on separate page) iatrogenic or traumatic lesions, catheter, incisions, etc.

   General petechiae, meconium stains or rashes ____ Bullae ____ Pigmentation ____ Vesicles ____
   Head shape ____ OFC ____ Fontanelles ____ Sutures ____ Scalp ____ Hair ____ Hair line ____ Eyes ____
   IPD ____ Nose ____ Choana ____ Philtrum ____ Brows ____ Frankfort line (eye–ear) ____ Ears ____
   Otic canal ____ Lobes ____ Tongue ____ Lips ____ Chin ____ Goiter ____ Other _____ Neck ____
   Web ____ Pterygia ____ Limbs ____ Joints ____ Creases ____ Chest (breast/nipples)/Back (spine) _____
   Hands/palms creases ____ Fingers (no.) ____ Print ____ Abdomen (umbilicus) _____ Feet/soles creases ____
   Toes (no.) ____ Prints ____ Perineum (anus) _____ Skin _____ Nails _____ External genitalia: male/
   female ____ Ambiguous ____ Body hair ____ Urethra patent ____ Scrotum ____ Labia ____ Size (clitoris/
   penis) ____ Other _____

Necropsy Form

Patient Record No.: _____   Date _____

---

7.   <u>Internal examination</u> size, color, shape, cut surface, normal? If not what _____

   <u>CNS (see 0–1)</u> General state of meninges, _____ base of brain _____ tentorium, _____ edema, _____ hemorrhage _____ location _____ and amount _____ infarcts _____

   <u>Heart (see 0–2)</u> situs _____ chambers _____ atria _____ R. ventricle _____ L. ventricle _____ Coronary sinus _____ Pulmonary veins _____ Valves _____ TV _____ PV _____ MV _____ AV _____ Coronary arteries _____ Ductus _____ Aorta _____ Renal art/veins _____ IVC and SVC _____ Carotid arteries _____ Larynx _____ Trachea _____ Bronchial tree _____ Thyroid _____ Thymus _____ Mediastinum _____ Thoracic pleura _____ Pericardial sac _____ R. lung _____ L. lung _____ Diaphragm _____ Ductus venosus _____ Liver (R/L): _____ Gallbladder _____ Pancreas (HBT) _____ Spleen(s) _____ Mesentery _____ Adrenals R/L _____ Kidneys R/L _____ Ureters R/L _____ Urinary bladder _____ Umbilical cord _____ Urethra _____ Prostate _____ Uterus _____ Fall. tubes _____ Cx/Vg _____ Ovary R/L _____ Testes R/L _____ Skel. muscle. (specify) _____ /Lymph nodes _____ Bones (specify) _____. Palate/tongue _____ Esophagus _____ Stomach _____ Pylorus _____ Duodenum _____ Ileocecum _____ Appendix _____ Colon _____ Rectum _____ Anus _____ Other _____.

   Review: situs of organs, R/O FB, TEF, CDH, hydronephrosis, anomalous venous return, thrombi in renal arteries/veins

   (See separate page for descriptions of abnormal findings and diagrams or photos)

   (see page _____)

---

8.   <u>Following pages</u>.   1. Microscopic findings (separate page)

      Maturation, describe anomalies

   2. The correlation of placental and maternal findings to necropsy diagnoses

      Comments, diagnoses (code)

   (see page _____)

109.8 Addendum: a simplified method for routine study of the major components of the conduction system of the heart in perinatal infants
D.J. deSa

The method described below is one that the author has found useful and has used routinely. It is not meant to supplant the very extensive procedures that are used by many cardiac pathologists, but it does have the advantage of being relatively simple and has yielded some interesting results. Those readers who desire a more extensive sampling are referred to standard texts (e.g. Hudson's review [30]).

109.8.2 SINUATRIAL NODE

The sinuatrial node lies at the summit of the right atrium near the junction of the point of entry of the superior vena cava and the crista terminalis. This area may be dissected and divided into parallel blocks taken transversely. The resulting blocks are usually small enough for several to be embedded in one cassette.

109.8.2 ATRIOVENTRICULAR NODE AND BUNDLE OF HIS

After fixation and removal of the free walls of both ventricles and atria, the interventricular and interatrial septa and the roots of the great vessels can be examined. The medial wall of the right atrium is cut at the opening of the coronary sinus and the cut is carried in an anterior and cephalad direction to include the roots of the aorta and pulmonary trunk. A second cut, parallel to the first, is made across the interventricular system just beyond the septal papillary muscle of the tricuspid valve (Figure 109.6). Anterior and posterior cuts at right angles to the first two cuts are made, to include the root of the great vessels anteriorly and through the posterior interventricular septum, to complete the block. The author has found it useful to photograph this block from both its right and left aspects at this point. Parallel slices are taken from this block in its long axis from the posterior aspect to the anterior aspect and placed in a sequential manner and photographed (Figure 109.7). The right ventricular surface is always placed on the right, and the left ventricular on the left. Each block can then be embedded, and their orientation can be checked with the photograph. The example illustrated is from the heart of a term infant with pulmonary hypertension, bronchopulmonary dysplasia, cardiac failure, and jaundice complicating intravenous hyperalimentation and the slices are of approximately 5-mm thickness. The necrotic myocardium is bilestained in this example. Smaller hearts do pose greater problems, but can be studied (Figure 109.8), after some practice.

The sections provide adequate sampling of the atrioventricular node and the bundle of His, and as all the material is embedded, serial sections can be studied if required.

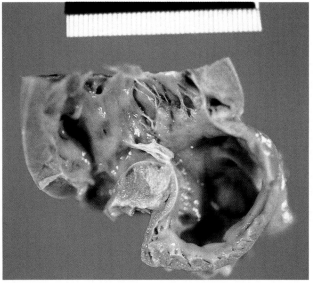

(a)

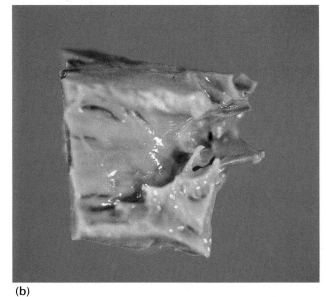

(b)

Figure 109.6 Two views of the dissected cardiac block used for studying the conduction system. The details are outlined in the text. This relatively large block of tissue is derived from a term infant who required ventilation and parenteral feeding all his life, and who had bronchopulmonary dysplasia, cholestasis and cardiac failure. (a) The view from the right ventricular aspect with septal leaflets of the tricuspid valve and the septal muscle of Lancisi. (b) The view of the block from the left ventricular aspect.

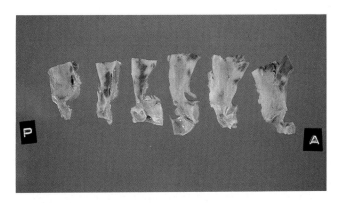

Figure 109.7 Parallel blocks taken as described in the text are shown. The infant is the same as in Figure 109.6. P = posterior aspect of block; A = anterior aspect of block. In each slice the right ventricular aspect is on the right. The necrotic myocardial fibres in this example are inadvertently but conveniently bile stained.

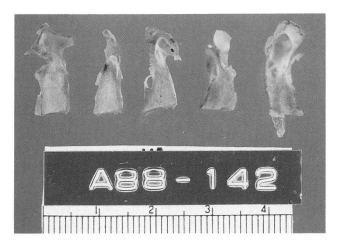

Figure 109.8 Blocked out septum in a 31-week-old infant. In this example, the blocks are oriented with those from the posterior aspect on the left, whereas those from the anterior aspect are on the right, but the right ventricular aspect is on the **left** of the block as viewed. This was done to demonstrate the small area of subendocardial hemorrhage near the atrioventricular node (second slice from left). (This infant also had a microscopic polycystic tumor of the atrioventricular node! Case presented by Dr D. Rosati, Canadian Congress of Laboratory Medicine, St John's, Newfoundland, June 1990.)

Procedure for removal of the petrous temporal bone

The scheme for examination of the petrous temporal bone, outlined in the following, offers a reasonable and practical approach for the routine laboratory.

After removal of the brain, the right petrous temporal bone is opened using strong bone-cutting scissors. Converging cuts are placed at the medial and lateral ends of the bone, and the bone can then be lifted away exposing the cavity [29]. The contents are inspected and sampled for microbiologic and virologic studies. With practice the bone can be opened through the tympanic cavity in a consistent fashion, allowing the labyrinth to be separated from the rest of the bone and affording an opportunity to examine the ossicles. In addition, the separated labyrinth is now more accessible to penetration by fixatives, and may be used for ultrastructural examination if so desired.

The left petrous temporal bone is removed *en bloc* from the skull with an external plane of cleavage that passes through the terminal portion of the external auditory canal and the temporalis muscle [31]. The specimen is fixed in formal saline for a week. The sample is subjected to X-irradiation using a portable Faxitron machine; horizontal blocks of tissue of 0.3 cm average thickness are cut through the undecalcified bone using a Buehler Isomet low-speed saw. These slices are taken parallel to a plane that joins the external auditory canal with the foramina of the eighth nerve. The slices can be examined visually before being decalcified and embedded in paraffin. This procedure shortens the length of time that is needed for decalcification, allowing better histological preparations. The radiologic preparations enable one to identify major defects in the labyrinth.

References

1. Byrne, J.M. (1983) Fetal pathology, Laboratory manual. *Birth Defects*, **19**, 1–48.
2. Valdes-Dapena, M. and Huff, D. (1983) *Perinatal Autopsy Manual*, Armed Forces Institute of Pathology, Washington, DC.
3. Winter, R., Knowles, S., Bieber, F. *et al.* (1988) *The Malformed Fetus and Stillborn*, Wiley, New York, p. 304.
4. Winter, R. and Baraister, M. (eds) (1990) *Multiple Anomalies Diagnostic Compendium*, Chapman & Hall, London.
5. Buyse, M. (ed.) (1990) *Birth Defects Encyclopedia*, Blackwell Scientific Boston.
6. Kalousek, D., Fitch, N. and Pardice, B. (1990) *Pathology of the Human Embryo and Previable Fetus*, Springer, New York.
7. Warburton, D., Byrne, J. and Canki, N. (1991) *Chromosome Anomalies and Prenatal Development: An Atlas*, Oxford University Press, Oxford.
8. Dimmick, J. and Kalousek, D. (eds) (1992) *Developmental Pathology of the Embryo and Fetus*, J.B. Lippincott, Philadelphia.
9. Merlob, P., Sivan, Y. and Reisner, S. (1984) Anthropomorphic measurements of the newborn infant. *Birth Defects*, **20**, 1–52.
10. Saul, R., Skinner, S. and Stevenson, R. *et al.* (1988) *Growth References from Conception to Adulthood*, Proc. Greenwood Genet. Center, Greenwood, SC. (Suppl. 1).
11. Hall, J., Froster–Iskernius, U. and Allanson, J. (1989) *Handbook of Normal Physical Measurements*, Oxford University Press, New York.
12. Aase, J. (1990) *Diagnostic Dysmorphology*, Plenum Press, New York.
13. Goodman, R. and Gorlin, R. (1983) *The Malformed Infant and Child*, Oxford University Press, Oxford.
14. Gruenwald, P. and Minh, H. (1961) Evaluation of body and organ weights in perinatal pathology II. Weight of body and placenta in surviving and in autopsied infants. *Am. J. Obstet. Gynecol.*, **82**, 312–19.

15. Phillipe, E. (1974) *Histopathologie Placentaire*, Masson, Paris, p. 27.
16. Gruenwald, P. and Minh, H. (1960) Evaluation of body and organ weights in perinatal pathology I. Normal standards derived from autopsies. *Am. J. Clin. Pathol.*, **34**, 247–53.
17. Streeter, G.L. (1920) *Contribution to Embryology XI*, No. 55, Carnegie Institute, Baltimore, pp. 143–70.
18. Gilles F.H. (1985) Perinatal neuropathology in, *Textbook of Neuropathology*, 1st edn (eds R. Davis and D. Robertson), Williams & Wilkins, Baltimore, MD, pp. 252–53.
19. Manchester, D.K. (1987) The dysmorphic infant, in *Current Pediatric Diagnosis and Treatment*, 9th edn (eds C. Kempe, H. Silver, D. O'Brien and V. Fulginiti) Appleton, & Lange, Norwalk, CT, p. 1054.
20. Kraus, F. (1991) Role of the pathologist in evaluation of infertility, in *Pathology of Reproductive Failure* (eds F. Kraus, I. Damjanov and N. Kaufman), Williams & Wilkins, Baltimore, MD, pp. 334–48.
21. Stillbirth and Neonatal Death Society (1991) *Miscarriage, Stillbirth and Neonatal Death*, SANDS, London.
22. Limbo, R. and Wheeler, S. (1990) *When a Baby Dies*, RTS, Resolve Through Sharing, Lutheran Hospital, LaCrosse, La Crosse, WI.
23. Cordero, J. (1992) Registries of birth defects and genetic diseases. *Pediatr. Clin. North Am.*, **39**, 65–75. [Author used modification of ICD-9 and Br. Paediatr. Assoc., CDC, Atlanta.]
24. International Clearinghouse of Birth Defects Monitoring System (1991) *Congenital Malformations, Worldwide*, ICBDMS, Elsevier, Amsterdam.
25. European Study of Congenital Anomalies and Twins (Eurocat): Central Registry, Institut d'Hygiène et d'Epidémiologie, 14 Rue J. Wytsman, 1050 Brussels, Belgium.
26. Donnelly, W. and Buchhoz, C. (1984) *Systematized Nomenclature of Medicine (SNOMED): Microglossary for Pediatrics, Pediatric Pathology and Perinatal Medicine*, CAP, Skokie, IL.
27. Buetow, S. (1992) The perinatal autopsy: its conduct and reporting in Australia. *Med. J. Aust.*, **156**, 492–94.
28. Chambers, H. (1992) The perinatal autopsy: a contemporary approach. *Pathology*, **24**, 45–55.
29. Morison, J.E. (1970) *Foetal and Neonatal Pathology*, 3rd edn, Butterworth, London, p. 563.
30. Hudson, R.E.B. (1991) The conducting system: Anatomy, histology and pathology in acquired heart disease. In *Cardiovascular Pathology*, 2nd edn. (ed. M. Silver) Churchill-Livingstone, New York, pp. 1367–427.
31. deSa, D.J. (1973) Infection and amniotic aspiration of middle ear in stillbirths and neonatal deaths. *Arch. Dis. Child.*, **48**, 872–80.

Further reading

American College of Obstetricians and Gynecologists (1989) *ACOG Antepartum Record*, copyright ACOG, 409 12th St SW, Washington, DC (4 page protocol).
Anonymous (1989) Joint study group – fetal abnormalities. *Arch. Dis. Child.*, **64**, 971–76.
Beckwith, J.B. (1989) The value of the pediatric postmortem examination. *Pediatr. Clin. North Am.*, **36**, 29–36.
de la Fuente, A., Dornseiffen, G., van Noort, G. and Laurini, R. (1988) Routine perinatal postmortem radiography in a peripheral pathology laboratory. *Virchows Arch. [A]*, **413**, 513–19.
Freeman R.K. and Poland, R.L. (eds) (1992) *Guidelines for Perinatal Care*, 3rd edn, American Academy of Pediatrics and American College of Obstetricians and Gynecologists, Washington, DC, and Elk Grove, IL, Appendix A: Personnel services, pp. 235–39; Appendix B: Maternal consultation/transfer, p. 241; Appendix C: Newborn consultation/transfer, p. 243; Appendix D: US requirement for patient transfer, pp. 245–47; Appendix E: Antepartum record, pp. 249–520.
Gilbert-Barness, G., Opitz, J. and Barness, L. (1989) The pathologists' perspective of genetic disease: malformation and dysmorphology. *Pediatr. Clin. North Am.*, **36**, 163–87.
Hanzlick, R. and Parrish, R. (1993) The failure of death certificates to record the performance of autopsies (letter). *JAMA*, **269**, 47.
Hey, E., Lloyd, D. and Wigglesworth, J. (1986) Classifying perinatal death: fetal and neonatal factors. *Br. J. Obstet Gynaecol.*, **93**, 1213–23.
Hutchins, G. (ed.) (1990) Perinatal and pediatric autopsies, in *Autopsy Performance and Reporting*, College of American Pathologists, Northfield, IL pp. 123–26
Joint Working Party (1988) *Report on Fetal and Perinatal Pathology*, Royal College of Obstetricians and Gynaecologists and Royal College of Pathologists, London.
Kozakewich, H., Fox. K., Plato, C. *et al.* (1992) Dermatoglyphics in sudden infant death syndrome, *Pediatr. Pathol.*, **12**, 637–51.
Lynch, H. and Hoden, R. (1990) *International Directory of Genetic Services*, March of Dimes, White Plains, NY.
McManus, B., Suvalsky, S. and Wilson, J. (1992) A decade of acceptable autopsy rates. *Arch. Pathol. Lab. Med.*, **116**, 1128–36.
Report of the Royal College of Pathologists Working Party (1990) Paediatric and perinatal pathology. *Bull. R. Coll. Pathol.*, **69**, 10–13.
Sobey, W. and Cardaci-Polizzotto, R. (1992) *Antepartal Screening of the Pregnant Woman*, 2nd edn, Series 2: Prenatal Care, Module 7, March of Dimes, White Plains, NY.
Society of Pediatric Pathology (USA) (1975) Questionnaire: curriculum content of medical school teaching development, embryo, fetal, neonatal and pediatric pathology.
Vance, R. (1992) Autopsies and attitudes (editorial). *Arch. Pathol. Lab. Med.*, **116**, 1111–12.
Wigglesworth, J. (1991) Quality of the perinatal autopsy. *Br. J. Obstet. Gynaecol.*, **98**, 617–23.

Computer databases

- OMIM, W.H. Welch Medical Library, Johns Hopkins University, Baltimore, MD.
- GEMS (epidemiology), Department of Human Genetics, University of Pittsburgh, Pittsburgh, PA.
- POSSUMS, Department of Genetics, Royal Children's Hospital, Parkville, Victoria, Australia.
- Medline, National Library of Medicine, Bethesda, MD.
- See reference 10 (other databases).
- See Winter, R. and Baraister, M. (eds) (1991) *Multiple Congenital Anomalies*, Chapman & Hall, London (Supplement, 1993, dysmorphology and neurogenetic databases, London).

110 TWO PIONEER PHYSICIAN–SCIENTISTS

S.F. Cahalane

Dr John W. Ballantyne, a Scot, and Sir Archibald Garrod, an Englishman, flourished a century ago. Each was a medical pioneer with compelling claims to remembrance in a work on fetal and neonatal pathology. It may be that their work is emerging from the near oblivion in which it has languished. Almost 25 years ago a biographical monograph on Ballantyne was published by Helen Russell [1], while Garrod's biography has been recently written by Alexander Bearn [2], both biographers being of the medical profession.

Ballantyne comprehensively recorded his observations on morphological abnormalities of the embryo, fetus and newborn infant. Garrod's lasting achievement was the recognition of the hereditary diathesis and the chemical individuality of man. Garrod was the forerunner of molecular genetics and Ballantyne the father of perinatal pathology. Each had crossed over the borderland of the other's domain: Ballantyne pondered the inheritance of malformation while Garrod recognized that some morphological abnormalities were inborn.

110.1 John William Ballantyne (1861–1923) and antenatal pathology

Around the turn of the last century Dr John Ballantyne was a familiar figure in Edinburgh. A slightly built, dapper, good humoured man with a modish walrus moustache, he walked briskly through her streets, squares and closes bound for hospital, laboratory, library, lecture theatre or 'kirk o' Sundays'.

Sprung on his father's side from lowland stock of high seriousness and professional botanical pursuits, his mother was of a Dutch family. His scientific bent was channelled into medicine through accompanying his uncle, a country doctor, on his rounds. Walking holidays in Europe gave him his early knowledge of the continent and its languages and this would later mature into familiarity with the great universities and medical centres.

Although formally an obstetrician he was at the same time a paediatrician and a pathologist, even the first perinatal pathologist. He sought, from meticulous dissections of hundreds of dead fetuses and newborn infants, in addition to clinical observations of thousands of maternities, the unravelling of antenatal pathology and teratology. These areas of knowledge were little understood, being either ignored or shrouded in myth and folklore. From the outset his devotion was to library and laboratory but he gave generously and charitably to the clinical needs of mothers and children in the Royal Maternity and other Edinburgh hospitals and dispensaries. His reading and writing were undertaken from 6 a.m. to 10 a.m., and thereafter clinical and laboratory work as well as teaching responsibilities occupied his day. He and his wife were childless and society seems to have had little attraction for them, or leastwise for him!

Ballantyne was born in Dalkeith and went to school and university in Edinburgh. Portents of his life's work were signalled by distinctions at his degree examinations in medicine, pathology, obstetrics and gynaecology. Had paediatrics been on the curriculum then, it too would surely have granted him further honours as at one time it seemed to be his chosen career and became the subject of the first of his three textbooks: *Diseases of Infancy* [3]. This work was a compendium of historical survey, practical advice on the approach to and examination of the sick child and a down to earth system-based primer on clinical appearance, diagnosis and treatment. There was a strong anatomical and physiological framework for this wide fabric. Punctilious indexing of his sources, a hallmark of his extensive writings, was evident from this beginning.

Thereafter, as Helen Russell [1] states in her biographical monograph, the focus of his endeavours was exploring the early stages of human development and their disorders. This led to the appearance in 1892 and 1895 of the two volumes of *The Diseases and Deform-*

Diseases of the Fetus and Newborn, 2nd edn, Edited by G.B. Reed, A.E. Claireaux and F. Cockburn. Published in 1995 by Chapman & Hall, London. ISBN 0 412 39160 0

ities of the Foetus [4]. His dedication of this work to Cesare Taruffi of Bologna, the historian of teratology, and Camille Dareste of Lyons, a leading contemporary teratologist, reflects his easy familiarity with current European thought in this area. A historical section reviews what was known about congenital malformations in the recorded annals of mankind. This ranges from cuneiform lists of these anomalies on clay tablets from Chaldean times to nineteenth century histological studies.

He personally related the exacting laboriousness of literature research and the benumbing deviations into blind alleys and mazes to which the pursuit of accuracy led him. Some indexing of sources was then available but he had none of the modern means of instant communication or literature searches. Yet he published three text books and probably some 400 original communications and invited articles. His publications from 1902 to his death in 1923 have not been catalogued, but he listed those before 1902 in volume 1 of *Antenatal Pathology and Hygiene* [5].

Many of the sources for his work were written in Latin but this did not pose a problem since it was then the lingua franca of scholars. If some of his correspondents did not understand English, or he their native tongues, they would resort to the language of Virgil, Horace and Cicero.

Perhaps Ballantynes's most valiant venture was in establishing and personally editing a quarterly journal named Teratologia, the first number of which appeared in 1894 [6]. This was the fruit of inspired thinking and he visualized it as a large repository of 19th century literature on teratology, in which would be included original articles, book reviews and abstracts of current papers. The concept won the approbation of prominent physicians on both sides of the Atlantic and the first issue was warmly welcomed by editorials in prestigious journals. None the less it failed after eight issues, for the want of 50 subscribers! It deserved a better fate! But, undaunted and undeterred in his belief that antenatal pathology had an important future, he immediately set about writing a lengthy paper on the history of the causes of monstrosities, which was published in 1895.

All of this was merely a prelude, a flexing of intellectual muscles, to his master work: the magnificent *Antenatal Pathology and Hygiene* published in two volumes (*The Foetus* and *The Embryo*) in 1902 and 1904 [5]. Helen Russell has justifiably stated that this established him among the pioneers of medicine. It was stamped with all the diligence and all the care for detail which had already marked his writing. But now the scale was vaster, its basic philosophy more authoritatively and trenchantly expressed. As in his other works there were polemical nuances, delivered in a measured mode and carrying the blazon of his absolute conviction that preventive medicine would not progress until the laws governing antenatal health were known. This work of inspiration and withal unremitting toil was presented in lucid clear-cut English.

The artist, W. Cathie, produced (as he had done for *Diseases and Deformities of the Foetus* [4]), water colour depictions of Ballantyne's whole mounted sections of abnormal fetuses. These offer further vividness to the author's prose description.

What we know of John Ballantyne's identification with Victorian women's affairs suggests that he would have sympathized with the objectives, if not the methods, of his contemporary Emmeline Pankhurst, the suffragette leader. He had genuine insights into the social problems of women, espousing their rights as mothers and as individuals. He actively supported the admission of women into medical schools and he paid a generous tribute to Dr Elizabeth Blackwell on the jubilee of her graduation as the first woman doctor. It can be taken that his wider engagement with the inequities of women in society stemmed from his recognition of their plight, particularly if poor, during pregnancy, parturition and the puerperium.

He lived to see his crusade for better antenatal care vindicated by the establishment of prematernity accommodation in The Royal Maternity Hospital, and later an antenatal outpatient clinic as well as a venereal disease clinic, all under his own supervision. His last published paper was a summation of his concepts of midwifery in the twentieth century [8].

Ballantyne's writings are rendered in a crisp English style that engages and carries the reader along. This is said by Russell [6] to reflect his devotion to the works of Johnson and Boswell. When we are also told that his great literary love was Dante we are at first surprised, then delighted. We wonder what dreams he may have dreamed of those doomed lovers Paula and Francesca, their stolen glances locked over the pages of a book. We can gratefully remember that the *Divine Comedy* influenced this man and lightened his own travail.

110.2 Archibald Garrod (1857–1936)

A molecular geneticist, not a student of the past, might require cogent persuasion that an almost forgotten London physician of 100 years ago was central to the concepts and development of his discipline. Indeed, Sir Archibald Edward Garrod might have permitted himself a sardonic smile at such a prophecy, even though, as I think likely, he knew that his ideas would last. It is also scarcely remembered that it was he who coined the term 'inborn errors of metabolism', and that the 'one gene one enzyme' concept was attributed to him, albeit inappropriately, by the Nobel laureates, Beadle and Tatum, in 1958. He was the lifelong proponent of the chemical individuality of man and other species.

Garrod was the quintessential establishment consultant physician of turn of the century London, honoured with a knighthood for his achievements and contributions to the broad field of medical education and administration. His special field of interest was, however, to his contemporaries, little more than a faddish preoccupation with a few rare conditions. He himself admitted that: 'Clinical medicine is not really my main interest, I am a wanderer down the bypaths of Medicine.' He was for many years a greatly respected consultant physician to St Bartholomew's Hospital and to the Hospital for Sick Children, Great Ormond Street. When the great Osler died, it was Garrod who was invited to succeed him in the most prestigious post of Regius Professor of Medicine at Oxford University. Garrod is the father of chemical pathology and, just a 100 years ago, he produced a handbook of pathology in colloboration with two colleagues at St Bartholomew's [9].

An accomplished linguist, he was familiar with and translated some classic Continental papers; in his early days his major interest was in rheumatism and rheumatoid arthritis, while his chemical background led him to explore the metabolic products of patients with gout.

Garrod published his first medical paper while a student at St Bartholomew's Hospital in 1884 [10], and scarcely a year passed without an important contribution from his pen until his last publication [11] in 1936, the year of his death.

His very first paper was written as a prize-winning essay in 1879, when he was an undergraduate in natural science at Oxford, and was entitled 'The Nebulae: a fragment of astronomical history'. While clearly not nebulous, there was nothing of the meteor's fire in his rise. Rather, he seems to have been an ever present, but little noticed star in the firmament of science for almost the whole of his professional life. Indeed, it might be said that a slow, steady beam marked the ascent of the Garrod family from archetypal 18th century Suffolk smallholders, through 19th century commerce and ultimately to quiet lambency in the intellectual and social ambience of Victorian London and the two great universities. Although a Huguenot origin has been mooted, the name would appear to refute this and suggests the quiet untrodden ways of immemorial shires. His father, his elder brother and he, all doctors, became Fellows of the Royal Society. Both his father and he were knighted, a distinction which early death probably denied the older brother. The First World War and its immediate aftermath robbed Garrod and his lady of their three soldier sons, leaving only his daughter, Dorothy, an archaeologist who would become the first woman professor at Cambridge.

When in the early 1900s mendelism was being rediscovered, Garrod recognized its application to the kindreds of alkaptonuria which he had collected at Great Ormond Street. With his contribution to the study of this disorder given to the Royal Medical and Chirurgical Society, he launched his epoch making concept of inborn errors of metabolism (1899) [12]. This was later seen to fulfil Kuhn's [13] postulates for a scientific revolution: 'a conceptual breakthrough, whose consequences continue to have the greatest theoretical and practical significance for physicians, biochemists and geneticists.'

There is a striking paradox at the heart of the perceptions of Garrod held by his contemporaries. He was honoured, and justly so, for his innovative organizational skills, his clinical teaching reforms and his espousal of chemical pathology as a medical specialty. At the same time, his life's work on inherited disease was scarcely acknowledged. Yet, this work was not carried out in any self-effacing obscurity. It was demonstrated in his daily teaching, described in medical journals, explained in two classical textbooks and expounded in named lectureships which he was invited to present. What underlay these contradictions? Was his work misunderstood? Was it flawed with any heterodoxy? None of these! Garrod's work on the biochemical individuality of man and other species was frequently simply not understood, often not comprehended by the doctors of science or of medicine to whom it was generously portrayed. Medical doctors were as interested in plant life as biologists were in human disease. There were notable exceptions in both groups, and with these he shared his thoughts and his work. It was not until 1908 that the Royal College of Physicians invited Garrod to deliver the important Croonian Lectures, which he entitled 'Inborn Errors of Metabolism' and which were published in the *Lancet* [14]. Bearn [2] emphasizes the failure of contemporary medicine to grasp the essence of these lectures, which, as he says, are 'now recognized as a landmark in medicine, biochemistry and genetics'. Garrod's own failure, if that be an appropriate term, was that he either did not or could not convince his contemporaries of the significance of his few rare diseases. Even he himself does not appear to have apprehended the coming revolution in molecular genetics.

The evolution of his thinking on alkaptonuria as a hereditary chemical imbalance has been chronicled by Bearn [2], including his successive demonstration of its occurrence among siblings, the importance of parental consanguinity and its simple recessive transmission. During his early days at Great Ormond Street he would relate, somewhat impishly, that he had tried to interest a male and female alkaptonuric in each other in order to demonstrate vertical descent of the disorder. At the Bradshaw lecture to the Royal College of Physicians in 1900, he elaborated his thoughts on cystinuria; this allowed him to generalize his ideas to other metabolic errors [15]. He was in contact with Osler in Baltimore for American cases and gave credit to Carl Huppert of Prague, who suggested interspecies differences in metabolizing drugs and infectious agents as being due to chemical individuality and who believed that the underlying mechanism rested in 'the structural differences of proteins in the body' [16].

In a paper of the first lecture on chemical pathology which he gave to students at St Bartholomew's in 1903, he said: 'The various families, genera, and species of animals and plants, differ as much from each other in their chemical structure and the products of their metabolism as in their anatomical structure and form [2].

When, in 1905, Bateson introduced the term 'genetics', it was too vague and elusive to be of great interest to Garrod [17]. In the years immediately prior to the First World War he appears to have wearied of the polemical battles between the Mendelians and the Ancestrians. When the War was over, and his three sons had failed to return, it is said that the fire had gone out of Garrod. Yet he had before him 7 years as Regius at Oxford (1920–1927) and time for tranquility and reflection. In 1931 he published his great book *The Inborn Factors in Disease* [18], and his last paper was published in 1936 [11], the year of his death. He had had time to read Asbjorn Folling's description of phenylketonuria in 1934, and to correspond briefly with him [2].

Archibald Garrod's report from Marlborough School in 1874 included this comment from his Headmaster: 'I wish he would continue to do his utmost in science, a subject in which he may certainly win distinction' [2].

References

1. Russell, H. (1971) *J.W. Ballantyne M.D., F.R.C.P. Edin.*, The Royal College of Physicians, Edinburgh.
2. Bearn, A.G. (1993) *Archibald Garrod and the Individuality of Man*, Clarendon Press, Oxford.
3. Ballantyne, J.W. (1891) *An Introduction to Diseases of Infancy: The Anatomy, Physiology and Hygiene of the Newborn Infant*, Oliver and Boyd, Edinburgh.
4. Ballantyne, J.W. (1892, 1985) *The Diseases and Deformities of the Foetus: An Attempt Towards a System of Antenatal Pathology*, 2 vols, Oliver and Boyd, Edinburgh.
5. Ballantyne, J.W. (1902, 1904) *Manual of Antenatal Pathology and Hygiene, The Foetus* (vol. 1), *The Embryo* (vol. 2), William Green, Edinburgh.
6. Ballantyne J.W. (ed.) (1894–1985) *Teratologia* (A Quarterly Journal of Antenatal Pathology), Williams and Norgate, London.
7. Ballantyne, J.W. (1895) *Teratogenesis: An Inquiry into the Causes of Monstrosities: Histories of the Theories of the Past*, Oliver and Boyd, Edinburgh.
8. Ballantyne, J.W. (1923) The new midwifery: preventive and reparative obstetrics. *BMJ*, i, 617–21.
9. Herringham, W.P., Garrod, A.E. and Gow, W.J. (1894) *A Handbook of Medical Pathology: For the Use of Students in the Museum of St Bartholomew's Hospital*, Baillière, Tindall and Cox, London.
10. Garrod, A.E. (1884) A visit to the leper hospital at Bergen (Norway). *St Bartholomew's Hosp. Rep.*, 30, 311–13 (abstract).
11. Garrod, A.E. (1936) Congenital porphyrinuria: a postscript. *Q. J. Med.*, 29, 473–80.
12. Garrod, A.E. (1899) A contribution to the study of alkaptonuria. *Med. Chir. Trans.*, 82, 369–94; *Proc. R. Med. Chir. Soc.*, N.S. 11, 130–35.
13. Kuhn, T.S. (1962) *The Structure of Scientific Revolutions*, University of Chicago Press, Chicago.
14. Garrod, A.E. (1908) The Croonian lectures on inborn errors of metabolism. *Lancet*, ii, 1–7, 73–79, 142–48, 214–20.
15. Garrod, A.E. (1900) The Bradshaw lecture on the urinary pigments in their pathological aspects. *Lancet*, ii, 1323–31.
16. Huppert, C.H. (1896) *In Die Erhaltung Der Arteigenschaften*, Carl Ferdinand Univesity Press, Prague.
17. Bateson, W. (1928) *Essays and Addresses*, Cambridge University Press, Cambridge, p. 93.
18. Garrod, A.E. (1931) *The Inborn Factors in Disease: An Essay*, Clarendon Press, Oxford.

INDEX

Editor's note
As well as using the index, the reader should refer to the minicontents for each chapter in Parts One to Six (see pages vii–xxviii). In addition there are several detailed appendices, for example, at the end of Chapter 36 on kidney disease, Chapter 74 on biochemical genetics and Chapter 77 on prenatally diagnosable mendelian disorders. Other chapters have extensive tables and detailed categories of various conditions, diseases and disorders.

Page entries in bold refer to figures and those in italic refer to tables. As a result of the trans-Atlantic nature of this book, all those entries that occur in both English and American chapters are spelt in the British form.

Abdomen,
  circumference 15, 890–1
    B-scan measurement 888
    for SGA 279
    ultrasound measurement 877, 890–1
  embryoscopy 1069
  ultrasound diagnosis of fetal anomalies
    927–9
  ultrasound imaging **887**
  viscera, trauma 313–14
  wall,
    anterior defect 927–9
    defects 605–6
      screening 1494–5
    prenatal ultrasonography 1495–6
Abdominal heterotaxy 500
Abnormalities, isolated, embryoscopy
  1070
ABO blood groups 192
ABO incompatibility 713
Abortion,
  habitual, definition 175
  malformation data *177*
  occult 227
  recurrent 167–73
    and antiphospholipid antibodies 344
    causes 168–9, 179–80
    chromosomal abnormalities 179
    chromosomal rearrangements *169*
    consanguinity studies 170
    cytogenetic causes 169–70
    definition 167, 175
    endocrine factors 171
    environmental exposure 172
    epidemiology 167–8
    HLA sharing 170
    immunotherapy 342–3
    infectious causes 172
    and pregnancy immunology 341–3
    uterine disorders 171–2
  spontaneous 163–6, 175
    after IVF 243
    autosomal trisomies *248*
    chromosomal abnormality types *247*
    cohort studies *168*
    cytogenetics 241–2
    definition 175
    emotional sequelae 180
    familial clustering 170
    frequency,
      in multiple gestation 208
      in twins 222
    HLA allele sharing 342
    IVF embryo 241

  maternal age 168–9
    in MC twins 206, 210–11
    in multiple pregnancy 206
    probability *168*
    prospective studies *168*
    retrospective studies *168*
    in smokers 356
    susceptibility locus gene 170
    as tissue source 390
    threatened, raised MSAFP 920
Abortion Act (1967) 1013
Abruptio placentae 303, 321, *1197*
  and amphetamine use 356
  and asphyxia 293–4
  and cocaine 358
  fetal death 269
  and hypoxia 1352
  and prematurity 8
  recurrent 276
Acardia–acephalus anomaly 404
Acardiac fetus 974
  normal twin prognosis 974
Accutane (isotretinoin) 401
  as teratogen 402–3
Acetylcholinesterase (AChE) testing of
  amniotic fluid 1033
Achondrogenesis 788–90, 933–4
  type II 795–7
Achondroplasia 788, 933–4
  homozygous 788
Acidaemia 280
Acidosis, perinatal 319
Acinar length **526**
Acoustic impedance 883–4
ACTH (adrenocorticotrophin) 694–5
  excess 699
  insensitivity to 702
Activin A 35
ADAML (late-amniotic deformities
  adhesion mutilation) complex 401, 404
Addiction,
  definition 353
  fetal effects 353
Addison's disease 1270
Adenoma sebaceum 844
Adenosine deaminase deficiency,
  replacement therapy 1508–9
Adenosine deaminase gene,
  deficiency **38**
  intron sites **41–2**
Adnexa uteri 319–21
Adoption 1010
Adrenal corticomedullary junction necrosis
  511–12

Adrenal gland,
  cells **695**
  haemorrhagic necrosis 817
  hyperplasia,
    congenital 703–4
    nodular cortical **817**
  hypoplasia 705
  in intrapartum asphyxia 299–301
Adrenal hyperplasia, congenital, external
  features *379*
Adrenal studies at autopsy 385
Adrenocorticotrophin, *see* ACTH
Adrenoleucodystrophy 1139
  neonatal 446
Advanced Diagnostic Research Corporation
  (ADR) scanner 873–4
AFAFP (amniotic fluid α-fetoprotein)
  1032–3
  elevation in NTD pregnancy 1033
AFP (α-fetoprotein) 151–2, 1032–3
  in neutral tube defects 1031
  in placental pathology 987
  screening, cost–benefit assessment 1034
Agent orange 90
Agyria 419, **421**
Aicardi syndrome 24
AIDS syndrome 106, 108
  and brain 445
  fetal defects 404
  perinatally acquired 748–9
  and pregnancy 1294
AIDS virus 348–9
  see also HIV
Air embolism 808
Airway, upper,
  muscles 1389
  reflexes 1389
Airway injury 806–7
Airways,
  count 525
  development 324
  reduced number and associated disorders
    533
Alagille syndrome 255, 566
Albumin, parenteral requirements 1431
Alcohol 26, 86, 355–6
  10-year study 355
  with cocaine 357
  fetal effects **1274–5**
  and fetal loss 172
  neonatal withdrawal signs *354*
  as teratogen 84, *181*, 403
Alcohol myopathy 774
Alcohol, *see* Fetal alcohol syndrome

Alder–Reilly anomaly 723
Aldosterone,
  biosynthetic defects *699*
  biosynthetic pathway **704**
  defective *705*
Alimentary tract 589–608
  development 589–91
  infections from 261
  Hirschsprung disease **600**
  inflammations 601–3
  in intrapartum asphyxia 302–3
  motor disorders 598–603
Allele specific oligonucleotide (ASO) probes
  1194–5
Allografts, annual number used in the USA
  389
Alloimmune hematologic disorders 343
Alloimmunization,
  maternal 342
  rhesus 1301–6
Alloreactive cells 1504
Alper disease 782
Alpers–Huttenlocher syndrome 449–50
Alpha satellite probes 1124
Alpha-fetoprotein, *see* AFP
Alpha-thalassaemia *see* Thalassaemia, α
Alphoid probe **1124**
Aluminium 1430
  skeletal deposition 819–20
Alveolar capillary dysplasia **542**
Alveolar epithelium, explant,
  4-day dexamethasone culture **394**
  electron micrographs **393**
Alveolar liquid homeostasis **545**
Alveolar period lung growth 523–4
Alveolar proteinosis, lung SP-A **546**
Alveoli,
  development 324–5
  increase **526**
  radial count **525**
Alzheimer type II astrocytes **448**
Ambroxol 1341
American Association of Tissue Banks
  (ATTB) 389
American Cell Type Repository 390
Amino acids,
  code degeneracy **33**
  disorders *1050*
    metabolic 1133, 1135–8
  metabolic block 1133
  plasma, biochemical test 1132
  in pregnancy 1275–6
  sequence, and protein structure 1187
  serum, neonatal concentration *1521*
  transport systems 12–13
  urine, neonatal concentration *1521*
Aminoacidurias 448
Aminopterin as teratogen 402
Amiodarone 967, 1263
Ammonia, blood, biochemical test 1132
Amniocentesis,
  additional risk in multiple pregnancy 972
  after fetal viability 1085
  back-up 973
  clinical significance of organisms 264
  comparison with CVS 1084–5
  decompression 1251
  'early' 1084–5
    technique and safety 1084
  early and late 1083–7
  fetal trauma 804–5
  for hydramnios 1085
  midtrimester,
    complications 1083–4
    technique and safety 1083

for mosaicism 243
in multiple gestation 972, 1084
results 1037
risk evaluation *1081*
safety and efficacy *1081*
therapeutic 974, 1085
for TORCH infections 263
ultrasound replacement 922
ultrasound-guided 1308
Amniocytes,
  cultured, as diagnostic test 1091
  technique 1095
  uncultured 1092
Amnioinfusion 1085, **1247**
  serial 1248
Amnion nodosum 318
Amnion rupture 401
  fetal defects 404
Amnion rupture sequence, external features
  379
Amnioreduction 1251
Amniotic band syndrome 206, **404**
Amniotic fluid 13
  drainage 1309–10
  examination for hydrops fetalis 712
  infections 101
  meconium-stained 322
    abnormal fetal heart rate pattern 1353
    detection 1352–3
    thick 1353
  pools in four quadrants 932
  skin cell culture 764–5
  ultrasound diagnosis of abnormalities
    932–3
  ultrasound views of quadrants **1244**
  ultrasound volume assessment 881, **891**,
    893, 932
  zygosity testing 201
Amniotic fluid AFP, *see* AFAFP
Amniotic fluid cell **1093**
Amniotic fluid index 932
  normal range **1245**
Amniotic fluid leak, hypoplastic lungs 535
Amniotic fluid volume,
  abnormal, and abnormal chromosomes
    248–9
  determinants 1243–4
  urinary tract anomaly diagnosis 629
Amniotic infection syndrome 387–8
Amphetamine,
  abuse 1272, 1274
  associated congenital anomalies *356*
  infant group study 356
  neonatal withdrawal signs *354*
Amplification refractory mutation system
  (ARMS) procedure **1178**
Amylopectinosis 569, 1142
Amyoplasia 202
Anabolism 1407–8
Anaemia,
  in donor twin 974
  neonatal 709–13
    due to haemorrhage 709–10
    and non-immune hydrops 1260
    of prematurity 713
Anaesthesia and fetal distress 297
Anaesthetics 90
Anal atresia 929
Analgesia 1375–6
Anaphase lag 58, 242, **243–4**
  possible causes 253–4
Anatomic disorders, and recurrent abortion
  171
Androgen insensitivity syndromes 683

Androgen receptor, X-linked genes 24
Androgenetic diploid 195
Androgenetic mole 187
Anencephaly 400, **416–17**, 920–**1**
  clinical pathology 700–1
  with rachischisis 416
  in twins 972
Anencephaly–spina bifida 25
Aneuploid chromosomes, origins 253–5
Aneuploid gametes, production by 21
  trisomic mother **228**
Aneuploid gestation with type I confined
  placental mosaicism **1109**
Aneuploid parents 230
Aneuploidy 58, 120
  cellular events and 249, 253
  defect mapping 256
  detection 1063, 1123–5
  maternal age effect *254*
  non-random, recurrent 169
  secondary, and parental chromosome
    abnormality 228–9
Aneuploidy syndromes 375
Angelman syndrome 23, 123, 1125, 1127
Angiomatosis 836
Angiomyxoma 987–8
Angiotensin 15
Angiotensin-converting enzyme inhibitors 86
Anhidrotic hypohidrotic ectodermal
  dysplasia 764
Anhydramnios, fetal kidneys **1247**
Aniridia gene, *Pax* mutation 48
Aniridia–Wilms' tumor 75
Aniridia–Wilms' tumor association 1125
Annular array transducer **886**
Annular pancreas 581
Anorchia 677
  and male pseudohermaphroditism 677
Anorectal malformations **603–4**
Anorectal sphincter **591**
Antenatal care, ultrasound role 877–82
Antenatal diagnosis, placental control 321
Antenatal Diagnosis Working Group 1041
Antenatal pathology 365–6
  special training 366
Antenatal steroid therapy 1340
Antepartum death, description 176
Antepartum tests, possible harm 889
Anthropomorphic data for gestational age
  assessment *383*
Anthropomorphic measurements 383, 385
  major *1541*
Antibiotic therapy and testing 1050
Antibodies, placental transport 737
Antibody-mediated immunity 734–7
Anticardiolipin 343
Anticoagulants, values *1282*
Antigen-specific immunocompetence 735
Antiphospholipid syndrome 343–4
α-Antitrypsin deficiency 566–7
  and lungs 554
Anxiety and screening 1034
Aorta, typical coarctations **489**
Aortic arch,
  development 466, **469**
  interrupted 485, **490**
  right, persistence 484
  stage 16, frontal reconstruction **472**
  stage 18, frontal reconstruction **472**
Aortic flow, prenatal and postnatal
  distribution **488**
Aortic stenosis, critical, ultrasound-guided
  therapy 1311–12
Aortic valve,
  atresia **492**

Aortic valve (contd)
  bicuspid 488–9, **491**, **496**
  fusion **491**
  stenotic, raphe **491**
Aortopulmonary window 490
Apgar score 9, 368
  outcome prediction 1365–6
  in perinatal distress 324
  in SGA **281**
Aplasia cutis congenita 213
Apnoea 1387–91
  central 1387
  management 1390–1
  mixed 1387
  obstructive 1387
  predisposing factors **1388**
  respiratory pauses **1388**
  sleep **1388**
Apnoeic episodes *370*
Apnoeic index **1391**
Apoptosis 132
Appendicitis 603
Apple-peel syndrome **597**
Appropriate for gestational age (AGA) 16
  neonatal morbidity incidence **281**
Aqueduct stenosis 24–5, 423, 924, 1317
Arcuate/uterine artery, Doppler imaging 887
Argininosuccinic aciduria 1137
Arnold–Chiari malformation 418, **420**, 450, 921
  ultrasound detection 1040
Arskin encephaly, unilateral renal agenesis *29*
Arterial flow studies, cardiac and extracardiac 981
Arterial wall structure **528**
Arteries,
  great,
    development 466, 469
    malformations 482, 484–8
    transposition 492–3
      corrected 495
    systemic 502
Arteriogram for lung artery 525, 527
Arteriosclerosis in pre-eclampsia **329**
Arteriovenous anastomosis 974
  in MC fetus **207**
Arteriovenous aneurysm 835–6
Artery–artery anastomoses 973
Arthrogryposis,
  congenita 773–4
  multiplex congenita 450–1
  myopathic 773
  neuropathic 772–3
  pathogenetic classification 772
Artificial insemination 1010
Ascites 262, 604–5
  in non-immune hydrops **1262**
Ascitic fluid collection 1317
Aspartame 90
Asphyxia 285
  biochemical markers 1369
  brain-stem damage 440
  intrapartum,
    causes 292–7
    pathology 298–5
    risk in twins 977
  neonatal 1365–7
  pathophysiology 1362–3
  perinatal,
    aetiology 1361
    neurological problems 1376
    and perinatal distress 321–2
    predisposing factors *293*

Asphyxiated infants, nutrition 1420
Asphyxiating thoracic dysplasia 792
Aspiration, ultrasound-guided 1308
Aspiration syndromes 808
Aspirin 90
  and placental circulation 15
Asplenia syndrome **496**, **500**, 503
  familial 501
Association, definition 27, 401
Associations 406–7
Asthma and SGA in infants 276
Astrocytes, hypertrophic **415**, **435**, 437, **438**
Astrogliosis 299
Asymmetric septal hypertrophy (ASH) 507, **509**
Ataxia telangiectasia 24, 65, 77, 764
Atelosteogenesis types 793
Atherosclerosis, risk factors 502
Atherosis 289
  acute 328–9, 345
Athyreosis 696–8
Atrial appendage, juxtaposition 502–3
Atrial natriuretic peptide 15
Atrial septal defect **495**
Atrioventricular block, complete 969
Atrioventricular canal defect,
  complete 495–6
  partial 495
Atrioventricular canal malformations 494–5
Atrioventricular node, mesothelioma 507, 509
Atrioventricular septum,
  defect 941–2, *943*, *945*, **962**
  echocardiography 958–9
Atrioventricular sulcus, embryonic rotation **474**
Atrioventricular valve 497
Atrium, left, opened **508**
Attenuation, in ultrasound 884
Auditory apparatus 819–21
Auditory brain-stem response 1403
Autism, in fragile X syndrome 1115
Autoantibodies 99–100
Autoimmune disease,
  antibodies 343
  vascular lesions 328–9
Autoimmune disorders 749–50
Autoimmune thrombocytopenia 1285–6
Autolysis,
  normal pattern 271
  post mortem 271–2
Autonomous embryonic development 33
Autopsy 381–8, 1529–30
  approach to *180*
  external examination 385
  family history in 376–7
  findings 376
  genetic implications 375–80
  internal examination 385
  microscopic examination 385
  for neonatal death 1378
  paediatric, block and trimming procedures **1538**
  permit 1530
  procedures and documentation 1532–3
  special methods *1542*
  surface feature examination *384–5*
Autopsy form 1548–9
Autoscanner, 13-week fetus **869**
Autosomal dominant disorders, recurrence risks 377
Autosomal dominant glomerulocystic kidney disease 619

Autosomal dominant mutations 24, 407
Autosomal dominant polycystic kidney disease 617–18, 927
Autosomal recessive disorders, recurrence risks 377
Autosomal recessive mutations 23–4, 407–8
Autosomal recessive polycystic kidney disease **616–17**, 927–8
Autosomal recessive syndromes, and hindbrain malformations 423
Autosomal trisomy 242
  non-mosaic **246**
  in spontaneous abortions *248*
Autosomes, in mosaicism 1101–2
Autoteratogenesis 31

B lymphocytes 100
B-cell system 730
B-scan devices, *see* Ultrasound
B-scan measurement 885–6
Back, embryoscopy 1069
Bacterial infections 347–8
Bacterial organisms 314
Ballantyne, J.W. 1553–4
Baller–Jerold syndrome 1070
Balloon valvoplasty 1311–12
Band counts for blood cells 720
Banker and Larroche lesions **433**
Barbiturates, neonatal withdrawal signs *354*
Bardet–Biedl syndrome 620, 1070
Bare lymphocyte syndrome *200*
Bartter syndrome 1248
Basal cell nevus syndrome 73
Basal energy expenditure 1422
Basal plate (placenta) 334
Batten–Spielmeyer–Vogt disease 723
Batten's disease,
  amniocyte test 1092–3
  DNA probe diagnosis 1094
  infantile, prenatal diagnosis 1094
  juvenile 1094
  late infantile 1094
Becker muscular dystrophy, structural and mutational phenotypes **44**
Beckwith–Wiedemann syndrome 24, 52, 73, 76, 247, 255, 334–5, 405, 574, 576
  and polyhydramnios 1498
  and Wilms' tumour 624
Beemer syndrome 791–2
Behavioral disorders 399
Bendectin 90, 804
Beneke technique 453
Benign tumours 831–54
Benzodiazepines, neonatal withdrawal signs *354*
Berlin definitions 26–7
Bernard–Soulier syndrome 1283
Beta-thalassaemia, *see* Thalassaemia, β
Bilateral rudimentary testes syndrome 677
Bile drainage 565
Bile ducts,
  extrahepatic, atresia 563–4, **565**
  intrahepatic, paucity **566**
Biliary structures, epithelium-lined 565
Biliary tree, extrahepatic **565**
Bilirubin,
  metabolic pathway 1453
  metabolism and physiology 1453–4
  photoisomerized conversion **1457**
Bilirubin oxidase 1458
Biochemical genetics 1131–58

Biochemical pregnancy 124
Biochemical tests,
  confirmatory 1095
  general 1132–3
Biochemistry,
  in prenatal diagnosis 1197
  uncertain, back-up 1095
Biological self-esteem, loss of 1014
Biometry at 15 weeks **905**
Biophysical profile 9, *893*
  in intrapartum asphyxia 303
  maturation assessment 16
  role understanding 892
  scoring *1367*
Biopsy,
  complications 825–6
  embryonic,
    at blastocyst stage 1056
    in early cleavage 1056
  fetal 1093–4, 1095
  heart 507
  muscle 771
  placental bed 278
  skin, for metabolic defect 1131
Biopsy, skin, fetal 758–9
Biotransformation variability 85
Biparietal diameter 15, 877–9
  at 15 weeks 912
  B-scan measurement 885–8
  imaging at 15 weeks **905**, 912
  measurement 879
    ultrasound **880**
  ultrasound use 1041
Birth 287–90
  assisted, trauma 309
Birth canal, infection exposure 105, 347
Birth defects 5, 366
  causes 23–6
  and family history 381
  idiopathic anomalies, prenatal deaths
    25–6
  multifactorial traits 25
  pathogenetic effects 26–7
  pathogenetic periods 27–9
  prenatal 23
  prevention 370
  recurrence risks 377, 382
Birth Defects Monitoring Program 5, 400
Birth injuries 369–70
Birth length 693
Birth place and malformations 400
Birth trauma 805–6
Birth weight 693
  measurement 278
  mortality risk measure 368
  relative risk 11
  standard **696**
Birthmark 836–7
Bladder,
  agenesis 627
  exstrophy 627
  fistula to urethra 627
  malformations 627–9
  obstructive lesions 628
  tumours 629
  ultrasound-guided aspiration 1309
Blalock–Taussig shunt 482, 514, 1481
Blastema, nodular renal 73
Blastocyst, implantation **123**
Blastocyst cavity 122
Blastocyst stage, embryonic biopsy 1056
Blastogenesis 25
  abnormalities 29
  defects 28

idiopathic defect associations 26
  timing 28
Blastopore, dorsal lip 35
Bleeding disorders, inherited 1284–5
Blighted ovum 163–4
Blocking antibodies 180, 339
Blood,
  chemical values in preterm infants *1521*
  coagulation 718
    normal values *1520*
  normal values *1518*
  reversed perfusion 973–4
Blood coagulability and thrombosis 1290
Blood culture at autopsy 385, 387
Blood flow,
  disturbances and thrombosis 1290
  insonation **885**
  through great vessels **487–8**
  ultrasound techniques 883, **885**
  velocity waveforms 980
Blood gas,
  cord values 1521
  tests 1132
  vaginal delivery values *1520*
Blood sample type 1049
Blood sampling 1514
  analysis 1515–16
  specific analyses 1516–17
  transportation 1514–15
Blood tests, for acute metabolic disease
  1132
Blood vessels 135
Bloom syndrome 24, 65, 72, 77, 764
Bochdalek hernia 930, 1319–20
Body composition *1408*
Bone marrow,
  neonatal counts *1520*
  transplantation, antigen recognition
    1506–7
Boomerang dysplasia 792–3
Borrelia burgdorferi 347
Botulism 775
Bourneville disease 544
Bowel,
  dilatation 929–30
  echogenicity, at 12 weeks **903**
  polyps 851
Brachial plexus palsy 310
Brachmann–de Lange syndrome 407
Bradyarrhythmias 966–7
  therapy 969
Bradycardia 321–2, **967**
  definition 1354
  terminal **1355**
Brain 413–63
  at 15 weeks, structural evaluation 913,
    915
  blood flow assessment 1368
  boundary zone infarction **437**
  cellular response maturation 416
  congenital tumours 451–3
  development 413–16
  examination after fixation 458
  function monitor trace 1403
  haemodynamic assessment 1400–2
    radioactive techniques 1401
  haemorrhage, Doppler prediction 1401
  haemorrhagic lesions 427–32
  hypoperfusion effects 511
  imaging at 9 weeks **901**
  inborn errors of metabolism 445–50
  infection products 262
  infections 440–5
  in Leigh disease **447**

malformations 416–23
  metabolism assessment 1368
  neonatal, imaging 1399–400
  neurophysiology 1402–4
  postmortem removal 453–4, 458
  relative weights *454*
  triploidy anomalies 195
  tuberous sclerosis 843
  ventricular dilatation 423
  'walnut' 448–9
  white matter,
    haemorrhage 428
    infarction 432, **434–5**
    lesions 432–7
    necrosis 432–3, **434–5**, 436
    scarring **436**
    slit-like defect **436**
Brain-sparing effect 894
Brain-stem lesions 1388
Brain-stem necrosis 437
Branched-chain organic acid disorders *1151*
Branchial cyst 846
Branchio-oto-renal syndrome, and renal
  hypoplasia 611
Breast milk,
  amphetamines in 356
  HIV infection 349
  and immune system 738–9
  infection transmission 347
Bridging veins 307
Brightness mode, *see* Ultrasound, B-scan
British Medical Ultrasound Society,
  historical collection 867, *869*
Bronchiolar epithelial damage 808
Bronchogenic cysts 89
Bronchopulmonary dysplasia 550–1, 553,
  809–10, 1396
Bronchopulmonary sequestration,
  extralobar 932
  intralobar 932
Bronchus, atresia 553–4, *555*
Brown, T.G. 868–9
Bruising 306
Budd–Chiari syndrome 562

Cachectin 68
Cadmium in cigarettes 356
Caesarean section 1345–6
  for HSV 110
  in multiple pregnancy 976
  placenta from 990
  for SGA infants 281
Calcium,
  intracellular 132
  recommended intravenous intake *1427*
  requirement of preterm infant 1428
Calcium : phosphorus ratio 1428
Call–Exner bodies 675–6
Caloric need 1421, 1422–3
Calorie : nitrogen ratio 1425
Campbell, S. **872**
Campomelic syndrome 27, **799–800**
Canadian Council on Health Facilities
  1515
Cancer,
  congenital *in situ* lesions 73–4
  developmental lesions 72–4
  embryonal and fetal milieu 68–9
  familial 72
  genetic epidemiology and ecogenetics 72
  malformation syndromes 75–6, 77
  and mutations 47–8
  predisposing gene defects 72
  risk in mutation syndromes 24

spontaneous regression and cytodifferentiation 68
teratologic predisposing conditions 74–7
Candida albicans 325, 443
Candida sp., perinatal infections 824–5
Candidiasis,
  fetal **104**
  neonatal 105, 549
Canicular lung growth 523–4
Capillary haemangiomatosis 542
Captopril 86
Caput succedaneum 306
Carbamoyl-phosphate synthetase deficiency 1136
Carbohydrate,
  metabolism disorders 1138–9, *1148*
  requirement of preterm infant 1423–4
Carbohydrate-deficient glycoprotein syndrome 448–50
Carbon dioxide challenge **1389**
Carcinogenesis,
  genetic models 70
  initiation–promotion model 67–8
  prenatal initiation 77–80
  transgenerational and parental factors 77–8
  transplacental 78–9
  'two-hit' hypothesis 49
Carcinogenic progression 67–8
Carcinogenic promotion 67
Carcinogens, chemical, and initiation 67
Cardiac, *see* Heart
Cardiac chambers, development 472, 474–6
Cardiac development, summary 480
Cardiac dysfunction 509–14
Cardiac jelly, arrangement **472**
Cardiac output 286
Cardiac septa, development 472, 474–6
Cardiac tube of stage 14 embryo **470**
Cardiac valves,
  development **473**, 476–7
  positions **493**
Cardiogenesis, major events **486**
Cardiolipin 344
Cardiomegaly 262, 814
Cardiomyopathy 505–6, **507–8**, 513
Cardiopulmonary bypass, history 1469
Cardiorespiratory function, normal 285–7
Cardiotocograph 889–90, 891–2
  description and interpretation 1354–6
  intrapartum 1354
  normal trace **892**
Cardiotocography,
  assessment before and during labour 891–2
  increased perinatal mortality 892
Cardiovascular causes of non-immune hydops 1259
Cardiovascular development, general features 465–6
Cardiovascular diseases at autopsy *507*
Cardiovascular malformations 480, 482, 484–505
  congenital, autopsy cases *487*
Cardiovascular system, infections 516
Carnegie Embryological Collection 465, 469
Carnegie staging of human embryos 465
Carpenter syndrome 1070
Cat faeces and parasitic infections 350
Catabolism 1408
Catecholamines, elevation 290, 292

Catheter,
  arterial line, complications 812–13
  cardiac complications 814
  foreign body emboli **813**
  KCH **1316**
  and thrombosis 1289
  venous lines 813
Caudal regression sequence 610
Cell,
  abnormal, proportions 1104–5
  dividing 1123
Cell adhesion molecules 131
Cell culture 56–7
Cell cycle 55, 1104
Cell death 132–3
  programmed 132–3
Cell engraftment 1503–6
  allogeneic **1504**
Cell migration 131
Cell populations, movements 133–5
Cell replication 131–3
Cell selection 1104–5
Cell separation methods 1061–3
Cell and tissue banks 390
Cell type,
  changes in metabolic disease, microscopy *1092*
  target selection 1059–61
Cell-mediated immunity 737
Cells,
  allocation to co-twins 202, 204
  culture and storage 390
Celosomias 605
Centers for Disease Control 400
Central core disease 778
Central Laboratory for Human Embryology, Seattle 389, 395
Central nervous system,
  infarction and cocaine 358
  in intrapartum asphyxia 298–9
  malformations 416
  perinatal 822–3
  tumours, incidence 451–2
  ultrasound fetal anomaly diagnosis 919–24
  ultrasound-guided aspiration 1308
Centromere division, premature 254
Centromere probe 1122–3, **1124**
Centromere separation 254
Centrum semiovale, sclerotic atrophy 436
Cephalohaematoma 304, 306–7
Cephalothoracopagus twins 218–19
Cerclage, efficacy 171
Cerebellar folial cortex, petechial haemorrhages **429**
Cerebellar sclerosis 440
Cerebellum,
  banana configuration 921–2
  cortical dysplasia, CMV infection 442
  cortical necrosis **441**
  haemorrhage 428
Cerebral arteries, infarction **437**
Cerebral cortex,
  formation 414
  haemorrhage 427–8
Cerebral hemispheres, regional development *414*
Cerebral lactic acidosis 423
Cerebral necrosis 437–8
Cerebral oedema **298**
Cerebral palsy 290, 323–4, 365
  and aminoacidurias 448
  and intrapartum asphyxia 1352
  and neonatal asphyxia 1367
  in twins 213

and vaginal bleeding 323
Cerebro-ocular dysplasia 421
Cerebro-ocular syndromes 421
Cerebrohepatorenal syndrome 405
Cerebrospinal fluid values, neonatal *1522*
Cerebrovascular monitoring, neonatal 1399–405
Cervical incompetence 171
  fetal infection 325
Cervical 'ripening' 289
Cervical viral and bacterial cultures in TORCH neonate 266
Cervicovaginal region, flora 325
Cervix,
  occlusion 1248
  papillary adenocarcinoma 685
  transvaginal ultrasound 975
  transverse septa 685
CFTR (cystic fibrosis transmembrane regulator),
  deletion 39
  lung explant culture 394
CFTR gene 42–4
  exons, domains and mutations **43**
  mutation by ethnic group **47**
  mutations causing cystic fibrosis **43**
Chagas disease 96
Charcot–Marie–Tooth syndrome 619, 784
CHARGE association, external features *379*
Chediak–Higashi syndrome 723, 765
  diagnosis 1093–4
Chemical mismatch cleavage analysis 1179–80
Chemical pregnancy 227
Chemicals,
  and IUGR 276
  teratogenic *181*
Chemoreceptor responses in apnoea 1388–9
Chiari malformations 418, 423
Chiasmata 56
Chickenpox, gestational, and TORCH 262
Chignon lesion 306
Child Abuse Prevention and Treatment Act 1384
Chimaerism 28, 58, 1503
  confined 248
  widespread 248
Chlorpromazine antibodies 343
Cholecystitis in parenteral nutrition 1439
Choledochal cyst 578, 848–9
Cholelithiasis 578
Cholestasis in newborn 563–6
Chondrodysplasia punctata 760
Chondrodysplasia punctata syndromes 798–9
Chondrodysplasias 31
  congenital 787–801
Chondroectodermal dysplasia 792
Chorangioma 36–7, 334–5
Chorangioma, large 304
Chorangiomatosis 335
Chorangiosis 335–6
  rule of tens 335
Chorioamnionitis 101, 106
  and abortion 179
  acute 325
  fungal 326
  histologic patterns 325
  in intrapartum asphyxia 305
  and meconium staining 323
  necrotizing 325–6

Chorioamnionitis (contd)
  and prematurity 8, 288
  prevalence 325
Chorioangioma 836–7, 983, 985
  cellular, normal MSAFP 989
  high MSAFP 989
Choriocarcinoma 69, 187, 675
  after invasive mole 190
  origin 191
Chorion frondosum 143
Chorion laeve 143, 321
Chorionic gonadotropin,
  beta (hCG), zone, discriminatory 897
  beta (hCG), zone, for vaginal probes
    897–8
  in Down syndrome 1037–8
Chorionic gonadotropin (hCG) 340, 987
  abnormality after partial mole removal
    194
  in Down syndrome 1037–8
  in partial hydatidiform mole 192, 194
  for pregnancy confirmation 165, 176
  raised, with mole 188
  recession curve abnormalities in residual
    trophoblastic disease 190
  synthesis 150
Chorionic plate 321
Chorionic sac,
  'double-ring' 899
  at week 5 898–9
  at week 6 899
  at week 7 899
Chorionic stroma, mosaicism 1106
Chorionic villus, in birth asphyxia 295
Chorionic villus sampling, see CVS
Chorionicity,
  determination 222
  triplet placentas 209
Chorionitis 349
Chorioretinitis 262, 265
Choroid plexus cysts 942, 947
Choroid plexus haemorrhage 432
Choroideremia 24
Christ–Siemens–Touraine syndrome 764
Chromatin fibre 55
Chromosomal abnormality 23, 25, 58,
    60–2
  and abnormal amniotic fluid volume
    248–9
  and congenital heart disease 961–2
  and early fetal loss 178–9
  and mortality 65–6
  in mosaicism 237, 242–6
  in newborn 242, 249
  types 247
  non-immune hydrops 1259–60
  parental, and secondary aneuploidy 228–9
  in perinatal deaths 242, 249
  in prenatally detected malformed fetuses
    252
  in prenatally diagnosed cystic hygroma
    252
  screening for 1036–40
  SGA infants 276
  spontaneous abortions 247
  structured, parental 228–9
  ultrasound findings 939
Chromosomal analysis,
  indications 179
  prenatal, in multiple pregnancy 221
Chromosomal mosaicism, parental 169–70
Chromosomal rearrangements,
  balanced 169
  in recurrent abortion 169
Chromosomal sex determination 664

Chromosome,
  acentric 58
  architecture 55
  autosomal disorders 62–3
  band 55
  banding 1121
  banding methods 57
  breakage 58
  breakage syndromes 65
  breakage/DNA repair–defect syndromes
    24
  cell lines 246
  critical regions 1125, 1127
  defects 4
  deletion 60
    detection methods 254–5
  dicentric 62
  disorders,
    first trimester diagnosis 951
    heterogeneous group 201
    and polyhydramnios 932
    screening 1024
    ultrasound diagnosis 939–53
  displacement 254
  duplications 62
  in situ methods 254
  inversion 61
  microdeletions 254
  mosaic defect, incidence 950
  mosaic rearrangement 1103–4
  mosaicism 1099–1121
  non-disjunction 119
    mechanisms 253–4
  normal complement 59
  prenatal studies 1074
  rearrangements in mosaicism 1103–4
  ring 62
  ring X 255
  screening,
    recommendations 1024–5
    selective 1024
  segregation in abnormal spermatogenetic
    meiosis 232
  structural changes 58
  structural rearrangement 1127–8
    cryptic and complex 1127
Chromosome 4, duplication from 1126
Chromosome 11 (46,XY, 11q+) 1126
Chromosome anomaly syndromes
    408–11
Chromosome libraries 1122
Chromosome painting 1122–3, 1125
  specific probe 1124
  techniques 1111
Chylothorax 931
  in non-immune hydrops 1262
  stent procedures 1317
  surgery 1259
Cigarettes, see Smoking
Circumferences, B-scan measurement 886
Circummargination 324
Circumvallate placenta 983–4
Circumvallation 324
Cirrhosis of liver, see Liver, cirrhosis
Cisterna vena magna, with trisomy 18
    942–3
Citrullinaemia 1136–7
Clastogens 58
Clavicles,
  at 15 weeks, structural evaluation 910
  fracture 311
Cleavage, early, embryonic biopsy 1056
Cleft lip,
  embryoscopy 1070

prenatal mortality rate 25
Cleft palate 25
Clinical Laboratory Improvement
  Amendments 1988 1518
Clinical molecular genetics 1187–95
Clinical risk index for babies (CRIB) 9,
  368
Clinicopathological information 1534
Clinodactyly at 28 weeks 945, 948
Clitoral cyst 685
Cloacal exstrophy 627
Clostridium botulinum 775
Cloverleaf skull 787
Club foot 400
CMV (cytomegalovirus),
  brain-stem section 107
  congenital infection 441–3
  infection,
    frequency in the USA 265
    intrauterine frequency 348
    maternal reinfection 348
    neonatal 1450
    neurologic sequelae 265
    occupational acquisition 265
    perinatal infections 825
    pneumonia 548–9
    in pregnancy 1295
    sensorineural sequelae in infections 108
    in TORCH 261, 265
    transplacental infection 108–9, 325, 348
CMV infection 442
CMV syndrome 348
Coagulation factors, congenital deficiencies
  718
Coagulopathy 319
Coarctation,
  of aorta 484–5
    surgery 1480
  prenatal and postnatal distribution 488
  of pulmonary artery 485
Cocaethylene 357
Cocaine 86
  abuse 357–9
  with alcohol 357
  as 'crack' or 'rock' 357
  'freebase' 357
  with heroin ('speedball') 357
  neonatal withdrawal signs 354
  in pregnancy 1272–4
  as 'snow' 357
  as sympathomimetic 357
  as teratogen 26, 359–60, 403
Cochrane Collaboration Pregnancy and
  Childbirth Module 890
Cockayne syndrome 764
Codons 40–1
  mutations 41
Cohnheim fetal rest theory 67, 73
Coiled membrane oxygenator 1472
Collagen gene,
  mutations 44, 47
  structure 45
Colon
  necrosis 1486
  small left 601
Colony-stimulating factor 1 (CSF-1) 340–1
Color blindness 24
Colostrum, contents 1409
Community genetic services 8
Complement system 739
Computed tomography for neonatal brain
  1399–400
Conception,
  products 163–6
    examination 164–5

Conceptual age, calculation 897
Conceptus,
  aborted, as tissue source 389–90
  age determination 176
  autopsy permit 1530
  definition 4
  developmental stages 3
  disturbances 365
  genetic impact in first trimester 4
  IVF 241
Conditional development 33, 35
Congenital, *see under Individual condition*
Congenital anomalies,
  changes 1974–84 *400*
  definition 399
  distribution 369
  and dysmorphology 399–411
  incidence 399–400
  metaphase preparation **1126**
  multifactorial disorders 399–400
  US incidence *400*
Congenital anomaly, severe 1376–7
Congenital cystic adenomatoid
  malformation 529, **531–2**
Congenital heart disease, *see* Heart,
  congenital disease
Congenital infections 347
Conjoined twins (CT), *see* Twins,
  conjoined
Connective tissue hamartomas and tumours
  838–41
Conradi–Hunermann syndrome 798
Consanguineous matings and recurrent
  abortion 170
Contact scanner 868–9, 870–1, 873–4
Contiguous gene syndromes 255, 1125
Continuous positive airway pressure 1391
Contraception 1009
Contraction stress test 891
Cor triatriatum 501–2
Cordocentesis 9, 1071–6
  complications 992–3
  conclusions 1074
  fetal infection risk 264
  fetal karyotype 940
  fetal platelet counts *1520*
  fetal trauma 805
  indications 1072–3
  informed consent 1074
  methods 1071–2
  midtrimester blood value *1519*
  midtrimester red cell and platelet values
  1519
  in multiple pregnancy 973, 1073
  pregnancy losses *1074*
  risks 1073–4
  for TORCH infections 264–5
  for varicella-zoster infection 265
Cornelia de Lange syndrome, external
  features 379
Coronary artery, left, origin 502
Coronary artery branches, distribution **486**
Coronary circulation 478
Corpus callosum,
  agenesis 25, 419, 924
    with trisomy 13 940–*1*
Corpus luteum function in recurrent
  abortion 171
Cortical acute necrosis **438**
Cortical haemorrhagic infarction **437**
Cortical organizing necrosis **438**
Corticotrophin-releasing hormone 287–9
Cortisol, biosynthetic production pathway
  699–700

Costochondral junction,
  autopsy studies 385
  in intrapartum asphyxia 303
Cow's milk preparations 1409–10
Cowden syndrome 73–*4*
Coxsackie encephalitis **444**
Coxsackievirus 443
CPM (confined placental mosaicism),
  see Mosaicism
Cranial nerves, injury 310
Cranioschisis 417
CRIB (clinical risk index for babies) 9, 368
Crown–head length, standard **696**
Crown–rump length *16*
  assessment, ultrasound 879–80
  measurement 383
  and yolk sac diameter **153**
Cryptorchidism 74
Curvature–thickness index, determination
  482
Curvilinear array transducer **886**
Cushing syndrome 1270
  congenital 699–700
CVS (chorionic villus sampling) 1055,
  1077–82, 1089–91
  at 9–12 weeks 1078
  complications 1080
  cultured, and amniocytes 1090–1
  in development disorders of twin
    pregnancy 220
  dichorionic 972
  difficulties 1081
  direct and culture methods 242
  early and late 1077–82
  early rubella infection 265
  experienced centers 1081
  fetal chromosome result discrepancies
    240
  in fetal defects 181
  fetal TORCH infection research 264
  fetal trauma 805
  for fragile X syndrome 1118
  indications 1079
  karyotyping 1101
  laboratory results interpretation 973
  and limb reduction defects 403
  liver metabolic disorders 569
  malformations 86
  microscopic assessment 1089–90
  monochorionic 972
  mosaicism 238, 240, 247, 1107–8
    classification 247
    fetal outcomes 247
  multiple pregnancy 972–3, 1078
  normal **1091**
  risk evaluation *1081*
  safety and efficacy *1081*
  sampling methods 1077–8
  technique 1095
  timing 1078–9
  for TORCH infections 264
  transabdominal versus transcervical
    1079–80
  zygosity testing 203
Cyanide in cigarettes 356
Cyanosis 510–11
Cyclic AMP, fetal lung explant **393**
Cyclic AMP mediating agents 1341
Cyclic neutropenia 721
Cyclins 132
Cyclopia/holoprosencephaly, prenatal
  mortality rate 25
Cyclosomus 401
Cysteine 1424

Cystic adenomatoid malformation 931–2
  associated structural defects 931–2
  types 931
Cystic dysplasia, renal 927
Cystic fibrosis 31, 365, 554, 556, 573,
  582–**4**
  carrier detection 1054
  genetic linkage analysis 182
  and meconium ileus 597–8
  mutations 42–4
  in pregnancy 1271–2
  screening 583, 1029
  and uniparental disomy 378
Cystic fibrosis transmembrane regulator
  gene, *see* CFTR gene
Cystic hygroma 513, 836, **837–8**
  at 18 weeks 949
  karyotypes by gestational age *253*
  prenatal cytogenetic diagnosis 258–9
  prenatally diagnosed chromosome
    abnormality *252*
  septated and non-septated types 951
  in Turner syndrome 949
Cystinosis 1143
Cystourethrogram 1464
Cysts 846–50
  aspiration 1308
  associated with vestigial remnant 846–7
Cytogenetic advances 1121
Cytogenetic analysis,
  CVS 1079
  material handling 179
Cytogenetic assessment of stillborn 273
Cytogenetic diagnosis, and fetal
  malformations 248–9
Cytogenetic factors in recurrent abortion
  167
Cytogenetic studies, at fetal autopsy 387
Cytogenetic studies of congenital leukaemia
  725
Cytogenetics 55–66
  abnormalities and cancer 77
  causes of recurrent abortion 169–70
  combination with molecular methods
    254–5
  complete hydatidiform mole 190
  fragile X syndrome 1117
  hydatidiform mole 190–1
  laboratory caution 1117
  molecular 1121–9
  newer techniques 257
  preimplantation IVF embryos 243
  reproductive loss 227–53
  of spontaneous abortion 241–2
  techniques 255
  see also Amniocentesis; CVS; Molecular
    cytogenetics
Cytokine therapy 1508
Cytokines 99, 106, 340–1, 737
Cytolysis and regression 68
Cytomegalovirus, *see* CMV
Cytopathic effects 348
Cytoplasmic vacuoles 723
Cytosine 37
Cytotrophoblast,
  extravillous 339
  increased **295**
Cytotrophoblastic cyst 983

Dallas criteria for myocarditis 507
Dandy–Walker malformation 29, 423, 563,
  924–5
  and hydrocephalus 1317
  with trisomy 13 940–*1*
  with trisomy 18 942–3

DART (Developmental and Reproductive Toxicology) database 91
Data reporting 1517–18
Data-gathering and autopsy 381
Decidual vessels, premature rupture 323
Deciduitis 325
Deformation,
  causes 405
  description 27, 375, 401
Deformity sequence 26
Del Castillo syndrome 679
Deletion, small, detection by gel electrophoresis 1176
Deletions, causing β-thalassaemia 1171
Delivery, mode, anomalies affecting 1345–6
Delivery anomalies,
  affecting location 1346
  affecting timing 1345
Delivery room,
  care 1363–4
  decision-making 1383–4
  ethics 1381–5
Demographic data 1049–50
Denaturing gradient gel electrophoresis 1178–9
Development, and disease 162
Developmental age 176–7
Developmental biochemical mechanisms and birth defects 399
Developmental challenges 4
Developmental disorders, prenatal diagnosis in twin pregnancy 220
Developmental encephaloclastic lesions 423–7
Developmental fetal period 269
Developmental fields 28–9
  defects 25
  definition 401
Developmental pathology 177
Developmental periods 28
  and malformation 399
Developmental stage, assessment 176–7
Developmental vestiges, tumors 67
Dextroamphetamine 356
Dextrocardia 500
Diabetes insipidus 703
Diabetes mellitus, maternal, see Maternal diabetes mellitus
Diabetic embryopathy 404
Diagnosable diseases, prenatally, 1198–222
Diamond–Blackfan syndrome 713
Diandric triploid 195
Diandry 195
Diaphragm, formation 1321
Diaphragmatic hernia 930–1, 943
  congenital 606, 1319
    associated anomalies 1320
    causing lung hypoplasia 537–8, 539
    embryology 1319–20
    postnatal diagnosis 1323
    postnatal management 1324
    prenatal diagnosis 1320, 1322–3
      cytogenetic 248
    prenatal management 1324
    prenatal surgery 1325–6
    survival probability 1323
Diastolic flow degree, Doppler imaging 888
Diastrophic dysplasia 794
Dicarboxylic aciduria 1134–5
Dicephalus twins 217
Diethylstilboestrol 804
  carcinogenicity 78
DiGeorge sequence 26

DiGeorge syndrome 135, 255, 402–3, 745–6, 750, 1125
  thymus transplant 1507, 1511
Digestive duplications 596
Digoxin 1259
Digoxin for fetal atrial flutter 968
Digyny 195
Dilantin (phenytoin), as teratogen 84
Diphenylhydantoin, as teratogen 403
Diphosphoglycerate mutase deficiency 714
Diploid mole 187
Diploid sperm 195
Diploid versus triploid status determination 196
Dipygus twins 218
Direct mutation detection 1194–5
Directive counselling 1008
Diseases, prenatally diagnosable, 1198–222
Disorganization gene (Ds) 48
Disproportion in labour 293
Disruption,
  description 26, 376
  teratogenic 26
  types 401
Disruption (secondary malformation) 401, 402–5
Disruption sequence 26
Disseminated intravascular coagulation 718, 1283
  causes 1288
Diuretic renogram 1464
DNA,
  amplification 1177–8
    pitfalls 1182
  analysis 1192–5
    in fetal defects 181
    tissue sample 1132
  base pair (bp) 1187
  chorionic cancer studies 192
  cleavage by restriction endonucleases 1182
  cleavage enzyme 1182
  complementarity 1187
  component function and mutation 40
  CVS 1079
  deletions 38–9, 40
  duplications 39
  enhancer regions 40–1
  genomic 1131
  genotyping 1025
  hydatidiform mole imprinting 196
  in situ hybridization 1121–2
  insertions 38–9
  intergenic 1187
  irradiation injury 79
  length mutations 1190
  linked polymorphisms 182
  mole studies 192
  mutation 37–45, 1190–1
    standardized nomenclature 1191
  mutation 'hotspots' 37
  nuclear, representation 34
  nucleic genetic code 33
  PCR amplified specific fragment 1193
  point mutations 1191
  polymorphisms 1191–2
    in prenatal diagnosis 1197
  recognition site 1192–3
  repair enzymes, inborn deficiency 72
  replication 55
  sample storage 182
  sequencing, in porphyria 1194
  Southern analysis 1192–3
  structure and function 1187–9
  technology impact 1052–3

tests for enzyme defects 1277
  transcriptional 32
  types 32, 40–1
  unit of length 1187
DNA fragments 1193
  after restriction enzyme digestion 1193
DNA linkage 1192
DNA probe 57, 1192
DNA probes,
  labeling 1121
  for mosaicism 1111
DNA viruses 113, 348
DNA–RNA hybridization probes 263
Dohle bodies 723
Donald, I. 867–70, 874, 999
Donor twin 213
Doppler,
  blood flow studies 979
  continuous wave 976, 980
    steerable 955
  continuous wave unit 887
  diastolic flow waveforms 887
  for hypoxic–ischaemic encephalopathy 1400–1
  imaging,
    colour, for chorioangioma 983
    cord abnormalities 988
  mapping,
    blood velocity waveforms 980
  color,
    abdominal 982
    transvaginal 980
  colour flow 955, 969
  umbilical artery 982
  measurement of umbilical arterial resistance index 278
  measurements, correlation with hormonal parameters 979
  pulsed wave 955, 969, 980
    evaluation, fetal heart rhythm 964
    potential hazard 882
  pulsed-flow testing, abnormal 330, 332
  technique for blood cell velocity 1400
  ultrasound 893–4
    attention to detail 888
    colour flow systems 887
    combination with B-scan device 887
    duplex systems 887
      commercial configurations 887
    instrumentation 886–7
    measurements 887–8
    in multiple pregnancy 976
      colour flow imaging 976
      pulsed 976
    pulsatile blood flow waveform 893–4
    studies 877
    velocity measurements 888
    see also ultrasound
Doppler devices, inadvisable in first trimester 881–2
Doppler effect 885
Doppler flow, abnormal, in intrapartum asphyxia 305
Doppler spectrum 886–7
  frequency shifts 887
  triplex scanning 887
Dorsal remnants 596
Dot–blot analysis, for β-thalassemia 1176–7
Double-inlet left ventricle 495, 497–8
Double-outlet left ventricle 494
Double-outlet right ventricle 492–3
Dowling–Meara epidermolysis bullosa 762

Down syndrome 62, 400, *535, 537, 945,* 947, 949
  abnormalities frequency *947*
  antenatal diagnosis 945
  atrioventricular septal defects 945
  chromosomal basis 1121
  chromosome abnormality 119–20
  clinodactyly 945
  congenital heart disease 945
  detection 1123
  detection rates *1036*
  duodenal atresia 945, **947**
  duodenal obstruction 929
  and dysmyelopoietic syndome 725–6
  hCG levels 1037–8
  incidence 945
  major anomalies 408–9
  maternal gamete production **228**
  mosaicism 1101–2, 1104
  MSAFP,
    low 1036–7
    screening 1031
  in multiple pregnancy 973
  nuchal tissue thickening 945, **950**
  prenatal screening 1023
  recurrence risk 169
  regular free, origin *254*
  robertsonian translocation 60
  SGA infant 276
  structural abnormality mapping 255
  triple test 945
Doxapram 1391
Doxorubicin, complications 516
Drash syndrome 50–1, 52, 73, 76, 621, 623
  and Wilms' tumour 624–5
Driscoll, S.G. 177
Drugs 26, 91, 112
  and AIDS virus 348
  antibodies to 343
  and fetal muscle 774
  and IUGR 276
  obstetrical complications 354–5
  and platelet function disturbances 719
  taken by mother, fetal effects *1273*
  teratogenic *181*
  and TORCH 262
Duchenne muscular dystrophy 24
  genetic linkage analysis 182
  intestinal wall 601
  structural and mutational phenotypes 44
Ductus arteriosus,
  absent 488
  development 469
  patent, in twins 972
  premature closure 543
Duodenal atresia *596*, 929, 945, 947
  prenatal cytogenetic diagnosis 248
Duodenal obstruction 929
Duodenal stenosis, congenital **596**
Dura, tearing by traction **309**
Dynamic mutation, in fragile X syndrome 1116–17
Dysmorphic evaluation 387–8
  anthropomorphic measurements *383*
  by autopsy 382
Dysmorphic lesions 387
Dysmorphogenesis, mechanisms 375–6
Dysmorphology 365
Dysmorphology syndrome,
  diagnosis 376
  external features 376
Dysmyelopoietic syndrome **725–6**
Dysplasia,
  description 27, 401

Schneckenbecken 790
  sequence 26
  thanatophoric 787–8
Dysplasia syndromes,
  metabolic 405
  non-metabolic 405
Dysraphism 417–18
Dyssegmental dysplasia **794**
Dystocia 293–4
  constriction ring 294
  and delivery mode 1345–6
Dystrophic epidermolysis bullosa 761, **763**
Dystrophin mutations and muscular dystrophy 44

Ears *378*, 403, 406
Ebstein anomaly 498–9
  surgery 1482
Echocardiogram,
  color-encoded M-mode **966–7**
  impact on expectant family 969
  impact on health care team 969
Echocardiography 955–70
  examination techniques 957–8
  fetal arrhythmia assessment 963–9
  indications *956*
  structural heart disease,
    diagnosis and management 955–95
    incidence *963*
  team approach 955–6
  two-dimensional and M-mode imaging 969
  utility *958, 960*
  Yale Center findings *963*
Echogenic bowel, and trisomy 21 249
Echovirus 443
Eclampsia, placental circulation 13
ECMO, *see* Extracorporeal membrane oxygenation
Ectopic pancreas 581
Ectopic pregnancy 165–6
EDRF (endothelium-derived relaxing factor) 15
Edwards syndrome 62
EEC (ectrodactyly, ectodermal dysplasia and cleft palate) syndrome 1070
Ehlers–Danlos syndrome, heart anomalies 505
Ehlers–Danlos syndrome VI 765
Eisenmenger syndrome 509, 514
Electroencephalography, for neurophysiology 1402–4
Electroencephalopathy 1367–8
Electrolyte requirement of preterm infant 1427–30
Electrolytes, tests 1132
Electromagnetic fields,
  paternal exposure 77
  and women 91
Electromechanical dissociation 511
Electron microscopy 181
  cell type involvement in metabolic disease *1092*
ELISA (enzyme-linked immunosorbent assay) 104
  rubella-specific methods 263
  Toxoplasma-specific 263
Elliptocytosis, hereditary 715
Ellis–van Creveld syndrome 792–3, 1070
  external features *379*
  manifestations 24
  and renal dysplasia 616
Embden–Meyerhof pathway 1347
  defects 714
Embolization of hydatidiform villi 189
Embryo,
  anatomic features, stage of occurrence *467*

arrested, CVS 973
biopsy,
  blastocyst stage 1056–7
  in early cleavage 1056
circulation and homeostasis 135–6
compaction 122
development progression **473**
early stage 127–8
examination 136
fluid composition comparisons **155**
folds 133–4
fusions *134*
growth deficient 25
heart components, terminology **466**
imaging 867–994
malformed, embryoscopy 1069–70
mechanics 135
median sections **466**
'nodular' 269
normal, embryoscopy 1067–9
partitions 134–5
preimplantation development 121–3
preimplantation stage in mouse **121**
relative specification 33
separations *134–5*
stage 14,
  heart reconstruction **477**
  transverse section **468**
stage 16,
  heart reconstruction **477**
  sagittal section **471**
  transverse section **468**
stage 18,
  heart reconstruction **478**
  transverse section **468**
stage 20, transverse section **468**
'stunted' 269
and yolk sac **146**
Embryogenesis 25, 28, 127–37
  fundamental developmental processes *129*
  gene product control 48
  molecular mechanism 33–7
  in teratology 85
  timing 28
Embryology, history 365
Embryoma 69
Embryonal carcinoma 675, 686
  cell lines 122
Embryonal rhabdomyosarcoma 686
Embryonic cavities, biochemical composition determination 150–2
Embryonic development, landmarks *87*
Embryonic disk **124, 145**
Embryonic induction *130*
Embryonic testicular regression syndrome 676–7
Embryonic timing 136
Embryoscopy,
  conclusions 1070
  diagnostic value 1070
  first trimester diagnosis 1065–70
  future prospects 1070
  indications 1070
  materials 1065
  methods 1065–7
  obstetric risk 1070
  principles 1065
  results 1067–9
  technique 1065–7
  transabdominal **1066–7**
  transcervical 1065–6
Embryotoxicity 399
Emery–Mithal radial alveolar count *525–6*
Emotional sequelae, abortion 180

Emphysema **808–9**
Enalapril 86
Encephalitis, HSV 110
Encephalocele 417–**18**, 922–**3**
  occipital **417**
Encephaloclastic developmental lesions
  423–7
Encephalomyopathies 782
Encephalopathy,
  hypoxic–ischaemic 321–2, 1367–9,
    1400–1
  pathophysiology 1361–2
  multilocular cystic 425–6, 427
Endochondromatosis 841
Endo-ophthalmitis, candidal 824–5
Endocardial fibroelastosis 490, 503, 506,
  508
Endocarditis 299–**300**
  marantic **300**
Endocardium, arrangement **472**
Endocrine disease, screening for 706
Endodermal sinus tumour 675, 686
Endogenous retroviral particles 347
Endogenous retrovirus 347
Endometrial penetration by molar villi 190
Endometritis 345
Endometrium in gestation 165
Endothelin 1 peptide (ET-1) 15
Endothelium-derived relaxing factor
  (EDRF) 15
Endovascular trophoblast invasion failure
  345
Energy deficiencies 1413–14
Enteric cysts and duplications 847–8
Enterogenous cysts 849
Enteroviral infections 105, 330
Enteroviruses 443–5, 1449–50
Environmental agents, and congenital
  anomalies 399
Environmental teratogens 175
Enzyme,
  abnormalities in pregnancy 1270–1
  assay sample 1131–2
  fetal defects 1277
Enzyme deficiency, inherited 1131
Enzyme deficiency syndromes 683
Enzyme replacement therapy 1508
Enzyme-linked immunosorbent assay, *see*
  ELISA
Enzymopathy in peroxisomal disorders
  1139
Eosinophilia 722
Eosinophils 720
  hereditary hypersegmentation 722
Epicardial coronaries, pattern **485**
Epidermolysis bullosa 761
  junctional 761, 763
Epidermolysis bullosa atrophicans inversa
  762
Epidural anaesthesia, monitoring 298
Epiloia 844
Epimorphic fields 29
Epispadias 686
Epithelial sheets, movements 133
Epulis,
  congenital **841**
  melanotic 841
Erb palsy 311
Erdheim cystic medial necrosis 24, 503,
  505
Erythema infectiosum 113, 265
Erythroblastosis fetalis 295, 343, 711–12
  causes 1454–5
  exchange transfusion 1456
  intrauterine management 1455

Erythrocytes,
  fetal, abnormalities *710*
  metabolic disorders 714–15
  metabolism in newborn and adult *714*
  neonatal 709–**10**
  nucleated 1060–1
Erythroid precursor cells **113–14**
Erythropoietin in hypoxia 292
Escherichia coli 1446–7
Estimate of gestational age (EGA) 15–16
  at fetal autopsy 382, 383, 385
  scoring systems 368
Estimated fetal weight (EFW),
  decrease in standard deviation score 279
  in IUGR 279
  for SGA 277
Estrogens, carcinogenicity 78
Ethanol 133
Ethical issues 17–19
Ethical and medicolegal considerations
  1315
Ethics 1010–11, 1018
  and antenatal screening 1041
Ethylnitrosourea, as carcinogen 78–9
Euchromatin 55
Eugenics 1002, 1010–11
Euploid gametes, production by Down
  syndrome mother **228**
European Committee for Ultrasound
  Radiation Safety 881
European Federation of Societies for
  Ultrasound in Medicine and Biology 881
Ewing's tumour 855
Examination, internal, guidelines *1536*
Exchange transfusion 814
Exocoelomic cavity **139**, 152, **154**
Exocoelomic fluid 151–2, **155–6**
Exocrine pancreas, congenital hypoplasia
  581–2
Exomphalos 927–8, 929
  associated structural defects 928
Exosurf 547
Exposures, teratogenic *181*
Extracellular matrix (ECM) 129–31
Extracorporeal membrane oxygenation
  (ECMO) 1375, 1469–78
  bypass physiology 1473–4
  bypass techniques 1471–3
  cases by diagnosis *1474*
  future modifications 1476
  indications 1469–70
  morbidity 1475
  mortality 1474
  neonatal diagnoses 1470
  neurodevelopmental follow-up 1475–6
  respiratory failure criteria 1470
  venoarterial circuit **1471**
Extracorporeal membrane oxygenators 811
Extraembryonic coelom 899
  embryoscopy **1067**
Extraembryonic structures, abnormalities
  163
Extrasystoles 964–5
Extremely low birth weight 7, 368
Extremely low-birth-weight infant,
  neurological problems 1376
Extremities,
  embryoscopy 1068
  malformed, embryoscopy 1069
Extrinsic growth retardation 275
Eye,
  imaging at week 15 **907**
  perinatal lesions 823–**4**
  triploidy anomalies 195
  tuberous sclerosis 843

Fabry disease 39, 765, **1144–5**
Face,
  at 11 weeks 907
  defects, embryoscopic diagnosis 1065–70
  in Down syndrome 947
  dysmorphology 358
  embryoscopy at 9 weeks **1068–9**
  paralysis 311
  terms used **1542**
  triploidy anomalies 193
  ultrasound findings, chromosomal
    anomaly *939*
Facial clefting, with trisomy 13 940–**1** 941
Facioscapulohumeral dystrophy with
  trisomy 18 777, 941
Factor VIII deficiency (haemophilia A),
  1284
Factor IX deficiency (haemophilia B),
  1284
Factor XIII deficiency 1285
Fallopian tubes, infections from 261
Falx,
  in fetal aging 906
  tears 307–8
Familial clustering and recurrent abortion
  170
Familial intrahepatic cholestasis *567*
Familial polyposis of colon 73–**4**
Familial risk factors for fetal heart disease
  956–7
Family tree symbols 377, **1541**
Fanconi anaemia 65, 77, 764
Fanconi syndrome 24
Farber disease **1144**, 1146
Fat,
  dietary, digestion and absorption 1412
  intravenous use, complications 1433–4
  requirement of preterm infant 1425–7
Fat content 277–8
Fat necrosis, subcutaneous 306
Fatty acid deficiency states 1413
Fatty acid metabolism, disorders 1029,
  1134
Fatty acid oxidation disorders 573
Fatty acids in pregnancy 1276
FC, *see* Persistent fetal circulation
Feet,
  at 13 weeks 907
  deformities, with trisomy 18 941
  embryoscopy at 9 weeks **1068**
  length by gestation week *1539*
  rockerbottom, in trisomy 18 941
  ultrasound findings, chromosomal
    anomaly *939*
Femur,
  at 12 weeks **902**
  fetal shortened **935**
  fracture 311
  ultrasound measurement 879–80
Fertilization 120–1, 663–4
  defects 28
  double, simultaneous **234, 236**
  failure 120–1
  in vitro (IVF) 228, 972, 1010, 1055, 1057
    preimplantation cytogenetics 241
    spontaneous abortion 241
Fetal abnormality,
  and chromosomal disease *939*
  classification *1347*
  intrapartum management 1345–9
  MSAFP rise 1034–5
  pregnancy termination 1014
    emotional feelings **1015–16**
      men **1017**
      women **1016**

Fetal abnormality, pregnancy termination (contd)
  ethical issues 1018
  parental needs 1017–18
  psychosocial sequelae 1014–16
  reproductive behaviour 1016–17
  structural, ultrasound diagnosis 919–38
Fetal acid–base assessment, biochemical principles 1357–8
Fetal acid–base status, continuous monitoring 1359
Fetal adrenal hormones 698–9
Fetal alcohol syndrome 26, 86, 135, 355, 401, **1274–5**
  frequent associated features 355
  major features 355
  occasional associated features 355
  and renal hypoplasia 611
  signs and symptoms 355
Fetal anaemia 113, 296–7
  therapy 1263
Fetal anorectal continence 591
Fetal anuria, in MZ twins 204, 206
Fetal aorta, Doppler studies 895
Fetal arrhythmias 964–9
  echocardiography 955–69
  team approach 968
  therapy 967–9
    risks 967
  Yale Center diagnosis 965
Fetal arteries, echocardiography **960–1**
Fetal artery thrombosis 295
Fetal assessment,
  aims 889–90
  antepartum tests 889
  behaviour 890
  cordocentesis 1072–3
  randomized trials 890
  technical and physiological bases of tests 889
Fetal autopsy report 387
Fetal bladder shunt 1316
Fetal blood, for haemoglobinopathies 181
Fetal blood changes, in metabolic disease 1094
Fetal blood films, technique 1096–7
Fetal blood flow 287
  in acute distress 322
Fetal blood gas, continuous monitoring 1359
Fetal blood sampling 1071–6, 1092–3, 1097
  clinical aspects 1358
  genodermatosis diagnosis 765
  intrapartum indications 1358
  for prenatal diagnosis in twins 220
  total pregnancy loss 1074
Fetal blood vessels 894
Fetal bone, research on 391–2
Fetal bone marrow, parvovirus damage 265
Fetal brain 912–13
Fetal brain death 390
Fetal breathing movements 893
  and oligohydramnios 933
Fetal cancer-suppressive effect 68–9
Fetal cardiac output 286
Fetal cell,
  isolation from maternal blood 1059–1064
  isolation study variables 1059
Fetal chromosome abnormalities 269
Fetal circulation 286–7, 1362–3
  Doppler studies 995
  persistent (PFC), see Persistent fetal circulation
  separation from maternal 981

Fetal congenital anomalies 269
Fetal cortisol biosynthetic defects 699
Fetal cystic kidneys 926–7
  causes 926
  differential diagnosis 926
Fetal death 269–73
  acute 386
  anatomic and ancillary studies 180–1
  assessment 180–1
  causes 269, **366**
  classification 269
  early,
    classifications 177
    pathology 177–8
  gross evaluation 270
  groups 386
  histologic evaluation 271–3
  infectious syndromes 104
  intrauterine duration 387–8
  laboratory studies 386–7
  mechanism determination 382
  mechanism evaluation 385–6
  metabolic diseases 273
  in multiple gestation 208
  perinatal autopsy percentages 368
  prevalence 269
  procedural considerations 180
  retention 269
  timing 271
  unexplained 269
Fetal distress,
  and anaesthesia 297
  chronic 386
  heart rate 1353
  intrapartum trauma 305–12
Fetal echocardiographic frequency and yield 963
Fetal electrocardiographic waveform 1359
Fetal enzyme defects 1277
Fetal gestational age and growth assessment 387–8
Fetal gonadoblastoid testicular dysgenesis 680
Fetal great arteries,
  origins, normal cross-sectional view 960
  transposition 961
  and maternal diabetes mellitus 963
Fetal growth 693–6
  guide 1537
  restriction 17
Fetal growth factors, integration 695–6
Fetal haematopoietic disease, therapy 1331–4
Fetal haematopoietic stem cell transplantation,
  in utero 1331–6
  rationale 1331–2
Fetal haemoglobin 296
  higher level 285
  oxygen affinity 285
Fetal haemolysis, graph detection **1456**
Fetal haemorrhage 321–2
Fetal heart 914–15
  abnormal 964
    early and accurate detection 955
    in trisomy 13 941
  beating at week 7 899
  blood flow through **287**
  evaluation by echocardiography 958–60
  normal long axis view **959**
  structure, function and rhythm, imaging 955
Fetal heart disease,
  epidemiology 956

  risk factors 956
Fetal heart failure 983
Fetal heart rate 891–2
  accelerations 1356
  admission test 1358
  decelerations 1356–7
  electrical monitoring 290–1
  intermittent auscultation 1353
  monitoring 1347
    continuous 1353–4
    indications 1351
  reactive 893
  variability 1355–6
Fetal immunologically mediated disease 343
Fetal infant mortality rates (FIMRs) 10, 366
Fetal infection 269
  immune response **735–6**
  and IUGR 276
Fetal injection 1310
Fetal intracranial circulation 894
Fetal liver biopsy 1093, 1097
Fetal loss, see Abortion; Reproductive loss
Fetal lung, morphological changes 290–1
Fetal lung maturity index 545
Fetal lymph node **734–5**
Fetal lymphocyte progenitors 1506
Fetal malformation,
  and oligohydramnios 933
  prognosis 1312–13
Fetal Management Board 956
Fetal measurement 890–1, 976
Fetal metabolism 1267–79
  maternal influences 1267–75
Fetal monitoring, intrapartum 1351–60
Fetal muscle biopsy 1093–4
Fetal nuchal translucency **950**
Fetal organ retrieval timing 390
Fetal origins of adult diseases 370
Fetal outcome evaluation, clinical signs 368
Fetal ovarian cysts 930
Fetal oxygen saturation 1359
Fetal oxygenation 285
Fetal pathology 367
Fetal period, placenta 11–17
Fetal physiology, cordocentesis 1073
Fetal plate, sonographic differential diagnosis 983
Fetal pleural effusion shunting 1317
Fetal pneumonia 510
Fetal prolonged exposure to drugs 354
Fetal renal arteries, Doppler studies 894
Fetal rest, and vaginal adenosis 78
Fetal rest theory 67, 73
Fetal rhabdomyoma 842
Fetal sampling, for thalassemia 1175
Fetal scalp blood monitoring 9, 1356–8
  in labour 290–1
Fetal size for dates, and oligohydramnios 933
Fetal skin 755–8
  biopsy 758–9, 1093, 1097
  damage by scarring 265
Fetal stem cell transplantation, reported clinical experience 1333
Fetal structural anomaly, cordocentesis investigation 1073
Fetal surgery,
  open 1326–9
  risks 1326–7
  shunts 1315–18
Fetal swallowing 1243
  and polyhydramnios 1248
Fetal testicular failure 676

Fetal thymus 723
Fetal tissue,
  culture and storage 390
  research 391–5
  sources 389–90
Fetal tone 893
Fetal TORCH infections, prevalence 325
Fetal tumours 271
  aspiration 1309
Fetal uniparental disomy, with confined
  placental mosaicism 1106, 1108
Fetal urinary tract, dilated, causes 925
Fetal uropathies, incidence 924
Fetal vasculitis 325
Fetal vasculopathy,
  large-vessel type 330–1
  small-vessel type 330, 332
Fetal viability, definition 17
Feticide, selective, in multiple pregnancy
  221–2
Fetomaternal haemorrhage 296, 324,
  709–10
Fetoplacental circulation 13
  blood distribution 288
  Doppler studies 893–4
Fetoplacental influences 1275–7
Fetoplacental insufficiency, investigation
  291
Fetoplacental unit 979
α-Fetoprotein, see AFP
Fetus,
  acoustic stimulation 1358
  anaemic,
    diagnosis 1302–4
    physiologic adaptations 1301–2
    treatment 1304–5
  at-risk,
    biophysical assessment 889–95
    identification and assessment 877–8
    ultrasound measurement 890–1
  autopsy history 381–2
  blood transfusion 1310
  CMV pneumonitis 109
  cocaine effects 358
  developmental assessment 126
  developmental outline 16
  direct therapy 1307–14
  direct vision 1312
  electrolyte infusion 1311
  fat content 277–9
  gross body movement 893
  growth curves 15–16
  growth regulation 15–16
  heroin addiction 360
  high-risk 1351
    groups 1240
    management 1239–42
  imaging 867–995
  immunologically mediated disease 343
  inflammation and healing 114–16
  intravascular transfusion 1257, 1304–5
  in labour 287–90
  labour effect 290–1
  large-for-dates, assessment 877
  maternal drug therapy 803–4
  maternal substance abuse effects 353–62
  maturation 16–17
  modified dissection 305
  mosaicism 1101–5
  non-stressed test 891
  'physiological hypoxia' 286
  physiological sleep 1355
  platelet infusion 1310–11
  protective factors 99–101

reactions to injury 17
respiratory airway infection 102
scar formation 115
small-for-dates, assessment 877
sonographically malformed (references)
  252
stimulation tests 1358–9
structural evaluation, from 6 to 16 weeks
  897–918
triploid 69,XXY 237
triploid, flow cytometry diagnosis 237
ultrasound measurements 877
urine output 1461
viral infection effects 1294
Fetus compressus 269
Fetus in fetu 218
Fetus papyraceus 202, 267, 270
  complications 206
Fibrin,
  pathologic deposition patterns 334
  perivillous 333–4
Fibrinogen, disorders 1285
Fibrinoid necrosis 333
Fibroblast,
  cultured 181
  lung 394
Fibroblastic proliferation 116
Fibrochondrogenesis 790
Fibroelastosis 480
Fibromatosis, infantile 839
Fibromatosis colli 840
Fibromuscular sclerosis 272
Fibronectin 129, 131, 733–4
  and prematurity 7
Fibrosis, congenital hepatic 562–3
Fibrous hamartoma,
  of infancy 838–9
  of kidney 840–1
  of liver 841
Fibrous xanthoma 846
Fick's principle 1401–2
Filter paper application 1049
Filter paper technology 1042
Fingers,
  6 days in culture,
    growth zone 392
    metachromasia loss 392
  at 11 weeks 906
  from 11 to 16 weeks, for teratogen study
    391
  at 12 weeks, in culture 391
  at 13 weeks 903
  fixed flexion 941, 943–4
FISH, see Fluorescence in situ hybridization
Flecainamide 967, 1259
Floaters in paraffin block 165
Flow cytometry,
  distinction between complete and partial
    hydatidiform moles 233
  in hydatidiform mole diagnosis 196
  for hydatidiform mole separation 232,
    239
  in partial mole prognosis 192–3
  ploidy and molar pregnancy diagnosis 239
Flow velocity waveforms, at 8 and 16
  weeks 980
Fluid requirements in preterm infant 1423
Fluorescence in situ hybridization (FISH)
  25, 1063, 1104
  applications 1123–8
  clinical experience 1125
  karyotypic abnormalities 1127
  marker chromosomes 1127–8
  prenatal diagnosis 1123–5

probe strategies 1124
probes 1124
Fluorescence-activated cell sorter 1062
  histogram 1062
Foam cell infiltration 328–9
Focal dermal hypoplasia 24
Folic acid deficiency 87–8
Folic acid for NTD prevention 380, 1032
Food, contaminated, and infections 347
Foot, length measurement 383
Forceps delivery and birth trauma 805
Forebrain malformations 419–23
Foregut, development 589
Forensic investigations, basic elements 371
Fowler's syndrome 425
Fracarro achondrogenesis 789–90
Fragile X syndrome 40, 60, 64–5, 1115–19
  cytogenetics 1117
  diagnosis 1117–18
  gene (FMR1) 1115
  genetics 1117
    molecular 1116–17
  inheritance 1116
  male features 1115–16
  prenatal diagnosis 1118
  site at Xq27.3 1118
Froehlich, L.A. 177
Fructose intolerance, hereditary 571, 1138,
  1148
Fructose metabolism 1138–9
Fructose-1,6-bisphosphatase deficiency
  1138, 1148
Fryne syndrome 606
Fujikura, T. 177
Fungal infection,
  neonatal 443
  in neonatal intensive care 102
Funisitis, peripheral 325–6

Galactosaemia 571–2, 1138–9, 1148,
  1410
  effect of treatment 1023
  in pregnancy 1272
  prenatal fetal damage 1023–4
  prenatal screening 1023–4
  tests 1045, 1048
α-Galactosidase deficiency 765
Galactosialidosis 1143
Gallbladder 577–8
Gallstones, increased risk in parenteral
  nutrition 1439
Gametes, genotyping 1055–6
Gametogenesis 28, 119–20, 228, 663
  imprinting in hydatidiform mole 196
Ganglioneuroblastoma 856
Ganglioneuroma 856
Ganglioneuromatosis 599
Ganglioside degradation 1144
Gangliosidosis 571, 1143–4
  G_{M1}, 1093, 1143–4
    fetal blood film 1093
    microscopic assessment 1090
  G_{M2} 444, 1143
Gardner syndrome 24, 73, 852
Garrod, A. 1554–6
Gas exchange 523
Gastric outlet obstruction 594–5
Gastro-oesophageal reflux 594
Gastroenteritis, intrauterine 312
Gastrointestinal defects and
  polyhydramnios 932
Gastrointestinal tract,
  abnormalities, in twins 972
  cysts and duplications 847–8

Gastrointestinal tract (contd)
  development *1418*
  perinatal therapy, complications 817–19
  upper, perforation 811
Gastroschisis 605, 927–8, 929
  and caesarean section 1346
  definition 1493
  and fetal growth 1494
  management 1498–1502
  ultrasonography **1496**
Gastrulation 124
  molecular events 35
Gaucher disease 37, 571, 573, 1053,
  1144–6
  non-sense mutation 42
  variants 1145
Gender, antenatal glucocorticoid therapy
  1338
Gene,
  abnormal structure and maldevelopment
    31
  'body maps' 52
  CFTR, *see* CFTR gene
  cloned 1122
  defect identification 1022
  expressed sequence tags 52
  locus 1187
  position effect 60
  and protein products *1190*
  regional expression 129
  single disorders, molecular pathology
    1191
  'spontaneous abortion susceptibility locus'
    170
  SRY 24
  and testicular differentiation 664
  WT1, *see* Wilms' tumour gene
  see also under Descriptive title
Gene probes, single 1122
Gene therapy 1334–5, 1508–10
'Genethics' 1001
Genetic aftercare 999
Genetic analysis 1063
Genetic anomalies, and non-immune
  hydrops 1260
Genetic carrier state, premarital screening 8
Genetic code *1188*
Genetic counselling 999, 1001, 1007–12
  for abdominal wall defects 1498
  art of 1007
  basic elements *1000*
  definition 1007–8
  diagnosis 1008
  directive or non-directive 1008
  in early fetal loss 182–3
  management 1001
  objects 1008
  options 1001
  prospective and retrospective 1008–9
Genetic definitions 32–3
Genetic diagnosis 1000
  preimplantation 1055–8
Genetic disease,
  categories 35
  expression 31
  transmission 31
Genetic disorders, prenatal diagnosis by
  cordocentesis 1073
Genetic epidemiology of cancer 72
Genetic linkage analysis, problems 182
Genetic screening 999–1000, *1002*,
  1021–30
  basic indications *1000*
  confirmatory tests 1000–1

diagnostic 'test' 1000
enumeration and research 1022
impact *1023*
implications 999–1003
individual well-being 1000
medical management 1022
methods and causes of death **1022**
for omphalocele 1498
optimal technology *1002*
preconceptual 1001
premarital 1002
and prenatal diagnosis *1002*
range and objectives 1022
reproductive and societal implications
  1001
unacceptable for mass 1054
see also Screening
Genetic services, financial audit 1010
Genetic technology 1011
Genetics,
  clinical, as team approach 1003
  developmental periods 999
  medical, scope 1003
  pathology and medical care, overview
    1240
  role 1007
  somatic cell 999
Genital ducts, internal, differentiation
  665–6
Genital herpes and TORCH 262
Genital tubercule **1069**
Genitalia,
  ambiguous 698
  at 15 weeks, structural evaluation **910**
  external,
    differentiation 666
    embryoscopy 1069
    in mixed gonadal dysgenesis *671–2*
  intrapartum trauma 310
  male, ambiguous in XXY fetus 195
Genitourinary malformations in Wilms'
  tumor 76
Genitourinary pathogens 325
Genitourinary system,
  injury 312
  ultrasound diagnosis of fetal anomalies
    924–7
  ultrasound-guided aspiration 1309
Genome, mapping 999
Genome Project 37
Genomic imprinting, differential, in
  hydatidiform mole 196
Genotype 1187
  and malformation 399
Germ cell tumours 675
Germinal cell aplasia 679
Germinal matrix haemorrhages **430**,
  432
Germinoma 675
Germline mosaicism 377, 380
Gestation,
  screening time frames 6
  villous population **142**
  weekly development **145**
Gestational age,
  body weight and length *456*
  calculation 897
  placenta and organ weight *456*
  smoothed curve measurement data
    455
  ultrasound establishment 879–81
Gestational history 382
Gestational sac, early, anatomy 141–7

Gestational tissues, early, examination
  165
Giant cell angioblastoma, congenital
  infiltrating 836
Giant cell transformation, associated
  conditions *563*
Giant cell transformation **564**
Gitter cell response 297
Glanzmann's thrombasthenia 719, 1283
Glial cells, degeneration 437
Gliosis 436–7
Glomerular cysts, in inherited malformation
  syndromes 619
α-Globin gene 39
  cluster deletions **1166**
  localization and organization **1165**
β-Globin gene,
  linkage analysis **1181**
  molecular pathology **1191**
  normal and mutated allele **1180**
β-Globin gene cluster,
  deletions **1174**
  restriction polymorphic sites **1181**
Glomus tumour 846
Glucocorticoid therapy 394
Glucocorticoids,
  antenatal,
    clinical studies *1338–9*
    in preterm labour 1340
  issues affecting efficacy 1338–40
Glucose,
  crossing placenta 1275
  in fetal metabolism 12
  metabolism in newborn 1410
  placental transfer 12
  requirement of preterm infant 1423
Glucose phosphate isomerase deficiency
  714
Glucose-6-phosphate dehydrogenase
  deficiency 714–15
Glutaric acidemia type II 24
Glutaric aciduria 1134–5
Glutathione, metabolic disorders 715
Glutathione synthetase deficiency 715
γ-Glutamylcysteine synthetase deficiency
  715
Glycogen storage diseases 569–71, 1141–3,
  1207, 1414
  diagnostic tests *1142*
  hepatic, tests *1142*
  type I 570
  type II 571
  type III 570, **572**
  type IV 569–71
  see also McArdle disease; Pompe disease;
    von Gierke disease
Glycogenosis 1141–3, *1148*
  infantile forms 780, 782
  type I *570*
  type II *570*
  type III *570*
  type IV *570*
Glycoprotein storage diseases *1156*
Glycoproteinoses 1146
Glycosaminoglycans 129
  decrease in organ culture 392
Goitres 697
Golaby–Rosen syndrome 1070
Goldenhar syndrome 402
  and renal hypoplasia 611
Gonadal chromosome abnormality
  228–9
Gonadal development and differentiation
  664–5

Gonadal dysgenesis 666–74
  46,XX pure 670
  46,XY pure 669–70
  asymmetric 670–2, 674
    with ovarian differentiation 670–1
    with testicular differentiation 671–3, 674
  mixed 671–3, 674
    dysplastic testis 672
    external genitalia 671
    gonadal constitution 671
    karyotype distribution 672
  symmetric 668–70
  and tumours 674–5
Gonadal mosaicism 229, 377
  and trisomy 233
Gonadoblastoma 670, 672–3, 674–5, 676
Gonadogenesis 28
Gonads,
  infarcts and catheterization 817
  teratoma 832–3
Graft-versus-host disease (GVHD) 332,
  749, 1503–4, 1505–6
Gram-negative organisms 824
Granular cell myoblastoma 841
Granulocyte–macrophage 340
Graves' disease 698
Group B streptococci 327, 1446
Growth-deficient embryo 25
Growth factors 133, 340
  receptors 130
Growth hormone 694
Growth-promoting factors in human milk
  1409
Guidelines for Perinatal Care 1513
Gunther disease 765
Gut hormones 1409
Guthrie, R., biographical sketch 1005–6
Guthrie neonatal screening cards 1192
Guthrie's blood test 1045
GVHD, see Graft-versus-host disease
Gyral scarring 438–9

Haem metabolism disorders 1154
Haem synthesis disorders 716–17
Haemangioendothelioma 574–5
Haemangioma 834–6
  in alcohol abuse 356
  capillary 834
  cavernous 834–5
  liver 835
  placental 835
Haematology, cordocentesis in 1072
Haematoma 569
  after venepuncture 1284
  nodular 307
Haematopoiesis, extramedullary 262
Haematopoietic diseases, congenital, in
  utero stem-cell transplantation 1331
Haematopoietic stem-cell transplantation,
  animal model data 1333
Haematopoietic system, embryology 709
Haemochromatosis 572–3
Haemoglobin 31
  abnormalities, screening 717
  electrophoresis 181
  normal 715–16
  in smaller twin 974
  synthesis disorders 715–17
Haemoglobin C syndrome 716
Haemoglobinopathies 1165–95
  prenatal diagnosis 717
Haemolysis, in immune hydrops 1257
Haemolytic anaemia 710–13
  immune 711–13

Haemolytic disease, history 1454–6
Haemolytic hyperbilirubinaemia, neonatal,
  management 1453–60
Haemolytic uraemic syndrome 328
Haemophilia 24
  and mutation 37
Haemophilia A and B 1284
Haemorrhage,
  antenatal 323
  antepartum, marker 208, 303
  brain lesions 427–32
  central nervous system 358
  in closed environment 325
  clot maturation 323
  extradural 304, 307
  fetal 323–4
  germinal matrix 430
  intracerebral 427–8
  intracranial 1288
  intrapartum 303
  intraventricular 370, 428, 430–2, 1288–9
  maternal 323–4
  periventricular 1400
  placental 323–4, 325
  pulmonary 57, 549
  retroplacental 303
  subaponeurotic 304, 306
  subarachnoid 427, 429
  subcapsular 569
  subdural 304, 307, 427
  subependymal 428, 431–2
  subperiosteal 304, 306–7
  subpial 427–8
Haemorrhagic disease of newborn 718,
  1286–8
Haemorrhagic endovasculitis 330
Haemorrhagic intracerebral involvement,
  pathogenesis 1362
Haemorrhagic white matter infarction 434
Haemosiderin-laden macrophages 431–2
Haemostasis,
  acquired defects 1285–90
  disorders 1282–3
  inherited deficiencies 1283–5
  neonatal development 1281–91
  screening test reference values 1283
    in preterm infants 1284
Hair–cartilage–hypoplasia syndrome 721
Halo lesion 325–6
Hamartoma 72–4, 834–46
  connective tissue 838–41
  lung 841
  of skeleton 841–2
Hamartoses 72–4
Hamster oocyte penetration technique 229
Hand,
  at 15 weeks, structural evaluation 909
  embryoscopy at week 9 1068
  ultrasound examination 935
Haploid, contribution of extra copies 232
Haplotype, inheritance 1503–4
Hardy–Weinberg law 46, 482
Harlequin ichthyosis 762
Harris–Benedict equations 1422
Hartnup's disease, in pregnancy 1272
hCG, see Chorionic gonadotropin
Head,
  abnormalities, in trisomy 18 942
  circumference 15
    at 15 weeks 912
    B-scan measurement 886
    increase at 18 months in PCP infants 361
    standard 696
    ultrasound measurement 877

injury sites 304
and intrapartum trauma 304, 306–8
lemon configuration 921–2
normal,
  at 15 weeks 905
  at 18 weeks 919
teratoma 833
ultrasound examination 935
ultrasound findings, chromosomal
  anomaly 939
Heart 465–521
  at 15 weeks, structural evaluation
    914–16
  abnormalities, interpretative guidelines
    517
  asymmetric hypertrophy 506–7, 509
  biopsy 507
  conduction system, study method 1550–1
  congenital disease,
    lung changes 542–3
    surgery 514–16
  congestive failure 509
    left-sided 513
    right-sided 511
  developing, external surface configuration
    475
  examination 516–17
  four-chamber view 957–8
    at 15 weeks 915
  genetic diseases 505–9
  great vessel d-transposition, surgery
    1480–1
  infection products 262
  in intrapartum asphyxia 299
  laterality malformations 498, 500–1
  malformations 262
  normal development 465–80
  perinatal, conduction system method
    826–7
  petechial haemorrhage 299
  reconstructed, right posterior lateral views
    476
  right-sided obstructive lesions, surgery
    1481–2
  situs inversus 498–9
  specimen preparation 516–17
  transplantation 515–16, 1479, 1483
  triploidy anomalies 195
  tuberous sclerosis 843
  tumours 507, 509
  in Turner syndrome 950
  two-dimensional imaging 957
  see also Cardiac
Heart beats in gestational aging 899
Heart block,
  congenital 503
    caesarean section 1346
Heart disease,
  congenital 400
    fetal management 960–2
    haemostatic defects 1289
    karyotype 955
    and maternal diabetes mellitus 963
    obstetrical care planning 955
    other structural abnormalities 955
    postnatal medical intervention planning
      955
    recurrence risk 377
    and structural malformations 961
    and trisomy 13 and 18 249
    and trisomy 18 249
    types 482
  identification 956–60
  in trisomy 18 941–2

Heart failure, and hydrops fetalis 513
Heart–lung transplantation 515–16
Heat production 1407–9
Hedgehogs, foxes, lumpers and splitters 1002
Heinz body anaemia 715
Hematoma, of umbilical cord **993**
Hemihypertrophy 73, 75
Hensen's node 35
Hepatic, *see* Liver
Hepatic microsomal monoxygenase system 85
Hepatitis,
  neonatal 563–4
  in pregnancy 1294
Hepatitis B 326
Hepatitis B antigenaemia 566
Hepatitis viruses 1297
Hepatoadrenal necrosis 110
Hepatoblastoma 576–7
Hepatocerebrorenal syndrome, *see* Zellweger hepatocerebrorenal syndrome
Hepatocyte growth factor, lung produced 535
Hepatosplenomegaly 262, 573
Hepatosteatosis, familial 573
Hereditary disorders, confusion with unexpected death 371–2
Hereditary exostosis 73
Hereditary multiple exostoses 841–2
Hereditary persistence of fetal hemoglobin 1173
Hereditofamilial cancers 71–2
Hermaphroditism 75, 680–4
  true *681–2*
Hernia uteri inguinalis 672, **674**
Heroin 91
  abuse 359–1
  with cocaine ('speedball') 357
  neonatal withdrawal signs *354*
  in pregnancy 1272, 1274
Herpes simplex virus, *see* HSV
Heterochromatin 55
  X and Y, determination 687
Heteroduplex **34**
Heterokaryotypia 203–4, 214, 241
Heteromorphism 58
Heterozygote detection 1053
Heterozygotes 60
Hexokinase deficiency 714
Hibernoma 845
High-resolution images 255
Hindbrain malformations 423
Hindgut, development 591
Hip dislocation 400
Hippocampal necrosis 438–9, 440
Hirschsprung disease 204, 598–9, **600**
Histidinaemia, in pregnancy 1272
Histiocytic tumours 846
Histiocytoma 846
Histiocytosis X 726–7
Histocompatibility antigens, inheritance 1503–4
Histogenesis 28
Histograms, giving ploidy 196
HIV (human immunodeficiency virus),
  congenital infection diagnosis 350
  infections 105–6, 108, 348–50
  neonatal testing 1051–2
  perinatal transmission 349
  in pregnancy 1297–8
  transmission 98–9, 106
  transplacental 328, 349
  see also AIDS virus

HLA (human leucocyte histocompatibility antigens) alleles, sharing 342
HLA antigens, in placenta 192
HLA sharing 339
  and abortion 170, 179–80, 341–2
HLA-G 340
Hofbauer cells 96, 106, 142
  HIV in 349
  as indication of metabolic disease 1090
Holoprosencephaly 216, 419–20, 924
  alcohol abuse 355
  alobar **941**
  Pax mutation 48
  in trisomy 13 940–1
Home births 9
Homeobox homeoproteins 37
Homeorrhesis 80
Homeotic genes, in development 48
Homocystinuria, in pregnancy 1272
Honeycomb lung 550
Horner syndrome 310
Horseshoe kidney 613
Host resistance model of Matsunaga 70
Housekeeping genes 31
Houston–Harris syndrome 788–**9**
Hox genes 35, 37
  patterns **129**
  transcription and intron length 48
HSV (herpes simplex virus),
  at delivery 105
  fetal evaluation 265
  infection 110, 325
  neonatal liver **111**
  liver **568**
  neonatal 1448–9
  pneumonia 548–**9**
  in pregnancy 1296–7
  smear preparation **112**
  in TORCH 261, 265, 327
  type II 445
Human embryonic and fetal tissue (HEFT), future developments 395
  in research 390–5
  uses 389–97
Human immunodeficiency virus, *see* HIV
Human leukocyte histocompatibility antigens (HLA) 1503–6
Human life, early links *1002*
Human papilloma virus (HPV) in pregnancy 1297
Human tissue for medical biology studies 391
Human trophic lymphocyte viruses 549
Humerus, intrapartum trauma 311
Humerus at 15 weeks **906**
Hunter, John and William 979
Hunter gene 1147
Hunter syndrome 24
Huntington disease or chorea,
  causative mutations 40
  genetic linkage analysis 182
Hurler disease 1143, 1146–7
  CVS **1091**
Hutterite population, pregnancy studies 342
Hyaline membrane disease, respiratory distress syndrome (RDS) *370*, 510, **547**, *1393*
Hyaline membranes,
  resolution 807
  yellow 811
Hybridization *in situ* 1121–2
  applications 1123–8
  methods 255
Hydatidiform change and karyotyping 950

Hydatidiform mole 985
  clinical presentation and diagnosis 187–8
  clinically silent 187
  complete 187–92
    at 8 weeks, microscopic view **188**
    at 9 weeks **189**
    at 10 weeks **188**
    androgenetic origin 191
    cistern **188–9**
    clinicopathologic features *197*
    cytogenetics 190, 232, **239**
    definition 187
    diagnostic triad 188
    flow cytometry diagnosis 196, **239**
    formation 232
    genetic background 190–2
    invasive **189–90**
    malignant potential 196
    origin 190–1
    pathologic anatomy 188–9
    presentation and diagnosis 187–8
    residual trophoblastic disease 190
    theoretical origin **239**
    unique paternal origin 191
    zygosity 192
  in fetal presence 187
  flow cytometry diagnosis 196
  and high MShCG levels 989
  intrauterine diagnosis 194
  invasive
    biologically non-invasive nature 190
    embolizing 190
  obstetric complications 187
  occurrence in twin 187
  partial 187, 192–6
    at 12 weeks **193**
    at 13 weeks **193**
    ascertainable embryo/fetus 192
    clinicopathologic features *197*
    cytogenetics 232, **234–5**, 237
    with dead fetus **194**
    definition 192
    embryo/fetus, late death 192, 195
    embryo/fetus in 195
    fertilization error 195
    fetal presence 187
    flow cytometry diagnosis 196
    follow-up 194
    genetics 195–6
    'large for dates' uterus 192
    origin **195**
    parental alleles **240**
    pathologic anatomy 193–4
    presentation and diagnosis 192–3
    prognosis 194–5
    prolonged retention after fetal death 195
    residual trophoblastic disease 194
    RFLPs 195
    triploid **234**, 237
    trophoblastic changes 193
    trophoblastic hyperplasia of syncytium **193**
    varied clinicopathologic spectrum 193
  postevacuation complications 187
  preoperative diagnosis 187
  sperm and egg genomic imprinting 196
  syndrome overlap 187
  in twin pregnancy 194
Hydatidiform transformation **987**
Hydatidiform vesicle, with central cistern **189**
Hydatidiform villi **188–9**
Hydramnios 1085
  complications 213–14

Hydranencephaly 262, 424–5
Hydrocephalus 423, **920**
  causes *425*
  drainage 1316–17
  posthaemorrhagic **430–1**
    Doppler detection 1401
  in twins 972
Hydrocephaly 262, *370*
  ultrasound detection 1040
Hydrocytosis 715
Hydronephros, congenital 612
Hydronephrosis,
  antibiotic prophylaxis 1465
  differential diagnosis *1462*
  neonatal evaluation 1463
  postnatal evaluation 1462–3
  prenatal intervention *1465*
  stent procedures 1317
  unilateral **925–6**
Hydrops fetalis,
  blood flow 304
  causes 513
  definition 1257
  in Down syndrome 949
  and fetal dead twin 213–14
  and fetal death 269
  β-glucuronidase deficiency 1093
  and infections 113
  liver **113**
  lung hypoplasia 533
  non-immune 962–3, 1257–64
    causes 712, *1258–9*
    cordocentesis 1073
    investigation 1260–1, *1262*
    maternal complications 1263–4
    prenatal therapy 1262–3
  postinfection 262
  in supraventricular tachycardia 968
  ultrasound findings, chromosomal
    anomaly *939*
Hydroxycorticosterone synthesis, defective
  705
Hymenal cyst 685
Hyperalimentation 1050
Hyperbilirubinaemia *370*
  indirect neonatal, causes *1454*
  phenobarbital for 1458
Hypercalcaemia 706
Hyperechoic bowel **903**
Hyperechoic chorionic sac **898**
Hyperganglionosis 599
Hyperglycaemia 585, 586, 702
Hyperglycinaemia, non-ketotic 1137–8
Hyperhaploidy 229, 232
Hyperkeratosis 760
Hypermagnesaemia 776
Hyperparathyroidism 705–6
Hyperplasia, and fetal growth 277
Hyperplastic decidual vasculopathy 328–9
Hypertension,
  and catheterization 817
  malignant 328
  and pre-eclampsia 344–5
  pregnancy-associated 206
  pregnancy-induced 343
Hypertensive disorders 344
  classification lack 345
Hypertensive pulmonary vascular disease
  509, 513–14
  arterial, stages of development **514**
  blood pressures **514**
Hyperthermia 88
  as teratogen 84, 405
Hyperthyroidism 344, 698

Hypertrophic subaortic stenosis 506
Hypertrophy, and fetal growth 277
Hyperviscosity 717–18
Hypervitaminosis A 417
Hypoglycaemia 282, 702
Hyponatraemia 12
Hypoparathyroidism 705
Hypoperfusion 509–11
Hypophosphatasia 800–1
Hypopituitarism 566
Hypoplasia in triploidy 195
Hypoplastic left heart syndrome 542,
  1482–3
Hypospadias 686
Hypotension 511
Hypothyroidism 206
  congenital 696
    screening 706
  tests 1045, *1048*
Hypotonia, congenital 779–80
Hypoxaemia 509–11
  hypotonic, neonatal, evaluation *1365*
  and IUGR 276
Hypoxia,
  blood flow 291
  evaluation 6, 9
  and fetal heart rate 1355–6
  fetal integrated response 291
  in utero, and congenital anomalies
    399
  intrauterine, pathophysiology 1351–2
Hypoxia injury 135
Hypoxic–ischaemic encephalopathy,
  Doppler detection 1400–1
  evaluation methods 1367–9
Hypoxic–ischaemic grey matter lesions
  437–40

ICE 10
  cause of death groups **11**
  infant death classification *11*
I-cell disease, *see* Mucolipidosis type II
Ichthyosiform erythroderma,
  bullous congenital 759
  non-bullous congenital 759
IgA,
  antibody responses 344
  in human milk 738
IgE 736–7
IgG,
  antibody responses 344
  in antiphospholipid syndrome 344
  fetal loss 344
  in gestation 98
  organism-specific 264
  parvovirus-specific 265
  placental transport 737
  replacement therapy 1503
  subclasses 735
  in TORCH syndrome 266
  transfer mechanism 12
IgG1 344
IgG2a 344
IgG4 344
IgM 181
  antibody responses 344
  organism-specific 264
  parvovirus-specific 265
  rubella-specific 265
  in TORCH syndrome 266
Ileum, cyst **847**
Imaging, in prenatal diagnosis 1197
Imaging techniques, comparison *1399*
Immaturity, and deaths 4

Immune deficiencies,
  primary 741–2
    congenital *742*
  secondary 748–9
Immune reactions 163
Immune system 729–53
  developing 96–7
  disorders 741–50
  functional anatomy 729
  laboratory evaluation 740–1
  ontogeny 729–30, 732–3
  organization and development 729–39
Immunity levels *100*
Immunization, for rubella 265
Immunodeficiencies, neonatal therapy
  1503–12
Immunodeficiency syndromes,
  bone marrow therapy 1507
  cell engraftment 1503
  neonatal clinical findings *741*
  treatment *1510–11*
Immunogenetics, complete hydatidiform
  mole 192
Immunoglobulins, *see* IgA; IgE; IgG; IgM
Immunohistochemical analysis 348
Immunohistochemical stains, for pregnancy
  confirmation 165
Immunological factors
  in abortion 341
  in human milk 1409
Immunology,
  in maternal–fetal syndromes 339–44
  and recurrent spontaneous abortion
    341–3
Immunomagnetic beads 1062–3
Immunotherapy,
  placebo effect 343
  for recurrent spontaneous abortion 342–3
Imperforate anus 25
Implantation 123–4
  defects 4
Imprinting 122–3, 1127
In vitro fertilization (IVF), *see* Fertilization,
  in vitro
Incontinentia pigmenti 24, 763
Indirect mutant gene tracking 1193–4
Indomethacin 1402, 1434
  fetal toxicity 1327
  gastrointestinal tract effects 818
  for polyhydramnios 1250–1
Infant feeding 1408–13
Infantile digital fibromatosis 839
Infantile fibromatosis 839
Infantile neuromuscular disorders 769–86
Infantile obstructive cholangiopathy 564
Infantile polycystic disease **562**
Infantile pyknocytosis 715
Infants,
  mortality rates *367*
  phencyclidine symptoms 361
  regressive tumors 68
Infants of diabetic mothers 16, 334
  metabolic disturbance 583–4
  pancreas **584**
  pattern of anomalies 27
Infection,
  antibodies 343
  antibody titers 181
  ascending 101–3
  bacterial 347–8
  brain cell migration defects 423
  congenital viral 748
  direct or indirect effects 346
  and fetal loss 345
  fetal and neonatal host responses 95–101

Infection (contd)
in utero 4
intrapartum 312
  and placenta 97–8
  routes 312
intrauterine 1073
and intravenous fat 1435
and leukopenia 720
localization 262
in maternal–fetal syndromes 345–50
neonatal bacterial 1445–8
neonatal viral 1448–50
and neutrophilia 722
and non-immune hydrops 1260
nosocomial 1447
parasitic 350
perinatal 824–15
placental 325–8
  diagnosis by examination 319
  and premature labour 288–9
  and prematurity 7
  protective maternal factors 98–9, 346
  protective mechanisms 95
  and recurrent abortion 172
  severe long-term sequelae 345
teratogenic *181*
transmissibility rate 103
transplacental 103–104, 328
viral 348–50
Infectious disruption 26, 401, 403–4
Infectious teratogenesis 261
Information processing 1531
Informed consent 1001
Inguinal hernia 698
Initiation, carcinogenic 67
Injection, inadvertent 297
Injury, ontogeny of reaction **69**
Inner cell mass (ICM), lineage analysis 122
Insulin and premature infant 1423
Insulin-like growth factor 1 (IGF1), and
  birth weight 280
Insulin-like growth factor 2 (IGF2) 76, 121
  gene 123
  gene mutations 52
Integrins 131
Intelligence quotient reduction in
  phencyclidine infants 361
Intensive care, neonatal 1373–9
Interdisciplinary evaluation of intrapartum
  trauma 305
Intercellular communication 130–1
Interferon-γ 341
  fetal loss 347
Interferons 68
Interleukin-2 (IL-2), and prematurity 7
Interleukin-3 (IL-3) 340
Interleukin-10 (IL-10) 341
International Collaborative Effort on
  Perinatal and Infant Mortality, *see* ICE
International Federation of Obstetrics and
  Gynaecology (FIGO) 1354
International Fetal Surgery Registry
  1316–17
International Neuroblastoma Staging
  System *857*
International Reference Preparation (IRP),
  First 898
International Skeletal Dysplasia Registry
  801
International Working Group on
  Congenital Anomalies 26–7, 399
International Workshop on Fetal Genetic
  Pathology 27
Interorbital distance at 15 weeks **907**
Interphase cells **1126**

Interphase genetics 1123–5
  centromeric probes for 1124
Interphase nuclei from non-dividing tissue
  1123
Intersex syndromes 680–4
Interventricular septum,
  changes **483**
  malformations 495, 497–8
  sections **483**
Intervillositis 325–6, **327**
Intervillous space 13, **150, 152,** 321
Intervillous thrombi 324
Intestine,
  atresia 596–7
    schematic representation **597**
  large 595–8
  polyps 24, 851
  pseudo-obstructions, chronic 599, 601
  rotation, abnormalities 595
  small 595–8
    volvulus 595
  stenosis 596–7
    schematic representation **597**
Intra-abdominal cystic mass 929–30
  causes *929*
Intra-acinar air space growth **526**
Intra-acinar artery **541**
Intracerebellar haematoma **429**
Intracerebral calcifications 262
Intracranial germ-cell tumours 452–3
Intracranial haemorrhage 1288
Intracranial lesions, identification 822
Intracranial pressure measurement 1402
Intrafetal vascular anastomoses 203
  clinical outcome *205–6*, 212
Intrafetal vascular anomalies,
  frequency 215
  in MC twins 209, 214
Intrafetal venous anomalies, placental fetal
  surface examination 222
Intramammary pathway **701**
Intraneural membranous cytoplasmic bodies
  444
Intrapartum asphyxia 298–5
  incidence 298
Intrapartum death, definition 176
Intrapartum events 285–317
Intrapartum fetal monitoring 1351–60
Intrapartum fetal stress 290
Intrapartum fetal surveillance methods
  1352–9
Intrapartum monitoring,
  anomalous fetus considerations 1347–8
  techniques 1347
Intrapartum pathology 300–7
Intrapartum trauma 305–12
  incidence 305–6
  superficial injury 306
Intrathoracic mass,
  major causes *930*
  ultrasound diagnosis 930–2
Intrauterine death,
  in confined placental mosaicism *1110*
  in multiple pregnancy 974–5
  raised MSAFP 920
Intrauterine device (IUD), infections
  102–3
Intrauterine growth retardation, *see* IUGR
Intrauterine hypoxia, pathophysiology
  1351–2
Intrauterine infection, cordocentesis 1073
Intrauterine transfusion 1304
Intravenous alimentation 814–15
  biliary lesions 815

fat embolism 815
Intravenous fat 1425–7
  altered pulmonary function 1433–5
  recommendations 1436
  use *1426*
Intraventricular haemorrhage 428, 430–2,
  1288–9
  antenatal steroids 7
Introns, donor and acceptor splice sites
  40–1, 42
Intubation, effects 819
Inulin, placental clearance 13
Inv gene, and left–right asymmetry 48
meta-Iodobenzylguanidine (MIBG) 858
Ionizing radiation, as risk factor 178
Irradiation,
  prenatal 79
  see also Radiation
Ischaemia 280
Ischaemic disruptions 401, 404
Ischaemic injury in twins 213, 221
Ischaemic myocardial necrosis 814
Ischiopagus twins 217
Islet cell,
  hyperplasia 584
  non-functioning, tumours 585
Isochromosomes 61
Isoimmune neonatal thrombocytopenic
  purpura 719
Isoimmunization 1085–6
Isotretinoin, *see* Accutane
Isovaleric acidaemia 1134
IUGR (intrauterine growth retardation)
  275–83
  aetiology 275–6
  alcohol abuse 355
  amino acid transfer 13
  antibody titers 181
  antiphospholipid antibodies 344
  biochemical assessment 280
  blood pressure 893
  causes *275*
  cellular effects 277
  chorioangioma 983
  in chromosomal disease 940
  chromosomal mosaicism 696
  cordocentesis 1072–3
  definitions 275
  detection 971
  diagnosis 276–7
  disproportionate 280
  in donor twin 974
  factor importance **369**
  in gastroschisis 1494–5
  growth rate downward inflection
  275
  heroin use 360
  intrinsic factors 276
  maternal factors 275–6
  in mosaicism *1109*
  multiple pregnancy 975–6
    size discordancy 976
  muscle in 774
  neonatal morbidity 280
  organ weights 277–8
  outcome 280–1
  placental biopsy 991–2
  placental mosaicism 336
  placental pathology 320
  proportionate 280
  singleton standards in multiple pregnancy
  975
  and smoking 356, 1275
  types 17

IUGR (contd)
ultrasonic measurement 277
ultrasound diagnosis 878
ultrasound findings, chromosomal
anomaly 939
vascular lesions 328
vascular pathophysiology 15
Ivemark syndrome 563, 591
IVF, see Fertilization, in vitro

Jarcho–Levin syndrome 800
Jaundice 564, 702
physiologic 1454
Jejunal atresia type I 597
Jejunoileal atresia 929
Jeune syndrome 563, 619, 792
external features 379
lung hypoplasia 533
and renal dysplasia 616
Johns Hopkins Hospital 482
Jordan's anomaly 723

Kallmann syndrome 24
Karnofsky's principle 86
Kartagener syndrome 498, 500
Karyogamy 28
Karyorrhexis 857
Karyotype description, symbols 60
Karyotype–phenotype correlations 1101
Karyotyping 57–8, 887
for abnormal echocardiogram 962
for chromosomal disease 940
cordocentesis for 940
for genetic sex determination 687
methods 1105
oligohydramnios and 933, 1246
for omphalocele 1498
on placental tissue 273
in polyhydramnios 1250
rapid 940
for recurrent abortion 169–70
Kasabach–Merritt syndrome 334, 574, 835
Keimbahn formation 28
Kennedy disease 1212
Kennedy's spinal and bulbar muscular
atrophy 1117
Keratin 31
Keratinization, disorders 759–61
Kernicterus 370, 445, 1455
intravenous fat risk 1435
Ketoaciduria, branched chain 1137
Kidney,
abnormalities,
of number 614
and oligohydramnios 933
and polyhydramnios 932
of position 613–14
agenesis 400, 610–11
bilateral, prenatal diagnosis 629
lung arteriograms 536
Ask–Upmark 611
circulatory disturbances 621
clear cell sarcoma 625
cystic 614–20, 926–7
associated syndromes 927
development 1461–2
and embryology 609–10
dilation, ultrasound assessment 926
duplication 614
dysplasia 271, 614–15, 616
aplastic 615
cystic, associated syndromes 650–1
with cysts 619
diffuse cystic 615
hypoplastic 615
lung arteriograms 536

multicystic 615
ectopy 613
crossed 613
fibrous hamartoma 840–1
from 12 to 14 weeks 909
glomerulocystic disease 618–19
hypoplastic 619
hereditary dysplasia 611
in heritable disorders and malformations
631–46
hypoplasia 611–12
infection 621
in intrapartum asphyxia 302
malformations 610
and maternal diabetes mellitus 963
in multiple anomaly syndromes 648–9
multicystic 614
perinatal therapy, complications 815–16,
817
polycystic 614
postnatal lesions associated with heritable
syndromes 653–7
rhabdoid tumour 625
supernumerary 614
tuberous sclerosis 843
tubular dysgenesis 612–13
tubule necrosis 302
tumours 621–5
unilateral multicystic dysplastic 927
Kidney–lung loop 534–5
Kleihauer test 296–7, 299
Kleihauer–Betke test 324, 710
Kline intervillous haemorrhage 296
Klinefelter syndrome 63–4, 74, 410, 678
Klippel–Trenauney syndrome 836
Klippel–Trenauney–Weber syndrome 1212
Klumpke paralysis 310
Kniest dysplasia 795–6
Knudsonian first hit 73
Knudson's 'two-hit' hypothesis 49, 69–71
Koch's postulates and teratology 84
Kostmann syndrome 721
Krabbe disease 1144–5

Laboratory evaluations 181
Laboratory support 1513–26
Laboratory tests,
anatomic pathology 1517
biochemistry 1516–17
haematology 1517
microbiology 1517
Labour 287, 289–92
augmentation 297–8
dysfunctional 293
induction 297–8
initiation mechanism 287
premature (preterm),
and cocaine 358
and heroin 360
onset 288
Lactic acidaemia 1152
Ladder diagram analysis 965
Lamellar body 544–5
Lamellar ichthyosis 759, 761
Laminectomy, posterior, and traction 309
Laminin 129, 131
Langer–Giedion syndrome 255, 788, 795–7
Laparoschisis 605
Laplace relation 472–3, 476, 480, 513
Large for gestational age (LGA) 16
Large molecule diseases, biochemical
investigation 1141–7
Laryngeal nerve palsy 311
Late-amniotic deformities adhesion
mutilation (ADAML) complex 401

Lead in cigarettes 356
Left heart syndrome 489–90
Leg, length measurement 383
Legal implications 1384
Leigh disease 446–7, 448, 782, 1388
Leiomyomata 171–2
Leptomeningitis, neonatal 443
Lesch–Nyhan syndrome 24
Lecithin : sphingomyelin (LS) ratio 16
Leucine zipper zone 49
Leucomalacia, periventricular 1400
Leukaemia 73
congenital acute 724–5
cytogenetic studies 725
granulocytic 724
Leukaemia inhibitory factor (LIF) 341
Leukaemogenesis after irradiation 79
Leukocytes,
bone marrow and pancreatic dysfunction
724
cytoplasmic abnormalities 723–4
neonatal 720–7
nuclear appendages 722
quantitative changes 720–1
values in term and preterm infants 1519
Leukoerythroblastic reaction 722
Leydig cell,
dysgenesis 680
in triploidy 195
Li–Fraumeni syndrome 72
Limbs,
bowing 935
defects,
after CVS 1080
embryoscopic diagnosis 1065–70
distal, vascular disruption 359
fracture 935
at birth 805
hypoplasia 262
identification and measurement 935
imaging at week 10 905–6
long-bone fractures 311
mineralization 935
reduction defects, and cocaine 358–9
triploidy anomalies 195
Limit dextrinosis 1141–2
Linear array transducer 886
Linear distances, B-scan measurement
885–6
Linkage analysis 1181
Lipid,
metabolism in newborn 1411–12
utilization defects 781–2
Lipid metabolism disorders 571–2
Lipidoses 1143–6, 1154–5
Lipoblastic tumours 844–6
Lipoblastomatosis 845
Lipoid hyperplasia 704
Lipoma, congenital 844–5, 846
Lipomatosis 845
Lipoprotein disorders 1153
Lissencephaly types 421
Listeria monocytogenes 325, 347, 443,
549, 1446–7
Listeriosis 102–3, 347–8
intrauterine 326
Lithium, as teratogen 88
Live donor organs 390
Liver,
autopsy studies 385
centrilobular necrosis 511–12, 814–15
cirrhosis 573–4
Indian 574
congenital anomalies 561–3

Liver (contd)
congestion **513**
cystic disease *562*
development and anomalies *561*
dysfunction, in parenteral nutrition
1436–7
fibrosis, congenital **562–3**, *617*
fibrous hamartoma *841*
haemangioma *835*
hereditary and metabolic disorders
569–70, **571–3**
in hypoxia *292*
in intrapartum asphyxia **301–2**
right and left lobes **301–2**
intrapartum trauma *311*
intravenous alimentation changes **814–15**
metastatic tumour *577*
necrosis *68–9*
perinatal,
infection *566–9*
normal histology *561*
in right-sided congestive heart failure *511*,
513
tissue handling for metabolic disease *569*
tumours *574–7*
vascular abnormalities *562*
Lobar emphysema, congenital **552–4**
Locus specific probe **1124**
London Dysmorphology database *25*
Long bones, at 15 weeks **906**, **912**
Long-acting thyroid stimulation (LATS)
698
Low birth weight,
and high MSAFP *1036*
mortality *366–8*
Low-birth-weight infant *1418–20*
gastrointestinal tract incomplete
development *1419*
nutritional support *1419–20*
parenteral nutrition intake *1420*
risks *6–8*
Lowe syndrome *24*
LSD *91*
Lumbosacral plexus injury *311*
Lung,
agenesis **528–9**
aplasia **528–9**
arterial angiogram, *post mortem* **300**
arteriogram *527*
arteriovenous malformation *532–3*
autopsy culture *385*, *387*
blood vessel development *525*
blood vessels to, development *528*
congenital structural anomalies *809*
development *1322*
agents affecting *1337*
disturbed growth *527–54*
echogenicity, at 12 weeks **903**
embryonic disturbed growth *527–33*
epithelium–mesenchyme interaction **525**
fetal disturbed growth *533–44*
fibroblasts *394*
fibrosis *549–50*
genetics *554*, *556*
hamartoma *841*
hypoplasia *375*, *533–4*
arteriogram **534**
and congenital lobar emphysema *554*
exclusion *300*
interstitial and intralobular injury,
evolution **550**
intralobar sequestration *529–30*
in intrapartum asphyxia *299–300*, *301*
microscopic appearance **324**
non-aerated *299*

non-surfactant aspects *1387*
normal growth *523–7*
perinatal/postnatal *544–54*
in persistent fetal circulation *539–42*
petechial haemorrhages *299*
prematurity *547*
prenatal maturation *1337–43*
in renal agenesis, arteriograms **536**
in renal dysplasia, arteriograms **536**
research on *392–5*
sequestration *529*
structure, quantitative assessment *525*,
527
surfactant developmental patterns **395**
surfactant system *544–7*
tissue, developmental processes *394*
tissue culture *392*
Lupus anticoagulant *343*
Lupus erythematosus *344*
vasculopathy **329**
Luteinizing hormone *340*
Lutembacher syndrome *495*
Lyme disease *347*
Lymphangiectasis *838*
Lymphangioma *836–8*
of extremities *838*
head and neck, *see* Cystic hygroma
intra-abdominal *838*
Lymphangiomatosis *543–4*, *838*
Lymphocytes *720*, *1060*
paternal *342*
third-party *342*
Lymphokines *340–1*, *347*
Lympholysis, 'starry-sky' *303*
Lymphopenia *721–2*
Lyonization, unequal, in MZ twinning **202**
Lysine metabolism disorders *1150*
Lysinuric protein intolerance *1272*
Lysosomal disease in muscle *780*
Lysosomal enzyme deficiencies *445*
Lysosomal storage diseases *1143*, *1154–5*
Lysyl hydroxylase deficiency *765*

M-mode imaging, *see* Ultrasound
McArdle disease *1142*
McKusick, V.A., *377*, *1022*, *1197*
Maceration,
categories *270*
description *269*
early changes *270*
evaluation pitfalls *271*
gross evaluation *270–1*
Macroabscesses *347*
Macrogenitosomia *699*
Macroglossia, in Down syndrome *947*
Macrophage infiltration of uterine arteries
328–9
Macrophages *733*
Macrosomia *76*, *334*, *877–8*, *990*
MacVicar, J. *867–8*, **869**
Mafucci syndrome *841*
Magnesium, recommended intravenous
intake *1427*
Magnetic resonance imaging, for neonatal
brain *1400*
Magnetic-activated cell sorter *1062*
Majewski syndrome **791**
Major histocompatibility antigens *733*
Major histocompatibility complex (MHC)
1503
expression on term placenta **340**
homozygosity and recurrent spontaneous
abortion *342*
molecules, trophoblast lack *347*

Malaria *96*
congenital *350*
Malformation *401–2*
and deaths *4–5*
description *26*, *375*
evaluation *182*
in heroin babies *361*
major *176*
in MC twins *209*
percentages *176–7*
and prenatal cytogenetic diagnosis *248–9*
primary *25*
and programmed cell death *132–3*
sequence *26*
surveillance *177*
Malformation syndrome(s) *375–6*
definition *401*
embryoscopy *1070*
Malnutrition,
and immunodeficiency *749*
intrauterine *281*
and perinatal mortality *367*
Malpresentation in multiple pregnancy *207*,
209
Mammary gland *701*
Mannitol, placental clearance *13*
Maple syrup urine disease *448–9*, *1133*,
1137
Marantic endocarditis *300*
Marden–Walker syndrome *450*
Marfan syndrome *24*
heart anomalies *505*
Marijuana *91*
neonatal withdrawal signs *354*
Marker chromosomes *1127–8*
non-satellite *1128*
Markers *7*
Maroteaux–Lamy disease *1143*, *1146*
Martin–Bell syndrome *64–5*
Master genes *31–3*
Mastitis, neonatal *701*
Maternal 'addictions' and IUGR *276*
Maternal age,
effect on autosomal trisomies *253*
effect in livebirth aneuploidy *254*
and MSAFP screening *1037*
risk in DZ twins *220*
and spontaneous abortion *168–9*
Maternal alloimmunization *342*
Maternal anaemia *206*
Maternal blood flow,
in intrapartum asphyxia *304*
reduced *278*
Maternal causes of intrapartum asphyxia
292
Maternal chromosomal set of 23,X *195*
Maternal circulating organisms *327*
Maternal diabetes mellitus *26*, *269*
fetal cardiomyopathy *36*
large placenta *334*
malformations *87*, *403*
external features *379*
intervention *380*
polyhydramnios *1250*
in pregnancy *1269*
protocol *963*
in recurrent abortion *171*
teratogenic *181*
vascular lesions *328–9*
see also Pancreas
Maternal dietary habits *262*
Maternal disease,
effects on pregnancy *343–4*
and pregnancy loss *4*
Maternal drug therapy and fetus *803–4*

Maternal factors,
   in fetal death 178, 269
   intrapartum asphyxia 291–3
   in IUGR 275–6
Maternal floor infarction 334
Maternal haemorrhage 323–4
Maternal health, risks in multiple
   pregnancy 206, 209
Maternal history 381–2
   forms 1544–5
   in TORCH neonate 266
Maternal hypertension 269
Maternal hyperthyroidism 1270
Maternal hypotension 297
Maternal hypothyroidism 1270
Maternal IgG and IgM studies in TORCH
   neonate 266
Maternal immune system 339
Maternal infection,
   and fetal loss 345–50
   timing and route 345–6
Maternal isovaleric acidaemia 1272
Maternal ITP, and neonatal
   thrombocytopenia 719
Maternal metabolic disorder 1269–72
Maternal occupational history 262
Maternal phenylketonuria 1271
   teratogenic 181, 403
Maternal plate, sonographic differential
   diagnosis 983
Maternal primary infection 348
Maternal pronucleus exclusion 232
Maternal race and malformations 400
Maternal risk,
   factors for fetal heart disease 956
   in fetal surgery 1327
   probability 1533
Maternal sedation and fetal heart rate
   1355
Maternal serum, see MS
Maternal serum α-fetoprotein, see MSAFP
Maternal substance abuse,
   fetal effects 353–62
   obstetrical complications 354
   typical 354
Maternal systemic lupus erythematosus and
   neonatal thrombocytopenia 719
Maternal T cells 341
Maternal thrombocytopenia, drug-induced,
   and neonatal thrombocytopenia 719
Maternal toxins 1272–5
Maternal vasculopathy 328–9, 330
Maternal vasoconstriction, sudden 357
Maternal weight gain and large placenta
   334
Maternal–fetal interface 339–40
   lymphocytes 347
   lymphokines 340–1
Maternal–fetal mirror syndromes 345
Maternal–fetal syndromes 339–52
   animal study problems 341
Matsunaga, E. 70
Maturation-promoting factor 132
May–Hegglin anomaly 723
MC (monochorionic) twins, see under
   Twins
Meckel diverticulum 595, 847
Meckel–Gruber syndrome 31, 407, 450,
   563, 927, 941, 1070
   AFP rise 1035
   external features 379
   genital anomalies 683
   and renal dysplasia 616
Meconium, and acute fetal death 386

Meconium aspiration 510
   and heroin use 360
Meconium aspiration syndrome 323,
   539–41
Meconium ileus 554, 582, 597–8
Meconium peritonitis 365, 582–3, 605,
   930
   cystic, at 28 weeks 930
Meconium plug syndrome 598
Meconium-stained amniotic fluid,
   and abnormal fetal heart rate pattern
   1353
   detection 1352–3
   thick 1353
Meconium staining 291, 322
   in heroin use 361
   and postmaturity 304
Mediastinal teratoma 833
Medical referral centers 8
Medicolegal implications of bone fractures
   819
Medicolegal investigations 370–1
Medium-chain acyl-CoA dehydrogenase
   (MCAD) deficiency 1134
MEDLINE database 25
Medulla, forceps lesion 310
Medullary cysts 619–20
Megacystis–microcolon–intestinal
   hypoperistalsis syndrome 601
Megaureter 626
Meiosis 56, 1187
   and aneuploidy 249, 253
   de novo mutation 254
Meiosis I 228
   errors 229
   in aneuploid spontaneous abortus 229
   excessive recombination 255
   non-disjunction 378
Meiosis II 229
   failed oogenetic 234–5
   non-disjunction 378
Meiotic configurations, complex 254
Meiotic errors in oogenesis 229
Meiotic segregation mechanisms in parental
   robertsonian translocation carrier 230–1
Melanin 31
MELAS 1140
Membrane haemosiderin 324
Membrane-limited transfer 12
Membranes, uterine position 320
Mendelian disease,
   prevalence 1022–3
   response to treatment 1022–3
Mendelian inheritance, genetic screening
   1002
Mendelian Inheritance in Man, McKusick,
   V.A. 377, 1022, 1197
Mendelian mutations 33–4
Mendelian phenotypes, inherited 1131
Mendes da Costa syndrome 762
Meningitis, pseudomonas 442–3
Meningomyelocele 921, 923
   delivery 1346
   as NTD 1031–2
Menkes' syndrome 765
Menstrual age 897
Mental handicap,
   in fragile X syndrome 1115
   see also Down syndrome, Intracerebral
   haemorrhage; Microcephaly; under
   Trisomy
MERRF 1140
Mesangial sclerosis, diffuse 620–1
Mesenchymal hamartoma 574–5

Mesenchymal layer 148
Mesenteric cysts 848
Mesoblastic nephroma 622, 840–1
Mesomelic dysplasia 935
Mesomelic dysplasia group 799
Mesonephric duct 609
Mesonephros 609
Mesothelial cysts 849
Mesothelial layer 148
Mesothelioma of atrioventricular node 507,
   509
Metabolic acidosis 291, 1132
Metabolic disorders,
   biochemical tests 1132
   clinical expression 1131
   fetal blood changes 1094
   histological and histochemical screen 1026
   inherited 1148–58
      clinical features 1413–14
      screening for 1025–6
   neonatal screening 1025–6
   in stillborn 273
   subsets 1147
Metabolic disruptions 401, 403
Metabolic dysplasia syndromes 405
Metabolic dysplasia/MCA (multiple
   congenital anomaly) syndromes 24
Metabolism, neonatal 1407–15
Metachromatic leucodystrophy 1144–5
Metaethics 18
Metal metabolism disorders 1154
Metalloporphyrins 1458
Metanephros 609
Metaphase preparation 1126
   multiple congenital abnormalities 1126
Metatrophic dysplasia 791
Methadone 361
   neonatal withdrawal signs 354
Methaemoglobinaemia 717
Methamphetamine 356
   as 'crystal' or 'ice' 356
Methylmalonate metabolism disorders 1152
Methylmalonic acidaemia 1133–4
Methylnitrosourea 124
Metropolitan Atlanta Congenital Defects
   Program 5
Microbiologic assessment of TORCH
   neonate 266
Microcephaly 265
   and alcohol abuse 355
   in cocaine use 358
Microdeletion syndromes 1125–7
Microgastria 591–2
Micrognathia,
   in trisomy 18 941
   at 18 weeks 945
Microscopic examination of fetus and
   placenta 272
Microtia-auriculo-facio-vertebral syndrome
   402
Microvilli 150, 153
Micturition, increased 212–13
Mid-arm to head circumference (MAC/HC)
   ratio 280
Midgut, development 589–91
Midgut hernia,
   physiologic 902–3
   in pregnancy dating 905–6
Midline as developmental field 401
Midwives 9
Miller–Dieker syndrome 253, 421, 1127,
   1225
Minerals,
   placental transfer 12
   requirement of preterm infant 1427–30

Minicore disease 778
Mirror syndromes 344–5
Miscarriage, definition 175
Mitochondria, DNA 55
Mitochondrial disorders 1140, 1152
Mitochondrial dysfunction 1132
Mitochondrial encephalomyopathy 446–7, 448
Mitochondriopathies 781–2
  biochemical defects 781
Mitosis 55–6, 1187
  abnormal early postzygotic 237–9, 240–1
  and aneuploidy 249, 253
Mitotic cycle 132
Mitotic non-disjunction 233, 237–8, 240–1
  possible causes 253–4
Mitotic–karyorrhexis index 856
Mitral atresia 497
Mitral orifice, double 496
Mitral regurgitation 506
Mitral ring, supravalvular 503
Mitral valve,
  cleft 495–6
  excess mobility effect 504
  floppy 503
  parachute 503–4
  straddling 499
Möbius syndrome 450
Mohr syndrome 1070
Molar pregnancy,
  flow cytometry diagnosis 237
  parental contributions 240
  and ploidy 237
Molecular analysis 273
Molecular composition, regional differences 125, 127–8
Molecular cytogenetics 1121–9
  techniques, conclusion 1128
Molecular embryology 136
Molecular genetics 1131–63
  clinical 1187–95
  complete hydatidiform mole 191–2
  and cytogenetics 254–5
  at fetal autopsy 387
  fragile X syndrome 1116–17
  hydatidiform mole 191–2
  for mitotic and meiotic event identification 248–9
  techniques 182, 610
Molecular heterogeneity 1191
Molecular pathology,
  single gene disorders 1191
  α-thalassaemia 1166–7
  β-thalassaemia 1171, 1173
Moles 28
Monitoring techniques in clinical practice 1404
Mono-oogonial twins 203
Monoamniotic (MA) twins, see Twins, monoamniotic
Monochorionic (MC) twins, see monochorionic
Monoclonal antibodies, for fetal trophoblast cells 1060
Monocytes 720
Monosomy 58, 119–20
Monosomy X, see Turner syndrome
Monotopic developmental field defects 401–2
Monotopic field defect, definition 401
Montana Medical Genetics Program 25
Montevideo units 289
Moral self-esteem, loss 1014
Morbidity prediction 282
Morgagni hernia 930

Morphogenesis 28
Morphometric analyses 143
Morphometric measurements 278, 280
Morquio disease 1143, 1146–7
Mortality rates, Japan and USA 10
Mosaic development 33
Mosaic pleiotropy 24
Mosaicism,
  in chorionic stroma (type II confined placental mosaicism or CPM) 1106
  classification in extraembryonic tissues 238, 240
  confined 1100
  confined placental 240, 336
    complete 240
    and fetal disomy 1106, 1108
    fetal loss 1110
    future directions 1111
    and IVF conceptuses 241
    in trisomy 16 1111
    types 1106–8
  CVS 238, 240, 247
    cases 1107–8
    classification 245
    fetal outcomes 245
  cytogenetics 237–8, 240–1, 242–6
  definition 1099
  in different tissues 1104
  fetal 1101
  generalized 1100
  germline 377, 380
  gonadal 229, 377
    and trisomy 233
  implications 1101–5
  involving autosomes 1101–2
  involving chromosomal rearrangements 1103–4
  molar 196
  origin 1099
  for polyploidy 1042–4
  preferentially expressed in certain tissues 1100
  pregnancy complications 1109
  ring X chromosome 253
  for sex chromosome abnormalities 1102
  technical aspects 1111
  tissue-specific 1100–1
  tissues for diagnosis 1105
  in trophoblast and stroma (type III CPM) 1106
  in trophoblast (type I CPM) 1106, 1109
  type I 240, 247
  type II 240, 247
  type III 240, 247
  type IV 247
  types 1100
Mosaicism (representation) 240, 241–4
MRC European Collaborative Study 1081
MRC Fetal Tissue Bank, uses 389
MRC Human Cytogenetic Registry 1101
mRNA, see RNA
MS biochemical markers 987, 989, 1031, 1039
MS chorionic gonadotropin (MShGC),
  in Down syndrome 1037
  raised, and hydatidiform mole 1035
  trophoblastic disorders 987
MS (maternal serum) screening 1031–44
  ultrasound role 1040–1
MS unconjugated estriol (MSuE3) 1038–9
MSAFP (maternal serum α-fetoprotein) 7
  and CVS 1078, 1080
  distribution overlap in spina bifida 1034
  interpretation 920

low 1036–7
  chromosomal abnormalities 1036–7
  in fetal defects 181
  screening in California 1038
  screening experience 1037
raised,
  extrafetal causes 1035
  fetal abnormalities 920–1
  increased fetal wastage 1036
  low birth weight 1036
  and maternal barrier breakdown 987
  in NTD 1033–4
  in placental and cord abnormalities 987, 989
  selected abnormalities 1035
  significance 1035–6
  in twin pregnancy 220
MSAFP screening 936
  timing 1033
MSAFP testing, ultrasound replacement 922–3
Mucolipidoses 572, 1146, 1156, 1214
Mucolipidosis II, microscopic assessment 1090, 1092
Mucolipidosis IV 1144
  cultured amniocyte test 1091
Mucopolysaccharidoses 572, 1146–7, 1157, 1214–15
  type I, Hurler 570
  type II, Hunter 570
  type VII, Sly 570
Mucosal immune system 737–9
  ontogeny 738
Müllerian aplasia 685
Müllerian duct suppressor 24
Müllerian fusion, incomplete 685
Müllerian inhibitory substance 128
Multidisciplinary pathology organization 1531, 1535
Multidrug use and postnatal abnormalities 359
Multifetal pregnancies, see Multiple pregnancy
Multifocal pacemakers 295
Multilocular cyst 624
Multilocular cystic encephalopathy 425–6, 427
Multilocular cystic nephroma 624
Multiple congenital anomaly (MCA) syndromes 24
Multiple marker screening 1039–40
  adverse outcome 1040
Multiple pregnancy 201–5
  amniocentesis 1084
  biology 201–3
  cervical assessment 979
  complications 206
  CVS 1078
  diagnosis 971
    at 18 weeks 971
  epidemiology 203
  fetal death,
    early, and retention 206
    single 69
  fetal measurement 976
  frequency 203
  high 971
  hydatidiform mole in 194
  intrauterine death 974–5
  labour and delivery 976–7
  late gestation at presentation 971
  low birth weight for gestational age and outcome 976
  malpresentation 207, 209

Multiple pregnancy (contd)
  monitoring and intervention 220–4
  one fetal death 269
  pathology 206–18
  perinatal death 207, 209
    cause 201
  perinatal disease 201
  placenta examination 222
  placental hemorrhage 324
  placentation 205–6
  prenatal chromosome analysis 221
  prenatal diagnosis 218, 220, 972–3
    controversy 972
  preterm delivery risk 975
  preterm labor 207
  preterm labour, prediction 975
  raised MSAFP 920
  selective reduction 972
    controversy 972
  specific pathologies 971
  ultrasound in 971–6
  uterine volume measurements 975
  see also Triplets; Twins
Mummification 270
Muscle,
  biopsy 771
  development disorders 771–2
  developmental relationships 772–4
  diseases due to exogenous agents 774–6
  in IUGR 774
  metabolic diseases 780–2
  normal development 769–70, 771
  tumours 842
Muscle-specific genes 48
Muscular dystrophy,
  Becker 777
  congenital 776
  Duchenne 24, 777
    genetic linkage analysis 182
    PCR amplification 1194
    structural and mutational phenotypes 44
Mutant genes, prevalence and genetic
  diseases 46–52
Mutation,
  in differentiation and oncogenesis 48
  direct detection 1194–5
  effects 41–2
  and embryonic development 47–8
  in β-thalassaemia 1168–70, 1174
Myasthenia gravis 344, 775
myc oncogenes 70–1
Mycoplasma cultures in stillborn 272
Mycoplasma infections 103
Myelination 415–16
Myelination glia 415
Myelocele 417–18
Myelomeningocele 417, 419
  lumbosacral, at 18 weeks 923
Myocardial injuries, surgery 515
Myocardial necrosis 511
Myocarditis 507–8
  viral and cardiomyopathy 506
Myocardium 507
  coagulation necrosis 515
  concentric layer rotation 479
  contraction band necrosis 515
  contraction banding 299
  growth 474–5
  left ventricle,
    myocyte nuclei count 481
    sections 481
  metabolism and cardiomyopathy 505
  reconstruction 479
  reflow necrosis 515

systolic time intervals 1359
Myocytes, histocytoid change 509
Myofibrillar degeneration 515
Myopathy,
  centronuclear 777, 779
  congenital 777, 779
  histiocytoid 510
  nemaline 777–8
Myosin, genetic abnormalities 507
Myositis,
  intrauterine 774–5
  lymphocytic 775
Myotonic dystrophy, infantile 776–7
Myxoma, atrial 509

Naevus,
  compound 844
  congenital giant pigmented 844
  intradermal 844–5
  intraepidermal 844
  junctional 844
Naevus flammeus 836–7
Nager syndrome 1070
Nasal polyps 850–1
Nasopharyngeal teratoma 833
National Association for Perinatal
  Addiction Research and Education 1272
National Bone Marrow Registry 1507
National Collaborative Perinatal Project
  427, 434, 1365
National Perinatal Study, USA 216
Natural killer cells 340, 733
Neck, teratoma 833
Necropsy, see Autopsy
Necrotizing enterocolitis (NEC) 302, 370,
  601–2, 603, 818–19, 1485–91
  barium contrast enema 1487–8, 1490
  complications 1489–90
  and early feeding 1417, 1420
  incidence and aetiology 1485
  intestinal stricture 1490
  surgical management indications 1488–9
Neglect and postnatal abnormalities 359
Neonatal adaptations 369
Neonatal adrenoleucodystrophy (ALD) 446
Neonatal approach to screening 1025–6
Neonatal asphyxia,
  morbidity and mortality 1366–7
  neurodevelopmental outcome 1365–7
Neonatal assessment 278, 280
  of TORCH neonate 266
Neonatal bacterial sepsis 1445–8
  etiology 1446
  prevention 1448
  risk factors 1445–6
Neonatal care, clinical categories 1394
Neonatal cerebrovascular monitoring
  1399–1405
Neonatal cholestasis 563–6
Neonatal convulsions 705, 1367
  aetiology 1368
Neonatal death,
  definition 174
  external examination 378
  external features of syndromes 379
  groups 4–5
  management 1377–8
  postbereavement care 1378
  and prematurity complications 401
Neonatal fungal infection 443
Neonatal haemolytic hyperbilirubinaemia,
  management 1453–60
Neonatal hepatitis 563–4

Neonatal hypoxic–ischaemic
  encephalopathy 1361–2
Neonatal identification of inherited
  metabolic disorders 1026
Neonatal immunodeficiencies 1503–12
Neonatal intensive care 1373–9
  prolonged survival effects 822–3
Neonatal intensive care unit (NICU) 8,
  368, 812
Neonatal 'intoxications' 1413
Neonatal iron storage disease 815
Neonatal jaundice, phototherapy 1457–8
Neonatal leptomeningitis 443
Neonatal measurements 1540
Neonatal metabolism 1407–15
  laboratory investigation 1026
Neonatal Network of the National Institute
  of Child Health and Human
  Development 1337
Neonatal neurological distress 1413
  initial investigations 1413
Neonatal obstructive uropathy 1461–8
Neonatal outcome 280
  evaluation, clinical signs 368
Neonatal parenteral nutrition 1417–43
Neonatal pathology, purposes 381
Neonatal resuscitation 1361–71
  management 1363–5
Neonatal screening 1025–6, 1045–54
  amended guidelines 1047
  choice of conditions and tests 1027
  consent 1052
  cost/benefits 1047
  costs 1049
  current issues 1051–2
  factors influencing 1027
  HIV testing 1051–2
  mass 1026
  organization 1046
  program organization 1046
  quality control issues 1051
  recommendations 1027
  results follow-up 1050–1
  results in Irish Republic 1027
  routine rescreening 1051
  specimen collection 1047, 1049–50
  system model 1046
  targeted 1051
  tests,
    in North America 1048
    selection criteria 1046–7
    timing 1047, 1049
    top ten 1047
  universal 1046–51
Neonatal screening record 1051
Neonatal services, organization 1373–4
Neonatal therapy 806–14
Neonatal thrombocytopenia 719–20
  causes 1286
Neonatal thrombocytosis 720
Neonatal thrombosis, treatment 1290
Neonatal transfer between hospitals 1050
Neonatal unit,
  ethical decisions 1376–7
  guidelines 1377
Neonatal viral sepsis 1448–50
Nephritis, hereditary tubulointerstitial
  619–20
Nephroblastoma 840
  cystic partially differentiated 624
  see also Wilms' tumour
Nephroblastomatosis 623
Nephrogenic rests 73, 662–3
Nephromegaly, congenital 612

Nephronophthisis, familial juvenile 619–20
Nephrosis, MSAFP screening 1035
Nephrotic syndrome,
    congenital 620–1
        Finnish-type 620–1
Nerve growth factor 861
Nerve plexus, injury 310
Nerve roots, lesions 310
Nerves, and intrapartum trauma 310–11
Nesidioblastosis **585**–6
Neural tube, at week 7 899
Neural tube closure 133
Neural tube defect, *see* NTD
Neuroblast, migration defects 419, 421,
    423
Neuroblastoma 577, 855–63
    associated disorders 858
    clinical features 858
    favourable versus unfavourable types *860*
    gross features and staging 857–8
    histologic evolution and classification
        856–7
    in situ 73, 859
    neonatal 859–61
    overt 859–60
    regression 68
    screened 860
    Shimada classification *856–7*
    stage IVS 860–1
    and Wilms' tumor 71–2
Neuroepithelial tumours 453
Neurofibroma,
    localized 842–3
    plexiform 842–3
Neurofibromatosis 24, **842**–3
    see also van Recklinghausen's
        neurofibromatosis
Neurofibromatosis type 1 (NFB1), mutation
    42
Neuromuscular diseases 450–1
    pathogenetic categorization 769
Neuromuscular transmission, disorders
    775–6
Neuronal ceroid lipofuscinosis 723
Neuronal intestinal dysplasia 599
Neurons,
    ferruginated **440**
    karyorrhectic **440**
Neuropathy,
    demyelinating 784
    motor–sensory **784**
    sensory 783–4
Neurosyphilis 112
Neurulation,
    mechanisms *133*
    secondary 413
Neutropenia 720–1
    congenital 721
    drug-induced immune 721
    immune-mediated 721
Neutrophilia 722
Neutrophils 720
    hereditary giant 722
    hereditary hypersegmentation 722
New England Regional Infant Cardiac
    Program *963*
Newborn,
    chromosomal abnormalities 242, *247, 249*
    classification **280**
    clinical events 702–6
    congenital heart disease, surgery 1479–84
    congenital myocarditis **107**
    drug withdrawal signs and symptoms *354*
    haemostasis development 1281–91

heroin withdrawal symptoms 360
HIV infection 106
host defence mechanism evaluation
    741
HSV infection 110–**11, 112**
immune system evaluation 740–1
infections acquired from mother or staff
    105
inherited metabolic diseases, clinical
    features 1413–14
innate immunity 733–4
internal haemorrhage 710
liver disease 1289
liver with HSV infection **111**
methadone withdrawal signs 361
neuroblastoma 859–61
parenteral nutrition indications *1419*
phencyclidine symptoms 361
protective factors 99–101
specific immunity 734–7
TORCH, unexpected, microbiologic
    assessment *266*
weights and lengths *454*
Nezelof syndrome 746
    thymus therapy 1508
Niemann–Pick disease 571, **1144**–6
    variants 1145
NIH Collaborative Perinatal Study,
    1959–66 8, 261
Nijmegen breakage syndrome 24
Nitric oxide synthase 15
Nitrofen, and diaphragm development 539
Nitrogen balance studies 1275–6
Nitrosoureas 78–9
Noggin 35
Non-denaturing electrophoresis, for
    β-thalassaemia 1175–6
Non-directive counselling 1008
Non-disjunction **1099**
Non-immune factors in recurrent abortion
    167
Non-traditional inheritance 377
Noonan syndrome 957
Normoblastaemia 271
Novel splice mutation **41**
NTD (neural tube defect) 417–18
    AFAFP rise 1033
    AFP testing 1023, 1032–4
    associated problems 1032
    confirmatory testing 1033
    definition and scope of problem
        1031–2
    detection rate *1034*
    diagnosis 922
    etiology 1032
    and folic acid deficiency 87–8
    identification 7
    intervention 380
    Pax mutation 48
    population screening 1033
    prenatal diagnosis 417
    prenatal mortality rate 25
    prevention 1032
    raised MSAFP 920
    recurrence risk 377, *1032*
    screening efficacy 1033–4
    in UK 400
    ultrasound diagnosis accuracy *924*
Nuchal cord, entanglement 305
Nuchal tissues, thickening, in Down
    syndrome 943, **948**
Nuclear Enterprises 871
Nuclear gene, structure **32**
Nuclear inclusion bodies 348

Nucleic acid,
    analysis 1192–3
    pathology 1190–2
    structure and function 1187–90
Nucleolus organizer regions (NORs) 57
Nucleolysis 271–2
Nucleosome 55
Nutrient availability 1267–9

Obesity and large placenta 334
Obstetrical practice, changes and fetal
    death timing 271
Obstructive uropathy 1461–8
    postnatal intervention indications 1465–7
Occipital osteodiastasis 308–9, 805
    unilateral or bilateral 308
Oedema, neonatal 702
OEIS complex 627
Oesophagus,
    atresias 592
    ciliated cells **590**
    congenital short 591
    congenital stenosis 592–3
    cyst 847
    development 591–3
    diverticula 593
    duplication 593
    parietal cysts 593
Oligohydramnios 881, 891, 932–3, 1244–8
    aetiology 1245
    causes *932*
    disruption 401, 404
    and 'stuck twin' 213
    therapies 1247–8
    in twin–twin transfusion syndome 974
    ultrasonographic questions *933*
Oligohydramnios sequence 406
Oligomeganephronia 611–**12**
Oligonucleotide molecular probes 180
Olive-coloured skin in maceration 270
Olivopontocerebellar atrophy 449–**50**
Ollier disease 841
Omenn syndrome 749
OMIM database 25
Omphalocele 25, *29*, 605, 943
    associated malformations 1494, 1497
    and caesarean section 1346
    chromosomal abnormalities **1497**
    definition 1493
    embryology and pathogenesis 1493–4
    management 1498–1502
    in MC twins 216–17
    prenatal pathology 1494
    ultrasonography **1496**
Oncogene-suppressor gene concept 70–1
Oncogenes, *ras* 70
Oncogenesis, and teratogenesis 69
Oncoproteins, Rb-1 binding **49**
Ontogeny 27–8
Oocytes, investigation methods 229
Oogenesis 119, 663
    abnormal 229
    error rates 229
Opioid for heroin withdrawal 361
Opitz–Frias syndrome 407
Opium, neonatal withdrawal signs *354*
Opsismodysplasia 790
Opsoclonus–myoclonus 858
Oral anticoagulants and nasal hypoplasia
    85
Oral contraceptives 90
Organ culture methods for teratogen study
    391

Organ immaturity, disorders and
complications *370*
Organ retrieval, cadaveric 390
Organ storage 390
Organic acid disorders *1131*
Organic acid metabolism, disorders
1133–5, *1149*
Organogenesis, *see* Embryogenesis
Organotypic culture 392
Ornithine carbamoyl transferase deficiency
449, 1136
Ornithine metabolism disorders *1150*
Oro-facio-digital syndrome type I 24
Osler–Weber–Rendu syndrome 532, 836
Ossification centres, *in utero*, appearance
1539
Osteoblast growth, 'pile-up' 305
Osteochondritis 112
Osteochondrodysplasias identifiable at birth
787–800
Osteochondromatosis 841–2
Osteochondroplasias, evaluation 272–3
Osteogenesis imperfecta 31
external features *379*
mutations 44, 46, 377
types 800
Osteomyelitis, fungal **106**
Osteopenia of prematurity 1436
Osteosarcoma 24
Ostium primum septal defect **496**
Oto-palato-digital syndrome type II 793–4
Outflow tract 469–72
developmental arrests 491–4
left ventricular, reconstruction **485**
rotation **484**
valves,
angle of line **484**
Ovarian differentiation 665
Ovary,
cysts 849–50, 930
follicular 849–50
inclusion 850
Ovum, differential genomic imprinting
196
Oxalate crystals 815–16, 817
Oxford Database of Perinatal Trials 890
Oxygen content curves 285–6
Oxygen dissociation curves 285–6
Oxygen gradient 285
Oxyhaemoglobin dissociation curves **1363**

Pachygyria 419, **421–2**
in Zellweger syndrome **446**
Palate,
at 12 weeks 907
at 15 weeks, structural evaluation **908**
Pallister–Killian syndrome 1100–1
Pancreas 581–7
β-cell tumour 585
congenital cysts 582
congenital malformations 581–2
polycystic disease 582
tumours 584–6
Pancreatic cysts 848
Panhypopituitarism 702
Panplacentitis 325, **327**
Papillary muscle, contraction banding **299**
Papillary pseudomucinous
cystadenocarcinoma 675
Paracentric chromosome inversion 61
Paracervical block 297
Paralogous genes 35
Parasagittal cortex, watershed lesions 823
Parasitic infections 350

Parasitic twin (PT), *see* Twin, parasitic
Parathyroid glands 705–6
Paraurethral cyst 685
Parental alcohol consumption 355
Parental assessment in first 6 months after
pregnancy termination 1015–16
Parental needs and management after
termination 1017–18
Parental origins,
of moles and chorionic cancers 192
of twins and triplets 192
Parental socioeconomic circumstances and
postnatal abnormalities 359
Parental–fetal bonding 1013
Parenteral fat emulsions *1426*
Parenteral nutrition,
calories 1422–3
catheter-associated infection 1433
catheter insertion complications 1433
complications *1420*, 1431–9
metabolic 1433–4, 1435–9
technical 1431, 1433
contraindications 1417
electrolytes and minerals *1427*
indications 1417–20
metabolic monitoring *1437–8*
neonatal 1417–43
requirements 1422–31
route of administration 1420–2
selection for 1417
therapy initiation 1431
total 566, **568**
Parenti–Fracarro syndrome 788
Parents, communication with 1381
Parturition, *see* Birth
Parvovirus 112–13
bone marrow infection **114**
in TORCH syndrome 265
Parvovirus B19 328
in pregnancy 1295–6
therapy lack 265
Patau syndrome 63, **420**
Patent ductus arteriosus 400, 486
shunt 1394
surgery 1479–80
Paternal history 381
Pathologist,
and family 381
participation 162
role and responsibility 163–4, 365–6
Pathology service, organization 1531–2
Pax genes, mutations 48
PCR (polymerase chain reaction) 104,
1055–6, 1063, 1122
amplified specific DNA fragment **1193**
analysis 1192–3
choriocarcinoma origin 191
cystic fibrosis gene **1194**
point mutation **1194**
hydatidiform mole origin 191
technical difficulties 263
for TORCH detection 263
PDGF-A (platelet-derived growth factor A)
121
Peak systolic velocity **981**
Pelger–Huët anomaly 722
Pena–Shokeir syndrome 450, 774
external features *379*
hypoplastic lungs **534**
Penis, agenesis and hypoplasia 685–6
Pentose phosphate pathway defects 714–15
Peri-implantation loss 227
Pericardial cysts 849
Pericardial effusion 262

Pericardium, development 480
Pericentric chromosome inversion 61
Perinatal asphyxia, aetiology 1361
Perinatal autopsy, extensive sampling 271
Perinatal care,
communication 1381
laboratory microtechniques *1516*
Perinatal death,
chromosome abnormalities 242
description 176
groups 4
increased 207, 209
and intrapartum trauma 305
in multiple pregnancy 207, 209
Perinatal distress, acute 321–3
Perinatal forensic pathology 370
Perinatal infections, clinically silent 262
Perinatal loss rate 971
Perinatal morbidity, and oligohydramnios
1246
Perinatal mortality,
audits 368
classifications 203, **1534**
comparisons 367
curves 368–9
and oligohydramnios 1245–6
rates **222**
SGA 280–1
Perinatal mortality rates in multiple
pregnancy 972
Perinatal networks 368
Perinatal period, genetics 999
Perinatal surveillance 9
Perinatal 'team' 7
Perinatal telencephalic leucoencephalopathy
437
Perineum, female, abnormalities 699–**700**
Periodic breathing 1389–**90**
Periostitis 112
Peripheral blood cell transfusions 1507
Peripheral cysts 849
Peripheral nerve, injury 310
Peripheral neural tumours, comparison *855*
Peripheral neuropathy 783–4
Peristaltic pump **990**
Peritoneal cavity 604–5
Periventricular cysts **436**
Periventricular haemorrhage 1400
Periventricular infarct, haemorrhagic 431,
434
Periventricular leucomalacia 432–3, **1362**,
1400
Perivillous fibrin 333–4
Perlman syndrome 24, 76
and Wilms' tumour 624–5
Peroxisomal disorders 446, *1139*, *1157*
electron microscopic assessment *1139*
functional 1139–80
group *1139*
Persistent fetal circulation 300–1, 510
hypoplastic lungs 539–42
types 540
Persistent müllerian duct syndrome 679
Persistent pulmonary hypertension of
newborn, *see* Persistent fetal circulation
Pet ownership 262
Petechial haemorrhages and acute fetal
death 386
Petrous temporal bone 819–21
Peutz–Jeghers polyp **850–1**
Peutz–Jeghers syndrome **851–2**
Phakoma 543–4
Pharmacology, cordocentesis 1073
Phased array transducer **886**

Phencyclidine 361
  in cigarettes 361
  neonatal withdrawal signs *354*
  use with other dugs 361
Phenogenesis 25, *28–9*
Phenotype analysis 23
Phenotype/genotype mapping for Down
  syndrome abnormalities 255
Phenylalanine,
  disorders *1149*
  metabolism **1028**
Phenylketonuria,
  bacterial inhibition assay 1005
  dietary treatment 1028
    failure to respond 1028
  female patients 1028
  mental handicap 448
  molecular basis 1028–9
  problem areas 1028
  screening 1027–9
  tests 1045, *1048*
  variant forms 1028
Phocomelia, and thalidomide 803–4
Phosphatidylcholine 344, *545*
Phosphatidylethanolamine 344
Phosphatidylserine 344
  antibodies to 344
Phosphoglycerate kinase deficiency 714
Phospholipids,
  antibody responses 344
  tissue 1412–13
Phosphorus,
  normal serum levels *1427*
  recommended intravenous intake *1427*
  requirement of preterm infant *1428*
Photographic documentation 180
  at autopsy 382
Phrenic nerve palsy 310
Phthisis bulbi 71
Physical disruption 26
Physicians for genetic counselling 1008
Physiologic herniation 902–3
  normal 928
Physiological umbilical hernia **1069**
Picker Ultrasonoscope **872**
Pigmented naevi 844
Pinealoblastoma 71
Pituitary concretions 822
Pituitary lesions 821–2
PLA1 (major antigen system) 343
Placenta,
  abnormal findings 319, 344
  abnormal shapes 320, 334
  at autopsy 386
  CD4 expression **349**
  choriocarcinoma 69
  chromosomal abnormalities 334
  chronic disease 328–34
  circumvallate 276
  CMV infection **349**
  compartmental diagram **321**
  decidua basalis 143, 320–1
  decidua vera plus decidua capsularis
    320–1
  dichorionic, separate or fused 222
  disorders 4
    and asphyxia 294–5
  drug metabolism 353–4
  dyfunction 328–4
  endogenous retrovirus particles 347
  enlarged **987**
  evaluation after fetal death 272
  examination,
    careful gross 320

  indications *319*
  purposes 336
  examination indications *1517*
  fetal death change evaluation 272
  fetal infection 262
  fetal transfer 12–13
  fibrin deposition 333–4
  gaseous exchange 285
  growth, guide *1537*
  haemangioma 835
  haematogenous infections 96–7
  haemorrhages 323–4, 357
  heterogeneous mass at 32 weeks **985**
  HIV infection 349
  HLA antigens 192
  iatrogenic lesions 992–4
  infarction 269, 303, 330, 344, 357
  infections 102–3, 325, **326–7**, 328
    histologic pattern **326**
  inflammation, chronic 327
  inspection in twin–twin transfusion
    syndrome 974
  insufficiency,
    organ weights **278**
    and prematurity 8
  intervillous thrombosis **986**
  in intrapartum asphyxia 303–5
  and intrapartum infections 97–8
  IUGR abnormalities 276
  large 334
  in late pregnancy 319–38
  lesions 320–1
  maldevelopment 334–6
  maternal blood-borne infections 96
  maternal substance abuse effects 353–62
  MC, vascular anastomoses, frequencies of
    205
  'membrane' 13, 319
  metabolic functions 13–15
  MHC expression **340**
  monochorionic,
    vascular anastomoses frequency *205*
    vascular arrangements 209
  mosaicism, confined, IUGR 336
  multiple pregnancy examination 222
  and neonatal anaemia 709
  nuclear inclusion bodies 348
  pathologic examination 994
  pathologic study 319
  pathology 347
    in twins 222
  perfusion–fixation **989–90**, **991**
  permeability 12
  Po_2 values **152**
  report 1543
  rubella-infected infant 348
  sampling areas 320
  and smoking 334, 357
  sonograms at 35 weeks **986**
  thrombosis 344
  tissue sampling 320
  TORCH neonate assessment 266
  transverse scan at 20 weeks' gestation **984**
  trophoblastic tumor 192
  ultrasound assessment 888
  uterine position 320
  villi **141**, **144**
  villous oedema 323
  weights 320, 334
  see also Villous tissue
Placenta membranacea 303
Placenta praevia,
  and asphyxia 295, 303
  indications 320

  transvaginal ultrasound 881
Placental abnormalities,
  high MSAFP 989
  location, size, echogenicity and number *983*
  prenatal diagnosis 982–9
  ultrasonographic assessment and
    classification 982–7
Placental anatomy,
  Doppler investigations 990–1
  experimental systems 989–92
Placental arteries, in hypoxia 292
Placental bed biopsy 278
Placental biopsy 991–2
  chromosomal defect karyotyping 940
Placental circulation,
  early 979–80
  experimental systems 989
  flow velocity waveforms **980**
  hemodynamics 979–80
  two-level resistance system 991
Placental collapse 989
Placental function and morphology,
  research history 979
Placental grading, classification system
  982–3
Placental lactogen,
  human 693
  maternal 693
Placental lesions, sonographic classification
  983
Placental localization, ultrasound use 881
Placental maturation and grading 982–3
Placental morphology, in multiple
  pregnancy 973–5
Placental mosaicism,
  confined,
    diagnosis 1100
    and fetal disomy 1106, 1108
    types *1106*
  fetal loss *1110*
  in trisomy 16 *1111*
Placental pathology, biochemical markers
  987, 989
Placental position 979
Placental structure and function 1275–7
Placental thromboses 984
Placental tissue, sonographic differential
  diagnosis *983*
Placental trauma 992
Placental villi, sampling 991
Placentation,
  abnormalities, and asphyxia 295
  in higher multiples 203–4
  MC, vascular anastomoses **212**
  monochorionic 971
    abnormal consequences 973–411
  monochorionic monoamniotic 973
  in multiple pregnancy 205–6
  in triplets 206
  in twinning 201–2
  by zygosity **201**, 205
Plasma cells 325
Platelet-derived growth factor A (PDGFA)
  121
Platelets,
  antibodies against 343
  disorders 718–20
  function disturbances 719
  in newborn 1282
  normal function 718–19
  problem management 1286
  transfusion 1286
  X-chromatin 722
  Y-chromatin 722

Platyspondylic lethal short-limbed dysplasia 790
Pleiotropy 23
Pleural effusion,
  bilateral **931**
  drainage 1308
Pleuritic fluid collection 1317
Pleuroamniotic shunt **1259**
Pleurosomus 401
Ploidy,
  and flow cytometry 196
  flow cytometry diagnosis **237**
  and molar pregnancy **237**
Pneumatosis intestinalis **1486–7**
Pneumocystis carinii, perinatal infections 825
Pneumocystis carinii pneumonia 549
Pneumocyte type II, freeze fracture **544**
Pneumonia, congenital 271, **548–9**
Pneumonitis 809
Pneumothorax 808
Point mutations 37–8, 42
  detection 1195
  network **38**
Poland syndrome 76, 135
Polio 443
Polyarteriolar lobe 554
Polycythaemia 510, 717
Polycythaemia in twin–twin transfusion syndrome 974
Polydactyly 24
  postaxial, at 28 weeks **942**
Polygenes 25
Polyhydramnios 881, 928, **1248–51**
  aetiology 1248–9
  amniotic pressure **1249**
  causes *932*
  with chorioangioma 983
  fetal complications 1249
  fetal hypoxaemia **1250**
  malformation incidence *932*
  malformation in twins 972
  maternal complications 1249
  in multiple pregnancy 206
  prevalence *932*
  in twin–twin transfusion syndrome 974
  ultrasound findings, chromosomal anomaly 940
Polymerase chain reaction, *see* PCR
Polymicrogyria 419, 421–2, **423–4**
  in CMV infection **441–2**
  pathogenesis 423
  in Zellweger syndrome **446**
Polymorphism,
  heterozygous 1191
  homozygous 1191
Polymorphism analysis **1179–81**
Polymorphonuclear inflammatory response 101
Polymyositis 775
Polypeptide gene products 42
Polyploidy 58
  mosaicism 1102–4
Polyposis coli **849–50**
Polyps 850–2
Polysomy 58
Polysplenia syndrome **496**
  familial 501
Polytopic developmental field defects 402
Polytopic field defect, definition 401
Pompe disease 780, 1141
  amniocyte test 1092
  deficiency masking 1132

heart anomalies 505–6
Ponderal index (PI) 278, 280–1
Porencephalic cysts 975
Porencephaly 262, 424–5
Pork and parasitic infections 350
Porphyria, erythropoietic 765
Porphyrin metabolism disorders *1154*
Portal fibrosis 568
POSSUM database 25
Postimplantation development 124
Postnatal life, birth defects 29
Potassium cardioplegia techniques 515
Potter cysts 616
Potter facies **406**
Potter oligohydramnios sequence 26, 401, 406
Potter syndrome 534, 614
PPROM, *see* Preterm premature rupture of the membranes
Prader–Willi syndrome 23, 123, 247, 255, 1125, 1127
  metaphase preparation **1126**
Pre-eclampsia 287
  adrenal gland in 299
  arteriosclerosis **327**
  and haemorrhage 301
  in hydatidiform mole 186, 190
  and hypertensive disease 344–5
  and vascular disease 326
Preacinar airways, development 324
Preconceptual nutritional evaluation 8–9
Preconceptual period 3–4
Preconceptual screening 8
Pregenesis 28
Pregnancy,
  adrenal gland disorder 1270
  after 42 weeks 304
  carbohydrate metabolic changes 1275
  chemical 227
  cocaine use,
    and structural malformations *360*
    vascular disruptions *360*
  confirmation 165, 176
  developmental stage assessment 174–5
  ectopic 165–6
  energy cost *1268*
  energy requirements 1267–8
  enzyme abnormalities 1270–1
  evaluation in bad perinatal outcome 336
  exposures 181
  extrauterine 139
  grief after loss 1013–14
  'high risk' 5
  hope for 1019
  immunology 339, 341–3
  innovative therapeutic approaches 162
  loss after fetal blood sampling *1074*
  mean energy cost *1267*
  mosaic complications *1109*
  nutrient intake variations 1268–9
  placental examination for diagnosis 336
  'polydrug' users 1272
  postdate and large placenta 334
  psychodynamics 1013
  risks 162
  schematic representations 145
  seroconversion in 350
  smoking complications 356
  termination,
    communication 1018
    for fetal abnormality 1014
    information on fetal abnormality 1018
    psychosocial sequelae 1014–16
    recognition of grief 1018

transvaginal view **139**
tubal 165–6
viral infection 1293–9
see also Multiple pregnancy
Pregnancy loss, *see* Abortion; Reproductive loss
Pregnancy outcome,
  placental examination assessment 319
  poor,
    risk of recurrence 319
    unexplained 319
Pregnancy trimester 4
first,
  abortion 163–4
  chromosomal disease diagnosis 951
  CVS benefits 1077
  infections 348
  prenatal diagnosis by embryoscopy 1065–70
  screening 1040
  ultrasound examination 878
  uteroplacental circulation 979
second,
  intrauterine death 975
  mole diagnosis 188
  ultrasound examination 878
third,
  intrauterine death 975
  ultrasound examination 878
Prehydatidiform core 188
Preimplantation diagnosis,
  future of 1057
  genetic 1055–8
  patient perspectives 1057
Preimplantation IVF embryo, cytogenetics 239
Premature birth 7
  ascending infections 97–8
  description 176
  endocrine profiles 288
  neurologic damage 323
  perinatal deaths 201
Premature rupture of membranes (PROM),
  lung hypoplasia 533
  and prematurity 8
Premature or sick infants, testing 1050
Prematurity,
  anaemia of 713
  definition 7
  factor importance 370
  lungs in 547
  in multiple gestation 206
  and subependymal haemorrhage 431
  surveys 8
  'trigger' 8
Prenatal care, lack in substance-abusing mother 354
Prenatal diagnosis 5–6, *1000*, 1010
  congenital diaphragmatic hernia 1320, 1322–3
  cytogenetic, fetal malformations 248–9
  definite familial diagnosis 1089
  disease compendium 1197–1236
  early 1007
  education importance 1041
  experienced center 1089
  first trimester, by embryoscopy 1065–70
  genetic 999
  and genetic screening *1002*
  guidelines 1024
  haemoglobinopathies 717
  implications 999–1003
  indications *1000*
  metabolic disorders 1131

Prenatal diagnosis (contd)
  midtrimester amniocentesis 1083
  multiple pregnancy 971
  non-traditional inheritance *1002*
  placental examination 319
  placental and umbilical cord abnormalities
    982–9
  and primary prevention 7
  programs 126, 162
  requirements for 1089
  sole diagnostic test 1094
  technologies 1123
  thalassaemia 1175–82
    α, 1181–2
    β, 1175–82
  triploid fetus **239**
  twin pregnancy 218, 220
  ultrasound role 877–8
  urinary tract abnormalities 629–30
Prenatal gene therapy,
  experimental studies 1335
  rationale 1334–5
Prenatal life, disorders peculiar to 163
Prenatal loss rates 242
Prenatal procedures, invasive, increasing
  use 992
Prenatal samples, handling and processing
  1525
Prenatal screening 5–6
  approach to 1023–4
  tests 6
  see also Doppler; Ultrasound
Prenatal surgery, congenital diaphragmatic
  hernia 1325–6
Prenatal therapy, complications 803–5
Prenatal tissue samples,
  histopathological investigation 1089–97
  investigation value 1094–5
  microscopic assessment 1089–97
  morphological experience 1089
  techniques 1095–6
  turnaround time 1095
Prenatal tolerance induction 1334
Prenatal urological intervention, indications
  1465
Preterm infant,
  intraventricular haemorrhage 1362
  mineral content *1408*
  nutritional requirements 1422–31
  pulmonary disease 1337
  respiratory problems 1387–97
  risks 6–8
  viability 1382–3
Preterm labour, prediction of 975
Preterm premature rupture of the
  membranes (PPROM) 1245–6, 1248
Primer specific amplification 1177–8
  for β-thalassaemia **1177–8**
Primitive canal defects 495
Primitive neuroectodermal tumour 855
Procainamide 967
Procoagulants, values *1281*
Procollagen 46
Production line hypothesis 251–2
Progesterone 90, 340
Prolactin 694
Proliferating cell nuclear antigen 857
Prolonged rupture of membranes,
  glucocorticoid therapy 1340
PROM, *see* Premature rupture of
  membranes
Prometaphase 55
  analysis 1121
Promoter regions and mutations **42**
Pronephros 609

Pronuclei, male and female, DNA 196
Propionate metabolism disorders *1152*
Propionic acidaemia 440, 1133–4
Prospective counselling 1008–9
Prostaglandin E treatment 811
Prostaglandins 340
Protein,
  average, amino acid content 1188
  disordered function 1022
  metabolism in newborn 1411
  requirement of preterm infant 1424–5
  structure and function 1187
  synthesis 1188
    first-stage 1188
Proto-oncogene activation 70
Protodiastolic notch **980**
Prune-belly sequence **406**, 628–9, 771
Pseudocyst 987
Pseudofollicular microcysts 301
Pseudoglandular lung growth 523
Pseudohermaphroditism,
  external genitalia **675**
  female 74, *682*
  male 682–3
    and anorchia 677
    dysgenetic 684
    with renal disease and Wilms' tumour
      684
Pseudomonas meningitis 442–3
Pseudomosaicism 241, 1106
Pseudoxanthoma elasticum, heart anomalies
  505
Psychoactive substances,
  abuse *353–62*
  classes *353*
Psychosocial sequelae,
  of pregnancy termination,
    after 2 years 1016
    for fetal abnormality 1014
Public health, and genetic screening 1000
Public health department, reports to 371
Pulmonary, *see* Lungs
Pulmonary air leak 807–8
Pulmonary artery,
  hypoplasia 540
  'precocious muscularization' **541**
Pulmonary artery flow, prenatal and
  postnatal distribution **488**
Pulmonary circulation 478, 480
Pulmonary haemorrhage 547, 549
Pulmonary hypertension 370
  neonatal 300
Pulmonary hypoplasia and oligohydramnios
  933
Pulmonary infections 811
Pulmonary lymphangiectasis, congenital
  543
Pulmonary surfactant composition 544–7
Pulmonary valve, raphe **491**
Pulmonary venous return,
  partial anomalous 501
  total anomalous 501
Pulmonary-derived renotrophin 535
Pulsatility index (PI) 888, 981, 1400
  increased 991
  values 981
Pump co-twin 214
Purine metabolism disorders 1140–1,
  1152–3
Pygopagus twins 217
Pyloric atresia 595
Pyloric stenosis, hypertrophic 594–5
Pyrimethamine, for toxoplasmosis 264

Pyrimidine metabolism disorders 1140–1,
  1152–3
Pyropoikilocytosis, hereditary 715
Pyruvate kinase deficiency 714
Pyruvate metabolism disorders 1135

Quadricuspid semilunar valve 490
Quadruplets, perinatal mortality rate
  972
Quazi syndrome 1070
Quintuplets, perinatal mortality rate 972

Rachischisis **416–17**
Radial nerve palsy 311
Radiation 26
  effects 89
  paternal exposure 79
  therapy 71
  see also Irradiation
Radiation disruptions 401–2
Radiography,
  at autopsy 382
  embryo and fetus 180–1
  in fetal death 272–3
Radioiodine and fetus 85
Radius,
  at 15 weeks 912
  aplasia *1218*
  at 20 weeks **944**
Raphe 488-9, **491**
ras oncogenes 70
ras proto-oncogene 73
Rb, *see* Retinoblastoma
Rb-1 gene 71
  binding sites 49
  mitosis 49–50
  retinoblast differentiation 50
Rb-1 protein,
  leucine zipper zone **49**
  oncoprotein binding **49**
Receptor-mediated endocyte uptake 12
Recessive mutant tumor suppressor gene
  196
Reciprocal translocations 228
Recombinant genes 61
Rectorrhagia 595
Red cell alloimmunization 1301
  management scheme **1303**
Red cell antigens, and recurrent abortion
  170
Red cell isoimmunization 1301
Red cells, circulating nucleated 323
Reflection, in ultrasound 883
Refsum syndrome 760, 784, 1139
Regional referral center, for antenatal and
  neonatal pathology 9
Registry of International Society of Fetal
  Medicine and Surgery 1345
Regulative development 33, 35
Regulatory genes 31–2
Regulatory proteins and cell lineage 35
Reifenstein syndrome 684
Relational pleiotropy 24
Renal, *see* Kidney
Repetitive mutations 39–40
Reporter compounds 1122
Reproduction,
  behaviour after termination 1016–17
  pattern change 1009
Reproductive failure 124
Reproductive health care system 8–9
Reproductive loss,
  causes 4
  chromosomally abnormal gestation 242

Reproductive loss (contd)
classification *177–8*
cytogenetic aspects 227–59
definition 227
early 175–86
  assessment of goals 183
  causes 178
  definition 175
  evaluation *182*
  genetic counselling 182–3
  morphology and pathology 176–80
  relative frequency 242
endocrinology 227
epidemiology 227
etiologic aspects 227
quantitative and etiologic aspects 227
recurrence risk 382
Reproductive medicine 1001
Reproductive options 1009–10
and genetic screening 1022
Reproductive organs,
female 684–5
male 685–6
Reproductive systems 663–91
Reproductive wastage 175
early 164–5
reporting 165
terminology 165
Rescreening 1051
Resistance index (RI) 888, **981**
Respirator therapy, complications 516
Respiratory distress, preventive agents
1337–8
Respiratory distress syndrome (RDS) 7,
101, 357, *370*, 1392–6
differential diagnosis *1392*
management 1394–6
prophylaxis 1374
surfactants for 544
Respiratory system,
neonatal therapy 806–11
ultrasound-guided aspiration 1308
Respiratory tract 523–60
Respiratory viruses 1450
Restriction endonuclease analysis, for
β-thalassemia 1175–6
Restriction enzymes 1192–3
DNA cleavage 1192–3
recognition sites **1193**
Restriction fragment length polymorphism
(RFLP) 1192
for abnormal syngamy 232
complete hydatidiform mole **191**
markers 1025
maternal and paternal contribution
diagnosis **240**
in partial hydatidiform mole **195**
site 37
testing for twin zygosity **204**
for zygosity testing 203–**4**
Resuscitation, dilemmas 1382
Reticular dysgenesis 721
Retinitis pigmentosa 24
Retinoblastoma 24, 71
mental handicap 255
paternal preconceptual carcinogenic
exposure 77
transcription mutation 48
'trilateral' 71
Retinoic acid 80, *130*, 133
Retinoic acid receptors 130–1
Retinoic acid syndrome 89
Retinol, human digit study 391
Retinopathy of prematurity 824
Retrolental fibroplasia 823

Retroperitoneal teratoma 834
Retroplacental haematoma 323–4, 985,
987
Retrospective counselling 1008–9
Retrovirus, endogenous 347
Rett syndrome 24
Reye syndrome *573*, 1132, 1134
Rhabdomyoma,
cardiac 299
  spider cell **506**
juvenile 842
myocardial 509
ventricular **510**
Rhabdomyosarcoma 73, *577*
congenital 686
Rhesus alloimmunization 1301–6
Rhesus D hydrops 4
Rhesus immunization 1455
cordocentesis diagnosis 1072
Rhesus incompatibility 711
Rheumatoid factor 99–100
Rhizomelic chondrodysplasia punctata,
types 799
Rhizomelic dysplasia 935
Ribs, in respiratory distress 819
Ribs five and six, disruption 303
Rickets 819
radiograph check 1427
Right heart syndrome 489–90
Rights in decisions 18
Riley–Day syndrome 783
Ring chromosomes 1103
Risk assessment 5, 376
Risk scores 5
RNA,
alternative splicing 33
coding for CG 150
maternal influence 35
processing 1188–9
ribosomal synthesis (rRNA) 56
translation **1189**
RNA viruses 348
Robertsonian translocations 60, 228–9,
230–1
sperm analysis *232*
Robin sequence 405–6
Rolland–Desbuquois dysplasia 794
Rothmund–Thomson syndrome 1070
Roviralta syndrome 594
Rubella 96
CNS involvement 440, 442
fetal infection 549
immunization 265
in pregnancy 1294–5
in TORCH 261, 264, 325
Rubella syndrome 348, 365, 401
Rubella vaccine 90
Rubinstein–Taybi syndrome 29, 408
Runting 332

Sacral defect with anterior meningocele 25
Sacrococcygeal teratoma 686, 831, **832**–3
Saldino–Noonan syndrome 791–2, 1070
Salla disease 1143, 1446
Sandhoff disease 1143–4
Sanfilippo syndrome 1146–7
types 1147
Scalp electrode monitoring 977
Schisis association 26
Schneckenbecken dysplasia 790
Schwachman–Diamond syndrome 721
Schwann cells 856
Score for neonatal acute physiology (SNAP)
9, 368

Screening,
abnormal results 1051
antenatal, ethical and other considerations
1041
automation 1030
for chromosomal abnormalities 1036–40
for chromosomal disorders 1021
computerization 1030
cost versus benefit 1029
for cystic fibrosis 1029
for endocrine disease 706
haemoglobin abnormalities 717
histological and histochemical *1026*
individual 1021
inherited metabolic disorders 1025
laboratory transit 1050
mass or population 1021
for neural tube defect 1032–4
normal results 1050
psychological aspects 1025
quality control measures 1029–30
results follow-up 1050–1
for β-thalassemia 1174–5
unsatisfactory specimens 1050
see also Genetic screening; Neonatal
screening
Segmental aneusomy 1125
Segregation types 60–1
Self-esteem, loss of 1014
Semiallograft 339
Semilunar valves,
development **483**
malformations 488–91
Seminiferous tubule dysgenesis 677–8
Seminoma 74
Septal chorionicity, prenatal diagnosis *221*
Septal defects 501
Septal membrane rolls 222
Septal membrane status 205
Septo-optic dysplasia 701–2
Septum, in fused DC,DA twins **210–11**
Sequence, description 26, 401
Sequence analysis **1180**–1
Sequences 405–6
Sequestrated lung segment 525
Serologic screening,
technical problems 262–3
for TORCH syndrome 262
Seropositive mothers 348
Severe combined immunodeficiency disease
742–4, 1140
Severe combined immunodeficiency–
adenosine deaminase deficiency
(SCID–ADA), gene therapy 395
Sex chromosome aneuploidies,
in females 63
in males 63–4
Sex chromosome abnormalities, and
mosaicism 1102
Sex chromosome aneuploidies, detection
1123
Sex chromosome complements, in fragile X
syndrome **1118**
Sex determination and differentiation 664
Sex reversal syndrome (46,XX males)
678–9
Sex-determining region Y 664
Sextuplets, perinatal mortality rate 972
Sexual development, dysgenetic gonads
74–5
Sexual intercourse and AIDS virus 348
SGA, *see* Small for gestational age
Sherman paradox 1117
Shock 511
Shone syndrome 503–**4**

Short bowel syndrome 370, 1490
  parenteral nutrition 1418
Short limb dysplasia, fetal identification
  933–4, 935
Short tandem repeats (STRs) 1181
Short-rib polydactyly syndromes 24, 791
Sialic acid storage disease 1090
  cell type involvement 1092
Sickle-cell disease 716
Sickle mutation, detection by restriction
  endonuclease digestion 1176
Sideroblastic anaemia, refractory 713
Siemens Vidoson 873
Silverman–Handmaker dysplasia 794
Simpson–Golabi–Behmel syndrome 23
Single copy probes 1124
Single gene disorder, molecular pathology
  1191
Single-strand conformation polymorphism
  analysis 1179
Sirenomelia 401–2, 610, 627
Sjögren–Larsson syndrome 760
Skeletal changes, perinatal 819–20, 821
Skeletal dysplasias, diagnosis 801
Skin,
  biopsy, for metabolic defect 1131
  bullous disorders 761–4
  chromosomal instability syndromes
    764–5
  colours in maceration 270
  compound naevus 844
  embryogenesis 755
  intradermal naevus 845
  laceration 306
  neonatal therapy 806
  postinfection 262
  reddening 270
  third trimester 758
  tuberous sclerosis 844
  weeks 8–15 955, 956–7
  weeks 15–24 757–8
Skin slipping, in maceration 270–1
Skinfold thickness 280
Skull,
  embryoscopy 1069
  triploidy anomalies 195
Skull fractures 308
  depressed 308
  linear 308
  transverse linear 308
Small-for-gestational age (SGA) 16
  causes 275
  definition 275
Small-for-gestational-age (SGA) infant,
  chromosomal abnormalities 276
  early morbidity 280
  intrapartum and neonatal complications
    281
  neonatal morbidity 280–1
  neurodevelopmental outcome 282
  perinatal mortality 280–1
  postnatal growth 282
  risk factors and clinical examination
    276–7
  spiral arteriole 279
Small molecule diseases, biochemical
  investigation 1132–3
Smith–Lemli–Opitz syndrome 23, 407–8,
  1070
  external features 379
  genital anomalies 683
Smith's Diasonograph 871–2
Smith's Recognizable Patterns of Human
  Deformation 377

Smith's Recognizable Patterns of Human
  Malformation 377
Smoking 26
  effect on marker screening 1040
  effects 356–7
  and fetal loss 172
  and IUGR 275–7, 1275
  neonatal withdrawal signs 354
  and perinatal mortality 367
  and spontaneous abortion 178
Social self-esteem, loss 1014
Sodium, placental transfer 12–13
Soldner, R. 873
Somatosensory evoked potential 1403–4
Somatostatin 695
'Sonic' hedgehog 1002
Sonoembryography, see Transvaginal
  sonography
Sonoembryology, see Transvaginal
  sonography
Southern analysis,
  autoradiograph 1192
  for fragile X syndrome 1118
Spaulding's sign 270
Spectral analysis 982
Spectroscopy, near infrared 1368–9,
  1401–2
Sperm,
  analysis in robertsonian translocations
    232
  binding, attachment and fusion 120
  capacitation 120
  differential genomic imprinting 196
  diploid 195
  hyperhaploid 229
  and structural defects 377
Spermatogenesis 119, 663
  abnormal 229, 232
Spermatogonia 56, 119
Spermicides 91
Spherocytosis, hereditary 715
Sphingolipid degradation 1144
Sphingolipidoses 1143–6
Spina bifida 417–18, 921–2
  AFAFP rise 1033
  ultrasound detection 1040–1
Spina bifida complex 400
Spina bifida cystica 417
  see also Meningomyocele
Spina bifida occulta 418
Spinal artery, thrombosis 823
Spinal cord,
  disruption, and forceps rotation 310
  insult 309
  and intrapartum trauma 308–10
  perinatal lesions 823
  postmortem removal 454, 458
  transection 805
Spinal dysraphism 417–18
Spinal muscular atrophy type I 450
Spine,
  at 15 weeks, structural evaluation 911
  birth trauma 309
  intact, with ventriculomegaly 923–4
  normal, with assessment by ultrasound 919–20
Spinomuscular atrophy 782–3
Spiral arteries,
  early 979
  lesions 330
  reconstruction 150
  transformation 139, 141, 147
Spiral arterioles,
  histopathology 345–6
  normal pregnancy 279

placental bed 345–6
SGA baby pregnancy 279
Spiramycin, for toxoplasmosis 264
Spleen,
  infarcts 817
  intrapartum trauma 311–12
Splice site mutations 41
Spondylocostal dysplasia 800
Spondyloepiphyseal dysplasia 796
  congenital lethal 798
Spondyloepiphyseal dysplasia congenita
  796–7
Spondylothoracic dysplasia 800
Squeeze mutations 44
Squeeze zones 42
SRY gene 24
Staphylococcus aureus 1446
Starling mechanism 511
Starvation, and IUGR 275–6
Status marmoratus 437, 440, 823
Stem cells 729–30
  in utero transplantation 1331–6
  role 1505
  transfusion 1263
Sterilization 1009–10
Steroid 21-hydroxylase defect 704–5
Steroid metabolism disorders 1158
Steroidogenesis 24
Steroids,
  and prematurity 7
  synthesis by adrenal tissue 699
Stillbirth 269
  ancillary studies 272–3
  definition 176
  external examination 378
  external features of syndromes 379
  'fresh' 269
  risks 126
Stillbirth and Neonatal Death Society
  1377–8
Stomach,
  perforation 595
  sonograph 1323
  teratoma 834
  ulcers 595–6
Stomatocytosis, hereditary 715
Strawberry skull,
  in trisomy 18 942
  at 18 weeks 946
Streak gonads 666, 667–8, 670
Streeter band 404
Streptococci, group B 325, 1446
Streptococcus agalactia 549
Stria of Nitabuch 334
Strudwick dysplasia 798
Stuck twin 213–14
  prognosis 214
  in twin-to-twin transfusion 206
Stuck twin syndrome 974, 1085
Sturge–Weber sequence/syndrome 408, 836
Subamniotic cyst 984
Subamniotic hematoma 984
Subarachnoid haemorrhage 427, 429
Subcapsular haemorrhage 569
Subchorial thrombosis 324
Subcortical leucomalacia 436
Subcortical necrosis 438, 440
Subdermal fibromatous tumour of Reye
  838–9
Subdural haemorrhage 427
Subependymal cysts 431–2
Subependymal haemorrhage 428, 431–2
Subpial haemorrhage 427–8
Substance abuse, effects 353–62

Sudden infant death syndrome (SIDS) 357
  and brain 451
  in drug abuse 354
  heroin abuse 360
  incidence in drug abuse 354
Sulcus, catenoidal shape 472–3
Sulfonamides, for toxoplasmosis 264
Sulphur amino acid disorders *1150*
Sunden, B. 870–1
Superior vena cava, persistent left 501–2
Suppressor cells 340
Suppressor genes 70
Supraventricular tachycardia **966**
Surface tension-reducing substance 544
Surfactant,
  aerosol therapy 810–11
  components in fetal lung 395
  composition 544
  lipids and proteins, hormonal influence
    545
  pulmonary 1393–4
    replacement therapy *1395*
  replacement 1340
    for preterm infant 1374–5
Surfactant protein A (SP-A), fetal lung
  explant 393–4
Surfactant-associated proteins **545**
Surgical pathologist 163
Surgical report: forms 1546–7
Survanta 547
Swyer syndrome 24, 669–70
Symmelia 216
Symphysis–fundal height 976
Symphysis–fundus measurement for SGA
  infant 276–7
Syncytiotrophoblast 148, 150, **153**, 339–40
  in CMV infection 348–9
  in partial hydatidiform mole 193
Syndactyly 132, *134*, 941, 1069
Syndrome, description 27
Syngamy 28, **234–6**
  abnormal 232, **234–6**
    analysis 232
Synthetic probes 191
Syphilis 96–7
  congenital 112, 325, **327**
    development 347
    increasing numbers 265
    pathology 347
  in TORCH syndrome 265–6
Systemic lupus erythematosus (SLE) 343
Systolic anterior motion of anterior mitral
  leaflet 507

T cells, role 1504–**5**
T lymphocytes 100, 332
T-cell system 730
Tachycardia,
  causes 1355
  supraventricular **966**
    therapy 968
  ventricular 966
    therapy 968–9
Tan–gray coloured skin in maceration 270
Tarui disease 1142
Taurine 1424
Taussig–Bing anomaly 493
Tay–Sachs disease 37
  carrier detection 1053–4, 1131–2, 1143–4
  insertional mutations **39**
  mutations in Ashkenazi Jews 47
  mutations causing 41
  prenatal screening 1023
Technologies, new 181–2

Telangiectasis, hereditary 836
Telemetry 1358
Telomeres 57
Tentorium, tears **307–8**
Teratogenesis,
  infectious 261
  and oncogenesis 69
Teratogenic disruption 26, 401, 402–3
Teratogenicity,
  criteria for proof *84*
  of drugs 354
Teratogens 26, 181
  agents *89*
  animal tests 85–6
  confirmation of disorders 8
  environmental 175
  exposure screening 8–**9**
  human *181*
  identification 83–5
  known 86–9
  possible *89*
  surveillance centers *5*
  time specificity of action *88*
  unlikely 89–*90*, 91
  windows of susceptibility 86
Teratologia 1554
Teratology 365, 399
  definitions 83
  information 91
Teratoma 271, 831–4
  congenital **452**
  as dysplasia 27
  gastric 834
  gonadal 832–3
  head and neck 833
  intracranial, prenatal diagnosis 453
  mediastinal 833
  nasopharyngeal **833**
  reproductive organs 686
  retroperitoneal 834
  sacrococcygeal 831, **832–3**
TERIS database 91
Terminal sac lung growth 523
Testicular differentiation 664–5
  chronology *665*
Testicular feminization 64
Testicular feminization syndrome 683–4
  incomplete 684
Testis,
  dysgenesis 675–80
    fetal testicular failure *676*
    and multiple malformation syndromes
      680
  dysplastic **672–3**
  perinatal haemorrhage and infarction 686
  perinatal tumours 686
Tests for conditions *in utero* and at birth
  1526
Tetralogy of Fallot 488, 490, **493–4**
Tetraploidy 237, 1103
Tetratology, information 91
TGF-α (transforming growth factor α)
  121–2, 134
  and cleft lip/palate 25
TGF-β (transforming growth factor β) 35,
  115, 121–2, 133–4
Thalassaemia, 31
  α syndromes 717
  carrier detection 1054
  causal mutations 41–2
  gene deletion 40
α-Thalassaemia 1165–7
  clinical aspects 1165–6
  hematologic findings 1165–6

molecular pathology 1166–7
mutations *1167*
  non-deletional *1167*
prenatal diagnosis 1181–2
β-Thalassaemia 1167–75
  carrier screening, implications 1174–5
  cells **717**
  clinical aspects 1167, 1171
  common mutant screening **1177**
  complex 1167–75
    clinical and molecular aspects 1173–4
  control 1182
  deletions **1171**
  detection, future prospects 1182–3
  heterogenicity 1174–5
  homozygous, birth rate fall in Sardinia
    1183
  molecular pathology 1171, 1173
  mutation,
    known, detection 1175–8
    unknown, detection 1178–81
  mutation frequencies *1172*
    in Asians *1173*
    in Mediterranean populations *1172*
  mutations,
    common mild **1174**
    known, diagnosis 1175–8
    unknown 1175
      diagnosis 1178–81
  mutations causing *1168–70*
  prenatal diagnosis 1175–82
  probe 1176
  in Sardinia, birth rate fall **1183**
  unknown origin 1175
Thalidomide 401, 774
  and phocomelia 803–4
  as teratogen 402
Thanatophoric dysplasia 787–8
Theca–luteal cysts 188, 192
Thermodisruptive anomalies 401, 405
Thermoregulation disturbance *370*
Thoracopagus CT 218–9
  embryonic disk arrangement **218**
Threshold phenomena 25
Thrombocytopenia 344, 1285–6
  and infection 719
  and intravenous fat 1435–6
  megakaryocytic hypoplasia 719–20
Thromboembolism **300**
Thromboplastins 213
Thrombosis 1289–90
Thrombotic disorders, inherited 1285
Thrombotic thrombocytopenic purpura 328
Thymic lobes,
  early **723**
  newborn **723**
Thymidine 37
Thymus,
  and cell transplantation 1504
  dysplastic **744**
  from hypoxic infant **733**
  in intrapartum asphyxia 303
  tissue sources 1508
  transplantations 1507–8
Thyroglossal cyst 846–7
Thyroglossal sinus **846**
Thyroid gland, hypoplasia, congenital
  696–7
Thyroid hormones for lung development
  1340–1
Thyroid status, biochemical assessment 697
Thyroid stimulator, human 698
Thyrotrophin 694
Thyroxine pathway **697**

Tibia at 15 weeks **906**
Time of flight absorbance 1369
Tissue,
  acoustic properties *884*
  ultrasonic pulse propagation **884**
Tissue engraftment 1503–6
Tissue phospholipids 1412–13
Tissue sampling, requirements 1533
Tissue specimens,
  inventory 163
  protocol limitations 163–4
Tissue-specific genes 31
  mutations 42–7
Toes at 13 weeks 907
TORCH (*toxoplasmosis, other, rubella, cytomegalovirus, herpes*), *see below*
TORCH antibody package 262
TORCH antigen detection 263
TORCH fetus,
  clinical features *261*
  neurologic deficits 263
  problems arising 261
TORCH infections,
  ascending from cervix 261
  detections 261–8
  fetal prevalence 325
  haematogenous spread 261
  screening 923
TORCH neonate, unexpected, microbiologic assessment 266
TORCH syndrome 104, 110, 181
  antigen detection 263
  clinical history 262
  fetal defects 403–4
  histologic examination, later pregnancy importance 264
  infections, detection 261–68
  invasive testing 263–4
  pathophysiology 261–2
  possible *in utero* therapy 266
  serologic screening 262–3
  specific infections 264–6
  ultrasound 263
  villous inflammation 325
  workplace health risks 266
Toriello–Higgins mutation *29*
Torticollis 840
Toxins,
  and fetal muscle 774
  and recurrent abortion 172
TOXNET (reference listing) 91
Toxoplasma gondii 350, 549
  in TORCH 261, 325
Toxoplasmosis 96
  brain-stem section **107**
  congenital **442–3**
    in France 264
  maternal therapy 264
  prevalence, in France 264
  in TORCH syndrome 264
Trace elements, recommended intravenous intakes *1430*
Tracheobronchial epithelium, diffuse coagulative necrosis 806–7
Tracheo-oesophageal fistula 400, *527–8*
Transabdominal CVS 1077
  safety and efficacy *1079–20*
Transabdominal embryoscopy **1066–7**
Transcervical CVS 1077
  safety and efficacy *1079–80*
Transcervical embryoscopy 1065–6
Transcobalamin II deficiency 713
Transcription 1188–9
Transcription factors 33, 35

Transcriptional DNA 40
  mutation effects 41–2
Transferrin receptor 1061
Transforming growth factor α, *see* TGF-α
Transforming growth factor β, *see* TGF-β
Transfusions 1050
Transitional mutations, mechanism of C to T 38
Translation 1188–9
Transplacental infections 328
Transplacental metastases 69
Transplacental oncogenesis 804
Transvaginal probe 897
Transvaginal sonography 897–900, **901–4**, 905–17
  advantages 881
  frequencies required 884
  in oligohydramnios 933
  structural evaluation,
    at 15 weeks 909, **910–15**
    from 6 to 16 weeks 897–918
  technical considerations 898
  week 8 of pregnancy **900**
  week 9 of pregnancy 903
    posterior contours **901**
  week 10 of pregnancy 905–6
    physiological herniation **902**
  week 11 of pregnancy 906–7
  weeks 12–14 907, 909
  weeks 15–16 909, 912
TRAP (twin reversed arterial perfusion) 202, 204, 973–4
  in MC twins 214
  prenatal diagnosis 221
Trauma, intrapartum 305–12
Treponema pallidum 549
Triage 'Q & A' 1531–2, *1535–6*
Tricuspid atresia 497
Tricuspid valve, cleft **496**
Triiodothyronine pathway **697**
Triose phosphate isomerase deficiency 714
Triple marker screening 1039, 1041
Triple X syndrome 63
Triplet gestation, membrane structure **901**
Triplet repeats 39–40
Triplets,
  perinatal mortality rate 972
  placenta chorionicity *209*
  placentation **208**
Triploid diandric conceptus 192
Triploid pregnancy, parental contributions **240**
Triploids, liveborn 232
Triploidy 28, 195, 950–1, 1102–3
  abnormality frequency *950*
  and abortion 179
  abortion in first trimester 951
  anomalies 195, 410
  external features *379*
  fetal karyotyping 962
  IUGR 276
  MSAFP rise 1035
  in partial mole 989
  in perinatal death 242
  poor outcome 951
  and renal hypoplasia 611
Trisomy conceptus, uniparental disomy **1110**
Trisomic zygote 'rescue' concept 1108, 1110–1, **1152**
Trisomies 28
Trisomy 58
  and gonadal mosaicism **233**
  triple marker screening *1039*
  and uniparental disomy 242, 247–8

Trisomy 13 63
  abnormalities *940–1*
    frequency *941*
  congenital heart disease 249
  detection 1123
  external features *379*
  fetal karyotyping 962
  incidence 940
  major anomalies 409–10
  in perinatal death 242
  and platelets 722–3
Trisomy 15 247
Trisomy 16 1108
  and confined placental mosaicism *1111*
  origins 253
Trisomy 18 62, 450
  abnormalities 941, *943*
  congenital heart disease 249
  detection 1123
  external features *379*
  fetal karyotyping 962
  finger overlapping **943–4**
  incidence 941
  interphase cells **1126**
  major anomalies 410
  in perinatal death 242
  screening for 1035
Trisomy 21,
  congenital heart disease 962
  see also Down syndrome
Trisomy X 63
Trophoblast **153, 321**
  as immunologic tissue 339
  and lymphokines 341
  and maternal immune response 339
  MHC lack 347
  molar, complications 189
  mosaicism 1106
  privileged site for infection 347
  receptors 341
  uterine arteries infiltration **328**
Trophoblast antigens 339
Trophoblast cells 1059–60
Trophoblast membrane 343
Trophoblast/lymphocyte cross-reactive antigen system 342
Trophoblastic disease 187–99
  residual 187, 190
    and choriocarcinoma 190
    and invasive mole 190
Trophoblastic hyperplasia 188–9, 192
  appearances 194
Trophoblastic infiltration 139
Trophoblastic layer 143, **145**, 148
Trophoblastic thickness **145**
Truncus arteriosus malformation 491–2
Tryptogram **1022**
Tuberculosis 96, 113–14
  placental granulomas **115**
  transplacental infection 114
Tuberous sclerosis 72–3, *74*, 509, 543–4, **619**, 843–4, 957
Tubular myelin **544–5**
Tumour,
  benign 831–54
  connective tissue 838–41
Tumour necrosis factor 68
  in abortion 123
Tumour necrosis factor α (TNF-α), fetal loss 347
Turner syndrome 28, 63, 75, 77, 566, 949–50
  AFAFP rise 1035
  chromosome abnormality 120, 253

Turner syndrome (contd)
and cystic hygroma 513
detection 1123–4
external features 379
FISH identification 1128
maternally derived (Xm) 253
neonatal 668–9
ovaries and genital tract **669**
satellite markers 1128
SGA infant 276
Twin,
donor 213
skull trauma **308**
stuck 213
vanishing 971
Twin pregnancy, MSAFP value 1033
Twin reversed arterial perfusion, see TRAP
Twin-to-twin transfusion 202, 204
acute reversed **213**
complications *205*, **207**
frequency 215
management 222
prenatal diagnosis 220–1
reversed perinatal 213
'stuck' twin 204
Twin–twin transfusion syndrome 710, 974,
1263
Twins 201–25, **900**
acardiac 214, 973–4
common malformations 972
with complete mole 192
congenital anomalies 216–17
conjoined (CT) 217–18
cephalothoracopagus *218*
classification *218–19*
prenatal diagnosis 221
separability 217
thoracopagus 217–8
craniopagus, types 217
disorders 201–25
disruptions 401, 405
dizygotic (DZ) 201–**2**
incidence 973
handicapping ethics 973
heart rate recording, external 977
and hydatidiform mole 194
mechanical problems in delivery 216
mono-oogonial 205
monoamniotic (MA) 215–16
cord complications **215**
outcomes *216*
monochorionic, diamniotic **900**
monochorionic (MC) 201
fetal growth 206
high prevalence 216
interfetal vascular anastomoses (IFVA)
and clinical outcomes 206
IVFA in 214
prenatal diagnosis and management of
complications 220–2
risks to 209
spontaneous abortion 206, **210–11**
vascular complications **207**, 209–15
monozygotic (MZ) 201–2
different degrees of severity of
phenotypic expression 204
discordancy and malformations **217**
etiological aspects 201
external features *379*
'flow-type' congenital heart disease 204
large zonal or organ lesions 204
phenotypic or genotypic discordance
causes 203–4

severity of non-chromosomal
malformations 204
tissue vasculogenic events 204
unequal X-chromosome inactivation 202
neurodevelopmental abnormalities 213
parasitic (PT) 202
pathology *209*
future of 222
perinatal death rates **220**
perinatal mortality rate 972
placental pathology 220
and prematurity 6
prenatal diagnosis 218, 220
of development disorders 220
second-delivered 211
sex ratios, by zygosity and placentation
202
small for gestational age 976
spontaneous abortion risk 220
third type 203
types **201**, **222**
unrecognized 971
mosaicism 1101
vascular anastomoses 973
zygosity determination by DNA RFLP
testing **204**
zygosity testing, concordance and
discordance 203–5
Tyrosinaemia 448
hereditary 571
Tyrosinaemia (type 1, hepatorenal) 1137
Tyrosinase-negative oculocutaneous
albinism 764
Tyrosine disorders *1149*

Uhl syndrome 503
Ulegyria 437–9
Ullrich–Turner syndrome 28, 410–11
Ultrasonic wave, amplitude 884
Ultrasound 91
A-scan 867–9
first-recorded image **868–9**
agenesis of corpus callosum detection 419
amniocentesis replacement 922
antenatal 181
B-scan devices 885–6
combination with Doppler device 887
hand-held probe 885
M-mode display 886
transducer types 885–6
B-scan measurements 885–6
calliper system calibration 885
brain scanning protocol *1404*
chromosomal disease diagnosis 939–53
clinical indications 879
clinical uses *883*
different types *883*
examination components 878
fetal age assessment 176
for fetal anomalies 248
fetal anomaly,
detection 936
in community-based population 936
diagnosis accuracy 935–6
structural, diagnosis 919–38
history 867–75
for hydatidiform mole 188
linear distances 885–6
M-mode display 886
M-mode imaging
dual chamber 964
fetal heart rhythm 964
in maternal serum screening 1040–1
measurement in pregnancy 890–1

in multiple pregnancy 971–95
potential pitfalls 971
for neonatal brain 1399
neurological haemorrhage and infarction
358
obstetric,
clinical indications 879
frequency used 885
overview 877–82
routine or selective 878–9
safety 881–2
services examination 878–9
'tiered' structure 878
timing 879
in oligohydramnios 1246
in partial hydatidiform mole 192–3
physics 883–8
in polyhydramnios 1250
possible adverse bioeffects 881
precision of diagnosis 936
prenatal 8
real-time
B mode 881
cross-sectional anatomy 883
real-time scanner 873–4
replacement of MSAFP testing 922–3
safety 881–2
serial measurement in IUGR 277
SGA 277
TORCH fetus 263
varicella-zoster infection 265
see also Doppler; Echocardiography;
Transvaginal sonography
Ultrasound-guided therapies 1308–12
Ultrastructural study 1195
Umbilical artery 893–4
absence 986, **988**
catheters 1421–2
Doppler imaging 887
Doppler mapping **982**
Doppler signal, normal **893**
in hypoxia 292
Umbilical circulation 980–2
Umbilical cord 34
abnormalities 269, 986–7, **988**
high MSAFP 989
imaging at 20 weeks 986
prenatal diagnosis 982, 986–7, **988**
anatomy, in vivo investigations 979–95
angiomyxoma 987–8
and asphyxia 295–6
at autopsy 386
blood pH 1369
braiding in twins **215**
damage by puncture 992–3, 994
entanglement 296, 305
entwining 222
haematoma 987, **992**
fetal damage 992
human cells 390
iatrogenic lesions, diagnosis 992, 994
identification in twins 222
inflammation 325–6
insertion, embryoscopy **1067**
intertwining risk 215
in intrapartum asphyxia 305
knots 296, 322
location 987
long 322
membranous vessel rupture 322
necrotizing phlebitis **327**
pathologic examination 994
prolapse 295–6
and hypoxia 1352

Umbilical cord (contd)
  prolapse compression 298
  rupture, and neonatal anaemia 709
  short 298
  teratoma 987
  trauma 992
  tumours 987
  velamentous insertion 987
  at week 13 **904**, 909
  at week 15, structural evaluation **916**
Umbilical vein, absence **988**
Umbilical vessels, superficial, lacerations 994
Unifactorial inherited disorders, identified by 1992 *1022*
Uniparental disomy 241, 247–9, 377–8, 380, **1110**, 1267
  as result of trisomy 242, 247–8
Uniparental disomy (representation) 250–1
Uniparental heterodisomy 378
Uniparental isodisomy 378
Unirenicular hypoplasia 611
United Network of Organ Sharing (UNOS) 389
University of Minnesota Biomedical Ethics 390
Urachal cyst and sinus 847
Urachus 610
  lesions 628
Urea cycle,
  disorders 31, 571, 1135–7, *1149*
  enzyme defects **1136**
  inborn errors 448
Ureaplasma urealyticum 387
Ureter,
  atresia 626
  duplication 625–6
  ectopy 626
  embryogenesis 1461
  malformations 625–6
  obstructive lesions 626–7
  stenosis 626
Ureterocele **626–7**, 926
Ureteropelvic junction obstruction 1465–6
Ureterovesical junction obstruction, postnatal intervention indications 1466–7
Ureterovesical membrane 1461
Urethra,
  atresia **926**
  posterior valves **628**
  tumours 629
Urinary reducing substances 1132–3
Urinary system, at 15 weeks, structural evaluation **912**
Urinary tract,
  calculus syndromes *652*
  dilated **925**
  disorders, treatment options 630
  in heritable disorders and malformations *631–46*
  malformations,
    in chromosomal abnormality syndromes *647*
    in multiple anomaly syndromes *648–9*
  obstruction, prenatal diagnosis 629–30
  obstructive lesions 1315–16
Urine, tests for acute metabolic disease *1132*
Urogenital ridge 609
Urogenital sinus 610
Urography, excretory 1464
USA, international mortality rank **10**
Uterine arteries,
  Doppler study **894–1**

macrophage infiltration 328
peak systolic velocity **980**
trophoblastic infiltration **328**
Uterine cavity, four quadrants 881
Uterine circulation 979
Uteroplacental arteries 139, **321**
  early 979
Uteroplacental circulation 13, 894, 979–80
  establishment 147–8
  in first trimester 979
Uteroplacental failure 285
Uteroplacental insufficiency 13
  chronic 295
  and hypoxia 1352
  investigation 291
Uteroplacental–fetal unit 12–13
Uterus,
  abnormalities, recurrent abortion 171–2
  activity **288**
  contractile wave 289–90
  contractilities and maternal blood flow **289**
  contractions,
    and blood flow 290
    type II dip **295**
  dysfunctional activity 293–4
  early radiograph **151**
  fibrillations **295**
  hypertonic contractions 293, **295**
  inefficient action 293
  myometrial contractions in labour 287, 289
  overefficient action 293
  placentation changes 139–41
  in pregnancy and labour **288**
  snowstorm appearance 985
Utilitarian theory 18

VACTER association 610
VACTERL association 406–7
VACTERL syndrome 592, 604, 929–30
Vagina,
  clear cell adenocarcinoma **686**
  endodermal sinus tumour 686
  obstructive lesions 685
  sarcoma botryoides 685
  transverse septa 685
Vaginal adenosis 73–4
  DES exposure 78
Vaginal delivery, placenta from 990
Valproic acid 89
Values for criteria in selection 19
Valve, malformed, fused commissure **491**
Valvuloplasty 516
Vanishing testis syndrome 677
Vanishing twin (VT) 202
  complications 206
Variable number of tandem repeats (VNTR) 39, 191
  analysis **1182**
Varicella-zoster embryopathy, congenital 443
Varicella-zoster infection and polymicrogyria **422**
Varicella-zoster virus 1296
  in TORCH syndrome 265
Vasa praevia 296
  ruptured 322, 324
Vascular anastomoses,
  frequencies in MC placentas *205*
  in MC placentation 212
Vascular anatomy of MC placentas 222
Vascular disruption 358–9, *360*, 404
Vascular insufficiency 15

Vascular naevi 836
Vascular ring 482, 484
Vasculopathy,
  decidual **329**
  fetal 330, **331–2**
  maternal 328–9, 330
Vasoactive intestinal polypeptide 858
VATER association 27, 402, 406–7, 528, 610
  external features *379*
  in maternal diabetes 403
VATER syndrome 26, 592, 604
VATERL-H syndrome 26
Veins,
  accessibility and parenteral nutrition 1421
  malformations 501–2
Velamentous vessels 296
Velo-cardio-facial syndrome 24
Venous flow studies, cardiac and extracardiac 981
Ventilation,
  assisted,
    pulmonary complications 807–9
    survival percentage **1341**
Ventilation increase 1389
Ventilatory responses in preterm infants **1388**
Ventral conjoining 217
Ventral remnants 595–6
Ventricle,
  left,
    dissection **479**
    double-inlet 495, **497–8**
    double-outlet **494**
    input abnormality **510**
    outflow tract **508**
  right, double-outlet 492–3
Ventricles, transverse sections **480**
Ventricular dilatation **508**
Ventricular ejection pathways **490**
Ventricular fibrillation 511
Ventricular rate, in tachycardia 966, 968
Ventricular septal defect (VSD) 400
  structural changes **542**
  surgery 1480
Ventricular septum,
  defect 941–2, *943*, 945
  and maternal diabetes mellitus 963
  echocardiography 959
Ventriculomegaly 923–4
Verapamil 1259
Verma–Naumoff syndrome 791
Vertebrae, fractures **309**
Vertebral column, and intrapartum trauma 308–10
Very low birth weight (VLBW) 368
  deaths 4
Very-low-birth-weight (VLBW) infant
  cerebrospinal fluid values *1522*
  difficulties 1417
Vesicoamniotic shunting 1248
Vestigial cysts 987
Vg-1 (transcription factor) 35
Video display screens 91
Villi,
  abscess 325
  after fetal death 272
  avascular 330–1
  branching at week 8 144
  hydatidiform change 192
  scalloping in partial moles 193
  at week 10 **144**

Villitis,
  chronic 1036
  in CMV infection 348
  with intrauterine infection **327**
Villitis of unknown etiology 325, **327**,
  332–3
Villous barrier, first trimester 148–50
Villous edema fluid 188
Villous infarction 330
Villous tissue,
  development 141–5
  see also Placenta
Villous tree,
  branching patterns 13–**14**
  infections 103
Villous trophoblastic syncytial knotting 330
Viral brain infection, intrauterine 440–3
Viral cultures at autopsy 387
Viral inclusions 325
Viral infection 348–50
  in fetal death 271
  and IUGR 276
Virilization in female 699
Virus,
  cytopathic effects 348
  infection effects on mother 1293–4
  infection in pregnancy 1293–9
  see also under Individual viruses
Visceral heterotaxy 500
Visual evoked potential 1403
Vitamin K 718, 1286–8
Vitamins,
  fetal concentrations 1276
  parenteral requirements *1429–30*
  transport systems 12
Vitellointestinal cyst 847
Vitellointestinal remnants 595–6
von Gierke disease 1141
von Recklinghausen's neurofibromatosis
  73–4, **842–3**
von Willebrand factor 1281
von Willebrand disease 1284–5

WAGR syndrome 50, 52, 73, 75, 255
  and Wilms' tumour 624–5
Walnut brain 448–9
Warfarin as teratogen 402
Water requirements in premature infant
  1423
Werdnig–Hoffmann disease 450–1, 783
Whipple's triad 585

Whitaker test 1464
WHO,
  breast feeding recommendations 349
  criteria for addiction 353
  screening definition 1031
  screening programmes 1031
  screening recommendations *1045*
WHO Science Group 390
WHO–CVS Registry, limb defects
  1080
Williams' syndrome 957
Wilms' tumour 622–3, 624–5
  in situ 73
  and malformations 624–5
  and neuroblastoma 71–2
  paternal occupation 77
  suppressor genes 71
  transcription mutation 48
  see also Nephroblastoma
Wilms' tumour gene (WT1),
  mutations in Drash syndrome 52
  oncogenesis 52
  teratogenesis and oncogenesis connection
    50–2
  zinc finger mutations 51
Wilson disease 572
Wiskott–Aldrich syndrome 744–5, 765,
  1503
  therapy 1511
Wolf–Hirschhorn syndrome 255, 1127
Wolff–Parkinson–White syndrome 503
Wolman disease 572, **1090**, *1092*, 1146
World Health Organization, *see* WHO

X chromosome,
  inactivation 122
    in twins 202–3
  long arm **34**
  short arm **34**
  unequal inactivation in MZ twins 204
X-inactive specific transcripts (XIST) 122
X-linked ichthyosis 760
X-linked infantile agammaglobulinaemia
  746–7, 748
X-linked mental retardation (handicap) 40,
  64–5
X-linked mutations 24
X-linked orofacial digital syndrome 423
X-linked recessive disorders 377
X-linked spina bifida sequence 26
Xenon as tracer 1401

Xeroderma pigmentosum 24, 72, 764
Xeroradiography 180–1
XIST (X-inactive specific transcripts) 122
XLMR mutations 24
XX male 64
XXX, in newborn *249*
XXY, in newborn *249*
XY female 64
XYY, in newborn *249*
XYY syndrome 64

Y factor 664
Y-linked mutations 24
Yale Fetal Cardiovascular Center *957*, *963*
Yolk sac 143, **146**
  canaliculi **149**
  definitive secondary 143
  development and disappearance 143,
    146–7
  diameter **153**
  embryoscopy 1067
  in fetal aging 899–900
  functions 150
  wall **149**
    section **147**
  at week 12 **902**

Zellweger cerebrohepatorenal syndrome 24,
  405, **422**, *446*, *573*, 782, 1089,
  1139–40
  and renal dysplasia 616
Zeugopod 29
Zinc finger Y factor 664
Zinc finger (ZnF),
  motifs 50
  mutations 50–1
Zollinger–Ellison syndrome 585, 586
Zygosity,
  concordance and discordance 205–7
  determination 222
Zygosity testing,
  in twins 203–5
  DNA RFLP method **202**
Zygotes,
  euploid diploid 245
  postzygotic mechanisms **238**
  triploid 232, *238*
  trisomic **245**
  uniparental disomy production
    mechanisms 242, 247